Understanding
Neuropsychiatric Disorders:
Insights from Neuroimaging

Understanding Neuropsychiatric Disorders: Insights from Neuroimaging

Edited by

Martha E. Shenton
Bruce I. Turetsky

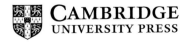

CAMBRIDGE
UNIVERSITY PRESS

CAMBRIDGE UNIVERSITY PRESS
Cambridge, New York, Melbourne, Madrid, Cape Town, Singapore,
São Paulo, Delhi, Dubai, Tokyo, Mexico City

Cambridge University Press
The Edinburgh Building, Cambridge CB2 8RU, UK

Published in the United States of America by
Cambridge University Press, New York

www.cambridge.org
Information on this title: www.cambridge.org/9780521899420

© Cambridge University Press 2011

First published 2011

Printed in the United Kingdom at the University Press, Cambridge

A catalog record for this publication is available from the British Library

Library of Congress Cataloging in Publication Data
Understanding neuropsychiatric disorders: insights from
neuroimaging / edited by Martha E. Shenton, Bruce I. Turetsky.
    p.   cm.
  Includes bibliographical references and index.
  ISBN 978 0 521 89942 0 (Hardback)
  1. Neurobehavioral disorders–Imaging.   I. Shenton, Martha
Elizabeth.   II. Turetsky, Bruce I., 1950–
  [DNLM: 1. Mental Disorders–diagnosis.   2. Diagnostic Imaging–
methods.   WM 141 U55 2010]
  RC473.B7U53 2010
  616.8–dc22   2010018055

ISBN 978 0 521 89942 0 Hardback

Contents

Contents

Contributors

Olusola Ajilore MD, PhD
Department of Psychiatry
University of Illinois at Chicago
Chicago, IL, USA

Jorge R. C. de Almeida MD, PhD
Department of Psychiatry
University of Pittsburgh School of Medicine
Pittsburgh, PA, USA

Nancy Andreasen MD, PhD
Department of Psychiatry
University of Iowa
Iowa City, IA, USA

Liana G. Apostolova MD, MSCR
Department of Neurology
David Geffen School of Medicine
University of California, Los Angeles
Los Angeles, CA, USA

Jan Booij MD
Department of Nuclear Medicine
University of Amsterdam
Amsterdam, The Netherlands

James Robert Brašić MD, MPH
The Russell H. Morgan Department of Radiology
and Radiological Science
The Johns Hopkins University School of Medicine
Baltimore, MD, USA

J. Douglas Bremner MD
Department of Psychiatry *and*
Department of Radiology
Emory University School of Medicine
Atlanta, GA, USA

Kathryn Handwerger Brohawn PhD
Department of Psychology
Tufts University
Medford, MA, USA

John O. Brooks III MD, PhD
Department of Psychiatry
David Geffen School of Medicine
University of California, Los Angeles
Los Angeles, CA, USA

Geraldo F. Busatto MD
Department of Psychiatry
University of São Paulo
São Paulo, SP, Brazil

Nicola Cascella MD
Department of Psychiatry and Behavioral Sciences
The Johns Hopkins University School of Medicine
Baltimore, MD, USA

Sandra Chanraud PhD
Department of Psychiatry and Behavioral Sciences
Stanford University School of Medicine
Stanford, CA, USA *and* Neuroscience Program
SRI International Menlo Park, CA, USA

José Alexandre de Souza Crippa MD, PhD
Department of Neuroscience and Behavioral Sciences
University of São Paulo
Ribeirão Preto, SP, Brazil

Raúl de la Fuente-Fernández MD
Division of Neurology
University of British Columbia
Vancouver, BC, Canada

Mony J. de Leon EdD
Department of Psychiatry
New York University School of Medicine
New York, NY, USA

Damiaan Denys MD, PhD
Department of Psychiatry
University of Amsterdam
Amsterdam,
The Netherlands

Martjin Figee MD
Department of Psychiatry
University of Amsterdam
Amsterdam, The Netherlands

Guido K. W. Frank MD
Department of Psychiatry
University of Colorado School of Medicine
Aurora, CO, USA

Joanna S. Fowler PhD
Department of Psychiatry
Mount Sinai School of Medicine
New York, NY, USA *and*
Medical Department
Brookhaven National Laboratory
Upton, NY, USA

Ajax George MD
Department of Radiology
New York University School of Medicine
New York, NY, USA

Alison M. Gilbert PhD
Department of Psychiatry
University of Pittsburgh School of Medicine
Pittsburgh, PA, USA

Andrew R. Gilbert MD
Department of Psychiatry
University of Pittsburgh School of Medicine
Pittsburgh, PA, USA

Mark W. Gilbertson PhD
Mental Health/Research Service
Manchester VA Medical Center
Manchester, NH, USA

Murray Grossman MD
Department of Neurology
University of Pennsylvania School of Medicine
Philadelphia, PA, USA

Bon-Mi Gu MSc
Interdisciplinary Program in Brain Science
Seoul National University College of Medicine
Seoul, Korea

John D. Herrington PhD
Center for Autism Research
Children's Hospital of Philadelphia
Philadelphia, PA, USA

Paul E. Holtzheimer III MD
Department of Psychiatry and Behavioral Sciences
Emory University School of Medicine
Atlanta, GA, USA

William Hu MD, PhD
Department of Neurology
University of Pennsylvania School of Medicine
Philadelphia, PA, USA

Do-Hyung Kang MD, PhD
Department of Psychiatry
Seoul National University College of Medicine
Seoul, Korea

Terence A. Ketter MD
Department of Psychiatry and Behavioral
Sciences Stanford University School of Medicine
Stanford, CA, USA

Marek Kubicki MD, PhD
Department of Psychiatry
VA Boston Healthcare System *and*
Department of Psychiatry
Brigham and Women's Hospital
Harvard Medical School
Boston, MA, USA

Anand Kumar MD
Department of Psychiatry
University of Illinois at Chicago
Chicago, IL, USA

Jun Soo Kwon MD, PhD
Interdisciplinary Program in Brain Science *and*
Department of Psychiatry
Seoul National University College
of Medicine
Seoul, Korea

Richard J. McClure PhD
Department of Psychiatry
University of Pittsburgh School of Medicine
Pittsburgh, PA, USA

Omar M. Mahmood PhD
Psychology Service
VA San Diego Healthcare System *and*
Department of Psychiatry
University of California, San Diego
San Diego, CA, USA

William M. Marchand MD
Department of Psychiatry
University of Utah School of Medicine
Salt Lake City, UT, USA

Graeme F. Mason PhD
Department of Psychiatry *and*
Department of Diagnostic Radiology
Yale University School of Medicine
New Haven, CT, USA

Sanjay J. Mathew MD
Department of Psychiatry and Behavioral Sciences
Baylor College of Medicine
Houston, TX, USA

Helen S. Mayberg MD
Department of Psychiatry and Behavioral Sciences
Emory University School of Medicine
Atlanta, GA, USA

Andreas Meyer-Lindenberg MD PhD
Department of Psychiatry and Psychotherapy
University of Heidelberg *and*
Central Institute of Mental Health
Mannheim, Germany

Nancy J. Minshew MD
Department of Psychiatry *and*
Department of Neurology
University of Pittsburgh School of Medicine
Pittsburgh, PA, USA

James W. Murrough MD
Department of Psychiatry
Mount Sinai School of Medicine
New York, NY, USA

Kanagasabai Panchalingam PhD
Department of Psychiatry
University of Pittsburgh School of Medicine
Pittsburgh, PA, USA

Godfrey D. Pearlson MD
Olin Neuropsychiatry Research Center
Institute of Living
Hartford, CT, USA *and*
Department of Psychiatry
Yale University School of Medicine
New Haven, CT, USA

Jay W. Pettegrew MD
Departments of Psychiatry, Neurology, Behavioral
and Community Health Sciences,
University of Pittsburgh School of Medicine *and*
Department of Bioengineering
University of Pittsburgh
Pittsburgh, PA, USA

Danielle L. Pfaff BA
Department of Psychology
Tufts University
Medford, MA, USA

Adolf Pfefferbaum MD
Neuroscience Program
SRI International
Menlo Park, CA, USA *and*
Department of Psychiatry and Behavioral Science
Stanford University School of Medicine
Stanford, CA, USA

Mary L. Phillips MD
Department of Psychiatry
University of Pittsburgh School of Medicine
Pittsburgh, PA, USA

Anne Lise Pitel PhD
Department of Psychiatry and Behavioral Science
Stanford University School of Medicine
Stanford, CA, USA

Roger K. Pitman MD
Department of Psychiatry
Massachusetts General Hospital
Harvard Medical School
Boston, MA, USA

Scott L. Rauch MD
Department of Psychiatry
McLean Hospital
Harvard Medical School
Belmont, MA, USA

Michael D. H. Rollin MD
Department of Psychiatry, Division of Child
and Adolescent Psychiatry, *and* The Children's
Hospital
University of Colorado
School of Medicine
Aurora, CO, USA

Henry Rusinek PhD
Department of Radiology
New York University School of Medicine
New York, NY, USA

Julia Sacher MD, PhD
PET Centre
Centre for Addiction and Mental Health
Toronto, ON, Canada

Andreia Santos PhD
Central Institute of Mental Health
Mannheim, Germany

Andrew J. Saykin PhD
Department of Radiology and Imaging Sciences
Indiana University School of Medicine
Indianapolis, IN, USA

Norbert Schuff PhD
Center for Imaging of Neurodegenerative Diseases
at the Veterans Affairs Medical Center *and*
Department of Radiology and Biomedical
Imaging
University of California San Francisco
San Francisco, CA, USA

Robert T. Schultz PhD
Department of Pediatrics
University of Pennsylvania School of Medicine *and*
Center for Autism Research
Children's Hospital of Philadelphia
Philadelphia, PA, USA

Alecia D. Dager Schweinsburg PhD
Department of Psychiatry
Yale University School of Medicine
New Haven, CT, USA

Brian C. Schweinsburg PhD
Department of Psychiatry
Yale University School of Medicine
New Haven, CT, USA

Martha E. Shenton PhD
VA Boston Healthcare System *and*
Department of Psychiatry
Brigham and Women's Hospital
Harvard Medical School
Boston, MA, USA

Lisa M. Shin PhD
Department of Psychology
Tufts University
Medford, MA, USA *and*
Department of Psychiatry
Massachusetts General Hospital
Harvard Medical School
Boston, MA, USA

David A. Silbersweig MD
Department of Psychiatry
Brigham and Women's Hospital
Harvard Medical School
Boston, MA, USA

Gwenn S. Smith PhD
Department of Psychiatry and Behavioral Sciences
The Johns Hopkins University School of Medicine
Baltimore, MD, USA

A. Jon Stoessl MD
Division of Neurology
University of British Columbia
Vancouver, BC, Canada

Stephen M. Strakowski MD
Department of Psychiatry
University of Cincinnati
Cincinnati, OH, USA

Edith V. Sullivan PhD
Department of Psychiatry and Behavioral Sciences
Stanford University School of Medicine
Stanford, CA, USA

Simon A. Surguladze MD, PhD
Institute of Psychiatry
King's College London
London, UK

Philip R. Szeszko PhD
Department of Psychiatry
The Zucker Hillside Hospital
Glen Oaks, NY, USA *and*
Albert Einstein College of Medicine
Bronx, NY, USA

Vanessa Taler PhD
Department of Radiology and Imaging Sciences
Indiana University School of Medicine
Indianapolis, IN, USA

Susan F. Tapert PhD
Psychology Service
VA San Diego Healthcare System *and*
Department of Psychiatry
University of California San Diego
San Diego, CA, USA

Panayotis K. Thanos PhD
National institute of Drug Abuse *and*
National Institute of Alcohol Abuse and
Alcoholism
Bethesda, MD, USA

Paul M. Thompson PhD
Department of Neurology
David Geffen School of Medicine
University of California Los Angeles
Los Angeles, CA, USA

Janet Treasure PhD, FRCP, FRCPsych
Institute of Psychiatry
Guys Campus
Kings College London
London, UK

Wai Tsui PhD
Department of Psychiatry
New York University School of Medicine
New York, NY, USA
and Nathan Kline Institute
Orangeburg, NY, USA

Bruce Turetsky MD
Department of Psychiatry
University of Pennsylvania School of Medicine
Philadelphia, PA, USA

Oliver Tüscher MD, PhD
Department of Neurology *and*
Department of Psychiatry and Psychotherapy
University of Freiburg
Freiburg, Germany

Nora D. Volkow MD
National institute of Drug Abuse *and*
National Institute of Alcohol Abuse and Alcoholism
Bethesda, MD, USA

Gene-Jack Wang MD
Department of Psychiatry
Mount Sinai School of Medicine
New York, NY, USA *and*

Medical Department
Brookhaven National Laboratory
Upton, NY, USA

Po W. Wang MD
Department of Psychiatry and Behavioral Sciences
Stanford University School of Medicine
Stanford, CA, USA

Jerzy Wegiel VMD, PhD
Department of Developmental Neurobiology
Institute for Basic Research
Staten Island, NY, USA

Thomas J. Whitford PhD
Department of Psychiatry
Brigham and Women's Hospital
Harvard School of Medicine
Boston, MA, USA *and*
Department of Psychiatry
Melbourne Neuropsychiatry Centre
University of Melbourne
Melbourne, Australia

Thomas Wisniewski MD
Department of Neurology
New York University School of Medicine
New York, NY, USA *and*
Department of Developmental Neurobiology
Institute for Basic Research
Staten Island, NY, USA

Dean F. Wong MD PhD
The Russel H. Morgan Department of Radiology and
Radiological Science
The Johns Hopkins University School of Medicine
Baltimore, MD, USA

Deborah A. Yurgelun-Todd PhD
Department of Psychiatry
Salt Lake City VA Healthcare System *and*
Department of Psychiatry
University of Utah School of Medicine
Salt Lake City, UT, USA

Daniel J. Zimmerman MD
Department of Neurology *and*
Department of Psychiatry and Psychotherapy
University of Freiburg
Freiburg, Germany

Preface

Historically, the opportunity to examine the inner workings of the human body was limited to the study of cadavers. In the past 30 years, medical imaging technology has provided researchers with a new window into the *living* human body. Advances in medical imaging technology have, in fact, truly revolutionized nearly every area of medicine. These advances include both dramatic improvements in image resolution and the development of novel imaging techniques, from computed axial tomography (CT), to positron emission tomography (PET), to single photon emission tomography (SPECT), to magnetic resonance imaging (MRI), including fMRI (functional MRI) and diffusion tensor imaging (DTI), to magnetic resonance spectroscopy (MRS), ultrasound, and magnetoencephalography (MEG) – all of which provide an unprecedented view, in exquisite detail, of anatomical structures and/or functions in the *living* human body.

One medical discipline that has been in the forefront of this revolution is neuropsychiatry (defined here as encompassing both psychiatry and behavioral neurology), where novel neuroimaging tools have been developed and applied to neuropsychiatric disorders in order to understand further the neuroanatomical and neurophysiological bases of mental illnesses and cognitive disorders, including Alzheimer's and Parkinson's diseases.

This book reviews important new findings about the role of brain abnormalities in neuropsychiatric disorders based on this new imaging technology. In considering the progress in this area, it is clear that initially the quest was to identify and characterize focal brain abnormalities in an effort to delineate further various psychiatric and neuropsychiatric syndromes. Here, as will be evident from the chapters that follow, much work has already been done to characterize brain pathology in disorders for which the etiologies are unknown, there are often no uniform or pathognomonic clinical symptoms, and there is often extensive overlap in clinical presentation across disorders.

More recently, the focus has shifted from the examination of a single brain region, or multiple discrete brain regions, implicated in a particular syndrome or disorder, to the examination of integrated brain systems. This is a common theme that can be followed throughout the chapters of this book. Specifically, the focus has shifted from investigating only gray matter of the brain to investigating the "other half" of the brain, white matter, and the neural networks involved in the pathophysiology of different neuropsychiatric disorders. Accordingly, we have moved from an appreciation that, for example, schizophrenia *is* a brain disorder – something that had been debated prior to the late 1980s – to a quest to understand the complex mechanisms underlying the neuropathology of schizophrenia. Thus there has been a shift from the "what" and "where" of brain regions implicated in neuropsychiatric disorders to an effort to understand the neural basis of clinical symptoms, or "how" abnormal brain regions produce the clinical picture of depression, or autism, or schizophrenia. These advances in neuroimaging are moving us towards a new understanding of neuropsychiatric disorders based on their underlying neurobiology. This will likely facilitate the diagnostic reclassification of these complex heterogeneous disorders, improve our ability to predict treatment outcome, and enhance our understanding of the genetic and environmental causes of these disorders.

The change in focus from discrete brain regions and gray matter to white matter and the integrated systems that underlie cognitive, behavioral, and emotional abnormalities has followed, closely, the advances and inroads made in imaging technology. Importantly, none of the insights into the neuropathology of neuropsychiatric disorders, to date, would have been possible without these advances. That is, without the tools to probe the brain, in vivo, we could not even have begun to ask questions about brain structure and function and their perturbations in neuropsychiatric disorders. There is now, however, a need to go beyond the technology and shift to more hypothesis- and model-driven approaches. These new approaches must not only elucidate the neural networks involved in complex disorders, but must also examine the inter-relationships among genetic variables, environmental stressors, behavioral, cognitive, social, and emotional factors, and the structural and functional integrity of the neural systems that underlie the symptomatology presently used to classify these disorders.

When we were first approached by Marc Strauss at Cambridge University Press to edit a book on neuroimaging and its contribution to what we know about neuropsychiatric disorders, we thought such a book was very timely, as we believe we are now at a critical juncture in terms of our knowledge of the living brain in both health and illness. Moreover, we believe that the most interesting and important findings are yet to come.

In the chapters that follow, the current status of neuroimaging is reviewed for each of the leading neuropsychiatric disorders. The "maturity" of this research and the breadth and depth of the available data vary considerably across disorders. In some cases, such as schizophrenia or mood disorders, neuroimaging findings are quite extensive, requiring separate chapters to review structural imaging (Proton MR and DTI), functional imaging (fMRI and PET/SPECT blood flow and metabolism studies), and molecular imaging (PET/SPECT receptor studies and MR spectroscopy). In other cases, such as autism spectrum disorders, the data are still relatively sparse and findings across imaging modalities are reviewed in a single chapter. Each disease section ends with a commentary from a luminary in the field, addressing the broad question: "What do we know and where are we going?" This was a feature that we decided to include very early in the editorial process. Given the broad scope of the book, we thought it important for a luminary to review each section, to provide a synthesis, and to comment more generally on the knowledge gleaned from these imaging techniques. The intended audience for this book is also broad and includes the clinical psychiatrist, the general practitioner, the psychiatry or neurology resident, the medical student, the PhD student in psychology or neuroscience, and/or the post-doctoral fellow interested in learning more about how neuroimaging tools lead to new discoveries about brain and behavior associations in neuropsychiatric disorders.

We wish to thank Marc Strauss, Richard Marley, and Nisha Doshi at Cambridge University Press for their assistance on all aspects of this book. We also wish to thank our spouses, George and Nancy, who kindly accepted our taking on, yet again, just one more task. Finally, we give our heartfelt thanks to all of the authors of the chapters in this book. These are leading investigators in their respective fields, who have graciously taken the time to offer their insights into neuropsychiatric disorders based on advances in neuroimaging. It goes without saying that, without them, this book would not exist.

Martha E. Shenton
Bruce I. Turetsky

Schizophrenia

Structural imaging of schizophrenia

Thomas J. Whitford, Marek Kubicki and Martha E. Shenton

Introduction

Emil Kraepelin, one of the founding fathers of the diagnostic concept of schizophrenia, argued that the disorder was underpinned by abnormalities in brain structure. In his 1899 textbook, Kraepelin wrote: "in dementia praecox [schizophrenia], partial damage to, or destruction of, cells of the cerebral cortex must probably occur" (Kraepelin, 1907). Since that time, an enormous amount of research has been undertaken with an eye to determining whether or not Kraepelin was correct. Until recently, the question of whether patients with schizophrenia (SZ) exhibit abnormalities in brain structure was more or less synonymous with the question of whether they exhibit abnormalities in gray matter (GM). The GM, so-called because of its grayish appearance in post-mortem tissue sections, is thought to consist primarily of neuron bodies, dendrites, axon terminals and other synaptic infrastructure and certain classes of neuroglia. Until recently, the vast majority of research aimed at investigating the neuroanatomical underpinnings of SZ has focused on GM. This is perhaps understandable, given that GM comprises both the brain's fundamental units of information processing (neurons) and the sites-of-action for most psychotropic medications (synapses). In recent years, however, a growing proportion of contemporary research has begun to focus on the "other half of the brain" (as wryly denoted by Fields, 2004), i.e. the white matter. The white matter (WM) is primarily constituted of myelinated axon sheaths, which form the infrastructure for signal transmission between spatially discrete populations of neurons. By way of analogy, just as the Internet is comprised of spatially disparate computers connected via electrical cabling, the brain is comprised of spatially disparate neurons connected via myelinated axons. Despite the

fact that the role of WM in facilitating and modulating communications between discrete brain structures makes it theoretically relevant with respect to the prevailing "connectivity" models of SZ (as discussed in the third section), it is only in the past decade that WM has become a major topic of interest in the SZ research community. A major factor underlying this increased interest has been the development of diffusion tensor imaging (DTI) as a mainstream neuroimaging technique. Unlike in conventional MRI, in which WM appears relatively homogeneous, DTI enables the visualization and quantification of fine WM structure. The development of DTI as a WM imaging technique, in combination with concurrent advances in the image quality afforded by conventional MRI, has meant that it has now become feasible to address the question of whether patients with SZ exhibit abnormalities in their GM, WM, or both (see Figure 1.1).

The primary aim of this chapter is to provide a review of the vast body of published research that has used either structural MRI or DTI to investigate for neuroanatomical abnormalities in SZ patients. The chapter also considers the implications of this research with respect to two fundamental questions relating to the neuropathology of SZ, namely: (1) what are the possible causes of the reported GM and WM abnormalities in patients with SZ, and (2) is there a causal relationship between these GM and WM abnormalities? The first section of this chapter provides a broad overview of the most consistent findings of the MRI studies that have investigated GM abnormalities in SZ patients. The second section provides a finer-grained analysis of the more than 50 published DTI studies that have investigated WM abnormalities in SZ.[1] This section also includes some discussion as to the physiological bases and clinical implications of

---

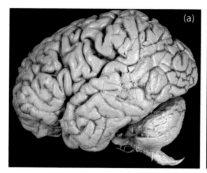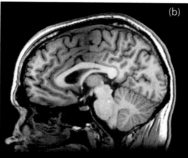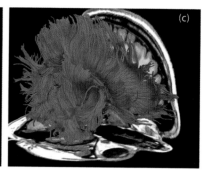

Figure 1.1 (a) A post-mortem specimen of the human brain. Image used with kind permission of Getty Images. (b) A structural magnetic resonance image (MRI) of the living human brain, showing a clear distinction between the gray and white matter. (c) Using diffusion tensor imaging (DTI) to image white matter in the living human brain. Note how that in contrast to panel (b) in which the WM appears largely featureless and homogeneous, DTI enables a far richer visualization of the macrostructural features of WM fiber bundles.

these WM abnormalities. Finally, in the third section, a speculative hypothesis is introduced which suggests how the GM abnormalities, WM abnormalities, hyper-dopaminergia and clinical profile characteristic of SZ could potentially arise from a single neuropathological mechanism.

MRI studies of GM abnormality in patients with schizophrenia: a review

In 2001, Shenton *et al.* published an influential review of the 190+ studies published to that point which had used MRI to investigate for neuroanatomical abnormalities in SZ patients. On the basis of the reviewed literature, Shenton *et al.* (2001) concluded that SZ patients, as a group, exhibit subtle but incontrovertible volumetric reductions in a number of GM structures. Specifically, the review reported consistent volumetric reductions in GM of the temporal cortex (especially the superior temporal gyrus), and the GM structures of the medial temporal lobe (esp. hippocampus), and moderately consistent reductions in the frontal cortex (esp. orbitofrontal), parietal cortex (esp. inferior parietal lobule) and basal ganglia (esp. striatum). Since Shenton's review, there has been an exponential increase in the number of MRI studies in SZ, such that there are currently more than 800 studies published in the literature.[2] Given the large number of studies, it is clear that providing a comprehensive review of the current MRI literature in SZ (as per Shenton *et al.*, 2001) would require the writing of an entire book, and as such is outside the scope of this chapter. Thus instead of providing a comprehensive review, this section aims to summarize the most consistent findings in the MRI literature by considering a selection of particularly illustrative studies.

SZ is associated with widely distributed GM abnormalities, which are observable with MRI

The past decade has seen enormous developments in both MRI acquisition and analysis technologies, with the development of 3 T magnets for human research and the rise of voxel-based morphometry as cases in point. In terms of identifying GM abnormalities associated with SZ, however, the findings of contemporary MR studies have, by and large, been consistent with the conclusions drawn by Shenton *et al.* (2001) almost a decade ago. It is now clear that SZ patients, on average, show abnormal volumetric GM reductions, observable with MRI, throughout a substantial proportion of the brain.[3] And whilst it is true that some GM regions have been more consistently reported as being volumetrically abnormal compared to others – with the language centers of the temporal cortex, the ganglia of the limbic lobe and the association areas of the parietal cortex being especially strongly implicated (Honea *et al.*, 2005; Glahn *et al.*, 2008; Pearlson and Marsh, 1999) – it is also true that almost every square millimeter of GM has been reported as being volumetrically reduced in SZ patients in at least one study. Thus it appears as though the GM pathology experienced in SZ is either not spatially localized (in contrast, for example, to the localized atrophy of the motor neurons in Amyotrophic Lateral Sclerosis), or that it is initially localized but spreads with illness progression.

GM abnormalities are observable early in the illness, and ostensibly pre-morbidly

The question of whether GM abnormalities are present in SZ patients at the time of their first psychotic episode has been the focus of a great deal of recent research, which has been motivated by at least two factors. First, it is hoped that gaining a better understanding of the dynamics of neuropathology will shed light onto both the nature of SZ and its underlying causes. Second, studying patients suffering from their first episode of schizophrenia (FES) allows us to address the issue as to whether the neuroanatomical abnormalities so consistently reported in patients with chronic SZ (CSZ patients) actually result from the neuroleptic medications that patients are typically exposed to, as opposed to anything fundamental to the disease process itself. This issue is particularly problematic in light of studies which have indicated that: (1) exposure to antipsychotic medication can influence brain structure in and of itself (see Scherk and Falkai, 2006, for a review), and (2) different classes of antipsychotics have differential effects on brain structure (Konopaske et al., 2008), making it difficult to covary for patients' neuroleptic exposure by converting the dosages of different medications into a common scale (such as the Chlorpromazine-Equivalent Scale). First-episode studies have attempted to address this issue by minimizing the confounding effects of medication exposure on brain structure by investigating patients who have had little or no exposure to neuroleptics.

Of the studies that have investigated for GM abnormalities in patients with FES, the majority have reported evidence of abnormal volumetric GM reductions. Furthermore, these reductions have, by and large, been observed in similar brain regions to those consistently identified as being structurally compromised in patients in the chronic phase of the illness (see reviews by Steen et al., 2006; Vita et al., 2006). However, on the whole, these studies have indicated that the neuroanatomical abnormalities exhibited by FES patients are both less severe and less widespread than the abnormalities exhibited by patients with chronic schizophrenia. Support for this point is provided by a recent meta-analysis by Ellison-Wright et al. (2008), who directly compared the extent of the GM reductions exhibited by CSZ patients in 20 voxel-based morphometry (VBM) studies to the reductions exhibited by FES patients in 9 VBM studies. The results of this meta-analysis indicated that the CSZ patients exhibited significantly more extensive GM reductions in the frontal cortex (esp. dorsolateral prefrontal cortex), temporal cortex (esp. superior temporal gyrus) and insular cortex, compared to the FES patients.

There is even some evidence suggesting that GM abnormalities may in fact precede the onset of psychotic symptoms in people who subsequently go on to develop schizophrenia. Pantelis et al. (2003), for example, compared the GM profiles of 23 people at "ultra-high risk" (UHR) for developing schizophrenia (based on genetic vulnerabilities, the presence of sub-clinical symptoms, and several other factors) who subsequently went on to develop psychosis (UHR-P) with 52 UHR people who subsequently did not go on to develop psychosis (UHR-NP). Pantelis et al. (2003) found that the UHR-P group exhibited lower GM volumes in hippocampal complex, superior temporal gyrus, inferior frontal cortex and cingulate gyrus compared to the UHR-NP group. Subsequent studies have also identified GM abnormalities in the para-cingulate cortex (Yücel et al., 2003), pituitary gland (Garner et al., 2005) and insular cortex (Borgwardt et al., 2007) in UHR groups (see Wood et al., 2008 for a review).

GM reductions are due to neuropil elimination as opposed to neuron death

There is now considerable evidence indicating that the GM abnormalities characteristically observed in SZ patients are not the result of (any substantial degree of) neuron death. For example, the brains of SZ patients have consistently been observed *not* to exhibit gliosis. Gliosis, which refers to the proliferation of astrocytes in damaged regions of the central nervous system (CNS), is a general feature of the immune system's response to necrotic cell death in the CNS (Pekny and Nilsson, 2005). Hence, the fact that the brains of SZ patients have consistently been found not to exhibit gliosis (e.g. Roberts et al., 1986) is evidence against the notion that SZ is associated with any substantial degree of neuron death via necrosis. However, the absence of gliosis does not exclude the possibility that SZ patients experience neuron death via apoptosis. Apoptosis, or programmed cell death, is not always associated with gliosis, as apoptotic cells typically alert immune cells prior to committing suicide, thus reducing the

3

non-specific immune response (Thompson, 1995). It is thus possible that the GM reductions characteristically exhibited by SZ patients are caused by increased levels of apoptosis. The empirical evidence does not, however, support this possibility. Pakkenberg (1993), for example, used optical microscopy to estimate the total number of neocortical neurons in the brains of 8 SZ patients and 16 controls. On the basis of this technique, Pakkenberg (1993) estimated that there was (on average) 22.06×10^9 neurons in the neocortex of the controls, and 22.12×10^9 neurons in the SZ patients – numbers that were essentially statistically identical ($p = 0.97$). The results of this study were subsequently replicated by Selemon and Goldman-Rakic (1999) in the prefrontal cortex. However, while Selemon and Goldman-Rakic (1999) did not find evidence of neuron death, they did find evidence of abnormally increased neuron density in SZ patients. They argued that since SZ patients typically show volumetric GM reductions compared to controls, the best explanation for this increase in neuron density was that "the distance between neurons diminished while the number of neurons is not changed" (p. 18). On the basis of this, they proposed the "reduced neuropil hypothesis", which argued that the increased neuron density and decreased GM volume exhibited by SZ patients resulted from the elimination of the neuropil (i.e. dendritic arbors and associated synaptic infrastructure) between neuron bodies. As will be discussed further, the idea that the volumetric GM reductions in SZ are caused by abnormal reductions in synaptic infrastructure has potential implications with respect to the WM abnormalities discussed later in the chapter.

GM abnormalities are likely progressive, at least over the initial years of illness

There is now a considerable amount of evidence to suggest that SZ patients experience progressive GM atrophy in the early stages of their illness (Whitford et al., 2006; Sun et al., 2009; Cahn et al., 2002; Salisbury et al., 2007; Kasai et al., 2003). In contrast, a smaller proportion of the studies on chronic SZ patients have reported progressive GM reductions above those experienced by matched healthy controls. A study by Gur et al. (1998) directly compared the degree of GM volume reduction that occurred in the frontal and temporal lobes over a 2–4-year follow-up interval in FES patients, CSZ patients and healthy

controls. The results showed that the FES patients experienced a significantly greater amount of progressive GM atrophy over the follow-up interval than did the CSZ patients, who on the whole did not experience more GM reductions than did the healthy controls. Similarly, Van Haren et al. (2008) compared the GM reductions over a 5-year period experienced by 96 SZ patients (aged between 16 and 56), and 113 matched controls. They reported that, over this 5-year interval, the most severe GM reductions were experienced by the youngest patients in the earliest stages of the illness, and that GM reductions experienced by the older patients were similar in degree to the reductions experienced by the healthy controls. Hence it appears that while SZ patients experience progressive GM reductions in the early stages of their illness, these reductions do not continue over patients' life spans, but rather decelerate with age to normal (or near-normal) levels. What factors might potentially underlie this curvilinear pattern of GM atrophy?

It has previously been suggested that the answer to this question might lie in the normative period of brain development that typically occurs during late adolescence to early adulthood (Feinberg, 1982; Keshavan et al., 1994), which is an age that corresponds to the typical age of onset for schizophrenia. Adolescence is a period of enormous structural change in the healthy human brain. In an influential study, Bourgeois and Rakic (1993) used electron microscopy to count the number of synapses in the visual cortex of macaque monkeys aged between 2.7 and 5 years (i.e. the period corresponding to their adolescence). Over this period, they observed the monkeys to lose approximately 5000 synapses per minute in the visual cortex alone. This staggering number could well have been even higher in the association cortices of these monkeys, given that the association cortices are among the last brain regions to mature (Yakovlev et al., 1967). The sheer scale of this "synaptic prune" (as it has been dubbed) suggests that its effects might be visible in humans with MRI. And indeed, a number of MRI studies have reported a period of accelerated GM volume loss in healthy people, beginning around 16 years of age and continuing until around 25–30 years of age (Whitford et al., 2007b; Pfefferbaum et al., 1994; Steen et al., 1997).

Given the sheer number of synapses thought to be eliminated in this periadolescent "synaptic prune", it seems reasonable to assume that even a minor

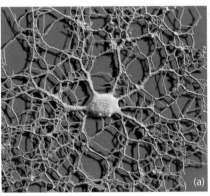
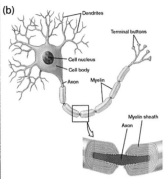
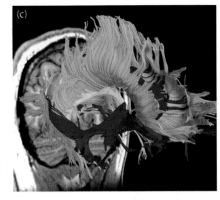

Figure 1.2 (a) An electron microscope image of an oligodendrocyte in rat optic nerve. Note the cell processes branching from the soma: these processes go on to form the myelin sheaths that insulate the axons of neighboring neurons. A single oligodendrocyte is capable of myelinating a single axon segment of up to 50 neurons. Image used with kind permission of Dr. Kachar at the Laboratory of Cell Structure and Dynamics at the National Institutes of Heath, and Dr. Wagner at the Department of Biology at the University of Delaware. (b) A schematic of the cellular features of a myelinated neuron. The primary purpose of myelin is thought to electrically insulate the axons and thus increase the transmission velocity of the action potential. Image used with kind permission of Prentice Hall. (c) Using DTI tractography to image the primary white matter fiber bundles of the brain. Myelinated axons connecting spatially disparate populations of neurons typically cluster together into large fiber bundles known as fascicles. This image illustrates the shape and trajectories of some of the major WM fiber bundles in the brain, including the corpus callosum (brown), cingulum bundle (purple), fornix (yellow), uncinate fasciculus (pink) inferior longitudinal fasciculus (green) and inferior fronto-occipital fasciculus (blue).

abnormality in the mechanisms underlying this process could potentially result in catastrophic consequences. Following this line of reasoning, Feinberg (1982) suggested that schizophrenia could arise because of an abnormality in this period of periadolescent brain maturation. A strength of Feinberg's (1982) theory is that it is able to explain why SZ patients only seem to exhibit progressive GM atrophy in the early stages of their illness. Specifically, if the GM atrophy exhibited by SZ patients is caused by an overly aggressive maturational period of synaptic pruning, then the end of this maturational period might be expected to result in an end to the progressive GM atrophy. The mechanisms underlying the synaptic "hyper-prune" hypothesized by Feinberg (1982) have implications with respect to the WM abnormalities reported in SZ patients (and summarized in the following section), and these implications are discussed further in the final section.

DTI studies of GM abnormality in patients with schizophrenia: a more detailed review

To reiterate from the first section, GM is thought to be constituted primarily of neuron bodies, dendrites, synaptic infrastructure and certain classes of

neuroglia (e.g. astrocytes). In contrast, white matter (the subject of this section) is thought to be primarily constituted of myelinated axon sheaths. More precisely, WM is thought to be constituted of the compacted cell membranes of a specialized class of neuroglia named oligodendrocytes (see Figure 1.2a). The processes of these oligodendrocytes (known as myelin) can ensheath short segments of the axons of several neighboring neurons (see Figure 1.2b), with a single oligodendrocyte (OL) capable of providing myelin sheaths for up to 50 axons. The hydrophobic phospholipid bilayer provides electrical insulation for the axon, which reduces ion leakage across the axon membrane, thus preserving the amplitude of the action potential and increasing the conduction velocity of the action potential as it travels along the myelinated axon segment (Baumann and Pham-Dinh, 2001). Thus it is clear that WM in the brain plays a crucial role in modulating the speed of communication between spatially disparate populations of neurons.

Axons with similar destinations often form large fiber bundles. These fiber bundles represent the "information highways" of the brain, along which travels the bulk of communication between populations of neurons separated by more than a few centimeters. Some of the most prominent fiber bundles in the brain include the corpus callosum (connecting the

5

cortices of the two cerebral hemispheres), the superior longitudinal fasciculus (connecting the parietal and temporal cortices with the prefrontal cortex), the inferior longitudinal fasciculus (connecting the temporal and occipital lobes), and the uncinate fasciculus (connecting the frontal and anterior temporal lobes) (see Figure 1.2c). Although WM constitutes approximately 40% of the total mass of the brain, it has only recently become the topic of much empirical investigation. One of the reasons for the recent increased interest in WM has been the advent of Diffusion Tensor Imaging (DTI), which enables a more precise visualization of the WM than afforded by conventional MRI. A second reason lies in the growing popularity of "connectivity" models of SZ, as discussed below.

SZ as a disorder of neural integration

The conceptualization of schizophrenia as a disorder defined by abnormal cognitive integration dates back at least as far as Bleuler (1911). Bleuler described the cardinal symptoms of schizophrenia (the name he coined to describe Kraepelin's "dementia praecox") as a "loosening of normal associations" between thoughts. In his 1911 treatise, Bleuler commented:

> Often ideas are only partially worked out, and fragments of ideas are connected in an illogical way to constitute a new idea … This results in associations which normal individuals will regard as incorrect, bizarre, and utterly unpredictable.

Bleuler's conceptualization of schizophrenia as a disorder of cognitive integration has heavily influenced the contemporary "connectivity" theories of schizophrenia, which have sought to describe the neural underpinnings of this cognitive disintegration.

The unifying tenet of "connectivity" theories of schizophrenia is the proposal that rather than being caused by normal interactions between pathological GM structures, schizophrenia instead arises from pathological interactions between pathological GM structures (Friston, 1999). The various connectivity theories differ, however, in terms of the specific mechanisms they propose as underlying this "pathological interaction". Feinberg (1982), as previously discussed, has suggested that this pathological interaction could arise from an abnormality in periadolescent brain development. Specifically, Feinberg (1982) suggested that in schizophrenia: "too many, too few

or the wrong synapses are eliminated", leading to "defects of neuronal integration" (p. 331). In a similar vein, Friston (1999) has argued that the fundamental neuropathology of schizophrenia lies in abnormal synaptic plasticity; that is, in the abnormal strengthening (and/or creation) and weakening (and/or elimination) of synapses in response to experience and development. Friston (1999) has argued that abnormalities in the processes underpinning the modulation of synaptic strength could lead to abnormal interactions between functionally specialized populations of neurons in SZ patients. In contrast, Crow (1998) has suggested that the aberrant neural interaction underlying schizophrenia is due to the fact that SZ patients do not exhibit the normative hemispheric specialization of the language centers. Specifically, Crow (1998) has suggested that the interhemispheric transmission delays associated with using both hemispheres to process language-related information could lead to abnormalities in neural timing and hence cognitive disintegration. And finally, Andreasen (1999) has emphasized the role of the thalamus and cerebellum in coordinating the development and maintenance of normative associations between cognitions originating in the prefrontal cortex. She has suggested that an abnormality in this coordination (or a "cognitive dysmetria", in her words) could cause SZ patients to "make abnormal associations between mental representations" (p. 785).

SZ as a disorder of neural integration arising from WM abnormalities

Bartzokis (2002) has offered a novel suggestion as to the underlying cause of the neural disintegration that is proposed to exist in patients with schizophrenia. Specifically, Bartzokis (2002) suggested that neural disintegration could arise from abnormalities in the periadolescent process of myelination. It has long been known that the normative developmental process of myelination continues well into the second decade of life, and that myelination of the association cortices are not complete until at least 30 years of age (Yakovlev et al., 1967). Given the aforementioned role that myelin plays in increasing the transmission velocity of neural signaling, Bartzokis (2002) proposed that an abnormality in the periadolescent process of myelination (particularly in the late-developing association cortices) could result in transmission delays, causing "a loss of the brain's ability to function normally by reducing its ability to maintain synchron-ous communication across functional neural net-works" (p. 678). In other words, Bartzokis suggested that abnormalities in the normative maturational pro-cesses of myelination could cause a breakdown in the synchronicity of neural activity between spatially dis-parate brain regions. This basic argument has also been proposed independently by other researchers (Fields, 2008; Walterfang et al., 2005).

Given the length of time that schizophrenia has been thought of as a disorder of neural integration, and given that WM constitutes the anatomical infra-structure for long-distance communication in the brain, it is in some ways surprising how little atten-tion WM has, until recently, received in the neuro-imaging literature. In another sense, however, this is perhaps understandable, given the aforementioned difficulties associated with studying WM via conven-tional imaging techniques such as structural MRI. The few studies which have used conventional MRI to investigate WM abnormalities in patients with SZ have produced equivocal results. Some studies have reported volumetric and/or morphometric WM abnormalities in patients with schizophrenia, including in the corpus callosum (Rotarska-Jagiela and Linden, 2008), inferior longitudinal fasciculus (O'Daly et al., 2007), and uncinate fasciculus (Park et al., 2004). Other studies have reported volumetric abnormalities in FES patients (e.g. Price et al., 2006), and at least one study has reported progressive volumetric WM atrophy over the first few years of illness in patients with FES (Whitford et al., 2007a). In contrast, however, several other published studies have failed to find evidence of volumetric or morphometric WM abnormalities in SZ patients (Cahn et al., 2002; Zahajszky et al., 2001; Hirayasu et al., 2001).

The development of DTI in the 1980s opened up new possibilities for the empirical investigation of WM in vivo. DTI differs from conventional MRI in that it is sensitive to spin dephasing associated with molecular movement. Specifically, DTI is sensitive to the random movement of water molecules that result from unpre-dictable thermal collisions, i.e. diffusion. DTI is based on the fact that the direction and extent of water diffusion in a given region of the brain provides clues as to the microstructure of the underlying tissue.

In brain tissue, the diffusion of water molecules is restricted by obstacles in the local environment, such as phospholipid membranes, myelin sheaths, macromolecules, etc. DTI relies on the fact that the

extent to which diffusion is restricted differs between the different tissues of the brain. In the ventricular cerebrospinal fluid (CSF), for example, there are rela-tively few obstacles to diffusion. As a result of this, water diffusion in the CSF is relatively unrestricted, and is consequently isotropic (i.e. spherical). In con-trast, in a WM fiber bundle, the dense and coherently aligned myelinated axons provide a considerable bar-rier to water diffusion, with water being more likely to diffuse parallel to the fiber bundle as opposed to perpendicular to it. By calculating the distance over which water diffuses from a given point in a given amount of time in a number of independent direc-tions, it is possible to construct a three-dimensional shape that best describes the shape of the water diffu-sion. The shape describing this diffusion is conven-tionally modeled as an ellipsoid (see Figure 1.3).

The assumption in DTI is that the shape and size of this ellipsoid provide information about the diffu-sivity of the underlying tissue. There are various ways in which the "shape" and "size" of a diffusion ellipsoid can be quantified, but the two indices most com-monly used in the literature are Fractional Anisotropy (FA) for shape, and Mean Diffusivity (MD) for size.

FA is a measure of the anisotropy (i.e. non-sphericity) of the diffusion ellipsoid. FA is generally calculated with the following formula:

$$FA = \sqrt{((\lambda 1 - \lambda 2)^2 + (\lambda 2 - \lambda 3)^2 + (\lambda 1 - \lambda 3)^2)} / \sqrt{2} \cdot \sqrt{(\lambda 1^2 + \lambda 2^2 + \lambda 3^2)}$$

FA can vary between values of zero and one, with isotropic (spherical; Figure 1.3a) diffusion having a value of zero and completely anisotropic (aspherical; i.e. planar (Figure 1.3b) or linear (Figure 1.3c)) diffu-sion having a value of 1 (see Figure 1.3b). In a WM fiber bundle, reduced FA is generally assumed to reflect damage to the myelin or axon membrane, reduced axonal packing density, and/or reduced axo-nal coherence (Kubicki et al., 2007).

MD, in contrast, is a measure of the size of the diffusion ellipsoid, i.e. the average displacement of water molecules as a result of diffusion in a given amount of time. MD is generally calculated with the following formula:

$$MD = (\lambda 1 + \lambda 2 + \lambda 3)/3 = \text{Trace}/3$$

MD is highest in tissues where there are few impediments to water diffusion (e.g. CSF), and lowest

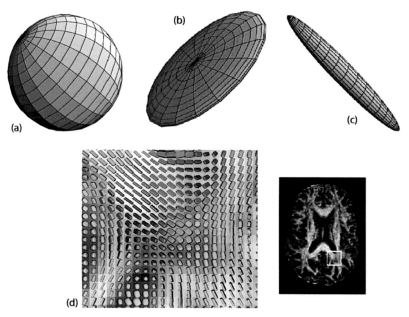

Figure 1.3 Diffusion ellipsoids come in many different shapes and sizes. Panel (a) illustrates the shape of the diffusion ellipsoid resulting from unrestricted water diffusion (i.e. isotropic). Isotropic diffusion is approximately what occurs in the fluid-filled ventricles where there are few obstacles to the diffusion of water. In the case of a WM fiber bundle, in contrast, the coherently aligned axon membranes and myelin sheaths constitute a significant obstacle to the diffusion of water. In this case, water will more readily diffuse parallel to the fiber bundle as opposed to perpendicular to it, and hence the resultant diffusion ellipsoid will be aspherical (i.e. anisotropic). An anisotropic diffusion ellipsoid can show either planar anisotropy (i.e. shaped like a disk as in panel (b)) or linear anisotropy (i.e. shaped like a cigar as in panel (c)). Mode is a measure of the linearity versus planarity of a diffusion ellipsoid. Panel (d) shows the variability in Mode between diffusion ellipsoids in the inferior fronto-occipital fasciculus of a healthy volunteer. Compare, for example, the "cigar-shaped" ellipsoids at the top left of the panel with the "disk-shaped" ellipsoids near the bottom left. Images used with the kind permission of Drs. Westin (panels a–c) and Kindlmann (panel d) at the Surgical Planning Laboratory, Department of Radiology, Brigham and Women's Hospital, and Harvard Medical School.

in tissues where diffusion is restricted at least one direction (e.g. WM). Although FA and MD are almost mathematically independent, they are often found to be inversely related in the brain (such that tissue showing high FA is generally found to show low MD), as the microstructural impediments that give rise to anisotropic diffusion also limit the maximal volume of the diffusion ellipsoid. Whilst FA and MD are the two indices that have been most commonly employed in the literature, a number of other indices – such as Mode (Ennis and Kindlmann, 2006), Inter-Voxel Coherence (Federspiel *et al.*, 2006), and Axial/Radial diffusivity (Song *et al.*, 2002) – have also been developed. As will be discussed further below, these novel indices are likely to play an important role in determining the microstructural underpinnings of the reported between-group differences in diffusivity.

Since 1998, when the first DTI study that investigated for WM abnormalities in SZ patients was published (Buchsbaum *et al.*, 1998), over 50 DTI studies have been published in the SZ literature. The methodologies and results of the DTI studies published to date are presented in Table 1.1. The remainder of this section summarizes the results of these studies, and discusses their implications with respect to the prevailing "connectivity" models of schizophrenia. This review aims to build on previously published reviews of the DTI literature, such as by Kubicki *et al.* (2007) and Kanaan *et al.* (2005).

Consistent findings in the DTI literature on SZ

As can be seen in Table 1.1, there have already been over 50 studies that have used DTI to investigate WM abnormalities in SZ patients, and this number is likely to increase dramatically in the next few years if recent publication trends are any guide. Some consistent results are already emerging, and these are summarized on a point-by-point basis in the following section. The following section also attempts to draw

Table 1.1 A summary of the studies published to date that have used DTI to investigate for white matter abnormalities in patients with schizophrenia. Acronyms: CSZ, chronic schizophrenia; FES, first-episode schizophrenia; EOS, early-onset schizophrenia; SPD, schizotypal personality disorder; nn, neuroleptic naïve; hall, with hallucinations; nonhall, without auditory hallucinations; CON, controls; EPI, echo-planar imaging; LSDI, line-scan diffusion imaging; FSE, fast spin-echo; ROI, region of interest; VBM, voxel-based morphometry; WM, white matter; FA, fractional anisotropy; MD, mean diffusivity; ADC, apparent diffusion coefficient; MTR, magnetization transfer ratio; IC, inter-voxel coherence; CC, corpus callosum; ILF, inferior longitudinal fasciculus; SLF, superior longitudinal fasciculus; FOF, frontal-occipital fasciculus; IFOF, inferior frontal-occipital fasciculus; SFOF, superior frontal-occipital fasciculus; RA, relative anisotropy

Study	Subjects	Acquisition details	Analysis method	Index	Significant groupwise differences (SZ relative to CON)	Significant clinical correlations
VOXEL-WISE/ MASS-ROI ANALYSIS						
Buchsbaum et al., 1998	5 CSZ, 6 CON	1.5T, LSDI, 7 directions, 7.3×2.7×1.8 mm, 6 slices	VBM (whole brain WM, p < 0.05 uncorrected, k = 116 voxels)	RA	Reduced RA in frontal WM and temporal WM, especially WM adjacent to putamen	–
Agartz et al., 2001	20 CSZ, 24 CON	1.5T, EPI, 20 directions, 1.8×1.8×4 mm, 22 slices	VBM (whole brain WM, p < 0.21 corrected, p(cluster) < 0.002)	FA	Reduced FA in splenium and forceps major	–
Foong et al., 2002	14 CSZ, 19 CON	1.5T, EPI, 7 directions, 2.5×2.5×5 mm, 12 slices	VBM (whole brain WM, p < 0.001 uncorrected, p(cluster) < 0.05 corrected)	FA, MD	No significant group-wise differences in FA or MD	–
Ardekani et al., 2003	14 CSZ, 14 CON	1.5T, EPI, 6 directions, 1.9×1.9×5 mm, 20 slices	VBM (whole brain WM, p < 0.01 uncorrected, k = 200 voxels)	FA	Widespread reductions in FA including in genu, midbody, splenium, inferior parietal lobule WM, superior and middle frontal gyrus WM, parahippocampal gyrus WM	–
Burns et al., 2003	30 CSZ, 30 CON	1.5T, EPI, 6 directions, 1.9×1.9×5 mm, 31 slices	VBM (ROIs in uncinate, arcuate and cingulum, p < 0.05 corrected)	FA	Reduced FA in arcuate fasciculus	–
Sun et al., 2003	30 CSZ, 19 CON	1.5T, EPI, 25 directions, 1.9×1.9×5 mm	ROIs in frontal, parietal, temporal and occipital WM, internal capsule, genu, splenium, and cingulum	FA	FA reductions in cingulum	–

Table 1.1 (cont.)

Study	Subjects	Acquisition details	Analysis method	Index	Significant groupwise differences (SZ relative to CON)	Significant clinical correlations
Hubl et al., 2004	13 CSZhall, 13 CSZnonhall, 13 CON	1.5T, LSDI, 6 directions, 1.8×1.7×5 mm, 12 slices	VBM (whole brain WM, $p < 0.05$ uncorrected, $k = 99$ voxels), and ROI analysis of significant clusters	FA	Widespread reductions in FA including in CC, arcuate fasciculus, uncinate fasciculus, ILF	CSZhall showed reduced FA relative to CON in the arcuate, uncinate and ILF. CSZhall showed increased FA relative to CSZnonhall in the arcuate, uncinate, ILF and CC
Park et al., 2004	23 CSZ, 32 CON	1.5T, LSDI, 6 directions, 1.7×1.3×4 mm, 31–35 slices	VBM (whole brain WM, $p < 0.005$ uncorrected, $k = 60$ voxels)	FA asymmetry	CSZ patients exhibited abnormally symmetrical FA in the cingulum, genu, internal capsule, uncinate and cerebral peduncle	–
Kubicki et al., 2005	21 CSZ, 26 CON	1.5T, LSDI, 6 directions, 1.7×1.3×4 mm, 31–35 slices	VBM (whole brain WM, $p < 0.005$ uncorrected, $k = 50$ voxels)	FA, MTR	Reduced FA in CC, cingulum, SFOF, IFOF, arcuate, internal capsule, fornix; Reduced MTR in CC, fornix, internal capsule, SFOF	–
Kumra et al., 2005	26 EOS, 34 CON	1.5T, EPI, 25 directions, 1.7×1.7×5 mm, 23 slices	VBM (whole brain WM, $p < 0.001$ uncorrected, $k = 100$ voxels)	FA	FA reductions in the cingulum	–
Buchsbaum et al., 2006	64 CSZ, 55 CON	3T, FSE, 12 directions, 1.6×1.6×3 mm, 28 slices	VBM (whole-brain WM, $p < 0.05$ (replication) and $p < 0.005$ (exploration))	FA	Widespread reductions in FA including in genu, SLF, cingulum, internal capsule, frontal WM, temporal WM	–
Federspiel et al., 2006	12 FES, 12 CON	1.5T, EPI, 6 directions, 3.8×3.8×5 mm, 12 slices	VBM (whole brain WM, $p < 0.02$ uncorrected, $k = 6$ voxels)	IC	Widespread reductions in IC including in CC, cingulum, SLF, internal	–

Study	Sample	Acquisition	Analysis	Measures	Findings	Correlations
					capsule. Increased IC in thalamic peduncle, optic radiation and external capsule.	
Hao et al., 2006	21 FES, 21 CON	1.5T, EPI, 13 directions, 1.7 × 1.7 × 4 mm, 30 slices	VBM (whole brain WM, $p < 0.001$ uncorrected, $k = 30$ voxels)	FA	Widespread reductions in FA including in the cingulum, SFOF, uncinate, insular WM, parahippocampal WM and precuneus WM	–
Jones et al., 2006	14 CSZ, 14 CON	1.5T, EPI, 2.5 × 2.5 × 2.5 mm	Tractography-derived analysis with seedpoints in the SLF, cingulum, uncinate and IFOF	FA, MD	Reduced FA in SLF	–
Douaud et al., 2007	25 EOS, 25 CON	1.5T, EPI, 60 directions, 2.5 × 2.5 × 2.5 mm, 60 slices	VBM (whole brain WM, $p < 0.05$ uncorrected, p(cluster) < 0.01 corrected)	FA, MD, axial and radial diffusivity	Reduced FA in corticospinal/pontine tracts, thalamic radiations, optic radiations, CC, arcuate fasciculus and brainstem WM. Reduced axial diffusivity and increased radial diffusivity across clusters	–
Mitelman et al., 2007	104 CSZ (51 w/ good outcome, 53 CSZ w/ poor outcome), 41 CON	EPI, 6 directions, 1.8 × 1.8 × 7.5 mm, 14 slices	Semi-automated placement of >100 ROIs throughout the WM	FA	Widespread reductions in FA including in internal capsule, thalamic radiations, cingulum, SLF, ILF	Positive correlations b/w PANSS-Positive scores and FA in internal capsule, FOF. Negative correlations b/w PANSS-Positive scores and FA in genu, cingulum and ILF, and b/w PANSS-Negative scores and FA in the internal capsule, SLF, CC, FOF

Table 1.1 (cont.)

Study	Subjects	Acquisition details	Analysis method	Index	Significant groupwise differences (SZ relative to CON)	Significant clinical correlations
Mori et al., 2007	42 CSZ, 42 CON	1.5T, EPI, 6 directions, 0.9×0.9×5 mm, 20 slices	VBM (whole-brain WM, $p < 0.001$ uncorrected)	FA	Widespread reductions in FA including in genu, splenium, cingulum, uncinate, frontal WM and temporal WM	–
Schlosser et al., 2007	18 CSZ, 18 CON	1.5T, EPI, 6 directions, 2.5×1.9×3 mm, 38 slices	VBM (whole brain WM, $p < 0.001$ uncorrected)	FA	Reduced FA in parahippocampal WM, cingulum and dorsolateral prefrontal WM	–
Seok et al., 2007	15 CSZhall, 15 CSZnonhall, 22 CON	1.5T, EPI, 32 directions, 1.72×1.72×2 mm, 45 slices	VBM (whole brain WM, $p < 0.001$ uncorrected, $k = 50$ voxels) and ROIs of significant clusters in the genu, cingulum, SLF, ILF and uncus WM	FA	Reduced FA in cingulum, SLF and cerebral peduncle	CSZhall showed increased FA relative to CSZnonhall in SLF. Positive correlation b/w hallucination severity and FA in SLF, and b/w PANSS-Positive score and FA in the SLF and cingulum
Shergill et al., 2007	33 CSZ, 40 CON	1.5T, EPI, 64 directions, 2.5×2.5×2.5 mm, 60 slices	VBM (whole brain WM, $p < 0.05$ uncorrected, $p(\text{cluster}) < 0.0001$)	FA	Reduced FA in SLF, ILF, genu	Propensity for auditory hallucinations associated with increased FA in the SLF, tapetum, cingulum and short fibers
White et al., 2007	14 EOS, 15 CON	3T, EPI, 12 directions, 2×2×2 mm	VBM (whole brain WM, $p < 0.001$ uncorrected)	FA, MD	Reduced FA in parahippocampal WM	–

Study	Subjects	Scanner/acquisition	Analysis method	Measure	Findings	Correlations
Cheung et al., 2008	25 FESnn, 26 CON	1.5T, EPI, 25 directions, 2.2×2.2×5 mm	VBM (whole brain WM, p < 0.05 FDR corrected); ROIs in genu and splenium of CC	FA	VBM: Reduced FA in splenium, FOF, ILF, internal capsule, precuneus WM, brainstem WM ROI: Reduced FA in splenium	–
Kyriakopoulos et al., 2008	19 EOS, 20 CON	1.5T, EPI, 64 directions, 1.9×1.9×2.5 mm, 60 slices	VBM (whole brain WM, p < 0.05 uncorrected, p(cluster) < 0.0025)	FA	FA reductions in parietal WM, splenium and cerebellar peduncle	No significant correlations b/w FA and PANSS-Positive or PANSS-Negative subscales
Seal et al., 2008	14 CSZ, 14 CON	3T, 28 directions, 1.9×1.9×2 mm, 50 slices	VBM (whole brain WM, p < 0.05 corrected)	FA, axial and radial diffusivity	Reduced FA in SLF, IFOF, uncinate, internal capsule	–
Szeszko et al., 2008	33 CSZ (doi <4.25yr), 30 CON	1.5T, EPI, 25 directions, 1.7×1.7×5 mm, 23 slices	VBM (whole brain WM, p < .001 uncorrected, k = 100 voxels)	FA	Reduced FA in uncinate, IFOF, SLF	Positive correlation b/w SADS-C+PD score (specifically auditory and visual hallucinations and delusions of control, mind-reading, persecution and reference) and FA in the IFOF. Negative correlation b/w FA in uncinate and SANS score (specifically alogia and affective flattening)
Schneiderman et al., 2009	35 CSZ, 33 CON; 23 FES, 15 CON	1.5T, EPI, 6 directions, 1.8×1.8×7.5 mm, 14 slices	Semi-automated placement of >50 ROIs throughout the WM	RA	SZ patients showed widespread reductions in FA including in the internal capsule, temporal-occipital WM, SFOF, and CC. The internal capsule and frontal anterior fasciculus showed differential patterns of aging in patients vs. controls	–

Table 1.1 (cont.)

Study	Subjects	Acquisition details	Analysis method	Index	Significant groupwise differences (SZ relative to CON)	Significant clinical correlations
CORPUS CALLOSUM						
Foong et al., 2000	20 CSZ, 25 CON	1.5T, EPI, 7 directions, 2.5×2.5×5 mm, 12 slices	ROIs in genu and splenium	FA, MD	Reduced FA and increased MD in splenium	No significant clinical correlations
Kumra et al., 2004	12 EOS, 9 CON	1.5T, FSE, 6 directions, 1.9×1.9×5 mm, 18 slices	ROIs in genu, splenium, frontal WM and occipital WM	FA	Reduced FA in frontal WM	No significant clinical correlations
Brambilla et al., 2005	67 CSZ, 70 CON	1.5T, EPI, 1.8×1.8×4 mm, 34 slices	ROIs in genu, midbody and splenium	ADC	Increased ADC in genu, midbody and splenium	Positive correlation b/w BPRS-Positive scores and ADC in genu
Price et al., 2005	20 FES, 29 CON	1.5T, EPI, 7 directions, 2.5×2.5×5 mm, 21 slices	ROIs in genu and splenium	FA, MD	No significant group-wise differences	–
Kanaan et al., 2006	33 SCZ, 40 CON	EPI, 64 directions, 2.5×2.5×2.5 mm, 60 slices	ROI in genu; tractography-derived analysis with genu ROI as seedpoint	FA	Reduced FA in genu with tractography-derived analysis method	–
Miyata et al., 2007	45 CSZ, 37 CON	3T, EPI, 12 directions, 1.7×1.7×3 mm, 40 slices	Tractography-derived analysis with seedpoints in the genu and splenium	FA, MD	No significant group-wise differences in FA or MD	No significant clinical correlations
Price et al., 2007	18 FEP, 21 CON	1.5T, EPI, 54 directions, 2.3×2.3×2.3 mm	Tractography-derived analysis with seedpoints in genu and splenium	FA	Reduced FA in genu and splenium	–
Friedman et al., 2008	40 FES, 39 CON; 40 CSZ, 40 CON	3T, FSE, 12 directions, 1.6×1.6×3 mm, 28 slices	ROIs in genu, splenium, forceps minor, forceps major and ILF	FA	Reduced FA in forceps minor, ILF	–

Study	Sample	Acquisition	Method	Measures	Findings	Correlations
Rotarska-Jagiela and Linden et al., 2008	24 CSZ, 24 CON	3T, EPI, 6 directions, 1.8×1.8×2 mm, 40 slices	Automated parcellation of CC into 9 segments	FA, MD	Reduced FA in genu (inferior and superior) and splenium	Positive correlations b/w PANSS-Positive scores and FA in genu, rostrum, midbody and isthmus. Negative correlations b/w PANSS-Positive scores and MD in isthmus and b/w PANSS-Negative scores and MD in midbody and isthmus
UNCINATE/ CINGULUM BUNDLE						
Kubicki et al., 2002	15 CSZ, 18 CON	1.5T, LSDI, 6 directions, 1.7×1.3×4mm, 31–35 slices	Semi-automated placement of ROI in uncinate	FA	No significant group-wise differences in FA	–
Kubicki et al., 2003	16 CSZ, 18 CON	1.5T, LSDI, 6 directions, 1.7×1.3×4mm, 31–35 slices	Semi-automated segmentation of cingulum	FA, MD	Reduced FA in cingulum	–
Fujiwara et al., 2007	42 CSZ, 24 CON	3T, EPI, 12 directions, 1.7×1.7×3 mm, 40 slices	Semi-automated placement of cingulum ROI	FA, FA asymmetry	Reduced FA in anterior and posterior cingulum. Loss of normal left > right FA asymmetry in the anterior cingulum	Negative correlation b/w FA in posterior cingulum and PANSS-Positive score
Gurrera et al., 2007	11 SPDnn, 8 CON	1.5T, LSDI, 6 directions, 1.7×1.3×4mm, 31–35 slices	Semi-automated placement of ROI in uncinate	FA, MD	Reduced FA in uncinate	–
Manoach et al., 2007	17 CSZ, 19 CON	3T, EPI, 72 directions, 2×2×2 mm, 64 slices	Semi-automated segmentation of cingulum; vertex-wise analysis (cingulum; $p < .05$ FDR corrected)	FA, FA asymmetry	Reduced FA in cingulum WM. CSZ patients showed abnormally large left > right FA asymmetry in the cingulum	–
Kendi et al., 2008	15 EOS, 15 CON	3T, EPI, 12 directions, 2×2×2 mm	Tractography-derived analysis with seedpoints in the fornix	FA, MD	No significant group-wise differences in FA or MD	No significant correlations b/w FA in fornix and SAPS, SANS or BPRS scores

Table 1.1 (cont.)

Study	Subjects	Acquisition details	Analysis method	Index	Significant groupwise differences (SZ relative to CON)	Significant clinical correlations
Nestor et al., 2008	25 CSZ, 28 CON	1.5T, LSDI, 6 directions, 1.7×1.3×4 mm, 31–35 slices	Tractography-derived analysis with seedpoints in cingulum and uncinate	FA	Reduced FA in cingulum	–
Price et al., 2008	19 FES, 23 CON	1.5T, EPI, 54 directions, 1.7×1.7×2.3 mm	Tractography-derived analysis with seedpoint in uncinate	FA, Probabilistic Index of Connectivity (PICo)	Reduced FA in uncinate	No significant correlations b/w FA or PICo and SAPS or SANS scores
Rosenberger et al., 2008	27 CSZ, 34 CON	1.5T, LSDI, 6 directions, 1.7×1.3×4 mm, 31–35 slices	Tractography-derived analysis with seedpoints in the uncinate, cingulum and IFOF	FA	Reduced FA in cingulum and IFOF	–
McIntosh et al., 2008	25 CSZ, 40 BPD, 49 CON	1.5T, EPI, 51 directions, 2.3×2.3×2.8 mm, 48 slices	Tractography-derived analysis with seedpoints in the uncinate and anterior thalamic radiations	FA	CON vs. CSZ: reduced FA in uncinate and anterior thalamic radiations. No significant differences b/w CSZ and BPD patients.	No significant correlations b/w FA and PANSS, YMRS or HDRS scores
Wang et al., 2004	21 CSZ, 20 CON	1.5T, EPI, 25 directions, 1.9×1.9×3 mm, 12 slices	ROIs in cingulum	FA	Reduced FA in cingulum. SCZ patients exhibited abnormally reduced left > right FA asymmetry in the cingulum	–
Kawashima et al., 2009	15 CSZ, 15 BPD (both within 4 yrs of first hospitalization), 15 CON	1.5T, LSDI, 6 directions, 1.7×1.3×4 mm, 31–35 slices	Semi-automated extraction of ROIs in uncinate and cingulum	FA, MD	Reduced FA in uncinate in SZ. BPD patients showed intermediate uncinate FA between SZ and CON	No significant correlations b/w FA in uncinate and PANSS subscale scores

FORNIX

Study	Sample	Acquisition	Analysis	Measures	Findings	Additional
Kuroki et al., 2006	24 CSZ, 31 CON	1.5T, LSDI, 6 directions, 1.7×1.3×4 mm, 31–35 slices	Tractography-derived analysis with seedpoints in the fornix	FA, MD	Reduced FA and increased MD in fornix	No significant correlations b/w FA or MD in fornix and SAPS or SANS scores
Takei et al., 2008	31 CSZ, 65 CON	1.5T, EPI, 6 directions	Tractography-derived analysis with seedpoints in the fornix	FA, MD	Reduced FA and increased MD in fornix	No significant correlations b/w FA in fornix and PANSS-Positive or Negative scores
Zhou et al., 2008	17 SCZ, 14 CON	1.5T, EPI, 13 directions, 1.9×1.9×4 mm, 30 slices	Tractography-derived analysis with seedpoints in fornix	FA	Reduced FA in fornix	No significant correlations b/w PANSS-Positive or Negative scores and FA in fornix

INTERNAL CAPSULE

Study	Sample	Acquisition	Analysis	Measures	Findings	Additional
Zou et al., 2008	21 CSZnn, 18 CON	1.5T, EPI, 12 directions, 1.6×1.6×3 mm	ROIs in internal capsule	FA, ADC	FA reduced in internal capsule	–

SUPERIOR/INFERIOR LONGITUDINAL FASCICULUS

Study	Sample	Acquisition	Analysis	Measures	Findings	Additional
Ashtari et al., 2007	23 EOS, 21 CON	1.5T, EPI, 15 directions, 2.5×2.5×2.5 mm, 50 slices	Tractography-derived analysis with seedpoints in the ILF and genu and VBM of extracted fibers ($p < 0.001$ FDR corrected, $k = 100$ voxels)	FA, MD, axial and radial diffusivity	Reduced FA, increased radial diffusivity and increased MD in the ILF	Patients w/ a history of visual hallucinations showed reduced FA in ILF relative to patients with no history
Karlsgodt et al., 2008	12 FES, 17 CON	1.5T, EPI, 6 directions, 2×2×2 mm, 75 slices	Semi-automated extraction of SLF; VBM (SLF, p(cluster) < 0.05)	FA	Reduced FA in SLF	–

Table 1.1 (cont.)

Study	Subjects	Acquisition details	Analysis method	Index	Significant groupwise differences (SZ relative to CON)	Significant clinical correlations
LOBAR WM						
Butler et al., 2006	17 CSZ, 21 CON	1.5T, EPI, 6 directions, 2×2×5 mm, 20 slices	ROIs in optic radiations, striate cortex WM, inferior parietal lobule WM, fusiform gyrus WM	FA	Reduced FA in optic radiations	–
Lim et al., 1999	10 CSZ, 10 CON	1.5T, EPI, 6 directions, 1.9×1.9×5 mm, 18 slices	Automated parcellation of whole-brain WM into 6 segments (L/R Prefrontal, Temperoparietal and Parieto-occipital)	FA	Reduced FA in Prefrontal WM	–
Minami et al., 2003	12 CSZ, 11 CON	1.5T, EPI, 1.9×1.9×6 mm	ROIs in frontal, temporal, parietal and occipital WM	FA	Reduced FA in the WM of all four ROIs	No significant correlations b/w PANSS-Positive or Negative scores and FA in any of the ROIs
Wolkin et al., 2003	10 CSZ	1.5T, EPI, 6 directions, 1.9×1.9×5 mm, 5 slices	ROIs in frontal WM	FA, MD	No control group	Negative correlation b/w frontal FA and SANS score

some tentative conclusions regarding the physiological underpinnings of the reported DTI abnormalities, and how they might relate to the GM abnormalities that were discussed in the first half of this chapter.

Fractional anisotropy is reduced in SZ patients, while mean diffusivity is increased

By far the most consistent finding in SZ patients, summarized in Table 1.1, is of FA reductions relative to matched healthy controls. Of the 56 studies that investigated group-wise differences in FA, all but 5 reported at least some evidence of FA reductions in SZ patients. In saying this, however, it should be noted that a sizeable proportion of the studies reported in Table 1.1 employed voxel-based analysis methods, which generally conduct thousands of statistical comparisons and have been criticized for their tendency to produce false-positive results, especially in the absence of stringent corrections for multiple comparisons (Davatzikos, 2004). The fact that statistically non-significant results are, in general, more difficult to publish than significant results could also be reason behind the scarcity of negative results in Table 1.1.

The second most consistent finding in SZ patients, summarized in Table 1.1, is of increased MD. In spite of the fact that MD was investigated in far fewer studies than was FA, MD increases were reported in the corpus callosum, inferior longitudinal fasciculus, and fornix. As mentioned previously, an inverse relationship is often observed between FA and MD, such that damage to a fiber bundle will typically result in regionally decreased FA but increased MD (Pfefferbaum and Sullivan, 2003). Thus, it is feasible that the abnormally reduced FA and increased MD simply reflect different indices of the same underlying neuropathology.

Diffusion anisotropy abnormalities in SZ patients are spatially widespread

Just as almost every gyrus and ganglion has been implicated as being structurally abnormal in the MRI literature (see above), diffusivity abnormalities have been reported in almost every major WM fiber bundle in SZ patients (see Table 1.1). This point is illustrated by Figure 1.4, in which the centroids of clusters of FA reductions from 20 VBM studies (12 chronic and 8 FES) are overlaid onto a single MR image. However, whilst it is true that the reported

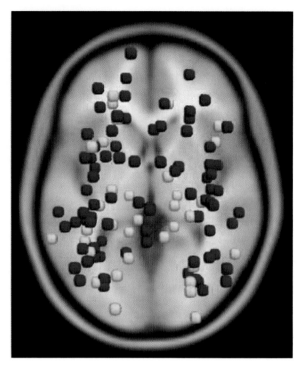

Figure 1.4 An illustration of the observed extent of the diffusion abnormalities exhibited by patients with schizophrenia. The colored dots represent the centers of voxel clusters for which SZ patients were found to exhibit reduced FA relative to matched controls in 12 VBM studies with chronic patients (pink dots) and 8 VBM studies with FES patients (yellow dots). As can be seen, all of the major WM fiber bundles have been implicated as being structurally abnormal by at least one VBM study. Image used with the kind permission of Eric Melonakos, Psychiatry Neuroimaging Laboratory, Department of Psychiatry, Brigham and Women's Hospital, and Harvard Medical School, and the Neuroscience Center, Brigham Young University.

diffusivity abnormalities have been widespread, it is also true that some fiber bundles have been more consistently found to be abnormal than have others, with the corpus callosum, uncinate fasciculus, cingulum bundle, and superior longitudinal fasciculus among the most consistently affected bundles.

One explanation for these results is simply that SZ is associated with diffuse WM abnormalities that affect most of the major fiber bundles. However, an alternative explanation (and one that will be revisited in a later section) is that the non-specificity of the DTI abnormalities is an artifact of studies lumping together patients with vastly different clinical profiles into a heterogeneous "schizophrenia group". In other words, it is possible that SZ patients with certain types of clinical symptoms (e.g. auditory hallucinations) will show quite different patterns of WM abnormality relative to patients experiencing other types of clinical symptoms (e.g. passivity experiences), but that these bundle-specific abnormalities are washed out when patients are lumped together into a catch-all diagnostic group. A third explanation lies in the fact that the methodologies used for DTI acquisition, processing and analysis have been largely unstandardized and thus vary considerably between research groups.

Irregular myelin may underpin the diffusion anisotropy abnormalities observed in SZ patients

There is evidence indicating that axonal membranes are the primary determinant of anisotropic water diffusion in WM fiber bundles (Beaulieu and Allen, 1994). Hence one possibility is that the reported FA reductions in SZ patients are due to these patients experiencing a pathological reduction in their number of axons. However, as discussed previously, the evidence suggests that SZ patients do not experience a significant amount of neuron death, but that their characteristic GM atrophy is more likely caused by a reduction in synaptic infrastructure and neuropil. Thus, if SZ patients do not show reduced numbers of neurons (and hence axons) relative to healthy controls, an alternative possibility is that the observed FA abnormalities are caused by damage to their myelin.

It has already been demonstrated that myelin abnormalities alone can result in substantial reductions in FA. In a recent study, Roy et al. (2007) observed disrupted normal oligodendrocyte development in mice by blocking the signaling of a necessary growth factor (Neuroregulin-1). While these transgenic mice showed no differences in the size or density of axons in the corpus callosum, they did show substantial reductions in myelin thickness and also marked reductions in FA. Intriguingly, these mice also showed abnormal increases in their levels of dopamine receptors and transporters, both of which are typical of SZ patients (Seeman and Kapur, 2000).

There is also evidence indicating that it is possible to distinguish between axonal damage and dysmyelination on the basis of the distinctive patterns of diffusivity abnormalities induced by these injuries. Specifically, Song et al. (2002) demonstrated that while the amount of diffusion perpendicular to the principal orientation of the optic nerve (which they termed "Radial Diffusivity") was increased in transgenic shiverer mice with severe dysmyelination, the amount of diffusion parallel to the tract ("Axial Diffusivity") was unaffected. Conversely, Song et al. (2003) demonstrated that axonal injury concurrent with myelin preservation resulted in a decrease in axial diffusivity but no change in radial diffusivity. These results are especially significant in the context of the study by Ashtari et al. (2007) (see Table 1.1), who found that schizophrenia patients exhibited abnormally increased Radial Diffusivity in the inferior longitudinal fasciculus, but no difference in Axial Diffusivity – indicating the presence of myelin abnormalities but the absence of axonal abnormalities. When taken in combination, the results of these studies suggest that myelin abnormalities are at least partially responsible for the FA reduction typically observed in SZ patients. These studies also illustrate the value of using novel indices of diffusivity in combination with the stalwart indices of FA and MD.

Evidence is equivocal as to whether WM abnormalities are present at FES

It is as yet unclear as to whether WM abnormalities are present in patients suffering from FES. The results of the FES studies summarized in Table 1.1 are equivocal. For example, Hao et al. (2006) reported widespread FA reductions in FES patients, including in the cingulum, inferior temporal gyrus WM and precuneus WM. Price et al. (2007) also reported abnormal FA reductions in the genu and splenium of FES patients, and Federspiel et al. (2006) reported widespread abnormal reduction in inter-voxel coherence in FES patients, including in the corpus, cingulum, and superior longitudinal fasciculus. On the other hand, Price et al. (2005, 2008) failed to find evidence of significant differences in FA between FES patients and controls in the corpus callosum and uncinate fasciculus, respectively. Friedman et al. (2008) also failed to find evidence of FA abnormalities in the inferior longitudinal fasciculus or the genu, splenium, forceps minor, or forceps major of the corpus in FES patients, but did report FA abnormalities in at least a subset of these regions of interest (ROIs) in patients with chronic schizophrenia.

The fact that FES patients have, as a whole, been found to exhibit fewer and less severe diffusion abnormalities compared to chronic patients suggests that the inferred WM abnormalities are progressive, at least over the initial years of illness. While this issue has not yet been empirically addressed by means of a longitudinal DTI study (although several studies have identified a negative correlation between age and diffusion anisotropy measures in SZ patients; e.g. Rosenberger *et al.*, 2008), it has been investigated using conventional MRI. For example, Whitford *et al.* (2007a) reported evidence that FES patients lost a significantly greater volume of WM in the uncinate fasciculus bilaterally over the first 2–3 years of their illness, relative to matched healthy controls. It would be informative if this finding could be replicated using DTI, especially in light of evidence from functional MRI which has indicated that frontotemporal connectivity is abnormal in SZ patients (Lawrie *et al.*, 2002).

Positive correlation between FA and psychotic symptoms in SZ patients

One interesting and consistently reported finding in the DTI literature is of a positive correlation between FA and the severity of psychotic symptoms in SZ patients. That is, the majority of those studies in Table 1.1 that reported a significant correlation between FA and psychotic symptom severity observed patients with higher FA values to show more severe psychotic symptoms relative to patients with lower FA values. Rotarska-Jagiela and Linden *et al.* (2008), for example, reported a positive correlation between FA in the corpus and patients' scores on the PANSS-Positive subscale. Similarly, Mitelman *et al.* (2007) reported a positive correlation between FA in the internal capsule and fronto-occipital fasciculus and PANSS-Positive subscale score (although to be fair they did also report a number of negative correlations). Hubl *et al.* (2004) compared SZ patients with auditory hallucinations to non-hallucinating patients and found that the hallucinating patients exhibited higher FA in the corpus, cingulum and arcuate fasciculus than non-hallucinators. Similarly, Seok *et al.* (2007) reported significantly higher FA values in the SLF in patients with auditory hallucinations compared with non-hallucinating patients. They also reported a positive correlation between FA in SLF and the severity of patients' hallucinations. Shergill *et al.* (2007) reported that the propensity for auditory hallucinations in patients with SZ was associated with increased FA in the superior longitudinal fasciculus. Finally, Szeszko *et al.* (2008) reported that higher FA in the inferior fronto-occipital fasciculus correlated with the severity of several psychotic symptoms including auditory hallucinations, delusions

of control, delusions of mind-reading, and persecutory delusions.

What is notable about the aforementioned studies is that they did not observe "highly symptomatic" patients to exhibit *abnormally* high levels of FA, i.e. relative to healthy controls. In contrast, of the two studies (Seok *et al.*, 2007; Hubl *et al.*, 2004) that directly compared the FA of "highly symptomatic" patients with that of healthy controls, both observed the "highly symptomatic" patients to have reduced FA in the ROIs they investigated. The FA of these regions was, however, significantly higher in the "highly symptomatic" patients relative to the "less symptomatic" patients.

What is the explanation for this seemingly paradoxical finding that the more floridly psychotic a SZ patient, the less severe their FA abnormalities? One possibility lies in the fact that patients with chronic SZ (who constituted the patient sample in the aforementioned studies) have typically received heavy exposure to neuroleptic medications over the course of their illness. This point is salient given that, in addition to reducing the severity of patients' psychotic symptoms, neuroleptic medications have been suggested to cause cerebral atrophy in and of themselves, and especially in the oligodendrocytes which constitute the bulk of the white matter (Konopaske *et al.*, 2008). Thus one possible explanation for the general finding that the more floridly psychotic SZ patients had less severe FA abnormalities than their less-psychotic counterparts could be that highly psychotic patients received less exposure to neuroleptic medications. Whilst this explanation must be considered seriously, especially in the absence of a study identifying a positive correlation between diffusion anisotropy and psychotic symptomatology in neuroleptic-naive SZ patients, it must also be borne in mind that at least two of the aforementioned studies (Seok *et al.*, 2007; Szeszko *et al.*, 2008) statistically controlled for patients' exposure to neuroleptic medications and still observed the positive correlation.

An alternative possibility lies with the "self-monitoring" theory of psychotic symptoms (Feinberg, 1978; Frith, 1992; Ford *et al.*, 2001). Broadly speaking, the "self-monitoring" theory argues that psychotic symptoms can arise when a person performs an action (either physical, such as moving one's hand, or mental, such as engaging in internal speech) without being aware of their intention to perform the action. This "failure of awareness" has been hypothesized to be caused by abnormalities in the "corollary discharges"

(CDs) that are sent from the brain regions involved in initiating the action (e.g. the premotor cortex, in the example of a hand movement) to the regions involved in processing the sensory consequences of that action (e.g. the parietal lobe, in the example of the hand movement; Frith *et al.*, 2000). It has previously been suggested by Whitford *et al.* (in press) that abnormalities in WM fiber bundles connecting the initiation and destination sites of CDs could underpin some psychotic symptoms. Specifically, if FA reductions resulting from dysmyelination were present in WM fiber bundles connecting the sites of CD initiation and destination, then the consequently slowed transmission velocity of the CDs could result in the CDs and the primary discharges reaching their respective destinations asynchronously. In the example of the hand movement, this could result in a person moving their hand before being aware of their intention to do so, which could lead to delusions of control (Frith and Done, 1989). The relevant point here is that a greater degree of dysmyelination (and a consequently slower transmission velocity), would not necessarily be expected to result in more severe psychotic symptoms. On the contrary, it is possible that primary discharges and CDs can only be integrated (even pathologically, as in the example of the delusion) if they arrive at their respective destinations within a certain critical time period. Thus if severe dysmyelination caused a CD to arrive at its destination too late to even be pathologically associated with its primary discharges, then rather than resulting in a psychotic symptom, this might instead trigger symptoms of psychomotor poverty, as the network might "freeze up": "much as a computer locks up when it cannot match signals sent at an incorrect rate" in the words of Andreasen (1999, p. 785). This might explain why the "highly psychotic" patients in the aforementioned studies exhibited FA values closer to normal that their "less-psychotic" counterparts. Testing this hypothesis could provide a fruitful avenue for future research, and emphasizes the importance of distinguishing between SZ patients on the basis of their symptom profiles, rather than simply lumping patients together into the catch-all diagnostic basket of "schizophrenia".

How do these findings relate to each other? A speculative hypothesis

If one thing is clear from the multitude of MRI and DTI studies reviewed in this chapter, it is that there is now a great deal of evidence indicating that SZ patients exhibit consistent (albeit subtle) and widespread abnormalities in both their GM and WM. An important question, then, is whether these GM and WM abnormalities have separate causes, or whether they share a common underlying pathology.

In this final section, a highly speculative theory is presented as to how a single mechanism could potentially underlie the GM abnormalities, WM abnormalities, hyperdopaminergia and psychotic features characteristic of schizophrenia.

The theory presupposes that schizophrenia arises because of some (currently incompletely understood) developmental trigger during late adolescence/early adulthood. This trigger (which may relate to the peripubertal increase in the levels of sex hormones; De Bellis *et al.*, 2001) causes the abnormal expression of a number of oligodendrocyte-related genes during the peripubertal myelination of the association cortices. The resulting myelin is structurally abnormal (Uranova *et al.*, 2007), and subsequently functionally abnormal in its ability to insulate axon membranes and increase the conduction velocity of action potentials. This disruption results in small but significant transmission delays in communications between spatially disparate GM regions. If this dysmyelination occurs in WM fiber bundles connecting the initiation and destination sites of certain corollary discharges (CDs), then this results in the CDs reaching their destination subsequent to the termination of their corresponding primary discharge. As discussed previously, this could lead to actions being performed in the absence of an awareness of an intention to act, which in turn could lead to internally generated actions being perceived as externally generated, and subsequently certain types of psychotic symptoms.

To speculate even further, it is possible that the brain's response to feedback indicating that internally generated, willed actions are not being executed as planned (i.e. due to them being perceived as externally generated) is to amplify the neural signal(s) involved in initiating the willed action. In this regard it is interesting to consider the role that dopamine is known to play in the initiation of motor actions (Jahanshahi and Frith, 1998).[4] To summarize, if the brain's response to the "feeling" that internally generated actions were not being executed as planned was to either increase its levels of dopamine or increase its sensitivity to dopamine (e.g. by increasing its number of dopamine receptors), then this could explain the hyperdopaminergia characteristically exhibited by SZ patients. Furthermore, this could also account for the fascinating results of Roy *et al.* (2007). As previously mentioned, Roy *et al.* (2007) disrupted normal oligodendrocyte development in mice by blocking the signaling of a necessary growth factor (Neuroregulin-1). The resultant transgenic mice exhibited significantly thinned myelin in the corpus callosum, significant FA reductions, significant nerve conduction delays and *significantly increased levels of dopamine receptors and transporters* in the limbic system, basal ganglia and cortex. In other words, by disrupting normal myelin formation, they were able to increase the sensitivity of the brains of these transgenic mice to dopamine – just as the brains of SZ patients have been shown to be hypersensitive to dopamine (Seeman and Kapur, 2000).

In addition to underpinning the hyperdopaminergia and psychosis associated with schizophrenia, the disruption in neural synchronization caused by myelin abnormalities could also potentially underlie the GM atrophy associated with the disease. It has previously been shown that one of the major factors influencing whether a synapse in the embryonic nervous system survives development is the synchrony of its activity relative to the activity of other synapses on the same neuron. Specifically, there is evidence that a synapse is more likely to be eliminated if it is asynchronously active relative to other synapses on the same neuron (Purves and Lichtman, 1980). If (a) similar mechanisms for synaptic elimination occur for the periadolescent "synaptic prune" as for embryonic development, and (b) dysmyelination does indeed result in disrupted neural synchrony in SZ patients, then this dysmyelination could result in the elimination of synapses that would otherwise have been preserved, i.e. a period of "hyper-pruning" in SZ patients (Bartzokis, 2002; Whitford *et al.*, in press). Such a reduction in the number of synapses and their associated infrastructure could potentially account for the GM atrophy typically observed in SZ patients, and would be consistent with the observation that SZ patients show an increase in neuron density but not a reduction in neuron number (Selemon and Goldman-Rakic, 1999).

Needless to say, this theory is extremely speculative and would benefit from a great deal more supporting empirical evidence. However, if nothing else, the theory provides an example of how GM and WM abnormalities that have been so consistently observed in SZ patients could feasibly be caused by a single underlying pathological mechanism.

Concluding comments

This chapter has attempted to summarize the findings of the 800+ structural MR studies and 50+ DTI studies that have investigated structural brain abnormalities in patients with schizophrenia. The chapter concludes with a potential mechanism by which the GM abnormalities (identified via MRI) and WM abnormalities (identified via DTI) that have been consistently reported in SZ patients could potentially result from a single underlying cause – namely, abnormal myelin development in the periadolescent period. Regardless of whether the hypothesis turns out to be correct, however, we suggest that it is important to consider both the mechanisms underlying the characteristic neuropathologies of schizophrenia and the relationship between these neuropathologies and the clinical features of the disease. Only by understanding these mechanisms will it become possible to target them directly with therapy – both pharmacological and psychological. For example, if dysmyelination was indeed shown to underlie the GM atrophy and hyperdopaminergia characteristic of schizophrenia, then targeting the root cause of this problem (e.g. with remyelinating medications such as those currently used in the treatment of multiple sclerosis; Stangel, 2004) could provide a useful adjunct to the presently available battery of antipsychotic medications. In contrast to the prevailing belief of 50 years ago, it is now clear – largely as a result of the MRI and DTI research discussed in this chapter – that there *is* a neuropathology of schizophrenia. The overriding challenge now is to understand the cause of this neuropathology. Once we are armed with this understanding, it may finally be possible to develop a targeted and comprehensive treatment strategy for this terrible disease that causes so much suffering to so many people.

Acknowledgments

Thomas Whitford is supported by an Overseas-Based Biomedical Training Fellowship from the National Health and Medical Research Council of Australia (NHMRC 520627), administered through the University of Melbourne. Marek Kubicki is supported by grants from the National Institutes of Health (R03 MH068464–0), the Harvard Medical School (Milton Award) and the National Alliance for Research on Schizophrenia and Depression. Martha Shenton is supported by grants from the National Institutes of Health (K05 MH 070047 and R01 MH 50747), the Department of Veterans Affairs (VA Merit Award, VA Research Enhancement Award Program and

VA Schizophrenia Research Center Grant), and the Boston Center for Intervention Development and Applied Research (CIDAR) funded through a center grant mechanism (P50 MH 080272). This work is also supported, in part, from the National Alliance for Medical Image Computing (NAMIC), funded by the National Institutes of Health through the NIH Roadmap Initiative for Medical Research (Grant U54 EB005149 to Kubicki and Shenton).

Box 1.1.   Summary

After more than 20 years of structural MRI and 10 years of DTI research, it is now clear that schizophrenia is associated with subtle yet widespread abnormalities in both the gray and white matter of the brain.

The evidence suggests that the widely documented gray matter abnormalities (most consistently reported in the temporal cortex, limbic system and association cortices) do not represent widespread neuron death, but are instead likely due to the elimination of synaptic infrastructure.

While less is known about the microstructural underpinnings of the white matter abnormalities (inferred with DTI), they are thought, at least in part, to be due to abnormalities in the developmental process of myelination.

Given the role that myelin is known to play in modulating the transmission velocity of action potentials, there has been growing interest in the idea that the cognitive disorganization and psychotic symptoms characteristic of schizophrenia could result from dysmyelination-induced transmission delays causing a discoordination in the activity of spatially disparate populations of neurons.

In light of studies indicating that the synchrony of synaptic activity is a major determinant of synaptic survival during development, it is also feasible that such dysmyelination-induced transmission delays could induce asynchronous synaptic activity and hence abnormal synaptic elimination during the normative periadolescent period of "synaptic pruning". Dysmyelination could also feasibly underpin the hyperdopaminergia characteristic of schizophrenia if it interfered with the neural circuitry underlying the generation and monitoring of willed actions.

While the ultimate role of myelin abnormalities in the etiology of schizophrenia remains largely unclear, the idea that schizophrenia could ultimately be a disorder of the white matter – with the well-documented gray matter abnormalities as a secondary consequence – is one that has the potential to radically change both the conceptualization of the disorder, and its treatment strategies.

References

Agartz I, Andersson J L and Skare S. 2001. Abnormal brain white matter in schizophrenia: a diffusion tensor imaging study. *Neuroreport* **12**, 2251–4.

Andreasen N C. 1999. A unitary model of schizophrenia: Bleuler's "fragmented phrene" as schizencephaly. *Arch Gen Psychiatry* **56**, 781–7.

Ardekani B A, Nierenberg J, Hoptman M J, Javitt D C and Lim K O. 2003. MRI study of white matter diffusion anisotropy in schizophrenia *Neuroreport* **14**, 2025–9.

Ashtari M, Cottone J, Ardekani B, *et al.* 2007. Disruption of white matter integrity in the inferior longitudinal fasciculus in adolescents with schizophrenia as revealed by fiber tractography. *Arch Gen Psychiatry* **64**, 1270–80.

Bartzokis G. 2002. Schizophrenia: breakdown in the well-regulated lifelong process of brain development and maturation. *Neuropsychopharmacology* **27**, 672–83.

Baumann N and Pham-Dinh D. 2001. Biology of oligodendrocyte and myelin in the mammalian central nervous system. *Physiol Rev* **81**, 871–927.

Beaulieu C and Allen P. 1994. Determinants of anisotropic water diffusion in nerves. *Mag Res Med* **31**, 394–400.

Bleuler E. 1911. *Dementia Praecox or the Group of Schizophrenias.* New York, NY: International Universities Press.

Borgwardt S, Riecher-Rössler A, Dazzan P, *et al.* 2007. Regional gray matter volume abnormalities in the at risk mental state. *Biol Psychiatry* **61**, 1148–56.

Bourgeois J P and Rakic P. 1993. Changes of synaptic density in the primary visual cortex of the macaque monkey from fetal to adult stage. *J Neurosci* **13**, 2801–20.

Brambilla P, Cerini R, Gasparini A, *et al.* 2005. Investigation of corpus callosum in schizophrenia with diffusion imaging. *Schizophr Res* **79**, 201–10.

Buchsbaum M, Tang C, Peled S, *et al.* 1998. MRI white matter diffusion anisotropy and PET metabolic rate in schizophrenia. *Neuroreport* **9**, 425–30.

Buchsbaum M S, Friedman J, Buchsbaum B R, *et al.* 2006. Diffusion tensor imaging in schizophrenia. *Biol Psychiatry* **60**, 1181–7.

Burns J, Job D, Bastin M E, *et al.* 2003. Structural disconnectivity in schizophrenia: a diffusion tensor magnetic resonance imaging study. *Br J Psychiatry* **182**, 439–43.

Butler P, Hoptman M, Nierenberg J, Foxe J, Javitt D and Lim K. 2006. Visual white matter integrity in schizophrenia. *Am J Psychiatry* **163**, 2011–3.

Cahn W, Pol H E, Lems E B, *et al.* 2002. Brain volume changes in first-episode schizophrenia: a 1-year follow-up study. *Arch Gen Psychiatry* **59**, 1002–10.

Cheung V, Cheung C, McAlonan G, *et al.* 2008. A diffusion tensor imaging study of structural dysconnectivity in never-medicated, first-episode schizophrenia. *Psychol Med* **38**, 877–85.

Crow T. 1998. Schizophrenia as a transcallosal misconnection syndrome. *Schizophr Res* **30**, 111–4.

Davatzikos C. 2004. Why voxel-based morphometric analysis should be used with great caution when characterizing group differences. *Neuroimage* **23**, 17–20.

De Bellis M, Keshavan M, Beers S, *et al.* 2001. Sex differences in brain maturation during childhood and adolescence. *Cereb Cortex* **11**, 552–7.

Douaud G, Smith S, Jenkinson M, *et al.* 2007. Anatomically related grey and white matter abnormalities in adolescent-onset schizophrenia. *Brain* **130**, 2375–86.

Ellison-Wright I, Glahn D, Laird A, Thelen S and Bullmore E. 2008. The anatomy of first-episode and chronic schizophrenia: an anatomical likelihood estimation meta-analysis. *Am J Psychiatry* **165**, 1015–23.

Ennis D and Kindlmann G. 2006. Orthogonal tensor invariants and the analysis of diffusion tensor magnetic resonance images. *Magn Reson Med* **55**, 136–46.

Federspiel A, Begré S, Kiefer C, Schroth G, Strik W and Dierks T. 2006. Alterations of white matter connectivity in first episode schizophrenia. *Neurobiol Dis* **22**, 702–9.

Feinberg I. 1978. Efference copy and corollary discharge: implications for thinking and its disorders. *Schizophr Bull* **4**, 636–40.

Feinberg I. 1982. Schizophrenia: caused by a fault in programmed synaptic elimination during adolescence? *J Psychiatr Res* **17**, 319–34.

Fields R. 2004. The other half of the brain. *Sci Am* **290**, 54–61.

Fields R. 2008. White matter in learning, cognition and psychiatric disorders. *Trends Neurosci* **31**, 361–70.

Foong J, Maier M, Clark C A, Barker G J, Miller D H and Ron M A. 2000. Neuropathological abnormalities of the corpus callosum in schizophrenia: a diffusion tensor imaging study. *J Neurol Neurosurg Psychiatry* **68**, 242–4.

Foong J, Symms M R, Barker G J, Maier M, Miller D H and Ron M A. 2002. Investigating regional white matter in schizophrenia using diffusion tensor imaging. *Neuroreport* **13**, 333–6.

Ford J M, Mathalon D H, Heinks T, Kalba S, Faustman W O and Roth W T. 2001. Neurophysiological evidence of corollary discharge dysfunction in schizophrenia. *Am J Psychiatry* **158**, 2069–71.

Friedman J, Tang C, Carpenter D, *et al.* 2008. Diffusion tensor imaging findings in first-episode and chronic schizophrenia patients. *Am J Psychiatry* **165**, 1024–32.

Friston K. 1999. Schizophrenia and the disconnection hypothesis. *Acta Psychiatr Scand Suppl* **395**, 68–79.

Frith C D. 1992. *The Cognitive Neuropsychology of Schizophrenia*. Hove, UK: Lawrence Erlbaum Associates.

Frith C D, Blakemore S and Wolpert D M. 2000. Explaining the symptoms of schizophrenia: abnormalities in the awareness of action. *Brain Res Rev* **31**, 357–63.

Frith C D and Done D J. 1989. Experiences of alien control in schizophrenia reflect a disorder in the central monitoring of action. *Psychol Med* **19**, 359–63.

Fujiwara H, Namiki C, Hirao K, *et al.* 2007. Anterior and posterior cingulum abnormalities and their association with psychopathology in schizophrenia: a diffusion tensor imaging study. *Schizophr Res* **95**, 215–22.

Garner B, Pariante C, Wood S, *et al.* 2005. Pituitary volume predicts future transition to psychosis in individuals at ultra-high risk of developing psychosis. *Biol Psychiatry* **58**, 417–23.

Glahn D, Laird A, Ellison-Wright I, *et al.* 2008. Meta-analysis of gray matter anomalies in schizophrenia: application of anatomic likelihood estimation and network analysis. *Biol Psychiatry* **64**, 774–81.

Gur R E, Cowell P, Turetsky B I, *et al.* 1998. A follow-up magnetic resonance imaging study of schizophrenia: relationship of neuroanatomical changes to clinical and neurobehavioral measures. *Arch Gen Psychiatry* **55**, 145–52.

Gurrera R, Nakamura M, Kubicki M, *et al.* 2007. The uncinate fasciculus and extraversion in schizotypal personality disorder: a diffusion tensor imaging study. *Schizophr Res* **90**, 360–2.

Hao Y, Liu Z, Jiang T, *et al.* 2006. White matter integrity of the whole brain is disrupted in first-episode schizophrenia. *Neuroreport* **17**, 23–6.

Hirayasu Y, Tanaka S, Shenton M E, *et al.* 2001. Prefrontal gray matter volume reduction in first episode schizophrenia. *Cerebral Cortex* **11**, 374–81.

Honea R, Crow T J, Passingham D and Mackay C E. 2005. Regional deficits in brain volume in schizophrenia: a meta-analysis of voxel-based morphometry studies. *Am J Psychiatry* **162**, 2233–45.

Hubl D, Koenig T, Strik W, *et al.* 2004. Pathways that make voices: white matter changes in auditory hallucinations. *Arch Gen Psychiatry* **61**, 658–68.

Jahanshahi M and Frith C. 1998. Willed action and its impairments. *Cogn Neuropsychol* **15**, 483.

Jones D K, Catani M, Pierpaoli C, *et al.* 2006. Age effects on diffusion tensor magnetic resonance imaging tractography measures of frontal cortex connections in schizophrenia. *Hum Brain Mapp* **27**, 230–8.

Kanaan R A, Kim J S, Kaufmann W E, Pearlson G D, Barker G J and McGuire P K. 2005. Diffusion tensor imaging in schizophrenia. *Biol Psychiatry* **58**, 921–9.

Kanaan R A, Shergill S S, Barker G J, *et al.* 2006. Tract-specific anisotropy measurements in diffusion tensor imaging. *Psychiatry Res* **146**, 73–82.

Karlsgodt K, van Erp T, Poldrack R, Bearden C, Nuechterlein K and Cannon T. 2008. Diffusion tensor imaging of the superior longitudinal fasciculus and working memory in recent-onset schizophrenia. *Biol Psychiatry* **63**, 512–8.

Kasai K, Shenton M E, Salisbury D F, *et al.* 2003. Progressive decrease of left Heschl gyrus and planum temporale gray matter volume in first-episode schizophrenia: a longitudinal magnetic resonance imaging study. *Arch Gen Psychiatry* **60**, 766–75.

Kawashima T, Nakamura M, Boiux S, *et al.* 2009. Uncinate fasciculus abnormalities in recent onset schizophrenia and affective psychosis: a diffusion tensor imaging study. *Schiz Res* **110**, 119–26.

Kendi M, Kendi A, Lehericy S, *et al.* 2008. Structural and diffusion tensor imaging of the fornix in childhood- and adolescent-onset schizophrenia. *J Am Acad Child Adolesc Psychiatry* **47**, 826–32.

Keshavan M S, Anderson S and Pettegrew J W. 1994. Is schizophrenia due to excessive synaptic pruning in the prefrontal cortex? The Feinberg hypothesis revisited. *J Psychiatr Res* **28**, 239–65.

Konopaske G, Dorph-Petersen K, Sweet R, *et al.* 2008. Effect of chronic antipsychotic exposure on astrocyte and oligodendrocyte numbers in macaque monkeys. *Biol Psychiatry* **63**, 759–65.

Kraepelin E, ed. 1907. *Textbook of Psychiatry.* London: Macmillan.

Kubicki M, McCarley R, Westin C F, *et al.* 2007. A review of diffusion tensor imaging studies in schizophrenia. *J Psychiatr Res* **41**, 15–30.

Kubicki M, Park H, Westin C F, *et al.* 2005. DTI and MTR abnormalities in schizophrenia: analysis of white matter integrity. *Neuroimage* **26**, 1109–18.

Kubicki M, Westin C F, Maier S E, *et al.* 2002. Uncinate fasciculus findings in schizophrenia: a magnetic resonance diffusion tensor imaging study. *Am J Psychiatry* **159**, 813–20.

Kubicki M, Westin C F, Nestor P G, *et al.* 2003. Cingulate fasciculus integrity disruption in schizophrenia: a magnetic resonance diffusion tensor imaging study. *Biol Psychiatry* **54**, 1171–80.

Kumra S, Ashtari M, Cervellione K, *et al.* 2005. White matter abnormalities in early-onset schizophrenia: a voxel-based diffusion tensor imaging study. *J Am Acad Child Adolesc Psychiatry* **44**, 934–41.

Kumra S, Ashtari M, McMeniman M, *et al.* 2004. Reduced frontal white matter integrity in early-onset schizophrenia: a preliminary study. *Biol Psychiatry* **55**, 1138–45.

Kuroki N, Kubicki M, Nestor P G, *et al.* 2006. Fornix integrity and hippocampal volume in male schizophrenic patients. *Biol Psychiatry* **60**, 22–31.

Kyriakopoulos M, Vyas N, Barker G, Chitnis X and Frangou S. 2008. A diffusion tensor imaging study of white matter in early-onset schizophrenia. *Biol Psychiatry* **63**, 519–23.

Lawrie S M, Buechel C, Whalley H C, Frith C D, Friston K J and Johnstone E C. 2002. Reduced frontotemporal functional connectivity in schizophrenia associated with auditory hallucinations. *Biological Psychiatry* **51**, 1008–11.

Lim K O, Hedehus M, Moseley M, de Crespigny A, Sullivan E V and Pfefferbaum A. 1999. Compromised white matter tract integrity in schizophrenia inferred from diffusion tensor imaging. *Arch Gen Psychiatry* **56**, 367–74.

Manoach D, Ketwaroo G, Polli F, *et al.* 2007. Reduced microstructural integrity of the white matter underlying anterior cingulate cortex is associated with increased saccadic latency in schizophrenia. *Neuroimage* **37**, 599–610.

McIntosh A M, Maniega S M, Lymer G K S, *et al.* 2008. White matter tractography in bipolar disorder and schizophrenia. *Biol Psychiatry* **64**, 1088–92.

Minami T, Nobuhara K, Okugawa G, *et al.* 2003. Diffusion tensor magnetic resonance imaging of disruption of regional white matter in schizophrenia. *Neuropsychobiology* **47**, 141–5.

Mitelman S, Torosjan Y, Newmark R, *et al.* 2007. Internal capsule, corpus callosum and long associative fibers in good and poor outcome schizophrenia: a diffusion tensor imaging survey. *Schizophr Res* **92**, 211–24.

Miyata J, Hirao K, Namiki C, *et al.* 2007. Interfrontal commissural abnormality in schizophrenia: tractography-assisted callosal parcellation. *Schizophr Res* **97**, 236–41.

Mori T, Ohnishi T, Hashimoto R, *et al.* 2007. Progressive changes of white matter integrity in schizophrenia revealed by diffusion tensor imaging. *Psychiatry Res* **154**, 133–45.

Nestor P, Kubicki M, Niznikiewicz M, Gurrera R, McCarley R and Shenton M. 2008. Neuropsychological disturbance in schizophrenia: a diffusion tensor imaging study. *Neuropsychology* **22**, 246–54.

O'Daly O, Frangou S, Chitnis X and Shergill S. 2007. Brain structural changes in schizophrenia patients with persistent hallucinations. *Psychiatry Res* **156**, 15–21.

Pakkenberg B. 1993. Total nerve cell number in neocortex in chronic schizophrenics and controls estimated using optical dissectors. *Biol Psychiatry* **34**, 768–72.

Pantelis C, Velakoulis D, McGorry P D, *et al.* 2003. Neuroanatomical abnormalities before and after onset of psychosis: a cross-sectional and longitudinal MRI comparison. *Lancet* **361**, 281–8.

Park H J, Westin C F, Kubicki M, *et al.* 2004. White matter hemisphere asymmetries in healthy subjects and in schizophrenia: a diffusion tensor MRI study. *Neuroimage* **23**, 213–23.

Pearlson G D and Marsh L. 1999. Structural brain imaging in schizophrenia: a selective review. *Biol Psychiatry* **46**, 627–49.

Pekny M and Nilsson M. 2005. Astrocyte activation and reactive gliosis. *Glia* **50**, 427–34.

Pfefferbaum A, Mathalon D H, Sullivan E V, Rawles J M, Zipursky R B and Lim K O. 1994. A quantitative magnetic resonance imaging study of changes in brain morphology from infancy to late adulthood. *Arch Neurol* **51**, 874–87.

Pfefferbaum A and Sullivan E V. 2003. Increased brain white matter diffusivity in normal adult aging: relationship to anisotropy and partial voluming. *Magn Reson Med* **49**, 953–61.

Price G, Bagary M S, Cercignani M, Altmann D R and Ron M A. 2005. The corpus callosum in first episode schizophrenia: a diffusion tensor imaging study. *J Neurol Neurosurg Psychiatry* **76**, 585–7.

Price G, Cercignani M, Bagary M, *et al.* 2006. A volumetric MRI and magnetization transfer imaging follow-up study of patients with first-episode schizophrenia. *Schizophr Res* **87**, 100–08.

Price G, Cercignani M, Parker G, *et al.* 2008. White matter tracts in first-episode psychosis: a DTI tractography study of the uncinate fasciculus. *Neuroimage* **39**, 949–55.

Price G, Cercignani M, Parker G J, *et al.* 2007. Abnormal brain connectivity in first-episode psychosis: a diffusion MRI tractography study of the corpus callosum. *Neuroimage* **35**, 458–66.

Purves D and Lichtman J W. 1980. Elimination of synapses in the developing nervous system. *Science* **210**, 153–7.

Roberts G, Colter N, Lofthouse R, Bogerts B, Zech M and Crow T. 1986. Gliosis in schizophrenia: a survey. *Biol Psychiatry* **21**, 1043–50.

Rosenberger G, Kubicki M, Nestor P, *et al.* 2008. Age-related deficits in fronto-temporal connections in schizophrenia: a diffusion tensor imaging study. *Schizophr Res* **102**, 181–8.

Rotarska-Jagiela A and Linden D. 2008. The corpus callosum in schizophrenia-volume and connectivity changes affect specific regions. *Neuroimage* **39**, 1522–32.

Roy K, Murtie J, El-Khodor B, *et al.* 2007. Loss of erbB signaling in oligodendrocytes alters myelin and dopaminergic function, a potential mechanism for neuropsychiatric disorders. *Proc Natl Acad Sci U S A* **104**, 8131–6.

Salisbury D, Kuroki N, Kasai K, Shenton M and McCarley R. 2007. Progressive and interrelated functional and structural evidence of post-onset brain reduction in schizophrenia. *Arch Gen Psychiatry* **64**, 521–9.

Scherk H and Falkai P. 2006. Effects of antipsychotics on brain structure. *Curr Opin Psychiatry* **19**, 145–50.

Schlösser R, Nenadic I, Wagner G, *et al.* 2007. White matter abnormalities and brain activation in schizophrenia: a combined DTI and fMRI study. *Schizophr Res* **89**, 1–11.

Schneiderman J S, Buchsbaum M S, Haznedar M, *et al.* 2009. Age and diffusion anisotropy in adolescent and adult patients with schizophrenia. *Neuroimage* **45**, 662–71.

Seal M, Yücel M, Fornito A, *et al.* 2008. Abnormal white matter microstructure in schizophrenia: a voxelwise analysis of axial and radial diffusivity. *Schizophr Res* **101**, 106–10.

Seeman P and Kapur S. 2000. Schizophrenia: more dopamine, more D2 receptors. *Proc Natl Acad Sci U S A* **97**, 7673–5.

Selemon L D and Goldman-Rakic P S. 1999. The reduced neuropil hypothesis: a circuit based model of schizophrenia. *Biol Psychiatry* **45**, 17–25.

Seok J, Park H, Chun J, *et al.* 2007. White matter abnormalities associated with auditory hallucinations in schizophrenia: a combined study of voxel-based analyses of diffusion tensor imaging and structural magnetic resonance imaging. *Psychiatry Res* **156**, 93–104.

Shenton M, Dickey C, Frumin M and McCarley R. 2001. A review of MRI findings in schizophrenia. *Schizophr Res* **49**, 1–52.

Shergill S, Kanaan R, Chitnis X, *et al.* 2007. A diffusion tensor imaging study of fasciculi in schizophrenia. *Am J Psychiatry* **164**, 467–73.

Song S, Sun S, Ju W, Lin S, Cross A and Neufeld A. 2003. Diffusion tensor imaging detects and differentiates axon and myelin degeneration in mouse optic nerve after retinal ischemia. *Neuroimage* **20**, 1714–22.

Song S, Sun S, Ramsbottom M, Chang C, Russell J and Cross A. 2002. Dysmyelination revealed through MRI as increased radial (but unchanged axial) diffusion of water. *Neuroimage* **17**, 1429–36.

Stangel M. 2004. Remyelinating and neuroprotective treatments in multiple sclerosis. *Expert Opin Investig Drugs* **13**, 331–47.

27

Steen R, Mull C, McClure R, Hamer R and Lieberman J. 2006. Brain volume in first-episode schizophrenia: systematic review and meta-analysis of magnetic resonance imaging studies. *Br J Psychiatry* **188**, 510–8.

Steen R G, Ogg R J, Reddick W E and Kingsley P B. 1997. Age-related changes in the pediatric brain: quantitative MR evidence of maturational changes during adolescence. *Am J Neuroradiol* **18**, 819–28.

Sun D, Stuart G, Jenkinson M, *et al.* 2009. Brain surface contraction mapped in first-episode schizophrenia: a longitudinal magnetic resonance imaging study. *Mol Psychiatry* **14**, 976–86.

Sun Z, Wang F, Cui L, *et al.* 2003. Abnormal anterior cingulum in patients with schizophrenia: a diffusion tensor imaging study. *Neuroreport* **14**, 1833–6.

Szeszko P, Robinson D, Ashtari M, *et al.* 2008. Clinical and neuropsychological correlates of white matter abnormalities in recent onset schizophrenia. *Neuropsychopharmacology* **33**, 976–84.

Takei K, Yamasue H, Abe O, *et al.* 2008. Disrupted integrity of the fornix is associated with impaired memory organization in schizophrenia. *Schizophr Res* **103**, 52–61.

Thompson C. 1995. Apoptosis in the pathogenesis and treatment of disease. *Science* **267**, 1456–62.

Uranova N, Vostrikov V, Vikhreva O, Zimina I, Kolomeets N and Orlovskaya D. 2007. The role of oligodendrocyte pathology in schizophrenia. *Int J Neuropsychopharmacol* **10**, 537–45.

van Haren N, Hulshoff Pol H, Schnack H, *et al.* 2008. Progressive brain volume loss in schizophrenia over the course of the illness: evidence of maturational abnormalities in early adulthood. *Biol Psychiatry* **63**, 106–13.

Vita A, De Peri L, Silenzi C and Dieci M. 2006. Brain morphology in first-episode schizophrenia: a meta-analysis of quantitative magnetic resonance imaging studies. *Schizophr Res* **82**, 75–88.

Walterfang M, Wood S, Velakoulis D, Copolov D and Pantelis C. 2005. Diseases of white matter and schizophrenia-like psychosis. *Aust N Z J Psychiatry* **39**, 746–56.

Wang F, Sun Z, Cui L, *et al.* 2004. Anterior cingulum abnormalities in male patients with schizophrenia determined through diffusion tensor imaging. *Am J Psychiatry* **161**, 573–5.

White T, Kendi A, Lehéricy S, *et al.* 2007. Disruption of hippocampal connectivity in children and adolescents with schizophrenia – a voxel-based diffusion tensor imaging study. *Schizophr Res* **90**, 302–7.

Whitford T J, Grieve S M, Farrow T F, *et al.* 2006. Progressive grey matter atrophy over the first 2–3 years of illness in first-episode schizophrenia: a tensor-based morphometry study. *NeuroImage* **32**, 511–9.

Whitford T J, Grieve S M, Farrow T F, *et al.* 2007a. Volumetric white matter abnormalities in first-episode schizophrenia: a longitudinal, tensor-based morphometry study. *Am J Psychiatry* **164**, 1082–9.

Whitford T J, Kubicki M and Shenton M E, in press. Diffusion tensor imaging (DTI), schizophrenia and discrete brain regions. *US Psychiatric Rev.*

Whitford T J, Rennie C J, Grieve S M, Clark C R, Gordon E and Williams L M. 2007b. Brain maturation in adolescence: concurrent changes in neuroanatomy and neurophysiology. *Human Brain Mapp* **28**, 228–37.

Wolkin A, Choi S, Szilagyi S, Sanfilipo M, Rotrosen J and Lim K. 2003. Inferior frontal white matter anisotropy and negative symptoms of schizophrenia: a diffusion tensor imaging study. *Am J Psychiatry* **160**, 572–4.

Wood S, Pantelis C, Velakoulis D, Yücel M, Fornito A and McGorry P. 2008. Progressive changes in the development toward schizophrenia: studies in subjects at increased symptomatic risk. *Schizophr Bull* **34**, 322–9.

Yakovlev P, Lecours A and Minkowski A. 1967. *Regional development of the brain early in life*. Boston, MA: Blackwell Scientific Publications, pp. 3–70.

Yücel M, Wood S, Phillips L, *et al.* 2003. Morphology of the anterior cingulate cortex in young men at ultra-high risk of developing a psychotic illness. *Br J Psychiatry* **182**, 518–24.

Zahajszky J, Dickey C, McCarley R, *et al.* 2001. A quantitative MR measure of the fornix in schizophrenia. *Schizophr Res* **47**, 87–97.

Zhou Y, Shu N, Liu Y, *et al.* 2008. Altered resting-state functional connectivity and anatomical connectivity of hippocampus in schizophrenia. *Schizophr Res* **100**, 120–32.

Zou L, Xie J, Yuan H, Pei X, Dong W and Liu P. 2008. Diffusion tensor imaging study of the anterior limb of internal capsules in neuroleptic-naive schizophrenia. *Acad Radiol* **15**, 285–9.

Endnotes

1. Given the length constraints of a book chapter, a fine-grained analysis of the DTI literature is more feasible than a similar analysis of the MRI literature.

2. One of the primary factors behind this rapid recent expansion in MRI research has been the development of voxel-based morphometry (VBM) as an MRI analysis method. In contrast to traditional region-of-interest (ROI) methodologies, in which specific brain structures are manually defined on MR images and the volumes of these structures statistically compared between groups (i.e. 1 statistical test per ROI), in VBM all MR images are warped into the same global shape, and group-wise statistical analyses are performed at every voxel in the

normalized images (i.e. thousands of statistical tests). A significant advantage of VBM, and undoubtedly a major reason behind its popularity, lies in the fact that it can be fully automated, and hence is a far less labor-intensive approach than traditional ROI methods. Another advantage of VBM lies in the fact that by investigating for structural abnormalities at every voxel in the brain, it is not constrained to comparing ROIs defined by potentially erroneous or incomplete prior hypotheses. Notwithstanding the strengths of the method, however, VBM has also been the subject of considerable criticism in the neuroimaging literature, with much of the criticism revolving around the validity of the warping algorithms, the danger of Type-I error inflation due to the vast numbers of statistical comparisons involved, and the negative connotations associated with the exploratory nature of an approach not guided by a-priori hypotheses.

3. It is important to emphasize the fact that the "GM abnormalities" reported here refer only to group-wise differences in brain structure between samples of SZ patients and samples of matched healthy controls. In other words, not every SZ patient has been found to exhibit these abnormalities in brain structure – the abnormalities are only apparent at the group level. Thus it is not possible to "diagnose" someone with SZ on the basis of an MR scan, as there is simply too great an overlap in the structural variance of the brains of healthy people relative to the brains of SZ patients. The hope, nonetheless, is that as the spatial resolution of MR images improves, and as advances continue in the post-processing of neuroimages, we will be able to use MR imaging, in conjunction with other biomarkers, to diagnose schizophrenia on the basis of biological features rather than on the basis of a symptom profile, as is currently used.

4. Consider, for example, the difficulties that patients with Parkinson's disease (who experience dopaminergic cell death in the substantia nigra and subsequently exhibit pathologically low levels of striatal dopamine) have in initiating willed motor actions.

Functional imaging of schizophrenia

Godfrey D. Pearlson

Introduction

Functional magnetic resonance imaging (fMRI) neuroimaging investigations in schizophrenia have been used for a variety of purposes. These include shedding light on the underlying pathophysiology of the illness, understanding the neural basis of characteristic symptoms, aiding with diagnostic classification, predicting treatment outcome, and understanding the effects of risk genes for the disorder.

Many of these efforts have been complicated by the fact that no central etiopathology is known for the disorder, which is non-uniform in clinical presentation, and overlaps symptomatically with other psychiatric disorders. As well, there are many associated challenges and confounds that add variance to functional imaging data in schizophrenia, including the fact that many patients are chronically ill and routinely take multiple medications known to affect functional brain response. Due to both positive and negative schizophrenia symptoms, they may be unwilling or unable to engage fully with test procedures, especially on complex tasks requiring sustained attention. Much of the existing functional MRI literature is based on blood oxygen level-dependent (BOLD) activation differences gathered during the performance of cognitive tasks, most often those on which patients are known characteristically to perform poorly outside of the scanner. Such an approach has undoubtedly been valuable and produced a large and rich literature. However, none of the fMRI abnormalities recorded in this manner to date has proved diagnostic, and as we discuss below, illness-related performance differences can introduce unavoidable confounds in such task designs. However, cognitive probe-based designs are not the only major approach used by functional MRI researchers in schizophrenia; some of the major paradigms are listed in Table 2.1.

Early functional imaging studies of psychiatrically ill patients, which used mainly single photon emission tomography (SPECT) or positron emission tomography (PET), examined individuals at rest. More recent investigators have argued persuasively that task conditions should be standardized and carefully specified, so that patients and controls could be more validly compared. Cognitive-based designs were generally chosen to accomplish this, so that particular brain regions or circuits could be specifically probed using "cognitive stress tests", based on tasks that were known in healthy volunteers to be dependent on the integrity of recognized neural circuits for their normal performance. This general approach has proved extremely useful and continues to be so, although interestingly, as we will review later, in recent years novel analysis methods have enabled much useful information to be extracted from the type of taskless design that was generally abandoned for PET imaging in the 1980s.

Cognitive task-based designs

Consistent with the task-directed strategy, the majority of functional imaging designs in schizophrenia patients have focused on cognitive task-based paradigms. This approach is a reasonable one since impaired cognition is a fundamental feature of schizophrenia, (the "dementia" of dementia praecox), that manifests early in the disorder, tends to endure, predicts instrumental functioning (Green, 1996), and is not fundamentally altered by any current antipsychotic medications (Harvey and Keefe, 2001). The dominant paradigm is the use of cognitive activation designs where cerebral BOLD measures are examined

Table 2.1 Simplified summary of types of MRI experiments commonly used to study schizophrenia

Probe/ domain	Examples	References
Cognitive task	Cognitive control	Ragland et al., 2007
	Working memory attention	Callicott et al., 2003b
	Response inhibition	Manoach, 2003
Social/ emotional task	Face processing	Marwick and Hall, 2008
	Emotion recognition	Baas et al., 2008
Core positive symptoms	Formal thought disorder	Assaf et al., 2007
	Auditory hallucinations	Hoffman et al., 2007
No task	Resting state	Jafri et al., 2009
	Default mode derived from cognitive paradigms	Garrity et al., 2008 Whitfield et al., 2009

in relation to specific cognitive task demands within a defined cognitive domain.

As reviewed by Ragland et al. (2007), investigators hewing to this approach generally choose functional tasks in which patients' behavior clearly distinguishes them from that of healthy controls – for example, working memory or attention, where many schizophrenia patients tend to be demonstrably impaired and have used fMRI designs that quantify between-group functional differences during task performance. For example, in comparing schizophrenia patients to healthy controls, working memory (WM) tasks such as the N-back and Sternberg paradigms show robust between-group differences in both behavior and activation in task-relevant circuits (that typically include dorsolateral prefrontal cortex, parietal regions, hippocampus). Patients may over- or under-activate relative to controls, for example as a function of task difficulty and WM load. A refinement of the above approach has been to choose parametric designs where a graded variety of task difficulties can be chosen, allowing

schizophrenia patients and controls to be compared either at equivalent levels of task difficulty, or at comparable levels of task performance. More sophisticated task analysis has, for example, compared low-performing controls to high-performing patients to help dissect intrinsic illness from performance factors.

More recent investigations have employed even more specific task paradigms derived from experimental cognitive neuroscience, that parse cognitive operations into distinct components; for example, working memory versus attention. Such improved designs also parametrically adjust, for example, working memory load or response inhibition components separately. Also, newer fMRI studies have transitioned from block design studies that average activity over multiple trials to event-related designs measuring activation during specific trials, yielding the ability to select for analysis only those encoding trials in a memory task that subsequently resulted in correct recognitions, for example.

Working memory tasks

Barch and Smith (2008) concluded both that working memory is a central, well-studied construct in cognitive science and that this domain is considered to be a core cognitive deficit in schizophrenia. Thus, among cognitive-based paradigms, working memory (using several varieties of stimulus sets including verbal and spatial material) has been the dominant functional MRI task studied in schizophrenia patients.

Working memory is commonly defined as the ability to hold information on-line and manipulate it for short periods of time (Baddeley, 1992), and has been extensively studied in humans and animals. Working memory is one exemplar of a related series of executive abilities, including planning and multi-tasking, all of which appear to be significantly impaired in many patients with schizophrenia (Silver et al., 2003). Working memory disturbances in schizophrenia are present in never-treated individuals, both acutely ill and chronic schizophrenia patients, and in unaffected first-degree relatives of patients (Meda, 2008). WM fMRI studies have largely focused anatomically on the dorsolateral prefrontal cortex (DLPFC), an area implicated in working memory studies of non-human primates (Friedman and Goldman-Rakic, 1994; Miller et al., 1996; Petrides, et al., 1995), as well as in human fMRI working memory tasks (D'Esposito *et al.*, 1999; Manoach *et al.*, 2003; Rypma and D'Esposito, 1999; Veltman *et al.*, 2003). Although DLPFC is a vital node in a distributed circuit subserving this task, other modules in the functional network relevant to the task are additional portions of frontal cortex, including ventrolateral prefrontal cortex (PFC), frontal pole and anterior cingulate cortex, as well as inferior parietal lobule (Manoach, 2003) and hippocampus (Glahn *et al.*, 2005; Meda, 2008).

Working memory tasks typically incorporate three epochs – encoding, maintenance, and recognition/retrieval – although all three epochs are not explicitly modeled separately in many task designs. There are disagreements in the literature examining healthy subjects as to relative DLPFC involvement in these various task phases (see for example Rypma and D'Esposito, 1999 vs. Veltman *et al.*, 2003).

Working memory deficits are clearly important in schizophrenia; patients exhibit deficits on working memory tasks of varied designs (Barch *et al.*, 1998; Cohen *et al.*, 1996; Goldberg *et al.*, 1998; Park and Holzman, 1992; Park *et al.*, 1999; Wexler *et al.*, 1998). Given the above-reviewed evidence for critical DLPFC involvement in normal task performance, fMRI studies in schizophrenia typically focus on patient/control activation differences in this region. Characteristics of the illness-related DLPFC abnormality are disputed; some studies report that schizophrenia patients show DLPFC *under-activation* compared to controls (Callicott *et al.*, 1998; Yurgelun-Todd *et al.*, 1996); others reveal *over-activation* (Callicott *et al.*, 2003a; Manoach *et al.*, 2000). These discrepant reports are likely dynamic rather than simply being "correct" vs. "incorrect"; the magnitude and direction of BOLD response depend on relative task difficulty and a given individual's baseline efficiency on a particular task (Callicott *et al.*, 2003a; Johnson *et al.*, 2006; Meda *et al.*, 2008). Thus the apparent discrepancy relates to task performance and task difficulty. In Callicott *et al.* (2003a), when patients' working memory performance was matched to that of controls, patients showed relative DLPFC over-activation; however, Manoach *et al.* (2000) found that at matched performance between-group activation was similar. A parsimonious explanation is that under conditions of equivalent task performance, schizophrenia patients activate DLPFC "inefficiently" and thus show greater working memory-related activation than do controls (Callicott *et al.*, 2000). Then, as task difficulty increases,

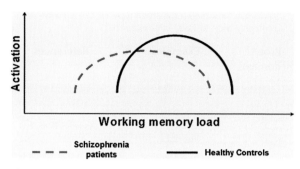

Figure 2.1 Conceptual model describing the hypothesized shape of neural response to increasing task load in the working memory network. The model predicts that schizophrenia patients and controls have similar load–response curves when dealing with increasing working memory load, but that patients' response curves are both *shifted to the left*, resulting in apparent over-activations at low loads and under-activations at high loads, as well as *flatter* in shape, reflecting reduced ability to modulate neural response with increasing task difficulty.

patients may disengage or begin performing poorly as they exceed their cognitive capacity, resulting in relative DLPFC under-activation (Callicott *et al.*, 2003a; Johnson *et al.*, 2006; Manoach *et al.*, 2000, 2003; Callicott *et al.*, 2000).

One way to summarize the above (see Figure 2.1) is that working memory load appears to be correlated with DLPFC activation in an inverted U-shaped curve.

Under the above explanatory scheme, the curve in schizophrenia compared to healthy controls appears to both be flatter and to be shifted towards the left, consistent with inefficient task-related BOLD response (Callicott, 2003b; Johnson *et al.*, 2006).

One can address these issues experimentally by examining activation across multiple levels of increasing memory load, which several studies accomplished using an N-back working memory task. For example, Callicott *et al.* (2000) showed increasing right PFC activation in schizophrenia with increased memory load across a circumscribed range of loads below capacity, and hypothesized by extension that activity might begin to decrease when WM capacity was exceeded, as previously shown in healthy control subjects (Callicott *et al.*, 1999). Perlstein *et al.* (2001) also employed a limited working memory load range, but found decreased right DLPFC activation at the highest load in patients compared with control subjects. Similarly, Jansma *et al.* (2004) exceeded WM capacity in patients using a 3-back load; compared with controls, schizophrenia patients showed increasing DLPFC activity as load increased up to capacity at the 3-back level, when activity dropped.

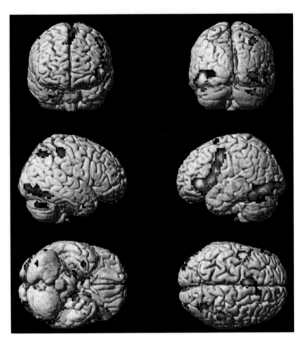

Figure 2.2 Sternberg item recognition paradigm (SIRP) showing the main effect of the encoding phase in 30 healthy control subjects.

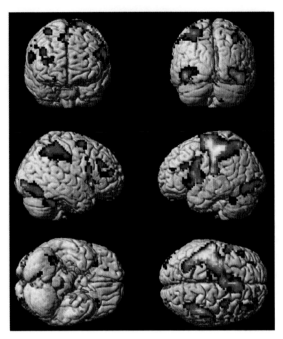

Figure 2.3 Sternberg item recognition paradigm showing the main effect of the recognition phase in the same 30 healthy control subjects as Figure 2.2.

N-back designs carry an inherent design problem, however. The steep difficulty gradient of the task limits studies of working memory load response to three working memory load levels. The 1-back level is relatively easy for all subjects, but the 3-back level exceeds working memory capacity in many patients and some healthy control subjects. This may explain downward trends in activation as one moves from the 2- to the 3-back condition. Also, patients are aware of their poor task performance at more difficult levels, and as a consequence can become demoralized and lose motivation and engagement with the task. In addition, N-back tasks tend to incorporate target stimuli as probes, conflating the separate working memory subprocesses of encoding, maintenance, and retrieval which are important to model separately, as they may both have differing underlying functional anatomy, and show differential impairment in schizophrenia.

For the above reasons, other investigators have used versions of the Sternberg Item Recognition Paradigm (Sternberg, 1966) to examine working memory (Manoach *et al.*, 1997, 2000, 2003; Veltman *et al.*, 2003, Johnson *et al.*, 2006; Meda *et al.*, 2008) (Figures 2.2 and 2.3), because working memory load can be increased more gradually and distinct task stages separated more easily.

Most recently, in selecting new working memory tasks to address remaining knowledge gaps for the Cognitive Neuroscience Treatment Research to Improve Cognition in Schizophrenia (CNTRICS) initiative, Barch *et al.* (2009) concluded that the two major constructs of interest for future working memory studies in schizophrenia were goal maintenance and interference control. They recommended use of the AX-Continuous Performance Task/Dot Pattern Expectancy task for the former, and the recent probes and operation/symmetry span tasks for the latter, for translation for use in clinical trials.

Despite the many working memory studies conducted in schizophrenia, several important questions remain to be addressed regarding the specific neural basis of impaired cognition in schizophrenia.

Is activation occurring in inappropriate regions, and if so why?

Irrespective of the working memory task employed, when examining task-related activation in schizophrenia vs. controls, several investigators (e.g. Glahn *et al.*, 2005; Ragland *et al.*, 2007), reviewing the N-back literature, comment generally on more diffuse/less punctuate DLPFC activation in schizophrenia, and more specifically on anterior medial and ventral frontal activation in patients that could be interpreted as task-inappropriate activation, representing reliance for "backup" on more functional neighboring regions. Some authors note a shift of the most highly activated DLPFC voxels in schizophrenia away from the area identified in healthy control subjects to immediately adjacent regions (Glahn et al., 2005). The explanation for this latter phenomenon could be based on aberrant functional connectivity, or even an anatomically based shift in functional localization. Currently these explanations ("wrong area" vs. "right area shifted to a different place") remain at the level of untested hypotheses, but ultimately testing them empirically may prove important for understanding the basis of the working memory-associated activation abnormalities in schizophrenia. A more recent quantitative meta-analysis (Minzenberg et al., 2009) sheds more light on this issue, and places it in a more general context, by examining published studies of prefrontal cortical dysfunction in schizophrenia across multiple tasks of executive cognition, of which working memory represents one subset. The major aim was to clarify whether aberrant frontal activation represents concurrent, overlapping dysfunction of several prefrontal region- and process-specific impairments, versus a more overarching dysfunction in a cognitive control network. The authors concluded that during executive task performance all groups activate a similar neural network, with critical nodes in the DLPFC and ACC, "consistent with the engagement of a general-purpose cognitive control network". Interestingly, in between-group analyses, patients had related activation reductions in left DLPFC, rostral/dorsal ACC, left thalamus, as well as in inferior/posterior cortical areas. Conversely, schizophrenia was associated with increased activation in several midline cortical areas which could be compensatory in nature, as suggested in an earlier paper (Glahn et al., 2005).

The role of context and a dissection of task phase

The observation of Johnson et al. (2006), of differential patient vs. control responsiveness to difficulty context, is consistent with a hypothesis that schizophrenia is associated with reduced ability to use context to guide task performance (Barch et al., 2001; Cohen et al., 1996; Ford et al., 2004; Henik et al., 2002; Servan-Schreiber et al., 1996). With regard to

clarifying specificity of deficits in working memory in schizophrenia to task phase, better study of the maintenance period between encoding and retrieval could isolate the precise nature and progression of working memory breakdown in schizophrenia. A recent paper provides one example of this. Driesen et al. (2008) compared prefrontal cortical activity during specific phases of working memory in controls and in schizophrenia using a spatial working memory task, similar to that used in non-human primates, at two levels of memory load, to better separate activation into encoding, maintenance, and response phases. While task accuracy was similar in the two groups, patients showed less prefrontal brain activation during maintenance and response phases, but not during encoding phases of working memory. The reduced prefrontal activity in patients during maintenance was related to a greater decay rate of activity over time.

In summary, abnormal working memory-related fMRI activation in schizophrenia occurs in a network, not a single region (DLPFC), and is affected by several factors. Activation during retrieval is abnormal, perhaps especially due to particular impairment of the maintenance period. The working memory network in patients seems less responsive to context and changing load demands, suggesting that both hyper- and hypoactivation are due to an inability to muster and allocate neural resources at context-appropriate levels. Finally, Johnson et al. (2006) argued for the need for future studies to analyze performance at the trial rather than the group level to characterize fully the relationship between neural activity and successful working memory performance.

An early, comprehensive approach was to consider that schizophrenia was predominantly a disease of DLPFC and that the working memory deficits in schizophrenia explained comprehensively other notable cognitive deficits as well as major positive symptoms of the disorder (e.g. for the latter argument see Cohen et al., 1996; Silver et al., 2003). However, brief reflection suggests difficulties with this approach. First, network-level understanding derived from cognitive neuroscience provides a more sophisticated explanation for circuit-wide abnormalities in schizophrenia, which is consistent with more recent understanding of how brain regions collaborate to support cognitive operations.

Independent component analysis (ICA) is one method used to identify such temporally coherent networks (Calhoun *et al.*, 2008). ICA is a data-driven approach which is especially useful for decomposing activation during complex cognitive tasks where multiple operations may occur simultaneously.

One insight derived from ICA is that the same region can participate simultaneously in concurrent cognitive operations during performance of complex multi-element cognitive tasks, such as simulated vehicle driving. The theme that disruption of neural circuits is an important part of the pathophysiology of schizophrenia will be taken up again in the concluding portion of this chapter.

Second, fMRI reveals that regions other than DLPFC, and not necessarily strongly connected to it, behave abnormally in schizophrenia. The anterior cingulate cortex (ACC) is one example of a brain region forming part of a network that is severely disrupted in schizophrenia. ACC activity in schizophrenia is abnormal across a wide range of cognitive operations that normally involve this region. These span both more complex cognitive paradigms such as the Stroop paradigm, involving conflict monitoring/cognitive interference, all the way to simpler tasks such as auditory oddball detection (Laurens *et al.*, 2005; Kiehl *et al.*, 2007). Response inhibition, error detection and conflict tasks in schizophrenia reliably elicit abnormal (usually deficient) ACC activation (Rubia *et al.*, 2001; Heckers *et al.*, 2004; Kerns *et al.*, 2005), consistent with known cognitive impairment in schizophrenia during tasks involving performance of error monitoring and conflict resolution. Interestingly, however, tasks that do not normally produce robust activation of ACC in healthy subjects, such as working memory paradigms, seem to inappropriately activate ACC in schizophrenia subjects, perhaps because they are invoking conflict situations not seen in healthy controls, as suggested by Ragland *et al.* (2007).

Positive-symptom-based approaches

Functional MRI studies in schizophrenia have utilized multiple approaches. Some investigators have started with obvious, active positive clinical symptoms, for example hallucinations, and attempted to identify the underlying circuitry. Although it is impossible to get patients to hallucinate "on cue", Sommer *et al.* (2008) reported that auditory verbal hallucinations were associated with activation in the right homologue of Broca's area and right superior temporal gyrus and

bilateral insula, supramarginal gyri, while Broca's area and left superior temporal gyrus were not activated. Hoffman *et al.* (2008) reported that fMRI maps of pre-hallucination periods revealed activation in the left anterior insula and in the right middle temporal gyrus, as well as deactivation in the anterior cingulate and parahippocampal gyri, possibly reflecting brain events triggering or increasing vulnerability to auditory/verbal hallucinations.

Indirect methods, not looking at activation during hallucination events, have been employed by other investigators. For example, Wible *et al.* (2009) examined data from the Sternberg working memory task in schizophrenia subjects during the task probe condition (during which subjects rehearsed stimuli). Patients with auditory hallucinations (relative to non-hallucinating subjects) showed decreased activity in superior temporal and inferior parietal regions, where activity also correlated with severity of hallucinations. Ford *et al.* (2009) examined patients during performance of an auditory target detection task, hypothesizing that hallucinating patients would show less auditory cortical activation to external acoustic stimuli in prespecified regions in primary and secondary auditory cortex, auditory association cortex, and middle temporal gyrus. Hallucinators had less activation to probe tones in left (but not right) primary auditory cortex (BA41). Overall, these studies implicate dysfunction of the auditory and language systems in the genesis of auditory hallucinations.

Because hallucinations are discrete, unpredictable events that are difficult to characterize directly in fMRI tasks, researchers interested in the neural basis of positive symptoms have tended to worked more with formal thought disorder, based on existing cognitive neuroscience knowledge. Formal thought disorder (FTD) in schizophrenia has been of considerable interest to researchers because of its resemblance to Wernicke's aphasia and the well-documented relationship between structural differences in schizophrenia in superior temporal gyrus in relationship to positive symptoms first described by Barta *et al.* (1990). Because it is hypothesized that FTD results from impaired semantic memory processing, Assaf *et al.* (2006) used an fMRI semantic object memory retrieval task in schizophrenia subjects and healthy controls and assessed symptom severity with the Thought Disorder Index (TDI). Participants viewed two words describing object features that either evoked (object recall) or did not evoke a semantic concept. Patients tended to over-recall objects for feature pairs that did not describe the same object. Functionally, activation in rostral anterior cingulate cortex (ACC) (an area that may function in choosing between alternatives, or in exclusion of inappropriate choices) in patients positively correlated with FTD severity during both correct recalled and over-recalled trials. Compared to controls, during object recall, patients over-activated bilateral ACC, temporo-occipital junctions, temporal poles and parahippocampi, right inferior frontal gyrus, and DLPFC, but under-activated inferior parietal lobules. Thus schizophrenia patients abnormally activated brain areas involved in semantic memory, verbal working memory, and initiation and suppression of conflicting responses, which were associated with semantic over-recall and FTD.

More recently, the same authors (Assaf *et al.*, 2009) better characterized the semantic object retrieval process by exploring the temporal sequence of and the relationship between the left and right hemispheres during the same fMRI semantic retrieval task described above in healthy individuals. They found an early activation of the right hemisphere that was closely followed by left hemisphere activation, to facilitate performance during word retrieval from semantic memory. Taken in conjunction with the above findings in both FTD and auditory hallucinations, these data as a whole are consistent with aberrant hemispheric lateralization, or a variant of the disconnection hypothesis underpinning these symptoms in schizophrenia.

Cognitive neuroscience tasks – Morris water task

Another task approach has been to use well-explored neuroscience paradigms developed originally in the animal research world, such as human versions of the hippocampally dependent Morris water task that assesses allocentric navigation, or three-dimensional mazes, that can be presented as virtual-reality tasks in the fMRI scanner. In this context, ecologic validity is the extent to which laboratory results or conditions are generalizable to real-world conditions. The majority of standard neuropsychological measures compromise ecologic validity for strong experimental control, but virtual-reality designs enable reintroduction of strong ecologic validity. Virtual reality (VR) has also been used to create and administer tasks for humans that are analogous to those used in non-humans

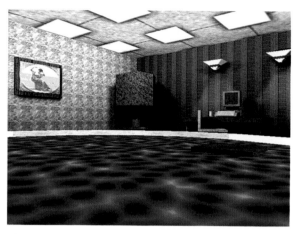

Figure 2.4 Screen shot of a virtual Morris water maze task adapted as a functional MRI paradigm. In the active phase of the task, subjects have to find a hidden platform beneath the surface of the virtual pool, by navigating using a joystick to the target based on memory cues in the environment. This task relies on hippocampus-based allocentric memory, which is impaired in schizophrenia patients (e.g. Foley *et al.*, 2010).

(for example, in rodent or primate studies), such as the Morris Water Maze Task (Figure 2.4). Because these paradigms have been extensively studied in the animal world, the translation to human fMRI can build immediately on this existing foundation. Astur *et al.* (Foley *et al.*, 2010; Carvalho *et al.*, 2006; Astur *et al.*, 2005) have pioneered the use of virtual-reality tasks for the fMRI environment in the form of simulation-based tasks that provide realistic environments in which to study complex naturalistic behaviours. Because it uses photorealistic graphics and excellent experimental control, VR can accomplish these goals, while providing a platform to assess performance in real-life scenarios that may be too complex or involved to examine via alternative methods (Kurtz *et al.*, 2007). Also, VR has been used to study complex paradigms, which are usually not amenable to direct measurement, in conjunction with fMRI. However, incorporating VR into the fMRI environment creates specific challenges related to the hardware (for example, the simulator must be non-magnetic and must not generate radio frequency signals that interfere with the fMRI scan).

Imaging emotional stimuli

Humans are social animals, and many brain areas are devoted to face processing and/or identifying the emotions of other individuals, as these stimuli are highly salient in social communication. As reviewed comprehensively by Marwick and Hall (2008), individuals with schizophrenia have marked difficulties in interpreting social cues from faces and manifest deficits in face identity recognition that are not fully attributable to problems with mnemonic or attentional factors. Schizophrenia patients have reduced functional activity compared to controls during matching of facial identity and emotion in the right fusiform gyrus (Quintana et al., 2003), an area known previously to be strongly implicated in processing facial identity as well as more generally in object processing.

Schizophrenia patients appear to show behavioral impairment in recognition of negative affect in particular (Hall et al., 2004), and related functional abnormalities in mesial temporal responses to facial affect, including reduced amygdala activation to fearful versus neutral faces, but also increased amygdala and parahippocampal activation to neutral faces (Surguladze et al., 2006; Holt et al., 2006; Aleman and and Kahn, 2005) that makes interpretation of the former observation more complex.

Introduction to imaging functional networks

Complex cognition arises not merely from the local processing in a single task-engaged brain region, but from widely distributed groups of brain regions (Fuster, 2006; Mesulam, 1998). In addition to the major, well-documented networks underlying, for example, working memory or focused attention, researchers were surprised to discover other sets of networks unrelated to tasks and even present at rest when no task was being performed (so-called "resting-state networks"). This resting state activity was initially discovered by observing a significant degree of low frequency correlations within contralateral motor, visual and auditory cortices, related to both blood flow and to BOLD activity (Biswal et al., 1997) mostly occurring at lower frequencies (Cordes et al., 2001). These phenomena are not merely local; temporal sampling of whole brain data at low rates reveals similar temporally coherent regions (Lowe et al., 1998).

This type of functional connectivity is often measured as inter-regional correlations among spontaneous fluctuations of hemodynamic activity during a "resting state" while participants lie passively in the MRI machine, but no active cognitive or behavioral

demands are imposed (Raichle et al., 2001). Initial identification of significant temporal inter-correlation among the precuneus/posterior cingulate, ventral anterior cingulate, and ventromedial prefrontal cortex (i.e. regions now defined as comprising the classic "default mode" of brain activity; see Figure 2.5) (Greicius et al., 2004) led to interest in locating additional functionally integrated neural networks during resting state. Further examination of resting state brain activity indeed identified numerous functionally connected circuits during rest, including classically described motor, sensory, language, and visual networks (Cordes et al., 2001). The brain is in "default mode" when a person is awake but resting quietly: this can be considered to represent brain "idling", nevertheless involving organized cognitive activity such as monitoring the internal and external environment. Studies applying independent component analysis (ICA; see below) or similar data-driven methods to resting-state fMRI data have identified additional discrete neural circuits comprised of brain regions often engaged by higher-order cognitive tasks, including fronto-cerebellar, parietal–cerebellar, fronto-parietal, and cingulo-opercular networks (Beckmann et al., 2005; Dosenbach et al., 2007; Fransson, 2006; Seeley et al., 2007). In sum, fMRI resting state research has found reproducible evidence for a "family" of 10 or more distinct networks engaged during rest (Beckmann et al., 2005; Calhoun et al., 2008; Damoiseaux et al., 2006; De Luca et al., 2005). Resting-state networks are also present during and modulated by cognitive task performance (where they are usually referred to as "default mode networks"; DMN). Such circuits are more generally termed "temporally coherent networks" (TCNs; Calhoun et al., 2008), and are robust, straightforwardly identified using ICA, and can be consistently identified at rest and during cognitive tasks. The "classic" DMN is highly metabolically active, being responsible for approximately 80% of brain energy metabolism. It participates in organized baseline brain "idling", and may represent self-reflection, focus on internal stimuli, stream of consciousness, or other activities (Gusnard et al., 2001); certainly it diminishes during task-related behaviors (Raichle et al., 2001) in a manner proportional to task difficulty (McKiernan et al., 2003). In general, the more effortful the cognitive task, the more the classic resting state/default mode network activity

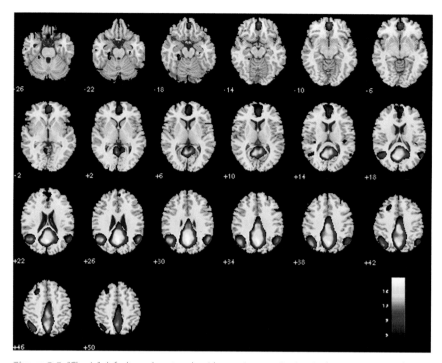

Figure 2.5 "Classic" default mode network, with prominent activation in the posterior cingulate/precuneus, derived using independent component analysis techniques from BOLD data collected during performance of an fMRI auditory oddball task. The default mode is always present and detectable using this analytic approach during performance of any cognitive paradigm, as well as at rest.

diminishes during task engagement (McKiernan *et al.*, 2007); in addition, multiple "families" of TCNs also show temporal and spatial modulation during cognitive tasks versus rest (Figure 2.6).

ICA and similar techniques are methods for recovering underlying signals from linear signal mixtures using higher-order statistics to determine a set of components that are maximally independent of each other. These are often used to identify TCNs. ICA also has the advantage of not requiring seed voxels or the use of temporal filtering (McKeown and Sejnowski, 1998). Broyd *et al.* (2009) review the pluses and minuses of these various approaches.

ICA is based on the assumption of spatially independent, temporally correlated, coherent brain networks, and is frequently used to examine the resting state. In addition to the strong temporal correlations *within* each network, ICA approaches can also be used to identify weak temporal correlations *among* the different components. The latter relationships, as we will review later, are used to assess functional network connectivity. ICA has been used to identify several temporally coherent networks present in healthy subjects either during rest or during the

performance of various tasks; of the 10 or so such networks emerging from such analyses, as noted above, one includes a predominance of signal from bilateral temporal lobe regions. This circuit has been used to reliably discriminate healthy controls from schizophrenia patients (Calhoun *et al.*, 2004).

Use of simple cognitive tasks and "task-free" approaches

Growing awareness of the default mode and TCNs in general had a significant effect on fMRI research in schizophrenia. Their use supplied a need because of problems inherent in the predominant strategy of focusing on the use of cognitive challenge tasks based in cognitive domains where schizophrenia patients are behaviorally impaired (such as working memory, as we reviewed earlier). Such problems include patients often not fully comprehending complex instructions and having problems performing tasks consistently in the scanner. They fatigue easily, have generally reduced concentration and attention, may be poorly motivated, distracted by illness symptoms such as hallucinations, and sedated from side effects of medications. Poor performance and abnormal

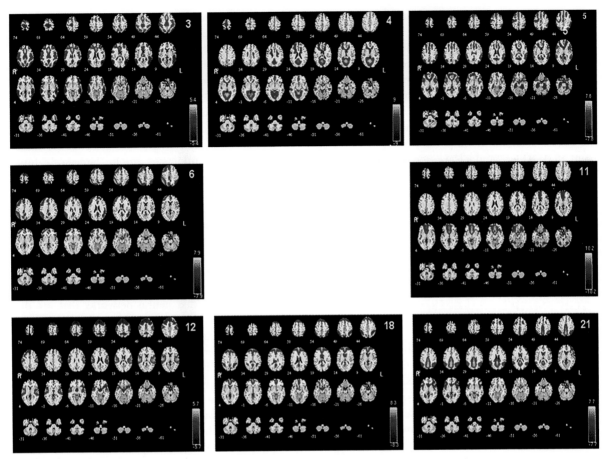

Figure 2.6 "Family" of several independent components ("networks") derived from a resting-state functional MRI scan. The "task" consisted of subjects resting quietly in the scanner for 5 min with eyes open, fixated on a crosshair. Temporally coherent networks were subsequently extracted using independent component analysis. Note that the lower right figure represents the "classical" default mode network portrayed in Figure 2.5, while the figure at the lower left represents the "temporal lobe" network.

task-related BOLD response are thus confounded in a "chicken and egg" situation which may be difficult to disambiguate. One solution to this problem is to use easy or minimal-effort paradigms where patients and controls perform at comparable levels of accuracy, or even at rest, when there is no task.

Such paradigms either use simple tasks such as the auditory oddball paradigm, or even "taskless" paradigms such as resting state/default mode, the latter of which require no cognitive effort on the part of the subject (e.g. Greicius *et al.*, 2004; Bluhm *et al.*, 2007; Garrity *et al.*, 2007). We and others have studied the auditory oddball detection (AOD) paradigm in detail using fMRI because it is a straightforward, simple task that activates multiple, diverse cortical and subcortical regions, and activation patterns are abnormal in most schizophrenia patients (although not specifically so;

despite the fact that patients can perform the task almost as well as healthy controls (i.e. generally as accurately if slightly slower; Kiehl *et al.*, 2005; Calhoun *et al.*, 2004, 2006a, 2006b, 2006c; Garrity *et al.*, 2007; Demirci *et al.*, 2009; Sui *et al.*, 2009). The electrophysiological parallel equivalent of the auditory oddball fMRI task is the well-known auditory oddball P300 paradigm, a well-recognized endophenotype or risk marker for schizophrenia, where activation patterns show strong heritability, which is minimally influenced by illness stage or antipsychotic medication, and tends to be abnormal in first-degree unaffected relatives of patients. As noted earlier, resting-state networks are also present during and modulated by cognitive task performance (as "default mode networks") in any cognitive task, including during the AOD paradigm.

This information was used by Garrity *et al.* (2007), who extracted default mode activity during performance of an auditory oddball task, and showed abnormalities in schizophrenia that correlated with both positive and negative illness symptoms. In a separate experiment that examined diagnostic discrimination between schizophrenia, psychotic bipolar disorder and healthy controls, an approach incorporating both the classic default and temporal lobe modes derived from an AOD task and a leave-one-out approach was able to achieve an average sensitivity and specificity of 90% and 95%, respectively (Calhoun *et al.*, 2008). This article showed the utility of the default mode as a diagnostic classifier even when two psychotic groups were included in the analysis.

Disturbed interactions between key circuits; functional network connectivity

As discussed above, complex cognition arises from task-related, widely distributed groups or networks of brain regions (Fuster, 2006; Mesulam, 1998) and in addition influences activity in other, non-task-related networks. For example, as noted above, in Calhoun *et al.* (2008), we examined temporally coherent networks revealed using ICA of fMRI data under two different conditions, during an auditory oddball task and rest. We found wide-ranging patterns of spatial and temporal changes in the networks, even for those not showing significant correlations with the oddball task. This differs from prior reports that non-task-related TCNs are unaffected by the task (Arfanakis *et al.*, 2000).

The profile and strength of such network-to-network influences, i.e. interactions across, rather than within, networks ("functional network connectivity"; FNC) turns out to contain useful information. ICA of fMRI is well-suited to characterize multiple functional networks, because by definition the brain regions in each component have the same profile hemodynamic signal change. Demirci *et al.* (2009) and Jafri *et al.* (2008) recently examined functional network connectivity in controls and schizophrenia patients during resting state alone or in addition to working memory and attention tasks.

For example, the Jafri *et al.* (2008) study, rather than deriving default mode from a cognitive task (even a simple one, such as the auditory oddball), used a classic resting-state paradigm where schizophrenia patients and matched healthy controls were imaged while alert with eyes open but performing no active task in the scanner. Rather than looking *within* each of the family of components derived by ICA, they looked at relationships *between* these circuits. Although there are strong temporal relationships within circuits, there often are weak temporal relationships, such as lags, among circuits.

These studies not only found evidence for measurable, directed influences among large-scale functional networks, but also found that a diagnosis of schizophrenia resulted in widespread disruption, greater dependency, and greater variability of network inter-relationships. Schizophrenia subjects showed significantly higher correlations than controls among many of the dominant resting-state networks. Thus, healthy adult brain function is characterized by the presence of distinct, directed relationships among numerous distributed neural networks that are disrupted in schizophrenia, possibly reflecting cortical processing deficiencies.

Several different functional networks identified through ICA of BOLD activation appear to be important indicators of schizophrenia pathophysiology. Emerging neural network research indicates that these circuits are commonly engaged across many tasks in both schizophrenia and control groups, including networks subserving complex focused attention, "brain idling", working memory/executive decision-making, set maintenance and language. These circuits are focused around four major anatomic hubs already implicated in schizophrenia, and suggest that illness-related deficits might arise from abnormalities in the quality or strength of functional connections among major nodes: (1) prefrontal–parietal, (2) cingulate–opercular, (3) temporal lobe, and (4) the classic "default mode" network. Therefore, an overarching hypothesis is that the "disconnection syndrome" in schizophrenia represents miscommunication and/or disconnection between these key networks, which can be best understood through analytic approaches that determine how structural or functional connectivity abnormalities underlie the well-documented cognitive deficits or symptomatic syndromes.

Imaging genomics

Over the past several years, new discoveries in the genetics of schizophrenia have begun to have more impact on functional neuroimaging research.

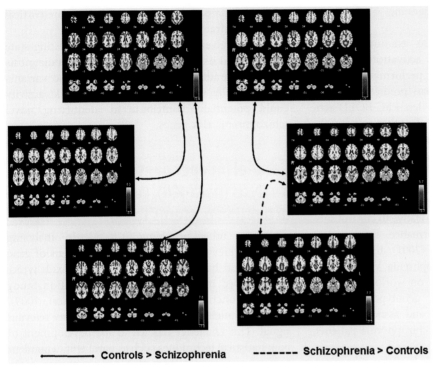

Controls > Schizophrenia   **Schizophrenia > Controls**

Figure 2.7 A hypothetical analysis illustrating differences between two diagnostic groups is portrayed. Within each "family", i.e. neural component/circuit shown in Figure 2.6, temporal correlations are by definition strong. The weaker temporal correlations among different families of circuits can be explored using functional network connectivity analyses as illustrated here.

The underlying normal function of most of these risk genes in the brain, and an overall understanding of how they may interact in leading to a common etiology or final common path of schizophrenia, is unknown. However, schizophrenia disease risk is likely mediated by two major genetic mechanisms (Allen *et al.*, 2009; Meyer-Lindenberg and Weinberger, 2006). The first mechanism consists of rare (not necessarily inherited) copy number variants in CNS-relevant genes. The second, probably more frequent mechanism fits into a "common disease common gene" schema of multiple, interacting gene variants of individually small effect, acting likely epistatically, but ultimately converging at molecular "bottlenecks". Through fast, inexpensive, replicable identification of risk genes for schizophrenia (especially chips that cover the entire human genome with millions of single nucleotide polymorphisms (SNPs)), more large-scale, testable, etiopathologic models of major mental illnesses have been advanced (Goldberg and and Weinberger, 2004; McDonald *et al.*, 2006; Meyer-Lindenberg and Weinberger, 2006, Pearlson and Folley, 2008a, 2008b), that trace plausible paths

from genes, through molecular and cellular biology, via brain systems, to overt behavior. (For potential complications in the use of such methods, see the section on parallel ICA.)

Obviously, schizophrenia risk genes did not evolve expressly to confer a predisposition to the disorder. Thus, once a potential schizophrenia risk gene is identified, an obvious step is to explore possible influences of normal SNP variants of the gene on normal brain structure or function. This helps provide a context for how dysfunction at the genetic level may have effects at a brain system level.

Starting with knowledge of working memory deficits in schizophrenia, Egan *et al.* (2001) quantified the effects of the well-known functional Val/Met COMT polymorphism in conjunction with an N-back working memory task in healthy subjects. There was a significant COMT genotype effect: Val/Val individuals had the lowest N-back performance and slowest reaction time, while Met/Met individuals had the highest performance. Similar effects were also seen in schizophrenia patients and their unaffected first-degree relatives. COMT genotype did not

41

influence attention or IQ, suggesting specificity to working memory.

Callicott *et al.* (2003a) also examined COMT genotype effects on PFC fMRI activation in similar diagnostic groups matched for performance, during the N-back task. Met allele load predicted a more efficient physiological response (less PFC BOLD activation) in the 2-back condition. In other words, "the group with relatively more cortical dopamine available at the synapse (i.e. Met homozygotes) had relatively greater behavioral 'bang' for its physiological 'buck', irrespective of diagnosis." In both cohorts, siblings and schizophrenia patients showed increased DLPFC activation (inefficiency) relative to control subjects, despite comparable performance. Further data from Meyer Lindenberg *et al.* (2001) and Winterer *et al.* (2003) suggest that schizophrenia Val homozygotes perform especially poorly on working memory tasks, illustrating that COMT genotype influences working memory performance and associated fMRI BOLD across normal subjects, schizophrenia patients, and first-degree relatives.

Analogously, the Disrupted in Schizophrenia-1 (DISC1) gene is expressed predominantly in the hippocampus; allelic variation at a $Ser^{704}Cys$ DISC1 SNP affects hippocampal function (and structure) in healthy subjects; the Ser allele is associated with altered hippocampal activation during several cognitive fMRI tasks (Callicott *et al.*, 2005). Pezawas *et al.* (2004) and Di Georgio *et al.* (2008) have shown a similar functional MRI role for a common variant of the putative schizophrenia risk gene, brain-derived neurotrophic factor (BDNF).

To summarize the above, Karlsgodt *et al.* (2008) concluded that the evidence across these and other studies implicates neurodevelopmental disruption of brain connectivity in schizophrenia that likely involves susceptibility genes affecting processes involved in the development of intra- and inter-regional connectivity. Similarly, Tan *et al.* (2007) conclude that these reports suggest a final common effect of risk genes on "macro-circuit stability and functional efficiency" as the pathophysiologic convergence underpinning the characteristic cognitive deficits in schizophrenia. They further suggest that patients engage larger networks of cortical regions during task performance consistent with "reduced signal-to-noise components and the recruitment of compensatory networks". They hypothesize how genes (such as COMT) that affect cortical dopamine signaling, and GRM3, which alters synaptic glutamate, may interact to modulate cortical processing strategies.

Finally, given the prior discussion of resting-state circuitry and its relevance to schizophrenia diagnosis in fMRI paradigms, determining the gene variants that normally contribute to default mode activity could potentially contribute to identifying novel schizophrenia risk genes.

Parallel independent component analysis (para-ICA); relating brain activation patterns to clusters of SNPs

There are other problems to tackle in analyzing large, complex data sets, such as the millions of gene variants and hundreds of thousands of voxels typically involved in a Genome Wide Association Study (GWAS)/functional imaging study (Pearlson, 2009). This multiplicity can rapidly overwhelm any relevant signal. This challenge has led to the development of new statistical techniques such as parallel independent component analysis (para-ICA), for analyzing high-dimensional, multi-modal data. Recent papers (Liu *et al.*, 2009a, 2009b) used this algorithm to identify simultaneously independent components of imaging and genetic modalities and the relationships between them.

Many relevant schizophrenia risk genes have yet to be identified, and require clusterwise or other agglomerative techniques to point the field towards reasonable but so-far unsuspected candidate genes. Finally, it is likely that certain demonstrable genetic influences on neural dysfunction may exert their effects epistatically, depending on the presence or absence of other genotypes' combined influence on brain structure/function. Therefore, without examining the genome, such effects would not be detected.

Para-ICA identifies "clusters" of SNPs that are functionally linked; it is likely that these represent SNPs with common interactions. The technique is an approach for revealing relationships between brain function and SNP groupings, i.e. to identify a combination of SNPs related to a functional brain network. This involves simultaneously solving three problems: revealing a set of specific independent brain functions, identifying independent SNP associations, and finding the relationship between SNP associations and brain functions. The resulting components extracted from fMRI data can be interpreted as networks of brain regions expressing functional changes in different subjects to different degrees. For instance, the value of a given component may distinguish healthy subjects from schizophrenia patients. Similarly, components extracted from SNP data are distinct linear combinations of SNPs that may affect certain genetic functionalities or phenotypes, or even represent clusters of physiologically interacting genes. These components are also expressed to different degrees in different subjects or under different conditions. Relationships between the two modalities can be assessed. For example, if an fMRI component is functionally related to a SNP component, i.e. if such a cluster of SNPs has functional consequences manifested in a specific fMRI brain network, then logically the expression pattern of these two components is correlated in all participants.

As proof of principle, from data derived from an fMRI auditory oddball task in only 43 healthy controls and 20 schizophrenia subjects (all Caucasian), the para-ICA approach was able to identify (Liu *et al.*, 2009b) a fronto-parietal fMRI component that significantly separated schizophrenia patients from healthy controls, and an associated 10-SNP component that also significantly separated the groups, that contained several known putative schizophrenia risk genes, including DISC1, CHRNA7 and the alpha-2 adrenergic receptor gene.

Future trends and conclusion

In summary, functional MRI activation tasks are becoming increasingly sophisticated and informative due to integration of cognitive neuroscience and genetic methods. Although most findings are still at the level of groups rather than individuals, the field is evolving towards what appear to be potentially useful clinical diagnostic tests. At the clinical level, current DSM-IV diagnoses are based on cross-sectional phenomenology and course, with no reference to neuroimaging. This will hopefully change with future editions of the DSM. Therefore, the question of the clinical specificity of brain imaging research findings will be examined more than at present, and may ultimately translate into a reclassification of psychiatric disorders, based on their biology.

As the fMRI field in general becomes more sophisticated, with faster integration of techniques from clinical neuroscience and the employment of novel analytic strategies, functional neuroimaging in schizophrenia becomes increasingly exciting. Some techniques have come full circle. The limitations of the initial resting, no-task nuclear medicine imaging studies in schizophrenia led to a functional MRI approach that focused heavily on cognitive challenge paradigms. With the relatively recent discovery that the default mode and resting state as measured in fMRI contain useful information, and that, moreover, these data distinguish schizophrenia patients from healthy controls, then approaches using simple cognitive tasks or no task at all are again recognized as informative.

Finally, the integration of functional MRI with genetic approaches is gathering momentum, with the sense that many exciting discoveries are on the horizon.

> **Box 2.1. Functional MRI investigations in schizophrenia: take-home points**
>
> Two variant major approaches to functional imaging:
> 1. "Traditional" approaches.
>   - Task probes derived from cognitive neuroscience, based on tasks in which schizophrenia patients perform poorly, thus "cognitive stress tests", in order to identify dysfunctional brain regions.
>   - Problematic in that task performance is inevitably confounded with diagnosis.
>   - Typical paradigms include working memory and executive function, but also diverse tasks including Morris water maze and facial recognition/emotional tasks.
> 2. "Recent, novel" approaches.
>   - Rely on simple task paradigms for example auditory oddball or no task (resting state).
>   - More likely to focus on neural networks rather than isolated brain regions.
>   - Use of independent component analysis (ICA) to identify temporally coherent brain networks.
>   - Focus on default mode circuitry, either extracted from task-related paradigms or derived from resting state data.
>   - Importance of functional network connectivity measurements.
>   - More straightforward integration of genetic approaches for example using parallel ICA analytic paradigms.

Funding and support

Dr. Pearlson is supported by the National Institute of Mental Health (2 R01 MH43775 MERIT Award, 5 R01 MH52886), National Institute on Drug Abuse

(1 R01 DA020709), National Institute on Alcohol Abuse and Alcoholism (1 R01 AA015615), and National Alliance for Research on Schizophrenia and Depression (Distinguished Investigator Award).

References

Aleman A, Kahn R S. 2005. Strange feelings: do amygdala abnormalities dysregulate the emotional brain in schizophrenia? *Prog Neurobiol* **77**, 283–98.

Allen A J, Griss M E, Folley B S, Hawkins K A and Pearlson G D. 2009. Endophenotypes in schizophrenia: A selective review. *Schizophr Res* **109**, 24–37.

Arfanakis K, Cordes D, Haughton V M, *et al.* 2000. Combining independent component analysis and correlation analysis to probe interregional connectivity in fMRI task activation datasets. *Magn Reson Imaging* **18**, 921–30.

Assaf M, Rivkin P R, Kuzu C H, *et al.* 2006. Abnormal object recall and anterior cingulate overactivation correlate with formal thought disorder in schizophrenia. *Biol Psychiatry* **59**, 452–9.

Assaf M, Jagannathan K, *et al.* 2009. Temporal sequence of hemispheric network activation during semantic processing: a functional network connectivity analysis. *Brain Cogn* **70**, 238–46.

Astur R S, St Germain S A, Baker E K, *et al.* 2005. fMRI hippocampal activity during a virtual radial arm maze. *Appl Psychophysiol Biofeedback* **30**, 307–17.

Baas D, Aleman A, Vink M, *et al.* 2008. Evidence of altered cortical and amygdala activation during social decision-making in schizophrenia. *Neuroimage* **40**, 719–27.

Baddeley A. 1992. Working memory. *Science* **255**, 556–9.

Barch D M, Berman M G, Engle R, *et al.* 2009. CNTRICS final task selection: working memory. *Schizophr Bull* **35**, 136–52.

Barch D M, Braver T S, Cohen A L, *et al.* 1998. Context processing deficits in schizophrenia. *Arch Gen Psychiatry* **50**, 280–8.

Barch D M, Carter C S, Braver T S, *et al.* 2001. Selective deficits in prefrontal cortex function in medication-naive patients with schizophrenia. *Arch Gen Psychiatry* **58**, 280–8.

Barch D M, and Smith E. 2008. The cognitive neuroscience of working memory: relevance to CNTRICS and schizophrenia. *Biol Psychiatry* **64**, 11–7.

Barta P E, Pearlson G D, Powers R E, *et al.* 1990. Auditory hallucinations and smaller superior temporal gyral volume in schizophrenia. *Am J Psychiatry* **147**, 1457–62.

Beckmann C F, DeLuca M, Devlin J T, *et al.* 2005. Investigations into resting-state connectivity using independent component analysis. *Phil Trans R Soc Lond B Biol Sci* **360**, 1001–13.

Biswal B B, Van Kylen J and Hyde J S. 1997. Simultaneous assessment of flow and BOLD signals in resting-state functional connectivity maps. *NMR Biomed* **10**, 165–70.

Bluhm R L, Miller J, Lanius R A, *et al.* 2007. Spontaneous low-frequency fluctuations in the BOLD signal in schizophrenic patients: anomalies in the default network. *Schizophr Bull* **33**, 1004–12.

Broyd S J, Demanuele C, Debener S, *et al.* 2009. Default-mode brain dysfunction in mental disorders: a systematic review. *Neurosci Biobehav Rev* **33**, 279–96.

Calhoun V D, Adali T, Giuliani N R, *et al.* 2006a. Method for multimodal analysis of independent source differences in schizophrenia: combining gray matter structural and auditory oddball functional data. *Hum Brain Mapp* **27**, 47–62.

Calhoun V D, Adali T, Kiehl K A, *et al.* 2006b. A method for multitask fMRI data fusion applied to schizophrenia. *Hum Brain Mapp* **27**, 598–610.

Calhoun V D, Adali T, Pearlson G D, *et al.* 2006c. Neuronal chronometry of target detection: fusion of hemodynamic and event-related potential data. *Neuroimage* **30**, 544–53.

Calhoun V D, Kiehl K A, Liddle P F, *et al.* 2004. Aberrant localization of synchronous hemodynamic activity in auditory cortex reliably characterizes schizophrenia. *Biol Psychiatry* **55**, 842–9.

Calhoun V D, Kiehl K A and Pearlson G D. 2008. Modulation of temporally coherent brain networks estimated using ICA at rest and during cognitive tasks. *Hum Brain Mapp* **29**, 828–38.

Callicott J H, Bertolino A, Mattay V S, *et al.* 2000. Physiological dysfunction of the dorsolateral prefrontal cortex in schizophrenia revisited. *Cereb Cortex* **10**, 1078–92.

Callicott J H, Egan M F, Mattay V S, *et al.* 2003a. Abnormal fMRI response of the dorsolateral prefrontal cortex in cognitively intact siblings of patients with schizophrenia. *Am J Psychiatry* **160**, 709–19.

Callicott J H, Mattay V S, Bertolino A, *et al.* 1999. Physiological characteristics of capacity constraints in working memory as revealed by functional MRI. *Cereb Cortex* **9**, 20–6.

Callicott J H, Mattay V S, Verchinski V A, *et al.* 2003b. Complexity of prefrontal cortical dysfunction in schizophrenia: more than up or down. *Am J Psychiatry* **160**, 2209–15.

Callicott J H, Ramsey N F, Tallent K, *et al.* 1998. Functional magnetic resonance imaging brain mapping in psychiatry: methodological issues illustrated in a study of working memory in schizophrenia. *Neuropsychopharmacology* **18**, 186–96.

Callicott J H, Straub R E, Pezawas L, *et al.* 2005. Variation in DISC1 affects hippocampal structure and function and increases risk for schizophrenia. *Proc Natl Acad Sci U S A* **102**, 8627–32.

Carvalho K N, Pearlson G D, Astur R S, *et al.* 2006. Simulated driving and brain imaging: combining behavior, brain activity, and virtual reality. *CNS Spectr* **11**, 52–62.

Cohen J D, Braver T S, O'Reilly R C, *et al.* 1996. A computational approach to prefrontal cortex, cognitive control and schizophrenia: recent developments and current challenges. *Phil Trans R Soc Lond B Biol Sci* **351**, 1515–27.

Cordes D, Haughton V M, Arfanakis K, *et al.* 2001. Frequencies contributing to functional connectivity in the cerebral cortex in "resting-state" data. *Am J Neuroradiol* **22**, 1326–33.

Damoiseaux J S, Rombouts S A, Barkhof F, *et al.* 2006. Consistent resting-state networks across healthy subjects. *Proc Natl Acad Sci U S A* **103**, 13 848–53.

De Luca M, Smith S, De Stefano N, *et al.* 2005. Blood oxygenation level dependent contrast resting state networks are relevant to functional activity in the neocortical sensorimotor system. *Exp Brain Res* **167**, 587–94.

Demirci O, Stevens M C, Andresen N C, *et al.* 2009. Investigation of relationships between fMRI brain networks in the spectral domain using ICA and Granger causality reveals distinct differences between schizophrenia patients and healthy controls. *Neuroimage* **46**, 419–31.

D'Esposito M, Postle B R, Ballard D, *et al.* 1999. Maintenance versus manipulation of information held in working memory: an event-related fMRI study. *Brain Cogn* **41**, 66–86.

Di Giorgio A, Blasi G, Sambataro F, *et al.* 2008. Association of the SerCys DISC1 polymorphism with human hippocampal formation gray matter and function during memory encoding. *Eur J Neurosci* **28**, 2129–36.

Dosenbach N U, Fair D A, Miezin F M, *et al.* 2007. Distinct brain networks for adaptive and stable task control in humans. *Proc Natl Acad Sci U S A* **104**, 11 073–8.

Driesen N R, Leung H C, Calhoun V D, *et al.* 2008. Impairment of working memory maintenance and response in schizophrenia: functional magnetic resonance imaging evidence. *Biol Psychiatry* **64**, 1026–34.

Egan M F, Goldberg T E, Kolachana B S, *et al.* 2001. Effect of COMT Val108/158 Met genotype on frontal lobe function and risk for schizophrenia. *Proc Natl Acad Sci U S A* **98**, 6917–22.

Foley B S, Astur R, Jagannathan K, *et al.* 2010. Anomalous neural circuit function in schizophrenia during a virtual Morris water task. *Neuroimage* **49**, 3373–84.

Ford J M, Gray M, Whitfield S L, *et al.* 2004. Acquiring and inhibiting prepotent responses in schizophrenia: event-related brain potentials and functional magnetic resonance imaging. *Arch Gen Psychiatry* **61**, 119–29.

Ford J M, Roach B J, Jorgensen K W, *et al.* 2009. Tuning in to the voices: a multisite FMRI study of auditory hallucinations. *Schizophr Bull* **35**, 58–66.

Fransson P. 2006. How default is the default mode of brain function? Further evidence from intrinsic BOLD signal fluctuations. *Neuropsychologia* **44**, 2836–45.

Friedman H R and Goldman-Rakic P S. 1994. Coactivation of prefrontal cortex and inferior parietal cortex in working memory tasks revealed by 2DG functional mapping in the rhesus monkey. *J Neurosci* **14**, 2775–88.

Fuster J M. 2006. The cognit: a network model of cortical representation. *Int J Psychophysiol* **60**, 125–32.

Garrity A G, Pearlson G D, McKiernan K, *et al.* 2007. Aberrant "default mode" functional connectivity in schizophrenia. *Am J Psychiatry* **164**, 450–7.

Glahn D C, Ragland J D, Abramoff A, *et al.* 2005. Beyond hypofrontality: a quantitative meta-analysis of functional neuroimaging studies of working memory in schizophrenia. *Hum Brain Mapp* **25**, 60–9.

Goldberg T E, Patterson K J, Taqqu Y, *et al.* 1998. Capacity limitations in short-term memory in schizophrenia: tests of competing hypotheses. *Psychol Med* **28**, 665–73.

Goldberg T E and Weinberger D R. 2004. Genes and the parsing of cognitive processes. *Trends Cogn Sci* **8**, 325–35.

Green M F. 1996. What are the functional consequences of neurocognitive deficits in schizophrenia? *Am J Psychiatry* **153**, 321–30.

Greicius M D, Srivastava G, Reiss A L, *et al.* 2004. Default-mode network activity distinguishes Alzheimer's disease from healthy aging: evidence from functional MRI. *Proc Natl Acad Sci U S A* **101**, 4637–42.

Gusnard D A, Akbudak E, Shulman G L, *et al.* 2001. Medial prefrontal cortex and self-referential mental activity: relation to a default mode of brain function. *Proc Natl Acad Sci U S A* **98**, 4259–64.

Hall J., Harris J M, Sprengelmeyer R, *et al.* 2004. Social cognition and face processing in schizophrenia. *Br J Psychiatry* **185**, 169–70.

Harvey P D and Keefe R S. 2001. Studies of cognitive change in patients with schizophrenia following novel antipsychotic treatment. *Am J Psychiatry* **158**, 176–84.

Heckers S, Weiss A P, Deckersbach T, *et al.* 2004. Anterior cingulate cortex activation during cognitive interference in schizophrenia. *Am J Psychiatry* **161**, 707–15.

Henik A, Carter C S, Salo R, *et al.* 2002. Attentional control and word inhibition in schizophrenia. *Psychiatry Res* **110**, 137–49.

Hoffman R E, Anderson A W, Varanko M, *et al.* 2008. Time course of regional brain activation associated with onset of auditory/verbal hallucinations. *Br J Psychiatry* **193**, 424–5.

Holt D J, Kunkel L, Weiss A P, *et al.* 2006. Increased medial temporal lobe activation during the passive viewing of emotional and neutral facial expressions in schizophrenia. *Schizophr Res* **82**, 153–62.

Jafri M J, Pearlson G D, Stevens M, *et al.* 2008. A method for functional network connectivity among spatially independent resting-state components in schizophrenia. *Neuroimage* **39**, 1666–81.

Jansma J M, Ramsey N F, van der Wee M J, *et al.* 2004. Working memory capacity in schizophrenia: a parametric fMRI study. *Schizophr Res* **68**, 159–71.

Johnson M R, Morris N A, Astur R S, *et al.* 2006. A functional magnetic resonance imaging study of working memory abnormalities in schizophrenia. *Biol Psychiatry* **60**, 11–21.

Karlsgodt K H, Sun D, Jimenez A M, *et al.* 2008. Developmental disruptions in neural connectivity in the pathophysiology of schizophrenia. *Dev Psychopathol* **20**, 1297–327.

Kerns J G, Cohen J D, MacDonald A W III, *et al.* 2005. Decreased conflict- and error-related activity in the anterior cingulate cortex in subjects with schizophrenia. *Am J Psychiatry* **162**, 1833–9.

Kiehl K A, Stevens M C, Laurens K R, *et al.* 2005. An adaptive reflexive processing model of neurocognitive function: supporting evidence from a large scale (n = 100) fMRI study of an auditory oddball task. *Neuroimage* **25**, 899–915.

Laurens K R, Kiehl K A, Ngan E T, *et al.* 2005. Attention orienting dysfunction during salient novel stimulus processing in schizophrenia. *Schizophr Res* **75**, 159–71.

Liu J, Kiehl K A, Pearlson G, *et al.* 2009a. Genetic determinants of target and novelty-related event-related potentials in the auditory oddball response. *Neuroimage* **46**, 809–16.

Liu J, Pearlson G, Windemuth A, *et al.* 2009b. Combining fMRI and SNP data to investigate connections between brain function and genetics using parallel ICA. *Hum Brain Mapp* **30**, 241–55.

Lowe M J, Mock B J and Sorensen J A. 1998. Functional connectivity in single and multislice echoplanar imaging using resting-state fluctuations. *Neuroimage* **7**, 119–32.

Manoach D S. 2003. Prefrontal cortex dysfunction during working memory performance in schizophrenia: reconciling discrepant findings. *Schizophr Res* **60**, 285–98.

Manoach D S, Gollub R L, Benson E S, *et al.* 2000. Schizophrenic subjects show aberrant fMRI activation of dorsolateral prefrontal cortex and basal ganglia during working memory performance. *Biol Psychiatry* **48**, 99–109.

Manoach D S, Greve D N, Lindgren K A, *et al.* 2003. Identifying regional activity associated with temporally separated components of working memory using event-related functional MRI. *Neuroimage* **20**, 1670–84.

Manoach D S, Schlaug G, Siewert B, *et al.* 1997. Prefrontal cortex fMRI signal changes are correlated with working memory load. *Neuroreport* **8**, 545–9.

Marwick K and Hall J. 2008. Social cognition in schizophrenia: a review of face processing. *Br Med Bull* **88**, 43–58.

McDonald C, Marshall N, Sham P C, *et al.* 2006. Regional brain morphometry in patients with schizophrenia or bipolar disorder and their unaffected relatives. *Am J Psychiatry* **163**, 478–87.

McKeown M J and Sejnowski T J. 1998. Independent component analysis of fMRI data: examining the assumptions. *Hum Brain Mapp* **6**, 368–72.

McKiernan K A, D'Angelo B R, Kaufman J N and Binder J R. 2006. Interrupting the "stream of consciousness": An fMRI investigation. *Neuroimage* **29**, 1185–9.

McKiernan K A, Kaufman J N, Kucera-Thomson J, *et al.* 2003. A parametric manipulation of factors affecting task-induced deactivation in functional neuroimaging. *J Cogn Neurosci* **15**, 394–408.

Meda S A, Bhattarai M, Morris N A, *et al.* 2008. An fMRI study of working memory in first-degree unaffected relatives of schizophrenia patients. *Schizophr Res* **104**, 85–95.

Mesulam M M. 1998. From sensation to cognition. *Brain* **121**, 1013–52.

Meyer-Lindenberg A, Poline J B, Kohn P D, *et al.* 2001. Evidence for abnormal cortical functional connectivity during working memory in schizophrenia. *Am J Psychiatry* **158**, 1809–17.

Meyer-Lindenberg A and Weinberger D R. 2006. Intermediate phenotypes and genetic mechanisms of psychiatric disorders. *Nat Rev Neurosci* **7**, 818–27.

Miller E K, Erickson C A, Desimone R, *et al.* 1996. Neural mechanisms of visual working memory in prefrontal cortex of the macaque. *J Neurosci* **16**, 5154–67.

Minzenberg M J, Laird A R, Thelen S, *et al.* 2009. Meta-analysis of 41 functional neuroimaging studies of executive function reveals dysfunction in a general-purpose cognitive control system in schizophrenia. *Arch Gen Psychiatry* **66**, 811–22.

Park S and Holzman P S. 1992. Schizophrenics show spatial working memory deficits. *Arch Gen Psychiatry* **49**, 975–82.

Park S, Puschel J, Sauter B H, *et al.* 1999. Spatial working memory deficits and clinical symptoms in schizophrenia: a 4-month follow-up study. *Biol Psychiatry* **46**, 392–400.

Pearlson G. 2009. Multisite collaborations and large databases in psychiatric neuroimaging: Advantages, problems, and challenges. *Schizophr Bull* **35**, 1–2.

Pearlson G D and Folley B S. 2008a. Endophenotypes, dimensions, risks: is psychosis analogous to common inherited medical illnesses? *Clin EEG Neurosci* **39**, 73–7.

Pearlson G D and Folley B S. 2008b. Schizophrenia, psychiatric genetics, and Darwinian psychiatry: An evolutionary framework. *Schizophr Bull* **34**, 722–33.

Perlstein W M, Carter C S, Noll D C, *et al.* 2001. Relation of prefrontal cortex dysfunction to working memory and symptoms in schizophrenia. *Am J Psychiatry* **158**, 1105–13.

Petrides M. 1995. Impairments on nonspatial self-ordered and externally ordered working memory tasks after lesions of the mid-dorsal part of the lateral frontal cortex in the monkey. *J Neurosci* **15**, 359–75.

Pezawas L, Verchinski B A, Mattay V S, *et al.* 2004. The brain-derived neurotrophic factor val66met polymorphism and variation in human cortical morphology. *J Neurosci* **24**, 10 099–102.

Quintana J, Wong T, Ortiz-Portillo E, *et al.* 2003. Right lateral fusiform gyrus dysfunction during facial information processing in schizophrenia. *Biol Psychiatry* **53**, 1099–112.

Ragland J D, Yoon J, Minzenberg M J, *et al.* 2007. Neuroimaging of cognitive disability in schizophrenia: search for a pathophysiological mechanism. *Int Rev Psychiatry* **19**, 417–27.

Raichle M E, MacLeod A M, Snyder A Z, *et al.* 2001. A default mode of brain function. *Proc Natl Acad Sci USA* **98**, 676–82.

Rubia K, Russell T, Bullmore E T, *et al.* 2001. An fMRI study of reduced left prefrontal activation in schizophrenia during normal inhibitory function. *Schizophr Res* **52**, 47–55.

Rypma B and D'Esposito M. 1999. The roles of prefrontal brain regions in components of working memory: effects of memory load and individual differences. *Proc Natl Acad Sci U S A* **96**, 6558–63.

Seeley W W, Menon V, Schtazberg A F, *et al.* 2007. Dissociable intrinsic connectivity networks for salience processing and executive control. *J Neurosci* **27**, 2349–56.

Servan-Schreiber D, Cohen J D and Steingard S. 1996. Schizophrenic deficits in the processing of context. A test of a theoretical model. *Arch Gen Psychiatry* **53**, 1105–12.

Silver H, Feldman P, Bilker W, *et al.* 2003. Working memory deficit as a core neuropsychological dysfunction in schizophrenia. *Am J Psychiatry* **160**, 1809–16.

Sommer I E, Diederen K M, Blom J D, *et al.* 2008. Auditory verbal hallucinations predominantly activate the right inferior frontal area. *Brain* **131**, 3169–77.

Sternberg S. 1966. High-speed scanning in human memory. *Science* **153**, 652–4.

Sui J, Adali T, Pearlson G D, *et al.* 2009. An ICA-based method for the identification of optimal FMRI features and components using combined group-discriminative techniques. *Neuroimage* **46**, 73–86.

Surguladze S, Russell T, Kucharska-Pietura K, *et al.* 2006. A reversal of the normal pattern of parahippocampal response to neutral and fearful faces is associated with reality distortion in schizophrenia. *Biol Psychiatry* **60**, 423–31.

Tan H Y, Callicott J H and Weinberger D R. 2007. Dysfunctional and compensatory prefrontal cortical systems, genes and the pathogenesis of schizophrenia. *Cereb Cortex* **17**, i171–81.

Veltman D J, Rombouts S A and Dolan R J. 2003. Maintenance versus manipulation in verbal working memory revisited: an fMRI study. *Neuroimage* **18**, 247–56.

Wexler B E, Stevens A A, Bowers A A, *et al.* 1998. Word and tone working memory deficits in schizophrenia. *Arch Gen Psychiatry* **55**, 1093–6.

Wible C G, Lee K, Molina I, *et al.* 2009. fMRI activity correlated with auditory hallucinations during performance of a working memory task: data from the FBIRN consortium study. *Schizophr Bull* **35**, 47–57.

Winterer G, Coppola R, Egan M F, *et al.* 2003. Functional and effective frontotemporal connectivity and genetic risk for schizophrenia. *Biol Psychiatry* **54**, 1181–92.

Yurgelun-Todd D A, Waternaux C M, Cohen B M, *et al.* 1996. Functional magnetic resonance imaging of schizophrenic patients and comparison subjects during word production. *Am J Psychiatry* **153**, 200–5.

Spectroscopic imaging of schizophrenia

Jay W. Pettegrew, Richard J. McClure and Kanagasabai Panchalingam

With all technological advances there is the initial infatuation followed by more thoughtful reassessment. In vivo, non-invasive magnetic resonance spectroscopy (MRS) has progressed along this trajectory over the past 20–30 years. While much of the initial excitement revolved around technological advances, case reports, and small clinical studies, now is a good time to engage in a thoughtful reassessment of the potential new insights and pitfalls provided by this technology. This review will attempt this assessment in the context of MRS findings in schizophrenia research.

The first part of the review will address fundamental technological considerations followed by a discussion of what molecular and metabolic information can be obtained from ^{31}P and ^{1}H MRS. This will be followed by a selective review of the literature to date on ^{31}P and ^{1}H MRS studies in schizophrenia.

High field methodological issues

The development of in-vivo MR spectrometers with higher magnetic fields potentially increases sensitivity; however, methodological issues limit the anticipated improvement in both sensitivity (signal to noise ratio) and spectral resolution (Fleysher et al., 2009). These methodological issues are discussed below.

Signal–noise ratio (SNR) following a 90 degree pulse along the rotating frame y-axis

The SNR improves with higher magnetic field (B_0). Under ideal conditions, one can calculate the theoretical SNR. For N nuclei of gyromagnetic ratio γ, the signal is approximated by $N\gamma^3 B_0^2$, and the noise detected by the receiver is approximated by $\gamma^{1/2} B_0^{1/2}$ to give SNR $\sim N\gamma^{5/2} B_0^{3/2}$ (Chandrakumar and Subramanian, 1987). However, for in-vivo studies above

1 MHz, the SNR increases are at best linear with B_0 (Hoult and Lauterbur, 1979). For a single voxel there is a 23–38% gain in SNR at 3.0 Tesla (T) compared to 1.5 T. For chemical shift imaging (CSI), there is a 23–46% gain in SNR at 3.0 T vs. 1.5 T (Gonen et al., 2001). At fields higher than 4.0 T, SNR is a function of location within a non-uniform sample and particular sample geometry (Ugurbil et al., 2003). Average SNR at 7.0 T is about 1.6-times that at 4.0 T.

B_0 inhomogeneity

The spread in B_0 due to inhomogeneity will result in a spread in ω_0, the resonance frequency in angular units for rotating frame, observable as line broadening.

$$v_0 = \gamma B_0 / 2\pi$$

$$2\pi v_0 = \omega_0$$

$$\omega_0 = \gamma B_0$$

$$\omega_0 + \Delta\omega = \gamma(B_0 + \Delta B),$$

where ΔB is inhomogeneity.

Radio frequency (RF) B_1 field inhomogeneity

An RF pulse applied along an axis orthogonal to the B_0 field (z-axis) will produce a tip (nutation) of the magnetic dipole moment and produce a magnetic dipole moment in the x–y plane. The resonance condition for the RF pulse is given by:

$$\omega_1 = \gamma B_1$$

where B_1 is the RF field.

The nutation angle (θ) is given by:

$$\theta = \gamma B_1 t_w$$

where t_w is the time the B_1 RF field is applied.

Understanding Neuropsychiatric Disorders, ed. M. E. Shenton and B. I. Turetsky. Published by Cambridge University Press.
© Cambridge University Press 2011.

A 90 degree nutation angle will produce the maximum projection in the x–y plane and therefore the maximum signal. At higher B_0 fields, there is more variation of the B_1 field in biological samples such as human brain, resulting in B_1 field inhomogeneity. Spread in the B_1 RF field will produce a spread in θ, resulting in a spread in the SNR. The estimated B_1 field inhomogeneity at 4.0 T is 23% compared to 42% at 7.0 T using the same size RF coils and identical acquisition parameters (Vaughan *et al.*, 2001).

^{1}H–^{31}P dipolar coupling

Similar considerations are important when considering the use of ^{1}H decoupled ^{31}P MRS to increase SNR; i.e. the lack of uniform ^{1}H decoupling RF power across a very inhomogeneous volume such as the human brain. This can lead to non-linear distortion of the true amplitude of the signal resonances (Li *et al.*, 1996). If spin–spin splitting resulting from ^{1}H (nucleus A) spin coupling with ^{31}P (nucleus B) is given by J_{AB}, then the decoupling field (B_2) should be large enough such that $\gamma B_2 >> J_{AB}$. Spread in B_2 RF field due to tissue inhomogeneity will result in a spread of the ^{1}H–^{31}P decoupling effect. In addition, due to the nuclear Overhauser effect (NOE), this will lead to a spread in SNR over the sample volume, especially for ^{31}P resonances, which can have positive or negative NOEs which can introduce significant confounds. NOE enhancements of Pi, PCr, and ATP (25%, 25%, and 10%, respectively) were measured in human brain in vivo by Murphy-Boesch *et al.* (1993). Reported in-vitro NOE enhancements (Barany and Glonek, 1984) of ^{31}P resonances are: sPME, PC (22%); Pi (11%); sPDE, GPC (22%), GPE (82%); PCr (0%); αATP (24%); βATP (11%); γATP (7%), and dinucleotide phosphates (120%). Therefore, the carefully determined in-vitro NOE enhancements for the in-vivo ^{31}P MRS observable metabolites ranges from 0 to 120%. This will introduce a significant confound into ^{1}H-decoupled ^{31}P MRSI quantitative results.

RF power requirements

In transverse electromagnetic coils, about 2 times more RF power is required at 7.0 T compared to 4.0 T for a 90 degree pulse for identical head coils. In addition, larger bandwidths are required at higher fields (Ugurbil *et al.*, 2003).

Phased array coil

Phased array coils provide uniform B_1 field and sensitivity. In 2D and 3D CSI methods, additional problems exist, such as B_0 and B_1 field inhomogeneities, because larger brain volumes are involved. This necessitates the availability of higher-order shims to improve B_0 field homogeneity.

Spectral resolution

At higher fields, there is improved resolution due to chemical shift dispersion. However, linewidths also increase with field due to chemical shift anisotropy effects, molecular dipole–dipole interactions, local B_0 fluctuations due to molecular motion (vibrations and rotations), tissue paramagnetic effects (blood vessels, tissue ferritin), susceptibility broadening due to tissue–air or tissue–bone interfaces, and the intrinsic B_0 inhomogeneity. A consideration of these parameters allows one to determine an optimal voxel size which enhances both spatial (SNR-limited) and spectral (chemical shift dispersion + line broadening-limited) resolution. Fleysher *et al.* (2009) have shown that spectral resolution improves very slowly with increasing B_0, and is proportional to $B_0^{0.2}$. The resolution of J-coupled multiplets (Hz units), however, decreases with a $B_0^{0.8}$ relationship. These two opposing factors limit the effective increase in spectral resolution with increasing B_0. Methods based on coherence transfer have been proposed that in the future could improve resolution even in magnetic fields with unknown spatiotemporal variation (Pelupessy *et al.*, 2009).

Summary

In order for MRS methods to be practically applied to clinical populations with sufficient statistical power (i.e., sufficiently large sample size), cost becomes a very important factor. The cost of MR instruments are roughly one million dollars per Tesla. Given the sizeable increase in acquisition, siting, and maintenance costs above 3.0–4.0 T, with little real improvement in critical factors such as spectral resolution, a strong economic case can be made for lower-field studies (1.5–4.0 T). In addition, molecular species with intermediate correlation times will be more reliably quantified at 1.5 T than 3.0–4.0 T and will be lost at fields higher than 4.0 T.

- ^{31}P and ^{1}H MRS are extremely powerful non-invasive molecular imaging techniques.
- The trend has been to employ higher and higher magnetic fields (B_0) to increase signal-to-noise and spectral resolution.
- However, inhomogeneities in both B_0 and RF (B_1) fields and magnetic susceptibility effects limit the anticipated improvement in both signal-to-noise and spectral resolution.
- For ^{31}P MRS, signal-to-noise also can be increased by ^{1}H-decoupling. However, inhomogeneity in the ^{1}H decoupling RF field across inhomogeneous brain tissue can lead to confounds in multi-voxel quantitation. In addition, the Nuclear Overhauser Effect (NOE) will further increase the signal-to-noise spread over the volume of the brain. Since the NOE of in-vivo ^{31}P MRS observable metabolites range from 0 to 120%, this can result in a significant confound.
- In order for ^{31}P–^{1}H MRS to gain wide clinical application, cost (purchase, site preparation, operating) becomes an important factor. At this time, fields above 4.0 Tesla provide insufficient improvement in critical factors such as spectral resolution to justify the significant increase in cost. In addition, important molecular species such as vesicles (synaptic and transport) and small phosphorylated proteins and peptides cannot be reliably quantified at fields much above 1.5 Tesla.

Quantifiable information from in-vivo ^{31}P MRS

In a proton-coupled in-vivo ^{31}P brain spectrum, the resonances that are reliably quantifiable include phosphomonoester (PME), inorganic orthophosphate (Pi), phosphodiester (PDE), phosphocreatine (PCr), γ-adenosine-5′-triphosphate (γATP), αATP, and βATP (see Figure 3.1). The freely mobile metabolites with short correlation times are predominantly intracellular, and are only exchanged very slowly with blood (McIlwain and Bachelard, 1985, p. 42). For example, there are no detectable arterio-venous differences for any of the acid-soluble metabolites measured by MRS, and after intravenous injection of ^{32}Pi isotope the labeling of acid-soluble metabolites peak at 12–24 h and at 3–4 days for phospholipids. Because

of this, the in-vivo ^{31}P MRS signal is not affected by brain vascular changes, unless the vascular changes result in changes in brain chemistry.

High-energy metabolites

The ^{31}P MRS resonances related to high-energy phosphate metabolism, Pi, PCr, and the nucleoside phosphate resonances are derived from small, rapidly tumbling molecules with short NMR correlation times. The simplest assignments are the Pi resonance, which is derived solely from inorganic phosphate (5 mmole P/g fresh tissue, rat) (mainly $H_2PO_4^{1-}$ and HPO_4^{2-} at physiologic pH), and the PCr resonance which is derived solely from PCr (3.2–5.0 μmole P/g fresh tissue). The nucleoside mono-, di-, and tri-phosphate (NMP, NDP, and NTP, respectively) resonances include contributions from adenosine, cytosine, guanosine, and uridine derivatives. The adenosine compounds are the predominant species in brain with a concentration of 10.0 mmole P/g fresh tissue; the concentrations of the other nucleotides (mmole P/g fresh tissue) are: guanine nucleotides 2.4; uridine nucleotides 2.4; and cytidine nucleotides 0.8 (McIlwain and Bachelard, 1985). The γATP resonance is made up of the terminal β-phosphate of NDPs and the terminal γ-phosphates of NTPs, predominantly ADP and ATP. The αATP resonance is made up of the nucleotide-coupled α-phosphates of NDPs and NTPs, predominantly ADP and ATP, but there also are contributions from dinucleotides, such as nicotine adenine diphosphate, as well as uridine diphospho-sugars (UDP-glucose 67 μmole/kg; Goldberg and O'Toole, 1969), and cofactors in membrane phospholipid synthesis such as cytidine-diphospho-choline (0.03 μmole/g tissue) (CDP-choline) and CDP-diacylglycerol. The difference in the αATP-γATP contribution (α-γ) provides a way to determine UDP-sugar and CDP-choline, CDP-diacylglycerol contributions. The middle (βATP) resonance is the simplest of the nucleoside resonances, being composed only of the middle β-phosphate of NTPs, mainly ATP. The linewidth of the PME and nucleoside phosphate resonances can be increased by increased intracellular levels of free Ca^{2+} or Mg^{2+} which form complexes with the phosphate groups, producing chemical exchange line broadening (Pettegrew et al., 1988). The intracellular pH is determined by the chemical shift difference between the PCr and Pi resonances (Petroff et al., 1985). The

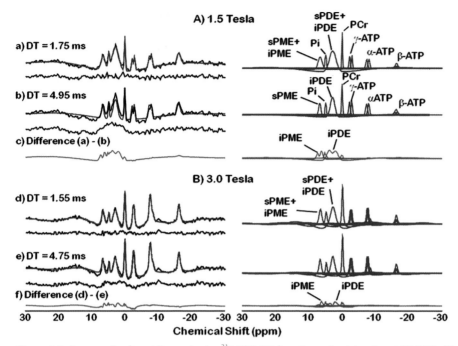

Figure 3.1 An example of modeling an in-vivo ^{31}P MRSI FID from the prefrontal region at (A) 1.5 T with DTs of (a) 1.75 ms and (b) 4.95 ms, and at (B) 3.0 T with DTs of (d) 1.55 ms and (e) 4.75 ms. The FT of the modeled FID superimposed on the acquired and residual are shown on the left and the individual peaks that make up the modeled FID are shown on the right for all DTs. The difference in the FT of the modeled FID (left) and in the individual peaks (right) between DT of 1.75 ms and 4.95 ms are shown for (c) 1.5 T and (f) 3.0 T. The intermediate correlation time peaks at 3.0 T (f) are marginally observable compared with 1.5 T (c). Abbreviations: DT, delay time; FID, free induction; FT, Fourier transform.

degree of intracellular di- and tri-valent cations can be estimated by the difference between the chemical shifts of ionized ends and esterified ends (Pettegrew et al., 1988).

Physiologic significance of PCr

There is an abundance of basic neuroscience literature dating back to the 1950s demonstrating that the major source of brain PCr utilization is repolarization of depolarized synapses (Kennedy and Sokoloff, 1957; Jansson et al., 1979; Sokoloff, 1991, 1993). PCr is a buffer for ATP and is consumed to maintain ATP levels as given in the creatine kinase (CrK) reaction below. Therefore, PCr levels provide a biomarker for functional activity of neural networks. Also, PCr linewidth can be a useful "internal standard" for B_0 homogeneity across the field of view provided susceptibility effects are minimal.

$$PCr + ADP + H^+ \underset{E.C.2.7.3.2}{\overset{CrK}{\rightleftharpoons}} Cr + ATP$$

Molecular composition of the PME and PDE resonances

The lineshape of the relatively broad in-vivo PME and PDE NMR spectral peaks is a superposition of various metabolites with PME and PDE moieties, which have different chemical shifts, and also includes the superposition of metabolites with different motional and/or rotational environments. This degree of mobility is characterized by a correlation time (τ_c), which is proportional to $1/T_2^*$, the spin–spin relaxation rate plus the static magnetic field (B_0) inhomogeneity. For example, the PME resonance is composed of freely mobile PMEs that have relatively short correlation times (sPME), including predominantly phosphocholine (PC) and phosphoethanolamine (PE). In-vitro concentrations as determined by careful freeze-clamped PCA tissue extraction and quantitation by high-resolution NMR (11.7 T) are PC $= 0.47 \pm 0.04$ µM/g tissue and PE $= 0.99 \pm 0.07$ µM/g tissue (Klunk et al., 1996). MRS in-vivo concentrations measured at 4.0 T are

51

PC $= 0.46 \pm 0.14$ mM/l tissue and PE $= 0.81 \pm 0.21$ mM/l tissue (Jensen *et al.*, 2002b). This demonstrates that there is good agreement between in-vivo and in-vitro MRS concentrations, with the in-vivo measurements having much higher variance. In-vivo MRS concentrations are often reported as mole percent, which correlates well with absolute concentrations and may yield a more accurate estimate of the relative change in disease state versus healthy control subjects (Klunk *et al.*, 1994). Inositol-1-phosphate, α-glycerol phosphate, phosphothreonine, and L-phosphoserine (L-PS) are present at lower concentrations (Glonek *et al.*, 1982; Pettegrew *et al.*, 1994). The PME resonance is also composed of less mobile molecules with PME moieties that have intermediate NMR correlation times (iPME), including phosphorylated proteins such as the phosphorylation of serine and threonine residues in proteins, and PMEs that are tightly coupled (in terms of MRS) to macromolecules (i.e. PMEs inserting into membrane phospholipids (Mason *et al.*, 1995)). Neuronal cytoskeletal proteins such as neurofilaments and the microtubule-associated protein tau are highly abundant in axons and exist in phosphorylated forms which would give rise to iPME signals. It is our contention that phosphorylated peptides and small proteins are observable as an iPME.

Therefore, the iPME resonance could monitor the phosphorylation–dephosphorylation state of proteins and indirectly monitor the protein kinase–protein phosphatase cascades in the brain which are influenced by brain neurotransmitter activity, especially glutamatergic (NMDA and AMPA, see below) and dopaminergic (D_1 and D_2) receptor activity. Multiple neurotransmitters acting through the second messengers cAMP, cGMP, and Ca^{2+} regulate the phosphorylation of dopamine-cAMP-regulated phosphoprotein molecular weight 32 kDa (DARPP-32) at the Thr^{34} site. Phosphorylation of DARPP-32 Thr^{34} is regulated through cAMP-stimulated protein kinase A and protein kinase G by various transmitters, principally dopamine through D_1 receptors but also by receptors for adenosine (A_{2A}), serotonin (5-HT), vasoactive intestinal peptide, and nitric oxide. Dephosphorylation of DARPP-32 Thr^{34} by protein phosphatase 2B (also known as calcinerin), a Ca^{2+}/calmodulin-dependent phosphatase, is activated by several transmitters, principally following Ca^{2+} influx produced by glutamate activity at *N*-methyl-D-aspartic acid

(NMDA) and $(\pm)\alpha$-amino-3-hydroxy-5-methyl isoxazole-4-propionic acid (AMPA) receptors, but also by dopamine D_2 receptors. The potency of dopamine receptor antagonists, whether typical or atypical, correlate with their potency as antagonists at the D_2 receptor (Creese and Hess, 1986; Seeman, 2002), and both typical and atypical neuroleptics increase the phosphorylation state of DARPP-32. Phosphorylated DARPP-32 inhibits a major brain phosphatase, protein phosphatase 1, which would secondarily increase the phosphorylation state of many brain proteins, including membrane channels and receptors. Loss of synapses, if they contain predominantly ionotropic glutamate receptors, could lead to an increased level of protein phosphorylation due to the mechanisms discussed. The level of DARPP-32 in bovine caudate is 2.5 μM (King *et al.*, 1984). However, the total level of all phosphoproteins in mammalian brain is 1.1 μM/g fresh tissue or 1.1 mmoles (McIlwain and Bachelard, 1985). A ^{1}H and ^{31}P study of one phosphoprotein, the 155-kDa phosphophoryn, revealed a ^{31}P line width of 34 Hz (Evans and Chan, 1994), which suggests that brain phosphoproteins could be observable by in-vivo ^{31}P MRS. The in-vivo ^{31}P MRS iPME line width observed in the chronic schizophrenia study is 75 Hz (Pettegrew *et al.*, unpublished observations). Therefore, we contend that brain phosphoproteins are detectable by in-vivo ^{31}P MRSI.

Likewise, the PDE resonance is composed of: (1) freely mobile PDEs (sPDE), glycerophosphocholine (GPC), and glycerophosphoethanolamine (GPE). In-vitro concentrations as determined by careful freeze-clamped PCA tissue extraction and quantitation by high-resolution NMR (11.7 T) are GPC $= 0.81 \pm 0.05$ μM/g tissue and GPE $= 0.93 \pm 0.06$ μM/g tissue (Klunk *et al.*, 1996). MRS in-vivo concentrations measured at 4.0 T are GPC $= 1.15 \pm 0.43$ mM/l tissue and GPE $= 0.74 \pm 0.30$ mM/l tissue (Jensen *et al.*, 2002b), and have relatively short correlation times in vivo (Glonek *et al.*, 1982; Pettegrew *et al.*, 1994); (2) less-mobile PDE moieties (iPDE) that have relatively intermediate correlation times and are part of small membrane phospholipid structures including micelles, synaptic vesicles and transport/secretory vesicles associated with the Golgi and endoplasmic reticulum (Pettegrew *et al.*, 1994; Murphy *et al.*, 1989; Kilby *et al.*, 1991; Gonzalez-Mendez *et al.*, 1984; de Kruijff *et al.*, 1979, 1980) or are tightly coupled to larger molecular structures (i.e., PDEs inserting into membrane phospholipid structures which would then give rise to a relative longer correlation time; Pettegrew *et al.*, 1994); and (3) partially mobile PDE moieties (lPDE) that have relatively long NMR correlation times and are part of the membrane phospholipid bilayer structure in myelin, external cell membranes and large organelle membranes such as the Golgi, endoplasmic reticulum, and nuclear membranes (Murphy *et al.*, 1989, 1992; McNamara *et al.*, 1994; Pettegrew *et al.*, 1994; Kilby *et al.*, 1991; Cerdan *et al.*, 1986; Seelig, 1978). A typical in-vivo ^{31}P brain spectrum would have negligible contribution from the long correlation time component unless the reacquisition delay time (DT) or echo time is of the order of 100 μs or less (Stanley *et al.*, 1994). Therefore, in a typical in-vivo ^{31}P MRSI study, the quantified PME and PDE would only include the short and intermediate correlation time contributions of PME and PDE resonances. Synaptic vesicles containing iPDE moieties are enriched in gray matter nerve terminals. Transport/secretory vesicles containing iPDE moieties are enriched in white matter axons. Although the exact molecular sources for the iPME and iPDE signals have not been definitely proven, tentative assignments to phosphorylated peptides and proteins (iPME), transport vesicles (iPDE, white matter), and synaptic vesicles (iPDE, gray matter) are supported by the available line width data presented above.

Physiologic significance of freely mobile PMEs and PDEs

The PME and PDE levels from the short NMR correlation time components provide a measure of membrane phospholipid metabolism. The sPME (i.e. PE, PC, and L-PS) are predominantly building blocks of phospholipids and, therefore, the relative concentrations of these metabolites are a measure of the active synthesis of membranes (Vance, 1988; Vance, 1991). This role for the water-soluble PME with short correlation times, such as PE and PC, has been demonstrated directly in an entorhinal cortical lesioned rat model of neural degeneration–regeneration in which high levels of these sPME are observed at the time and site of neuritic sprouting (Geddes *et al.*, 1997). I1P predominantly reflects phospholipase C (PLC) activity directed towards phophatidylinositol. Sources of PE, PC and L-PS are: (1) phosphorylation of their respective bases by kinases; (2) PLC cleavage of their respective phospholipids; and (3) phosphodiesterase

cleavage of their respective PDE, such as GPC and GPE. The PME are broken down by phosphatases to release Pi and the constituent base. Water-soluble sPDE, such as GPE and GPC, are the major products of membrane phospholipid degradation (Vance, 1988; Vance, 1991), which again has been demonstrated directly in an entorhinal cortical lesioned rat model of neural degeneration–regeneration in which high levels of GPE and GPC are observed at the site and time of neuronal membrane breakdown (Geddes *et al.*, 1997). The sPDE are products of phospholipase $A_1 + A_2$ activity toward their phospholipids, and are converted to their respective PME by PDE phosphodiesterase activity. In spite of their high abundance in the brain, the physiological function of the water-soluble sPDE remains unknown. Methods to reliably quantify the sPME, sPDE, iPME and iPDE by in-vivo ^{31}P MRSI at 1.5 T have been published (Stanley and Pettegrew, 2001).

PCr – a biomarker for exaggerated synaptic elimination in schizophrenia

There is in-vivo ^{31}P MRS-based evidence for exaggerated synaptic elimination in schizophrenia subjects (Pettegrew *et al.*, 1991) reviewed in McClure *et al.* (1998), especially in the dorsolateral prefrontal cortex (DPFC). DPFC undergoes synaptic elimination in humans during late adolescence to young-adult life, which is the same time frame as the usual onset of clinical symptoms in schizophrenia.

Synaptic elimination should result in an increased percentage of non-synaptic components (glial cell bodies and processes; neuronal cell bodies and processes without synapses), and a decrease in the highest energy-consuming component, i.e. the synapse, in a given brain voxel. There is evidence to suggest this would result in an elevation of high-energy phosphates. Research on anesthetic agents shows that synaptic activity in a normal awake "steady-state" is enough to drive high-energy phosphate levels below that which would occur in inactive neurons. Several studies have shown that anesthesia causes an elevation of PCr and ATP in parallel to the decrease in neuronal activity (McCandless and Wiggins, 1981). This is consistent with the studies of Jansson *et al.* (1979), who showed that PCr and ATP levels are lower in isolated cerebral nerve endings than in whole brain. Unlike nerve tissue in general, synaptosomes preferentially utilize endogenous PCr and ATP

53

stores. Jansson *et al.* (1979) conclude that synaptic transmission primarily depends on local stores of high-energy phosphates, rather than on the availability of glucose per se.

Demonstration of synaptic elimination in human brain development by ³¹P MRS

We have recently demonstrated (Goldstein *et al.*, 2009) the correlation of molecular biomarkers of membrane phospholipid turnover (sPME/sPDE) and PCr with structural and cognitive changes observed in human brain development, as illustrated in Figure 3.2. ³¹P and ¹H MRSI and neuropsychological examination of 105 healthy subjects (ages 6–18 years) at 1.5 T in an axial slice containing (left and right) DPFC, basal ganglia (BG), STC, IPC, centrum semi-ovale (CS), and OC; the time period of synaptic elimination was observed to be from 9.5 to 12 years, as reflected by change in gray matter volume and changes in sPME/sPDE. Note that *N*-acetyl aspartate (NAA) levels are less sensitive to the structural changes associated with synaptic elimination. Low levels of PCr prior to 9.5 years of age probably reflect the utilization of ATP and by extension PCr in membrane phospholipid synthesis (295 moles of ATP per mole of dipalmitoylphosphatidylcholine) and cholesterol synthesis (276 moles of ATP per mole of cholesterol). Following synaptic elimination, there is a marked increase in PCr levels in keeping with reduced numbers of synapses and/or reduced synaptic activity and decreased utilization of PCr for membrane synthesis.

Summary

³¹P MRS is ideally suited to investigate high-energy phosphate and membrane phospholipid metabolism in brain. In addition, resonances proposed to measure membraneous vesicles such as synaptic and transport vesicles are quantifiable at 1.5 T and to a lesser extent at 3.0 T, but are lost at 4.0 T and above. The high-energy phosphate PCr is a potential molecular biomarker for synaptic activity and indirectly of synaptic number. Finally, the potential exists to measure phosphorylated proteins and peptides which indirectly monitor protein kinase and protein phosphatase activity at 1.5 T, but probably not at fields above 3.0 T. Given the above and given the pivotal roles high-energy phosphate and membrane phospholipid metabolism, synaptic/transport

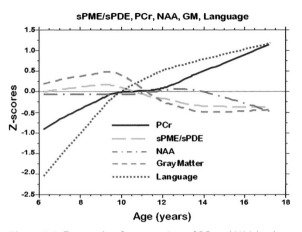

Figure 3.2 Z-score plots for comparison of PCr and NAA levels, sPME/sPDE ratio, gray matter percent, and composite language cognitive scores with age of healthy volunteers.

vesicles and protein kinase/protein phosphatase activity play in brain function and structure, it is clear that ³¹P MRS is an attractive modality for brain studies.

Quantifiable information from in-vivo ¹H MRS

N-Acetyl groups with short correlation times (sNA), total creatine (PCr + Cr (Cr$_t$)), and trimethylamines (TMA) are the predominant short correlation time metabolites observed by in-vivo ¹H MRS studies. NAA and NAAG are the major contributors to sNA; however, metabolites with short correlation times such as sialic acids and UDP-*N*-acetyl sugars could contribute (see below). An example of quantifying a ¹H MRS spectrum using LC model fitting is shown in Figure 3.3.

Both PCr and Cr contribute to the total creatine (Cr$_t$) resonance, so this resonance is not a preferred measure for high-energy phosphate metabolism. The TMA resonance of the in-vivo ¹H MR spectrum is comprised of freely mobile metabolites (Miller, 1991), including GPC (1.15 ± 0.43 mmole/l tissue) and PC (0.46 ± 0.14 mmole/l tissue) (Jensen *et al.*, 2002b), and to a much lesser degree choline (10–60 nmole/g) (McIlwain and Bachelard, 1985, p. 415), acetylcholine (7 nmole/g) (McIlwain and Bachelard, 1985, p. 416), carnitine (150 nmole/g) (Makar *et al.*, 1995), and acetyl-L-carnitine (15 nmole/g).

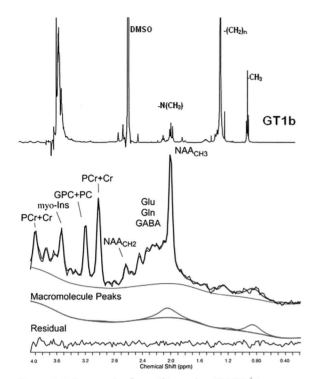

Figure 3.3 An example of quantifying a short TE MRSI ^{1}H spectrum of a healthy individual using LC Model fitting. The acquired spectrum with no line broadening is superimposed on the modeled and baseline spline function, and the residual is below. The quantified macromolecule signal is indicated in a separate trace. A high-resolution (11.7 T) spectrum of GT1b ganglioside is shown at the top.

NAA, which is second to glutamate in terms of total brain concentration of free amino acids, accounts for approximately 85–90% of the [1]H *N*-acetyl methyl resonance at 2.01 ppm, and NAAG contributes to the remaining 10–15% (Koller *et al.*, 1984; Frahm *et al.*, 1991; Pouwels and Frahm, 1997). Rat brain NAA levels rapidly increase from birth to adolescence (3 months). Both NAA and NAAG are localized exclusively in mature neurons and neuronal processes, and not in mature glia (Tallan *et al.*, 1956; Koller *et al.*, 1984; Birken and Oldendorf, 1989; Urenjak *et al.*, 1993). NAA is formed in neuronal mitochondria from acetyl-CoA and aspartate by the membrane bound enzyme L-aspartate *N*-acetyltrans-ferase, an enzyme found in brain but not in other tissue such as heart, liver and kidney (Goldstein, 1959, 1969; Knizley, 1967; Truckenmiller *et al.*, 1985). The neuronal synthesis of NAA is directly coupled to glucose and energy metabolism in the human brain. Monoclonal antibody studies show NAA to be localized to neurons with intense staining of the perikarya and proximal dendrites and axons (Simmons *et al.*, 1991). The neuronal immunoreactivity does not correspond to primary neurotransmitter characteristics. Approximately 30% of neurons do not appear to contain appreciable amounts of NAA. After formation in neuronal mito-chondria, NAA undergoes regulated release into the extracellular space and is hydrolyzed by aspartoacy-lase (amidohydrolase II), which is found in oligo-dendrocytes rather than astrocytes (Bhakoo *et al.*, 2001). The aspartate that is released is taken up by neurons and recycled into NAA (Baslow, 2003). Most of the acetyl groups that are released are taken up and metabolized by oligodendrocytes or astro-cytes where they are oxidized, converted into acetyl-CoA, or incorporated into membrane lipids, including myelin. Potential roles for NAA include a storage form of aspartate or acetate, oligodendroglia myelin formation, and a molecular water pump to remove metabolic water from metabolically active neurons (Baslow, 2003).

In-vitro versus in-vivo ^{1}H MRS values for NAA

In general, in-vivo spectroscopy studies have consist-ently reported higher concentration values of brain NAA as measured by the [1]H *N*-acetyl methyl reson-ance at 2.01 ppm (7.9–16.6 mmole/kg wet weight, average concentration 10.3 mmole/kg wet weight) than those reported using gas chromatography (5.5 mmole/kg wet weight) (Tallan, 1957; Nadler and Cooper, 1972), or high-resolution NMR of human biopsy brain tissue (5–6 mmole/kg wet weight; 5.97 ± 0.26 mmole/kg wet weight gray matter, 3.99 ± 0.20 mmole/kg weight white matter; 5.87 mmole/kg wet weight frontal) (Perry *et al.*, 1971). There are several factors that may account for the discrepancy, including breakdown of NAA during tissue removal and extraction, such that in-vitro values will be lower than in-vivo values. How-ever, with careful, freeze-clamped extraction methods (Glonek *et al.*, 1982; Pettegrew *et al.*, 1990), break-down is not a likely cause for the differences (see discussion of in-vivo versus in-vitro concentrations of PME and PDE). Other *N*-acetyl groups with short correlation times such as *N*-acetyl sugars, including UDP-*N*-acetyl sugars, could contribute to the sNA resonance, especially under pathological conditions, such as observed in chronic schizophrenia in which there is membrane repair and especially if there is repair of gangliosides (enriched in synaptosomal

55

membranes), since UDP-*N*-acetyl sugars are used in ganglioside synthesis.

Evidence indicates that gangliosides are specifically localized in neurons (Lowden and Wolfe, 1964), and are enriched in synaptic membranes (Whittaker, 1966; Wiegandt, 1967). The levels of gangliosides in human brain cerebral gray matter (1.45–1.68 mmoles/100 g dry weight) and cerebral white matter (0.28–0.37 mmoles/100 g dry weight) have been determined by Eeg-Olofsson *et al.* (1966). The levels of gangliosides are developmentally regulated. In rat brain, ganglioside levels start to increase by post-natal day 5 and peak at approximately post-natal day 20 (Suzuki, 1966). Hess *et al.* (1976) report that human neurons contain six times more sialic acid groups than rat brain. Sialo proteins also contain sialic acid and could contribute up to 15% of the total brain protein (McIlwain and Bachelard, 1985, p. 316). Gangliosides are synthesized by the sequential transfer of sialic acids and neutral sugars by membrane-bound glycosyl transferases and sialyl transferases located in regions of the Golgi apparatus that generally correspond to the order of sugar addition; i.e. initial sugar additions in the *cis* Golgi and terminal additions in the distal *trans* Golgi. CMP-*N*-acetylneuramic acid is used by sialyl transferases, and UDP-*N*-acetyl galactosamine and UDP-*N*-acetylglucosamine are used by glycosyl transferases (Merrill and Sandhoff, 2002, pp. 390–3). UDP-*N*-acetyl glucosamine and UDP-*N*-acetyl galactosamine levels have been observed to increase sevenfold in human tumor cells grown in tissue culture (Shedd *et al.*, 1993), suggesting that under conditions of enhanced ganglioside synthesis, UDP-*N*-acetyl sugar levels can increase several fold. Ganglioside biosynthesis also involves *O*-acetylation of sialic acid and *N*-deacetylation of the 5-amino group of sialic acid. Synthesized gangliosides are incorporated into the outer leaflet of the plasma membrane, especially the synaptosomal membrane, by vesicle-mediated transport (Merrill and Sandhoff, 2002).

Glutamate is the most abundant amino acid in the brain (781–125 μmole/100 g; McIlwain and Bachelard, 1985, p. 155), and plays a major role as an excitatory neurotransmitter in the cerebral cortex (Erecinska and Silver, 1990), which is rich in glutamatergic neurons; all cortical efferents and cortico-cortical connections are glutamatergic. Synaptic-released glutamate is taken up by surrounding glia and converted into glutamine (215–560 μmole/100 g; McIlwain and Bachelard, 1985, p. 155) by glutamine synthase [EC 6.3.1.2]. The glutamine is then released by glia and taken up by the pre-synaptic neurons and converted into glutamate by mitochondrial glutaminase [EC 3.5.1.2]. This glutamate–glutamine cycle increases with brain activity and is coupled with glucose utilization and lactate production in glia. The in-vivo concentration of glutamate is much higher than glutamine, which suggests that the majority of the in-vivo ^{1}H MRS observable glutamate is metabolic glutamate and not synaptic glutamate. In addition, glutamate, glutamine, and GABA cannot be reliably quantified at field strengths below 4.0 T, and even at 4.0 T are more convincing quantified by 2D J-resolved, single-voxel MRS (Onger *et al.*, 2008).

Summary

The in-vivo ^{1}H MRS spectrum contains three major resonance regions. The trimethylamine region is composed primarily of the membrane phospholipid precursor PC and breakdown product GPC with much smaller contributions from choline, acetylcholine, carnitine, and acetyl-L-carnitine. PC and GPC cannot be reliably separated and quantified by in-vivo ^{1}H MRS even at 7.0 T. Therefore, this ^{1}H resonance region is confounded and in-vivo interpretation is controversial. The *N*-acetyl region is predominantly comprised of NAA, but there are likely contributions by other in-vivo *N*-acetyl containing molecules, such as *N*-acetyl sugars found in ganglioside metabolism, which need to be considered.

The in-vivo ^{1}H MRS region referred to as total creatine contains both the labile high-energy PCr and its breakdown product, creatine. PCr and Cr cannot be reliable separated and quantified even at 7.0 T, so the interpretation is highly confounded.

Finally, glutamate and glutamine are difficult to reliably quantify at field strengths below 4.0 T, and even at 4.0 T and higher are more convincingly quantified by 2D J-resolved MRS, which requires a single-voxel approach. In addition, a majority of the glutamate resonance comes from metabolic glutamate and not neurotransmitter glutamate.

^{31}P MRS findings in schizophrenia

Many neurochemical, neuropathological and functional imaging studies have implicated the frontotemporal neural networks in schizophrenia (for review, see McClure *et al.*, 1998; Weickert and Kleinman,

- ^{31}P MRS

  ^{31}P MRS provides quantitation of molecular species related to membrane phospholipid metabolism (sPME, sPDE) and high-energy phosphate metabolism (PCr, ATP, ADP, Pi). In addition, at 1.5 Tesla, membrane vesicles (synaptic, transport) and phosphorylated proteins and peptides can be quantified.

  A major source of ATP consumption in brain is the repolarization of depolarized synaptic membranes. Since PCr is a buffer for ATP, via the creatine kinase reaction, levels of PCr potentially provide a surrogate measure of synaptic activity.

- ^{1}H MRS

  N-Acetyl groups with short correlation times (sNA, predominantly N-acetylaspartate), total creatine (PCr + Cr combined), and trimethylamines (GPC + PC combined) are the predominant metabolites observable by in-vivo ^{1}H MRS. Since the creatine and trimethylamine resonances contain both precursors and products, informative metabolic information is lacking. Other minor resonances include glutamate, glutamine, myo-inositol, GABA, taurine, NAAG, lactate and aspartate.

  Under some circumstances, sialic acids and UDP-acetyl sugars could make observable contributions to the sNA resonance region.

  In-vivo concentration of glutamate is much higher than glutamine, suggesting that the majority of in-vivo observable glutamate is metabolic glutamate and not synaptic vesicle glutamate. Glutamate, glutamine and GABA cannot be reliably quantified by in-vivo ^{1}H MRS at fields below 4.0 Tesla and even at 4.0 Tesla are more convincingly quantified by 2D J-resolved, single-voxel techniques.

1998). Our 1991 PME and PDE results (Pettegrew et al., 1991) were interpreted as consistent with either neurodegeneration or exaggerated synaptic elimination with reduced utilization of βATP secondary to reduced frontal lobe activity. In one subject, these findings were present 2 years prior to the onset of illness (Keshavan et al., 1991). Since our 1991 paper, over 175 ^{31}P and ^{1}H MRS studies in schizophrenia have been conducted, and most of these studies continue to demonstrate alterations in indices of membrane phospholipid metabolism which is remarkable given the non-uniform MRS and clinical methodological procedures used. Findings related to high-energy phosphate levels have been more variable (for reviews see McClure et al., 1998; Keshavan et al., 2000; Fukuzako, 2001; Stanley, 2002). Table 3.1 provides a list of ^{31}P MRS findings and characteristics of the studies conducted after these reviews. Tables 3.2–3.4 summarize the results from these ^{31}P MRS studies.

Important factors contributing to inconsistent membrane phospholipid and high-energy phosphate results among schizophrenia studies are: (1) diverse patient cohorts with small sample size, i.e. medication-naive, first-episode vs. chronic schizophrenia cohorts; (2) different brain region(s) studied; (3) methodological issues, e.g. sensitivity, field strength, localization techniques, resolution of metabolites, and quantitation methods (Stanley et al., 2000).

The finding of reduced PME levels in the dorsolateral prefrontal cortex reported in our 1991 study (Pettegrew et al., 1991) has been replicated in most studies; however, increased PDE in the DPFC has not been consistently demonstrated in more recent studies. Examination of the reasons for this helps to illustrate the issues that need to be considered in ^{31}P MRS studies in schizophrenia. Medication-naive, first-episode cohorts provide the gold standard for MRS studies of the molecular underpinnings of schizophrenia. Chronic schizophrenia cohorts are much more diverse, with several confounds that may affect membrane phospholipid and high-energy phosphate metabolism such as cognitive status, length of illness, number of episodes, age, and type of antipsychotic medication. Clinical differences may account for some of the inconsistency, but methodological differences most likely account for the inconsistency of reported PDE levels in the prefrontal region. Our 1991 study was conducted at 1.5 T, localized to the DPFC, and quantitated by Lorentzian curve fitting. Smesny et al. (2007), however, report a reduction in PDE levels in the right prefrontal cortex. This is likely due to the contribution of both intermediate and short correlation time PDEs to the quantitation of PDE in the Pettegrew et al. (1991) paper. Smesny used a quantitation method that removed the "mobile phospholipid" (MP) resonance (similar to the iPDE). Potwarka et al. (1999) reported that the MP increased in the frontal cortex of schizophrenia patients, and that this also may artificially increase the PDE peak. The Potwarka et al. (1999) study was done at 1.5 T

Table 3.1 Phosphorus in-vivo MRS findings in schizophrenia

Study	Cohort	Brain region(s)	Method	Field (Tesla)	Metabolite changes SZ vs. control subjects
Pettegrew *et al.* (1991)	**11 FEAN SZ** (7M, 4F) Age 24.4 ± 1.8 yrs (SEM) **10 Controls** (6M, 4F) Age 24.1 ± 1.8 yrs (SEM)	DPFC	Surface coil localized single voxel, approximately 20 cm^3	1.5	Decreased PME; Increased PDE
Fukuzako *et al.* (1996)	**31 CH SZ** (22M, 9F) Age 31 yrs **31 Controls** (22M, 9F) Age 31 yrs	2 voxels averaged R and L TL	2D CSI 3×3×4 cm^3	2	Increased PDE in R and L TL; Decreased βATP in L TL
Fukuzako *et al.* (1999)	**17 FEAN SZ** (10M, 7F) Age 23.1 yrs **17 Controls** (10M, 7F) Age 22.5 yrs	2 voxels averaged R and L TL	2D CSI 3×3×4 cm^3	2	Decreased PME in TL; Increased PDE in TL
Potwarka *et al.* (1999)	**11 CH SZ** (10M, 1F) Age 45.7 ± 6.2 yrs **11 Controls** (10M, 1F) Age 45.0 ± 7.5 yrs	R and L PFC, MC, POC	2D CSI ^{1}H decoupled 27 cm^3	1.5	Increased MP in PFC; Decreased PC and PI in PFC
Klem *et al.* (2001)	**14 HR for SZ** (4M, 10F) Age 16.7 ± 1.9 yrs **14 Controls** Age 16.9 ± 2.6 yrs (4M, 10F)	R and L PFC	ISIS 2.8×2.8×5 cm^3	1.5	Increased PDE in PFC; Decreased PME/PDE
Jensen *et al.* (2002a)	**11 CH SZ** (11M) Age 42.2 ± 8.5 yrs 6 olazapine, 2 conventional, 1 clozapine, 1 Quelipine, 1 ziprasidone **11 Controls** (11M) Age 42.9 ± 7.4 yrs	R and L PFC, ACC, POC, PC, Thalamus, Hippocampus, Cerebellum	3D CSI 15 cm^3	4	GPE decreased in ACC, RPFC, L Thalamus; GPE increased in L Hippocampus and L Cerebellum PE; GPC decreased in RPFC; PC decreased in ACC
Riehemann *et al.* (2002)	**72 CH SZ** Divided into 3 groups for study of pH effects of medication **Study A: 51 CH SZ** (31M, 20F) Age = 34.9 ± 12 yrs 29 received haloperidol, 14 received atypical clozapine; 8 drug-free for at least 1 week **Study B: 8 CH SZ** (5M, 3F) Age = 35.8 ± 12.8 yrs 2 scans, first drug-free 7.5 days, second, 20.6 ± 11.1 days classical drug	R and L PFC	ISIS Studies A and B: 39.2 ± 0.6 cm^3	1.5	Clozapine lowered intracellular pH in the PFC

Table 3.1 (cont.)

Study	Cohort	Brain region(s)	Method	Field (Tesla)	Metabolite changes SZ vs. control subjects
	treatment; **Study C: 13 CH SZ** (6M, 7F) Age 42.2 ± 9.5 yrs. 3 MR scans, first drug-free at least 3 days; second after 2 weeks on classical haloperidol, third scan after 2 weeks on atypical olanzapine **32 Controls** (19M, 13F) Age 37.1 ± 11.5 yrs				
Yacubian *et al.* (2002)	**18 AN SZ** (9M, 9F) Age 29.4 ± 9.3 35 SZ drug-free for at least 2 weeks (21M, 14F) Age 32.1 ± 9.3 yrs **35 Controls** (15M, 20F) Age 29.8 ± 8.6 yrs	LPFC	ISIS 2.8×2.8×5 cm^3	1.5	PDE decreased in LPFC of AN SZ
Jayakumar *et al.* (2003)	**20 AN SZ** (15M, 5F) Age 27.0 ± 7.5 yrs **30 Controls** (21M, 9F) Age 29.4 ± 8.3 yrs	R and L BG	ISIS 2.5×2.5×5 cm^3	1.5	PME/PDE and PME/ total phosphorus increased in L and R BG
Keshavan *et al.* (2003)	**11 HR for SZ** (8M, 8F) Age 15.4 ± 2.1 yrs **37 Controls** (29M, 8F) Age 14.2 ± 2.7 yrs	L and R PFC	2D CSI 4.5×4.5×3.0 cm^3	1.5	sPME decreased in PFC; sPME/sPDE increased in PFC. These changes were more prominent in HR subjects with Axis I psychopathology.
Rzanny *et al.* (2003)	**18 HR for SZ** (8M, 10F) Age 16.0 ± 2.5 yrs **19 Controls** (8M, 10F) Age 16.8 ± 3.2 yrs	R and L DPFC	ISIS 2.8×2.8×5.0 cm^3	1.5	PDE increased PME/PDE decreased βNTP decreased
Jensen *et al.* (2004)	**15 FE SZ** (10 AN) (13M, 2F) Age 22.5 ± 3.4 yrs 4 taking atypical antipsychotics 1 taking a typical antipsychotic **15 Controls** (13M, 2F) Age 22.1 ±3.0 yrs	R&L PFC, ACC, POC, PC, Thalamus, Cerebellum	3D CSI 15 cm^3 ^{31}P metabolite levels corrected for voxel gray and white matter and CSF content	4.0	GPC, PC, βATP, Pi increased in ACC
Puri *et al.* (2004)	**15 Violent SZ** (15M) Age 37.1 ± 12.4 yrs **13 Controls** Age 37.0 ± 10.6 yrs	Cerebrum	ISIS 7×7×7 cm^3	1.5	βNTP increased in Cerebrum

Table 3.1 (cont.)

Study	Cohort	Brain region(s)	Method	Field (Tesla)	Metabolite changes SZ vs. control subjects
Shirayama et al. (2004)	11 CH SZ (11M) Age 28.6 ± 8.6 yrs 15 Controls (15M) Age 28.4 ± 8.1 yrs	PFC	ISIS 3.5×4.5×7.0 cm^3 (Prior knowledge curve fitting)	2.0	GPC decreased in PFC
Theberge et al. (2004b)	9 CH SZ (9M) Age 41 ± 7 yrs all taking typical antipsychotics 8 Controls (9M) Age 43 ± 9 yrs	L ACC L Thalamus	^{31}P 3D CSI ^{1}H STEAM (TE = 20 ms) ^{31}P metabolite levels corrected for voxel CSF content	4.0	Correlated ^{1}H metabolites with ^{31}P metabolites PE vs. Gln positive correlation in L ACC; GPC vs. NAA negative correlation in L Thalamus.
Gangadhar et al. (2006)	19 AN SZ (11 had developmental reflexes) (15M, 4F) Age 27.4 ± 7.4 yrs 26 Controls (18M, 8F) Age 30.1 ± 8.7 yrs	R and L BG	ISIS 2DCSI 2.5×2.5×5.0 cm^3	1.5	PCr/total ATP ratio in the BG was lowest in those patients who had developmental reflexes.
Jayakumar et al. (2006)	12 AN SZ (10M, 2F) Age 28.7 ± 8.8 yrs 13 Controls (6M, 7F) Age 29.6 ± 9.4 yrs	R and L Caudate	ISIS 2D CSI 2.5×2.5×5.0 cm^3	1.5	L Caudate reduced PCr; L and R Caudate reduced volume. L Caudate PCr vs. L Caudate volume negative correlation.
Jensen et al. (2006)	12 FE SZ (11M, 1F) Age 23.2 ± 3.6 yrs 11 Controls (9M, 2F) Age 22.2 ± 3.4 yrs	Frontal Lobe (averaged voxels) Fronto-temporal-striatal (averaged voxels)	3D CSI 5.4 cm^3 ^{31}P metabolite levels corrected for voxel gray and white matter and CSF content	4.0	In fronto-temporal-striatal region βATP increased in white matter and decreased in gray matter. No differences were found in frontal-lobes.
Smesny et al. (2007)	12 FEAN SZ (7M, 5F) Age 32.2 ± 9.7 yrs 19 SZ (8M, 11F) Age 40.2 ± 11.5 yrs Off antipsychotic medication for at least 2 weeks (32.5 ± 59 days) Treatment before wash out Olanzapine (n = 7), Risperidone (n = 5), Haloperidol (n = 7) 31 Controls (15M, 16F) Age 37.2 ± 11.3 yrs	R and L PFC medial temporal (including hippocampus) caudate nucleus, thalamus, ACC	2D CSI 21 cm^3	1.5	PME, PDE, PCr and Pi reduced in R and L PFC; factor analysis of changes showed a characteristic spatial pattern of changes. No significant medication × voxel interactions found between ANFE SZ and AN SZ groups.

Table 3.1 (cont.)

Study	Cohort	Brain region(s)	Method	Field (Tesla)	Metabolite changes SZ vs. control subjects
Puri et al. (2008)	15 Violent SZ (15M) 12 Controls (9M) Medication (not reported)	Cerebrum	ISIS $7\times7\times7$ cm^3 MP removed in quantitation method	1.5	βATP reduced in Cerebrum No change in PME, PDE, MP

Abbreviations. ACC, anterior cingulate cortex; AN, antipsychotic naive; BG, basal ganglia; 2DCSI, 2-dimensional chemical shift imaging, FE, first episode; ISIS, image-selected in-vivo spectroscopy; L, left; MP, mobile phospholipid; MO, motor cortex; PC, posterior cingulate; POC, parieto-occipital; R, right; SEM, standard error of the mean; SZ, schizophrenia subjects; TE, time of echo; TL, temporal lobe.

Table 3.2 Phosphorus MRS phospholipid and high-energy metabolite findings of studies from Table 3.1. Studies that did not compare schizophrenia subjects to control subjects were not included in this table. Violent schizophrenia subjects were considered a separate subgroup and were not included in this table. Findings reported as ratios to other metabolites are not included

Metabolites	First episode and/or antipsychotic naive Number of studies Increased	Decreased	Partial volume correction	First episode Number of studies Increased	Decreased	Partial volume correction	Chronic Number of studies Increased	Decreased	Partial volume correction
Phospholipid
PME	1	3	4N		1	1Y		2	1N, 1Y
PDE	2	2	4N		1	1Y	2	2	3N, 1Y
iPDE							1		1N
High-Energy
βATP				1		1Y		1	1N
PCr		2	1Y, 1N	1	1	2Y			
Pi		1	1N		1	1Y		1	1N

Table 3.3 Summary of phosphorus MRS phospholipid metabolite findings

10 Studies	3 FEAN 2 AN 1 FE 4 CH	2 with partial volume correction	5 decreased PME, 2 increased PME
		8 no partial volume correction	4 decreased PDE, 5 increased PDE 1 increased iPDE

Table 3.4 Summary of phosphorus MRS high-energy metabolite findings

6 Studies	1 FEAN 1 AN 2 FE 2 CH	3 with partial volume correction	1 decreased βATP, 1 increased βATP
		3 no partial volume correction	3 decreased PCr, 1 increased PCr 2 decreased Pi, 1 increased Pi

61

with a [1]H-decoupled ^{31}P chemical shift method providing resolution of the PME (PE and PC) and PDE (GPE and GPC) resonances. Note that [1]H-decoupled ^{31}P spectra would greatly enhance (82%) the GPE contribution to the PDE resonance. Although resolution of the PME and PDE resonances is desirable, studies at higher field strength provide partial resolution of these peaks. Studies at 1.5 T by Volz et al. (2000) and Smesny et al. (2007) report a decrease in PDE after removal of the MP component. Studies at higher field strength (3.0 or 4.0 T) have greatly reduced MP contributions to the ^{31}P spectrum due to chemical shift anisotropy effects. Studies of schizophrenia subjects at higher field report no change in PDE (Jensen et al., 2006) in the frontal brain region. In summary, the reported increase in prefrontal PDE (Pettegrew et al., 1991) could have been due to an increase in iPDE and not sPDE. The Smesny et al. (2007) ^{31}P MRS study is an example of chemical shift imaging which simultaneously samples multiple brain regions providing data on molecular changes throughout regions of interest. The echo-planar spectroscopic imaging (EPSI) protocol (Ulrich et al., 2007) is another technological advance which improves the acquisition of ^{31}P MRS data.

Evidence for altered membrane phospholipid metabolism in subjects at high risk for schizophrenia and antedating first break episodes has been obtained by Keshavan et al. (2003) and Rzanny et al. (2003). Both studies report a reduction in the ratio sPME/sPDE for high-risk subjects versus controls, although compared to controls Keshavan et al. (2003) reported significantly reduced sPME but not sPDE, whereas Rzanny et al. (2003) reported a significant increase in sPDE, but no significant reduction in sPME. Keshavan et al. (2003) reported increased iPDE levels in the high-risk subjects whereas Rzanny et al. (2003) reported decreased broad component values in the high-risk subjects. However, the quantification methods were different for the two studies, and therefore the results are not entirely compatible.

Puri and colleagues have examined forensic schizophrenia cohorts by ^{31}P MRS (Puri et al., 2004, 2008). Puri et al. (2008) examined a $7 \times 7 \times 7$ cm^3 central voxel with ^{31}P ISIS, quantified by AMARES/ MRUI software (prior knowledge with the first 1.92 ms removed to analyze only short correlation metabolites) then modeled in time domain. The short correlation components were subtracted from the original spectrum to give a "broad component", whose area is fitted by Gaussian function and compared to the total short correlation metabolites and reported as a percentage. No change was observed for the "broad component" of forensic schizophrenia patients 57.9% (SEM 5.6) vs. controls 57.7% (SEM 6.0). (Note, the same quantitation method was not used for short correlation time metabolites or intermediate correlation time metabolites.) Puri and coworkers (2008) did not find support for membrane alterations in forensic schizophrenia patients. However, the clinical samples in the Puri studies are quite different from those reported in FEAN and chronic schizophrenia studies.

Shirayama et al. (2004) reported increased GPC in schizophrenia males ($n=11$) with no change in high-energy metabolites. The study was done at 2.0 T and quantitated by curve-fitting with prior knowledge.

Yacubian et al. (2002) reported reduced PDE in drug-naive schizophrenia subjects ($n=18$) compared to controls ($n=35$) and medicated schizophrenia subjects ($n=35$). Voxel size was $2.8 \times 2.8 \times 5$ cm^3 at 1.5 T quantitated by a convolution difference procedure with baseline correction. This quantitation method includes a baseline roll, which is removed by operator interaction.

^{1}H MRS findings

Most of the in-vivo ^{1}H MRS findings in schizophrenia focus on changes in NAA, the largest resonance in ^{1}H MRS spectra. As mentioned above, the NAA resonance contains N-acetyl moieties in addition to NAA, such as NAAG and N-acetyl sugars. Two other prominent resonances are the trimethylamine resonance (PC, GPC, a small amount of choline, acetylcholine, L-carnitine, and acetyl-L-carnitine), often labeled Cho, and total creatine resonance (PCr + creatine); however, ^{31}P MRS is best-suited for obtaining quantitative results of PC, GPC, and PCr metabolites. ^{1}H MRS acquisition with long (272 ms) echo times (TE) simplify the spectra to these three resonances. ^{1}H MRS acquisition using short TE (20 ms) produces resonances for additional metabolites, i.e. glutamate, glutamine, and myo-inositol (MI). Acquisition at higher field (4.0 T) is needed to separately quantify the complex resonances of glutamate and glutamine, even with prior knowledge quantification methods, such as the commercially available

LC Model. Most of the ^{1}H MRS studies reported in the literature focus on one or two localized regions of the brain; however, with advances in acquisition methods such as magnetic resonance spectroscopic imaging (MRSI), multiple regions can be acquired in times comparable to single voxel experiments. Examining multiple regions in the same cohort should help clarify the regional relationship of metabolite changes found in single-voxel studies. Longitudinal studies are needed to examine heterochronous regional changes in subjects at various stages of the disease. Reviews of methodological advances in ^{1}H MRS by Stanley *et al.* (2000) and Dager *et al.* (2008) provide a more detailed discussion of technical issues such as increasing signal-to-noise ratio, resolution of resonances, lipid suppression, and uniform magnetic field.

Reviews of ^{1}H MRS findings in schizophrenia provide a starting point for our review of selected literature reports of ^{1}H MRS findings in schizophrenia (Keshavan *et al.*, 2000; Steen *et al.*, 2005; Abbott and Bustillo, 2006; Dager *et al.*, 2008). Table 3.5 lists ^{1}H MRS findings and characteristics of the studies conducted after these reviews. Tables 3.6 and 3.7 summarize the results from these ^{1}H MRS studies. Steen *et al.* (2005) report a meta-analysis of 64 ^{1}H MRS studies and focus on NAA levels. The meta-analysis found a robust reduction of NAA levels in gray and white matter in frontal lobes in both first-episode and chronic schizophrenia subjects compared to controls. A robust reduction in hippocampal NAA was also found. Structural MRI studies reveal volumetric reductions in these areas (Shenton *et al.*, 2001). Abbott and Bustillo (2006) reviewed proton studies of schizophrenia between June 2004 and September 2005 and concluded that abnormalities in Glu and Gln findings were consistent with the glutamatergic excitotoxic process. Progress has been made in regard to improving Glu and Gln quantitation at 4.0 T (Onger *et al.*, 2008); however, separation of Glu and Gln resonances, the origin of the Glu and Gln resonance (i.e. metabolic pool versus synaptic glutamate recycling), and possible medication effects remain problematic in interpreting these results in the context of glutamatergic dysfunction in schizophrenia. Paz *et al.* (2008) review the literature supporting a glutamatergic-centered hypothesis of pathophysiological events in schizophrenia, and in particular evidence of the neurodevelopmental timing of cognitive abilities in the PFC involving dopamine–glutamate interactions that do not mature until post-puberty. Neurodevelopmental timing of synaptic elimination and membrane repair are best obtained by ^{31}P MRSI as discussed above, and recently demonstrated in control subjects 6–18 years old (Goldstein *et al.*, 2009).

Stanley *et al.* (2007) explored the reduction of NAA in the DLPFC of first-episode, antipsychotic-naive (FEAN) schizophrenia subjects compared to healthy controls. The FEAN were divided by age into early onset ($n=8$, 17.5 ± 2.1 years) and adult onset ($n=10$, 28.0 ± 4.6 years) groups. Early-onset FEAN demonstrated a 13% reduction in NAA compared to age-matched healthy controls; adult-onset did not show significant reduction in NAA in the left DLPFC. Symptom severity was not different in the early-onset versus adult-onset FEAN subjects.

^{1}H MRS findings reported after the reviews mentioned above include the following studies. No changes in Glu/Gln were found in the anterior cingulate and parieto-occipital cortex ($2 \times 2 \times 2$ cm^3 nominal voxel at 4.0 T) of chronic schizophrenia subjects compared with controls (Onger *et al.*, 2008). No changes in short TE ^{1}H MRS metabolites were seen in the right and left medial temporal cortex (largely consisting of the anterior hippocampus) ($2 \times 2 \times 2$ cm^3 nominal voxel at 3.0 T) in treatment-naive and chronic schizophrenia subjects compared to controls; however, *myo*-inositol levels correlated with cumulative antipsychotic dose in a subgroup of the treated subjects (Woods *et al.*, 2008). A study of the DLPFC in first-episode and chronic schizophrenia subjects demonstrated a correlation of NAA levels of the left DLPFC (3.375 cm^3 voxel size, 1.5 T) with verbal learning and memory (Ohrmann *et al.*, 2007). Adult siblings of schizophrenia subjects free of psychopathology indicated elevated MRS glutamate levels in the medial frontal lobes ($2.5 \times 2.5 \times 2.5$ cm^3 nominal voxel, 3.0 T), and stratification by glutamate levels in the sibling group indicated a difference between the high- and low-glutamate subjects in performance on the Continuous Performance Test (CPT) (Purdon *et al.*, 2008). Tang *et al.* (2007) have reported correlations of NAA levels and diffusion tensor imaging (DTI) anisotropic indices of chronic schizophrenia subjects compared with controls in the left medial temporal region white matter (CSI data nominal voxel $1.0 \times 0.9 \times 0.9$ cm^3 at 3.0 T, three slices were obtained to cover DLPFC and occipital white matter tracts in addition to the medial temporal region). A short TE

Table 3.5 Proton in-vivo MRS findings in schizophrenia

Study	Cohort	Brain region(s)	Method	Field (Tesla)	Metabolite changes SZ vs. Control subjects
Delamillieure et al. (2004)	**5 with deficit SZ** **17 without deficit SZ** **21 Controls**	R and L Medial PFC	STEAM TE = 30 ms 8.0 cm^3	1.5	Positive correlation between R MPFC NAA/Cr and Stroop tests performance in deficit SZ
O'Neill et al. (2004)	**11 child and adolescent SZ** (7M, 4F) Age 12.3 ± 3.8 yrs (7–18 yrs) **20 Controls** (10M, 10F) Ages 11.7 ± 2.9 yrs (6.8–16.3 yrs)	Mean of R and L PFC; ACC; Thalamus; Striatum	3DMRSI TE = 272 ms nominal voxel 1.2 cm^3 ^{1}H metabolite levels corrected for voxel gray and white matter and CSF content	1.5	PCr + Cr higher in ACC PC + GPC + Choline higher in ACC, PFC, and caudate head
Theberge et al. (2004a)	**19 FEAN SZ** (14M, 5F) Age 25 ± 8 yrs	L ACC and L Thalamus	STEAM TE = 20 ms nominal voxel 1.5 cm^3 ^{1}H metabolite levels corrected for voxel gray and white matter and CSF content	4.0	Effect of duration of untreated illness, duration of prodromal symptoms, and duration of untreated psychosis. PC + GPC + Choline positively correlated with DUP in L ACC and L Thalamus
Tibbo et al. (2004)	**20 HR for SZ** (7M, 13F) Age 16.4 ± 2.0 yrs **22 Controls** (9M, 13F) Age 16.7 ± 1.7 yrs	R medial PFC	STEAM TE = 20 ms 2.5 cm^3	3.0	Glu + Gln/PCr+Cr decreased in R medial PFC
Ende et al. (2005)	**14 SZ** (12M, 2F) Age 38.9 ± 7.3 yrs **14 Controls** (8M, 6F) Age 35.6 ± 3.7 yrs	Cerebellum, Pons, Dentate Nucleus	PRESS TE = 135 ms 2.1×2.1×1.5 cm^3	1.5	NAA significantly lower in cerebellar cortex and cerebellar vermis. Showed no difference in gray and white matter and CSF content in SZ vs. controls.
Jakary et al. (2005)	**22 SZ** (22M) Age 34.5 ± 9.4 yrs 36% on typical and 64% on atypical antipsychotics **22 Controls** (22M) Age 36.4 ± 11.3 yrs	L and R Thalamus (mediodorsal, anterior)	3D MRSI TE = 135 ms 0.8×0.8×1.5 cm^3 0.9 cm^3 ^{1}H metabolite levels corrected for voxel gray and white matter and CSF content	1.5	Decreased NAA in mediodorsal and anterior thalamus

Table 3.5 (cont.)

Study	Cohort	Brain region(s)	Method	Field (Tesla)	Metabolite changes SZ vs. Control subjects
Miyaoka et al. (2005)	15 with GS (+) SZ (7M, 9F) Age 32.5 ± 10.7 yrs 70.5% on atypical antipsychotics 15 without GS (–) SZ (8M, 7F) Age 34.0 ± 11.0 yrs 69.3% on atypical antipsychotics 15 Controls (8M, 7F) Age 41.7 ± 14.7 yrs	L hippocamus L BG, vermis of cerebellum	PRESS TE = 30 ms 8 cm^3	1.5	GS(+) vs. GS(–) SZ: NAA/Cr and MI/Cr reduced in hippocampus, and MI/Cr reduced in LBG; GS(+) SZ vs. controls: NAA/Cr and MI/Cr reduced in hippocampus and LBG; GS (+) vs. controls: MI/Cr reduced in vermis of cerebellum; GS (–) vs. control: NAA/Cr reduced in hippocampus
Ohrmann et al. (2005)	18 FEAN SZ (13M, 6F) Age 29.3 ± 11.2 yrs 21 CH SZ (15M, 6F) Age 29.7 ± 7.4 yrs 95% on atypical antipsychotics 21 Controls (13M, 8F) Age 28.0 ± 6.8 yrs	DLPFC	Fast spin echo single voxel	1.5	In DLPFC, CH SZ vs. Controls and CH SZ vs. FE SZ: NAA, Glx, and Cr reduced; FE SZ vs. Controls: reduced Cr and Cho
Rowland et al. (2005)	10 Controls (10M) Age 24.7 ± 3.4 yrs 3 MR scans (before, while loading, and with maintenance dose of ketamine or placebo)	R and L ACC	STEAM TE = 20 ms 8 cm^3	4.0	Gln increased from ketamine infusion in Controls
Szulc et al. (2005)	14 CH SZ (10M, 4F) Age 32.0 ± 7.2 yrs MR scans after 7 day washout and after 4 weeks of risperidone	Frontal lobe, TL, Thalamus	Single-voxel PRESS TE = 35 ms 8 cm^3	1.5	Risperidone treatment increased NAA and MI in the Thalamus; Risperidone treatment improved PANSS scores Positive correlation of NAA levels with positive PANSS scale before treatment in the frontal lobe and negatively in the temporal lobe. Positive correlation of Glx/Cr with negative PANSS scale in the temporal lobe

Table 3.5 (cont.)

Study	Cohort	Brain region(s)	Method	Field (Tesla)	Metabolite changes SZ vs. Control subjects
Terpstra et al. (2005)	**13 CH SZ** (8M, 5F) Age 26 ± 5 yrs **9 Controls** (4M, 5F) Age 25 ± 5 yrs	ACC	STEAM TE = 5 ms 8 cm^3 and 17 cm^3	4.0	No significant GSH differences
Van Elst et al. (2005)	**21 CH SZ** (13M, 8F) Age 28.5 ± 1.4 yrs All on atypical antipsychotics **32 Controls** (23M, 10F) Age 28.2 ± 1.0 yrs	L DLPFC L Hippocampus	PRESS TE = 30 ms 2×2×2 cm^3	2.0	Increased Glu and Gln in L DLPFC, increased Glu in L Hippocampus
Marenco et al. (2006)	**54 healthy individuals** genotyped at SNP rs6465084k	R and L DLPFC, Cingulate, CS, hippocampus, OC	2D MRSI Spinecho TE = 280 ms 0.75×0.75×0.75 cm^3	3.0	Decreased NAA/Cr in R DLPFC in subjects with SNP rs6465084
Tanaka et al. (2006)	**14 CH SZ** (10M, 4F) Age 29.4 ± 4.1 yrs approximately 70% on atypical antipsychotics **13 Controls** (10M, 3F) Age 29.5 ± 4.1 yrs	L frontal lobe	PRESS TE = 30 ms 1.5×1.5×1.5 cm^3	1.5	Decreased NAA In L frontal lobe; NAA negative correlation with WCST perseveration errors
Wood et al. (2006)	**46 FE SZ** (29M, 15F) Age 21.6±3.2 yrs all treated with atypical antipsychotics at time of scan Entry MR examination, subjects then followed longitudinally with clinical tests, antipsychotic medication given at the time of the MR examination	L DLPFC L MTL	PRESS TE = 135 ms 1.5×1.5×1.5 cm^3	1.5	NAA/Cr in L DLPFC correlated positively with Global Assessment of Functioning score; This suggests L DLPFC NAA/Cr is a predictor of poor outcome.
Aydin et al. (2007)	**12 FE SZ** (8M, 4F) Age 25.5 ± 5.8 yrs 83% given atypical antipsychotics before MR scan shortly after hospitalization, 2 subjects AN **14 Controls** (9M, 5F) Age 25.2 ± 5.4 yrs **16 CH SZ** (11M, 5F) Age 29.3 ± 11.4 yrs Most were on atypical antipsychotics **14 Controls** (9M, 5F) Age 28.9 ± 10.2 yrs	Corpus Callosum	STEAM	1.5	NAA reduced in FE SZ, CH SZ, and combined SZ; NAA negatively correlated with BPRS and SAPS in combined SZ; FE SZ did not show correlations of NAA with BPRS or SAPS

Table 3.5 (cont.)

Study	Cohort	Brain region(s)	Method	Field (Tesla)	Metabolite changes SZ vs. Control subjects
Chang et al. (2007)	**23 CH SZ** Age 66.3 ± 7.2 yrs **22 Controls** 70.0 ±5.3 yrs	R and L frontal white matter, OC white matter, temporal white matter	Double spin echo sequence TE = 30 ms	4.0	SZ had increased Cho [probably GPC] in R temporal white matter; decreased NAA in all white matter regions measured; decreased Cr in R frontal; increased Glx in R frontal, L temporal, and occipital; decreased mI in L frontal, R frontal, and R temporal
Molina et al. (2007)	**11 CH SZ** (11M) Age 36.7 ± 5.8 yrs 82% on atypical antipsychotics 13 Type I Bipolar Age 37.8 ± 6.7 yrs **10 Controls** Age 27.2 ± 4.9 yrs	R and L DLPFC	PRESS TE = 136 ms 3.0×1.5×1.5× cm^3	1.5	NAA decreased in DLPFC of both CH SZ and Type I Bipolar; more marked in SZ than in Type I Bipolar
Ohrmann et al. (2007)	**15 FEAN SZ** (10M, 5F) Age 27.0 ± 6.9 yrs **20 CH SZ** (14M, 6F) Age 30.3 ± 7.3 yrs 95% on atypical antipsychotics **20 Controls** (13M, 7F) Age 28.1 ± 6.5 yrs	L DLPFC	STEAM TE = 20 ms 3.375 cm^3	1.5	In L DLPFC NAA reduced in CH SZ patients compared with controls, NAA reduced in CH SZ compared with FEAN SZ; Cr and Glx reduced in CH SZ compared to controls and to FEAN SZ. CR reduced in FEAN SZ compared with controls. Cho reduced in CH SZ compared to controls. Medication had no significant impact on metabolite levels in CH SZ
Rothermundt et al. (2007)	**6 CH SZ** (high S100B, 6M) Age 23.8 ± 4,4 yrs **6 CH SZ**	L amygdala/ anterior hippocampus	STEAM TE = 20 ms 33.75 mm^3 ^{1}H metabolite levels	1.5	Serum S100B concentration, assay of astroglial activation and MRS

67

Table 3.5 (cont.)

Study	Cohort	Brain region(s)	Method	Field (Tesla)	Metabolite changes SZ vs. Control subjects
	(low S100B, 5M, 1F) Age 26.8 ± 4.9 yrs **12 Controls**		corrected for voxel gray and white matter and CSF content		ml concentration were compared. Those SZ with increased S100B had increased MI.
Shimizu et al. (2007)	**19 CH SZ** (11M, 8F) Age 40.4 ±13.1 yrs 84% on atypical antipsychotics **18 Controls** (12M, 6F) Age 34.9 ± yrs	PCG, L and R MTL	PRESS TE = 144 ms 15×15×15 mm^3	1.5	Reduced NAA/Cr ratio in PCG; Controls showed negative correlation of NAA/Cr vs. age, SZ subjects did not
Stanley et al. (2007)	**15 FEAN SZ** **3 Schizoaffective** (8 early-onset (5M, 3F) Age 17.5 ± 2.1 yrs **27 younger Controls** (18M, 9F) Age 18.3 ± 3.0 yrs **10 adult-onset** (8M, 2F) Age 28.0 ± yrs) **34 older Controls** (21M, 13F) Age 28.5 ± 4.9 yrs	L DLPFC	STEAM TE = 20 ms 20×20×20 mm^3 ^{1}H metabolite levels corrected for voxel gray and white matter and CSF content	1.5	In L DLPFC of FEAN SZ, NAA decreased; NAA and GPC + PC positively correlated with age in FEAN SZ; NAA decreased in L DLPFC of early-onset FEAN SZ compared with age matched controls whereas NAA levels in adult-onset FEAN SZ compared with age-matched controls were not significantly different
Tang et al. (2007)	**40 CH SZ** Age 38.7 ± 11.4 yrs 76% on atypical antipsychotics **42 Controls** Age 43.3 ± 20.2 yrs	L and R DLPFC and OCC white matter, MTL white matter ROI included 1–3 voxels averaged	PRESS 2DCSI TE = 30 ms 10×5×5 mm^3 (MTL and OCC white matter); 10×9×9 mm^3 (DLPFC white matter)	3.0	Reduced NAA in L and R MTL white matter; NAA and DTI-anisotropy indices correlated in L MTL white matter
Theberge et al. (2007)	**16 FEAN SZ** (14M, 2F) Age 25 ± 8 yrs **16 Controls** longitudinal study, SZ MR examinations before and after 10 months and 30 months of atypical antipsychotic treatment; Controls MR examinations at	L ACC; L Thalamus, parietal, temporal	STEAM TE = 20 ms 10×10×15 mm^3	4.0	GLN levels higher in L ACC and L Thalamus in FEAN SZ; L Thalamic levels of Gln significantly reduced after 30 months; in SZ, limited gray-matter reductions seen at 10 months; widespread gray-matter loss at 30 months; Parietal

Table 3.5 (cont.)

Study	Cohort	Brain region(s)	Method	Field (Tesla)	Metabolite changes SZ vs. Control subjects
	baseline and 30 months				and temporal lobe gray matter loss at 30 months
Wood et al. (2007)	**15 CH SZ** (15M) Age 31.8 ± 7.5 13 on atypical antipsychotics, 2 antipsychotic-free **14 Controls** (15M) Age 33.5 ± 8.5	R and L Dorsal and Rostral ACC	PRESS TE = 30 ms 6.5 cm^3	3.0	CH SZ decreased NAA in both R and L Dorsal and Rostral ACC
Ongur et al. (2008)	**17 SZ** (10M, 7F) Age 41.8 ± 9.8 yrs **15 Bipolar** (7M, 8F) Age 36.3 ± 11.6 **21 Controls** (11M, 10F)	ACC, POC	PRESS modified for 2D J-resolved ^{1}H MRS; TE = 30–500 ms 10 ms increments; 20×20×20 mm^3	4.0	Gln/Glu significantly higher in ACC and POC in BP, but not SZ compared with controls; NAA in ACC significantly lower in SZ compared with controls. Percent gray matter positively correlated with MRS measures
Bustillo et al. (2008)	**32 SZ** (26M, 6F) Age 24.7 ± 6.9 yrs 15 were antipsychotic-free at baseline, 17 received minimal treatment **21 Controls** (18M, 3F) Age 24.7 ± 5.3 yrs Longitudinal, SZ scanned every 6 months up to 2 years, 16 SZ on haloperidol 16 SZ on quetiapine	L Caudate; L PFC L OC R Cerebellum	PRESS TE = 40 ms 12.6 cm^3 except L Caudate 6 cm^3 ^{1}H metabolite levels corrected for voxel gray and white matter and CSF content	1.5	No change in slope for NAA vs. study timepoint for haloperidol vs quetiapine
Purdon et al. (2008)	**15 HR for SZ** (siblings) (2M, 13F) Age 46.3 ± 6.1 yrs **14 Controls** (3M, 11F) Age 43.5 ± 6.8 yrs	Medial frontal cortex	STEAM TE = 20 ms R and L	3.0	HR group showed higher variability in Glu. HR and Controls were grouped by high and low Glu levels. More HR subjects were in the high Glu group. CPT test scores were lower for high Glu HR subjects
Scherk et al. (2008)	**9 FE SZ** **19 euthymic bipolar 1 disorder**	L Hippocampus	Spin echo TE = 30 ms 10×10×35 mm^3	1.5	Participants grouped by SNP genotype of SNAP-25 gene (an

69

Table 3.5 (cont.)

Study	Cohort	Brain region(s)	Method	Field (Tesla)	Metabolite changes SZ vs. Control subjects
	10 OCD 17 Controls				integral part of the vesicle docking and fusion machinery that controls neurotransmitter release). SNAP-25 protein in hippocampus of SZ and BD found to be reduced at autopsy; NAA/Cho reduced for CC vs. TT SNPs
Wood *et al.* (2008)	**15 FEAN SZ** (12M, 3F) Age 20.0 ± 4.0 **19 FE SZ** (12M, 7F) Age 19.5 ± 4.0 treated with atypical antipsychotics **19 Controls** (12M, 3F)	R and L Anterior Hippocampus	PRESS TE = 30 ms 20×20×20 mm^3 ^{1}H metabolite levels corrected for voxel gray and white matter and CSF content	3.0	No metabolite changes due to treatment status. Also, none found in 7 participants that were followed longitudinally (scanned at 12 weeks)
Ongur *et al.* (2009)	**15 CH SZ** (8M, 7F) Age 42.9 ± 9.8 yrs **15 bipolar manic** (7M, 8F) Age 36.3 ± 11.6 yrs **22 Controls** (12M, 10 F) Age 34.9 ± 10.0 yrs	ACC and POC	PRESS modified for 2D J-resolved ^{1}H MRS; TE = 30–500 ms in 10 ms increments; 20×20×20 mm^3	4.0	Cr [PCr + Cr] levels reduced in SZ ACC and POC

Abbreviations: ACC, anterior cingulate cortex; AN, antipsychotic naive; CPT, Continuous Performance Test; DLPFC, dorsolateral prefrontal cortex; DUP, duration of untreated psychosis; DUI, duration of untreated illness; DPS, duration of prodromal symptoms; FE, first episode; GS, Gilbert's syndrome; HR, high risk; MPFC, medial prefrontal cortex; MTL, medial temporal lobe; OC, occipital cortex; OCD, obsessive–compulsive disorder; PCG, posterior cingulate gyrus; POC, parieto-occipital cortex; PRESS, point-resolved spectroscopy; SNP, single nucleotide polymorphisms; STEAM, simulated acquisition mode; SZ, schizophrenia; TE, time of echo.

Table 3.6 Proton MRS metabolite findings of studies from Table 3.5. Studies reporting findings as ratios of NAA to total creatine were not included. Findings limited to total creatine, or choline were not included

	First episode antipsychotic naive			First episode			Chronic		
	Number of studies		Partial volume correction	Number of studies		Partial volume correction	Number of studies		Partial volume correction
Metabolite	Increased	Decreased		Increased	Decreased		Increased	Decreased	
NAA		1	1Y		1	1N		9	7N, 2Y
Glu							1		1N
Gln	1		1Y				1		1N
Glu + Gln							1	1	1N, 1Y

Table 3.7 Summary of proton MRS metabolite findings

13 Studies	2 FEAN	5 with partial volume correction	12 decreased NAA
	2 mixed FEAN and Chronic	8 with no partial volume correction	1 increased Glu
			2 increased Gln
	1 mixed FE and Chronic		1 increased, 1 decreased
	8 Chronic		Glu + Gln

^{1}H MRS study (Aydin *et al.*, 2007) of the corpus callosum, a major inter-hemispheric white matter tract, in first-episode and chronic schizophrenia subjects compared with controls showed reduction in NAA in the corpus callosum of first-episode and chronic schizophrenia subjects combined. NAA levels in the corpus callosum of first-episode and chronic schizophrenia subjects combined correlated with severity of psychotic symptoms.

A longitudinal study ($1.0 \times 1.0 \times 1.5$ cm^3 at 4.0 T) of the anterior cingulate and thalamus region in first-episode schizophrenia subjects compared with controls was conducted at 10 months and 34 months after the first examination (Theberge *et al.*, 2007). Anterior cingulate and thalamic glutamine levels were higher in the schizophrenia cohort compared with controls at baseline. Thalamic glutamine levels were reduced at 30 months. Widespread gray-matter loss was seen at 30 months. A longitudinal single voxel (nominal 6 cm^3 at 1.5 T, 4 regions, left caudate, frontal and occipital lobes, and right cerebellum) ^{1}H MRS study (Bustillo *et al.*, 2008) of minimally treated schizophrenia patients examined at 6-month intervals up to 2 years showed no significant changes in NAA levels due to antipsychotic medication.

Future recommendations

1. All future studies should include quantitative neuromorphometric data so the quantitative neuromolecular data can be corrected for partial volume effects. There is little benefit in obtaining neuromolecular data that are confounded by structural changes such as atrophy.
2. All future studies should have well-defined clinical populations using validated, standardized diagnostic, clinical, and neuropsychological instruments (such as the NIMH consensus panel developed MATRICS).

Box 3.3. Selective review of ^{31}P and ^{1}H MRS studies in schizophrenia

- ^{31}P MRS studies in schizophrenia
  sPME and sPDE findings have been fairly consistent in schizophrenia subjects and are more likely related to disease trait. sPME and sPDE levels reflect alterations in membrane phospholipid metabolism which could alter the neurodevelopmentally controlled program of synaptic development and elimination.
  PCr findings are more variable in schizophrenia subjects, i.e. are probably more state-dependent, and probably reflect synaptic numbers and/or synaptic activity.
- ^{1}H MRS studies in schizophrenia
  Reduction in brain levels of NAA or NA-containing molecules appear to be the most robust of the ^{1}H MRS findings in schizophrenia.
  However, the reduced levels of NAA (or NA-containing molecules) coincide with loss of gray matter volume in the same areas and therefore could merely reflect brain atrophy.

3. The possibility to measure synaptic activity by PCr levels, estimate the number of synaptic and transport vesicles, and phosphorylated proteins and peptides by ^{31}P MRSI needs to be pursued in future studies.
4. Given the greatly increased cost and technical issues associated with higher magnetic fields, there needs to be compelling scientific and clinical justification for studies at field strengths above 3.0 T. If the information content obtained/cost is too small, the technology will not likely be widely available and therefore will have limited impact on the field of schizophrenia.

References

Abbott C and Bustillo J. 2006. What have we learned from proton magnetic resonance spectroscopy about schizophrenia? A critical update. *Curr Opin Psychiatry* **19**, 135–9.

Aydin K, Ucok A and Cakir S. 2007. Quantitative proton MR spectroscopy findings in the corpus callosum of patients with schizophrenia suggest callosal disconnection. *Am J Neuroradiol* **28**, 1968–74.

Barany M and Glonek T. 1984. Identification of diseased states by phosphorus-31 NMR. In Gorenstein D G (Ed.) *Phosphorus-31 NMR, Principles and Applications.* New York, NY: Academic Press, pp. 511–5.

Baslow M H. 2003. *N*-acetylaspartate in the vertebrate brain: metabolism and function. *Neurochem Res* **28**, 941–53.

Bhakoo K K, Craig T J and Styles P. 2001. Developmental and regional distribution of aspartoacylase in rat brain tissue. *J Neurochem* **79**, 211–20.

Birken D L and Oldendorf W H. 1989. *N*-Acetyl-L-aspartic acid: a literature review of a compound prominent in ^{1}H-NMR spectroscopic studies of brain. *Neurosci Biobehav Rev* **13**, 23–31.

Bustillo J R, Rowland L M, Jung R, *et al.* 2008. Proton magnetic resonance spectroscopy during initial treatment with antipsychotic medication in schizophrenia. *Crit Rev Neurobiol* **33**, 2456–66.

Cerdan S, Subramanian V H, Hilberman M, *et al.* 1986. 31P NMR detection of mobile dog brain phospholipids. *Magn Reson Med* **3**, 432–9.

Chandrakumar N and Subramanian S. 1987. Coherence transfer. In *Modern Techniques in High Resolution FT-NMR.* New York, NY: Springer-Verlag New York Inc.

Chang L, Friedman J, Ernst T, Zhong K, Tsopelas N D and Davis K. 2007. Brain metabolite abnormalities in the white matter of elderly schizophrenic subjects: implication for glial dysfunction. *Biol Psychiatry* **62**, 1396–404.

Creese I and Hess E J. 1986. Biochemical characteristics of D1 dopamine receptors: relationship to behavior and schizophrenia. *Clin Neuropharmacol* **9(Suppl 4)**, 14–6.

Dager S R, Corrigan N M, Richards T L and Posse S. 2008. Research applications of magnetic resonance spectroscopy to investigate psychiatric disorders. *Top Magn Reson Imaging* **19**, 81–96.

de Kruijff B, Rietveld A and Cullis P R. 1980. ^{31}P-NMR studies on membrane phospholipids in microsomes, rat liver slices and intact perfused rat liver. *Biochim Biophys Acta* **600**, 343–57.

de Kruijff B, Verkley A J, van Echteld C J, *et al.* 1979. The occurrence of lipidic particles in lipid bilayers as seen by ^{31}P NMR and freeze–fracture electron-microscopy. *Biochim Biophys Acta* **555**, 200–09.

Delamillieure P, Constans J M, Fernandez J, Brazo P and Dollfus S. 2004. Relationship between performance on the Stroop test and *N*-acetylaspartate in the medial prefrontal cortex in deficit and nondeficit schizophrenia: preliminary results. *Psychiatry Res* **132**, 87–9.

Eeg-Olofsson O, Kristensson K, Sourander P and Svennerholm L. 1966. Tay-Sach's Disease. A generalized metabolic disorder. *Acta Paed Scand* **55**, 546–62.

Ende G, Hubrich P, Walter S, *et al.* 2005. Further evidence for altered cerebellar neuronal integrity in schizophrenia. *Am J Psychiatry* **162**, 790–2.

Erecinska M and Silver I A. 1990. Metabolism and role of glutamate in mammalian brain. *Prog Neurobiol* **35**, 245–96.

Evans J S and Chan S I. 1994. Phosphophoryn, a biomineralization template protein: pH-dependent protein folding experiments. *Biopolymers* **34**, 507–27.

Fleysher R, Fleysher L, Liu S and Gonen O. 2009. On the voxel size and magnetic field strength dependence of spectral resolution in magnetic resonance spectroscopy. *Magn Reson Imaging* **27**, 222–32.

Frahm J, Michaelis T, Merboldt K D, Hanicke W, Gyngell M L and Bruhn H. 1991. On the *N*-acetyl methyl resonance in localized ^{1}H NMR spectra of human brain *in vivo*. *NMR Biomed* **4**, 201–04.

Fukuzako H. 2001. Neurochemical investigation of the schizophrenic brain by in vivo phosphorus magnetic resonance spectroscopy. *World J Biol Psychiatry* **2**, 70–82.

Fukuzako H, Fukuzako T, Hashiguchi T, Kodama S, Takigawa M and Fujimoto T. 1999. Changes in levels of phosphorus metabolites in temporal lobes of drug-naive schizophrenic patients. *Am J Psychiatry* **156**, 1205–08.

Fukuzako H, Fukuzako T, Takeuchi K, *et al.* 1996. Phosphorus magnetic resonance spectroscopy in schizophrenia: correlation between membrane phospholipid metabolism in the temporal lobe and positive symptoms. *Prog Neuropsychopharmacol Biol Psychiatry* **20**, 629–40.

Gangadhar B N, Jayakumar P N, Venkatasubramanian G, Janakiramaiah N and Keshavan M S. 2006. Developmental reflexes and 31P Magnetic Resonance Spectroscopy of basal ganglia in antipsychotic-naive schizophrenia. *Prog Neuropsychopharmacol Biol Psychiatry* **30**, 910–3.

Geddes J W, Panchalingam K, Keller J N and Pettegrew J W. 1997. Elevated phosphocholine and phosphatidyl choline following rat entorhinal cortex lesions. *Neurobiol Aging* **18**, 305–08.

Glonek T, Kopp S J, Kot E, Pettegrew J W, Harrison W H and Cohen M M. 1982. P-31 nuclear magnetic resonance analysis of brain: the perchloric acid extract spectrum. *J Neurochem* **39**, 1210–9.

Goldberg N D and O'Toole A G. 1969. The properties of glycogen synthetase and regulation of glycogen biosynthesis in rat brain. *J Biol Chem* **244**, 3053–61.

Goldstein F B. 1959. Biosynthesis of *N*-acetyl-l-aspartic acid. *J Biol Chem* **234**, 2702–06.

Goldstein F B. 1969. The enzymatic synthesis of *N*-acetyl-L-aspartic acid by subcellular preparations. *J Biol Chem* **244**, 4257–60.

Goldstein G, Panchalingam K, McClure R J, *et al.* 2009. Molecular neurodevelopment: An *in vivo* ^{31}P–^{1}H MRSI study. *J Int Neuropsychol Soc* **15**, 671–83.

Gonen O, Gruber S, Li B S, Mlynarik V and Moser E. 2001. Multivoxel 3D proton spectroscopy in the brain at 1.5 versus 3.0 T: signal-to-noise ratio and resolution comparison. *Am J Neuroradiol* **22**, 1727–31.

Gonzalez-Mendez R, Litt L, Koretsky A P, von Colditz J, Weiner M W and James T L. 1984. Comparison of ^{31}P NMR spectra of *in vivo* rat brain using convolution difference and saturation with a surface coil. Source of the broad component in the brain spectrum. *J Magn Reson* **57**, 526–33.

Hess H H, Bass N H, Thalheimer C and Devarakonda R. 1976. Gangliosides and the architecture of human frontal and rat somatosensory isocortex. *J Neurochem* **26**, 1115–21.

Hoult D I and Lauterbur P C. 1979. The sensitiivty of the zeugmatographic experiment involving human samples. *J Magn Reson* **34**, 425–33.

Jakary A, Vinogradov S, Feiwell R and Deicken R F. 2005. *N*-acetylaspartate reductions in the mediodorsal and anterior thalamus in men with schizophrenia verified by tissue volume corrected proton MRSI. *Schizophr Res* **76**, 173–85.

Jansson S E, Harkonen M H and Helve H. 1979. Metabolic properties of nerve endings isolated from rat brain. *Acta Physiol Scand* **107**, 205–12.

Jayakumar P N, Gangadhar B N, Subbakrishna D K, Janakiramaiah N, Srinivas J S and Keshavan M S. 2003. Membrane phospholipid abnormalities of basal ganglia in never-treated schizophrenia: a 31P magnetic resonance spectroscopy study. *Biol Psychiatry* **54**, 491–4.

Jayakumar P N, Venkatasubramanian G, Keshavan M S, Srinivas J S and Gangadhar B N. 2006. MRI volumetric and 31P MRS metabolic correlates of caudate nucleus in antipsychotic-naive schizophrenia. *Acta Psychiatr Scand* **114**, 346–51.

Jensen J E, Al Semaan Y M, Williamson P C, *et al.* 2002a. Region-specific changes in phospholipid metabolism in chronic, medicated schizophrenia: (31)P-MRS study at 4.0 Tesla. *Br J Psychiatry* **180**, 39–44.

Jensen J E, Drost D J, Menon R S and Williamson P C. 2002b. *In vivo* brain ^{31}P-MRS: measuring the phospholipid resonances at 4 Tesla from small voxels. *NMR Biomed* **15**, 338–47.

Jensen J E, Miller J, Williamson P C, *et al.* 2004. Focal changes in brain energy and phospholipid metabolism in first-episode schizophrenia: 31P-MRS chemical shift imaging study at 4 Tesla. *Br J Psychiatry* **184**, 409–15.

Jensen J E, Miller J, Williamson P C, *et al.* 2006. Grey and white matter differences in brain energy metabolism in first episode schizophrenia: 31P-MRS chemical shift imaging at 4 Tesla. *Psychiatry Res* **146**, 127–35.

Kennedy C and Sokoloff L. 1957. An adaptation of the nitrous oxide method to the study of the cerebral circulation in children; normal values for cerebral blood flow and cerebral metabolic rate in childhood. *J Clin Invest* **36**, 1130–7.

Keshavan M S, Pettegrew J W, Panchalingam K S, Kaplan D and Bozik E. 1991. Phosphorus 31 magnetic resonance spectroscopy detects altered brain metabolism before onset of schizophrenia. *Arch Gen Psychiatry* **48**, 1112–3.

Keshavan M S, Stanley J A, Montrose D M, Minshew N J and Pettegrew J W. 2003. Prefrontal membrane phospholipid metabolism of child and adolescent offspring at risk for schizophrenia or schizoaffective disorder: an *in vivo* ^{31}P MRS study. *Mol Psychiatry* **8**, 316–23.

Keshavan M S, Stanley J A and Pettegrew J W. 2000. Magnetic resonance spectroscopy in schizophrenia: methodological issues and findings – Part II. *Biol Psychiatry* **48**, 369–80.

Kilby P M, Bolas N M and Radda G K. 1991. 31P-NMR study of brain phospholipid structures in vivo. *Biochim Biophys Acta* **1085**, 257–64.

King M M, Huang C Y, Chock P B, *et al.* 1984. Mammalian brain phosphoproteins as substrates for calcineurin. *J Biol Chem* **259**, 8080–3.

Klemm S, Rzanny R, Riehemann S, *et al.* 2001. Cerebral phosphate metabolism in first-degree relatives of patients with schizophrenia. *Am J Psychiatry* **158**, 958–60.

Klunk W E, Xu C, Panchalingam K, McClure R J and Pettegrew J W. 1996. Quantitative ^{1}H and ^{31}P MRS of PCA extracts of postmortem Alzheimer's disease brain. *Neurobiol Aging* **17**, 349–57.

Klunk W E, Xu C J, Panchalingam K, McClure R J and Pettegrew J W. 1994. Analysis of magnetic resonance spectra by mole percent: comparison to absolute units. *Neurobiol Aging* **15**, 133–40.

Knizley H. 1967. The enzymatic synthesis of *N*-acetyl-L-aspartic acid by a water-insoluble preparation of a cat brain acetone powder. *J Biol Chem* **242**, 4619–22.

Koller K J, Zaczek R and Coyle J. 1984. *N*-acetyl-aspartyl-glutamate: regional levels in rat brain and the effects of brain lesions as determined by a new HPLC method. *J Neurochem* **43**, 1136–42.

Li C W, Negendank W G, Murphy-Boesch J, Padavic-Shaller K and Brown T R. 1996. Molar quantitation of hepatic metabolites in vivo in proton-decoupled, nuclear Overhauser effect enhanced 31P NMR spectra localized by three-dimensional chemical shift imaging. *NMR Biomed* **9**, 141–55.

Lowden J A and Wolfe L S. 1964. Studies on brain gangliosides. III Evidence for the location of gangliosides specifically in neurones. *Can J Biochem* **42**, 1587–94.

Makar T K, Cooper A J, Tofel-Grehl B, Thaler H T and Blass J P. 1995. Carnitine, carnitine acetyltransferase, and glutathione in Alzheimer brain. *Neurochem Res* **20**, 705–11.

Marenco S, Steele S U, Egan M F, *et al.* 2006. Effect of metabotropic glutamate receptor 3 genotype on *N*-acetylaspartate measures in the dorsolateral prefrontal cortex. *Am J Psychiatry* **163**, 740–2.

Mason R P, Trumbore M W and Pettegrew J W. 1995. Membrane interactions of a phosphomonoester elevated early in Alzheimer's disease. *Neurobiol Aging* **16**, 531–9.

McCandless D W and Wiggins R C. 1981. Cerebral energy metabolism during the onset and recovery from halothane anesthesia. *Neurochem Res* **6**, 1319–26.

McClure R J, Keshavan M S and Pettegrew J W. 1998. Chemical and physiologic brain imaging in schizophrenia. In Buckley P F (Ed.) *The Psychiatric Clinics of North America Schizophrenia*, Philadelphia: W.B. Saunders, pp. 93–122.

McIlwain H and Bachelard H S. 1985. *Biochemistry and the Central Nervous System*. Edinburgh: Churchill Livingstone.

McNamara R, Arias-Mendoza F and Brown T R. 1994. Investigation of broad resonances in ^{31}P NMR spectra of the human brain *in vivo*. *NMR Biomed* **7**, 237–42.

Merrill A H J and Sandhoff K. 2002. Sphingolipids: metabolism and cell signaling. In Vance D E and Vance J E (Eds) *Biochemistry of Lipids, Lipoproteins and Membranes*. New York, NY: Elsevier, pp. 390–407.

Miller B L. 1991. A review of chemical issues in ^{1}H NMR spectroscopy: *N*-acetyl-L-aspartate, creatine and choline. *NMR Biomed* **4**, 47–52.

Miyaoka T, Yasukawa R, Mizuno S, *et al.* 2005. Proton magnetic resonance spectroscopy (1H-MRS) of hippocampus, basal ganglia, and vermis of cerebellum in schizophrenia associated with idiopathic unconjugated hyperbilirubinemia (Gilbert's syndrome). *J Psychiatr Res* **39**, 29–34.

Molina V, Sanchez J, Sanz J, *et al.* 2007. Dorsolateral prefrontal N-acetyl-aspartate concentration in male patients with chronic schizophrenia and with chronic bipolar disorder. *Eur Psychiatry J Assoc Eur Psychiatrists* **22**, 505–12.

Murphy-Boesch J, Stoyanova R, Srinivasan R, *et al.* 1993. Proton-decoupled 31P chemical shift imaging of the human brain in normal volunteers. *NMR Biomed* **6**, 173–80.

Murphy E J, Bates T E, Williams S R, *et al.* 1992. Endoplasmic reticulum: the major contributor to the PDE peak in hepatic ^{31}P-NMR spectra at low magnetic field strengths. *Biochim Biophys Acta* **1111**, 51–8.

Murphy E J, Rajagopalan B, Brindle K M and Radda G K. 1989. Phospholipid bilayer contribution to ^{31}P NMR spectra *in vivo*. *Magn Reson Med* **12**, 282–9.

Nadler J V and Cooper J R. 1972. N-acetyl-L-aspartic acid content of human neural humours and bovine peripheral nervous tissues. *J Neurochem* **19**, 313–9.

O'Neill J, Levitt J, Caplan R, *et al.* 2004. 1H MRSI evidence of metabolic abnormalities in childhood-onset schizophrenia. *Neuroimage* **21**, 1781–9.

Ohrmann P, Siegmund A, Suslow T, *et al.* 2007. Cognitive impairment and in vivo metabolites in first-episode neuroleptic-naive and chronic medicated schizophrenic patients: a proton magnetic resonance spectroscopy study. *J Psychiatr Res* **41**, 625–34.

Ohrmann P, Siegmund A, Suslow T, *et al.* 2005. Evidence for glutamatergic neuronal dysfunction in the prefrontal cortex in chronic but not in first-episode patients with schizophrenia: a proton magnetic resonance spectroscopy study. *Schizophr Res* **73**, 153–7.

Ongur D, Jensen J E, Prescot A P, *et al.* 2008. Abnormal glutamatergic neurotransmission and neuronal–glial interactions in acute mania. *Biol Psychiatry* **64**, 718–26.

Ongur D, Prescot A P, Jensen J E, Cohen B M and Renshaw P F. 2009. Creatine abnormalities in schizophrenia and bipolar disorder. *Psychiatry Res* **172**, 44–8.

Paz R D, Tardito S, Atzori M and Tseng K Y. 2008. Glutamatergic dysfunction in schizophrenia: from basic neuroscience to clinical psychopharmacology. *Eur Neuropsychopharmacol* **18**, 773–86.

Pelupessy P, Rennella E and Bodenhausen G. 2009. High-resolution NMR in magnetic fields with unknown spatiotemporal variations. *Science* **324**, 1693–7.

Perry T L, Hansen S, Berry K, Mok C and Lesk D. 1971. Free amino acids and related compounds in biopsies of human brain. *J Neurochem* **18**, 521–8.

Petroff O A C, Prichard J W, Behar K L, Alger J R, den Hollander J A and Shulman R G. 1985. Cerebral intracellular pH by ^{31}P nuclear magnetic resonance spectroscopy. *Neurology* **35**, 781–8.

Pettegrew J W, Keshavan M S, Panchalingam K, *et al.* 1991. Alterations in brain high-energy phosphate and membrane phospholipid metabolism in first-episode, drug-naive schizophrenics. A pilot study of the dorsal prefrontal cortex by *in vivo* phosphorus 31 nuclear magnetic resonance spectroscopy. *Arch Gen Psychiatry* **48**, 563–8.

Pettegrew J W, Panchalingam K, Klunk W E, McClure R J and Muenz L R. 1994. Alterations of cerebral metabolism in probable Alzheimer's disease: a preliminary study. *Neurobiol Aging* **15**, 117–32.

Pettegrew J W, Panchalingam K, Withers G, McKeag D and Strychor S. 1990. Changes in brain energy and phospholipid metabolism during development and aging in the Fischer 344 rat. *J Neuropathol Exp Neurol* **49**, 237–49.

Pettegrew J W, Withers G, Panchalingam K and Post J F. 1988. Considerations for brain pH assessment by ^{31}P NMR. *Magn Reson Imaging* **6**, 135–42.

Potwarka J J, Drost D J, Williamson P C, *et al.* 1999. A 1H-decoupled 31P chemical shift imaging study of medicated schizophrenic patients and healthy controls. *Biol Psychiatry* **45**, 687–93.

Pouwels P J and Frahm J. 1997. Differential distribution of NAA and NAAG in human brain as determined by quantitative localized proton MRS. *NMR Biomed* **10**, 73–8.

Purdon S E, Valiakalayil A, Hanstock C C, Seres P and Tibbo P. 2008. Elevated 3T proton MRS glutamate levels associated with poor Continuous Performance Test (CPT-0X) scores and genetic risk for schizophrenia. *Schizophr Res* **99**, 218–24.

Puri B K, Counsell S J, Hamilton G, *et al.* 2004. Cerebral metabolism in male patients with schizophrenia who have seriously and dangerously violently offended: a 31P magnetic resonance spectroscopy study. *Prostag Leukotri and Ess Fatty Acids* **70**, 409–11.

Puri B K, Counsell S J, Hamilton G, Bustos M and Treasaden I H. 2008. Brain cell membrane motion-restricted phospholipids in patients with schizophrenia who have seriously and dangerously violently offended. *Prog Neuropsychopharmacol Biol Psychiatry* **32**, 751–4.

Riehemann S, Hubner G, Smesny S, Volz H P and Sauer H. 2002. Do neuroleptics alter the cerebral intracellular pH value in schizophrenics? A (31)P-MRS study on three different patient groups. *Psychiatry Res* **114**, 113–7.

Rothermundt M, Ohrmann P, Abel S, *et al.* 2007. Glial cell activation in a subgroup of patients with schizophrenia indicated by increased S100B serum concentrations and elevated *myo*-inositol. *Prog Neuropsychopharmacol Biol Psychiatry* **31**, 361–4.

Rowland L M, Bustillo J R, Mullins P G, *et al.* 2005. Effects of ketamine on anterior cingulate glutamate metabolism in healthy humans: a 4-T proton MRS study. *Am J Psychiatry* **162**, 394–6.

Rzanny R, Klemm S, Reichenbach J R, *et al.* 2003. 31P-MR spectroscopy in children and adolescents with a familial risk of schizophrenia. *Eur Radiol* **13**, 763–70.

Scherk H, Backens M, Zill P, *et al.* 2008. SNAP-25 genotype influences NAA/Cho in left hippocampus. *J Neural Transm* **115**, 1513–8.

Seelig J. 1978. 31P nuclear magnetic resonance and the head group structure of phospholipids in membranes. *Biochim Biophys Acta* **515**, 105–40.

Seeman P. 2002. Atypical antipsychotics: mechanism of action. *Can J Psychiatry – Rev Can Psychiatrie* **47**, 27–38.

Shedd S F, Lutz N W and Hull W E. 1993. The influence of medium formulation on phosphomonoester and UDP-hexose levels in cultured human colon tumor cells as observed by ^{31}P NMR spectroscopy. *NMR Biomed* **6**, 254–63.

Shenton M E, Dickey C C, Frumin M and McCarley R W. 2001. A review of MRI findings in schizophrenia. *Schizophr Res* **49**, 1–52.

Shimizu E, Hashimoto K, Ochi S, *et al.* 2007. Posterior cingulate gyrus metabolic changes in chronic schizophrenia with generalized cognitive deficits. *J Psychiatr Res* **41**, 49–56.

Shirayama Y, Yano T, Takahashi K, Takahashi S and Ogino T. 2004. In vivo 31P NMR spectroscopy shows an increase in glycerophosphorylcholine concentration without alterations in mitochondrial function in the prefrontal cortex of medicated schizophrenic patients at rest. *Eur J Neurosci* **20**, 749–56.

Simmons M L, Frondoza C G and Coyle J T. 1991. Immunocytochemical localization of *N*-acetyl-aspartate with monoclonal antibodies. *Neuroscience* **45**, 37–45.

Smesny S, Rosburg T, Nenadic I, *et al.* 2007. Metabolic mapping using 2D 31P-MR spectroscopy reveals frontal and thalamic metabolic abnormalities in schizophrenia. *Neuroimage* **35**, 729–37.

Sokoloff L. 1991. Measurement of local cerebral glucose utilization and its relation to local functional activity in the brain. *Adv Exp Med Biol* **291**, 21–42.

Sokoloff L. 1993. Function-related changes in energy metabolism in the nervous system: localization and mechanisms. *Keio J Med* **42**, 95–103.

Stanley J A. 2002. In vivo magnetic resonance spectroscopy and its application to neuropsychiatric disorders. *Can J Psychiatry* **47**, 315–26.

Stanley J A and Pettegrew J W. 2001. Post-processing method to segregate and quantify the broad components underlying the phosphodiester spectral region of *in vivo* 31-P brain spectra. *Magn Reson Med* **45**, 390–6.

Stanley J A, Pettegrew J W and Keshavan M S. 2000. Magnetic resonance spectroscopy in schizophrenia: methodological issues and fIndings – Part I. *Biol Psychiatry* **48**, 357–68.

Stanley J A, Vemulapalli M, Nutche J, *et al.* 2007. Reduced *N*-acetyl-aspartate levels in schizophrenia patients with a younger onset age: a single-voxel 1H spectroscopy study. *Schizophr Res* **93**, 23–32.

Stanley J A, Williamson P C, Drost D J, *et al.* 1994. Membrane phospholipid metabolism and schizophrenia: an *in vivo* ^{31}P-MR spectroscopy study. *Schizophr Res* **13**, 209–15.

Steen R G, Hamer R M and Lieberman J A. 2005. Measurement of brain metabolites by 1H magnetic resonance spectroscopy in patients with schizophrenia: a systematic review and meta-analysis. *Crit Rev Neurobiol* **30**, 1949–62.

Suzuki K. 1966. The pattern of mammalian brain gangliosides III. Regional and developmental differences. *J Neurochem* **12**, 969–79.

Szulc A, Galinska B, Tarasow E, *et al.* 2005. The effect of risperidone on metabolite measures in the frontal lobe, temporal lobe, and thalamus in schizophrenic patients. A proton magnetic resonance spectroscopy (1H MRS). *Pharmacopsychiatry* **38**, 214–9.

Tallan H H. 1957. Studies on the distribution of *N*-acetyl-L-aspartic acid in brain. *J Biol Chem* **224**, 41–5.

Tallan H H, Moore S and Stein W H. 1956. *N*-acetyl-L-aspartic acid in brain. *J Biol Chem* **219**, 257–64.

Tanaka Y, Obata T, Sassa T, *et al.* 2006. Quantitative magnetic resonance spectroscopy of schizophrenia: relationship between decreased *N*-acetylaspartate and frontal lobe dysfunction. *Psychiatry and Clin Neurosci* **60**, 365–72.

Tang C Y, Friedman J, Shungu D, *et al.* 2007. Correlations between Diffusion Tensor Imaging (DTI) and Magnetic Resonance Spectroscopy (1H MRS) in schizophrenic patients and normal controls. *BMC Psychiatry* **7**, 25.

Terpstra M, Vaughan T J, Ugurbil K, Lim K O, Schulz S C and Gruetter R. 2005. Validation of glutathione quantitation from STEAM spectra against edited 1H NMR spectroscopy at 4T: application to schizophrenia. *Magma* **18**, 276–82.

Theberge J, Al Semaan Y, Drost D J, *et al.* 2004a. Duration of untreated psychosis vs. *N*-acetylaspartate and choline in first episode schizophrenia: a 1H magnetic resonance spectroscopy study at 4.0 Tesla. *Psychiatry Res* **131**, 107–14.

Theberge J, Al Semaan Y, Jensen J E, *et al.* 2004b. Comparative study of proton and phosphorus magnetic resonance spectroscopy in schizophrenia at 4 Tesla. *Psychiatry Res* **132**, 33–9.

Theberge J, Williamson K E, Aoyama N, *et al.* 2007. Longitudinal grey-matter and glutamatergic losses in first-episode schizophrenia. *Br J Psychiatry* **191**, 325–34.

Tibbo P, Hanstock C, Valiakalayil A and Allen P. 2004. 3-T proton MRS investigation of glutamate and glutamine in adolescents at high genetic risk for schizophrenia. *Am J Psychiatry* **161**, 1116–8.

Truckenmiller M E, Namboodiri M A A, Brownstein M J and Neale J H. 1985. *N*-Acetylation of L-aspartate in the nervous system: differential distribution of a specific enzyme. *J Neurochem* **45**, 1658–62.

Ugurbil K, Adriany G, Andersen P, *et al.* 2003. Ultrahigh field magnetic resonance imaging and spectroscopy. *Magn Reson Imaging* **21**, 1263–81.

Ulrich M, Wokrina T, Ende G, Lang M and Bachert P. 2007. ^{31}P-{^{1}H} Echo-planar spectroscopic imaging of the human brain in vivo. *Magn Reson Med* **57**, 784–90.

Urenjak J, Williams S R, Gadian D G and Noble M. 1993. Proton nuclear magnetic resonance spectroscopy unambiguously identifies different neural cell types. *J Neurosci* **13**, 981–9.

Van Elst L T, Valerius G, Buchert M, *et al.* 2005. Increased prefrontal and hippocampal glutamate concentration in schizophrenia: evidence from a magnetic resonance spectroscopy study. *Biol Psychiatry* **58**, 724–30.

Vance D E. 1991. Phospholipid metabolism and cell signalling in eucaryotes. In Vance D E and Vance J E (Eds) *Biochemistry of Lipids, Lipoproteins and Membranes, Volume 20*. New York, NY: Elsevier, pp. 205–40.

Vance J E. 1988. Compartmentalization of phospholipids for lipoprotein assembly on the basis of molecular species and biosynthetic origin. *Biochim Biophys Acta* **963**, 70–81.

Vaughan J T, Garwood M, Collins C M, *et al.* 2001. 7T vs. 4T: RF power, homogeneity, and signal-to-noise comparison in head images. *Magn Reson Med* **46**, 24–30.

Volz H R, Riehemann S, Maurer I, *et al.* 2000. Reduced phosphodiesters and high-energy phosphates in the frontal lobe of schizophrenic patients: a (31)P chemical shift spectroscopic-imaging study. *Biol Psychiatry* **47**, 954–61.

Weickert C S and Kleinman J E. 1998. The neuroanatomy and neurochemistry of schizophrenia. In Buckley P F (Ed.) *The Psychiatric Clinics of North America Schizophrenia*. Philadelphia: W.B. Saunders, pp. 57–75.

Whittaker V P. 1966. Some properties of synaptic membranes isolated from the central nervous system. *Ann N Y Acad Sci* **137**, 982–98.

Wiegandt H. 1967. The subcellular localization of gangliosides in the brain. *J Neurochem* **14**, 671–4.

Wood S J, Berger G E, Lambert M, *et al.* 2006. Prediction of functional outcome 18 months after a first psychotic episode: a proton magnetic resonance spectroscopy study. *Arch Gen Psychiatry* **63**, 969–76.

Wood S J, Berger G E, Wellard R M, *et al.* 2008. A 1H-MRS investigation of the medial temporal lobe in antipsychotic-naive and early-treated first episode psychosis. *Schizophr Res* **102**, 163–70.

Wood S J, Yucel M, Wellard R M, *et al.* 2007. Evidence for neuronal dysfunction in the anterior cingulate of patients with schizophrenia: a proton magnetic resonance spectroscopy study at 3 T. *Schizophr Res* **94**, 328–31.

Yacubian J, de Castro C C, Ometto M, *et al.* 2002. 31P-spectroscopy of frontal lobe in schizophrenia: alterations in phospholipid and high-energy phosphate metabolism. *Schizophr Res* **58**, 117–22.

Neuroreceptor imaging of schizophrenia

Dean F. Wong, James Robert Brašić and Nicola Cascella

Introduction

Since the development of neuroreceptor positron emission tomography (PET) imaging in the 1980s, the application of this novel in-vivo technology has revolutionized the study of schizophrenia for pathophysiology and drug development. This now-coined "molecular imaging" in schizophrenia has a historical root in the very basis of in-vivo neuroreceptor imaging with PET and single-photon emission computed tomography (SPECT). Indeed, the first successful imaging study in 1983 in living human brain was with a radiolabeled antipsychotic, spiperone (Spiroperidol), labeled with [11C]-methyl iodine (Wagner *et al.*, 1983), and later with [18F]. This was followed with the isotopic labeling of [11C]-raclopride (i.e. no change in the chemical structure or pharmacology), also an antipsychotic and D_2/D_3 dopamine (DA) antagonist. Both unlabeled spiperone and raclopride have been studied for their potential therapeutic value for schizophrenia in clinical trials. Although neither of these antipsychotics was used clinically, their radiolabeled PET analogs led the way for studying D_2-like dopamine receptors, and opened up the entire field of studying neuroreceptors as essentially a new subspecialty of neuroimaging with tremendous application in neuropsychiatry. These two radiotracers were quickly shown to be displaceable by unlabeled marketed antipsychotics such as haloperidol (Haldol), which led ultimately to dopamine D_2/D_3 occupancy studies (see below), and guidance of therapeutic drug dose levels now being visualized in human brain. Most importantly, they illustrate the merging of basic psychopharmacology, CNS nuclear medicine methodology, and in-vivo neuropsychiatric applications.

Following these initial dopamine imaging studies, there was increased interest in the serotonin system, which also is believed to be relevant in schizophrenia symptomatology and potentially in treatment. Many antipsychotics starting with clozapine (Clozaril) and subsequently risperidone (Risperdal) and olanzapine (Zyprexa) have both serotonin and dopamine binding properties. Hence, the development of molecular imaging of the serotonin sites was a natural progression, which is described below.

Molecular imaging of dopamine in schizophrenia

Considerable lines of evidence converge to confirm that alterations in the density, distribution, and function of dopamine D_2/D_3 receptors in the brain play a role in the pathophysiology of schizophrenia (Wong and Brašić, 2005). The dopamine hypothesis of schizophrenia proposes that schizophrenia results from dysfunction of dopaminergic neurotransmission in the brain (Carlsson, 1999; Carlsson *et al.*, 1999), and can be tested with the aid of molecular imaging tools. An early application of dopamine D_2 PET imaging was to measure absolute receptor density (B_{max}). Early studies included [11C]-3-*N*-methylspiperone ([11C]-NMSP) in schizophrenia.

The observation that the positive symptoms of schizophrenia are alleviated when 60–80% of dopamine D_2/D_3 receptors in the brain are occupied by antipsychotic drugs as demonstrated by PET (Gründer *et al.*, 2003; Wong *et al.*, 2002) represented a major advance in the development of novel drugs to treat people with schizophrenia. PET/SPECT receptor occupancy allows determination of the likely optimal dose of dopamine D_2 receptor blocking drugs to produce a therapeutic effect with minimal adverse effects (Wong and Brašić, 2005).

Understanding Neuropsychiatric Disorders, ed. M. E. Shenton and B. I. Turetsky. Published by Cambridge University Press.
© Cambridge University Press 2011.

Table 4.1 Imaging studies of dopamine neurotransmission in schizophrenia: observations and possible mechanisms

Site	Observation	Salient and related findings	Possible mechanism
D_2 (striatum)	Elevations with [^{11}C]-NMSP (butyrophenone)	Varied post-mortem changes, internalization, monomer elevation	Decreased tonic DA
	No change (benzamides) except following AMPT using [^{123}I]-IBZM or [^{11}C]-raclopride	Due to competition with intra-synaptic DA or dimer configuration, unmasking of D_2 due to intrasynaptic DA removal with AMPT	Increased phasic DA Decreased tonic DA
DDC (striatum)	Elevation with [^{18}F]-fluorodopa	Majority of imaging studies	Decreased tonic DA
DA (striatum) release after AMP challenge	Elevation with [^{123}I]-IBZM or [^{11}C]-raclopride	Majority of imaging studies	Increased phasic DA
DA (striatum) release after ketamine challenge	Elevation with [^{11}C]-raclopride Elevation with [^{11}C]-FLB457	Glutamate antagonist stimulates hypoglutamatergic state	Increased phasic DA
Prefrontal D_1	Decrease with [^{11}C]-SCH23390	One published imaging study	Unknown
ACCX D_2	Decrease with [^{11}C]-FLB457	Post-mortem tyrosine hydroxylase immunoreactive changes	Unknown

[^{11}C]-NMSP, (3-N-[^{11}C]methylspiperone; DDC, dopa decarboxylase; DA, dopamine; AMPT, α-methylparatyrosine; AMP, amphetamine; [^{11}C]-FLB457, ((S)-N-((1-ethyl-2-pyrrolidinyl)methyl)-5-bromo-2[^{11}C], 3-dimethoxybenzamide); [^{11}C]-SCH23390, [^{11}C]-(R)-(+)-7-chloro-8-hydroxy-3-methyl-1-phenyl-2,3,4,5-tetrahydro-1H-3-benzazepine; ACCX, anterior cingulate cortex. (Adapted from Wong (2002b), with permission.)

Cognition (i.e. working memory) is related to D_1, for example, so the role of dopamine is relevant to all domains of schizophrenia psychopathology. All are developed below.

Imaging tools for D_2/D_3 dopamine

As mentioned earlier, the development of molecular imaging studies resulted from the successful radiolabeling of the dopamine receptor antagonists, raclopride and spiperone, in the mid 1980s, consistent with the investigation of post-synaptic dopamine (DA) D_2-like receptors (Table 4.1). The study of the binding of D_2-like DA receptors is typically made by a single PET or SPECT scan at high specific activity (low mass, non-pharmacologic, injected intravenously) to measure the so-called binding potential, which is a product of the receptor density and the binding affinity (Innis et al., 2007).

This imaging has been accomplished using two main classes of radiotracers. The first class of radiotracers to visualize D_2 or D_3 receptors in the brain includes butyrophenones such as [^{11}C]-NMSP and [^{18}F]-spiperone. The second class of radiotracers to visualize D_2-like receptors in the brain includes radiolabeled benzamides such as [^{11}C]-raclopride (Figure 4.1). More recently, imaging of extrastriatal D_2/D_3 receptors has been enabled with [^{18}F]-fallypride ([^{18}F]-FP) (Figure 4.2) and [^{11}C]-FLB457 (Nyberg et al., 2002), or iodine-123 [^{123}I]-iodobenzamide (IBZM).

Estimation of absolute dopamine D_2-like receptors
Density

The original studies in the 1970s to examine abnormalities in dopamine and dopamine receptors in schizophrenia could only be carried out in post-mortem brain tissue of patients. These studies mostly showed elevation of D_2 dopamine receptors in schizophrenia using in-vitro test tube techniques, where homogenates of tissue or X-ray film of the receptor distribution (autoradiography) were employed. However, since these studies were all done in post-mortem

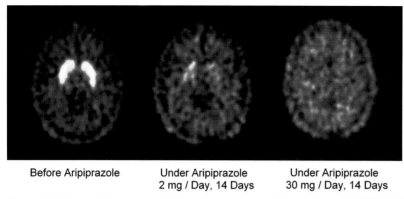

Before Aripiprazole | Under Aripiprazole 2 mg / Day, 14 Days | Under Aripiprazole 30 mg / Day, 14 Days

Figure 4.1 Representative transversal images from positron emission tomography (PET) with [^{11}C]-raclopride, a radiotracer for striatal D$_2$/D$_3$ receptors in the brain, of a healthy adult volunteer without medication (*left*) and after treatment for 14 days with either 2 mg (*middle*) or 30 mg (*right*) aripiprazole (Abilify). The baseline study (*left*) demonstrates marked uptake of the radiotracer in the striatum (caudate nucleus and putamen) indicating a high density of striatal D$_2$/D$_3$ receptors. After treatment with 2 mg aripiprazole for 14 days, approximately 70% of the D$_2$/D$_3$ receptors in the striatum are occupied by aripiprazole so the radiotracer uptake is markedly reduced (*middle*). After treatment with 30 mg aripiprazole for 14 days, almost all of the D$_2$/D$_3$ receptors in the striatum are occupied by aripiprazole so the radiotracer uptake is almost completely blocked (*right*). These results confirm that aripiprazole occupies the D$_2$/D$_3$ receptors in the striata of healthy adults in a dose-dependent manner, and that clinical doses of the drug lead to almost complete saturation of striatal D$_2$/D$_3$ receptors. (Modified from Yokoi *et al.*, 2002, with permission.)

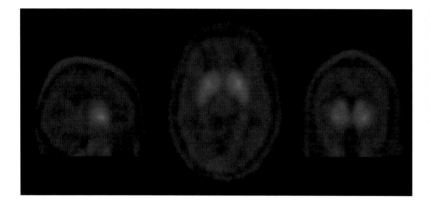

Figure 4.2 Representative sagittal (*left*), tranversal (*middle*), and coronal (*right*) images from positron emission tomography (PET) with [^{18}F]-fallypride ([^{18}F]-FP), a radiotracer for extrastriatal D$_2$/D$_3$ receptors in the brain, of a 24-year-old man with his first episode of schizophrenia treated with aripiprazole until 78 h before the tomography. The average striatal D$_2$/D$_3$ receptor occupancy was 82%. At the moment of tomography the aripiprazole serum concentration was 106 ng/mL. (From Gründer *et al.*, 2008, with permission.)

tissue, it was not possible to verify what the potential effects of medication or post-mortem change might be on these elevations of dopamine D$_2$ receptors. In particular, since these tissue samples looked only at the surface receptor protein, with any endogenous dopamine rinsed away in the in-vitro procedures, there were some inherent disadvantages of using this method. With the advent of the first PET studies in humans in 1983 (Wagner *et al.*, 1983), there was an opportunity to study living humans where not only the diagnosis could be more readily confirmed, but also drug exposure could be established through drug screening and the use of outside informants. While this is still something of a controversial area, the original measurements of the dopamine receptors in schizophrenia began with measuring absolute receptor density (B_{max}), not simply the binding potential (B_{max}/K_D). The first studies by Wong *et al.* (1986) and Farde *et al.* (1986) used a saturation procedure which required at least two or more PET scans to establish independently the measurement of the receptor density (B_{max}) and the binding affinity. Therefore, some discussion about the methodology for measuring receptor density, which is still employed, is given below (Innis *et al.*, 2007).

The measurement of absolute B_{max} can be carried out by performing two brain scans with the administration of [^{11}C]-raclopride or [^{11}C]-NMSP, after a known potent dose of an unlabeled (non-radioactive) D$_2$-like DA receptor antagonist, such as unlabeled raclopride (former) itself or haloperidol (in the latter), respectively, to reduce some of the binding of the first scan. Following some additional mathematical modeling, these results then provide an estimate of the B_{max} and the binding affinity. These results correspond to those from autoradiography studies or in-vitro homogenate studies (although not exactly in absolute units). Subsequently, simplified studies involving single high-specific activity scans (radiotracer mass injections of typically under 20 µg) were carried out to estimate the binding potential (BP); that is, the ratio of the B_{max} to K_D. Nonetheless, in order to mathematically separate these variables of B_{max} and K_D, it is necessary to carry out receptor saturation studies with varying unlabeled mass injections. In general, the absolute B_{max} studies have tended to show elevations ranging from small to large, and as much as a threefold increase with [11C]-NMSP, a butyrophenone. Although B_{max} elevations have been consistently shown with [11C]-NMSP, no significant changes have been demonstrated with B_{max} using benzamides such as [11C]-raclopride. Interestingly (see below), one of the characteristics of these benzamides is that they are also quite susceptible to endogenous dopamine, and recently have gained popularity for measuring the effect of pharmacologic challenges or psychological stress that alter endogenous dopamine levels. Some have suggested that the differences in B_{max} between raclopride and NMSP could be attributed to the preferential affinity for a monomer versus a dimer form of the dopamine receptor in the case of [11C]-NMSP, and possibly receptor internalization and susceptibility to endogenous neurotransmitter for [11C]-raclopride. Regardless of the reasons for the differences, meta-analysis has shown that there is a small (12%) significant elevation of striatal D_2 receptors with an effect size of 0.51, and there is an association between increased D_2 receptor density and positive symptoms.

Imaging neuroreceptor systems following pharmacological challenges

Pharmacological challenges are one of the most promising areas in in-vivo neuronal receptor imaging to alter neurotransmitters levels. The most successful approaches have been with the dopaminergic system using amphetamine, methylphenidate or cocaine to increase, or α-methyl-para-tyrosine (AMPT) to decrease intra-synaptic dopamine when given before PET scans. These techniques have shown that intra-synaptic dopamine is increased on average in drug-free schizophrenia (Laruelle et al., 1996; Breier et al., 1997) following the administration of amphetamine. Elevations of baseline dopamine D_2 receptors have been shown using AMPT administration, where schizophrenia subjects appear to have more dopamine available than controls, although both are decreased compared to non-treated AMPT subjects (as evidenced by elevated [11C]-raclopride binding; Abi-Dargham et al., 2000).

Subjects with schizophrenia may demonstrate abnormally elevated intra-synaptic levels of dopamine in the phasic state due to elevated DA, as evidenced by amphetamine challenge. Pharmacological challenges in the imaging of schizophrenia also include tools to evaluate the mechanisms of actions of treatments that may effect DA release and could become a potential imaging biomarker just as is D_2 receptor occupancy (see below).

Methodology for measuring intra-synaptic dopamine

In the 1990s, an important behavior of radiolabeled benzamides was discovered. Specifically, [123I]-IBZM, [11C]-raclopride, and more recently [18F]-fallypride (Figure 4.2) and [11C]-FLB 457, show DA receptor binding potential changes in the presence of a pharmacologic challenge that can elicit increased or decreased levels of intra-synaptic DA. In the case of increased intra-synaptic DA, challenges with dopaminergic agents, including oral and IV methylphenidate (Ritalin) as well as amphetamines, have been employed. Investigators have shown that these radiolabeled benzamides can have a reduced binding in the presence of an IV amphetamine challenge (0.2–0.3 mg/kg body weight), and significantly greater decreases in binding potentials in patients with schizophrenia in contrast to healthy normal control volunteers (Laruelle et al., 1996; Abi Dargham et al., 2004; Breier et al., 1997; Wong et al., 2003). There is still some controversy about the meaning of these decreases in binding potential (Munro et al., 2006a, 2006b; Oswald, et al., 2005). One mystery is that the radiotracer does not return to baseline as one might expect after psychostimulant challenge. Instead, the baseline continues to be depressed for many hours following a continuous infusion of [11C]-raclopride, sometimes exceeding 6 h. This implies other factors than intra-synaptic dopamine release alone (Carson et al., 1997), suggesting potential heterogeneity in DA response to challenges with stimulants. The reduction in occupancy has been hypothesized to be due to the increased intrasynaptic dopamine, but also a change of the affinity state (e.g. as D_2 at high and low states) could be envisioned. What may be most justifiable is that there is an increase in occupancy of the D_2/D_3 receptors due to DA that competes directly with the radiolabeled benzamides (Wong et al., 2006). An observed heterogeneity in DA release may be related to clinical heterogeneity in schizophrenia, as at least one study has shown that dopamine release is greater in patients with more positive symptoms during PET scanning (Nozaki et al., 2009). Furthermore, one other neuropsychiatric disorder, Tourette's syndrome, has also demonstrated significant elevations of dopamine release after IV amphetamine challenge and [^{11}C]-raclopride PET (Singer et al., 2002, Wong et al., 2008). These also seem to be greater with Tourette's syndrome patients who additionally have comorbid obsessive–compulsive disorder, suggesting that clinical heterogeneity may have a role in dopamine release differences.

Dopamine depletion

Another procedure used for measuring changing intrasynaptic dopamine is dopamine depletion. This has been carried out with reserpine in animal studies, or with AMPT (a drug which is approved in humans for pheochromocytoma). Such challenges have allowed the demonstration of elevation in binding potential presumably due to competition with intrasynaptic DA. These measures allow an estimate of basal synaptic dopamine. One study (Abi-Dargham et al., 2000) demonstrated the elevation of binding potential following AMPT. The elevation of binding is greater in people with schizophrenia, and patients with greater elevations showed better improvement in positive symptoms following antipsychotic treatment. This is consistent not only with an increase in baseline intra-synaptic dopamine in schizophrenia, but also is consistent with elevated D_2 receptor densities. These findings support the results of a meta-analysis that shows a small but significant elevation of D_2 receptors (a few percent) in schizophrenia by PET or SPECT imaging (Laruelle, 1998).

Dopa decarboxylase pre-synaptic measures

Dopamine precursor imaging using [^{18}F]-fluorodopa or [^{11}C]-dopa can reflect dopa decarboxylase (DDC) rates of activity, or represent some measure of dopamine pre-synaptic function. Several studies (more than 6) have shown that the [^{18}F]-fluorodopa binding is higher in patients with schizophrenia (e.g. Reith et al., 1994). Such increased [^{18}F]-fluorodopamine (FDOPA) turnover has been shown in at least 5 of 6 PET studies. These striatal findings are among the most consistent in schizophrenia imaging and are consistent with the concept of increased tonic dopamine and elevated phasic dopamine suggested by Grace in 1991 (Wong, 2002a, 2002b).

Dopamine transporter imaging

The dysfunction in dopaminergic neurotransmission in the pathobiology of schizophrenia may be tied to having several synaptic/neuronal sites. The dopamine transporter in schizophrenia has been studied using SPECT imaging with [^{123}I]-CIT (Martinez et al., 2001; Laruelle et al., 2000), but no significant changes have been detected.

Extrastriatal dopamine receptor imaging

Recently, higher-affinity radiopharmaceuticals of the D_2-like receptors, such as [^{18}F]-fallypride (Buchsbaum et al., 2006) (Figure 4.2) and [^{11}C]-FLB457 (Muhkerjee et al., 2001, 2002, 2004, 2005; Nyberg et al., 2002; Yasuno et al., 2004), have allowed PET and SPECT imaging of extrastriatal dopamine D_2-like receptors in cortical regions in human brain. Some PET/SPECT studies have been carried out showing decreases or no change. Some studies have suggested decreased binding in the thalamus, and in the cingulate cortex, temporal cortex (Davidson and Heinrichs, 2003), and amygdala. Absolute receptor density has not yet been carried out, as it has been in the case of striatal D_2 receptors and may be more technically challenging given the lower cortical than striatal D_2 density.

D_1 receptor imaging

Some PET studies have reported associations between D_1 receptor density in dorsolateral prefrontal cortex, and impairments in working memory performance and negative symptoms. However, there are limitations of these studies of the D_1 receptor in that the radiotracers ([^{11}C]-SCH 23390 and [^{11}C]-NNC 112) are not selective for D_1 receptors, but also bind to 5-HT$_{2A}$ receptors. Thus, further radiotracer development is needed for the D1 receptor site.

Serotonin imaging

Serotonin is the second major neurotransmitter system studied in schizophrenia. This has mostly been motivated in part by theories of the mechanisms of action of atypical antipsychotics. However, the study of serotonin is also relevant given the psychotic symptomatology from the hallucinogenic effects of chemically similar lysergic acid diethylamide (LSD).

Serotonin (5-HT$_{2A}$) imaging studies of 5-HT$_{2A}$ receptors

5-HT$_{2A}$ receptors were originally imaged in human brain with non-selective radiotracers such as [^{11}C]-3-N-methylspiperone (NMSP), which has affinity for both striatal D$_2$-like DA and for 5-HT$_{2A}$ cortical receptors (Wong *et al.*, 1984). [^{18}F]-altanserin has also been used with ketamine challenge to study 5-HT transmission (Matusch *et al.*, 2007). Post-mortem studies have found decreased 5-HT$_{2A}$ binding in the prefrontal cortex, but some PET studies in drug-free or drug-naive patients with schizophrenia have found normal or increased 5-HT$_{2A}$ receptor binding (Talvik-Lofti *et al.*, 2000; Erritzoe *et al.*, 2008). One study demonstrated significant decreases in prefrontal cortex in drug-naive schizophrenic patients (Hurlemann *et al.*, 2005), while other studies have shown recently some elevations (Zanardi *et al.*, 2001). Recent studies in drug-naive schizophrenia have shown depressions (Erritzoe, *et al.*, 2006, 2008; Rasmussen *et al.*, 2010).

Serotonin transporter (SERT) imaging

Initial studies of SERT were carried out with less-selective SPECT radiotracers, such as [^{123}I]-β-carbomethoxy-3-β-(4-iodophenyl)-tropane ([^{123}I]-β-CIT), and more selective [^{11}C]-3-amino-4-(2-dimethylaminomethylphenylthio) benzonitrile ([^{11}C]-(DASB)), which labeled SERT in the midbrain and where no differences were found (Frankle *et al.*, 2005). This is despite the fact that some post-mortem studies have shown decreases in SERT in frontal cortex and in cingulate cortex (Joyce *et al.*, 1993; Laruelle *et al.*, 1993).

Glutamate system imaging

Glutamate, the excitatory neurotransmitter, likely has multiple roles in the pathogenesis and pathology of schizophrenia. A "glutamate hypothesis" has developed in schizophrenia related to some extent to

dopamine. A prevailing theory is that a hypoglutamatergic state (possibly in frontal cortical regions) contributes to the hyperdopaminergic state seen in the striatum PET DA studies described above. If this hypothesis is confirmed, this may help explain the evidence for elevated amphetamine-induced dopamine release in some studies with schizophrenia (see below). NMDA antagonists which affect the phencyclidine (PCP) site (an ion channel), such as ketamine (Ketalar), which allow the possibility of measuring blood flow and dopamine release changes, are being actively studied. Imaging one site of the NMDA receptor channel, the PCP site, in thalamic and other regions in healthy humans was done with *N*-(1-naphthyl)-N′-(3-[^{123}I]iodophenyl)-N-methylguanidine ([^{123}I]-CNS-1261). This binds to the thalamic PCP site. This binding was reduced by ketamine, which also binds to the PCP site. Initial studies did not show differences in patients compared to controls, but clozapine did reduce the binding of the [^{123}I]-CNS-1261. This suggests that clozapine may exert some of its action through the glutamate system. As negative symptoms were increased in these studies, one possibility is that reductions of glutamate may lead to negative symptoms. Also, blockade of the NMDA receptor by glutamate antagonists may precipitate positive symptoms, as has been shown by the human administration of ketamine (Abi-Dargham *et al.*, 2000; Krystal *et al.*, 2005). [^{123}I]-CNS-1261 in patients with schizophrenia (both unmedicated and those under antipsychotic treatment) was unchanged compared to healthy controls. Treatment with first-generation antipsychotics did not alter NMDA receptor binding.

Ketamine challenge may stimulate hallucinations in schizophrenia, and hence has been considered to be a potential human model. Also, imaging studies with ketamine infusion have significantly reduced the binding of [^{11}C]-FLB457 in the posterior cingulate/retrosplenial cortices. This may suggest intrasynaptic DA release. This has further been supported by primate microdialysis studies (Adams *et al.*, 2002). Simultaneously, ketamine-induced psychotic symptoms were measured with imaging and suggested that cortical DA mechanisms may relate to ketamine-induced psychotic-like symptoms. This study showed that psychotomimetic doses of *s*-ketamine decreased the in-vivo binding of [^{11}C]-raclopride while eliciting psychotic-like symptoms. Dopamine release in the ventral striatum also correlated with heightened mood (euphoria and grandiosity). This provided additional evidence that the glutamate NMDA receptor may contribute to psychotic symptoms. Indeed, even in normal volunteers, studies have suggested evidence for ketamine-induced symptoms (Krystal *et al.*, 2005). These dopamine release effects, while not greater than those with IV amphetamine, were similar to the clinical symptomatology seen in schizophrenia. Thus, there is evidence of this relationship between indirect NMDA antagonists and dopamine release. These challenge studies with NMDA antagonists may simulate a hypoglutamatergic state, the subsequent effects on dopamine release, and may relate to positive symptoms.

PET/SPECT imaging in CNS drug development

Neuroreceptor imaging has a major role in aiding how to administer a clinically effective drug dose that minimizes dose-dependent side effects. At a given dose, plasma concentrations of antipsychotic drugs vary widely because of large inter-individual differences including absorption, metabolism, and excretion. PET and SPECT have been used extensively to document the relationships between receptor occupancy and plasma concentrations of the antipsychotic medication under study. PET occupancy measures have now reached the status almost of biomarkers, and are often critical in decision-making in the development of new antipsychotics. Determination of the appropriate occupancy level for various classes of drugs is vital to streamlining drug development. These studies have also helped to elucidate the mechanism of action of some psychotropic drugs, including some of the newer-generation antipsychotics, including the study of serotonin occupancy.

D$_2$ receptor occupancy and effects of antipsychotic medication

Lars Farde and collaborators (Farde *et al.*, 1988, 1990; Reith *et al.*, 1994; Wong 2002a, 2002b) demonstrated that clinically effective doses of typical neuroleptics occupy D$_2$-like dopamine receptors in the range between 65 and 90% in patients with schizophrenia. This so-called "therapeutic window" of D$_2$ receptor occupancy was predictive for sufficient treatment response, and a plateau of about 80% occupancy for extrapyramidal side effects (EPS) was confirmed,

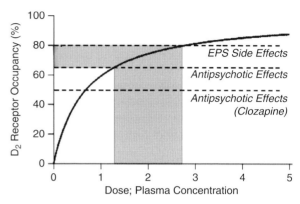

Figure 4.3 Relationship between striatal D$_2$ receptor occupancy and clinical effects. (From Farde *et al.*, 1988, with permission.)

especially for first-generation antipsychotics (Figure 4.3). Generally, the incidence of EPS increases in a dose-dependent manner, and also applies for most of the second-generation antipsychotics, including olanzapine and risperidone. Overall, striatal D$_2$ occupancy increases to levels that are associated with a higher incidence of EPS for both first- and second-generation antipsychotics.

Some exceptions include clozapine and quetiapine, which occupy a maximum of 60–70% of striatal D$_2$-like dopamine receptors even at extremely high plasma concentrations. For example, 24 h after the last administration of quetiapine, a significant occupancy of striatal D$_2$ receptors is no longer detectable as determined by PET. These particular characteristics of clozapine and quetiapine are most likely due to their low D$_2$ affinity. Thus, the tolerability and safety of these drugs is limited by other mechanisms rather than EPS.

A novel approach to the treatment of schizophrenia is that some antipsychotics act as dopamine stabilizers, and may provide beneficial therapeutic effects for the positive symptoms without the significant EPS, even with receptor occupancy exceeding 80% (Carlsson, 1999; Gründer *et al.*, 2003; Wong and Brašić, 2005). Aripiprazole (Abilify) is a relatively recent example of a dopamine stabilizer occupying as many as 95% of available dopamine D$_2$ receptors in patients under chronic treatment (Gründer *et al.*, 2003; Wong and Brašić, 2005). These dopamine stabilizers likely produce beneficial effects with minimal adverse effects by exhibiting both weak partial agonism and antagonism for dopamine D$_2$ receptors (Gründer *et al.*, 2003; Wong and Brašić, 2005). Aripiprazole (Abilify) leads to complete saturation of striatal D_2 receptors, as demonstrated in PET studies (Yokoi *et al.*, 2002), where efficiency occurs closer to 90% occupancy, perhaps due to the partial DA agonism. A review of Proof of Concept in CNS drug development and other uses of neuroreceptor imaging can be reviewed in (Wong *et al.*, 2009).

Box 4.1. Summary box

- Alterations in the density, the distribution, and the function of dopamine D_2/D_3 receptors in the brain play a role in the pathophysiology of schizophrenia.
- The dopamine hypothesis of schizophrenia proposes that schizophrenia results from dysfunction of dopaminergic neurotransmission in the brain.
- The positive symptoms of schizophrenia are alleviated when 60–80% of dopamine D_2 receptors in the brain are occupied by antipsychotic drugs as demonstrated by positron emission tomography (PET) and single photon emission computed tomography (SPECT).
- PET/SPECT neuroreceptor occupancy facilitates the determination of the likely optimal dose of dopamine D_2 receptor blocking drugs to produce a therapeutic effect with minimal adverse effects.
- The study of the binding of neuroreceptors is typically made by a single PET or SPECT scan to measure the binding potential (BP), the ratio of the receptor density (B_{max}) to the radioligand equilibrium dissociation constant (K_D), the inverse of the affinity of ligand binding, as follows:

$$BP = \frac{B_{max}}{K_D} = B_{max} \times \frac{1}{K_D} = B_{max} \times \text{affinity}$$

- Increased striatal dopamine D_2 receptor density is associated with the positive symptoms of schizophrenia.
- Some people with schizophrenia have abnormally elevated intra-synaptic levels of dopamine in the phasic, excited state.
- People with schizophrenia exhibit greater [^{18}F]-fluorodopa binding in the striatum. This finding suggests elevations of dopamine in both tonic, resting, and phasic, excited, states in schizophrenia.
- Serotonin (5-HT$_{2A}$) receptors are reduced in the prefrontal cortex of drug-naive people with schizophrenia.
- Clinically effective doses of typical neuroleptics occupy 65–90% of the D_2-like dopamine receptors in patients with schizophrenia. When more than 80% of D_2-like dopamine receptors are occupied, there is a marked risk of extrapyramidal side effects (EPS).

Acknowledgments

Grant support in part from: K24, DA00412, and MH078175 (DFW) Special Thanks for help from Ayon Nandi, MS, and discourse with Gerhard Grunder, MD.

References

Abi-Dargham A, Kegeles L S, Zea-Ponce Y, *et al.* 2004. Striatal amphetamine-induced dopamine release in patients with schizotypal personality disorder studied with single photon emission computed tomography and [123I]iodobenzamide. *Biol Psychiatry* **55**, 1001–06.

Abi-Dargham A, Rodenhiser J, Printz D, *et al.* 2000. Increased baseline occupancy of D_2 receptors by dopamine in schizophrenia. *Proc Natl Acad Sci U S A* **97**, 8104–09.

Adams B W, Bradberry C W and Moghaddam B. 2002. NMDA antagonist effects on striatal dopamine release: microdialysis studies in awake monkeys. *Synapse* **43**, 12–8.

Breier A, Su T P, Saunders R, *et al.* 1997. Schizophrenia is associated with elevated amphetamine-induced synaptic dopamine concentrations: evidence from a novel positron emission tomography method. *Proc Natl Acad Sci U S A* **94**, 2569–74.

Buchsbaum M S, Christian B T, Lehrer D S, *et al.* 2006. D2/D3 dopamine receptor binding with [F-18]fallypride in thalamus and cortex of patients with schizophrenia. *Schizophr Res* **85**, 232–44.

Carlsson A. 1999. Birth of neuropsychopharmacology – impact on brain research. *Brain Res Bull* **50**, 363.

Carlsson A, Waters N and and Carlsson M L. 1999. Neurotransmitter interactions in schizophrenia – therapeutic implications. *Biol Psychiatry* **46**, 1388–95.

Carson R E, Breier A, de Bartolomeis A, *et al.* 1997. Quantification of amphetamine-induced changes in [11C]raclopride binding with continuous infusion. *J Cerebr Blood Flow and Metab* **17**, 437–47.

Davidson L L and Heinrichs R W. 2003. Quantification of frontal and temporal lobe brain-imaging findings in schizophrenia: a meta-analysis. *Psychiatry Res* **122**, 69–87.

Erritzoe D, Rasmussen H, Kristiansen K, *et al.* 2006. Serotonin 2A binding in neuroleptics-naïve schizophrenic patients and healthy controls using PET and [18-F]altanserin. *NeuroImage* **31**, T44–186 [Abstract].

Erritzoe D, Rasmussen H, Kristiansen K T, *et al.* 2008. Cortical and subcortical 5-HT2A receptor binding in neuroleptic-naive first-episode schizophrenic patients. *Neuropsychopharmacology* **33**, 2435–41.

Farde L, Hall H, Ehrin E and Sedvall G. 1986. Quantitative analysis of D2 dopamine receptor binding in the living human brain by PET. *Science* **231**, 258–61.

Farde L, Wiesel F A, Halldin C and Sedvall G. 1988. Central D2-dopamine receptor occupancy in schizophrenic patients treated with antipsychotic drugs. *Arch Gen Psychiatry* **45**, 71–6.

Farde L, Wiesel F A, Stone-Elander S, *et al.* 1990. D2 dopamine receptors in neuroleptic-naive schizophrenic patients. A positron emission tomography study with [11C]raclopride. *Arch Gen Psychiatry* **47**, 213–9.

Frankle W G, Narendran R, Huang Y, *et al.* 2005. Serotonin transporter availability in patients with schizophrenia: a positron emission tomography imaging study with [11C]DASB. *Biol Psychiatry* **57**, 1510–6.

Grace A A. 1991. Phasic versus tonic dopamine release and the modulation of dopamine system responsivity: a hypothesis for the etiology of schizophrenia. *Neuroscience* **41**, 1–24.

Gründer G, Carlsson A and Wong D F. 2003. Mechanism of new antipsychotic medications: occupancy is not just antagonism. *Arch Gen Psychiatry* **60**, 974–7.

Gründer G, Fellows C, Janouschek H, *et al.* 2008. Brain and plasma pharmacokinetics of aripiprazole in patients with schizophrenia: An [18F]fallypride PET study. *Am J Psychiatry* **165**, 988–95.

Hurlemann R, Boy C, Meyer P T, *et al.* 2005. Decreased prefrontal 5-HT2A receptor binding in subjects at enhanced risk for schizophrenia. *Anat Embryol (Berl)* **210**, 519–23.

Innis R B, Cunningham V J, Delforge J, *et al.* 2007. Consensus nomenclature for in vivo imaging of reversibly binding radioligands. *J Cereb Blood Flow Metab* **27**, 1533–9.

Joyce J N, Shane A, Lexow N, Winokur A, Casanova M F and Kleinman J E. 1993. Serotonin uptake sites and serotonin receptors are altered in the limbic system of schizophrenics. *Neuropsychopharmacology* **8**, 315–36.

Krystal J H, Abi-Saab W, Perry E, *et al.* 2005. Preliminary evidence of attenuation of the disruptive effects of the NMDA glutamate receptor antagonist, ketamine, on working memory by pretreatment with the group II metabotropic glutamate receptor agonist, LY354740, in healthy human subjects. *Psychopharmacology (Berl)* **179**, 303–9.

Laruelle M. 1998. Imaging dopamine transmission in schizophrenia. A review and meta-analysis. *Q J Nucl Med* **42**, 211–21.

Laruelle M, Abi-Dargham A, Casanova M F, Toti R, Weinberger D R and Kleinman J E. 1993. Selective abnormalities of prefrontal serotonergic receptors in schizophrenia: a postmortem study. *Arch Gen Psychiatry* **50**, 810–8.

Laruelle M, Abi-Dargham A, van Dyck C H, Gil R and D'Souza C D. 1996. Single photon emission computerized tomography imaging of amphetamine-induced dopamine release in drug-free schizophrenic subjects. *Proc Natl Acad Sci U S A* **93**, 9235–40.

Laruelle M, Abi-Dargham A, van Dyck C, *et al.* 2000. Dopamine and serotonin transporters in patients with schizophrenia: an imaging study with [(123)I]beta-CIT. *Biol Psychiatry* **47**, 371–9.

Martinez D, Gelernter J, Abi-Dargham A, *et al.* 2001. The variable number of tandem repeats polymorphism of the dopamine transporter gene is not associated with significant change in dopamine transporter phenotype in humans. *Neuropsychopharmacology* **24**, 553–60.

Matusch A, Hurlemann R, Rota Kops E, *et al.* 2007. Acute *S*-ketamine application does not alter cerebral [18F]altanserin binding: a pilot PET study in humans. *J Neural Transm* **114**, 1433–42.

Mukherjee J, Christian B T, Dunigan K A, *et al.* 2002. Brain imaging of 18F-fallypride in normal volunteers: blood analysis, distribution, test-retest studies and preliminary assessment of sensitivity to aging effects on dopamine D_2/D_3 receptors. *Synapse*, **46**, 170–88.

Mukherjee J, Christian B T, Narayanan T K, Shi B and Collins D. 2005. Measurement of D-amphetamine-induced effects on the binding of dopamine D_2/D_3 receptor radioligand, ^{18}F-fallypride in extrastriatal brain regions in non human primates using PET. *Brain Res* **1032**, 77–84.

Mukherjee J, Christain B T, Narayanan T K, Shi B and Mantil J. 2001. Evaluation of dopamine D_2 receptor occupancy by clozapine, risperidone and haloperidol in vivo in the rodent and nonhuman primate brain using ^{18}F-fallypride. *Neuropsychopharmacology*, **25**, 476–88.

Mukherjee J, Shi B, Christian B T, Chattopadhyay S, and Narayanan T K. 2004. ^{11}C-fallypride: radiosynthesis and preliminary evaluation of a novel dopamine D_2/D_3 receptor PET radiotracer in non-human primate brain. *Bioorg Med Chem* **12**, 95–102.

Munro C A, McCaul M E, Oswald L M, *et al.* 2006a. Striatal dopamine release and family history of alcoholism. *Alcohol Clin Exp Res* **30**, 1143–51.

Munro C A, McCaul M E, Wong D F, *et al.* 2006b. Sex differences in striatal dopamine release in healthy adults. *Biol Psychiatry* **59**, 966–74.

Nozaki S, Kato M, Takano H, *et al.* 2009. Regional dopamine synthesis in patients with schizophrenia using L-[beta-11C]DOPA PET. *Schizophr Res* **108**, 78–84.

Nyberg S, Olsson H, Nilsson U, Maehlum E, Halldin C and and Farde L. 2002. Low striatal and extra-striatal D2 receptor occupancy during treatment with the atypical antipsychotic sertindole. *Psychopharmacology (Berl)* **162**, 37–41.

Oswald L M, Wong D F, McCaul M, *et al.* 2005. Relationships among ventral striatal dopamine release, cortisol secretion, and subjective responses to amphetamine. *Neuropsychopharmacology* **30**, 821–32.

Rasmussen H, Erritzoe D, Andersen R, *et al.* 2010. Decreased frontal serotonin 2A receptor binding in antipsychotic-naïve patients with first-episode schizophrenia. *Arch Gen Psychiatry* **67**, 9–16.

Reith J, Benkelfat C, Sherwin A, *et al.* 1994. Elevated dopa decarboxylase activity in living brain of patients with psychosis. *Proc Natl Acad Sci U S A* **91**, 11 651–4.

Singer H S, Szymanski S, Guiliano J, *et al.* 2002. Elevated intrasynaptic dopamine release in Tourette's syndrome measured by PET. *Am J Psychiatry* **159**, 1329–36.

Talvik-Lotfi M, Nyberg S, Nordström A L, *et al.* 2000. High 5HT2A receptor occupancy in M100907-treated schizophrenic patients. *Psychopharmacology (Berl)* **148**, 400–03.

Wagner H N, Jr, Burns H D, Dannals R F, *et al.* 1983. Imaging dopamine receptors in the human brain by positron tomography. *Science* **221**, 1264–6.

Wong D F. 2002a. In vivo imaging of D2 dopamine receptors in schizophrenia: the ups and downs of neuroimaging research. *Arch Gen Psychiatry* **59**, 31–4.

Wong D F. 2002b. [Erratum] In vivo imaging of D2 dopamine receptors in schizophrenia: the ups and downs of neuroimaging research. *Arch Gen Psychiatry* **59**, 440.

Wong D F, Potter W Z and Brašić J R. 2002. Proof of concept: functional models for drug development in humans. In Davis K L, Charney D, Coyle J T and Nemeroff C (Eds) *Neuropsychopharmacology: The Fifth Generation of Progress*. Baltimore, MD: Lippincott Williams and Wilkins, pp. 457–73.

Wong D F and Brašić J R. 2005. Progress in the neuropsychiatry of schizophrenia. *Psychiatric Times* **22**(3), 57–60.

Wong D F, Gjedde A, Wagner H N, Jr, *et al.* 1986. Quantification of neuroreceptors in the living human brain. II. inhibition studies of receptor density and affinity. *J Cerebr Blood Flow Metab* **6**, 147–53.

Wong D F, Kuwabara H, Schretlen D J, *et al.* 2006. Increased occupancy of dopamine receptors in human striatum during cue-elicited cocaine craving. *Neuropsychopharmacology* **31**, 2716–27. Erratum in: *Neuropsychopharmacology* 2007; **32**, 256.

Wong D F, Brašić J R, Singer H S, *et al.* 2008. Mechanisms of dopaminergic and serotonergic neurotransmission in Tourette Syndrome: clues from an *in vivo* neurochemistry study with PET. *Neuropsychopharmacology* **33**, 1239–51.

Wong D F, Maini A, Rousset O G and Brašić J R. 2003. Positron emission tomography: a tool for identifying the effects of alcohol dependence on the brain. *Alcohol Res Health* **27**, 161–73.

Wong D F, Tauscher J and Gründer G. 2009. The role of imaging in proof of concept for CNS drug discovery and development. *Neuropsychopharmacology*, **34**, 187–203.

Wong D F, Wagner H N Jr, Dannals R F, *et al.* 1984. Effects of age on dopamine and serotonin receptors measured by positron tomography in the living human brain. *Science* **226**, 1393–6.

Yasuno F, Suhara T, Okubo Y, *et al.* 2004. Low dopamine d(2) receptor binding in subregions of the thalamus in schizophrenia. *Am J Psychiatry* **161**, 1016–22.

Yokoi F, Gründer G, Biziere K, *et al.* 2002. Dopamine D2 and D3 receptor occupancy in normal humans treated with the antipsychotic drug aripiprazole (OPC 14597): a study using positron emission tomography and [11C] raclopride. *Neuropsychopharmacology* **27**, 248–59.

Zanardi R, Artigas F, Moresco R, *et al.* 2001. Increased 5-hydroxytryptamine-2 receptor binding in the frontal cortex of depressed patients responding to paroxetine treatment: a positron emission tomography scan study. *J Clin Psychopharmacol* **21**, 53–8.

Chapter 5

Neuroimaging of schizophrenia: commentary

Nancy Andreasen

As demonstrated in the previous four chapters, neuroimaging technologies have revolutionized our capacity to study schizophrenia and our understanding of its neural substrates and neural mechanisms. At the end of the first decade of the twenty-first century, it seems appropriate to take stock of how far we have in fact come.

The "Dark Ages" of schizophrenia research

When I began my career as a schizophrenia researcher in the mid 1970s, we had no way to directly study the malfunctioning organ that was producing the illness: the brain. In fact, it did not occur to most psychiatrists that the brain was the organ that they should study! The field of "biological psychiatry" was engaged in a fruitless examination of peripheral metabolites, such as platelet monoamine oxidase – a very remote window into the brain. As a young student of schizophrenia, I instead chose to study language and cognition, because they seemed to me to be a better window, since they at least clearly reflected the functional activity of the brain.

When I saw my first Computerized Tomography (CT) scan around this time, however, it was clear to me that this kind of technology offered enormous potential for studying schizophrenia, since it could permit us to make quantitative brain measurements using case-control designs. Because it required radiation exposure, however, and because our Insitutional Review Board was convinced that we would not learn anything about schizophrenia by conducting brain measurements, the honor of conducting the first CT study of schizophrenia was captured by the Northwick Park group in England (Johnstone *et al.*,

1976). The early CT studies firmly established that schizophrenia is a brain disorder with a measurable structural component that can be observed at the gross anatomic level when groups of patients are pooled together, averaged, and compared with normal volunteer control subjects. Measurement techniques were primitive, however. The principal measurement generated from CT, the ventricular brain ratio (VBR), was produced using a planimeter! And it was an extremely crude index of overall brain tissue loss – at that time typically referred to as "atrophy". Nonetheless, CT studies yielded many useful findings. Structural brain abnormalities were shown to be present from the outset, and ventricular enlargement was associated with poor pre-morbid functioning, negative symptoms, poor response to treatment, and cognitive impairment (Johnstone *et al.*, 1976; Weinberger *et al.*, 1980; Andreasen *et al.*, 1982).

The "Middle Ages"

By the early 1980s, a thrilling new imaging technology emerged: Magnetic Resonance Imaging (MRI). Seeing the enormous promise of MRI, with its beautiful anatomical resolution, I resolved to conduct the first quantitative MR study of schizophrenia (or any mental illness) and in that study reported a selective decrease in the frontal cortex, in addition to smaller cerebral and intra-cranial size, in a group of 38 patients with schizophrenia and 39 normal controls (Andreasen *et al.*, 1986). We suggested that this combination of findings was consistent with a neurodevelopmental process in which the brain failed to grow normally, rather than with a neurodegenerative process. We also resolved to abandon our planimeter, to collaborate with colleagues with expertise in computer science and biomedical engineering, and to write dedicated software custom-designed for rapid quantitative image analysis of MR data (Cohen *et al.*, 1992; Andreasen *et al.*, 1992; Cizadlo *et al.*, 1997).

A floodgate was opened. Now, some 25 years later, the family of MR technologies has expanded to include structural MR (sMR), diffusion tensor imaging (DTI), functional MR (fMR), and magnetic resonance spectroscopy (MRS). In addition, positron emission tomography (PET) permits us to do quantitative measurements of regional cerebral blood flow (rCBF) and receptor occupancy. An abundance of sophisticated software packages, many of them employing elegant statistical techniques, is available to facilitate rapid and automated image processing (Gold *et al.*, 1998; Worsley *et al.*, 1992; Arndt *et al.*, 1996). As demonstrated in this book as a whole, neuroimaging has become a major psychiatric research tool that is being applied to a broad range of diseases and to fundamental questions of cognitive neuroscience. Eight hundred papers have now been published on sMR abnormalities in schizophrenia alone. Thousands of papers have been published using neuroimaging technologies to study various mental illnesses.

The modern era

What have we learned about schizophrenia since the dawn of the neuroimaging era some 35 years ago? And what opportunities are in our future?

1. *We have moved from the use of crude indices of generalized tissue loss, such as the VBR, to increasingly refined measurements of specific cortical and subcortical brain regions, and our models for describing the nature of the brain dysfunction in schizophrenia have become increasingly more sophisticated.*

During the "middle ages" of imaging research, we moved from asking "Can schizophrenia be localized in the *brain*?" to "Can schizophrenia be *localized* in the brain?" Psychiatry had traded the ego, id, and super ego for the prefrontal cortex, the temporal lobes, and subcortical regions such as the thalamus or basal ganglia. It had joined hands with neurology, neuropsychology, and cognitive neuroscience. Early in the modern era investigators tended to emphasize the study of specific brain regions in relation to cognitive functions and illness symptoms (e.g. Shenton *et al.*, 1992). The prefrontal cortex was the ruler of

"executive functions"; it mediated processes such as working memory, decision-making, and goal initiation; it was potentially linked to negative symptoms. The temporal cortex and its subregions ruled over language and components of memory, and was potentially linked to positive symptoms such as auditory hallucinations. And so on. While this approach was valuable, because it reduced the nearly overwhelming complexity of the brain to manageable "concept bites", it also led to oversimplified models. As described in the chapters on structural and functional imaging, the field has now advanced to more complex network and connectivity models that more realistically capture the way that the brain actually works.

2. *There is now a relatively widespread consensus that schizophrenia should be conceptualized as a neurodevelopmental disorder. The finer details of "when?" and "how?" are still being parsed, however.*

The issue of "when" turns on the question of whether the initial hit occurs in the perinatal period, whether it occurs during adolescence, or whether it occurs in both time periods as a "two hit hypothesis". The two time periods are typically referred to as "early neurodevelopment" or "late neurodevelopment". The current prevailing opinion tends to favor "late neurodevelopment" occurring during the timeframe of adolescence, particularly because it gives more leverage on the "how" question. sMR studies of normal individuals have enhanced our understanding of the brain changes that occur during childhood, adolescence, young adulthood, and later life. These have documented the expansion of white matter (WM) during adolescence/young adulthood and the coincident pruning of gray matter (GM) (Sowell *et al.*, 2001). This information, combined with the characteristic age of onset of schizophrenia during this time period, suggests that overpruning could be a potential mechanism that could explain the occurrence of the brain abnormalities that have been shown to be present in first-episode patients (Feinberg, 1982).

The time course of brain changes after onset is less well characterized in the sMR literature, due chiefly to the inherent difficulty in executing the appropriate design: a prospective longitudinal study of first-episode patients that examines these patients over the lifetime trajectory of the illness. While some evidence suggests that most of the tissue loss occurs early in the illness and does not progress, the data addressing this topic are limited by small samples (usually only 15–30 subjects) and short time periods (usually 1–5 years) (DeLisi, 2008; Cahn *et al.*, 2002; Whitford *et al.*, 2006). Given that some patients show cognitive and clinical decline during the 5–20 years after onset, it is plausible to hypothesize that these changes could be accompanied by (and are presumably due to) ongoing brain tissue loss during later stages of the illness as well.

Achieving clarity on this issue is handicapped, however, by the ambiguous meaning of the term "neurodevelopmental". In some usages it refers to a time period (e.g. perinatal, adolescent). In other usages it refers to a process (e.g. formation of synapses, spines, and dendritic arbors; neuronal migration; myelination). Some of these processes are linked to time periods (e.g. neuronal migration during fetal development), while others are ongoing throughout life (e.g. synapse formation as an ongoing neuroplastic process that is driven by learning and memory). In the instance when the process is ongoing throughout life, it could be argued that brain changes measured during the later phases of the illness (or during later phases of life in normal individuals) are due to aberrations in neurodevelopment – i.e. a failure in any of the various mechanisms that drive and regulate neuroplasticity. In this instance, the boundary between neurodevelopmental processes and neurodegenerative processes (when used to refer to brain changes occurring in mid- and late-life) is blurred. Perhaps we should limit the meaning of the term "neurodegeneration" to demonstrable neuronal loss, as is implied in Chapter 1.

3. *Functional imaging has come of age with the advent of fMR, as a consequence of interdisciplinary collaborations that include psychologists, cognitive neuroscientists, basic neuroscientists, psychiatrists, statisticians, radiologists, biomedical engineers, and geneticists.*

The technical challenges of positron emission tomography (PET), the need for a cyclotron and a radiochemist, and design limitations imposed by repeated radiation exposure prevented this functional imaging modality from becoming widely available. Nonetheless, PET research laid the foundations of functional imaging research in psychiatry. Most of the fundamental problems inherent in functional imaging were first worked out in the world of PET: methods for correcting for multiple comparisons in correlated voxels, identification of appropriate sample sizes, selection of tasks that were suitable for both patients and controls, and addressing between-group differences in task performance (e.g. Andreasen *et al.*, 1996). PET was used to explore many facets of cognition and emotion in schizophrenia, providing multiple "ready-made" task designs that could be adapted to fMR.

While few sites have PET scanners, everyone has an MR scanner, and the advent of fMR opened up opportunities to do functional imaging studies to a broad range and a large number of investigators.

Chapter 2 nicely summarizes the various issues that have been confronted and experimental designs that have been developed in the fMR world. In an interesting twist of direction, functional imaging – which began by studying the resting state using fluorodeoxyglucose (FDG) or O^{15} water and PET, has now come full circle: the study of REST (Random Episodic Silent Thought) is now perceived as a valuable experimental pursuit for tapping into self-referential thought and primary process thinking; both of these components of cognition are of interest to students of schizophrenia (Andreasen *et al.*, 1995). As described in Chapter 2, the introduction of Independent Component Analysis (ICA) has also introduced a novel exploratory statistical tool that can be used to integrate disparate data domains, such as fMR and genetics or fMR and structural imaging.

4. *MR Spectroscopy (MRS) is a promising technology whose potential is still developing.*

Unlike structural and functional imaging, spectroscopic imaging is still not widely used in schizophrenia research, although a great deal of preliminary work has been done to suggest its promise. As Chapter 3 makes clear, MRS research requires a reasonable knowledge of biochemistry, physical chemistry, and physics. Furthermore, for many applications, access to high-field MR equipment is needed, and this equipment is neither widely available nor easy to use even when it is available. Nonetheless, MRS offers exciting opportunities for studying the biochemical mechanisms of diseases such as schizophrenia. However, most of its potential is as yet unrealized.

5. *PET neuroreceptor imaging has provided an empirical scientific basis for determining drug mechanisms and drug doses.*

This field is another one that is not for the faint-hearted or mathematically disadvantaged. Those without access to cyclotrons, radiochemists, and a large, well-trained interdisciplinary research team will not be able to conduct PET neuroreceptor research. However, the fields of psychiatry and neuropsychopharmacology have benefited greatly from this work. Thanks to PET research pioneered at Hopkins, the Karolinska Institute, and Brookhaven, we now have methods for doing in-vivo pharmacology. This work is technically challenging, in that it requires developing radioligands that cross the blood–brain barrier and are safe, easy to measure, and informative. Once developed, such ligands can be used to ask basic questions about distribution of receptors in the living human brain; for example, what is the distribution and density of extrastriatal D2 receptors? how does that distribution compare with other types of dopamine receptors? These ligands can be used to address pathophysiological questions; for example, do first-episode neuroleptic-naive patients have a higher or lower density of D2 receptors than normal controls? Perhaps most important in terms of clinical applications, they can be used to measure receptor occupancy at variable doses of medication in order to study dose–response curves. This latter application has been the most fruitful. We now have empirical data that define the therapeutic window for many of our most commonly used neuroleptic medications.

The future

Imaging technologies have become mature enough to address fundamental questions about the brain mechanisms of schizophrenia. In a sense there have been more limitations in experimental design and analysis than in the technologies themselves. For example, most studies examine chronic patients who have received large amounts of neuroleptic medications and are on neuroleptics at the time that imaging data are collected. We do not know the extent to which these data are compromised by neuroleptic effects, but we now have some evidence that these medications can change both brain structure and function (Dorph-Petersen et al., 2005; Lieberman et al., 2005; Miller et al., 2001). Optimally the field needs more studies of neuroleptic-naive patients and matched controls who are studied using longitudinal rather than cross-sectional designs, so that we can dissect medication effects from disease effects. Such studies are at present done very infrequently, for several reasons. First, such patients are difficult to find and to retain in research

studies. Second, the payoff is slow because the initial results will not be available for 3–5 years, and perhaps longer. Third, funding mechanisms are not designed to support this type of work, since funding occurs in 5-year segments, and yet a period of 10 years is needed for the recruitment and follow-up of an adequate sample size, given the scarcity of such patients.

The rapid growth of spinoffs in the MR world suggests that this technology is likely to continue to develop, and that these new developments will continue to be applied to the study of schizophrenia. In the world of MRS, a future goal is to develop the MR sequences and the analysis tools for conducting whole-brain MRS. In the world of sMR, goals include improved measurement of actual fiber tracts with DTI and improved resolution of GM imaging for visualization of cellular alignment. In the world of fMR, goals include methods to measure blood flow and metabolism rather than the BOLD effect.

Acknowledgments

This paper was written with support from the following grants MHCRC: Neurobiology and Phenomenology of the Major Psychoses (MH43271); Phenomenology and the Classification of Schizophrenia (5R01MH031593); MR Imaging in the Major Psychoses (5R01MH040856); Training in the Neurobiology of Schizophrenia and evaluation with DTI (Magnotta K award); and BRAINS Morphology and Image Analysis (5R01NS050568).

References

Andreasen N C, Arndt S, Cizadlo T, et al. 1996. Sample size and statistical power in ^{15}O H$_2$O studies of human cognition. *Journal of Cerebral Blood Flow and Metabolism* **16**, 804–16.

Andreasen N C, Cohen G C, Harris G, Parkkinen J, Rezai K and Swayze V W. 1992. Image processing for the study of brain structure and function: Problems and programs. *Journal of Neuropsychiatry and Clinical Neuroscience* **4**, 125–33.

Andreasen N C, Nasrallah H A, Dunn V, et al. 1986. Structural abnormalities in the frontal system in schizophrenia: A magnetic resonance imaging study. *Archives of General Psychiatry* **43**, 136–44.

Andreasen N C, O'Leary D S, Cizadlo T, A et al. 1995. Remembering the past: Two facets of episodic memory explored with positron emission tomography. *American Journal of Psychiatry* **152**, 1576–85.

Andreasen N C, Olsen S A, Dennert J W and Smith M R. 1982. Ventricular enlargement in schizophrenia: Relationship to positive and negative symptoms. *American Journal of Psychiatry* **139**, 297–302.

Arndt S, Cizadlo T, Andreasen N C, Heckel D, Gold S and O'Leary D. 1996. Tests for comparing images based on randomization and permutation methods. *Journal of Cerebral Blood Flow and Metabolism* **16**, 1271–9.

Cahn W, Hulshoff Pol H E, Lems E B, *et al.* 2002. Brain volume changes in first-episode schizophrenia: A 1-year follow-up study. *Archives of General Psychiatry* **59**, 1002–10.

Cizadlo T, Harris G, Heckel D, *et al.* 1997. An automated method to quantify the area, depth, and convolutions of the cerebral cortex from MR data: (BRAINSURF). *Neuroimage* **5**, 402.

Cohen G, Andreasen N C, Alliger R, *et al.* 1992. Segmentation techniques for the classification of brain tissue using magnetic resonance imaging. *Psychiatric Research: Neuroimaging* **45**, 33–51.

DeLisi L E. 2008. The concept of progressive brain change in schizophrenia: Implications for understanding schizophrenia. *Schizophrenia Bulletin* **34**, 312–21.

Feinberg I. 1982. Schizophrenia: Caused by a fault in programmed synaptic elimination during adolescence? *Journal of Psychiatric Research* **17**, 319–34.

Dorph-Petersen K A, Pierri J N, Perel J M, Sun Z, Sampson A R, and Lewis D A. 2005. The influence of chronic exposure to antipsychotic medications on brain size before and after tissue fixation: A comparison of haloperidol and olanzapine in macaque monkeys. *Neuropsychopharmacology* **30**, 1649–61.

Gold S, Christiansen B, Arndt S, *et al.* 1998. Functional MRI statistical software packages: A comparative analysis. *Human Brain Mapping* **6**, 73–84.

Johnstone E C, Frith C D, Crow T J, Husband J and Kreel L. 1976. Cerebral ventricular size and cognitive impairment in chronic schizophrenia. *Lancet* **2**, 924–6.

Lieberman J A, Tollefson G D, Charles C, *et al.* 2005. Antipsychotic drug effects on brain morphology in first-episode psychosis. *Archives of General Psychiatry* **62**, 361–70.

Miller D D, Andreasen N C, O'Leary D S, Watkins G L, Boles Ponto L L and Hichwa R D. 2001. Comparison of the effects of risperidone and haloperidol on regional cerebral blood flow in schizophrenia. *Biological Psychiatry* **49**, 704–15.

Shenton M E, Kikinis R, Jolesz F A, *et al.* 1992. Abnormalities of the left temporal lobe and thought disorder in schizophrenia: A quantitative magnetic resonance imaging study. *New England Journal of Medicine* **327**, 604–12.

Sowell E R, Thompson P M, Tessner K D and Toga A W. 2001. Mapping continued brain growth and gray matter density reduction in dorsal frontal cortex: Inverse relationships during postadolescent brain maturation. *Journal of Neuroscience* **21**, 8819–29.

Weinberger D R, Cannon-spoor E, Potkin S G and Wyatt R J. 1980. Poor premorbid adjustment and CT scan abnormalities in chronic schizophrenia. *American Journal of Psychiatry* **137**, 1410–3.

Whitford T J, Grieve S M, Farrow T F, *et al.* 2006. Progressive grey matter atrophy over the first 2–3 years of illness in first-episode schizophrenia: A tensor-based morphometry study. *Neuroimage* **32**, 511–9.

Worsley K, Evans A, Marrett S, and Neelin P. 1992. A three-dimensional statistical analysis for CBF activation studies in human brain. *Journal of Cerebral Blood Flow and Metabolism* **12**, 900–18.

Mood Disorders

Structural imaging of bipolar illness

Stephen M. Strakowski

Introduction

Bipolar disorder is a common psychiatric condition, affecting up to 3% of the world's population (Angst, 1998; Narrow *et al.*, 2002), and it is the sixth leading cause of disability worldwide (Murray and Lopez, 1996). Although bipolar disorder is defined by the occurrence of mania (type I disorder) or hypomania (type 2 disorder), in fact, the symptoms of bipolar disorder include affective instability, neurovegetative abnormalities, cognitive impairments, psychosis, and impulsivity. The likely neural basis of these symptoms, based on neuroimaging and other studies, has produced models of bipolar disorder that focus on dysfunction within so-called anterior limbic brain networks (Strakowski *et al.*, 2004, 2005, 2007; Adler *et al.*, 2006a; Brambilla *et al.*, 2005). These networks consist of iterative prefrontal–striatal–pallidal–thalamic circuits that are modulated by amygdala and other limbic structures to direct social and emotional behaviors. An example of one such anterior limbic network model is provided in Figure 6.1 and is based on work that has been reviewed previously (Strakowski *et al.*, 2005, 2007; Adler *et al.*, 2006a). Indeed, recent advances in neuroimaging techniques, particularly those based on magnetic resonance imaging (MRI) and spectroscopy, have revolutionized the study of bipolar neurophysiology, leading to a proliferation of studies attempting to clarify the neural substrates of bipolar disorder.

One approach toward evaluating and extending functional neuroanatomic models of bipolar disorder is to use brain imaging to determine whether structural brain abnormalities within relevant networks can be identified. Structural imaging is ultimately limited by the fact that intact or abnormal structure does not guarantee normal function or dysfunction, respectively. Nonetheless, the presence of structural abnormalities in bipolar disorder helps to reinforce and extend possible neuroanatomic models that might underlie the condition. Additionally, structural imaging may identify brain regions of interest to direct functional and neurochemical (e.g. spectroscopic) imaging, thereby potentially improving the power of these latter studies.

Since a number of recent reviews and meta-analyses of structural imaging of bipolar disorder have been published (e.g. McDonald *et al.*, 2004; Strakowski *et al.*, 2005, Konarski *et al.*, 2008; Kempton *et al.*, 2008), we will not exhaustively review prior work in this chapter. Instead, we will focus on recent structural neuroimaging studies that specifically address regions of interest in the proposed anterior limbic network model (Figure 6.1). Given the predominance of MRI in structural imaging of psychiatric disorders, we will focus on this imaging modality.

Anterior limbic network and bipolar disorder

To begin, we will review the network model illustrated in Figure 6.1. A major component of this network is the ventral prefrontal–striatal–pallidal–thalamic loop. It is well recognized that the prefrontal cortex (PFC) is a heterogeneous structure in which specific regions of PFC topographically map to specific regions of striatum, globus pallidus and thalamus, thereby providing relatively independent circuits that iteratively evaluate internal and external stimuli and direct various behavioral outputs (Mega *et al.*, 1997; Ongür and Price, 2000; Tekins and Cummings, 2002). In the model in Figure 6.1, ventromedial (orbitofrontal) and ventrolateral prefrontal cortices map to

Understanding Neuropsychiatric Disorders, ed. M. E. Shenton and B. I. Turetsky. Published by Cambridge University Press.
© Cambridge University Press 2011.

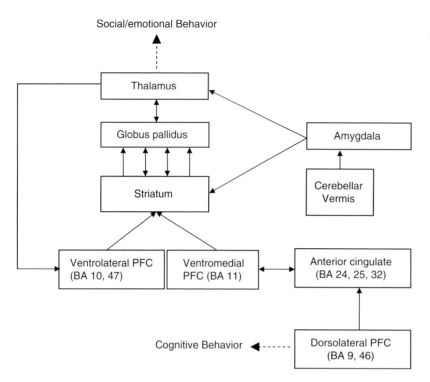

Social/emotional Behavior

Figure 6.1 Graphical representation of the anterior limbic network. PFC, prefrontal cortex; BA, Brodmann Area(s).

corresponding portions of the striatum (these circuits are combined in this model for simplicity, but are actually relatively distinct portions of a larger integrated network) that then connect through the corresponding locations on the globus pallidus and thalamus, only to connect back to the originating prefrontal area (Tekin and Cummings, 2002). This circuit is innervated through each of the components from diverse brain regions providing both processed and unprocessed external and internal data, which it then iteratively processes to produce emotional responses and social behavior (Tekins and Cummings, 2002). We hypothesize that the output from this iteration in bipolar patients is disturbed, leading to the affective instability and inappropriate interpersonal behavior that characterize mania and depression (Adler *et al.*, 2006a, Strakowski *et al.*, 2005). The amygdala nuclei and their extensions provide critical inputs into the network, which can be thought of simplistically as setting an "emotional tone" over the iterations. One could posit that if this "thermostat" is set incorrectly, maladaptive behaviors (e.g. mania) result. Although the cerebellum has been primarily viewed as an error detector within motor networks in order to provide coordinated intentional

motion, in fact the midline cerebellum (the vermis) is known to innervate the amygdala and modulate affective functions (Schmahmann *et al.*, 2007). Consequently, the vermis can be hypothesized to potentially perform a similar function (error detection) within these emotional networks consistent with the cerebellum's function in iterative prefrontal–striatal–pallidal–thalamic motor networks. Again, disruption of this function can produce erratic emotional behavior (Schmahmann *et al.*, 2007). The affective symptoms of bipolar disorder can then be posited to result from dysfunction within several or all of these integrated brain regions.

The anterior limbic network also connects to the anterior cingulate, which appears to integrate ventral and dorsal prefrontal neural streams (Yamasaki *et al.*, 2002). Indeed, these ventral and dorsal streams appear to inversely affect each other's function (Mayberg *et al.*, 1999; Yamasaki *et al.*, 2002). Consequently, if the anterior limbic network is dysfunctional, it might disrupt cognitive networks, resulting in the cognitive impairments exhibited in bipolar disorder (Bearden *et al.*, 2001). This brief review of the anterior limbic model of bipolar disorder provides an overview of more extensive discussions published elsewhere

(Adler *et al.*, 2006a; Strakowski *et al.*, 2005, 2007). A question arising from this discussion *vis-à-vis* neuroimaging is: "Do structural imaging studies identify abnormalities within this network in bipolar disorder, both to support and extend the neuroanatomic substrate of this model?" We will now focus on studies of the structures identified in Figure 6.1 to address this question.

Prefrontal cortex

The prefrontal cortex (PFC) is a functionally and histologically heterogeneous brain region in which specific regions topographically map to corresponding and specific regions within the striatum to initiate the iterative networks previously described (Tekins and Cummings, 2002). Functionally, then, the PFC modulates a wide variety of executive, emotional, social, and cognitive behaviors (Tekins and Cummings, 2002; Voorn *et al.*, 2004). Classic morphometric MRI approaches, in which specific structural boundaries are used to define specific regions of interest (ROIs), do not work well within the PFC, due to variability in sulcal and gyral landmarks among individuals, as well as variability within those landmarks in the anatomic boundaries of specific prefrontal functions. Consequently, many imaging studies of PFC have delineated relatively large ROIs (e.g. all gray matter anterior to the genu of the corpus callosum) that almost certainly lack functional specificity (Strakowski *et al.*, 2005). It is perhaps no surprise, then, that studies comparing bipolar to healthy subjects that examine large prefrontal regional volumes are equivocal (Strakowski *et al.*, 2005; Konarski *et al.*, 2008). However, in all cases, when differences have been reported, prefrontal volumes in bipolar subjects are smaller than in healthy subjects (e.g. Sax *et al.*, 1999, Coffman *et al.*, 1990). Moreover, Lyoo *et al.* (2006) found decreased cortical thickness in bipolar compared with healthy subjects, a finding that is consistent with the decreased prefrontal gray and white matter density observed in bipolar subjects by Haznedar and colleagues (2005). In order to interpret the clinical meaning of these putative findings, Sax *et al.* (1999) observed that decreased prefrontal volumes were associated with worse performance on an attentional task, and Haldane *et al.* (2008) found a lack of the healthy correlation between inhibitory control and prefrontal structure in bipolar disorder. These findings suggest that structural measurements

of even large, functionally non-specific prefrontal regions may inform performance on cognitive measures. Lyoo *et al.* (2006) found that the thickness of PFC was inversely correlated with the duration of illness, providing a potential marker of illness progression. In the end, however, these volumetric studies of large prefrontal areas are too few and the measures too non-specific to adequately inform neuroanatomic models of bipolar disorder.

To address this limitation, investigators have used two approaches. One is to define smaller prefrontal subregions based on sulcal and gyral landmarks within the PFC. As noted, subject variability limits the specificity of this approach as well, although presumably these smaller volumes are more likely to be functionally homogeneous than the overall, large prefrontal "slabs" reviewed previously. A second approach is to abandon landmarks and use a voxel-wise approach, similar to methods employed in fMRI research. This latter approach places subjects' brains into a common stereotactic framework and can then combine subjects within groups for comparisons without having to specifically delineate prefrontal subregions a priori (see Figure 6.3, for example). The trade-off with this method is that, virtually by definition, it is exploratory, which limits the statistical power of many studies due to relatively small samples. Nonetheless, with these approaches, investigators have evaluated some of the specific brain regions of interest in our anterior limbic model of bipolar disorder: namely, ventral (orbitofrontal), dorsolateral and anterior cingulate prefrontal cortices.

Ventral (orbitofrontal) prefrontal cortex

The ventral PFC (primarily within Brodmann areas (BA) 10, 11 and 47) appears to be responsible for integrating emotional and social behaviors, so that dysfunction within these prefrontal regions is likely to produce symptoms seen in bipolar disorder (Tekins and Cummings, 2002; Strakowski *et al.*, 2005; Blumberg *et al.*, 2006). Unlike the studies of larger prefrontal regions, studies of ventral PFC have more consistently reported gray matter decreases in bipolar compared with healthy subjects. Specifically, when comparing bipolar and healthy subjects using volumetric (ROI) approaches, although Chang *et al.* (2005) found no differences in an adolescent sample, three studies in adult patients observed smaller gray matter volumes in bipolar than healthy subjects

(Lopez-Larson *et al.*, 2002; Nugent *et al.*, 2006; Blumberg *et al.*, 2006). However, in contrast to the gray matter findings, these latter three studies reported increased white matter volume (Nugent *et al.*, 2006), decreased white matter volume (Blumberg *et al.*, 2006), and no white matter differences (Lopez-Larson *et al.*, 2002) between bipolar and healthy subjects. Consequently, decreases in the ventrolateral prefrontal cortex appear to reflect reduced gray matter. Additionally, both Nugent *et al.* (2006) and Blumberg *et al.* (2006) found that increased gray matter volumes were associated with increased medication exposure, suggesting that medication confounds may minimize some of the differences observed between healthy and bipolar subjects, as the latter are almost always receiving psychotropic medications in these studies.

Voxel-based morphometry (VBM) has generally supported the ROI findings, as several studies have observed reductions in ventral prefrontal cortical gray matter volumes or density (Wilke *et al.*, 2004; Farrow *et al.*, 2005; Lyoo *et al.*, 2004; Frangou *et al.*, 2005; Nugent *et al.*, 2006). Again, gray matter abnormalities were not observed in adolescent patients using VBM by Dickstein *et al.* (2005; although they were reported by Wilke *et al.*, 2004), nor in first-episode patients (Adler *et al.*, 2007). In another study, Adler *et al.* (2005) actually reported increased gray matter volume using VBM in the ventrolateral PFC of early-course bipolar patients. They suggested that these two latter early-course studies (Adler *et al.*, 2005, 2007), coupled with the findings in adolescents (Dickstein *et al.*, 2005; Chang *et al.*, 2005) and contrasted with older patients, supports a hypothesis that ventral gray matter volumes may decrease over time during the course of bipolar disorder. Supporting this notion, Brambilla *et al.* (2001a) and Lopez-Larson *et al.* (2002) found that gray matter volumes

were inversely associated with duration of bipolar illness. Blumberg *et al.* (2006) also found that the decline in ventral prefrontal cortical volume in young bipolar patients appeared to be more rapid than that in healthy subjects. Together, these studies suggest that progressive changes in ventral PFC may be associated with the early progression of bipolar disorder in which euthymic intervals become progressively shorter with each affective episode (Angst and Sellaro, 2000; Roy-Byrne *et al.*, 1985; Kraepelin, 1921; see Figure 6.2). However, whether the changes in ventral PFC precede the clinical progression, or instead result from recurring affective episodes, is not known.

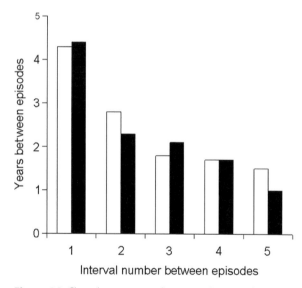

Figure 6.2 Chart demonstrating decreasing duration of intervals between successive affective episodes during the early course of bipolar disorder from two studies: white bar, Kraepelin (1921); black bar, Roy-Byrne *et al.* (1985).

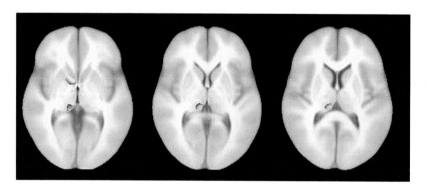

Figure 6.3 This image presents an example of voxel-based morphometry. In this contrast, 19 healthy and 28 bipolar subjects were compared in which significant differences were defined as $p<0.01$ for a cluster of 25 voxels. Orange areas indicate ares of reduced gray matter density in the bipolar subjects (Strakowski *et al.*, unpublished data).

Anterior cingulate cortex

The cingulate gyrus is located in cerebral midline beginning inferiorly to the genu of the corpus callosum (the subgenual prefrontal cortex, SGPFC, BA 25) and proceeding along the corpus callosum superiorly and posteriorly through the rostral anterior cingulate (BA 24) and dorsal anterior cingulate (BA 32). The SGPFC is heavily connected with limbic structures and, as the anterior cingulate is then followed superiorly and posteriorly, it appears to become progressively less connected to ventral brain regions associated with affective regulation and more connected to cognitive (dorsal) cortex. Consequently, the subgenual and anterior cingulate cortices appear to integrate cognitive and affective (dorsal and ventral) brain functions, modulating and integrating emotional and "logical" behavior (Devinsky et al., 1995). Given the dysregulation of these functions in bipolar disorder, the anterior cingulate plays potentially a central role in neuroanatomic models of the condition (Figure 6.1). Moreover, the subregions of anterior cingulate can be relatively consistently defined (even though it is not likely that there are distinct functional boundaries within these anatomic areas), so that there are a number of structural imaging studies examining this brain area in bipolar disorder.

Drevets et al. (1997) first reported that patients with bipolar disorder (and unipolar depression) and a family history of affective illness exhibited smaller left SGPFC volumes than healthy subjects. This finding was replicated by Hirayasu et al. (1999) and Koo et al. (2008) in combined samples of patients with first-episode psychotic affective (bipolar and unipolar) disorders, and in bipolar disorder by Sharma et al. (2003) and Haznedar et al. (2005). However, two other studies have not found differences in the SGPFC between healthy and bipolar subjects (Brambilla et al., 2002; Sanchez et al., 2005). It is likely that these different findings reflect differences in patient sampling and imaging approaches, although all of these studies used ROI methods. Although somewhat equivocal, these studies suggest that SGPFC abnormalities may occur, perhaps non-specifically, in bipolar and unipolar depressed patients with familial affective illness. Indeed, a meta-analysis of SGPFC studies found this decrease to be greatest on the left in unipolar, rather than bipolar, patients who also had a family history of affective illness (Hajek et al., 2008).

Additionally, the study by Koo et al. (2008) suggested that SGPFC volumes decrease over time, more so in patients who fail to improve with treatment than in treatment responders.

Similar findings have been observed in the remainder of the anterior cingulate. Most investigators found decreases in the ACC volumes, thickness or density in bipolar compared with healthy subjects (Wilke et al., 2004; Kaur et al., 2005; Farrow et al., 2005; Lyoo et al., 2004, 2006; Lochhead et al., 2004; Yatham et al., 2007; Chiu et al., 2008), although Sassi et al. (2004) found no differences and Javadapour et al. (2007) actually found an increase ACC volume in bipolar disorder. In a first-episode sample, Strakowski et al. (1993) also observed no differences between bipolar and healthy subjects in cingulate volume. However, since Farrow et al. (2005) found that anterior cingulate volumes decreased in bipolar patients during the first two years of illness, together, these studies may reflect a finding similar to that observed in ventral PFC: namely, that the anterior cingulate volume decreases with illness progression or duration. Complicating this story are two studies, using VBM methods, that have reported increased anterior cingulate gray matter volumes in bipolar versus healthy subjects (Adler et al., 2005; Frangou et al., 2002).

Together, these studies suggest decreases in some regions of the ACC in bipolar disorder, particularly in people with a family history of affective illness. These decreases may reflect progressive tissue losses in these brain areas during the course of bipolar illness. Additionally, a recent study by Fornito et al. (2008) found evidence of developmental abnormalities in the cingulate in bipolar disorder. Together, these findings converge with those of ventral PFC to suggest an underlying substrate of structural changes and perhaps developmental abnormalities in prefrontal areas in bipolar disorder. These specific prefrontal areas modulate mood, affect, and social interactions consistent with the symptoms of bipolar illness.

Dorsolateral PFC

The dorsolateral prefrontal cortex (DLPFC; BA 9, 10, 46) manages cognitive function, in particular working memory and attention, as well as the integration of cognitive processes to provide executive modulation of cognitive behavior. Patients with bipolar disorder express cognitive impairments, particularly during

- Prefrontal cortex's role in healthy brain:
  Ventral prefrontal (orbitofrontal) cortex – initiates iterative prefrontal–striatal–pallidal–thalamic circuit to modulate social/emotional behavior.
  Anterior cingulate cortex – integrates cognitive and emotional iterative networks (i.e. ventral and dorsal streams).
  Dorsolateral prefrontal cortex – initiates iterative prefrontal–striatal–pallidal–thalamic circuit to modulate cognitive behavior.
- Prefrontal cortex's relevance to bipolar disorder:
  Ventral prefrontal cortex – dysfunction leads to loss of emotional homeostasis and impulsive erratic behavior.
  Anterior cingulate cortex – dysfunction may lead to loss of inhibitory control.
  Dorsolateral prefrontal cortex – dysfunction leads to cognitive impairments, particularly in memory and attention.
- Prefrontal structural MRI findings – summary:
  Ventral prefrontal cortex – decreased gray matter volumes in bipolar versus healthy subjects that may progress with illness duration.
  Anterior cingulate cortex – decreased volumes, particularly in subgenual cingulate, that may progress with illness duration.
  Dorsolateral prefrontal cortex – equivocal changes that may be secondary to primary "emotional" cortex.

mood episodes, that may persist to a lesser degree into euthymia (Bearden *et al.*, 2001). These cognitive studies suggest possible involvement of the DLPFC in the neuroanatomic substrate of this illness.

Several studies observed decreased DLPFC gray matter volumes using both ROI and VBM methods in bipolar versus healthy subjects (Lopez-Larson *et al.*, 2002; McIntosh *et al.*, 2004; Frangou *et al.*, 2005; Dickstein *et al.*, 2005), although others have not (Schlaepfer *et al.*, 1994; Adler *et al.*, 2005, 2007; Chang *et al.*, 2005). Relatively speaking, there has been less attention to DLPFC in the study of bipolar disorder, as the focus has been more commonly directed toward areas of the prefrontal cortex thought to modulate mood (i.e. ventral PFC). The results of these studies of DLPFC are clearly equivocal. One could hypothesize that a primary abnormality in ventral and anterior cingulate cortical regions underlies bipolar disorder, consistent with mood symptoms

defining the condition, with reciprocal, secondary changes in cognitive (dorsal) brain. Indeed, as Mayberg *et al.* (1999) have demonstrated, the ventral and dorsal prefrontal cortices are inversely connected so that dysfunction in one leads to dysfunction in the other. Yamasaki *et al.* (2002) have suggested that anterior cingulate modulates these reciprocal interactions. Consequently, in our functional neuroanatomic model of Figure 6.1, we hypothesize that abnormalities observed in DLPFC are secondary, reflecting primary dysfunction within emotional (ventral) brain. Clearly, neuroanatomic studies cannot ultimately disentangle these considerations, as this work falls within the realm of functional (fMRI) and chemical (MRS) neuroimaging.

Striatum

Within our anterior limbic model, the prefrontal cortical areas project to the striatum (Figure 6.1). The striatum can be divided into dorsal and ventral divisions. The dorsal striatum consists of the caudate nucleus and the putamen. These two structures share a common embryology and histology and, in fact, the head of the caudate fuses with the anterior putamen (Bonelli *et al.*, 2006). The ventral striatum is comprised of the olfactory tubercle and the nucleus accumbens; the latter in particular shares histology with the dorsal striatum and is not actually a distinct nucleus (Voorn *et al.*, 2004). However, ultimately, a sharp distinction between ventral and dorsal striatum is probably imprecise (Voorn *et al.*, 2004).

The striatum serves as input nuclei into the larger basal ganglia system (which is comprised of the striatum plus globus pallidus and substantia nigra) (Bonelli *et al.*, 2006). The striatum receives diffuse input from the cerebral cortex, amygdala and hippocampus, as well as thalamus (Bonelli *et al.*, 2006). The ventral striatum and ventral caudate receive cortical input from brain areas consistent with a role in affective and reward processes, whereas the remaining caudate appears to modulate cognitive processes (Bonelli *et al.*, 2006; Voorn *et al.*, 2004). The putamen receives sensorimotor cortical fibers (Yelnik, 2002). Consequently, the striatum appears to provide the first-level processing of prefrontal information, and this input is then further modulated within the effector components of the basal ganglia (e.g. globus pallidus; Bonelli *et al.*, 2006; Yelnik, 2002; Voorn *et al.*, 2004). With its central location within the anterior limbic networks previously mentioned, the striatum has garnered some interest in the study of the neuroanatomy of bipolar disorder.

A number of studies identified striatal enlargement in subjects with bipolar disorder relative to healthy subjects (see Strakowski *et al.*, 2005 or Konarski *et al.*, 2008 for review). Specifically, enlargement was noted in studies of bipolar adolescents (Wilke *et al.*, 2004; DelBello *et al.*, 2004), adult first-episode patients (Strakowski *et al.*, 2002a), and adults with multiple affective episodes (Aylward *et al.*, 1994; Strakowski *et al.*, 1999; Sax *et al.*, 1999; Frangou *et al.*, 2002, 2005). Noga and colleagues (2001) observed increased caudate volumes in both bipolar subjects and their unaffected monozygotic twins. The first-episode and twin studies suggest this abnormality may predate illness onset and not simply reflect medication effects, since, notably, conventional antipsychotic use has been observed to enlarge striatum (Chakos *et al.*, 1994).

However, there are also a number of studies that did not observe striatal enlargement in bipolar relative to healthy subjects, including first-episode (Strakowski *et al.*, 1993), adolescent (Chang *et al.*, 2005) and adult (McIntosh *et al.*, 2004) samples. Moreover, even among the positive studies, when separately measured, enlargement was variably noted in caudate or putamen, but typically not both (Konarski *et al.*, 2008). We recently examined striatal volumes in 8–12-year-old children of bipolar parents (who did not meet criteria for bipolar disorder themselves) and matched children of healthy parents and found no differences between groups, although the number of subjects was relatively small (Singh *et al.*, 2008). A meta-analysis of most of these studies of striatal volumes found no differences between healthy and bipolar subjects (Kempton *et al.*, 2008). Some of these discrepancies may be explained by a study from Hwang and colleagues (2006). Although they did not observe striatal volume differences between bipolar and healthy subjects, they did report subtle shape differences in the anterior and ventral surfaces of the striatum, particularly on the right.

Although equivocal, there are enough positive studies of striatal enlargement in bipolar disorder that suggest anatomic abnormalities occur in this brain structure. However, these abnormalities may be subtle and limited to small regions of the ventral striatum and antero-ventral caudate/putamen, resulting in discrepant studies. In contrast, studies in unipolar depression often report decreased striatal volumes, and this difference between bipolar and unipolar depressive disorders has been suggested to potentially distinguish these conditions (Strakowski, 2002; Strakowski *et al.*, 2002b; Konarski *et al.*, 2008). Together, this work suggests that additional investigation is warranted into striatal dysfunction and morphometry as a potential component of the functional neuroanatomy of bipolar disorder, using more sophisticated or higher-resolution approaches (e.g. Hwang *et al.*, 2006).

Globus pallidus

The globus pallidus is the primary output structure of the basal ganglia. It is heavily connected to the striatum and, within the pallidus, integrated with the ventral tegmental area and substantia nigra, so that convergence across the segregated prefrontal–striatal pathways may occur, perhaps so that the relatively independent iterative networks can "inform" one another (Yelnik, 2002; Bonelli *et al.*, 2006). Additionally, the globus pallidus has both internal and external segments that send differently valenced (i.e. inhibitory versus excitatory) information to the thalamus, which then relays the information back to the cortex (Haber and McFarland, 2001). This portion of the basal ganglia circuit may inhibit unwanted or unsuccessful behaviors (Haber and McFarland, 2001). Although obviously closely linked to the striatum and serving in a critical output role within this network, the globus pallidus has been less studied with morphometric MRI in bipolar disorder than the striatum.

In their recent meta-analysis of five studies, Kempton *et al.* (2008) observed enlargement of the globus pallidus in bipolar compared with healthy subjects (effect size 1.09, $p = 0.052$). Brambilla *et al.* (2001b), among these studies, did not specifically observe significant globus pallidus enlargement, but noted older patients (>36 years of age) exhibited enlargement compared with younger patients, consistent with two studies in pediatric bipolar disorder that did not observe globus pallidus enlargement (DelBello *et al.*, 2004; Ahn *et al.*, 2007). Consequently, enlargement of this subcortical structure may reflect age or duration of illness effects. Coupled with the studies in striatum, together these findings suggest structural abnormalities within the basal ganglia in

99

bipolar disorder: namely, relative enlargement or shape abnormalities. Whether any of these potential abnormalities exist prior to illness onset (as suggested by Noga *et al.*, 2001, but not Singh *et al.*, 2008) or develop over time (e.g. Brambilla *et al.*, 2001b) requires additional longitudinal work.

Thalamus

The thalamus is a subcortical structure that is actually comprised of a number of distinct subregions and nuclei that, typically, are difficult to resolve using current imaging methods. Consequently, measurements tend to involve the entire multinuclear structure. Processed information from the globus pallidus topographically maps onto distinct subregions of the thalamus, much like the prefrontal cortical mapping onto the striatum. As noted, the thalamus then relays information back to the originating prefrontal cortical area, as well as to the basal ganglia, providing feedback loops critical to iterative information processing and behavioral responses (Haber and McFarland, 2001). For the regions of interest in this discussion, specifically the "emotional" ventral PFC, brain networks appear to map predominantly onto the medial dorsal nucleus of the thalamus. Although historically often simply considered a relay station between subcortical and cortical structures, in fact, through its feedback connections, extensive connections to sensory and motor brain areas, and both reciprocal and non-reciprocal corticothalamic connections, the thalamus is likely to be further modulating processed information received from the globus pallidus in order to refine behavioral outputs (Haber and McFarland, 2001).

To date, those studies that examined thalamic structure in bipolar disorder have primarily been negative, as few studies reported differences in thalamic volumes between bipolar and healthy subjects (see Konarski *et al.*, 2008 for summary), and when differences have been observed, they have included both decreases (Lochhead *et al.*, 2004; Frangou 2005; Haznedar *et al.*, 2005; McIntosh *et al.*, 2004) and increases (Strakowski *et al.*, 1999; McIntosh *et al.*, 2001). Indeed, a meta-analysis of three studies (Kempton *et al.*, 2008) found no difference in thalamic volumes between healthy and bipolar subjects. In total, studies to date do not provide support for the presence of structural abnormalities of the thalamus in bipolar disorder.

Amygdala

Although by necessity the amygdala is treated as a unitary structure in morphometric MRI studies, due to the current spatial resolution limits of MRI, it is actually a collection of nuclei located in the medial temporal lobe that is connected with a number of other brain structures (e.g. basal nucleus of the stria terminalis), sometimes referred to as the "extended amygdala". The amygdala appears to modulate both emotional and cognitive functions, although it is clearly involved in managing the "fight or flight" (fear) response in lower animals (and humans). It is known to be activated in a number of affective processes, from studies of induced sadness (Posse *et al.*, 2003) to recognizing fearful faces (Adolphs, 2008). As noted in our anterior limbic model of bipolar disorder, we simplistically view the amygdala as setting an emotional tone over the iterative prefrontal–striatal–pallidal–thalamic iterative circuits; indeed, ablation or injury to the amygdala produces a state of emotional indifference and lassitude (Mega *et al.*, 1997). Given its central role in emotional modulation and processing, it is no surprise that the amygdala has received considerable attention in neuroimaging studies of bipolar disorder.

In general, these studies have used ROI approaches, as the boundaries of the amygdala nuclei (as a group) can be relatively easily delineated at the current resolution of MRI. In one of the earlier studies, we performed an ROI analysis of the amygdala in bipolar compared with healthy subjects, within the context of a larger analysis of anterior limbic structures (Strakowski *et al.*, 1999). We found the amygdala to be enlarged in the bipolar group, which was a relatively novel finding as brain regions tend to be smaller in psychiatric patients in general (e.g. Strakowski, 2002; Honea *et al.*, 2005) than in healthy subjects. Concurrently, Altshuler *et al.* (1998 preliminary report; 2000 final report) were also measuring amygdala volumes in patients with bipolar disorder, schizophrenia, and healthy subjects, and they also reported amygdala enlargement in the bipolar subjects compared with both other groups. Moreover, they found no differences in hippocampal volumes in bipolar compared with healthy subjects (which is generally observed across studies; see Konarski *et al.*, 2008 for review), although they did find smaller hippocampal volumes in patients with schizophrenia. A meta-analysis of studies comparing these patient

- Subcortical structures' role in healthy brain:
  Striatum – first-level processing of prefrontal information, integrating sensory and other cortical input.
  Globus pallidus – second-level processing from striatum converging information and providing output from basal ganglia.
  Thalamus – third-level processing to modulate basal ganglia output in order to refine behavior and provide feedback to prefrontal cortex.
  Amygdala – modulates fear and other emotional states, setting "emotional tone" over mood networks.
- Subcortical structures' relevance to bipolar disorder:
  Striatum – dysfunction disrupts integration of cortical and limbic information, disturbing emotional homeostasis.
  Globus pallidus – dysfunction disrupts convergence of cortical information, disturbing emotional homeostasis.
  Thalamus – dysfunction disrupts initiation of behavioral responses to processed basal ganglia information.
  Amygdala – dysfunction leads to abnormal emotional tone; injury can cause lassitude and emotional indifference.
- Subcortical structural MRI findings – summary:
  Striatum – may be enlarged or abnormally shaped in bipolar disorder, findings equivocal.
  Globus pallidus – enlarged in bipolar disorder, which may reflect effects of illness progression.
  Thalamus – structurally does not differ between bipolar and healthy subjects.
  Amygdala – volumes are decreased in bipolar adolescents, although in bipolar adults volumes are similar to or larger than healthy subjects. Difference may reflect developmental abnormalities in bipolar disorder.

groups supported the conclusion that the hippocampus is larger in bipolar than schizophrenic patients (Kempton *et al.*, 2008). These two studies led to a hypothesis that amygdala enlargement coupled with normal hippocampal volumes might be relatively unique to bipolar disorder, and might distinguish bipolar and schizophrenic patients (Altshuler *et al.*, 2000). Moreover, differences in age-related changes in amygdala growth reported by Chen *et al.* (2004) suggested that this enlargement might represent

a developmental anomaly in bipolar disorder. However, in contrast, Doty *et al.* (2008) reported age-related reductions in amygdala volumes, and a recent study by Geller *et al.* (2009) also suggests that stressful life events may impact amygdala volumes, perhaps interacting with and disrupting development in bipolar children. Moreover, lithium exposure has been associated with increased amygdala volume (Foland *et al.*, 2008). Subsequent attempts to replicate the findings of amygdala enlargement in bipolar disorder have been mixed, at least in adults with bipolar disorder. Indeed, in a meta-analysis of studies of amygdala volumes in bipolar adults, Pfeiffer *et al.* (2008) concluded that there were no differences between the bipolar and healthy subjects. In contrast, studies in pediatric bipolar disorder have consistently found decreased amygdala volumes as compared with healthy children, supported by meta-analysis (Pfeiffer *et al.*, 2008).

Together, the combined results imply an abnormal underdevelopment or atrophy of amygdala in childhood bipolar disorder that may be normalized or over-grown during adolescence. However, in the absence of longitudinal measurements within subjects, and with the potentially confounding influences of lithium and life events, this speculation cannot be directly supported. Moreover, there is a dearth of histological studies to even begin to suggest what abnormalities in development could account for these volumetric changes. Nonetheless, given the function of the amygdala in affective modulation, clearly more research into its development and function during the early progression of bipolar disorder is warranted.

Cerebellum

The cerebellum has been recognized for perhaps centuries as a critical component of fine motor control. Specifically, the cerebellum seems to coordinate movement by serving an error detection function, preventing over- and under-shooting of intentional movement, thereby ensuring fine motor control (Jueptner and Weiller, 1998). Studies in animal models suggest that the cerebellum participates in emotional behavior, motor learning and fear conditioning (Sacchetti *et al.*, and 2005), consistent with findings of emotional dysregulation in patients with cerebellar abnormalities (Schmahmann, 2004). In particular, lesions in the cerebellar vermis are associated with affective symptoms, leading Schmahmann

(2004) to hypothesize that the vermis is the "limbic cerebellum". Because the histological structure of the cerebellum is relatively uniform throughout, it suggests that this brain structure serves a consistent role in all of the neural networks that it modulates; in other words, the cerebellum may serve an error-detector role in iterative prefrontal–striatal–pallidal–thalamic networks that control mood similarly to its role in prefrontal–striatal–pallidal–thalamic networks that control movement. Consequently, Schmahmann (2004) hypothesizes that impairments in cerebellar function produce dysmetria in movement, in cognition or in emotional behavior, depending on which part of the cerebellum is injured. Given that the emotional dysregulation in bipolar disorder could be interpreted as emotional dysmetria, it is reasonable to consider abnormalities within the midline cerebellum as potentially playing a role. With these considerations in mind, several investigators examined the cerebellar vermis in bipolar patients using structural MRI.

DelBello and colleagues (1999) were the first to report cerebellar vermis abnormalities in bipolar disorder. Specifically, they observed that, although the vermis in first-episode bipolar patients did not differ from healthy subjects, in multiple-episode patients the vermis (specifically vermal area 3) was smaller and its size was inversely associated with the number of depressive episodes. In a separate study, this same group again found decreased volumes in multiple-episode bipolar patients in vermal area 3, as well as area 2, although they noted an association with antidepressant exposure, suggesting a possible treatment effect (Mills et al., 2005). Monkul and colleagues (2008) similarly observed a smaller vermis (area 2) size in pediatric bipolar patients, with an inverse correlation between vermal size and the number of previous affective episodes. Brambilla et al. (2001c) observed smaller vermal size in bipolar patients with familial illness, although not in patients more generally, compared with healthy subjects; they did not separate first- and multiple-episode patients, however. Moorhead et al. (2007) also recently reported significantly greater progressive decreases in the cerebellum over a four-year period in bipolar compared with healthy subjects. Although the decreases were in the left lobe of the cerebellum, rather than the midline, these changes may reflect similar processes. Taken together, these findings suggest that the cerebellar vermis may be smaller in bipolar patients after repeated affective episodes or antidepressant exposure

(or both). This interpretation suggests progressive atrophy in the cerebellar vermis, and perhaps cerebellum more generally, consistent with the findings in PFC mentioned previously.

White matter

Of course, the brain regions of interest in the anterior limbic network do not simply float in space, but are connected through white matter tracts. These tracts pass from the PFC posteriorly to the basal ganglia, thalamus and back, comprising much of the periventricular structure of the brain. Although direct measurements of these white matter tracts are few, in fact, one of the more established findings in bipolar disorder is lateral ventricular enlargement (see Kempton et al., 2008, for meta-analysis), which might reflect a decrease in periventricular white matter, in the very connections that constitute the anterior limbic model. One question arising from these reports of lateral ventricular enlargement in bipolar disorder is whether increased ventricles are present at illness onset or instead reflect changes during the course of illness. To address this, we examined lateral ventricular volumes in bipolar patients at the time of their first-episode and compared them to patients with multiple episodes and healthy subjects (Strakowski et al., 2002a). We found that first-episode patients' ventricular volumes were virtually identical to matched healthy subjects, whereas ventricular enlargement was noted in the multiple-episode patients. Since the periventricular gray matter structures were either similar to or larger in the patients than healthy subjects, ventricular enlargement likely reflected decreases in white matter. Supporting these suggestions, the corpus callosum, which represents a significant part of the periventricular white matter, was recently observed in a meta-analysis to be reduced in size in bipolar disorder compared with healthy subjects (Arnone et al., 2008). Moreover, Strakowski et al. (2002a) found that ventricular volumes were correlated with the number of prior manic episodes, which, like the changes in cerebellar vermis and prefrontal cortex, might reflect a neuroanatomic basis for the early course progression in bipolar disorder (Figure 6.2).

Further support for white matter abnormalities in bipolar disorder arises from a number of recent studies that used diffusion tensor imaging (DTI) techniques to examine white matter structure in bipolar

Table 6.1 Differences in fractional anisotropy values in bipolar and healthy subjects from recent reports

Study	Bipolar subjects N	Healthy subjects N	Direction	Location
McIntosh et al., 2008	40	49	dec	Uncinate fasciculus, anterior thalamic radiation
Versace et al., 2008	31	25	inc	Left uncinate fasciculus, left optic radiation, right anterothalamic radiation
			dec	Right uncinate fasciculus
Wang et al., 2008a	42	42	inc	Anterior cingulum
			none	Posterior cingulum
Wang et al., 2008b	33	40	dec	Anterior and middle corpus callosum
Bruno et al., 2008	36	28	dec	Inferior and and middle temporal, middle occipital regions.
Frazier et al., 2007*	10	8	dec	Bilateral superior frontal, left orbital frontal, right corpus callosum.
Yurgelun-Todd et al., 2007	11	10	inc	Genu of corpus callosum
Houenou et al., 2007	16	16	none	Fiber tracts between subgenual cingulate and and amygdala
Adler et al., 2006b*	11	17	dec	Superior–frontal
Beyer et al., 2005	14	21	none	Orbital frontal, superior and and middle frontal
Haznedar et al., 2005	40**	36	inc	Right anterior frontal
			dec	Fronto-occipital anterior fasciculus
Adler et al., 2004	9	9	dec	Prefrontal white matter

dec, bipolar subjects with significantly decreased FA versus healthy subjects; inc, bipolar subjects with significantly increased FA versus healthy subjects; none, non-significant differences between groups.
*Subjects were children and adolescents; **included a range of bipolar spectrum patients.

disorder. These studies have fairly consistently observed differences in fractional anisotropy (FA) in bipolar compared with healthy subjects (see Table 6.1), supporting the suggestion that ventricular changes may reflect abnormalities in white matter in bipolar disorder. FA provides a measure of water movement in the brain and is believed to increase with increasing tissue organization (e.g. in the presence of well-defined and organized white matter tracts). Therefore, decreases in FA might suggest a loss of "bundle coherence" in these regions, whereas increases could suggest a loss of healthy variability. Increases in FA in bipolar compared with healthy subjects were reported in 4/12 studies, whereas 8/12 observed decreases (Table 6.1). Some studies observed increases in FA in some brain areas with decreases in other regions, suggesting regional specificity to the finding. However, many of these studies were hampered by small numbers of subjects. Nonetheless, abnormalities in the structure of white matter in brain regions that potentially represent disruption of tracts involved within the anterior limbic network may occur in bipolar disorder.

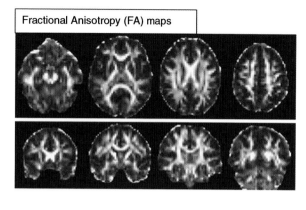

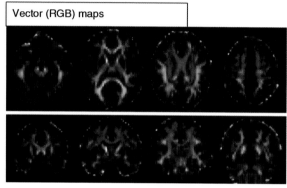

Figure 6.4 Examples of diffusion tensor imaging illustrating distribution of fractional anisotropy (brighter represents higher values) and vector maps in which red is left–right, blue is inferior–superior and green is anterior–posterior (diffusion has been calculated in 30 directions).

Finally, perhaps the most robust neuroimaging finding in bipolar disorder is the presence of signal hyperintensities observed with T_2-weighted MRI, predominantly in white matter. In a recent meta-analysis, Kempton *et al.* (2008) found that bipolar patients had approximately a threefold increased risk of hyperintensities than healthy subjects. A number of brain locations were involved supporting this increased risk including deep white matter, subcortical gray matter, both hemispheres (although right > left), frontal and parietal lobes. The specific histopathological basis of these hyperintensities has remained elusive, but these findings further suggest abnormalities in white matter in bipolar disorder.

Summary and conclusions

In this review, we examined studies of structural MRI abnormalities in brain regions that comprise an anterior limbic model of bipolar disorder. Perhaps

the most consistent theme among these studies is that replicating imaging findings in bipolar disorder has often been difficult (Kempton *et al.*, 2008; Konarski *et al.*, 2008; Strakowski *et al.*, 2005). Nonetheless, when framed within the context of a specific functional neuroanatomic model of bipolar disorder, a number of findings do appear to support the notion that structural brain abnormalities may exist consistent with that model. Additionally, in several brain regions there is a suggestion of progressive or developmental changes that might either reflect or underlie the early progression of the course of bipolar disorder.

From these and other considerations, several approaches for future research using structural MRI techniques are suggested. First, longitudinal studies are needed to clarify how brain structures change within individual patients, with particular regard to the corresponding course of illness. It will be important to determine if changes precede or follow affective episodes, for example. Additionally, given the dynamic nature of bipolar disorder, brain regions that are changing in structure may be more likely to localize etiological factors for the illness. Second, more sophisticated measures, such as DTI tractography or shape analyses, may more consistently define the subtle structural abnormalities that are likely in bipolar disorder and that may be missed with less-specific measures. Third, studies in young patients are critical given the typical adolescent onset of bipolar disorder and early course progression, but must be framed within the context of understanding normal brain developmental changes in healthy subjects; this approach has not been used frequently to date. Fourth, integrating structural imaging with functional and neurochemical (e.g. magnetic resonance spectroscopy or proton emission tomography) are the only ways to move morphometric imaging from high-priced and sophisticated phrenology to a better understanding of the neural basis of bipolar disorder. It is critical that we move our imaging research from "where" to "how" with these types of integrations. Indeed, finally, as our understanding and identification of genetic risk factors in this illness increase, integrating genetic and neuroimaging techniques likely will provide the most powerful means for untangling the neurophysiological basis of bipolar disorder (e.g. Chepenik *et al.*, 2009).

There is little doubt that neuroimaging, including structural MRI, has changed the way we think about studying bipolar disorder and other psychiatric illnesses. The constant acceleration in advances of neuroimaging technologies guarantees that we will be able to increasingly better understand brain function, in health and illness, in living human beings in the future. The neuroanatomic substrate underlying bipolar disorder, as suggested by the studies reviewed in this chapter, represents a starting point. The future for further advances and finally defining the neural basis of bipolar disorder remains bright and provides hope that we will soon be able to develop better treatments that truly improve the lives of people affected by this illness.

References

Adler C M, Adams J, DelBello M P, et al. 2006b. Evidence of white matter pathology in bipolar disorder adolescents experiencing their first episode of mania: A diffusion tensor imaging study. *Am J Psychiatry* **163**, 322–4.

Adler C M, DelBello M P, Jarvis K, Levine A, Adams J and Strakowski S M. 2007. Voxel-based study of structural changes in first-episode patients with bipolar disorder. *Biol Psychiatry* **61**, 776–81.

Adler C M, DelBello M P and Strakowski S M. 2006a. Brain network dysfunction in bipolar disorder. *CNS Spectrums* **11**, 312–20.

Adler C M, Holland S K, Schmithorst V, et al. 2004. Abnormal frontal white matter tracts in bipolar disorder: A diffusion tensor imaging study. *Bipolar Disord* **6**, 197–203.

Adler C M, Levine A D, DelBello M P, Strakowski S M. 2005. Changes in gray matter volume in patients with bipolar disorder. *Biol Psychiatry* **58**, 151–7.

Adolphs R. 2008. Fear, faces, and the human amygdala. *Curr Opin Neurobiol* **18**, 166–72.

Ahn M S, Breeze J L, Makris N, et al. 2007. Anatomic brain magnetic resonance imaging of the 4 basal ganglia in pediatric bipolar disorder. *J Affect Disord* **104**, 147–54.

Altshuler L L, Bartzokis G, Grieder T, Curran J and Mintz J. 1998. Amygdala enlargement in bipolar disorder and hippocampal reduction in schizophrenia: An MRI study demonstrating neuroanatomic specificity. *Arch Gen Psychiatry* **55**, 663–4.

Altshuler L L, Bartzokis G, Grieder T, et al. 2000. An MRI study of temporal lobe structures in men with bipolar disorder and schizophrenia. *Biol Psychiatry* **48**, 147–62.

Angst J. 1998. The emerging epidemiology of hypomania and bipolar II disorder. *J Affect Disord* **50**, 143–51.

Angst J and Sellaro R. 2000. Historical perspectives and natural history of bipolar disorder. *Biol Psychiatry* **48**, 445–57.

Arnone D, McIntosh A M, Chandra P and Ebmeier K P. 2008. Meta-analysis of magnetic resonance imaging studies of the corpus callosum in bipolar disorder. *Acta Psychiatr Scand* **118**, 357–62.

Aylward E H, Roberts-Twillie J V, Barta P E, et al. 1994. Basal ganglia volumes and white matter hyperintensities in patients with bipolar disorder. *AmJ Psychiatry* **151**, 687–93.

Bearden C E, Hoffman K M, Cannon T D. 2001. The neuropsychology and neuroanatomy of bipolar affective disorder: A critical review. *Bipolar Disord* **3**, 106–50.

Beyer J L, Taylor W D, MacFall J R, et al. 2005. Cortical white matter microstructural abnormalities in bipolar disorder. *Neuropsychopharmacology* **30**, 2225–9.

Blumberg H P, Krystal J H, Bansal R, et al. 2006. Age, rapid-cycling, and pharmacotherapy effects on ventral prefrontal cortex in bipolar disorder: A cross-sectional study. *BiolPsychiatry* **59**, 611–8.

Bonelli R M, Kapfhammer H P, Pillay S S and Yurgelun-Todd D A. 2006. Basal ganglia volumetric studies in affective disorder: What did we learn in the last 15 years? *J Neural Transmission* **113**, 255–68.

Brambilla P, Glahn D C, Balestrieri M and Soares J C. 2005. Magnetic resonance findings in bipolar disorder. *Psychiatr Clin North Am* **28**, 443–67.

Brambilla P, Harenski K, Nicoletti M, et al. 2001a. Differential effects of age on brain gray matter in bipolar patients and healthy individuals. *Neuropsychobiology* **43**, 242–7.

Brambilla P, Harenski K, Nicoletti M A, et al. 2001b. Anatomical MRI study of basal ganglia in bipolar disorder patients. *Psychiatry Res* **106**, 65–80.

Brambilla P, Harenski K, Nicoletti M, et al. 2001c. MRI study of posterior fossa structures and brain ventricles in bipolar patients. *J Psychiatr Res* **35**, 313–22.

Brambilla P, Nicoletti M A, Harenski K, et al. 2002. Anatomical MRI study of subgenual prefrontal cortex in bipolar and unipolar subjects. *Neuropsychopharmacology* **27**, 792–9.

Bruno S, Cercignani M and Ron M A. 2008. White matter abnormalities in bipolar disorder: A voxel-based diffusion tensor imaging study. *Bipolar Disord* **10**, 460–8.

Chang K, Barnea-Goraly N, Karchemskiy A, Simeonova D I, et al. 2005. Cortical magnetic resonance imaging findings in familial pediatric bipolar disorder. *Biol Psychiatry* **58**, 197–203.

Chen B K, Sassi R, Axelson D, et al. 2004. Cross-sectional study of abnormal amygdala development in adolescents and young adults with bipolar disorder. *Biol Psychiatry* **56**, 399–405.

Chakos M H, Lieberman J A, Bilder R M, et al. 1994. Increase in caudate nuclei volumes of first-episode schizophrenic patients taking antipsychotic drugs. *Am J Psychiatry* **151**, 1430–6.

Chepenik L G, Fredericks C, Papademetris X, *et al.* 2009. Effects of the brain-derived neurotrophic growth factor Val66Met variation on hippocampus morphology in bipolar disorder. *Neuropsychopharmacology* **34**, 944–51.

Chiu S, Widjaja F, Bates M E, *et al.* 2008. Anterior cingulate volume in pediatric bipolar disorder and autism. *J Affect Disord* **105**, 93–9.

Coffman J A, Bornstein R A, Olson S C, Schwarzkopf S B and Nasrallah H A. 1990. Cognitive impairment and cerebral structure by MRI in bipolar disorder. *Biol Psychiatry* **27**, 1188–96.

DelBello M P, Strakowski S M, Zimmerman M E, Hawkins J M and Sax K W. 1999. MRI analysis of the cerebellum in bipolar disorder: A pilot study. *Neuropsychopharmacology* **21**, 63–8.

DelBello M P, Zimmerman M E, Mills N P, Getz G E and Strakowski S M. 2004. Magnetic resonance imaging analysis of amygdala and other subcortical brain regions in adolescents with bipolar disorder. *Bipolar Disord* **6**, 43–52.

Devinsky O, Morrell M J and Vogt B A. 1995. Contributions of anterior cingulate cortex to behaviour. *Brain* **118**, 279–306.

Dickstein D P, Milham M P, Nugent A C, *et al.* 2005. Frontotemporal alterations in pediatric bipolar disorder: Results of a voxel-based morphometry study. *Arch Gen Psychiatry* **62**, 734–41.

Doty T J, Payne M E, Steffens D C, Beyer J L, Krishnan K R and LaBar K S. 2008. Age-dependent reduction of amygdala volume in bipolar disorder. *Psychiatry Res* **163**, 84–94.

Drevets W C, Price J L, Simpson J R Jr, *et al.* 1997. Subgenual prefrontal cortex abnormalities in mood disorders. *Nature* **386**, 824–7.

Farrow T F, Whitford T J, Williams L M, Gomes L and Harris A W. 2005. Diagnosis-related regional gray matter loss over two years in first episode schizophrenia and bipolar disorder. *Biol Psychiatry* **58**, 713–23.

Foland L C, Altshuler L L, Sugar C A, *et al.* 2008. Increased volume of the amygdala and hippocampus in bipolar patients treated with lithium. *Neuroreport* **19**, 221–4.

Fornito A, Malhi G S, Lagopoulos J, *et al.* 2008. Anatomical abnormalities of the anterior cingulate and paracingulate cortex in patients with bipolar I disorder. *Psychiatry Res* **162**, 123–32.

Frangou S. 2005. The Maudsley Bipolar Disorder Project. *Epilepsia* **46** (Suppl 4), 19–25.

Frangou S, Hadjulis M, Chitnis X, Baster D, Donaldson S and Raymont V. 2002. The Maudsley Bipolar Disorder Project: Brain structural changes in bipolar I disorder. *Bipolar Disor* **4**(Suppl 1), 123–4.

Frazier J A, Breeze J L, Papdimitriou G, *et al.* 2007. White matter abnormalities in children with and at risk for bipolar disorder. *Bipolar Disord* **9**, 799–809.

Geller B, Harms M P, Wang L, *et al.* 2009. Effects of age, sex, and independent life events on amygdala and nucleus accumbens volumes in child bipolar I disorder. *Biol Psychiatry* **65**, 432–7.

Haber S and McFarland N R. 2001. The place of the thalamus in frontal cortical–basal ganglia circuits. *Neuroscientist* **7**, 315–24.

Hajek T, Kozeny J, Kopecek M, Alda M and Höschl C. 2008. Reduced subgenual cingulate volumes in mood disorders: A meta-analysis. *J Psychiatry Neurosci* **33**, 91–9.

Haldane M, Cunningham G, Androutsos C and Frangou S. 2008. Structural brain correlates of response inhibition in Bipolar Disorder I. *J Psychopharmacol* **22**, 138–43.

Haznedar M M, Roversi F, Pallanti S, *et al.* 2005. Fronto-thalamo-striatal gray and white matter volumes and anisotropy of their connections in bipolar spectrum illnesses. *Biol Psychiatry* **57**, 733–42.

Hirayasu Y, Shenton M E, Salisbury D F, *et al.* 1999. Subgenual cingulate cortex volume in first-episode psychosis. *Am J Psychiatry* **156**, 1091–3.

Honea R, Crow T J, Passingham D and Mackay C E. 2005. Regional deficits in brain volume in schizophrenia: A meta-analysis of voxel-based morphometry studies. *Am J Psychiatry* **162**, 2233–45.

Houenou J, Wessa M, Douaud G, *et al.* 2007. Increased white matter connectivity in euthymic bipolar patients: Diffusion tensor tractography between the subgenual cingulate and the amygdalo-hippocampal complex. *Mol Psychiatry* **12**, 1001–10.

Hwang J, Lyoo I K, Dager S R, *et al.* 2006. Basal ganglia shape alterations in bipolar disorder. *Am J Psychiatry* **163**, 276–85.

Javadapour A, Malhi G S, Ivanovski B, Chen X, Wen W and Sachdev P. 2007. Increased anterior cingulate cortex volume in bipolar I disorder. *Aust N Z J Psychiatry* **41**, 910–6.

Jueptner M and Weiller C. 1998. A review of differences between basal ganglia and cerebellar control of movements as revealed by functional imaging studies. *Brain* **121**, 1437–49.

Kaur S, Sassi R B, Axelson D, *et al.* 2005. Cingulate cortex anatomical abnormalities in children and adolescents with bipolar disorder. *Am J Psychiatry* **162**, 1637–43.

Kempton M J, Gedes J R, Ettinger U, Williams S C R and Grasby P M. 2008. Meta-analysis, database, and meta-regression of 98 structural imaging studies in bipolar disorder. *Arch Gen Psychiatry* **65**, 1017–32.

Konarski J Z, McIntyre R S, Kennedy S H, Rafi-Tari S, Soczynska J K and Ketter T A. 2008. Volumetric neuroimaging investigations in mood disorder: Bipolar disorder versus major depressive disorder. *Bipolar Disord* **10**, 1–37.

Koo M S, Levitt J J, Salisbury D F, Nakamura M, Shenton M E and McCarley R W. 2008. A cross-sectional and longitudinal magnetic resonance imaging study of cingulate gyrus gray matter volume abnormalities in first-episode schizophrenia and first-episode affective psychosis. *Arch Gen Psychiatry* **65**, 746–60.

Kraepelin E. 1921. *Manic-Depressive Insanity and Paranoia* (transl. R M Barclay), G M Robertson, Ed. Edinburgh: E. and S. Livingstone; reproduced in the series "The Classic of Psychiatry and Behavioral Sciences Library", E T Carlson, Ed. Birmingham, AL: Gryphon Editions, Inc., p. 138.

Lochhead R A, Parsey R V, Oquendo M A and Mann J J. 2004. Regional brain gray matter volume differences in patients with bipolar disorder as assessed by optimized voxel-based morphometry. *Biol Psychiatry* **55**, 1154–62.

Lopez-Larson M P, DelBello M P, Zimmerman M E, Schwiers M L and Strakowski S M. 2002. Regional prefrontal gray and white matter abnormalities in bipolar disorder. *Biol Psychiatry* **52**, 93–100.

Lyoo I K, Kim M J, Stoll A L, *et al.* 2004. Frontal lobe gray matter density decreases in bipolar I disorder. *Biol Psychiatry* **55**, 648–51.

Lyoo I K, Sung Y H, Dager S R, *et al.* 2006. Regional cerebral cortical thinning in bipolar disorder. *Bipolar Disord* **8**, 65–74.

Mayberg H S, Liotti M, Brannan S K, *et al.* 1999. Reciprocal limbic–cortical function and negative mood: Converging PET findings in depression and normal sadness. *Am J Psychiatry* **156**, 675–82.

McDonald C, Zanelli J, Rabe-Hesketh S, *et al.* 2004. Meta-analysis of magnetic resonance imaging brain morphometry studies in bipolar disorder. *Biol Psychiatry* **56**, 411–7.

McIntosh A M, Forrester A, Lawrie S M, *et al.* 2001. A factor model of the functional psychoses and the relationship of factors to clinical variables and brain morphology. *Psychol Med* **31**, 159–71.

McIntosh A M, Job D E, Moorhead T W, *et al.* 2004. Voxel-based morphometry of patients with schizophrenia or bipolar disorder and their unaffected relatives. *Biol Psychiatry* **56**, 544–52.

McIntosh A M, Maniega S M, Lymer G K, *et al.* 2008. White matter tractography in bipolar disorder and schizophrenia. *Biol Psychiatry* **64**, 1088–92.

Mega M S, Cummings J L, Salloway S and Malloy P. 1997. The limbic system: An anatomic, phylogenetic, and clinical perspective. *J Neuropsychiatr Clin Neurosci* **9**, 315–30.

Mills N P, Delbello M P, Adler C M and Strakowski S M. 2005. MRI analysis of cerebellar vermal abnormalities in bipolar disorder. *Am J Psychiatry* **162**, 1530–2.

Monkul E S, Hatch J P, Sassi R B, *et al.* 2008. MRI study of the cerebellum in young bipolar patients. *Prog Neuropsychopharmacol Biol Psychiatry* **32**, 613–9.

Moorhead T W, McKirdy J, Sussmann J E, *et al.* 2007. Progressive gray matter loss in patients with bipolar disorder. *Biol Psychiatry* **62**, 894–900.

Murray C J L and Lopez A D. 1996. *The Global Burden of Disease: Summary*. Cambridge, MA, Harvard School of Public Health Monograph.

Narrow W E, Rae D S, Robins L N and Regier D A. 2002. Revised prevalence estimates of mental disorders in the United States: Using a clinical significance criterion to reconcile 2 surveys' estimates. *Arch Gen Psychiatry* **59**, 115–23.

Noga J T, Vladar K and Torrey E F. 2001. A volumetric magnetic resonance imaging study of monozygotic twins discordant for bipolar disorder. *Psychiatry Res* **106**, 25–34.

Nugent A C, Milham M P, Bain E E, *et al.* 2006. Cortical abnormalities in bipolar disorder investigated with MRI and voxel-based morphometry. *Neuroimage* **30**, 485–97.

Ongür D and Price J L. 2000. The organization of networks within the orbital and medial prefrontal cortex of rats, monkeys, and humans. *Cerebral Cortex* **10**, 206–19.

Pfeiffer J C, Welge J, Strakowski S M, Adler C M and DelBello M P. 2008. Meta-analysis of amygdala volumes in children and adolescents with bipolar disorder. *J Am Acad Child Adolesc Psychiatry* **47**, 1290–9.

Posse S, Fitzgerald D, Gao K, *et al.* 2003. Real-time fMRI of temporolimbic regions detects amygdala activation during single-trial self-induced sadness. *Neuroimage* **18**, 760–8.

Roy-Byrne P P, Post R M, Uhde T W, Porcu T and Davis D. 1985. The longitudinal course of recurrent affective illness: life chart data from research patients at the NIMH. *Acta Psychiatr Scand* **71** (suppl 317), 1–34.

Sacchetti B, Scelfo B and Strata P. 2005. The cerebellum: Synaptic changes and fear conditioning. *Neuroscientist* **11**, 217–27.

Sanches M, Sassi R B, Axelson D, *et al.* 2005. Subgenual prefrontal cortex of child and adolescent bipolar patients: A morphometric magnetic resonance imaging study. *Psychiatry Res* **138**, 43–9.

Sassi R B, Brambilla P, Hatch J P, *et al.* 2004. Reduced left anterior cingulate volumes in untreated bipolar patients. *Biol Psychiatry* **56**, 467–75.

Sax K W, Strakowski S M, Zimmerman M E, *et al.* 1999. Frontosubcortical neuroanatomy and the Continuous Performance Test in mania. *Am J Psychiatry* **156**, 139–41.

107

Schlaepfer T E, Harris G J, Tien A Y, *et al*. 1994. Decreased regional cortical gray matter volume in schizophrenia. *Am J Psychiatry* **151**, 842–8.

Schmahmann J D. 2004. Disorders of the cerebellum: Ataxia, dysmetria of thought, and the cerebellar cognitive affective syndrome. *J Neuropsychiatry Clin Neurosci* **16**, 367–78.

Schmahmann J D, Weilburg J B and Sherman J C. 2007. The neuropsychiatry of the cerebellum – insights from the clinic. *Cerebellum* **6**, 254–67.

Sharma V, Menon R, Carr T J, Densmore M, Mazmanian D and Williamson P C. 2003. An MRI study of subgenual prefrontal cortex in patients with familial and non-familial bipolar I disorder. *J Affect Disord* **77**, 167–71.

Singh M K, Delbello M P, Adler C M, Stanford K E and Strakowski S M. 2008. Neuroanatomical characterization of child offspring of bipolar parents. *J Am Acad Child Adolesc Psychiatry* **47**, 526–31.

Strakowski S M. 2002. Differential brain mechanisms in bipolar and unipolar disorders: Considerations from brain imaging. In Soares J C (Ed) *Brain Imaging in Affective Disorders*. New York, NY: Marcel Dekker, Inc.

Strakowski S M, Wilson D R, Tohen M, Woods B T, Douglass A W and Stoll A L. 1993. Structural brain abnormalities in first-episode mania. *Biol Psychiatry* **33**, 602–09.

Strakowski S M, DelBello M P, Sax K W, *et al*. 1999. Brain magnetic resonance imaging of structural abnormalities in bipolar disorder. *Arch Gen Psychiatry* **56**, 254–60.

Strakowski S M, DelBello M P, Zimmerman M E, *et al*. 2002a. Ventricular and periventricular structural volumes in first- versus multiple-episode bipolar disorder. *Am J Psychiatry* **159**, 1841–7.

Strakowski S M, Adler C and DelBello M P. 2002b. Comparison of morphometric magnetic resonance imaging findings in bipolar disorder and unipolar depression. *Bipolar Disorders* **4**, 80–8.

Strakowski S M, Adler C M, Holland S K, Mills N P and DelBello M P. 2004. A preliminary fMRI study of sustained attention in unmedicated, euthymic bipolar disorder. *Neuropsychopharmacology* **29**, 1734–40.

Strakowski S M, DelBello M P and Adler C M. 2005. The functional neuroanatomy of bipolar disorder. *Molecular Psychiatry* **10**, 105–16.

Strakowski S M, Adler C M and DelBello M P. 2007. Metabolic dysfunction within the anterior limbic network in bipolar disorder: A model for studying new treatments. *Neuropsychiatria i Neuropsychologia (Neuropsychiatry and Neuropsychology; Poland)* **1**, 5–14.

Tekins S and Cummings J L. 2002. Frontal–subcortical neuronal circuits and clinical neuropsychiatry: An update. *J Psychosom Res* **53**, 647–54.

Versace A, Almeida J R, Hassel S, *et al*. 2008. Elevated left and reduced right orbitomedial prefrontal fractional anisotropy in adults with bipolar disorder revealed by tract-based spatial statistics. *Arch Gen Psychiatry* **65**, 1041–52.

Voorn P, Vanderschuren L J M J, Groenewegen H J, Robbins T W and Pennartz C M A. 2004. Putting a spin on the dorsal–ventral divide of the striatum. *Trends Neurosci* **27**, 468–74.

Wang F, Jackowski M, Kalmar J H, *et al*. 2008a. Abnormal anterior cingulum integrity in bipolar disorder determined through diffusion tensor imaging. *Br J Psychiatry* **192**, 126–9.

Wang F, Kalmar J H, Edmiston E, *et al*. 2008b. Abnormal corpus callosum integrity in bipolar disorder: A diffusion tensor imaging study. *Biol Psychiatry* **64**, 730–3.

Wilke M, Kowatch R A, DelBello M P, Mills N P and Holland S K. 2004. Voxel-based morphometry in adolescents with bipolar disorder: First results. *Psychiatry Res* **131**, 57–69.

Yamasaki H, LaBar K S and McCarthy G. 2002. Dissociable prefrontal brain systems for attention and emotion. *Proc Natl Acad Sci U S A* **99**, 11 447–51.

Yatham L N, Lyoo I K, Liddle P, *et al*. 2007. A magnetic resonance imaging study of mood stabilizer- and neuroleptic-naïve first-episode mania. *Bipolar Disord* **9**, 693–7.

Yelnik J. 2002. Functional anatomy of the basal ganglia. *Movement Disord* **17**, S15–21.

Yurgelun-Todd D A, Silveri M M, Gruber S A, Rohan M L and Pimentel P J. 2007. White matter abnormalities observed in bipolar disorder: A diffusion tensor imaging study. *Bipolar Disord* **9**, 504–12.

Functional imaging of bipolar illness

William M. Marchand and Deborah A. Yurgelun-Todd

Introduction

Bipolar disorder (BD) is a complex neuropsychiatric disorder characterized by cognitive, emotional and motor symptoms. Multiple neuroimaging modalities have been applied to patients with bipolar disorder; nevertheless, the underlying neurobiology remains poorly understood. Data acquired with increasingly sophisticated functional neuroimaging techniques in combination with advances in neuroscience have the potential to enhance our understanding of the neuropathy of this illness. Further, these studies may provide a means of assessing those brain functional abnormalities associated with a specific phase of illness and those consistent across mood states, thus differentiating brain changes which are trait markers from those functional changes related to mood state. Moreover, functional neuroimaging is being incorporated into the development of biomarkers that may aid in clinical diagnosis and treatment selection.

The number of functional imaging studies reported in the literature has increased dramatically in recent years. Comparison of these studies is complicated by several factors. These include the fact that patient groups have been studied with significant differences in clinical variables, such as comorbidity, duration of illness and current treatment. Also, many different activation paradigms have been used for functional magnetic resonance imaging (fMRI) studies and some metabolism and blood flow studies have been conducted at rest. Nonetheless, a review of functional imaging studies may provide insights into the neurobiology of this disorder.

Since bipolar illness is a disorder characterized by dysregulation of affect as well as changes in cognitive function, it is likely that the underlying neuropathology involves the neural systems involved in the production and regulation of affect. Several different models

have been proposed in conceptualizing the neurobiological changes underlying affective changes in mood disorders. For example, there has been an interest in examining mood disorders in light of disruption in brain reward circuitry, given that these disorders have notable disturbances in motivated behavior (Salamone, 2007). A second approach has been to examine the relationship between stress, the hypothalamic–pituitary–adrenal (HPA) axis and brain responses and mood changes, a perspective that has been of particular relevance to depression (Nestler *et al.*, 2002). However, the neurobiological model that appears to best address both depressed and manic states is to consider mood changes as a disruption of interactive brain groups defined as either ventral or dorsal networks (Davidson, 1998; Blumberg *et al.*, 2000; Mayberg, 1997; Yurgelun-Todd and Ross, 2006). Considerable evidence suggests that two neural systems are critical in human affect generation and modulation. The first of these is a ventral system which includes the ventral prefrontal cortex (VPFC), amygdala, insula, ventral striatum, thalamus, orbitofrontal cortex (OFC), ventral anterior cingulate, and brainstem nuclei. This ventral system is responsible for the perception of emotional stimuli, generation of an affective state, and production of an autonomic response. In contrast, the dorsal system, which includes the dorsolateral prefrontal cortex (DLPFC), medial prefrontal cortex, dorsal anterior cingulate and hippocampus, is responsible for effortful regulation of affective state (Phillips *et al.*, 2003).

Mood dysregulation in bipolar disorder could theoretically occur as a result of dysfunction in the dorsal or ventral system or both. Dysregulation of the ventral system could result in the pathologic mood states of mania and depression at the level of affect generation. Impairment in the dorsal system could result in mood episodes as a result of inadequate regulation. In this chapter, we review functional neuroimaging findings in the dorsal and ventral systems, as well as in other brain regions.

Dorsal system

Dorsolateral prefrontal cortex

The DLPFC (BA 9 and 46/middle frontal gyrus) is involved in executive functions including shifting attention, working memory, and voluntary response inhibition. The mid-dorsolateral frontal cortex is involved with visual working memory tasks (Stern et al., 2000) and regulation of emotional responses (Goel and Dolan, 2003; Liotti et al., 2000; Levesque et al., 2003). Thus, the DLPFC could be associated with both cognitive and emotional symptoms of BD.

Multiple studies have reported DLPFC functional abnormalities in BD. An ^{18}F-FDG PET study found decreased glucose metabolism in the left dorsal anterolateral PFC, which correlated with the total Hamilton Depression Rating Scale score (Baxter et al., 1989). Many fMRI studies have reported DLPFC abnormalities in BD.

Among the fMRI studies that have examined homogeneous depressed groups, increased activation has been reported in response to both motor (Marchand et al., 2007a) and emotional (Malhi et al., 2004b) paradigms. However, decreased activation in response to an emotional paradigm has also been reported (Altshuler et al., 2008). In regard to DLPFC function in the euthymic state, increased activation has been reported by studies using motor (Marchand et al., 2007b) and emotional (Lagopoulos and Malhi, 2007) tasks, while decreased activation has been reported in response to cognitive (Frangou, 2005; Frangou et al., 2008; Strakowski et al., 2005; Monks et al., 2004; Lagopoulos et al., 2007; Malhi et al., 2007a) and emotional (Jogia et al., 2008) paradigms. The only study of mania (Elliott et al., 2004) reported increased activation in response to an emotional task. In regard to treatment response, one study found that with medication for depression, left PFC metabolism increased significantly and the percentage change in the Hamilton scale score correlated with the percentage change in metabolism (Baxter et al., 1989). Another study (Benedetti et al., 2007), using a cognitive activation paradigm, found that for sleep deprivation combined with light therapy, treatment response was related to changes in bilateral DLPFC, and genotype of the promoter for the serotonin transporter influenced baseline neural responses in this region.

Taken together, these studies provide compelling evidence of DLPFC dysfunction in BD, and some evidence of functional change related to treatment response in this region. DLPFC functional abnormalities appear to exist across depressed, manic, and euthymic mood states. The strongest evidence is in the euthymic state, for which nine separate studies have demonstrated abnormalities. A particularly compelling finding is that all six studies using cognitive paradigms that have studied the euthymic state report decreased activation in this region.

Medial frontal cortex

A ^{99m}Tc-HMPAO SPECT study (Culha et al., 2008) found the mean regional cerebral blood flow (rCBF) values of the bipolar euthymic patients were significantly lower than those of the controls in the bilateral medial frontal cortex. In regard to fMRI studies, increased activation in depression (Malhi et al., 2004b) has been reported in response to an emotional task. Cognitive tasks have revealed increased (Monks et al., 2004; Lagopoulos et al., 2007) and decreased (Malhi et al., 2007a) activation in euthymia. Finally an fMRI study using a facial affect recognition task (Jogia et al., 2008) found that following lamotrigine monotherapy, patients demonstrated increased right medial frontal activation. At this time, the evidence for medial frontal dysfunction in BD is limited in comparison to other frontal regions, and results are variable.

Hippocampus

An ^{18}F-FDG PET study (Drevets et al., 2002) found left hippocampus metabolism was increased in BD depressives, relative to a control group. A few fMRI studies have reported hippocampal functional abnormalities (Lagopoulos and Malhi, 2007; Lawrence et al., 2004; Altshuler et al., 2008). Mood state-specific results indicate increased activation in depression in response to a cognitive task (Altshuler et al., 2008), and in euthymia in response to an emotional task (Lagopoulos and Malhi, 2007).

Anterior cingulate cortex

The anterior cingulate cortex (ACC) is involved in normal sadness (Liotti et al., 2000), and the detection of unfavorable outcomes, response errors, response conflict, and decision uncertainty (Ridderinkhof *et al.*, 2004). Further, as discussed above, the dorsal ACC is part of the system involved with effortful regulation of affect, while the ventral ACC is part of the system which produces affect. Many studies suggest ACC dysfunction in BD; however, in many cases, dorsal and ventral segments are not clearly differentiated in reports. Thus, we have included all studies reporting abnormal ACC function in BD in this section.

An ^{18}F-FDG PET study (Dunn *et al.*, 2002) found that the Beck Depression Inventory psychomotor–anhedonia symptom cluster correlated with higher glucose metabolism in the anterior cingulate in bipolar depressed medication-free subjects. Also, a ^{15}O-H$_2$O PET study found brain activity in mania was increased in the left dorsal anterior cingulate (Blumberg *et al.*, 2000). Abnormal ACC function has also been reported in multiple fMRI studies (Killgore *et al.*, 2008; Lennox *et al.*, 2004; Chen *et al.*, 2006; Malhi *et al.*, 2004b, 2007a; Lagopoulos *et al.*, 2007; Monks *et al.*, 2004; Gruber *et al.*, 2004; Marchand *et al.*, 2007b). A study of mania revealed decreased activation in response to an emotional task (Lennox *et al.*, 2004). Depression studies using emotional paradigms (Malhi *et al.*, 2004b; Chen *et al.*, 2006) have shown increased ACC activation. Studies of euthymic subjects have revealed increased activation using motor tasks (Marchand *et al.*, 2007b) and decreased activation using cognitive tasks (Malhi *et al.*, 2007a; Lagopoulos *et al.*, 2007; Monks *et al.*, 2004). In regard to treatment, a ^{99m}Tc-exametazime SPECT study found that manic relapse after lithium withdrawal was associated with increased perfusion of the superior anterior cingulate (Goodwin *et al.*, 1997).

Ventral system

Ventral prefrontal cortex

An ^{18}F-FDG PET study (Ketter *et al.*, 2001) using the Continuous Performance Test (CPT) revealed increased metabolism in the left ventrolateral prefrontal cortex (VLPFC) for the entire BD group, and increased right VLPFC metabolism for the euthymic-only subgroup. Among fMRI studies of homogeneous mood state, cognitive tasks have revealed increased (Strakowski *et al.*, 2004; McIntosh *et al.*, 2008) and decreased (Lagopoulos *et al.*, 2007; Frangou, 2005; Frangou *et al.*, 2008; Monks *et al.*, 2004) activation in euthymia. However, studies using emotional paradigms (Lagopoulos and Malhi,

2007; Malhi *et al.*, 2005; Jogia *et al.*, 2008) have consistently demonstrated decreased activation in euthymia. In mania, an emotional task revealed increased activation (Elliott *et al.*, 2004), while a cognitive paradigm revealed decreased activation (Blumberg *et al.*, 2003a). All three studies of depression have reported increased activation using emotional (Malhi *et al.*, 2004b; Chen *et al.*, 2006) and cognitive (Blumberg *et al.*, 2003a) tasks. Further, Drapier and colleagues (2008) studied 20 remitted bipolar I disorder patients, 20 of their unaffected first-degree relatives, and 20 controls using fMRI and an N-back working memory task. Unaffected relatives demonstrated abnormal activity in the left VLPFC regions, which the authors conclude suggests that left prefrontal hyperactivation during working memory represents a potential neurobiological endophenotype for the illness.

As with the DLPFC, studies suggest VPFC dysfunction occurs across all phases of illness, including euthymia. Further, there is evidence of consistent decreased activation in euthymia and increased activation in depression in response to emotional tasks. Finally, one study suggests increased activation in depression in response to a cognitive paradigm as well.

Orbitofrontal cortex

A ^{15}O-H$_2$O PET study found that manic subjects had decreased right OFC activation during word generation and decreased orbitofrontal activity during rest (Blumberg *et al.*, 1999). As with other frontal regions, a variety of fMRI tasks have demonstrated abnormal functioning. Of the investigations of homogeneous mood state, one study using an emotional paradigm (Altshuler *et al.*, 2008) found some OFC regions with increased and decreased activation in depression. A recent investigation of newly diagnosed bipolar patients demonstrated that bipolar patients produced increased orbitofrontal activation relative to controls early in the response to happy face stimuli, suggesting that the duration of increased response in this region may be time limited (Yurgelun-Todd and Killgore, in preparation). However, only decreased activation has been reported in mania using cognitive (Altshuler *et al.*, 2008) and emotional (Altshuler *et al.*, 2005; Elliott *et al.*, 2004) tasks. Finally, a ^{99m}Tc-exametazime SPECT study found that manic relapse after lithium withdrawal was associated with increased perfusion of the left OFC (Goodwin *et al.*, 1997). In summary, studies to date indicate OFC dysfunction in depression

(a)

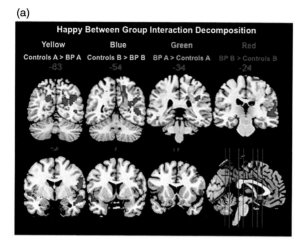

(b)

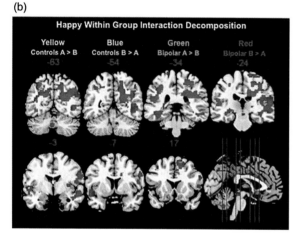

Figure 7.1a,b Bipolar patients differed significantly in the pattern of early- (block A) versus late- (block B) stage activation in response to a passive happy face perception task during acquisition of fMRI data. Within the bipolar sample, contrasts between the two blocks showed significantly different temporal activation of regions of the orbitofrontal cortex for early-stage (block A) and late-stage (block B) responses. Bipolar patients also showed greater activation across widespread posterior cortical regions involved in visual processing and memory for the same contrast for late-stage (block B) relative to early-stage (block A). Relatively limited areas of activation were evident for the control group when activation was contrasted for the two time blocks.

and mania. Of particular interest is the fact that all studies (three fMRI and one PET) of mania report decreased OFC activation using both cognitive and emotional paradigms.

Insula

An ^{18}F-FDG PET study (Dunn et al., 2002) found the Beck Depression Inventory psychomotor–anhedonia symptom cluster correlated with lower absolute metabolism in the right insula in bipolar depressed subjects. Another project using ^{18}F-FDG PET and a CPT (Ketter et al., 2001) found increased right insula metabolism in euthymic subjects as compared to controls. Functional MRI studies have revealed increased insula activation in mania (Lennox et al., 2004) and depression (Malhi et al., 2004b) in response to emotional tasks, and in euthymia in response to a cognitive task (Strakowski et al., 2004). Additionally, one study (Benedetti et al., 2007) suggests treatment may impact insula activation.

Amygdala

Two ^{18}F-FDG PET studies have reported amygdala abnormalities in BD. One, using an auditory CPT (Ketter et al., 2001), revealed increased metabolism in the right amygdala among BD depressed subjects, and the other (Drevets et al., 2002) found left amygdala metabolism was increased in BD depressives. In the later study (Drevets et al., 2002), BD subjects were also imaged during remission, and amygdala metabolism remained elevated in remitted subjects not taking mood-stabilizing drugs, but was within the normal range in subjects taking mood stabilizers.

A number of fMRI studies have also reported abnormal amygdala function in BD (Malhi et al., 2005; Lagopoulos and Malhi, 2007; Malhi et al., 2004b, 2007b; Altshuler et al., 2005; Lennox et al., 2004; Lawrence et al., 2004; Yurgelun-Todd et al., 2000; Mitchell et al., 2004; Strakowski et al., 2004). Those that have reported results from homogeneous mood states have revealed increased (Altshuler et al., 2005) and decreased (Lennox et al., 2004) activation in response to emotional tasks during mania. One study reported increased activation in response to an emotional task during depression (Malhi et al., 2004b). During euthymia, increased (Lagopoulos and Malhi, 2007) and decreased (Malhi et al., 2005) activation has been found in response to emotional tasks and increased activation has been reported in response to a cognitive task (Strakowski et al., 2004).

In one of the few functional connectivity studies done in BD, Foland and colleagues (2008) studied 9 bipolar manic and 9 control subjects using fMRI and an emotional faces paradigm and functional connectivity analyses to evaluate the hypothesis that VLPFC modulation of the amygdala was altered in bipolar subjects when manic. The degree to which the VLPFC regulated amygdala response during these tasks was assessed using a psychophysiological interaction (PPI) analysis. Compared with healthy subjects, manic patients had a significantly reduced VLPFC regulation of amygdala response during the emotion labeling task (an increased BOLD response in the amygdala and a decreased BOLD response in VLPFC). The authors conclude that these findings, taken in context with previous fMRI studies of bipolar mania, suggest that reductions in inhibitory frontal activity in these patients may lead to increased reactivity of the amygdala.

Ventral striatum and globus pallidus

Multiple functional imaging studies indicate basal ganglia dysfunction in BD. We have included the globus pallidus in this section with the striatum, since both are integral components of the frontal subcortical circuitry. An HMPAO SPECT study (Benabarre et al., 2004) using visual analysis of images found decreases of blood flow among five patients in the basal ganglia.

With regard to abnormalities in specific basal ganglia structures, reports have indicated dysfunction in both the striatum (caudate, putamen and nucleus accumbens) and globus pallidus. Two ^{18}F-FDG PET studies have reported striatal dysfunction in BD. One, using an auditory CPT task (Ketter et al., 2001), revealed that depressed subjects compared to controls exhibited increased metabolism in the caudate, putamen and nucleus accumbens. Another (Dunn et al., 2002), found Beck Depression Inventory (BDI) psychomotor–anhedonia symptom cluster correlated with lower absolute metabolism in right anteroventral caudate/putamen in bipolar depressed subjects. An HMPAO SPECT study of a group of mixed mood state bipolar subjects (Benabarre et al., 2005) found increased striatal profusion associated with deficits in memory and attention. Finally, a ^{15}O-H$_2$O PET study (Blumberg et al., 2000) revealed that brain activity in mania was increased in the left head of the caudate.

Further, many fMRI studies have demonstrated striatal dysfunction (Strakowski et al., 2005; Malhi et al., 2004a, 2005, 2007a, 2007b; Killgore et al., 2008; Chen et al., 2006; Lawrence et al., 2004; Adler et al., 2004; Caligiuri et al., 2003, 2006; Marchand et al., 2007a; McIntosh et al., 2008). Studies of euthymia have revealed increased activation in response to motor (Caligiuri et al., 2006; Marchand et al., 2007a) and cognitive tasks (Adler et al., 2004), as well as decreased activation in response to

emotional (Malhi et al., 2005, 2007b) and cognitive (Malhi et al., 2007a; Strakowski et al., 2005) tasks. However, striatal activation is increased in mania in response to motor (Caligiuri et al., 2006) and emotional (Malhi et al., 2004a) tasks, as well as in depression in response to motor (Caligiuri et al., 2003; Marchand et al., 2007a) and emotional tasks (Chen et al., 2006). Further, one fMRI study (Benedetti et al., 2007) of bipolar depression suggests that treatment response is related to changes in activation in the bilateral caudate.

To date, three fMRI studies implicate the globus pallidus in the neurobiology of BD. Increased activation has been reported in response to a motor task in mania (Caligiuri et al., 2003). In depression, increased activation has been reported in response to an emotional task (Malhi et al., 2004b), and decreased activation in response to a motor task (Caligiuri et al., 2006).

In summary, there is compelling evidence of dysfunction of the striatum in BD and some evidence of abnormalities in the globus pallidus. Of particular interest is the pattern of consistent increased striatal activation demonstrated in both depression and mania.

Thalamus

One ^{18}F-FDG PET study using an auditory CPT task (Ketter et al., 2001) revealed increased metabolism in the thalamus in BD. Studies using fMRI have found increased (Adler et al., 2004) and decreased (Malhi et al., 2007a) activation in response to cognitive tasks, and decreased activation in response to emotional (Malhi et al., 2005) tasks in euthymia. One study found increased activation in mania in response to an emotional task (Malhi et al., 2004a). Three studies suggest relatively compelling evidence of consistent increased activation in depression in response to emotional (Malhi et al., 2004b; Chen et al., 2006) and motor (Caligiuri et al., 2003) tasks. Finally, one study (Jogia et al., 2008), which used fMRI during a sad facial affect recognition task to study 12 euthymic bipolar subjects, revealed that following lamotrigine monotherapy, patients demonstrated increased right thalamus activation.

Other brain regions

Prefrontal cortex

Specific subregions of the prefrontal cortex were discussed above. Here, we provide a more generalized review of functional abnormalities of the PFC in BD. For the entire PFC, at least 31 studies of adults have reported prefrontal functional abnormalities in BD in either the depressed, manic, or euthymic state. Further, another seven studies have reported frontal abnormalities in studies combining individuals with different mood states (Yurgelun-Todd *et al.*, 2000; Lawrence *et al.*, 2004; Killgore *et al.*, 2008; Roth *et al.*, 2006, Mitchell *et al.*, 2004; Ketter *et al.*, 2001).

Among those studies reporting findings related to specific mood states, 10 (Benabarre *et al.*, 2004; Ketter *et al.*, 2001; Baxter *et al.*, 1989; Ito *et al.*, 1996; Rubin *et al.*, 1995; Marchand *et al.*, 2007a; Altshuler *et al.*, 2008; Malhi *et al.*, 2004b; Chen *et al.*, 2006; Blumberg *et al.*, 2003a) have reported findings during bipolar depression. Six (Benabarre *et al.*, 2004; Ketter *et al.*, 2001; Baxter *et al.*, 1989; Ito *et al.*, 1996; Rubin *et al.*, 1995; Altshuler *et al.*, 2008) reported decreased activation, and five (Malhi *et al.*, 2004b; Chen *et al.*, 2006; Blumberg *et al.*, 2003a; Marchand *et al.*, 2007a; Altshuler *et al.*, 2008) reported increased activation (one study reported both increased and decreased activation). Seven studies (Rubin *et al.*, 1995; Blumberg *et al.*, 1999; Altshuler *et al.*, 2005, 2008; Elliott *et al.*, 2004, Blumberg *et al.*, 2003a; Hariri *et al.*, 2003) have reported findings during mania, and all have reported decreased activation. In regard to the euthymic state, 20 studies have reported abnormal activation (Malhi *et al.*, 2005, 2007a, 2007b; Matsuo *et al.*, 2007; Curtis *et al.*, 2001; Adler *et al.*, 2004; Marchand *et al.*, 2007b; Frangou, 2005; Frangou *et al.*, 2008; Jogia *et al.*, 2008; Lagopoulos *et al.*, 2007; Strakowski *et al.*, 2004, 2005; Monks *et al.*, 2004; Culha *et al.*, 2008; Ketter *et al.*, 2001; Blumberg *et al.*, 2003a; Drapier *et al.*, 2008; Lagopoulos and Malhi, 2007; McIntosh *et al.*, 2008). Of these, 10 have reported increased (Curtis *et al.*, 2001; Adler *et al.*, 2004; Marchand *et al.*, 2007b; Lagopoulos and Malhi, 2007; Monks *et al.*, 2004; Ketter *et al.*, 2001; Drapier *et al.*, 2008; McIntosh *et al.*, 2008; Lagopoulos *et al.*, 2007; Strakowski *et al.*, 2004) and 14 decreased (Malhi *et al.*, 2005, 2007a, 2007b; Matsuo *et al.*, 2007; Frangou, 2005; Frangou *et al.*, 2008; Jogia *et al.*, 2008; Lagopoulos *et al.*, 2007; Strakowski *et al.*, 2004, 2005; Monks *et al.*, 2004; Culha *et al.*, 2008; Blumberg *et al.*, 2003a; Lagopoulos and Malhi, 2007) activation (some studies have reported increased and decreased PFC activation). Thus, reviewing all studies that have reported PFC function reveals compelling evidence of dysfunction in BD in multiple regions and all mood states.

Posterior cingulate

Functional abnormalities in posterior cingulate cortex have been identified using fMRI. In mania, an emotional task revealed increased activation (Lennox *et al.*, 2004), while in depression decreased activation has been demonstrated using cognitive (Marchand *et al.*, 2007a) and increased activation using emotional (Chen *et al.*, 2006) tasks. Studies of euthymia have shown decreased activation using emotional (Malhi *et al.*, 2007b) and cognitive (Malhi *et al.*, 2007a) tasks. Further, abnormalities in unspecified cingulate regions have also been reported using fMRI (Altshuler *et al.*, 2008; Malhi *et al.*, 2007b; Jogia *et al.*, 2008) and ^{99m}Tc-HMPAO SPECT (Culha *et al.*, 2008).

Finally, two studies suggest that treatment may impact cingulate function. An fMRI study of sleep deprivation combined with light therapy for bipolar depression (Benedetti *et al.*, 2007) revealed that treatment response was associated with changes in bilateral cingulate activation. Another fMRI study (Haldane *et al.*, 2008), using working memory and facial affect tasks, found lamotrigine monotherapy compared to baseline was associated with increased cingulate activation.

Taken together, studies that have reported cingulate findings indicate dysfunction across all mood states, as well as treatment likely impacting on cingulate function. In regard to the ACC, all three studies of euthymia have shown decreased activation in response to cognitive paradigms. There is also evidence of consistent ACC hyperactivation in depression in response to emotional tasks, and consistent decreased PCC activation in euthymia in response to both emotional and cognitive tasks.

Primary motor cortex and SMA

Several fMRI studies have demonstrated primary motor cortex and supplementary motor area (SMA) dysfunction in BD. In studies of mania, increased primary motor cortex activation has been reported in response to cognitive (Monks *et al.*, 2004) and motor (Caligiuri *et al.*, 2004) tasks. For depression, decreased activation has been reported in response to emotional tasks (Malhi *et al.*, 2004b), and in the euthymic phase, increased activation has been reported in response to a cognitive (Monks *et al.*, 2004) and decreased activation in response to an emotional (Malhi *et al.*, 2007a) task. For the SMA, increased activation in response to a motor task has been reported during depression (Caligiuri *et al.*, 2004). In addition to the studies above, studies suggest treatment may impact primary motor and SMA cortical function. A study (Silverstone *et al.*, 2005) using fMRI and word generation and verbal memory tasks found that, after lithium treatment, the mean BOLD signal decreased significantly in the left precentral gyrus and the left SMA. Another study (Jogia *et al.*, 2008) used fMRI during a sad facial affect recognition task, and found that after lamotrigine monotherapy, patients demonstrated reduced right and increased left precentral activation. A study of bipolar depression treated with sleep deprivation combined with light therapy (Benedetti *et al.*, 2007) found that treatment response was related to changes in activation in the bilateral PFC. In summary, these studies suggest functional abnormalities in the primary motor cortex in all phases of illness. Both cognitive and motor studies suggest consistent activation of M1 in mania. Some evidence also suggests that treatment impacts M1 function.

Parietal cortex

Three fMRI studies have demonstrated functional abnormalities of somatosensory cortex in BD. Studies have shown decreased S1 activation in the euthymic state in response to a cognitive paradigm (Malhi *et al.*, 2007a), and increased activation during euthymia in response to a cognitive paradigm (Strakowski *et al.*, 2004). Also, a treatment study (Benedetti *et al.*, 2007) reported that response was related to changes in activation in the right postcentral cortex. In regard to other parietal regions, fMRI has demonstrated decreased activation of the inferior parietal lobule in depression (Malhi *et al.*, 2004b) in response to an emotional task and increased activation in euthymia has been demonstrated using PET (Ketter *et al.*, 2001). Further, one treatment study reported changes in inferior parietal lobule (IPL) activation (Lawrence *et al.*, 2004). In euthymia, decreased (Monks *et al.*, 2004) and increased (Adler *et al.*, 2004) precuneus activation has been reported in response to a cognitive task. Further, treatment-related changes in activation have also been reported in this region (Lawrence *et al.*, 2004; Benedetti *et al.*, 2007). More generalized abnormalities in parietal regions have also been reported. A ^{99m}Tc-HMPAO SPECT study (Culha *et al.*, 2008) reported that the mean regional cerebral blood flow values of the bipolar euthymic patients were significantly lower

than those of the controls in bilateral parietal regions. Another HMPAO SPECT investigation (Benabarre *et al.*, 2005) also reported decreased left parietal profusion, in this case associated with deficits in working memory and attention. One fMRI study (Strakowski *et al.*, 2004) reported increased activation in the right superior and inferior parietal gyrus in euthymic bipolar patients compared to controls. A treatment study (Benedetti *et al.*, 2007) of bipolar depression reported that treatment response was related to changes in activation in bilateral parietal regions. These studies provide some evidence of parietal dysfunction in BD as well as changes related to treatment.

Occipital cortex

A few studies have reported functional abnormalities in the occipital cortex in BD. Two HMPAO SPECT studies have reported occipital abnormalities in BD; one (Benabarre *et al.*, 2005) found increased bilateral occipital profusion associated with deficits in executive dysfunction, and the other (Culha *et al.*, 2008) found that mean rCBF values of bipolar euthymic patients were significantly lower than those of the controls in the bilateral occipital regions. Functional MRI studies have found occipital increased (Adler *et al.*, 2004; Strakowski *et al.*, 2005) and decreased (Malhi *et al.*, 2007a) activation in response to cognitive tasks in euthymia. Finally, increased activation of right lingual cortex has been reported in depression in response to an emotional task (Chen *et al.*, 2006).

Temporal cortex

Considerable evidence suggests temporal dysfunction in BD. An IMP SPECT study (Gyulai *et al.*, 1997) revealed ^{123}I-IMP distribution in the anterior part of the temporal lobes was asymmetric in both depression/dysphoria and mania/hypomania, but not in euthymia. An HMPAO SPECT study (Migliorelli *et al.*, 1993) found that manic patients showed significantly lower blood flow in the basal portion of the right temporal lobe compared with normal control subjects, but another (O'Connell *et al.*, 1995) found an increase in the temporal lobe CBF of manic patients using ^{123}I-IMP SPECT. An ^{18}F-FDG PET study (Dunn *et al.*, 2002) found Beck Depression Inventory psychomotor–anhedonia symptom cluster correlated with lower absolute metabolism in right temporal cortex in bipolar depressed subjects. In

Activation during Viewing of Fearful Facial Affect
Positive Regression with Age: Chronic Patients

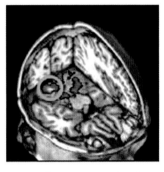

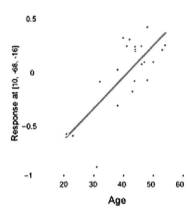

Response at [10, -68, -16]

Age

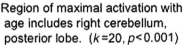

Region of maximal activation with age includes right cerebellum, posterior lobe. (k=20, p<0.001)

Figure 7.2 Chronic bipolar patients showed significant BOLD activation in the right cerebellum associated with increasing age during the viewing of a passive fearful face perception task. These results suggest that with increasing age bipolar patients rely increasingly on cerebellar regions for processing visual affective stimuli.

contrast, another investigation (Dye *et al.*, 1999) used a PET verbal fluency paradigm to compare remitted BD patients to controls and schizophrenics, and found a similar pattern of relative reduction of rCBF in the superior temporal cortex bilaterally without any significant between-group differences. Another ^{99m}Tc-HMPAO SPECT study (Culha *et al.*, 2008) found that the mean rCBF values of the bipolar euthymic patients were significantly lower than those of the controls in the bilateral medial–basal temporal cortex. Finally, an HMPAO SPECT study (Benabarre *et al.*, 2005) found increased bilateral temporal profusion associated with deficits in memory and executive function among BD subjects.

Additionally, several fMRI studies have reported temporal activation abnormalities (Strakowski *et al.*, 2005; Monks *et al.*, 2004; Adler *et al.*, 2004, Malhi *et al.*, 2004b, 2007a, 2007b; Mitchell *et al.*, 2004; McIntosh *et al.*, 2008; Chen *et al.*, 2006; Frangou *et al.*, 2008; Roth *et al.*, 2006; Lawrence *et al.*, 2004; Lagopoulos *et al.*, 2007; Jogia *et al.*, 2008). In regard to mood state, parahippocampal dysfunction has been reported in depression (Malhi *et al.*, 2004b) in response to a cognitive task. During euthymia, decreased (Lagopoulos *et al.*, 2007; Malhi *et al.*, 2007a) and increased (Strakowski *et al.*, 2004) activation has been shown in response to cognitive tasks as well as increased activation in response to emotional tasks (Malhi *et al.*, 2007b; Jogia *et al.*, 2008). Finally, treatment has been reported to impact temporal activation in two studies (Jogia *et al.*, 2008; Benedetti *et al.*, 2007).

Cerebellum

One HMPAO SPECT study (Benabarre *et al.*, 2005) found decreased cerebellar profusion associated with deficits in memory and executive function. An ^{18}F-FDG PET study (Ketter *et al.*, 2001) found that for a heterogeneous BD group, in terms of mood state compared to controls, there was increased metabolism in the cerebellum. Further, a comparison of the 10 euthymic subjects to controls also revealed increased cerebellar metabolism. Investigators using fMRI have found increased cerebellar activation in depression (Malhi *et al.*, 2004b) in response to an emotional task, and decreased activation in euthymia in response to emotional (Malhi *et al.*, 2005, 2007a) and cognitive (Strakowski *et al.*, 2005) tasks. Additionally, a recent study (Figure 7.2) showed significant BOLD activation in the right cerebellum associated with increasing age during a passive fearful face perception task. Authors suggest that as bipolar individuals grow older, they use their cerebellar regions more for processing visual affective information (Yurgelun-Todd and Killgore, in preparation).

Hypothalamus and midbrain

Two fMRI studies have suggested increased activation of the hypothalamus; one (Strakowski *et al.*, 2004) among euthymic, and one (Malhi *et al.*, 2004b) among depressed subjects. Two fMRI studies have also found abnormalities in the midbrain of bipolar subjects. The first (Lawrence *et al.*, 2004) found that a mixed group of bipolar subjects exhibited decreased activation compared to controls in the bilateral mid-brain in response to intense happy facial expression. The second (Malhi et al., 2007a) studied euthymic bipolar subjects and found that positive affect achieved greater activation among controls in the midbrain.

Bipolar II studies

Only two studies have examined brain function in bipolar II disorder. A ^{15}O-H$_2$O PET study using a novel motor sequence task (Berns et al., 2002) found that comparison subjects activated the superior parietal lobe and SMA in response to the introduction of the new sequence. In contrast, BD subjects did not display this activation pattern; instead, a widespread limbic network was activated in response to the new sequence. In the other study, Ketter et al. (2001) used an auditory CPT task during ^{18}F-FDG PET. Comparison of the bipolar I to bipolar II group revealed increased metabolism among the bipolar I cohort in the subgenual ACC, right middle frontal and right inferior parietal lobule regions.

Pediatric studies

Relative to the number of adult studies, few pediatric BD functional imaging studies have been completed. However, this area of investigation has expanded significantly in recent years.

Dorsal system

Several fMRI studies suggest abnormal functioning of prefrontal regions in pediatric BD. In a mixed group in regard to mood state, increased DLPFC activation was reported (Nelson et al., 2007) in response to a visual attention task. Two studies of euthymia report decreased (Pavuluri et al., 2008) and increased (Chang et al., 2004) activation in the DLPFC in response to cognitive tasks. Three studies have reported ACC dysfunction using fMRI and working memory (Chang et al., 2004), emotional faces (Dickstein et al., 2007), and color word matching (Pavuluri et al., 2008) paradigms. Finally, a comorbidity study (Adler et al., 2005) revealed that ADHD comorbidity was associated with less activation in the anterior cingulate.

Ventral system

A study of a mixed mood state cohort and event-related fMRI showed that BD subjects, compared to controls, had increased neural activation in the orbitofrontal cortex when successfully encoding angry faces (Dickstein et al., 2007). Two studies indicate VLPFC dysfunction in euthymic pediatric BD subjects. The first (Pavuluri et al., 2008) found less activation in right rostral VLPFC in response to a color word matching paradigm and the second (Chang et al., 2004) found greater VLPFC activation in response to a cognitive task. Finally, a study of comorbidity (Adler et al., 2005) revealed that ADHD was associated with less activation in the ventrolateral prefrontal cortex compared to BD subjects without ADHD.

As with adult studies, dysfunction of the amygdala has been reported in pediatric studies. One (Pavuluri et al., 2008) using fMRI and a color word matching paradigm found that patients with bipolar disorder demonstrated greater activation of the left amygdala. The other (Rich et al., 2008) studied 33 bipolar and 24 control subjects using fMRI and a task of face emotion identification and functional connectivity analyses. Compared to healthy subjects, BD subjects had significantly reduced connectivity between the left amygdala and two regions: right posterior cingulate/precuneus and right fusiform gyrus/parahippocampal gyrus. Deficits were evident regardless of mood state and comorbid diagnoses. The authors conclude that BD youth exhibit deficient connectivity between the amygdala and temporal association cortical regions previously implicated in processing facial expressions and social stimuli.

Amygdala dysfunction has also been reported in a study (Chang et al., 2008) of lamotrigine treatment. Blocks of negatively and neutrally valenced emotional pictures were presented during scanning. Activation in bilateral amygdalae for negative minus neutral pictures was correlated with Children's Depression Rating Scale scores. Clinical improvement was correlated with decreased right amygdalar activation. The authors conclude that adolescents with BD treated with lamotrigine demonstrated less amygdalar activation when viewing negative stimuli as depressive symptoms improved.

A study of adolescents with bipolar depression using a color-naming Stroop task found increased activation in the left putamen in the bipolar disorder group compared to controls (Blumberg et al., 2003b). Another investigation (Chang et al., 2004) of euthymic male subjects with BD performing a 2-back visuospatial working memory task and an affective task found that for the visuospatial working memory task, subjects with BD had greater activation in the left putamen. In viewing positively valenced pictures, subjects with BD had greater activation in the bilateral caudate. Lastly, an event-related fMRI study (Dickstein et al., 2007) of a mixed affective state cohort showed that PBD subjects, compared to controls, had increased neural activation in the striatum.

Two studies have reported thalamic dysfunction in pediatric BD. The first (Blumberg et al., 2003b) studied 10 adolescents with bipolar depression and 10 healthy comparison subjects using a color-naming Stroop task during event-related fMRI. They found increased activation in the left thalamus in the bipolar disorder group compared to controls. The second (Chang et al., 2004) studied 12 euthymic male subjects with BD and 10 age-, sex- and IQ-matched healthy controls. Subjects underwent fMRI at 3 T while performing a 2-back visuospatial working memory task and an affective task with positively, neutrally, or negatively valenced pictures. For the visuospatial working memory task, subjects with BD had greater activation in the left thalamus. In viewing positively valenced pictures, subjects with BD had greater activation in the bilateral thalamus. Finally, a study (Chang et al., 2004) of euthymic male subjects with BD found that in viewing negatively valenced pictures, subjects with BD had greater activation in the right insula.

Other brain regions

One project (Nelson et al., 2007) used event-related fMRI and a visual attention and response flexibility task. On correctly performed change trials relative to correctly performed go trials, BD patients generated significantly more activity in the left primary motor cortex than did healthy controls, even though performance levels did not differ across groups. Another study (Chang et al., 2004) of euthymic male subjects found that for a visuospatial working memory task, controls had greater activation in the cerebellar vermis. Finally, a study found that ADHD comorbidity was associated with greater activation in the middle temporal gyrus as well as in the posterior parietal cortex (Adler et al., 2005).

Summary of pediatric studies

Functional imaging studies of pediatric BD to date have found evidence of abnormalities of the dorsal and ventral emotional control systems as well as in other brain regions also implicated in adult BD. At this time it is unknown whether pediatric bipolar disorder is the result of the same neuropathology as the adult condition. The fact that functional brain abnormalities have been found in the same regions among children and adolescents with BD as among adults could suggest similar underlying neuropathology. Nonetheless, it is unclear whether findings in either pediatric or adult studies represent primary neurobiology or a final common pathway. Thus, it is possible that the pediatric form of the illness might have different primary pathology but the same final common pathways as the adult disorder. Further studies will be needed to disambiguate this issue. However, it is encouraging that studies are now being done with the aim of beginning to elucidate functional brain abnormalities associated with pediatric BD.

Dorsal and ventral emotional control systems

As discussed above, the dorsal emotional control system, which includes the dorsolateral prefrontal cortex, medial prefrontal cortex, dorsal anterior cingulate and hippocampus, is responsible for effortful regulation of affective state (Phillips et al., 2003). Impairment of this system could theoretically result in mood episodes as a result of deficient modulation of affective states generated in the ventral system.

The studies reviewed above provide compelling evidence of dorsal system dysfunction in BD. The strongest evidence is for DLPFC dysfunction. Studies have reported functional abnormalities in depression (Marchand et al., 2007a; Malhi et al., 2004b; Altshuler et al., 2008) and mania (Elliott et al., 2004). Further, nine studies (Marchand et al., 2007b; Lagopoulos and Malhi, 2007; Frangou, 2005; Frangou et al., 2008; Strakowski et al., 2005; Monks et al., 2004; Lagopoulos et al., 2007; Malhi et al., 2007a; Jogia et al., 2008) indicate that functional abnormalities persist in the euthymic state. Interpretation of activation patterns is complex because abnormalities have been demonstrated using cognitive (Frangou, 2005; Frangou et al., 2008; Strakowski et al., 2005; Monks et al., 2004; Lagopoulos et al., 2007; Malhi et al., 2007a), emotional (Malhi et al., 2004b; Lagopoulos and Malhi, 2007; Jogia et al., 2008; Elliott et al., 2004) and motor (Marchand et al., 2007a, 2007b) paradigms, and many paradigms have only been used in one mood state. Nonetheless, most fMRI studies (8 of 13) report decreased DLPFC

Activation during Viewing of Fearful Facial Affect
Negative Regression with Age: Chronic Patients

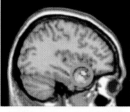

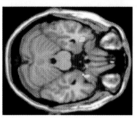

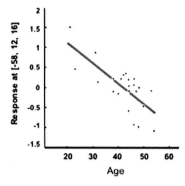

Region of maximal activation with age includes left frontal lobe, inferior frontal gyrus. ($k=20$, $p<0.001$)

Figure 7.3 Chronic bipolar patients showed significant BOLD activation in the left inferior frontal gyrus associated negatively with increasing age during the viewing of a passive fearful face perception task. Significant activation for this regression was also seen for the inferior right frontal gyrus. In contrast to the results in Figure 7.2, these findings suggest that with increasing age bipolar patients show decreasing reliance on frontal regions for processing visual affective stimuli.

activation in BD. If only the studies using cognitive and emotional paradigms are considered, then 73% (8 of 11) report decreased activation. Therefore, while variable results have been reported, these studies suggest that impaired DLPFC function could contribute to a lack of dorsal system regulation of affect in BD. Further, three studies (Nelson *et al.*, 2007; Pavuluri *et al.*, 2008; Chang *et al.*, 2004) have reported functional abnormalities in pediatric BD in this region, suggesting this dysfunction may represent core neuropathology rather than occur as a consequence of repeated mood episodes or treatment.

Studies to date have also provided evidence of abnormalities in other components of the dorsal system. Several studies suggest medial frontal (Culha *et al.*, 2008; Malhi *et al.*, 2007a, 2004b; Monks *et al.*, 2004; Lagopoulos *et al.*, 2007) and hippocampal (Drevets *et al.*, 2002; Lagopoulos and Malhi, 2007; Lawrence *et al.*, 2004; Altshuler *et al.*, 2008) dysfunction in BD; however, activation patterns have been variable.

The studies reviewed in this chapter also provide compelling evidence of ventral system dysregulation in BD. Functional abnormalities have been reported in the VPFC, OFC, insula, amygdala, striatum and thalamus.

Ventral prefrontal cortical dysfunction has been demonstrated using PET (Ketter *et al.*, 2001) and fMRI in mania, depression and euthymia (Strakowski *et al.*, 2004; McIntosh *et al.*, 2008; Lagopoulos *et al.*, 2007; Frangou, 2005; Frangou *et al.*, 2008; Monks

et al., 2004; Lagopoulos and Malhi, 2007; Malhi *et al.*, 2004b, 2005; Jogia *et al.*, 2008; Elliott *et al.*, 2004; Blumberg *et al.*, 2003a; Chen *et al.*, 2006). Activation patterns have been variable; however, all three studies of depression (Malhi *et al.*, 2004b; Chen *et al.*, 2006; Blumberg *et al.*, 2003a) report increased activation, and one (Elliott *et al.*, 2004) of two studies (Elliott *et al.*, 2004; Blumberg *et al.*, 2003a) of mania also reported hyperactivation. VPFC dysfunction has also been demonstrated in first degree relatives of bipolar subjects (Drapier *et al.*, 2008) and pediatric BP subjects (Pavuluri *et al.*, 2008; Chang *et al.*, 2004). Interestingly, increasing age of adult chronic BP subjects has been shown to be associated with decreased BOLD activation in the left and right inferior frontal gyrus during a passive fearful face perception task, suggesting that activation of this region may be related to duration of illness (Yurgelun-Todd and Killgore, in preparation) (see Figure 7.3). Taken together, these studies indicate that VPFC abnormalities likely play a critical role in the neurobiology of BD. Similarly, several studies have indicated OFC dysfunction. A particularly interesting finding is that only decreased activation has been reported during mania using PET (Blumberg *et al.*, 1999) and fMRI (Altshuler *et al.*, 2005, 2008; Elliott *et al.*, 2004). In regard to the insula, fMRI studies have revealed increased insula activation in mania (Lennox *et al.*, 2004), depression (Malhi *et al.*, 2004b), and in euthymia (Strakowski *et al.*, 2004). An ^{18}F-FDG PET study

(Ketter *et al.*, 2001) also found increased right insula metabolism in euthymic subjects as compared to controls; however, another (Dunn *et al.*, 2002) found BDI psychomotor–anhedonia symptom cluster correlated with lower absolute metabolism in the right insula in bipolar depressed subjects. Multiple studies (Ketter *et al.*, 2001; Drevets *et al.*, 2002; Malhi *et al.*, 2004b, 2005, 2007b; Lagopoulos and Malhi, 2007; Altshuler *et al.*, 2005; Lennox *et al.*, 2004; Lawrence *et al.*, 2004; Yurgelun-Todd *et al.*, 2000; Mitchell *et al.*, 2004; Strakowski *et al.*, 2004) suggest amygdala dysfunction in BD, but activation patterns have been variable. There is compelling evidence of increased striatal activation in depression (Ketter *et al.*, 2001; Caligiuri *et al.*, 2003; Marchand *et al.*, 2007a; Chen *et al.*, 2006) and mania (Blumberg *et al.*, 2000; Caligiuri *et al.*, 2006; Malhi *et al.*, 2004a), although results in euthymia have been variable (Caligiuri *et al.*, 2006; Marchand *et al.*, 2007a; Adler *et al.*, 2004; Malhi *et al.*, 2005, 2007a, 2007b; Strakowski *et al.*, 2005). Three studies of pediatric BD also report hyperactivation (Blumberg *et al.*, 2003b; Chang *et al.*, 2004; Dickstein *et al.*, 2007). Finally, studies also suggest hyperactivation of the thalamus in depression (Malhi *et al.*, 2004b; Chen *et al.*, 2006; Caligiuri *et al.*, 2003) and mania (Malhi *et al.*, 2004a), with variable results (Adler *et al.*, 2004, Malhi *et al.*, 2005, 2007a) in euthymia. Two pediatric studies also report increased thalamic activation (Blumberg *et al.*, 2003b; Chang *et al.*, 2004).

Although some results are variable, multiple functional imaging studies using cognitive, emotional and motor tasks clearly demonstrate dysfunction of both the dorsal and ventral emotional regulation systems in BD. With regard to the dorsal system, decreased activation of the DLPFC may indicate an impairment of effortful regulation of affect. Functional abnormalities in the ventral system could occur either as a result of, or in addition to, attenuated dorsal system modulation. These studies provide preliminary evidence that hyperactivation of the VPFC, striatum and thalamus occur in both mania and depression, while decreased OFC activation is associated with mania.

Other brain regions

The focus of the chapter has been on the dorsal and ventral emotional control systems. Nonetheless, the review provides considerable evidence of dysfunction in other brain regions including temporal, posterior cingulate, motor, parietal, occipital, and cerebellar regions. While an in-depth discussion of these abnormalities is beyond the scope of this review, these findings suggest that multiple cortical and subcortical regions are impacted by this illness.

Limitations of current research

The functional neuroimaging studies reported in the literature have provided important insights into the neurobiology of bipolar disorder. Nonetheless, BD is a complex illness which is difficult to study using neuroimaging methods. Thus, the interpretation of results requires recognition of some inevitable confounding variables.

One potential confound is that BD subjects sometimes do not perform as well as normal controls on cognitive tasks (Gruber *et al.*, 2004; Strakowski *et al.*, 2005). It has been pointed out that if task performance differs between groups, then differences in brain activation may reflect a diminished ability of the patients to complete the task, instead of actual differences in brain function (Strakowski *et al.*, 2004). Also, functional neuroimaging studies of bipolar patients who are experiencing a mood episode may reveal differences in brain activation from healthy subjects, which represent epiphenomena of that mood state but are not a trait of bipolar disorder (Strakowski *et al.*, 2004). Thus it will be important for future studies to disambiguate trait versus mood state abnormalities. Finally, subtle variations in mood state may be a confound. For example, similar but slightly different results have been found comparing mild to severe bipolar depression (Ketter *et al.*, 2001).

Findings related to medication and treatment

The potential impact of treatment on functional studies reviewed herein is a significant concern. Most studies have examined medicated subjects, which introduces a significant potential confound. However, due to the nature of the illness, it is extremely difficult, and some would say unethical, to study unmedicated subjects.

One approach to this problem is to utilize second-level regression analyses to determine whether medication has impacted the findings of the study. For example, a study revealed that patients off antipsychotic or mood-stabilizing medication exhibited greater activation compared with patients on these medications in the bilateral MI, right thalamus and right SMA (Caligiuri *et al.*, 2003). In another study, BD subjects treated with antipsychotics or mood-stabilizing medications exhibited lower BOLD responses in M1 and SMA (Caligiuri *et al.*, 2004).

Conclusions and future directions

Despite the limitations described above, the emergence of functional neuroimaging methodologies has provided an opportunity to greatly enhance our understanding of the neurobiology of bipolar disorder. Results to date suggest that further functional neuroimaging studies are warranted, and also suggest some potential directions for future investigations.

Perhaps the most compelling argument is for additional studies to disambiguate the precise mechanisms by which dorsal and ventral emotional control circuitry dysfunction contributes to the expression of mood symptoms and cycling in bipolar disorder. One approach is the utilization of functional connectivity methods. For example, two studies have already provided insights into the mechanisms of amygdala

dysfunction in BD. In one of these, Foland and colleagues (2008) studied 9 bipolar manic and 9 control subjects using fMRI and an emotional faces paradigm and functional connectivity analyses to evaluate the hypothesis that VLPFC modulation of the amygdala was altered in bipolar subjects when manic. The degree to which the VLPFC regulated amygdala response during these tasks was assessed using a psychophysiological interaction analysis. Compared with healthy subjects, manic patients had a significantly reduced VLPFC regulation of amygdala response during the emotion labeling task (increased BOLD response in the amygdala and a decreased BOLD response in VLPFC). The authors conclude that these findings, taken in context with previous fMRI studies of bipolar mania, suggest that reductions in inhibitory frontal activity in these patients may lead to an increased reactivity of the amygdala. In the other, Rich and colleagues (2008) studied 33 bipolar and 24 control subjects using fMRI and a task of face emotion identification and functional connectivity analyses. Compared to healthy subjects, BD subjects had significantly reduced connectivity between the left amygdala and

---

Box 7.1. Functional imaging studies of bipolar disorder – summary of key findings

Although studies are difficult to compare because of different populations and methodologies, there is consistent evidence of abnormalities of function in both the dorsal and ventral emotional control systems in response to a variety of activation paradigms.

- Abnormal activation of the dorsal system, which provides conscious regulation of affect.
  - Dorsolateral prefrontal cortex in depression, euthymia and mania.
  - Anterior cingulate in depression, mania and euthymia.
  - Medial frontal cortex in depression and euthymia.
  - Hippocampus in depression and euthymia.
- Abnormal activation of the ventral system, which perceives emotional stimuli, generates affective state and produces an autonomic response.
  - Ventral prefrontal cortex in depression, euthymia and mania.
  - Insula in depression, euthymia and mania.
  - Amygdala in depression, euthymia and mania.
  - Striatum in depression, euthymia and mania.
  - Thalamus in depression, euthymia and mania.
  - Orbitofrontal cortex in depression and mania.
  - Globus pallidus in depression and mania.

Other brain regions in which several studies have demonstrated abnormalities of activation.
  - Various prefrontal subregions in depression, euthymia and mania.
  - Temporal lobe in depression, euthymia and mania.
  - Posterior cingulate in depression, euthymia and mania.
  - Primary motor cortex in depression, euthymia and mania.
  - Cerebellum in depression and euthymia.

two regions: right posterior cingulate/precuneus and right fusiform gyrus/parahippocampal gyrus. Deficits were evident regardless of mood state and comorbid diagnoses. The authors conclude that BD youth exhibit deficient connectivity between the amygdala and temporal association cortical regions previously implicated in processing facial expressions and social stimuli. These encouraging results suggest future studies evaluating connectivity between the dorsal and ventral system as well as between regions within each system may provide important information in regard to emotional dysregulation in BD. Other promising areas include studies combining functional imaging and genetics as well as those combining functional imaging and structural methods, such as diffusion tensor imaging.

References

Adler C M, Delbello M P, Mills N P, Schmithorst V, Holland S and Strakowski S M. 2005. Comorbid ADHD is associated with altered patterns of neuronal activation in adolescents with bipolar disorder performing a simple attention task. *Bipolar Disord* **7**, 577–88.

Adler C M, Holland S K, Schmithorst V, Tuchfarber M J and Strakowski S M. 2004. Changes in neuronal activation in patients with bipolar disorder during performance of a working memory task. *Bipolar Disord* **6**, 540–9.

Altshuler L L, Bookheimer S Y, Townsend J, *et al.* 2005. Blunted activation in orbitofrontal cortex during mania: A functional magnetic resonance imaging study. *Biol Psychiatry* **58**, 763–9.

Altshuler L, Bookheimer S, Townsend J, *et al.* 2008. Regional brain changes in bipolar I depression: A functional magnetic resonance imaging study. *Bipolar Disord* **10**, 708–17.

Baxter L R Jr, Schwartz J M, Phelps M E, *et al.* 1989. Reduction of prefrontal cortex glucose metabolism common to three types of depression. *Arch Gen Psychiatry* **46**, 243–50.

Benabarre A, Vieta E, Martin F, *et al.* 2004. Clinical value of 99mTc-HMPAO SPECT in depressed bipolar I patients. *Psychiatry Res* **132**, 285–9.

Benabarre A, Vieta E, Martinez-Aran A, *et al.* 2005. Neuropsychological disturbances and cerebral blood flow in bipolar disorder. *Aust N Z J Psychiatry* **39**, 227–34.

Benedetti F, Bernasconi A, Blasi V, *et al.* 2007. Neural and genetic correlates of antidepressant response to sleep deprivation: A functional magnetic resonance imaging study of moral valence decision in bipolar depression. *Arch Gen Psychiatry* **64**, 179–87.

Berns G S, Martin M and Proper S M. 2002. Limbic hyperreactivity in bipolar II disorder. *Am J Psychiatry* **159**, 304–06.

Blumberg H P, Leung H C, Skudlarski P, *et al.* 2003a. A functional magnetic resonance imaging study of bipolar disorder: State- and trait-related dysfunction in ventral prefrontal cortices. *Arch Gen Psychiatry* **60**, 601–09.

Blumberg H P, Martin A, Kaufman J, *et al.* 2003b. Frontostriatal abnormalities in adolescents with bipolar disorder: Preliminary observations from functional MRI. *Am J Psychiatry* **160**, 1345–7.

Blumberg H P, Stern E, Martinez D, *et al.* 2000. Increased anterior cingulate and caudate activity in bipolar mania. *Biol Psychiatry* **48**, 1045–52.

Blumberg H P, Stern E, Ricketts S, *et al.* 1999. Rostral and orbital prefrontal cortex dysfunction in the manic state of bipolar disorder. *Am J Psychiatry* **156**, 1986–8.

Caligiuri M P, Brown G G, Meloy M J, *et al.* 2003. An fMRI study of affective state and medication on cortical and subcortical brain regions during motor performance in bipolar disorder. *Psychiatry Res* **123**, 171–82.

Caligiuri M P, Brown G G, Meloy M J, *et al.* 2004. A functional magnetic resonance imaging study of cortical asymmetry in bipolar disorder. *Bipolar Disord* **6**, 183–96.

Caligiuri M P, Brown G G, Meloy M J, *et al.* 2006. Striatopallidal regulation of affect in bipolar disorder. *J Affect Disord* **91**, 235–42.

Chang K, Adleman N E, Dienes K, Simeonova D I, Menon V and Reiss A. 2004. Anomalous prefrontal–subcortical activation in familial pediatric bipolar disorder: A functional magnetic resonance imaging investigation. *Arch Gen Psychiatry* **61**, 781–92.

Chang K D, Wagner C, Garrett A, Howe M and Reiss A. 2008. A preliminary functional magnetic resonance imaging study of prefrontal–amygdalar activation changes in adolescents with bipolar depression treated with lamotrigine. *Bipolar Disord* **10**, 426–31.

Chen C H, Lennox B, Jacob R, *et al.* 2006. Explicit and implicit facial affect recognition in manic and depressed States of bipolar disorder: A functional magnetic resonance imaging study. *Biol Psychiatry* **59**, 31–9.

Culha A F, Osman O, Dogangun Y, *et al.* 2008. Changes in regional cerebral blood flow demonstrated by 99mTc-HMPAO SPECT in euthymic bipolar patients. *Eur Arch Psychiatry Clin Neurosci* **258**, 144–51.

Curtis V A, Dixon T A, Morris R G, *et al.* 2001. Differential frontal activation in schizophrenia and bipolar illness during verbal fluency. *J Affect Disord* **66**, 111–21.

Davidson R J. 1998. Anterior electrophysiological asymmetries, emotion, and depression: Conceptual and methodological conundrums. *Psychophysiology* **35**, 607–14.

Dickstein D P, Rich B A, Roberson-Nay R, *et al.* 2007. Neural activation during encoding of emotional faces in pediatric bipolar disorder. *Bipolar Disord* **9**, 679–92.

Drapier D, Surguladze S, Marshall N, *et al.* 2008. Genetic liability for bipolar disorder is characterized by excess frontal activation in response to a working memory task. *Biol Psychiatry* **64**, 513–20.

Drevets W C, Price J L, Bardgett M E, Reich T, Todd R D and Raichle M E. 2002. Glucose metabolism in the amygdala in depression: Relationship to diagnostic subtype and plasma cortisol levels. *Pharmacol Biochem Behav* **71**, 431–47.

Dunn R T, Kimbrell T A, Ketter T A, *et al.* 2002. Principal components of the Beck Depression Inventory and regional cerebral metabolism in unipolar and bipolar depression. *Biol Psychiatry* **51**, 387–99.

Dye S M, Spence S A, Bench C J, *et al.* 1999. No evidence for left superior temporal dysfunction in asymptomatic schizophrenia and bipolar disorder. PET study of verbal fluency. *Br J Psychiatry* **175**, 367–74.

Elliott R, Ogilvie A, Rubinsztein J S, Calderon G, Dolan R J and Sahakian B J. 2004. Abnormal ventral frontal response during performance of an affective go/no go task in patients with mania. *Biol Psychiatry* **55**, 1163–70.

Foland L C, Altshuler L L, Bookheimer S Y, Eisenberger N, Townsend J and Thompson P M. 2008. Evidence for deficient modulation of amygdala response by prefrontal cortex in bipolar mania. *Psychiatry Res* **162**, 27–37.

Frangou S. 2005. The Maudsley Bipolar Disorder Project. *Epilepsia* **46** (Suppl 4), 19–25.

Frangou S, Kington J, Raymont V and Shergill S S. 2008. Examining ventral and dorsal prefrontal function in bipolar disorder: A functional magnetic resonance imaging study. *Eur Psychiatry* **23**, 300–08.

Goel V and Dolan R J. 2003. Reciprocal neural response within lateral and ventral medial prefrontal cortex during hot and cold reasoning. *Neuroimage* **20**, 2314–21.

Goodwin G M, Cavanagh J T, Glabus M F, Kehoe R F, O'Carroll R E and Ebmeier K P. 1997. Uptake of 99mTc-exametazime shown by single photon emission computed tomography before and after lithium withdrawal in bipolar patients: Associations with mania. *Br J Psychiatry* **170**, 426–30.

Gruber S A, Rogowska J and Yurgelun-Todd D A. 2004. Decreased activation of the anterior cingulate in bipolar patients: An fMRI study. *J Affect Disord* **82**, 191–201.

Gyulai L, Alavi A, Broich K, Reilley J, Ball W B and Whybrow P C. 1997. I-123 iofetamine single-photon computed emission tomography in rapid cycling bipolar disorder: A clinical study. *Biol Psychiatry* **41**, 152–61.

Haldane M, Jogia J, Cobb A, Kozuch E, Kumari V and Frangou S. 2008. Changes in brain activation during working memory and facial recognition tasks in patients

with bipolar disorder with Lamotrigine monotherapy. *Eur Neuropsychopharmacol* **18**, 48–54.

Hariri A R, Mattay V S, Tessitore A, Fera F and Weinberger D R. 2003. Neocortical modulation of the amygdala response to fearful stimuli. *Biol Psychiatry* **53**, 494–501.

Ito H, Kawashima R, Awata S, *et al.* 1996. Hypoperfusion in the limbic system and prefrontal cortex in depression: SPECT with anatomic standardization technique. *J Nucl Med* **37**, 410–4.

Jogia J, Haldane, M., Cobb, A., Kumari, V. and Frangou S. 2008. Pilot investigation of the changes in cortical activation during facial affect recognition with lamotrigine monotherapy in bipolar disorder. *Br J Psychiatry* **192**, 197–201.

Ketter T A, Kimbrell T A, George M S, *et al.* 2001. Effects of mood and subtype on cerebral glucose metabolism in treatment-resistant bipolar disorder. *Biol Psychiatry* **49**, 97–109.

Killgore W D, Gruber S A and Yurgelun-Todd D A. 2008. Abnormal corticostriatal activity during fear perception in bipolar disorder. *Neuroreport* **19**, 1523–7.

Lagopoulos J, Ivanovski B and Malhi G S. 2007. An event-related functional MRI study of working memory in euthymic bipolar disorder. *J Psychiatry Neurosci* **32**, 174–84.

Lagopoulos J and Malhi G S. 2007. A functional magnetic resonance imaging study of emotional Stroop in euthymic bipolar disorder. *Neuroreport* **18**, 1583–7.

Lawrence N S, Williams A M, Surguladze S, *et al.* 2004. Subcortical and ventral prefrontal cortical neural responses to facial expressions distinguish patients with bipolar disorder and major depression. *Biol Psychiatry* **55**, 578–87.

Lennox B R, Jacob R, Calder A J, Lupson V and Bullmore E T. 2004. Behavioural and neurocognitive responses to sad facial affect are attenuated in patients with mania. *Psychol Med* **34**, 795–802.

Levesque J, Eugene F, Joanette Y, *et al.* 2003. Neural circuitry underlying voluntary suppression of sadness. *Biol Psychiatry* **53**, 502–10.

Liotti M, Mayberg H S, Brannan S K, Mcginnis S, Jerabek P and Fox P T. 2000. Differential limbic–cortical correlates of sadness and anxiety in healthy subjects: implications for affective disorders. *Biol Psychiatry* **48**, 30–42.

Malhi G S, Lagopoulos J, Owen A M, Ivanovski B, Shnier R and Sachdev P. 2007a. Reduced activation to implicit affect induction in euthymic bipolar patients: an fMRI study. *J Affect Disord* **97**, 109–22.

Malhi G S, Lagopoulos J, Sachdev P S, Ivanovski B and Shnier R. 2005. An emotional Stroop functional MRI study of euthymic bipolar disorder. *Bipolar Disord* **7** (Suppl 5), 58–69.

Malhi G S, Lagopoulos J, Sachdev P S, Ivanovski B, Shnier R and Ketter T. 2007b. Is a lack of disgust something to fear? A functional magnetic resonance imaging facial emotion recognition study in euthymic bipolar disorder patients. *Bipolar Disord* **9**, 345–57.

Malhi G S, Lagopoulos J, Sachdev P, Mitchell P B, Ivanovski B and Parker G B. 2004a. Cognitive generation of affect in hypomania: An fMRI study. *Bipolar Disord* **6**, 271–85.

Malhi G S, Lagopoulos J, Ward P B, *et al.* 2004b. Cognitive generation of affect in bipolar depression: An fMRI study. *Eur J Neurosci* **19**, 741–54.

Marchand W R, Lee J N, Thatcher G W, *et al.* 2007a. A functional MRI study of a paced motor activation task to evaluate frontal–subcortical circuit function in bipolar depression. *Psychiatry Res* **155**, 221–30.

Marchand W R, Lee J N, Thatcher J, Thatcher G W, Jensen C and Starr J. 2007b. A preliminary longitudinal fMRI study of frontal–subcortical circuits in bipolar disorder using a paced motor activation paradigm. *J Affect Disord* **103**, 237–41.

Matsuo K, Kouno T, Hatch J P, *et al.* 2007. A near-infrared spectroscopy study of prefrontal cortex activation during a verbal fluency task and carbon dioxide inhalation in individuals with bipolar disorder. *Bipolar Disord* **9**, 876–83.

Mayberg H S. 1997. Limbic–cortical dysregulation: A proposed model of depression. *J Neuropsychiatry Clin Neurosci* **9**, 471–81.

Mcintosh A M, Whalley H C, Mckirdy J, *et al.* 2008. Prefrontal function and activation in bipolar disorder and schizophrenia. *Am J Psychiatry* **165**, 378–84.

Migliorelli R, Starkstein SE, Teson A, *et al.* 1993. SPECT findings in patients with primary mania. *J Neuropsychiatry Clin Neurosci* **5**, 379–83.

Mitchell R L, Elliott R, Barry M, Cruttenden A and Woodruff P W. 2004. Neural response to emotional prosody in schizophrenia and in bipolar affective disorder. *Br J Psychiatry* **184**, 223–30.

Monks P J, Thompson J M, Bullmore E T, *et al.* 2004. A functional MRI study of working memory task in euthymic bipolar disorder: Evidence for task-specific dysfunction. *Bipolar Disord* **6**, 550–64.

Nelson E E, Vinton D T, Berghorst L, *et al.* 2007. Brain systems underlying response flexibility in healthy and bipolar adolescents: An event-related fMRI study. *Bipolar Disord* **9**, 810–9.

Nestler E J, Barrot M, Dileone R J, Eisch A J, Gold S J and Monteggia L M. 2002. Neurobiology of depression. *Neuron* **34**, 13–25.

O'Connell R A, Van Heertum R L, Luck D, *et al.* 1995. Single-photon emission computed tomography of the brain in acute mania and schizophrenia. *J Neuroimaging* **5**, 101–04.

Pavuluri M N, O'Connor M M, Harral E M and Sweeney J A. 2008. An fMRI study of the interface between affective and cognitive neural circuitry in pediatric bipolar disorder. *Psychiatry Res* **162**, 244–55.

Phillips M L, Drevets W C, Rauch S L and Lane R. 2003. Neurobiology of emotion perception I: The neural basis of normal emotion perception. *Biol Psychiatry* **54**, 504–14.

Rich B A, Fromm S J, Berghorst L H, *et al.* 2008. Neural connectivity in children with bipolar disorder: Impairment in the face emotion processing circuit. *J Child Psychol Psychiatry* **49**, 88–96.

Ridderinkhof K R, Ullsperger M, Crone E A and Nieuwenhuis S. 2004. The role of the medial frontal cortex in cognitive control. *Science* **306**, 443–7.

Roth R M, Koven N S, Randolph J J, *et al.* 2006. Functional magnetic resonance imaging of executive control in bipolar disorder. *Neuroreport* **17**, 1085–9.

Rubin E, Sackeim H A, Prohovnik I, Moeller J R, Schnur D B and Mukherjee S. 1995. Regional cerebral blood flow in mood disorders: IV. Comparison of mania and depression. *Psychiatry Res* **61**, 1–10.

Salamone J D. 2007. Functions of mesolimbic dopamine: Changing concepts and shifting paradigms. *Psychopharmacology (Berl)* **191**, 389.

Silverstone P H, Bell E C, Willson M C, Dave S and Wilman A H. 2005. Lithium alters brain activation in bipolar disorder in a task- and state-dependent manner: An fMRI study. *Ann Gen Psychiatry* **4**, 14.

Stern C E, Owen A M, Tracey I, Look R B, Rosen B R and Petrides M. 2000. Activity in ventrolateral and mid-dorsolateral prefrontal cortex during nonspatial visual working memory processing: Evidence from functional magnetic resonance imaging. *Neuroimage* **11**, 392–9.

Strakowski S M, Adler C M, Holland S K, Mills N and Delbello M P. 2004. A preliminary FMRI study of sustained attention in euthymic, unmedicated bipolar disorder. *Neuropsychopharmacology* **29**, 1734–40.

Strakowski S M, Adler C M, Holland S K, Mills N P, Delbello M P and Eliassen J C. 2005. Abnormal FMRI brain activation in euthymic bipolar disorder patients during a counting Stroop interference task. *Am J Psychiatry* **162**, 1697–705.

Yurgelun-Todd D A, Gruber S A, Kanayama G, Killgore W D, Baird A A and Young A D. 2000. fMRI during affect discrimination in bipolar affective disorder. *Bipolar Disord* **2**, 237–48.

Yurgelun-Todd D A, and Ross A J. 2006. Functional magnetic resonance imaging studies in bipolar disorder [review]. *CNS Spectr* **11**, 287–97.

Chapter 8

Molecular imaging of bipolar illness

John O. Brooks III, Po W. Wang and Terence A. Ketter

Introduction

Investigation of the pathophysiology of psychiatric disorders includes molecular, cellular, and behavioral studies that go from "bench to bedside" and back again, with basic, translational, and clinical studies informing one another (chapter 14 in Goodwin and Jamison, 2007). For example, the serendipitous discovery of the clinical utility of medications that affect monoaminergic neurotransmission in mood, anxiety, and psychotic disorders led to extensive studies of the roles of monoamines in the pathophysiology of these conditions.

Bipolar disorders are a heterogeneous group of conditions characterized by diverse mood, anxiety, and psychotic symptoms, so it is understandable that their pathophysiology is complex. Consequently, neurochemical studies have included assessments of both intercellular signaling (i.e. neurotransmitters such as monoamines, acetylcholine, and amino acids) and intracellular signaling (e.g. signal transduction and amplification, mitochondrial function, and control of genetic expression). Intercellular (neuronal surface receptor) effects, such as the serotonergic and noradrenergic actions of antidepressants, the antidopaminergic actions of antipsychotics, and the pro-gamma-aminobutyric acid (GABAergic) and antiglutamatergic actions of anticonvulsants, as well as the intracellular actions of the mood stabilizers lithium and valproate, are relevant to the underlying neurochemistry of bipolar disorder (Table 8.1).

Neuroimaging studies of bipolar disorder have assessed the neuroanatomy, and increasingly the neurochemical anatomy of this illness. For example, functional neuroimaging studies of bipolar disorder have provided evidence of neuroanatomical and biochemically non-specific functional corticolimbic dysregulation in euthymic (Brooks *et al.*, 2009a), manic (Brooks *et al.*, 2010), and depressed phases (Ketter *et al.*, 2001; Brooks *et al.*, 2009b) of bipolar disorder. Advances in neuroimaging technology have increasingly allowed the assessment of regional neurochemical alterations that support the hypothesis of specific neurochemical corticolimbic dysregulation in bipolar disorder. This chapter focuses on translational studies that integrate neurochemical and neuroanatomical information to better understand the pathophysiology of bipolar disorders.

Corticolimbic dysregulation

The hypothesis of corticolimbic network dysregulation (Mayberg, 1997; Strakowski *et al.*, 2005; Adler *et al.*, 2006; Brooks *et al.*, 2009a) has been invoked as an explanation for bipolar symptoms. Figure 8.1 provides a graphic depiction of network linkages across brain regions that have been implicated in the pathology of bipolar disorder.

There are three major frontal–subcortical circuits that constitute the corticolimbic network: dorsolateral prefrontal, lateral orbitofrontal, and anterior cingulate. We shall describe the neuroanatomy of each and then organize the subsequent review of cerebral neurochemistry accordingly.

Dorsolateral prefrontal and orbitofrontal circuits

The dorsolateral prefrontal subcortical circuit originates in Brodmann's Areas (BA) 9 and 10 of the anterior frontal lobe. From BA 9 and 10, neurons project to the caudate nucleus and then directly to the mediodorsal globus pallidus interna and indirectly to the dorsal globus pallidus externa (Mega and Cummings, 1994).

Understanding Neuropsychiatric Disorders, ed. M. E. Shenton and B. I. Turetsky. Published by Cambridge University Press.

Table 8.1 Neurochemicals and neurochemical anatomic studies

Neurochemical group	Neurochemicals	Interventions	Imaging
Monoamines	5-HT, NE	Antidepressants	PET
	DA	Antipsychotics	PET
Amino acids	GABA	VPA, BZD	MRS
	Glutamate	LTG	MRS
Other	Acetylcholine	Anticholinergics	MRS
Second messengers	Inositol	Lithium, inositol	MRS
	Choline	Choline	MRS

Note: 5-HT, serotonin; NE, norepinephrine; DA, dopamine; GABA, gamma-aminobutyric acid; VPA, valproic acid; BZD, benzodiazepine; LTG, lamotrigine; PET, positron emission tomography; MRS, magnetic resonance spectroscopy.

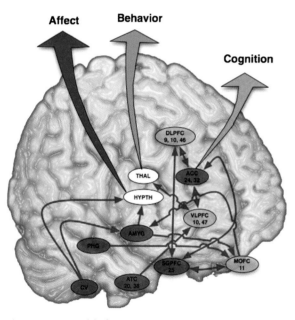

Figure 8.1 A model of corticolimbic dysregulation in bipolar disorder. Areas and connections generally associated with increased activity in bipolar disorder are depicted in red and those with decreased activity in blue. Such color-coding represents consensus data, though some findings vary. Cerebral regions are overlaid upon a surface rendering of the brain, yielding a simpler figure, but requiring readers to impute locations of subcortical structures. Appropriate numbers for Brodmann's areas are provided. ACC, anterior cingulate cortex; AMYG, amygdala; ATC, anterior temporal cortex; CV, cerebellar vermis; DLPFC, dorsolateral prefrontal cortex; HYPTH, hypothalamus; MOFC, medial orbital prefrontal cortex; PHG, parahippocampal gyrus; SGPFC, subgenual prefrontal cortex; THAL, thalamus; VLPFC, ventrolateral prefrontal cortex. With permission from Brooks et al. (2009a).

The dorsal globus pallidus externa projects to the lateral subthalamic nucleus from which fibers terminate in the globus pallidus interna and substantia nigra pars reticulata. The output from both structures terminates in the ventral anterior and mediodorsal thalamus, which in turn project back to BA 9 and 10. According to Mega and Cummings (1994), the dorsolateral prefrontal circuit receives afferent projections from BA 46 and 7a, and has efferent projections to BA 46 and 8.

The orbitofrontal circuit (Mega and Cummings, 1994), which originates laterally in BA 10 and 11, projects to the ventromedial caudate, which in turn projects to the mediodorsal globus pallidus interna as well as the substantia nigra pars reticulata. The globus pallidus and the substantia nigra projections go to the ventral anterior thalamus and the magnocellular division of the mediodorsal thalamus. The circuit is completed through the projections of the thalamus to the lateral orbitofrontal cortex.

Anterior cingulate circuit

The anterior cingulate circuit originates in BA 24 of the anterior cingulate, which provides input to the ventral striatum (ventromedial caudate, ventral putamen, nucleus, accumbens, and olfactory tubercle). From the ventral striatum, there are projections to the rostromedial globus pallidus interna, ventral pallidum, and the rostrodorsal substantia nigra. The ventral pallidum provides projections to the magnocellular mediodorsal thalamus, which completes the circuit by projecting back to the anterior cingulate.

Neuroimaging modalities

Several techniques have been developed that allow for non-invasive assessment of neurochemistry. Ligand-specific positron emission tomography (PET) and

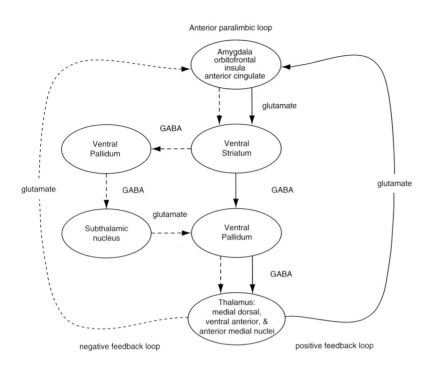

Anterior paralimbic loop

Amygdala
orbitofrontal
insula
anterior cingulate

glutamate

GABA

Ventral
Pallidum

Ventral
Striatum

glutamate

glutamate

GABA

GABA

Subthalamic
nucleus

glutamate

Ventral
Pallidum

GABA

Thalamus:
medial dorsal,
ventral anterior, &
anterior medial nuclei

negative feedback loop

positive feedback loop

Figure 8.2 Limbic basal ganglia–thalamocortical circuits. Solid lines indicate positive feedback loop, and dashed lines indicate negative feedback loop. GABA, inhibitory gamma-aminobutyric acid interneuron connections. Glutamate, excitatory glutamatergic projection neuron connections. Adapted from Alexander *et al.* (1990).

single photon emission computed tomography (SPECT) permit regional measurement of monoamines and other neurochemicals, which are thought to be crucial to affective processes. The origins of monoaminergic innervation derive from the brainstem and project to prefrontal and paralimbic circuits. The raphe nuclei serve as the origins for serotonin, locus ceruleus for norepinephrine, and substantia nigra and ventral tegmental area for dopamine.

Proton magnetic resonance spectroscopy (^{1}H-MRS), which is a form of magnetic resonance technology, allows non-invasive, limited resolution imaging of concentrations of diverse cerebral metabolites, including amino acids, cystolic choline, and *N*-acetyl aspartate (NAA). Metabolite concentrations are reported in either absolute or relative (compared to creatine) terms. Neurochemical signals detected by MRS often reflect components that are not directly related to neurotransmission. For example, although choline is an acetylcholine precursor and itself involved in second messenger cascades, ^{1}H-MRS choline peaks represent total cellular choline stores. The predominant component of these peaks is likely from cell membranes (phospholipids) rather than acetylcholine. Similarly, NAA is an amino acid that is involved in amino acid metabolism and fatty acid and protein synthesis, but is broadly distributed in

diverse brain regions, and mature neurons; NAA may reflect neuronal density and integrity. In contrast to monoamines, these metabolites are more diffusely distributed, but the components related to neurotransmission can have important regional differences. For example, excitatory glutamatergic neurons project between components of diverse circuits, including the circuit described in Figure 8.2. In contrast, inhibitory GABAergic neurons project within components of such circuits.

MRS also permits measurement of concentrations of cerebral gamma-aminobutyric acid (GABA) and glutamate, which are the main inhibitory and excitatory amino acid neurotransmitters, respectively. Measures of glutamate are somewhat complicated because glutamate exists in both metabolic and neurotransmitter pools. In addition, the glutamine and glutamate peaks overlap, so that some studies report combined glutamine/glutamate concentrations.

^{1}H-MRS allows for the measurement of concentrations of inositol (stored as *myo*-inositol), which is involved in signal transduction and may itself have antidepressant effects. Inositol depletion may contribute to the pathophysiology of mood disorders, and some data suggest that administration of inositol yields modest benefits in patients with mood disorders (Agam *et al.*, 2002).

Phosphorus-31 magnetic resonance spectroscopy (^{31}P-MRS) permits measurement of concentrations of cerebral phospholipids, including phosphomonoesters, phosphodiesters, inorganic phosphate, high-energy phosphates and related compounds such as phosphocreatine. Phosphomonoesters consist of phosphoethanolamine, phosphocholine, phosphoserine, and sugar phosphates such as inositol-1-monophosphate; phosphodiesters consist of glycerophosphocholine, glycerophosphoethanolamine, and mobile phospholipids. Phosphomonoesters and phosphodiesters include cell membrane precursors and degradation products, respectively, and are related to intracellular signaling and membrane phospholipid changes proposed in bipolar disorder. Phosphocreatine is considered a high-energy phosphate buffer.

Dorsolateral prefrontal and orbitofrontal circuit neurochemistry

Monoamines

There have been numerous findings of peripheral serotonergic dysfunction in bipolar disorder, including decreased serotonergic reuptake in platelets (Marazziti et al., 1993; Stahl et al., 1983). A high-sensitivity study of serotonin transporter binding potential in unmedicated, depressed patients with bipolar disorder revealed *increased* serotonin transporter binding potential (consistent with increased serotonin transporter concentrations or decreased endogenous serotonin concentrations) in medial prefrontal cortex, as well as insula and dorsal cingulate cortex (Cannon et al., 2006). A subsequent study of unmedicated patients (Oquendo et al., 2007) did not replicate these findings, and found evidence of *decreased* serotonin transporter binding potential (consistent with decreased serotonin transporter concentrations or increased endogenous serotonin concentrations) in insula, thalamus, and anterior cingulate. The contradictory findings could reflect variations in subject samples or the differences in derivation of estimates of binding potential. Other researchers, however, have reported increased prefrontal serotonin transporter binding potential in patients with unipolar depression who attempted suicide (Meyer et al., 1999).

The role of the dopaminergic system in bipolar disorder has not been the focus of many studies. There is evidence of reduced dopamine D_1 receptor binding potential (consistent with decreased dopamine D_1 receptor concentrations or increased endogenous dopamine concentrations) in the frontal cortex of unmedicated bipolar patients compared to controls (Suhara et al., 1992).

NAA

NAA and NAA/creatine findings exhibit regional variation in bipolar disorder patients. One study of pediatric bipolar disorder patients compared to controls reported decreased NAA in left dorsolateral prefrontal cortex (Olvera et al., 2007), as was reported in some studies of adult bipolar disorder (Sassi et al., 2005; Winsberg et al., 2000). One study found that medial and orbitofrontal NAA was decreased in bipolar disorder patients relative to controls (Cecil et al., 2002); however, other studies have found little or no differences between bipolar disorder patients and controls in medial frontal cortex (Cecil et al., 2003; Hamakawa et al., 1999), or frontal/prefrontal regions (Bertolino et al., 2003; Brambilla et al., 2005; Castillo et al., 2000; Dager et al., 2004; Hajek et al., 2008; Michael et al., 2003; Scherk et al., 2007). One study reported a difference between bipolar type I and type II patients regarding left dorsolateral NAA/Creatine (Winsberg et al., 2000), but another study did not find such differences (Hamakawa et al., 1999). In addition, there does not appear to be a relation between illness duration and prefrontal NAA (Brambilla et al., 2005; Hamakawa et al., 1999; Sassi et al., 2005). Prefrontal NAA appear to be unrelated to degree of depression in bipolar disorder as measured by Hamilton Depression Rating Scale scores (Hamakawa et al., 1999), nor does it appear to differ between hypomanic patients and control subjects (Malhi et al., 2007).

Because lithium has neurotrophic properties and may increase NAA, it could mask NAA deficits in patients with bipolar disorders, although the evidence is unclear. A four-week lithium monotherapy trial similarly increased prefrontal, temporal, parietal and occipital NAA in depressed adult bipolar I disorder patients and healthy controls, but cerebral NAA did not correlate with blood lithium concentrations (Moore et al., 2000b). In contrast, in primarily depressed adult bipolar I and bipolar II disorder patients, lithium for a mean of 3.6 months and valproate for a mean of 1.4 months failed to alter NAA (Friedman et al., 2004). In adult healthy volunteers, lithium administration for four weeks failed to alter dorsolateral prefrontal NAA (Brambilla et al., 2004).

Glutamate and GABA

Findings regarding glutamate and glutamate/creatine suggest differences in specific prefrontal regions. Relative to healthy controls, glutamate or glutamate/creatine in bipolar disorder patients was increased in prefrontal (Castillo *et al.*, 2000; Cecil *et al.*, 2002) and dorsolateral prefrontal (Michael *et al.*, 2003) regions, but not medial prefrontal regions (Cecil *et al.*, 2002). Port *et al.* (2008) reported decreased glutamate in bilateral frontal white matter. However, one study of medication-free bipolar disorder patients did not find prefrontal differences in glutamate (Frey *et al.*, 2007b). One small study reported preliminary evidence of increased GABA-A receptor binding (consistent with increased GABA-A receptor concentrations or decreased endogenous GABA-A concentrations) in BA 9 in bipolar disorder patients relative to controls (Dean *et al.*, 2001).

Choline

Studies consistently report the absence of choline differences in dorsolateral prefrontal cortex between bipolar disorder patients and healthy controls (Amaral *et al.*, 2006; Bertolino *et al.*, 2003; Brambilla *et al.*, 2005; Cecil *et al.*, 2002; Michael *et al.*, 2003; Sassi *et al.*, 2005; Winsberg *et al.*, 2000; Molina *et al.*, 2007; Scherk *et al.*, 2007). Although there is one report of decreased choline in medial prefrontal regions of bipolar disorder patients relative to control subjects (Cecil *et al.*, 2002), other studies have not found any difference (Dager *et al.*, 2004; Hamakawa *et al.*, 1999; Hajek *et al.*, 2008). Choline and choline/creatine do not appear to be related to illness duration in dorsolateral prefrontal (Brambilla *et al.*, 2005) or medial prefrontal (Hamakawa *et al.*, 1999) cortices.

Emerging data suggest possible medication effects on choline. In depressed adult bipolar I disorder patients, lithium monotherapy yielded antidepressant effects and decreased prefrontal choline (Moore *et al.*, 1999). In contrast, in primarily depressed adult bipolar I and bipolar II disorder patients, lithium administration for a mean of 3.6 months and valproate for a mean of 1.4 months failed to alter gray or white matter or regional choline (Friedman *et al.*, 2004). Also, in children and adolescents during manic or mixed episodes, anterior cingulate choline/creatine did not change with acute (one week trial) adjunctive lithium and did not correlate with serum lithium concentrations (Davanzo *et al.*, 2001). Finally, in

healthy adult volunteers, lithium administration for four weeks failed to alter dorsolateral prefrontal choline (Brambilla *et al.*, 2004). Patients taking lithium on a chronic basis, compared to those who did not, had similar basal ganglia choline/creatine (Kato *et al.*, 1996) and choline (Hamakawa *et al.*, 1998), medial prefrontal choline (Hamakawa *et al.*, 1999), temporal choline/creatine (Wu *et al.*, 2004), and anterior cingulate choline/creatine (Moore *et al.*, 2000a), and serum lithium concentrations were not related to basal ganglia or occipital choline/creatine (Sharma *et al.*, 1992).

Myo-inositol

Some studies have reported increased *myo*-inositol/creatine in the dorsolateral prefrontal regions of bipolar disorder patients (Cecil *et al.*, 2002; Winsberg *et al.*, 2000), although this finding was not replicated in studies of pediatric bipolar disorder patients (Olvera *et al.*, 2007; Chang *et al.*, 2003). A more recent study of medication-free bipolar disorder patients also failed to detect any difference between *myo*-inositol levels compared to healthy controls. There is no evidence of *myo*-inositol differences in bipolar disorder patients in medial prefrontal (Cecil *et al.*, 2002; Hajek *et al.*, 2008) or fronto temporal regions (Silverstone *et al.*, 2002).

Emerging data suggest possible medication effects on *myo*-inositol and *myo*-inositol/creatine in bipolar disorder patients. Lithium inhibits inositol monophosphatase and thus depletes inositol. In depressed bipolar I disorder patients, lithium monotherapy yielded about a 30% decrease in prefrontal *myo*-inositol in patients who were generally still depressed at days 5–7; the decrease persisted at weeks 3–4 when patients were generally improved (Moore *et al.*, 1999). The authors proposed that the temporal dissociation between *myo*-inositol decreases and clinical improvement suggested that short-term *myo*-inositol depletion per se was not related to lithium antidepressant effects. In contrast, in adult healthy volunteers, lithium administration for four weeks failed to alter dorsolateral prefrontal *myo*-inositol (Brambilla *et al.*, 2004). Moreover, in a more sensitive paradigm in which lithium amplified amphetamine-induced phosphomonoester increases, a similar effect was not detected for *myo*-inositol/creatine (Silverstone *et al.*, 1999). In contrast, in one study

129

of primarily depressed adult bipolar I and bipolar II disorder patients, lithium for a mean of 3.6 months, but not valproate for a mean of 1.4 months, increased gray matter *myo*-inositol (Friedman *et al.*, 2004).

Creatine and phosphocreatine

Early work revealed decreased prefrontal phosphocreatine in bipolar II patients (independent of mood state) compared to healthy controls (Kato *et al.*, 1995; Deicken *et al.*, 1995), but failed detect such differences in bipolar I patients (Kato *et al.*, 1992, 1993). Decreased prefrontal phosphocreatine in bipolar II patients could reflect decreased creatine or creatine phosphokinase activity, increased intracellular magnesium, or mitochondrial dysfunction (Kato *et al.*, 1994). In bipolar disorder patients, phosphocreatine appears to be decreased in the left prefrontal region during depression (Kato *et al.*, 1995) and the right prefrontal region in mania (Kato *et al.*, 1995) and euthymia (Kato *et al.*, 1995; Deicken *et al.*, 1995). A study of medication-free euthymic bipolar I disorder and bipolar II disorder patients did not detect any differences in prefrontal phosphocreatine (Kato *et al.*, 1998).

Bipolar disorder patients may have lower creatine and phosphocreatine in the dorsolateral prefrontal cortex compared to control subjects (Frey *et al.*, 2007b), although not all studies report such a finding (Scherk *et al.*, 2007). However, in bipolar depression there is evidence of increased creatine and phosphocreatine in bipolar disorder patients relative to controls (Frye *et al.*, 2007b).

There are limited data regarding the effect of oral creatine administration on cerebral creatine. In healthy volunteers, creatine 20 g/d for 4 weeks yielded increased gray matter, cerebellum, white matter, thalamus and overall creatine; these changes were reversed on repeat scans at least three months after creatine was discontinued (Dechent *et al.*, 1999). In healthy volunteers, creatine 8 g/d for 5 days yielded attenuation of mathematical calculation task-induced mental fatigue and cerebral oxygenated hemoglobin increases (Watanabe *et al.*, 2002).

There are few data regarding medication effects on creatine. In depressed bipolar I disorder patients, lithium monotherapy yielded antidepressant effects by weeks 3–4, but did not alter prefrontal, temporal, parietal, or occipital creatine at days 5–7 or weeks 3–4

(Moore *et al.*, 1999). In primarily depressed adult bipolar I and bipolar II disorder patients, lithium for a mean of 3.6 months and valproate for a mean of 1.4 months did not affect cerebral creatine (Friedman *et al.*, 2004). In bipolar disorder patients lithium, valproate, antidepressant, and benzodiazepine therapy were not related to medial prefrontal creatine (Hamakawa *et al.*, 1999). Bipolar disorder patients who were taking antipsychotics, compared to those who were not, did not exhibit changes in medial prefrontal creatine (Hamakawa *et al.*, 1999).

Phosphomonoesters

Euthymic patients diagnosed with bipolar disorder type I appear to have decreased prefrontal phosphomonoesters, consistent with abnormal phospholipid metabolism and resultant alterations in signal transduction (Manji and Lenox, 2000). Indeed, several studies have revealed decreased prefrontal phosphomonoesters in euthymic bipolar I patients compared to healthy controls (Kato *et al.*, 1992, 1993, 1994a, 1994b), depressed bipolar disorder patients (Kato *et al.*, 1992, 1994a), and manic patients (Kato *et al.*, 1991, 1993). Curiously, one previous study from the same research group did not find decreased prefrontal phosphomonoesters in euthymic patients and found increased prefrontal phosphomonoesters in manic patients (Kato *et al.*, 1991). In addition, Deicken and associates found that euthymic medication-free bipolar I disorder patients had decreased prefrontal phosphomonoesters compared to controls (Deicken *et al.*, 1995).

In studies that have included bipolar type II disorder, findings have been less consistent. Some studies have not found any differences between prefrontal phosphomonoesters in euthymic type II patients compared to healthy controls (Kato *et al.*, 1994a, 1994b), nor have they reported differences across affective episodes (Kato *et al.*, 1994a). Interestingly, there is some evidence of *increased* phosphomonoesters in depressed and hypomanic bipolar II patients compared to healthy controls (Kato *et al.*, 1994a). Studies that have combined medicated bipolar I and bipolar II patients have provided varied results, ranging from non-significant decreases in prefrontal phosphomonoesters in euthymic BD patients relative to healthy controls (Kato *et al.*, 1994b) to non-significant increases in another (Kato *et al.*, 1995). Considering studies thus far, it appears that prefrontal phosphomonoester differences may be unique to bipolar disorder type I.

In a meta-analysis of phosphomonoester findings in bipolar disorder, the authors concluded that phosphomonoesters were lower in euthymic bipolar disorder patients than controls and patients with bipolar depression had higher phosphomonoesters than did euthymic bipolar disorder patients (Yildiz et al., 2001).

Phosphodiesters

Phosphodiesters have been the focus of less research than phosphomonoesters. This difference in focus may reflect the general lack of findings of differences between bipolar disorder patients and controls. For example, two studies reported that euthymic bipolar I disorder patients compared to healthy controls had similar prefrontal phosphodiesters (Kato et al., 1992, 1993), but another reported increased bilateral prefrontal phosphodiesters (Deicken et al., 1995). A meta-analysis that included the four published studies of phosphodiesters concluded that levels were similar for bipolar disorder patients and healthy controls (Yildiz et al., 2001).

Summary

There are a number of potential neurochemical alterations in the dorsolateral prefrontal circuit that are related to the clinical expression of bipolar disorder. Relative to healthy controls, bipolar disorder patients could have an increased medial prefrontal serotonin transporter binding potential during depression. However, this finding was not replicated, and there is some evidence of decreased serotonin transporter binding potential in the insula. There is limited evidence of decreased dopamine transporter binding potential in the frontal cortex. Currently, it appears that monoaminergic alterations in the dorsolateral prefrontal circuit of bipolar disorder patients are debatable.

Explanations of the neurochemical pathology of bipolar disorder that involve neuronal integrity in the prefrontal cortex are not strongly supported by the current state of findings. Consistent with neuroimaging findings using other modalities (e.g. cerebral glucose metabolism, gray matter density), there have been several reports of decreased NAA concentrations in prefrontal cortex. However, these findings were often not replicated, and there is a lack of evidence for concordance between NAA levels in prefrontal cortex and affective state or illness duration.

Glutamatergic transmission appears impaired in bipolar disorder patients, although findings are again somewhat inconsistent. As with NAA levels, glutamine/glutamate concentrations could vary in dorsolateral prefrontal cortex, but are less likely to vary in medial prefrontal cortex. Even this conclusion is called into question by several recent studies that have failed to replicate these findings.

Many studies of choline and the choline/creatine ratio have failed to find differences in between bipolar disorder patients and controls regarding elements of the dorsolateral prefrontal and orbitofrontal circuits. This lack of relation is consistent with failures to find relations between choline and choline/creatine ratios and illness duration.

Studies of *myo*-inositol differences in the dorsolateral prefrontal and orbitofrontal circuit in bipolar disorder patients have been equivocal. Some studies have suggested dorsolateral differences in which bipolar disorder patients have exhibited higher *myo*-inositol levels than controls, but other studies have failed to replicate these findings.

Differences in creatine and phosphocreatine may be confined to bipolar disorder type I. There is a lack of support for such differences between type II patients and controls or across different mood states of bipolar type II. With bipolar type I, however, there is substantial evidence of alterations of phosphocreatine in prefrontal regions. These findings have largely centered on decreased phosphocreatine in dorsolateral prefrontal cortex during mania and depression and even some evidence of differences during euthymia. Although findings have been largely consistent, they have derived mainly from the work of one research group, and need to be replicated by other investigators.

Phosphomonoesters, which could reflect alterations in signal transduction, appear to be decreased in euthymic and depressed bipolar disorder type I patients. Studies of samples of heterogeneous type I and II patients and homogeneous type II patients have not detected prefrontal alterations in phosphomonoesters. Phosphodiesters have been the focus of too few studies to draw firm conclusions.

There are numerous unanswered questions about neurochemical changes associated with bipolar disorder in the dorsolateral prefrontal and orbitofrontal circuits. Thus far, findings suggest that NAA and creatine would be more fruitful measures to explore for neurochemical alterations of dorsolateral pre-frontal/orbitofrontal circuits.

Anterior cingulate circuit neurochemistry

Monoamines

An early post-mortem study in bipolar disorder patients who committed suicide found a significant 55% mean decrease in the major serotonin metabolite hydroxyindolacetic acid (HIAA) in the temporal cortex (Young *et al.*, 1994). A PET study using [^{18}F]-setoporone did not find any evidence of differential serotonin 5-HT$_2$ receptor binding potential when comparing depressed patients (some of whom were diagnosed with bipolar disorder) and control subjects (Meyer *et al.*, 1999). A study with a small ($n = 4$) number of depressed bipolar disorder patients who had relatives with a mood disorder suggested that serotonin 5-HT$_{1A}$ receptor binding potential was reduced in the hippocampus and amygdala relative to control subjects (consistent with decreased serotonin 5-HT$_{1A}$ receptor concentrations or increased endogenous serotonin; Drevets *et al.*, 1999). A subsequent PET study using a different radioligand ([^{11}C]-3-amino-4-(2-dimethylamino-methyl-phenylsulfanyl)-benzonitrile11; [^{11}C]-DASB) revealed decreased serotonin transporter binding capacity (consistent with decreased serotonin transporter concentrations or increased endogenous serotonin) in the thalamus, dorsal cingulate and insula (Cannon *et al.*, 2006). Moreover, more recently, a study of serotonin transporter binding in medication-free depressed children diagnosed with bipolar disorder compared to healthy controls revealed that bipolar disorder was associated with decreased serotonin transporter binding potential (consistent with decreased serotonin transporter concentrations or increased endogenous serotonin) in the anterior cingulate, amygdala, hippocampus, thalamus, and putamen (Oquendo *et al.*, 2007).

Bipolar disorder patients with current mood episodes with psychotic features (manic more than depressed) exhibit increased dopamine D$_2$ receptor binding (consistent with increased dopamine D$_2$ receptor concentrations or decreased endogenous dopamine) in the caudate, which correlates with ratings of psychosis (Pearlson *et al.*, 1995). In depressed patients

with bipolar disorder type II, baseline dopamine D$_2$ receptor binding did not differ from control subjects, but responders after sleep deprivation had decreased basal ganglia D$_2$ receptor binding (consistent with decreased dopamine D$_2$ receptor concentrations or increased endogenous dopamine; Ebert *et al.*, 1994). This finding suggests that enhanced dopamine release may be associated with sleep deprivation antidepressant response. Striatal dopamine transporter density in bipolar disorder patients may be higher than controls in the right posterior putamen and the left caudate (Amsterdam and Newberg, 2007). There does not appear to be evidence of differential dopamine D$_1$ receptor binding in the striatum (Suhara *et al.*, 1992). However, some studies have reported increased vesicular monoamine transporter protein (consistent with decreased monoaminergic receptor concentrations or increased endogenous monoamines) in the thalamus and ventral brainstem of bipolar disorder patients compared to controls (Zubieta *et al.*, 2000, 2001).

Glutamate

Relative to control subjects, glutamate was increased in basal ganglia of bipolar disorder patients (Castillo *et al.*, 2000). Some studies have found no evidence of changes in glutamate levels in the anterior cingulate (Davanzo *et al.*, 2001; Dager *et al.*, 2004; Frey *et al.*, 2007b). However, a recent study found that, compared to control subjects, melancholic depressed bipolar patients exhibited increased glutamate levels in the anterior cingulate (Frye *et al.*, 2007b). In a study of acute mania, the glutamate/glutamine was elevated in the anterior cingulate (Ongür *et al.*, 2008). Even with variability of findings, a recent review concluded that there is likely abnormal glutamatergic transmission in the hippocampus (Ng *et al.*, 2009). Interestingly, post-mortem studies of bipolar disorder patients have reported diffuse abnormalities of glutamatergic neurons in the anterior cingulate (Benes *et al.*, 2000) and hippocampus (Frey *et al.*, 2007a).

GABA

GABA levels tend to be increased in certain regions. One study found that GABA was increased in left insula and tended to be increased in left cingulate (but not in other regions) in BD patients compared to controls (Dager *et al.*, 2004). Another study found that bipolar disorder patients tended to have increased medial prefrontal/anterior cingulate GABA/creatine compared to healthy controls (Wang *et al.*, 2006). Regulation of GABA activity could explain the activity of some medications used to treat bipolar disorder (Ketter and Wang, 2003).

NAA

Findings regarding cerebral NAA levels have been variable. Several studies have failed to report alterations of NAA levels in the anterior cingulate of bipolar disorder patients (Amaral *et al.*, 2006; Bertolino *et al.*, 2003; Dager *et al.*, 2004; Davanzo *et al.*, 2001).

An early study reported that first-episode psychosis patients (about half of whom were diagnosed with bipolar disorder) exhibited decreased temporal NAA/Creatine (Renshaw *et al.*, 1995). A later study, however, failed to detect a difference in NAA levels between bipolar disorder patients and controls (Moore *et al.*, 2000a).

Examination of deeper temporal complexes has provided different results than consideration of the temporal lobe as a whole. Relative to controls, patients with familial bipolar disorder exhibited decreased hippocampal NAA (Deicken *et al.*, 2003), and NAA/creatine was decreased in the hippocampus of non-familial bipolar disorder patients (Bertolino *et al.*, 2003). Also, first-episode affective psychosis patients, who were also depressed or manic, exhibited decreased NAA/creatine in hippocampus but not other regions (Blasi *et al.*, 2004). In a post-mortem study, BD patients (most of whom had had psychotic symptoms) exhibited decreased superior temporal cortex NAA, which is consistent with the notion that temporal lobe NAA deficits may be a common feature of psychotic disorders (Nudmamud *et al.*, 2003).

Other structures have demonstrated alterations in NAA or NAA/creatine. For example, a recent study reported bilaterally increased NAA in the head of caudate in bipolar disorder patients compared to controls (Port *et al.*, 2008). Studies of the basal ganglia have reported that bipolar disorder patients compared to controls had decreased (Frye *et al.*, 2007a), increased (Sharma *et al.*, 1992), or similar (Bertolino *et al.*, 2003; Hamakawa *et al.*, 1999; Kato *et al.*, 1995; Ohara *et al.*, 1998) basal ganglia NAA/creatine. One study found increased NAA in medication-free bipolar disorder patients compared to controls in left putamen (Dager *et al.*, 2004). In the thalamus, NAA was found to be increased in bipolar disorder patients relative to control subjects in one study (Deicken *et al.*, 2001), but similar in another (Dager *et al.*, 2004); NAA/creatine in the thalamus has also been found to be similar (Bertolino *et al.*, 2003).

Choline

Choline and choline/creatine in the anterior cingulate of bipolar disorder patients compared to that of healthy controls have been found to be increased (Moore *et al.*, 2000a) or similar (Amaral *et al.*, 2006; Bertolino *et al.*, 2003; Davanzo *et al.*, 2001; Scherk *et al.*, 2007). However, in a recent study, manic and hypomanic bipolar disorder patients were found to have somewhat lower levels of choline in the anterior cingulate than euthymic bipolar disorder patients (Malhi *et al.*, 2007). Temporal (Renshaw *et al.*, 1995; Wu *et al.*, 2004) and hippocampal (Bertolino *et al.*, 2003; Deicken *et al.*, 2003) choline has been found to be similar between bipolar disorder patients and controls. Choline and creatine have been found to be decreased in the head of the right caudate (Port *et al.*, 2008).

Myo-inositol

In the anterior cingulate, findings regarding *myo*-inositol/creatine are variable, with some data suggesting an increase (Davanzo *et al.*, 2001), and other data indicating no difference (Moore *et al.*, 2000a). *Myo*-inositol has also been found to be elevated in the head of the left caudate in medication-free patients diagnosed with bipolar disorder (Port *et al.*, 2008). Also, in adult healthy volunteers, acute (one-week trial) lithium monotherapy did not alter temporal *myo*-inositol/creatine (Silverstone *et al.*, 1999).

Creatine and phosphocreatine

Anterior cingulate creatine appears to be similar in bipolar disorder patients compared to control subjects (Davanzo *et al.*, 2001; Ongür *et al.*, 2008; Hajek *et al.*, 2008). Although one study did find evidence of increased creatine in the hippocampus of bipolar disorder patients compared to controls (Bertolino *et al.*, 2003), another study reported decreased hippocampal creatine (Deicken *et al.*, 2003). Bipolar disorder patients who were taking antipsychotics compared to those who were not had increased basal ganglia creatine (Hamakawa *et al.*, 1999).

Euthymic medication-free bipolar I disorder patients appear to be similar to control subjects with respect to temporal lobe phosphocreatine (Deicken *et al.*, 1995a, 1995b). Although a later study did not find gray matter differences in phosphocreatine between bipolar disorder patients and controls, it did reveal an inverse relation between white matter phosphocreatine and scores on the Hamilton Depression Rating Scale (Dager *et al.*, 2004).

Phosphomonoesters

Lithium inhibits inositol monophosphatase (Hallcher and Sherman, 1980), so lithium could affect phosphomonoesters (PMEs), which have a limited (about 10%) inositol phosphate component (Gyulai *et al.*, 1984). If lithium increases phosphomonoesters, this could be related to lithium inhibiting conversion of inositol-1-phosphate to inositol. In six manic bipolar disorder patients, lithium failed to significantly alter prefrontal PMEs (Kato *et al.*, 1993). In healthy volunteers, lithium administration for one week failed to significantly alter left temporal phosphomonoesters (Silverstone *et al.*, 1996; 1999), but in a more sensitive paradigm lithium amplified amphetamine-induced phosphomonoester increases (Silverstone *et al.*, 1999). Euthymic bipolar disorder patients taking chronic lithium therapy compared to those taking chronic valproate therapy had similar temporal phosphomonoesters (Silverstone *et al.*, 2002).

Phosphodiesters

There have been few reports of phosphodiesters in the anterior cingulate circuit in bipolar disorder. There is one report of similar levels of phosphodiesters in the temporal lobe of bipolar disorder patients compared to controls (Deicken *et al.*, 1995). It is likely, then, that any differences in phosphate metabolism in the anterior cingulate circuit related to bipolar disorder may be at most subtle.

Summary

Neurochemical changes in components of the anterior cingulate circuit appear more consistent than those that have been reported for the dorsolateral prefrontal and orbitofrontal circuits. Perhaps not surprisingly, alterations in monaminergic transmission appear relatively reliable. In particular, decreased serotonin 5-HT$_2$ receptor and 5-HT transporter binding potential in

the thalamus, dorsal cingulate, and insula have been reported as well as decreased serotonin transporter binding potential during bipolar depression in the anterior cingulate, amygdala, hippocampus, putamen, and thalamus. Dopaminergic transmission in the putamen and caudate appears to be affected in bipolar disorder, though primarily during affective episodes.

Glutamate may be altered in the anterior cingulate, basal ganglia, and hippocampus. These findings are further supported by reported associations with mood state and post-mortem studies. Abnormalities of glutamatergic transmission support the contention that the anterior cingulate circuit is intimately involved in affective regulation in bipolar disorder, and are consistent with antiglutamatergic properties of some medications used in the treatment of bipolar disorders (Ketter and Wang, 2003).

NAA levels may be unaltered in the anterior cingulate, but temporal structures including the hippocampus appear to exhibit decreased NAA and NAA/creatine. In addition, there is growing evidence of altered NAA or NAA/creatine associated with bipolar disorder in the thalamus, caudate, and basal ganglia.

Choline levels in the anterior cingulate appear to be increased or similar relative to controls. Interestingly, there is also evidence of decreased choline levels in the anterior cingulate in manic and hypomanic patients compared to euthymic bipolar disorder patients. Choline levels in the hippocampus appear to be similar in bipolar disorder patients and controls.

Alterations of *myo*-inositol levels associated with elements of the anterior cingulate circuit do not appear reliable, although alterations within the anterior cingulate and caudate are possible.

Phosphate metabolism in the anterior cingulate circuit of bipolar disorder patients does not appear to be grossly disrupted. Although there are a few reports of altered phosphocreatine in the hippocampus and phosphodiesters in the temporal lobe, these findings have not been replicated.

Conclusions

The neurochemistry of corticolimbic circuits presents additional challenges for clarifying the neurochemical basis of dysregulation that has been observed in functional neuroimaging studies. In contrast to the growing consensus of cerebral metabolic or cerebral blood flow dysregulation in euthymic (Brooks *et al.*, 2009a), depressed (Brooks *et al.*, 2009b; Ketter *et al.*, 2001),

Dorsolateral prefrontal circuit
  Originates in BA 9 and 10.
  Projects through the caudate to the mediodorsal globus pallidus.
  Eventually terminates in the ventral anterior and mediodorsal thalamus.
  Receives afferent projections from BA 46.
Orbitofrontal prefrontal circuit
  Originates in BA 10 and 11.
  Projects to ventromedial caudate, then through globus pallidus interna.
  Terminates in the mediodorsal thalamus.
Anterior cingulate circuit
  Originates in BA 24.
  Projects to ventral striatum and then to rostro-medial globus pallidus interna.
  Terminates in magnocellular mediodorsal thalamus.

Dorsolateral and orbitofrontal prefrontal circuits
  Data do not support the notion that neuronal integrity explains the pathology of bipolar disorder.
  Glutamatergic transmission is likely to be impaired.
  Creatine and phosphocreatine differences have only been found in bipolar disorder type I.
  Phosphomonoesters may only be decreased in bipolar disorder type I.
Anterior cingulate circuit
  There appear to be glutamatergic abnormalities associated with bipolar disorder.
  GABA levels are increased.
  Findings with NAA have been variable.
  Creatine levels appear to be similar to controls.

and manic (Brooks *et al.*, 2010; Drevets *et al.*, 1997) phases of bipolar disorder, the findings in neurochemical studies are more variable.

Nevertheless, neurochemical dysregulation may be present, such as glutamatergic transmission in the anterior cingulate, basal ganglia, and hippocampus, and future studies may have success in determining the associations between other neurochemical abnormalities and clinical presentations of bipolar disorder. Additional studies that control bipolar subtype, mood state, medications, and other individual differences, such as illness severity, may provide a more detailed picture of neurochemical dysregulation. If patterns of neurochemical dysregulation were defined for bipolar disorder, attempts could be made to validate them as biomarkers of treatment success.

References

Adler C M, DelBello M P and Strakowski S M. 2006. Brain network dysfunction in bipolar disorder. *CNS Spectr* **11**, 312–20.

Agam G, Shamir A, Shaltiel G and Greenberg M L. 2002. *Myo*-inositol-1-phosphate (MIP) synthase: A possible new target for antibipolar drugs. *Bipolar Disord* **4** Suppl 1, 15–20.

Alexander G E, Crutcher M D and DeLong M R. 1990. Basal ganglia–thalamocortical circuits: Parallel substrates for motor, oculomotor, "prefrontal" and "limbic" functions. *Prog Brain Res* **85**, 119–46.

Amaral J A, Tamada R S, Issler C K, *et al.* 2006. A 1HMRS study of the anterior cingulate gyrus in euthymic bipolar patients. *Hum Psychopharmacol* **21**, 215–20.

Amsterdam J D and Newberg A B. 2007. A preliminary study of dopamine transporter binding in bipolar and unipolar depressed patients and healthy controls. *Neuropsychobiology* **55**, 167–70.

Benes F M, Todtenkopf M S, Logiotatos P and Williams M. 2000. Glutamate decarboxylase(65)-immunoreactive terminals in cingulate and prefrontal cortices of schizophrenic and bipolar brain. *J Chem Neuroanat* **20**, 259–69.

Bertolino A, Frye M, Callicott J H, *et al.* 2003. Neuronal pathology in the hippocampal area of patients with bipolar disorder: A study with proton magnetic resonance spectroscopic imaging. *Biol Psychiatry* **53**, 906–13.

Blasi G, Bertolino A, Brudaglio F, *et al.* 2004. Hippocampal neurochemical pathology in patients at first episode of affective psychosis: A proton magnetic resonance spectroscopic imaging study. *Psychiatry Res* **131**, 95–105.

Brambilla P, Stanley J A, Nicoletti M A, *et al.* 2005. 1H magnetic resonance spectroscopy investigation of the dorsolateral prefrontal cortex in bipolar disorder patients. *J Affect Disord* **86**, 61–7.

Brambilla P, Stanley J A, Sassi R B, *et al.* 2004. 1H MRS study of dorsolateral prefrontal cortex in healthy individuals before and after lithium administration. *Neuropsychopharmacology* **29**, 1918–24.

Brooks J O, Hoblyn J C and Ketter T A. 2010. Metabolic evidence of corticolimbic dysregulation in bipolar mania. *Psychiatry Res* **181**, 136–40.

Brooks J O, Hoblyn J C, Woodard S A, Rosen A C and Ketter T A. 2009a. Corticolimbic metabolic dysregulation in euthymic older adults with bipolar disorder. *J Psychiatr Res* **94**, 32–7.

Brooks J O, Wang P W, Bonner J C, *et al.* 2009b. Decreased prefrontal, anterior cingulate, insula, and ventral striatal metabolism in medication-free depressed outpatients with bipolar disorder. *J Psychiatr Res* **43**, 181–8.

Cannon D M, Ichise M, Fromm S J, *et al.* 2006. Serotonin transporter binding in bipolar disorder assessed using [11C]DASB and positron emission tomography. *Biol Psychiatry* **60**, 207–17.

Castillo M, Kwock L, Courvoisie H and Hooper S R. 2000. Proton MR spectroscopy in children with bipolar affective disorder: Preliminary observations. *Am J Neuroradiol* **21**, 832–8.

Cecil K M, DelBello M P, Morey R and Strakowski S M. 2002. Frontal lobe differences in bipolar disorder as determined by proton MR spectroscopy. *Bipolar Disord* **4**, 357–65.

Cecil K M, DelBello M P, Sellars M C and Strakowski S M. 2003. Proton magnetic resonance spectroscopy of the frontal lobe and cerebellar vermis in children with a mood disorder and a familial risk for bipolar disorders. *J Child Adolesc Psychopharmacol* **13**, 545–55.

Chang K, Adleman N, Dienes K, Barnea-Goraly N, Reiss A and Ketter T. 2003. Decreased *N*-acetylaspartate in children with familial bipolar disorder. *Biol Psychiatry* **53**, 1059–65.

Dager S R, Friedman S D, Parow A, *et al.* 2004. Brain metabolic alterations in medication-free patients with bipolar disorder. *Arch Gen Psychiatry* **61**, 450–8.

Davanzo P, Thomas M A, Yue K, *et al.* 2001. Decreased anterior cingulate *myo*-inositol/creatine spectroscopy resonance with lithium treatment in children with bipolar disorder. *Neuropsychopharmacology* **24**, 359–69.

Dean B, Pavey G, McLeod M, Opeskin K, Keks N and Copolov D. 2001. A change in the density of [(3)H] flumazenil, but not [(3)H]muscimol binding, in Brodmann's Area 9 from subjects with bipolar disorder. *J Affect Disord* **66**, 147–58.

Dechent P, Pouwels P J, Wilken B, Hanefeld F and Frahm J. 1999. Increase of total creatine in human brain after oral supplementation of creatine-monohydrate. *Am J Physiol* **277**, R698–704.

Deicken R F, Eliaz Y, Feiwell R and Schuff N. 2001. Increased thalamic *N*-acetylaspartate in male patients with familial bipolar I disorder. *Psychiatry Res* **106**, 35–45.

Deicken R F, Fein G and Weiner M W. 1995a. Abnormal frontal lobe phosphorus metabolism in bipolar disorder. *Am J Psychiatry* **152**, 915–8.

Deicken R F, Pegues M P, Anzalone S, Feiwell R and Soher B. 2003. Lower concentration of hippocampal *N*-acetylaspartate in familial bipolar I disorder. *Am J Psychiatry* **160**, 873–82.

Deicken R F, Weiner M W and Fein G. 1995b. Decreased temporal lobe phosphomonoesters in bipolar disorder. *J Affect Disord* **33**, 195–9.

Drevets W C, Frank E, Price J C, *et al.* 1999. PET imaging of serotonin 1A receptor binding in depression. *Biol Psychiatry* **46**, 1375–87.

Drevets W C, Price J L, Simpson J R, *et al.* 1997. Subgenual prefrontal cortex abnormalities in mood disorders. *Nature* **386**, 824–7.

Ebert D, Feistel H, Kaschka W, Barocka A and Pirner A. 1994. Single photon emission computerized tomography assessment of cerebral dopamine D2 receptor blockade in depression before and after sleep deprivation – Preliminary results. *Biol Psychiatry* **35**, 880–5.

Frey B N, Andreazza A C, Nery F G, *et al.* 2007a. The role of hippocampus in the pathophysiology of bipolar disorder. *Behav Pharmacol* **18**, 419–30.

Frey B N, Stanley J A, Nery F G, *et al.* 2007b. Abnormal cellular energy and phospholipid metabolism in the left dorsolateral prefrontal cortex of medication-free individuals with bipolar disorder: An in vivo 1H MRS study. *Bipolar Disord* **9** Suppl 1, 119–27.

Friedman S D, Dager S R, Parow A, *et al.* 2004. Lithium and valproic acid treatment effects on brain chemistry in bipolar disorder. *Biol Psychiatry* **56**, 340–8.

Frye M A, Thomas M A, Yue K, *et al.* 2007a. Reduced concentrations of *N*-acetylaspartate (NAA) and the NAA–creatine ratio in the basal ganglia in bipolar disorder: A study using 3-Tesla proton magnetic resonance spectroscopy. *Psychiatry Res* **154**, 259–65.

Frye M A, Watzl J, Banakar S, *et al.* 2007b. Increased anterior cingulate/medial prefrontal cortical glutamate and creatine in bipolar depression. *Neuropsychopharmacology* **32**, 2490–9.

Goodwin F K and Jamison K R. 2007. *Manic-Depressive Illness* (2nd ed.). New York, NY: Oxford University Press.

Gyulai L, Bolinger L, Leigh J S, Barlow C and Chance B. 1984. Phosphorylethanolamine – The major constituent of the phosphomonoester peak observed by 31P-NMR on developing dog brain. *FEBS Lett* **178**, 137–42.

Hajek T, Bernier D, Slaney C, *et al.* 2008. A comparison of affected and unaffected relatives of patients with bipolar disorder using proton magnetic resonance spectroscopy. *J Psychiatry Neurosci* **33**, 531–40.

Hallcher L M and Sherman W R. 1980. The effects of lithium ion and other agents on the activity of *myo*-inositol-1-phosphatase from bovine brain. *J Biol Chem* **255**, 10 896–901.

Hamakawa H, Kato T, Murashita J and Kato N. 1998. Quantitative proton magnetic resonance spectroscopy of the basal ganglia in patients with affective disorders. *Eur Arch Psychiatry Clin Neurosci* **248**, 53–8.

Hamakawa H, Kato T, Shioiri T, Inubushi T and Kato N. 1999. Quantitative proton magnetic resonance spectroscopy of the bilateral frontal lobes in patients with bipolar disorder. *Psychol Med* **29**, 639–44.

Kato T, Hamakawa H, Shioiri T, *et al.* 1996. Choline-containing compounds detected by proton magnetic resonance spectroscopy in the basal ganglia in bipolar disorder. *J Psychiatry Neurosci* **21**, 248–54.

Kato T, Murashita J, Kamiya A, Shioiri T, Kato N and Inubushi T. 1998. Decreased brain intracellular pH measured by 31P-MRS in bipolar disorder: A confirmation in drug-free patients and correlation with white matter hyperintensity. *Eur Arch Psychiatry Clin Neurosci* **248**, 301–6.

Kato T, Shioiri T, Murashita J, Hamakawa H, Inubushi T and Takahashi S. 1994a. Phosphorus-31 magnetic resonance spectroscopy and ventricular enlargement in bipolar disorder. *Psychiatry Res* **55**, 41–50.

Kato T, Shioiri T, Murashita J, *et al.* 1995. Lateralized abnormality of high energy phosphate metabolism in the frontal lobes of patients with bipolar disorder detected by phase-encoded 31P-MRS. *Psychol Med* **25**, 557–66.

Kato T, Shioiri T, Takahashi S and Inubushi T. 1991. Measurement of brain phosphoinositide metabolism in bipolar patients using in vivo 31P-MRS. *J Affect Disord* **22**, 185–90.

Kato T, Takahashi S and Inubushi T. 1992. Brain lithium concentration by 7Li- and 1H-magnetic resonance spectroscopy in bipolar disorder. *Psychiatry Res* **45**, 53–63.

Kato T, Takahashi S, Shioiri T and Inubushi T. 1993. Alterations in brain phosphorus metabolism in bipolar disorder detected by in vivo 31P and 7Li magnetic resonance spectroscopy. *J Affect Disord* **27**, 53–9.

Kato T, Takahashi S, Shioiri T, Murashita J, Hamakawa H and Inubushi T. 1994b. Reduction of brain phosphocreatine in bipolar II disorder detected by phosphorus-31 magnetic resonance spectroscopy. *J Affect Disord* **31**, 125–33.

Ketter T A, Kimbrell T A, George M S, *et al.* 2001. Effects of mood and subtype on cerebral glucose metabolism in treatment-resistant bipolar disorder. *Biol Psychiatry* **49**, 97–109.

Ketter T A and Wang P W. 2003. The emerging differential roles of GABAergic and antiglutamatergic agents in bipolar disorders. *J Clin Psychiatry* **64** Suppl 3, 15–20.

Malhi G S, Ivanovski B, Wen W, Lagopoulos J, Moss K and Sachdev P. 2007. Measuring mania metabolites: A longitudinal proton spectroscopy study of hypomania. *Acta Psychiatr Scand* **434**(Suppl), 57–66.

Manji H K and Lenox R H. 2000. Signaling: Cellular insights into the pathophysiology of bipolar disorder. *Biol Psychiatry* **48**, 518–30.

Marazziti D, Lenzi A, Raffaelli S, Falcone M F, Aglietti M and Cassano G B. 1993. A single electroconvulsive treatment affects platelet serotonin uptake in bipolar I patients. *Eur Neuropsychopharmacol* **3**, 33–6.

Mayberg H S. 1997. Limbic–cortical dysregulation: A proposed model of depression. *J Neuropsychiatry Clin Neurosci* **9**, 471–81.

Mega M S and Cummings J L. 1994. Frontal–subcortical circuits and neuropsychiatric disorders. *J Neuropsychiatry Clin Neurosci* **6**, 358–70.

Meyer J H, Kapur S, Houle S, *et al.* 1999. Prefrontal cortex 5-HT2 receptors in depression: An [18F]setoperone PET imaging study. *Am J Psychiatry* **156**, 1029–34.

Michael N, Erfurth A, Ohrmann P, *et al.* 2003. Acute mania is accompanied by elevated glutamate/glutamine levels within the left dorsolateral prefrontal cortex. *Psychopharmacology (Berl)* **168**, 344–6.

Molina V, Sánchez J, Sanz J, *et al.* 2007. Dorsolateral prefrontal N-acetyl-aspartate concentration in male patients with chronic schizophrenia and with chronic bipolar disorder. *Eur Psychiatry* **22**, 505–12.

Moore C M, Breeze J L, Gruber S A, *et al.* 2000a. Choline, *myo*-inositol and mood in bipolar disorder: A proton magnetic resonance spectroscopic imaging study of the anterior cingulate cortex. *Bipolar Disord* **2**, 207–16.

Moore G J, Bebchuk J M, Hasanat K, *et al.* 2000b. Lithium increases N-acetyl-aspartate in the human brain: In vivo evidence in support of bcl-2's neurotrophic effects? *Biol Psychiatry* **48**, 1–8.

Moore G J, Bebchuk J M, Parrish J K, *et al.* 1999. Temporal dissociation between lithium-induced changes in frontal lobe *myo*-inositol and clinical response in manic-depressive illness. *Am J Psychiatry* **156**, 1902–08.

Ng W X, Lau I Y, Graham S and Sim K. 2009. Neurobiological evidence for thalamic, hippocampal and related glutamatergic abnormalities in bipolar disorder: A review and synthesis. *Neurosci Biobehav Rev* **33**, 336–54.

Nudmamud S, Reynolds L M and Reynolds G P. 2003. N-acetylaspartate and N-acetylaspartylglutamate deficits in superior temporal cortex in schizophrenia and bipolar disorder: A postmortem study. *Biol Psychiatry* **53**, 1138–41.

Ohara K, Isoda H, Suzuki Y, *et al.* 1998. Proton magnetic resonance spectroscopy of the lenticular nuclei in bipolar I affective disorder. *Psychiatry Res* **84**, 55–60.

Olvera R L, Caetano S C, Fonseca M, *et al.* 2007. Low levels of *N*-acetyl aspartate in the left dorsolateral prefrontal cortex of pediatric bipolar patients. *J Child Adolesc Psychopharmacol* **17**, 461–73.

Ongür D, Jensen J E, Prescot A P, *et al.* 2008. Abnormal glutamatergic neurotransmission and neuronal–glial interactions in acute mania. *Biol Psychiatry* **64**, 718–26.

Oquendo M A, Bongiovi-Garcia M E, Galfalvy H, *et al.* 2007. Sex differences in clinical predictors of suicidal acts after major depression: A prospective study. *Am J Psychiatry* **164**, 134–41.

Pearlson G D, Wong D F, Tune L E, *et al.* 1995. In vivo D2 dopamine receptor density in psychotic and nonpsychotic patients with bipolar disorder. *Arch Gen Psychiatry* **52**, 471–7.

Port J D, Unal S S, Mrazek D A and Marcus S M. 2008. Metabolic alterations in medication-free patients with bipolar disorder: A 3T CSF-corrected magnetic resonance spectroscopic imaging study. *Psychiatry Res* **162**, 113–21.

Renshaw P F, Yurgelun-Todd D A, Tohen M, Gruber S and Cohen B M. 1995. Temporal lobe proton magnetic resonance spectroscopy of patients with first-episode psychosis. *Am J Psychiatry* **152**, 444–6.

Sassi R B, Stanley J A, Axelson D, *et al.* 2005. Reduced NAA levels in the dorsolateral prefrontal cortex of young bipolar patients. *Am J Psychiatry* **162**, 2109–15.

Scherk H, Backens M, Schneider-Axmann T, *et al.* 2007. Cortical neurochemistry in euthymic patients with bipolar I disorder. *World J Biol Psychiatry* 1–10.

Sharma R, Venkatasubramanian P N, Bárány M and Davis J M. 1992. Proton magnetic resonance spectroscopy of the brain in schizophrenic and affective patients. *Schizophr Res* **8**, 43–9.

Silverstone P H, Hanstock C C, Fabian J, Staab R and Allen P S. 1996. Chronic lithium does not alter human *myo*-inositol or phosphomonoester concentrations as measured by 1H and 31P MRS. *Biol Psychiatry* **40**, 235–46.

Silverstone P H, Hanstock C C and Rotzinger S. 1999. Lithium does not alter the choline/creatine ratio in the temporal lobe of human volunteers as measured by proton magnetic resonance spectroscopy. *J Psychiatry Neurosci* **24**, 222–6.

Silverstone P H, Wu R H, O'Donnell T, Ulrich M, Asghar S J and Hanstock C C. 2002. Chronic treatment with both lithium and sodium valproate may normalize phosphoinositol cycle activity in bipolar patients. *Hum Psychopharmacol* **17**, 321–7.

Stahl S M, Woo D J, Mefford I N, Berger P A and Ciaranello R D. 1983. Hyperserotonemia and platelet serotonin uptake and release in schizophrenia and affective disorders. *Am J Psychiatry* **140**, 26–30.

Strakowski S M, Delbello M P and Adler C M. 2005. The functional neuroanatomy of bipolar disorder: A review of neuroimaging findings. *Mol Psychiatry* **10**, 105–16.

Suhara T, Nakayama K, Inoue O, *et al.* 1992. D1 dopamine receptor binding in mood disorders measured by positron emission tomography. *Psychopharmacology (Berl)* **106**, 14–8.

Wang P W, Sailasuta N, Chandler R A and Ketter T A. 2006. Magnetic resonance spectroscopic measurement of cerebral gamma-aminobutyric acid concentrations in patients with bipolar disorders. *Acta Neuropsychiatrica* **18**, 120–6.

Watanabe A, Kato N and Kato T. 2002. Effects of creatine on mental fatigue and cerebral hemoglobin oxygenation. *Neurosci Res* **42**, 279–85.

Winsberg M E, Sachs N, Tate D L, Adalsteinsson E, Spielman D and Ketter T A. 2000. Decreased dorsolateral prefrontal *N*-acetyl aspartate in bipolar disorder. *Biol Psychiatry* **47**, 475–81.

Wu R H, O'Donnell T, Ulrich M, Asghar S J, Hanstock C C and Silverstone P H. 2004. Brain choline concentrations may not be altered in euthymic bipolar disorder patients chronically treated with either lithium or sodium valproate. *Ann Gen Hosp Psychiatry* **3**, 13.

Yildiz A, Sachs G S, Dorer D J and Renshaw P F. 2001. 31P Nuclear magnetic resonance spectroscopy findings in bipolar illness: A meta-analysis. *Psychiatry Res* **106**, 181–91.

Young L T, Warsh J J, Kish S J, Shannak K and Hornykeiwicz O. 1994. Reduced brain 5-HT and elevated NE turnover and metabolites in bipolar affective disorder. *Biol Psychiatry* **35**, 121–7.

Zubieta J K, Huguelet P, Ohl L E, *et al.* 2000. High vesicular monoamine transporter binding in asymptomatic bipolar I disorder: Sex differences and cognitive correlates. *Am J Psychiatry* **157**, 1619–28.

Zubieta J K, Taylor S F, Huguelet P, Koeppe R A, Kilbourn M R and Frey K A. 2001. Vesicular monoamine transporter concentrations in bipolar disorder type I, schizophrenia, and healthy subjects. *Biol Psychiatry* **49**, 110–6.

Structural imaging of major depression

Anand Kumar and Olusola Ajilore

Introduction

An important step in our understanding of the pathophysiology of mood disorders has been made with the advent of neuroimaging. Studies exploring structural changes in the brain associated with unipolar major depression have identified key regions that may underlie the pathogenesis, course, and prognosis of major depression. This chapter will review structural imaging findings in major depression focusing on MRI methodologies such as volumetric analysis, shape analysis, magnetization transfer, and diffusion tensor imaging. We will first examine morphological changes associated with major depression. Then we will discuss white matter changes such as signal hyperintensities and microstructural alterations identified by novel MR-based techniques. We will also explore the pathological and cognitive correlates, as well as the clinical significance of these structural findings.

Cerebral cortex

Initial studies showing neuroanatomical changes associated with major depression explored global cortical alterations, typically characterized by evidence of volume loss. An early qualitative study demonstrating cortical changes showed greater cerebral sulcal and temporal sulcal atrophy in addition to larger ventricles (Rabins *et al.*, 1991). Global gray matter volume losses have been associated with major depression and correlated with clinical variables, such as illness duration (Lampe *et al.*, 2003). Other global structural characteristics have been associated with major depression. For example, patients with major depression are less likely to display left–right asymmetries seen in control subjects (Kumar *et al.*, 2000b).

While earlier studies have demonstrated global cortical volumetric changes, a number of studies using a variety of methods have shown significant specific reductions in frontal regions. For example, depressed patients were more likely to have decreased frontal lobe volumes compared to control subjects (Kumar *et al.*, 2000a). There has been a specific focus on two frontal lobe regions: anterior cingulate (AC) and orbitofrontal cortex (OFC). One of the first papers to implicate the OFC in geriatric depression using simple volumetric measurements demonstrated reduced total OFC volume in elderly depressed patients (Lai *et al.*, 2000). These findings have been more accurately detailed in a study using MRI-based parcellation of the prefrontal cortex into seven distinct subregions (Ballmaier *et al.*, 2004b) (Figure 9.1). In this study, elderly depressed patients exhibited decreased gray matter volumes of the bilateral AC, OFC, and gyrus rectus (medial OFC). There were also white matter reductions in AC and gyrus rectus. In a paper using cortical pattern-matching, which allows for standardization among individual subjects, bilaterally decreased OFC volume was demonstrated in elderly depressed patients (Ballmaier *et al.*, 2004a). Interestingly, this decrease in volume was associated with an increase in gray matter, which may reflect an imbalance of gray matter to white matter in depressed patients. Focusing specifically on late-onset geriatric depression, Ballmaier *et al.* used cortical pattern-matching to identify right temporal and right parietal gray matter deficits, expanding typical structural findings outside of frontal regions (Ballmaier *et al.*, 2007). In a comprehensive volumetric analysis of multiple cortical and subcortical regions, Andreescu and colleagues (2008) identified 17 out of 24 regions of decreased volumes associated with geriatric depression. These regions included frontal cortical areas, gyrus

Understanding Neuropsychiatric Disorders, ed. M. E. Shenton and B. I. Turetsky. Published by Cambridge University Press.
© Cambridge University Press 2011.

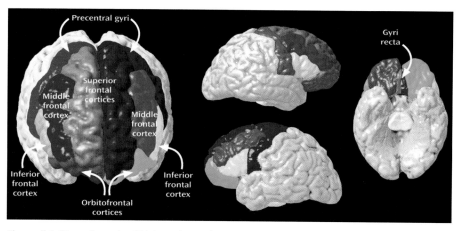

Figure 9.1 Three-dimensional high-resolution shape representations detailing the parcellation of prefrontal cortex subregions. With permission from Ballmaier *et al.*, 2004b.

rectus, hippocampus, amygdala, putamen, pallidum, thalamus, and temporal areas.

There have been some studies to examine gender differences in volumetric changes. For example, left AC volumes have been shown to be smaller in depressed males compared to depressed females, while amygdala volumes are smaller only in depressed females compared to controls (Hastings *et al.*, 2004). In a geriatric depression study, depressed men demonstrated lower frontal gray matter volumes compared to depressed women (Lavretsky *et al.*, 2004).

Hippocampus

In addition to prefrontal cortical regions, the hippocampus has been the focus of a great deal of research into structural brain changes in major depression. In a study of depressed women, bilateral hippocampal volumes were significantly smaller compared to controls and hippocampal volumes were correlated with the duration of depression (Sheline *et al.*, 1996). Similar hippocampal volume decreases have also been seen in geriatric depression (Steffens *et al.*, 2000). These studies suggest that chronicity of depression is related to hippocampal volume reduction. This notion is also confirmed in a study comparing first-episode medication-naive depressed patients with multiple-episode depression patients. In this study, MacQueen *et al.* (2003) found that only multiple-episode depressed patients had significant volume reductions compared to controls. In addition, they found a significant association between depression duration and hippocampal volume consistent with

previous reports. A more refined examination of the relationship between depression duration and hippocampal volume decreases was done by Sheline *et al.* (2003). Hippocampal volume loss was specifically related to length of time *untreated* during a depressive episode (Sheline *et al.*, 2003). In line with the relationship between hippocampal volumes and antidepressant treatment, remitted patients no longer on medication and medication-naive depressive patients still have smaller posterior hippocampal volumes, suggestive of a trait characteristic (Neumeister *et al.*, 2005). Posterior hippocampal changes were also seen in a study by Maller *et al.* (2007).

The neurocognitive correlates of hippocampal volume loss associated with major depression was explored in a study showing a significant association with persistent memory deficits (O'Brien *et al.*, 2004; Hickie *et al.*, 2005b). Hippocampal volume loss has also been correlated with impairment in executive function (Frodl *et al.*, 2006). Thus, volume changes in the hippocampus may underlie some of the cognitive symptoms of major depression.

In addition to volumetric analysis, there have been attempts for more detailed characterization of hippocampal changes associated with major depression. In a study using high-dimensional brain mapping, hippocampal shape was analyzed. The authors of that study found that hippocampal surface deformation in depressed patients involved the subiculum (Posener *et al.*, 2003). The subiculum has also been implicated in another shape analysis study of hippocampal morphology that showed specific contractions in CA1–CA3 cell fields associated with geriatric depression (Ballmaier *et al.*, 2007). This study also distinguished changes specific to late-onset geriatric depression (left CA1 and subiculum contractions) compared to early-onset cases, and found correlations between these morphological changes and memory deficits. Another shape analysis that also confirmed lateralized effects showed left hippocampal deformations noted in depressed patients compared to control subjects. In contrast to what was observed with hippocampal volume data, remitted depressed subjects were undifferentiated from controls, suggestive of a state characteristic (Zhao *et al.*, 2008).

Basal ganglia

The basal ganglia are another major locus of structural changes in major depression. Depressed patients have smaller putamen volumes compared to controls (Husain *et al.*, 1991). Both caudate and putamen volumes have been shown to be significantly reduced in depressed patients and related to the age of first depressive episode (Parashos *et al.*, 1998). In a study excluding subjects that were positive for cerebrovascular risk factors, striatal volume differences were not seen between depressed patients and control subjects (Lenze and Sheline, 1999). No differences in basal ganglia volumes were shown in another study comparing depressed patients and control subjects (Pillay *et al.*, 1998). However, the authors found that left caudate volumes had a significant negative relationship to baseline depression severity scores. A similar finding was noted by Lacerda *et al.*, who found no volume differences between depressed patients and control subjects, but did find a significant negative correlation between left putamen volumes and illness duration (Lacerda *et al.*, 2003). In a paper using three-dimensional surface mapping, bilateral reduced caudal volumes were found in geriatric depressed patients compared to control subjects, with caudal volume reduction correlated with disease severity (Butters *et al.*, 2008). Reduced caudate volumes may be limited to gray matter according to a study by Kim and colleagues (2008). While most studies have focused on depression in older depressed patients, there is a one report of smaller basal ganglia volumes associated with pediatric major depression in medication-naive patients (Matsuo *et al.*, 2008). The literature on neurocognitive correlates of basal ganglia volume in major depression is sparse. However, there is one study that showed that reduced right caudate volumes

appear to at least partially mediate psychomotor slowing seen in geriatric depression (Naismith *et al.*, 2002).

Amygdala

The first report of amygdalar volumes found a decrease in amygdala core nuclei volumes in depressed patients (Sheline *et al.*, 1998). In a study of treatment-resistant depressed patients, amygdalar asymmetries with left larger than right occurred in depressed patients, but not control subjects (Mervaala *et al.*, 2000). Smaller left amygdalar volumes were found in depressed patients with subjective memory complaints in a report from von Gunten *et al.* (2000). Depressed patients also had smaller left amygdalar volumes in a functional MRI study by Siegle *et al.* (2003). Bilateral amygdalar volume reductions were noted in a study of pediatric major depression (Rosso *et al.*, 2005). In contrast to most studies demonstrating a decrease in structural volumes, in the amygdala, *larger* volumes have also been seen in depressed patients compared to controls (Frodl *et al.*, 2002). This has been replicated in a study of young depressed women who had 13% larger amygdalar volumes compared to control subjects (Lange and Irle, 2004). A study comparing depressed patients, remitted depressed patients, and controls demonstrated bilateral enlarged amygdala volume in acutely depressed patients compared to remitted patients and controls, indicative of a state characteristic (van Eijndhoven *et al.*, 2008).

In an effort to clarify the divergent data described above, Hamilton *et al.* reviewed the literature of amygdalar volume changes in major depression in a recent meta-analysis (2008). They found that overall there was no significant difference between depressed patients and control subjects. However, there was a great deal of variability in the data secondary to medication exposure in the studies analyzed. Unmedicated depressed subjects tended to have smaller volumes, compared to medicated depressed subjects with increased volumes.

Clinical significance

In order to understand the functional significance of these structural changes seen in major depression, studies have been performed correlating functional impairment with the severity of volumetric findings. Taylor and colleagues looked at the relationship between structural changes and functional disability.

They showed that smaller OFC volumes, along with increased cognitive impairment, in elderly depressed patients are significantly correlated with impairment in basic activities of daily living (Taylor *et al.*, 2003c). Volumetric changes have also been correlated with clinical features of major depression. Lavretsky *et al.* demonstrated that AC volumes have also been associated with apathy in geriatric depression (2007).

The functional and clinical significance of the changes described above have been examined in studies that focus on treatment response and remission rates associated with neuroimaging findings. In patients who did not respond to fluoxetine treatment, gray matter volumes were negatively correlated with depression severity (Pillay *et al.*, 1997). Lower volumes in frontotemporal regions have also been associated with treatment-resistance in elderly depressed patients (Simpson *et al.*, 2001). In one of the few prospective studies examining neuroanatomical changes associated with major depression, decline in gray matter density was seen in hippocampus, AC, left amygdala and right dorsolateral prefrontal cortex in depressed patients compared to controls over a three-year period (Frodl *et al.*, 2008b). Frodl *et al.* also found lower rates of gray matter decline in remitted patients. In addition, lower hippocampal volumes have also been associated with higher rates of recurrence in male depressed patients (Kronmuller *et al.*, 2008).

There have been a few genetic correlations of hippocampal volume loss in major depression. For example, the l/l genotype for the serotonin transporter gene (5HTTLPR) has been associated with smaller hippocampal volumes in depressed patients compared to controls (Frodl *et al.*, 2004, 2008a). In addition, smaller caudate volumes have been associated with the short allele of the 5HTT gene (Hickie *et al.*, 2007).

White matter hyperintensities

One of the early links between major depression and structural brain changes was first shown in studies that demonstrated a consistent radiological finding of white-matter hyperintensities (WMH) on magnetic resonance imaging (MRI). WMH are regions of increased signal intensity, especially on T_2-weighted images, commonly associated with geriatric depression. They are typically found in subcortical, periventricular, and deep white matter regions. One of the first studies associating WMH with major depression was done by Coffey *et al.* (1988). They showed that

approximately two-thirds of elderly depressed patients referred for electroconvulsive therapy (ECT) had evidence of subcortical white matter disease. In a subsequent study where elderly depressed patients were compared with age-matched controls, the depressed patients demonstrated more severe WMH more often (Coffey *et al.*, 1990). WMH appear to be more associated with late-onset elderly depression compared to early-onset depression in the elderly (Figiel *et al.*, 1991; Salloway *et al.*, 1996). This has been confirmed in later studies which have shown that these subcortical WMH in elderly depressed patients tended to be more severe in late-onset depression versus early-onset cases and controls (Tupler *et al.*, 2002; Murata *et al.*, 2001), suggestive of complementary pathways for early-onset as compared to late-onset cases. There have been attempts to localize WMH associated with depression. Studies of WMH in major depression have demonstrated that frontal regions are particularly important (Taylor *et al.*, 2003a). In particular, WMH in the left frontal deep white matter and left putamen appear to be associated with geriatric depression (Greenwald *et al.*, 1998).

While many studies often control for cerebrovascular risk factors, there has been a considerable effort to examine the specific role of cerebrovascular risk factors for WMH in depression. Some studies demonstrate that cerebrovascular risk factors are important for the expression of WMH in geriatric depression. An early study which excluded subjects with cerebrovascular risk factors found no predominance of WMH in depressed subjects compared to control subjects. However, they did find a significant correlation between age and depression and WMH number (Lenze *et al.*, 1999). In a study by Greenwald *et al.*, hypertensive depressed patients had significantly more subcortical and deep white matter hyperintensities compared to depressed patients with normal blood pressures (Greenwald *et al.*, 2001). Deep WMH and subcortical hyperintensities were associated with hypertension and diabetes in another study of depressed patients (Hickie *et al.*, 2005a).

However, the role of cerebrovascular risk factors is more complex than initially conceptualized. In a study that excluded subjects with hypertension, diabetic or ischemic heart disease, elderly depressed patients had larger frontal WMH volumes compared to elderly controls (Firbank *et al.*, 2004). In a more recent study that matched elderly depressed subjects and control subjects for vascular risk factors, depressed subjects had significant increases in WMH in specific regions (superior longitudinal fasciculus, fronto-occipital fasciculus, uncinate fasciculus, extreme capsule and inferior longitudinal fasciculus) compared to control subjects (Sheline *et al.*, 2008). Taken together, these studies indicated that major depression, independent of vascular risk factors, is associated with WMH.

Despite the confusion from the associative studies discussed above, further evidence for the role of cerebrovascular risk factors comes from pathological studies. Neuropathological correlates of WMH have been examined to better characterize what these white matter lesions actually represent. Initial pathological studies indicated that periventricular hyperintensities in geriatric depression are due to dilated perivascular spaces, oligemic demyelination, and ischemic demyelination (Thomas *et al.*, 2002, 2003).

Genetic factors also play a role in the association of WMH with major depression. One of the first studies to show such a role for genetic factors demonstrated an increased prevalence of longitudinal increases in WMH in elderly depressed patients with the apolipoprotein-E (APOE) epsilon 4 allele (Lavretsky *et al.*, 2000). APOE epsilon 4 was also implicated in a study showing a significant correlation between having the allele and subcortical lesion volumes in depressed patients (Steffens *et al.*, 2003). More recently, the BDNF Val66-Met polymorphism has been shown to be associated with more WMH in elderly depressed and control subjects (Taylor *et al.*, 2008b). The l/s genotype of the serotonin transporter gene (5HTTLPR) was associated with higher WMH volumes in elderly depressed patients (Steffens *et al.*, 2008).

The clinical significance of WMH in major depression is characterized by treatment response, disease severity, and cognitive performance. WMH associated with major depression has been associated with poorer treatment-response (both ECT and pharmacotherapy) in a number of studies (Hickie *et al.*, 1995; Simpson *et al.*, 1997, 1998; Steffens *et al.*, 2001; Iosifescu *et al.*, 2006). Elderly depressed patients that achieved remission after antidepressant treatment had lower WMH volume increases compared to those who did not respond (Taylor *et al.*, 2003b). There is one study that showed no association with the presence or absence of WMH in elderly depressed patients treated with sertraline (Salloway *et al.*, 2002); however, most studies support the notion of treatment resistance in association with WMH burden.

Not only do WMH have implications for treatment response, they also appear to be related to prognosis and disease progression. It has been shown that depressed subjects with WMH have more severe depressive episodes and a more severe longitudinal course (Heiden *et al.*, 2005; O'Brien *et al.*, 1998). Further evidence of greater disease severity associated with WMH come from studies demonstrating that in younger depressed patients, periventricular WMH are more prevalent in cases of depression with a history of suicidality (Ehrlich *et al.*, 2004). This finding has also been replicated with an older adult sample (Pompili *et al.*, 2008). Even mortality has been associated with deep WMH in elderly depressed patients (Levy *et al.*, 2003).

The neurocognitive consequences of WMH have been demonstrated in studies showing impaired executive function in geriatric depression (Lesser *et al.*, 1996) and impaired performance on memory and naming tasks (Kramer-Ginsberg *et al.*, 1999). Specifically, geriatric depressed patients with subcortical hyperintensities have been found to have problems with semantic encoding and learning efficiency (Jenkins *et al.*, 1998). One study examining WMH regional localization and cognitive performance found periventricular WMH associated with delayed recall after distraction, basal ganglia hyperintensities associated with impaired category production, and pontine WMH related to psychomotor speed (Simpson *et al.*, 1997). WMH also predicted chronicity of depression and subsequent cognitive decline in a longitudinal study by Hickie *et al* (Hickie *et al.*, 1997). Another focus on localization suggests that basal ganglia WMH are particularly related to depression severity and cognitive impairment (Agid *et al.*, 2003). WMH in elderly depression is also associated with cognitive decline and even dementia according to a study by Steffens *et al.* (2007). WMH are also associated with functional decline associated with geriatric depression as demonstrated by a Japanese study of elderly patients (Sonohara *et al.*, 2008). In a study by Steffens *et al.*, impairment in the activities of daily living (ADLs) was significantly correlated with the volume of white-matter lesions (Steffens *et al.*, 2002).

In an interesting case study indicating possible causality, the longitudinal increase in WMH volume was associated with onset of major depression in one elderly subject compared to 12 subjects who did not develop depression and had significantly less longitudinal change in WMH volume over the study period (Nebes *et al.*, 2002). This intriguing finding has been further explored in a longitudinal study that demonstrated higher WMH volumes significantly increases the risk of developing depression (OR = 1.3, 95% CI 1.1–1.7) (Godin *et al.*, 2008).

While data from volumetric studies and WMH studies have been presented separately, there have been some attempts to study how these findings may be related. The interaction of WMH and decreased OFC volume was demonstrated in a study of Lee *et al.* This study showed that decreases in OFC volume (left, right, and total) were negatively associated with the degree of subcortical white-matter lesions (Lee *et al.*, 2003). This suggests that disruption in white matter tracts connecting frontal–subcortical circuits might lead to functionally significant abnormalities in the OFC. However, in a path analysis study, it was shown that volumetric changes and WMHs likely represent distinct pathological processes that co-exist in major depression (Kumar *et al.*, 2002).

Magnetization transfer imaging

Magnetization transfer (MT) imaging is a method to examine the biophysical properties of the brain parenchyma by means of MR imaging (Barbosa *et al.*, 1994; Eng *et al.*, 1991; Grossman, 1994; Henkelman *et al.*, 2001). MT allows for the measurement of white matter microstructural integrity and can detect abnormalities in normal-appearing white matter. Water protons produce the signal used to create MT images, as well as other forms of MRI. MT imaging, however, utilizes the fact that there are two classes of water in biological tissues: water bound to macromolecules (bound water) and free water. The free water signal is the main contributor to MRI; bound water contributes less to the signal, secondary to its wide frequency band distribution. An "off-resonance" saturation pulse is utilized to minimize the exchange between the two water pools, thereby minimizing the contribution of the bound water pool to the MR signal. In the MT imaging protocol, two images are acquired at every slice location within an organ. The signal of the MT acquisition is reduced compared to the control acquisition in every tissue region having water protons that exchange between the free and bound states. Therefore, a magnetization transfer ratio (MTR) image can then be created, reflecting the difference in signal intensity between the two images. In the white matter, myelin-related proteins are the main macromolecular contributors in MT imaging. Decreases in MT ratios are associated with findings in multiple sclerosis, which is characterized by demyelination and underlying axonal transections (Bjartmar *et al.*, 1999; Grossman, 1994; van Waesberghe *et al.*, 1999). In gray matter, decreases in MT ratios are less clear, but may represent abnormalities in the macromolecular protein pool.

There have been two studies which have used MT to probe white matter changes associated with geriatric depression. Kumar *et al.* (2004) found lower MT ratios in the genu and splenium of the corpus callosum, right caudate and putamen, and occipital lobes in elderly depressed patients compared to controls. These findings were echoed in a later study of geriatric depression finding lower MT ratios in multiple left hemispheric regions such as anterior and posterior cingulate, insular, subcallosal, middle occipital lobe and the thalamus (Gunning-Dixon *et al.*, 2008). These studies further implicate white matter abnormalities in the pathophysiology of major depression.

Diffusion tensor imaging

An imaging technique that has been useful for the study of white matter integrity and brain microstructural changes is diffusion tensor imaging (DTI). DTI works on the principle that water diffuses randomly in unrestricted environments resulting in isotropic movement (or equal movement in all directions). This movement is restrained in white matter tracts, thus water diffusion tends to move along the axis of axon sheath, leading to anisotropy. One of the ways DTI can be quantified is fractional anisotropy (FA), which represents a measure of directional coherence and in white matter tracts, the degree of structural alignment. Another quantification technique measures the average diffusion of water in a voxel and can be expressed as the apparent diffusion coefficient (ADC). Several studies have used to DTI to examine microstructural changes in white matter that appears normal using more conventional MRI techniques.

In one of the first studies to use DTI to examine white matter abnormalities associated with major depression, Taylor *et al.* (2001) found that in geriatric depressed patients and controls, brain regions with hyperintensities demonstrated higher ADC and lower FA compared to normal regions. While this first study of DTI in geriatric depression demonstrated no differences between depressed patients and controls, a later report from Nobuhara and colleagues found that geriatric depression patients had widespread regions of lower FA in frontal and temporal white matter

(Nobuhara *et al.*, 2006), but no differences in parietal or occipital white matter were seen. In addition, they found that higher frontal white matter FA below the AC–PC line was significantly correlated with lower scores on the Hamilton Rating Scale for Depression. Consistent with WMH associations, DTI has other clinical correlates as demonstrated by a study showing that diastolic blood pressure is negatively correlated with FA in anterior cingulate (Hoptman *et al.*, 2008). The theme of regional specificity has been echoed in other studies. For example, in elderly depressed patients, Bae *et al.* (2006) demonstrated lower FA in the white matter of the right anterior cingulate cortex, bilateral superior frontal gyri, and left middle frontal gyrus. Similar regions were affected in a study by Yang *et al.* (2007) demonstrating lower FA in frontal and temporal white matter. Lower FA has also been demonstrated in elderly depressed patients in remission after their first episode (Yuan *et al.*, 2007). The first demonstration of lower FA associated with major depression in a non-geriatric population was done in a study published by Ma *et al.* In their brief report, depressed patients (mean age = 28.9 years) had lower FA in the white matter of the middle frontal gyrus, left occipitotemporal gyrus, and the subgyral and angular gyri of the parietal lobe (Ma *et al.*, 2007). Although these results were suggestive that similar white matter alterations occur in younger depressed patients, later work from the same group showed that, unlike older depressed patients, lower FA was not correlated with illness severity or course (Li *et al.*, 2007). A more recent study in non-elderly depressed did show an association between low FA in the anterior limb of the internal capsule and severity of illness (Zou *et al.*, 2008).

The white matter disruptions detected by DTI are not just correlated with WMH and disease severity, they have also been shown to have implications for treatment. In an early study using DTI to detect white matter changes associated with major depression, Alexopoulos *et al.* found microstructural white matter abnormalities lateral to the anterior cingulate were associated with low remission rates after 12 weeks of citalopram treatment (Alexopoulos *et al.*, 2002, 2008). This association with low remission rates has been replicated in a recent study using sertraline (Taylor *et al.*, 2008a). It is interesting to note that while lower FA was associated with poor remission to oral anti-depressant treatment, FA has been shown to *increase* in response to ECT treatment. Nobuhara *et al.* demonstrated that lower frontal white matter FA seen in elderly depressed patients increased within two weeks after the cessation of ECT treatment. Although the authors found lower FA in temporal white matter, FA in that region did not change in response to ECT treatment (Nobuhara *et al.*, 2004).

In addition to being an indicator of treatment resistance and response, changes assessed by DTI have also been associated with cognitive functions. For example, it has been associated with poor performance on executive function as measured by the Stroop task (Murphy *et al.*, 2007). Thus, white matter alterations detected by DTI have implications for neuropsychological sequelae seen in major depression.

Summary

Structural imaging studies in major depression have identified volume alterations in prefrontal cortex, hippocampus, amygdala, and basal ganglia structures. In addition, white matter hyperintensities have been seen in periventricular, deep white matter and subcortical regions in association with major depression. More subtle white matter alterations have been detected with DTI and MT, suggestive of microstructural abnormalities, even in normal-appearing white matter. The neuroanatomical changes seen in major depression appear to be modified by genetic and environmental factors, such as polymorphisms, gender, and comorbidity. The changes described above have functional and clinical significance in terms of having an impact on cognitive function, disease severity, and treatment response. While these studies have been important for the neuroanatomical localization of major depression, further work is needed to understand how derangements in these brain regions contribute to clinical picture of depression, and how they may provide targets for better and more effective treatments.

> **Box 9.1.** Structural imaging findings associated with major depression
>
> - Volumetric decreases in prefrontal cortex, hippocampus, amygdala and basal ganglia
> - White matter hyperintensities in periventricular, subcortical and deep white matter regions
> - White matter alterations in normal-appearing white matter detected by DTI and MT
>
> Clinical and functional associations with structural imaging abnormalities
>
> - Cognitive and functional impairment
> - Treatment resistance and lower remission rates
> - Genetic polymorphisms

References

Agid R, Levin T, Gomori J M, Lerer B and Bonne O. 2003. T2-weighted image hyperintensities in major depression: Focus on the basal ganglia. *Int J Neuropsychopharmacol* **6**, 215–24.

Alexopoulos G S, Kiosses D N, Choi S J, Murphy C F and Lim K O. 2002. Frontal white matter microstructure and treatment response of late-life depression: A preliminary study. *Am J Psychiatry* **159**, 1929–32.

Alexopoulos G S, Murphy C F, Gunning-Dixon F M, *et al.* 2008. Microstructural white matter abnormalities and remission of geriatric depression. *Am J Psychiatry* **165**, 238–44.

Andreescu C, Butters M A, Begley A, *et al.* 2008. Gray matter changes in late life depression – A structural MRI analysis. *Neuropsychopharmacology* **33**, 2566–72.

Bae J N, MacFall J R, Krishnan K R, Payne M E, Steffens D C and Taylor W D. 2006. Dorsolateral prefrontal cortex and anterior cingulate cortex white matter alterations in late-life depression. *Biol Psychiatry* **60**, 1356–63.

Ballmaier M, Narr K L, Toga A W, *et al.* 2007. Hippocampal morphology and distinguishing late-onset from early-onset elderly depression. *Am J Psychiatry* **165**, 229–37.

Ballmaier M, Sowell E R, Thompson P M, *et al.* 2004a. Mapping brain size and cortical gray matter changes in elderly depression. *Biol Psychiatry* **55**, 382–9.

Ballmaier M, Toga A W, Blanton R E, *et al.* 2004b. Anterior cingulate, gyrus rectus, and orbitofrontal abnormalities in elderly depressed patients: An MRI-based parcellation of the prefrontal cortex. *Am J Psychiatry* **161**, 99–108.

Barbosa S, Blumhardt L D, Roberts N, Lock T and Edwards R H. 1994. Magnetic resonance relaxation time mapping in multiple sclerosis: Normal appearing white matter and the "invisible" lesion load. *Magn Reson Imaging* **12**, 33–42.

Bjartmar C, Yin X and Trapp B D. 1999. Axonal pathology in myelin disorders. *J Neurocytol* **28**, 383–95.

Butters M A, Aizenstein H J, Hayashi K M, *et al.* 2008. Three-dimensional surface mapping of the caudate nucleus in late-life depression. *Am J Geriatr Psychiatry* **17**, 4–12.

Coffey C E, Figiel G S, Djang W T, Cress M, Saunders W B and Weiner R D. 1988. Leukoencephalopathy in elderly depressed patients referred for ECT. *Biol Psychiatry* **24**, 143–61.

Coffey C E, Figiel G S, Djang W T and Weiner R D. 1990. Subcortical hyperintensity on magnetic resonance imaging: A comparison of normal and depressed elderly subjects. *Am J Psychiatry* **147**, 187–9.

Ehrlich S, Noam G G, Lyoo I K, Kwon B J, Clark M A and Renshaw P F. 2004. White matter hyperintensities and their associations with suicidality in psychiatrically hospitalized children and adolescents. *J Am Acad Child Adolesc Psychiatry* **43**, 770–6.

Eng J, Ceckler T L and Balaban R S. 1991. Quantitative 1H magnetization transfer imaging in vivo. *Magn Reson Med* **17**, 304–14.

Figiel G S, Krishnan K R, Doraiswamy P M, Rao V P, Nemeroff C B and Boyko O B. 1991. Subcortical hyperintensities on brain magnetic resonance imaging: A comparison between late age onset and early onset elderly depressed subjects. *Neurobiol Aging* **12**, 245–7.

Firbank M J, Lloyd A J, Ferrier N and O'Brien J T. 2004. A volumetric study of MRI signal hyperintensities in late-life depression. *Am J Geriatr Psychiatry* **12**, 606–12.

Frodl T, Meisenzahl E, Zetzsche T, *et al.* 2002. Enlargement of the amygdala in patients with a first episode of major depression. *Biol Psychiatry* **51**, 708–14.

Frodl T, Meisenzahl E M, Zetzsche T, *et al.* 2004. Hippocampal and amygdala changes in patients with major depressive disorder and healthy controls during a 1-year follow-up. *J Clin Psychiatry* **65**, 492–9.

Frodl T, Schaub A, Banac S, *et al.* 2006. Reduced hippocampal volume correlates with executive dysfunctioning in major depression. *J Psychiatry Neurosci* **31**, 316–23.

Frodl T, Zill P, Baghai T, *et al.* 2008a. Reduced hippocampal volumes associated with the long variant of the tri- and diallelic serotonin transporter polymorphism in major depression. *Am J Med Genet B Neuropsychiatr Genet* **147B**, 1003–07.

Frodl T S, Koutsouleris N, Bottlender R, *et al.* 2008b. Depression-related variation in brain morphology over 3 years: Effects of stress? *Arch Gen Psychiatry* **65**, 1156–65.

Godin O, Dufouil C, Maillard P, *et al.* 2008. White matter lesions as a predictor of depression in the elderly: The 3C-Dijon study. *Biol Psychiatry* **63**, 663–9.

Greenwald B S, Kramer-Ginsberg E, Krishnan K R, Ashtari M, Auerbach C and Patel M. 1998. Neuroanatomic localization of magnetic resonance imaging signal hyperintensities in geriatric depression. *Stroke* **29**, 613–7.

Greenwald B S, Kramer-Ginsberg E, Krishnan K R, *et al.* 2001. A controlled study of MRI signal hyperintensities in older depressed patients with and without hypertension. *J Am Geriatr Soc* **49**, 1218–25.

Grossman R I. 1994. Magnetization transfer in multiple sclerosis. *Ann Neurol* **36** Suppl, S97–9.

Gunning-Dixon F M, Hoptman M J, Lim K O, *et al.* 2008. Macromolecular white matter abnormalities in geriatric depression: A magnetization transfer imaging study. *Am J Geriatr Psychiatry* **16**, 255–62.

Hamilton J P, Siemer M and Gotlib I H. 2008. Amygdala volume in major depressive disorder: A meta-analysis of magnetic resonance imaging studies. *Mol Psychiatry* **13**, 993–1000.

Hastings R S, Parsey R V, Oquendo M A, Arango V and Mann J J. 2004. Volumetric analysis of the prefrontal cortex, amygdala, and hippocampus in major depression. *Neuropsychopharmacology* **29**, 952–9.

Heiden A, Kettenbach J, Fischer P, *et al.* 2005. White matter hyperintensities and chronicity of depression. *J Psychiatr Res* **39**, 285–93.

Henkelman R M, Stanisz G J and Graham S J. 2001. Magnetization transfer in MRI: A review. *NMR Biomed* **14**, 57–64.

Hickie I, Naismith S, Ward P B, *et al.* 2005a. Vascular risk and low serum B12 predict white matter lesions in patients with major depression. *J Affect Disord* **85**, 327–32.

Hickie I, Naismith S, Ward P B, *et al.* 2005b. Reduced hippocampal volumes and memory loss in patients with early- and late-onset depression. *Br J Psychiatry* **186**, 197–202.

Hickie I, Scott E, Mitchell P, Wilhelm K, Austin M P and Bennett B. 1995. Subcortical hyperintensities on magnetic resonance imaging: Clinical correlates and prognostic significance in patients with severe depression. *Biol Psychiatry* **37**, 151–60.

Hickie I, Scott E, Wilhelm K and Brodaty H. 1997. Subcortical hyperintensities on magnetic resonance imaging in patients with severe depression – A longitudinal evaluation. *Biol Psychiatry* **42**, 367–74.

Hickie I B, Naismith S L, Ward P B, *et al.* 2007. Serotonin transporter gene status predicts caudate nucleus but not amygdala or hippocampal volumes in older persons with major depression. *J Affect Disord* **98**, 137–42.

Hoptman M J, Gunning-Dixon F M, Murphy C F, *et al.* 2008. Blood pressure and white matter integrity in geriatric depression. *J Affect Disord* **115**, 171–6.

Husain M M, McDonald W M, Doraiswamy P M, *et al.* 1991. A magnetic resonance imaging study of putamen nuclei in major depression. *Psychiatry Res* **40**, 95–9.

Iosifescu D V, Renshaw P F, Lyoo I K, *et al.* 2006. Brain white-matter hyperintensities and treatment outcome in major depressive disorder. *Br J Psychiatry* **188**, 180–5.

Jenkins M, Malloy P, Salloway S, *et al.* 1998. Memory processes in depressed geriatric patients with and without subcortical hyperintensities on MRI. *J Neuroimaging* **8**, 20–6.

Kim M J, Hamilton J P and Gotlib I H. 2008. Reduced caudate gray matter volume in women with major depressive disorder. *Psychiatry Res* **164**, 114–22.

Kramer-Ginsberg E, Greenwald B S, Krishnan K R, *et al.* 1999. Neuropsychological functioning and MRI signal hyperintensities in geriatric depression. *Am J Psychiatry* **156**, 438–44.

Kronmuller K T, Pantel J, Kohler S, *et al.* 2008. Hippocampal volume and 2-year outcome in depression. *Br J Psychiatry* **192**, 472–3.

Kumar A, Bilker W, Jin Z and Udupa J. 2000a. Atrophy and high intensity lesions: Complementary neurobiological mechanisms in late-life major depression. *Neuropsychopharmacology* **22**, 264–74.

Kumar A, Bilker W, Lavretsky H and Gottlieb G. 2000b. Volumetric asymmetries in late-onset mood disorders: An attenuation of frontal asymmetry with depression severity. *Psychiatry Res* **100**, 41–7.

Kumar A, Gupta R C, Albert T M, Alger J, Wyckoff N and Hwang S. 2004. Biophysical changes in normal-appearing white matter and subcortical nuclei in late-life major depression detected using magnetization transfer. *Psychiatry Res* **130**, 131–40.

Kumar A, Mintz J, Bilker W and Gottlieb G. 2002. Autonomous neurobiological pathways to late-life major depressive disorder: Clinical and pathophysiological implications. *Neuropsychopharmacology* **26**, 229–36.

Lacerda A L, Nicoletti M A, Brambilla P, *et al.* 2003. Anatomical MRI study of basal ganglia in major depressive disorder. *Psychiatry Res* **124**, 129–40.

Lai T, Payne M E, Byrum C E, Steffens D C and Krishnan K R. 2000. Reduction of orbital frontal cortex volume in geriatric depression. *Biol Psychiatry* **48**, 971–5.

Lampe I K, Hulshoff Pol H E, Janssen J, Schnack H G, Kahn R S and Heeren T J. 2003. Association of depression duration with reduction of global cerebral gray matter volume in female patients with recurrent major depressive disorder. *Am J Psychiatry* **160**, 2052–4.

Lange C and Irle E. 2004. Enlarged amygdala volume and reduced hippocampal volume in young women with major depression. *Psychol Med* **34**, 1059–64.

Lavretsky H, Ballmaier M, Pham D, Toga A and Kumar A. 2007. Neuroanatomical characteristics of geriatric apathy and depression: A magnetic resonance imaging study. *Am J Geriatr Psychiatry* **15**, 386–94.

Lavretsky H, Kurbanyan K, Ballmaier M, Mintz J, Toga A and Kumar A. 2004. Sex differences in brain structure in geriatric depression. *Am J Geriatr Psychiatry* **12**, 653–7.

Lavretsky H, Lesser I M, Wohl M, Miller B L, Mehringer C M and Vinters H V. 2000. Apolipoprotein-E and white-matter hyperintensities in late-life depression. *Am J Geriatr Psychiatry* **8**, 257–61.

Lee S H, Payne M E, Steffens D C, *et al.* 2003. Subcortical lesion severity and orbitofrontal cortex volume in geriatric depression. *Biol Psychiatry* **54**, 529–33.

Lenze E, Cross D, McKeel D, Neuman R J and Sheline Y I. 1999. White matter hyperintensities and gray matter lesions in physically healthy depressed subjects. *Am J Psychiatry* **156**, 1602–7.

Lenze E J and Sheline Y I. 1999. Absence of striatal volume differences between depressed subjects with no comorbid medical illness and matched comparison subjects. *Am J Psychiatry* **156**, 1989–91.

Lesser I M, Boone K B, Mehringer C M, Wohl M A, Miller B L and Berman N G. 1996. Cognition and white matter hyperintensities in older depressed patients. *Am J Psychiatry* **153**, 1280–7.

Levy R M, Steffens D C, McQuoid D R, Provenzale J M, MacFall J R and Krishnan K R. 2003. MRI lesion severity and mortality in geriatric depression. *Am J Geriatr Psychiatry* **11**, 678–82.

Li L, Ma N, Li Z, *et al.* 2007. Prefrontal white matter abnormalities in young adult with major depressive disorder: A diffusion tensor imaging study. *Brain Res* **1168**, 124–8.

Ma N, Li L, Shu N, *et al.* 2007. White matter abnormalities in first-episode, treatment-naive young adults with major depressive disorder. *Am J Psychiatry* **164**, 823–6.

MacQueen G M, Campbell S, McEwen B S, *et al.* 2003. Course of illness, hippocampal function, and hippocampal volume in major depression. *Proc Natl Acad Sci U S A* **100**, 1387–92.

Maller J J, Daskalakis Z J and Fitzgerald P B. 2007. Hippocampal volumetrics in depression: The importance of the posterior tail. *Hippocampus* **17**, 1023–7.

Matsuo K, Rosenberg D R, Easter P C, *et al.* 2008. Striatal volume abnormalities in treatment-naive patients diagnosed with pediatric major depressive disorder. *J Child Adolesc Psychopharmacol* **18**, 121–31.

Mervaala E, Fohr J, Kononen M, *et al.* 2000. Quantitative MRI of the hippocampus and amygdala in severe depression. *Psychol Med* **30**, 117–25.

Murata T, Kimura H, Omori M, *et al.* 2001. MRI white matter hyperintensities, (1)H-MR spectroscopy and cognitive function in geriatric depression: A comparison of early- and late-onset cases. *Int J Geriatr Psychiatry* **16**, 1129–35.

Murphy C F, Gunning-Dixon F M, Hoptman M J, *et al.* 2007. White-matter integrity predicts stroop performance in patients with geriatric depression. *Biol Psychiatry* **61**, 1007–10.

Naismith S, Hickie I, Ward P B, *et al.* 2002. Caudate nucleus volumes and genetic determinants of homocysteine metabolism in the prediction of psychomotor speed in older persons with depression. *Am J Psychiatry* **159**, 2096–8.

Nebes R D, Reynolds C F, III, Boada F, *et al.* 2002. Longitudinal increase in the volume of white matter hyperintensities in late-onset depression. *Int J Geriatr Psychiatry* **17**, 526–30.

Neumeister A, Wood S, Bonne O, *et al.* 2005. Reduced hippocampal volume in unmedicated, remitted patients with major depression versus control subjects. *Biol Psychiatry* **57**, 935–7.

Nobuhara K, Okugawa G, Minami T, *et al.* 2004. Effects of electroconvulsive therapy on frontal white matter in late-life depression: A diffusion tensor imaging study. *Neuropsychobiology* **50**, 48–53.

Nobuhara K, Okugawa G, Sugimoto T, *et al.* 2006. Frontal white matter anisotropy and symptom severity of late-life depression: A magnetic resonance diffusion tensor imaging study. *J Neurol Neurosurg Psychiatry* **77**, 120–2.

O'Brien J, Ames D, Chiu E, Schweitzer I, Desmond P and Tress B. 1998. Severe deep white matter lesions and outcome in elderly patients with major depressive disorder: Follow up study. *BMJ* **317**, 982–4.

O'Brien T J, Lloyd A, McKeith I, Gholkar A and Ferrier N. 2004. A longitudinal study of hippocampal volume, cortisol levels, and cognition in older depressed subjects. *Am J Psychiatry* **161**, 2081–90.

Parashos I A, Tupler L A, Blitchington T and Krishnan K R. 1998. Magnetic-resonance morphometry in patients with major depression. *Psychiatry Res* **84**, 7–15.

Pillay S S, Renshaw P F, Bonello C M, Lafer B C, Fava M and Yurgelun-Todd D. 1998. A quantitative magnetic resonance imaging study of caudate and lenticular nucleus gray matter volume in primary unipolar major depression: Relationship to treatment response and clinical severity. *Psychiatry Res* **84**, 61–74.

Pillay S S, Yurgelun-Todd D A, Bonello C M, Lafer B, Fava M and Renshaw P F. 1997. A quantitative magnetic resonance imaging study of cerebral and cerebellar gray matter volume in primary unipolar major depression: Relationship to treatment response and clinical severity. *Biol Psychiatry* **42**, 79–84.

Pompili M, Innamorati M, Mann J J, *et al.* 2008. Periventricular white matter hyperintensities as predictors of suicide attempts in bipolar disorders and unipolar depression. *Prog Neuropsychopharmacol Biol Psychiatry* **32**, 1501–07.

Posener J A, Wang L, Price J L, *et al.* 2003. High-dimensional mapping of the hippocampus in depression. *Am J Psychiatry* **160**, 83–9.

Rabins P V, Pearlson G D, Aylward E, Kumar A J and Dowell K. 1991. Cortical magnetic resonance imaging changes in elderly inpatients with major depression. *Am J Psychiatry* **148**, 617–20.

Rosso I M, Cintron C M, Steingard R J, Renshaw P F, Young A D and Yurgelun-Todd D A. 2005. Amygdala and hippocampus volumes in pediatric major depression. *Biol Psychiatry* **57**, 21–6.

Salloway S, Boyle P A, Correia S, *et al.* 2002. The relationship of MRI subcortical hyperintensities to treatment response in a trial of sertraline in geriatric depressed outpatients. *Am J Geriatr Psychiatry* **10**, 107–11.

Salloway S, Malloy P, Kohn R, *et al.* 1996. MRI and neuropsychological differences in early and late-onset geriatric depression. *Neurology* **46**, 1567–74.

Sheline Y I, Gado M H and Kraemer H C. 2003. Untreated depression and hippocampal volume loss. *Am J Psychiatry* **160**, 1516–8.

Sheline Y I, Gado M H and Price J L. 1998. Amygdala core nuclei volumes are decreased in recurrent major depression. *Neuroreport* **9**, 2023–8.

Sheline Y I, Price J L, Vaishnavi S N, *et al.* 2008. Regional white matter hyperintensity burden in automated segmentation distinguishes late-life depressed subjects from comparison subjects matched for vascular risk factors. *Am J Psychiatry* **165**, 524–32.

Sheline Y I, Wang P W, Gado M H, Csernansky J G and Vannier M W. 1996. Hippocampal atrophy in recurrent major depression. *Proc Natl Acad Sci U S A* **93**, 3908–13.

Siegle G J, Konecky R O, Thase M E and Carter C S. 2003. Relationships between amygdala volume and activity during emotional information processing tasks in depressed and never-depressed individuals: An fMRI investigation. *Ann N Y Acad Sci* **985**, 481–4.

Simpson S W, Baldwin R C, Burns A and Jackson A. 2001. Regional cerebral volume measurements in late-life depression: Relationship to clinical correlates, neuropsychological impairment and response to treatment. *Int J Geriatr Psychiatry* **16**, 469–76.

Simpson S, Baldwin R C, Jackson A and Burns A S. 1998. Is subcortical disease associated with a poor response to antidepressants? Neurological, neuropsychological and neuroradiological findings in late-life depression. *Psychol Med* **28**, 1015–26.

Simpson S W, Jackson A, Baldwin R C and Burns A. 1997. 1997 IPA/Bayer Research Awards in Psychogeriatrics. Subcortical hyperintensities in late-life depression: Acute response to treatment and neuropsychological impairment. *Int Psychogeriatr* **9**, 257–75.

Sonohara K, Kozaki K, Akishita M, *et al.* 2008. White matter lesions as a feature of cognitive impairment, low vitality and other symptoms of geriatric syndrome in the elderly. *Geriatr Gerontol Int* **8**, 93–100.

Steffens D C, Bosworth H B, Provenzale J M and Macfall J R. 2002. Subcortical white matter lesions and functional impairment in geriatric depression. *Depress Anxiety* **15**, 23–8.

Steffens D C, Byrum C E, McQuoid D R, *et al.* 2000. Hippocampal volume in geriatric depression. *Biol Psychiatry* **48**, 301–09.

Steffens D C, Conway C R, Dombeck C B, Wagner H R, Tupler L A and Weiner R D. 2001. Severity of subcortical gray matter hyperintensity predicts ECT response in geriatric depression. *J ECT* **17**, 45–9.

Steffens D C, Potter G G, McQuoid D R, *et al.* 2007. Longitudinal magnetic resonance imaging vascular changes, apolipoprotein E genotype, and development of dementia in the neurocognitive outcomes of depression in the elderly study. *Am J Geriatr Psychiatry* **15**, 839–49.

Steffens D C, Taylor W D, McQuoid D R and Krishnan K R. 2008. Short/long heterozygotes at 5HTTLPR and white matter lesions in geriatric depression. *Int J Geriatr Psychiatry* **23**, 244–8.

Steffens D C, Trost W T, Payne M E, Hybels C F and MacFall J R. 2003. Apolipoprotein E genotype and subcortical vascular lesions in older depressed patients and control subjects. *Biol Psychiatry* **54**, 674–81.

Taylor W D, Kuchibhatla M, Payne M E, *et al.* 2008a. Frontal white matter anisotropy and antidepressant remission in late-life depression. *PLoS ONE* **3**, e3267.

Taylor W D, MacFall J R, Steffens D C, Payne M E, Provenzale J M and Krishnan K R. 2003a. Localization of age-associated white matter hyperintensities in late-life depression. *Prog Neuropsychopharmacol Biol Psychiatry* **27**, 539–44.

Taylor W D, Payne M E, Krishnan K R, *et al.* 2001. Evidence of white matter tract disruption in MRI hyperintensities. *Biol Psychiatry* **50**, 179–83.

Taylor W D, Steffens D C, MacFall J R, *et al.* 2003b. White matter hyperintensity progression and late-life depression outcomes. *Arch Gen Psychiatry* **60**, 1090–6.

Taylor W D, Steffens D C, McQuoid D R, *et al.* 2003c. Smaller orbital frontal cortex volumes associated with functional disability in depressed elders. *Biol Psychiatry* **53**, 144–9.

Taylor W D, Zuchner S, McQuoid D R, *et al.* 2008b. The brain-derived neurotrophic factor VAL66MET polymorphism and cerebral white matter hyperintensities in late-life depression. *Am J Geriatr Psychiatry* **16**, 263–71.

Thomas A J, O'Brien J T, Barber R, McMeekin W and Perry R. 2003. A neuropathological study of periventricular white matter hyperintensities in major depression. *J Affect Disord* **76**, 49–54.

Thomas A J, Perry R, Barber R, Kalaria R N and O'Brien J T. 2002. Pathologies and pathological mechanisms for white matter hyperintensities in depression. *Ann N Y Acad Sci* **977**, 333–9.

Tupler L A, Krishnan K R, McDonald W M, Dombeck C B, D'Souza S and Steffens D C. 2002. Anatomic location and laterality of MRI signal hyperintensities in late-life depression. *J Psychosom Res* **53**, 665–76.

van Eijndhoven P, van Wingen G, van Oijen K, *et al.* 2008. Amygdala volume marks the acute state in the early course of depression. *Biol Psychiatry* **65**, 812–8.

van Waesberghe J H, Kamphorst W, De Groot C J, *et al.* 1999. Axonal loss in multiple sclerosis lesions: Magnetic resonance imaging insights into substrates of disability. *Ann Neurol* **46**, 747–54.

von Gunten A, Fox N C, Cipolotti L and Ron M A, 2000. A volumetric study of hippocampus and amygdala in depressed patients with subjective memory problems. *J Neuropsychiatry Clin Neurosci* **12**, 493–8.

Yang Q, Huang X, Hong N and Yu X. 2007. White matter microstructural abnormalities in late-life depression. *Int Psychogeriatr* **19**, 757–66.

Yuan Y, Zhang Z, Bai F, *et al.* 2007. White matter integrity of the whole brain is disrupted in first-episode remitted geriatric depression. *Neuroreport* **18**, 1845–9.

Zhao Z, Taylor W D, Styner M, Steffens D C, Krishnan K R and Macfall J R. 2008. Hippocampus shape analysis and late-life depression. *PLoS ONE* **3**, e1837.

Zou K, Huang X, Li T, *et al.* 2008. Alterations of white matter integrity in adults with major depressive disorder: A magnetic resonance imaging study. *J Psychiatry Neurosci* **33**, 525–30.

Chapter 10

Functional imaging of major depression

Simon A. Surguladze and Mary L. Phillips

Major depressive disorder (MDD) remains one of the most debilitating psychiatric illnesses worldwide, with an estimated lifetime prevalence of 16% (Kessler *et al.*, 2003). By the year 2020, MDD is predicted to become the second-largest cause of disability after ischemic heart disease, is amongst leading causes of disability-adjusted life years (World Health Organization, 1999), and is associated with lost productivity, physical morbidity, and suicide (Üstün and Chatterji, 2001). Unfortunately, each depressed episode increases the risk for subsequent episodes (Solomon *et al.*, 1997; Mueller *et al.*, 1999). Early identification and diagnosis of MDD is therefore crucial to help target appropriate treatment interventions as early as possible in the illness history for individuals suffering from this debilitating illness.

The recent research agenda for DSM-V has emphasized a need to translate basic and clinical neuroscience research findings into a new classification system for all psychiatric disorders based upon pathophysiologic and etiological processes (Charney and Babich, 2002; Hasler *et al.*, 2004, 2006; Phillips and Frank, 2006). These pathophysiologic processes involve complex relationships between genetic variables, environmental stressors, and abnormalities in neural systems supporting neuropsychological function and behavior, that may be represented as *biomarkers* of a disorder (e.g. Kraemer *et al.*, 2002), and, in turn, be used to help improve diagnostic accuracy of illnesses such as MDD. Examination of the functional integrity of neural systems supporting key cognitive and emotion processing abnormalities that characterize MDD is therefore a first stage toward identifying biomarkers of MDD.

Studies in MDD have been consistent in reporting impaired performance on executive control tasks,

such as tasks involving cognitive flexibility, problem-solving, planning and monitoring (Austin *et al.*, 1992; Veiel, 1997; Dalla *et al.*, 1995; Beats *et al.*, 1996; Moreaud *et al.*, 1996); as well as episodic and declarative memory (for meta-analysis see Zakzanis *et al.*, 1998). Studies have also highlighted negative emotional information processing bias in individuals with MDD. For example, cognitive theories of MDD propose negatively biased associative processing, especially negative self-referent information underlying the dysfunctional assumptions that predispose a person to depression (Beck *et al.*, 1979; Teasdale, 1988). Depressed individuals with MDD are also poor in interpersonal functioning (Libet and Lewinson, 1973; Gotlib and Whiffen, 1989), which may in part be due to faulty appraisal of socially salient stimuli. Studies have demonstrated that depressed individuals with MDD are impaired in recognition of facial expressions of emotion, accompanied by negative reactions to others' emotions (Persad and Polivy, 1993), together with a negative perceptual bias, i.e. recognizing significantly more sadness (Gur *et al.*, 1992; Bouhuys *et al.*, 1999), or less happiness (Suslow *et al.*, 2001; Surguladze *et al.*, 2004) in facial expressions compared with healthy volunteers. There are further reports that the negative attentional bias to facial expressions may persist during remission (Koschack *et al.*, 2003; Bhagwagar *et al.*, 2004), and may be found in first-degree relatives of depressed patients (Masurier *et al.*, 2007). Therefore, it has been suggested that increased sensitivity to recognition of negative facial expressions may represent a familial vulnerability factor for MDD (Masurier *et al.*, 2007).

In this chapter we focus on recent developments in functional neuroimaging that have highlighted functional abnormalities in key neural regions and

Understanding Neuropsychiatric Disorders, ed. M. E. Shenton and B. I. Turetsky. Published by Cambridge University Press.
© Cambridge University Press 2011.

neural systems underlying different executive control and emotional processes that are impaired in MDD. These studies have contributed to a better understanding of the neural mechanisms underlying MDD, and in turn have begun to help identify potential biomarkers of MDD.

We first briefly describe neural systems supporting normal emotion processing and executive control. We then turn to findings from studies that employed functional neuroimaging techniques to examine functional neural abnormalities during rest, executive control and emotional challenge in individuals with MDD during depressed episode. There is, however, a growing consensus that abnormalities that are persistent rather than episodic or state features of a disorder can be more readily used to identify those individuals with the disorder (e.g. Kraemer *et al.*, 1994). We therefore examine the extent to which neuroimaging abnormalities may persist during recovery from depressed episodes in individuals with a history of MDD. We next describe findings from studies that employed pharmacological challenge paradigms to examine the likely neurotransmitter dysfunction underpinning these neural system abnormalities in MDD. We then move to describe new directions in functional neuroimaging of MDD, including functional neuroimaging studies that have examined the nature of functional neuroimaging abnormalities in child and adolescent MDD, functional neuroimaging abnormalities in late-life MDD, and studies that examined the extent to which functional neuroimaging abnormalities are present in healthy individuals at familial risk of developing MDD. We also examine the newer neuroimaging analysis techniques that can be employed in the study of MDD, including functional and resting-state connectivity analyses. We conclude with an integration of the major findings from these studies that have led to the development of neural models of MDD and highlight the key neural system functional abnormalities that may represent potential biomarkers of MDD.

Neural systems for emotion processing and executive control

An increasingly large number of functional neuro-imaging studies implicate a network of predominantly subcortical, anterior limbic regions in processing different emotional stimuli, including dorsal and ventral striatal regions, amygdala, hippocampus and anterior insula (Calder *et al.*, 2001; Hariri *et al.*, 2002; Haxby *et al.*, 2000; Phillips *et al.*, 1997; Sprengelmeyer *et al.*, 1998; Surguladze *et al.*, 2003). While a variety of different emotional stimuli have been used to examine neural activity associated with emotion processing, some of the most commonly used stimuli for this purpose are facial expressions of different positive and negative emotions because of their importance as highly salient social signals of emotional states, the correct recognition of which is crucial for social interaction (Phillips *et al.*, 2003a, 2003b). Other widely employed emotional stimuli include the photographs of emotional and non-emotional pictures from the International Affective Picture System (IAPS; Lang *et al.*, 2001), or emotional words.

The nature of neural systems implicated in emotion regulation remains less well-studied. However, neural systems supporting cognitive control (referring to a combination of planning, working memory, inhibitory control, strategy development, and cognitive flexibility; Stuss and Levine, 2002) have been widely examined, and mapped to a lateral prefrontal cortical system, comprising dorsolateral and ventrolateral prefrontal cortices (DLPFC and VLPFC), important for cognitive and executive function (e.g. Monchi *et al.*, 2001) and the hippocampus, important for memory (Zola-Morgan *et al.*, 1991). We recently developed a neural model of emotion regulation that emphasizes the roles of two major neural systems for emotion regulation that necessarily include cognitive control processes (Phillips *et al.*, 2008). Here, we highlight roles of voluntary and automatic subprocesses supporting emotion regulation. We indicate that voluntary emotion regulation subprocesses include voluntary behavioral control, voluntary attentional control, and voluntary reappraisal of emotional content, that are associated with dorsal and lateral prefrontal cortical regions, including bilateral DLPFC and VLPFC, bilateral dorsomedial prefrontal cortex (MdPFC), and bilateral dorsal anterior cingulate gyrus (ACG). In contrast, we indicate that medial prefrontal cortical regions, including bilateral subgenual ACG, bilateral orbitofrontal cortex (OFC), left rostral ACG, bilateral MdPFC, midline dorsal ACG, and contributing roles of the hippocampus and parahippocampus, are more implicated in the different subprocesses associated with automatic emotion regulation, including automatic behavioral control, automatic attentional control, and automatic cognitive change.

While few studies have specifically focused on examination of neural systems during emotion regulation per se in individuals with MDD, a relatively large number of functional neuroimaging studies have examined neural systems supporting emotion processing and executive control in this population. We next examine findings from these studies and from functional neuroimaging studies that examined functional neural abnormalities during rest, in individuals with MDD. We first focus on studies that examined individuals with MDD during depressed episodes and then describe findings from studies that examined these individuals after treatment and during remission.

Neuroimaging studies of the depressed episode

In this section, we describe findings from studies that employed positron emission tomography (PET) and single photon emission tomography (SPET) to examine abnormalities in metabolism or blood flow during rest.

Studies examining metabolism and blood flow at rest in MDD

A number of PET studies have provided evidence for reduced metabolism in multiple regions within DLPFC and MdPFC prefrontal cortex together with ACG in MDD during depressed episodes (Baxter et al., 1985, 1989; Biver et al., 1994; Martinot et al., 1990). Furthermore, metabolism in the ACG has been found to negatively correlate with the severity of depression (Kimbrell et al., 2002). Reduced activity in DLPFC during rest during depressed episodes in MDD has also been replicated in a more recent SPET study (Gonul et al., 2004).

Other studies have implicated medial prefrontal cortex and ACG in depressed episode in MDD. One study reported reduced resting state glucose metabolism in subgenual ACG (Drevets et al., 1997). Subsequent studies, however, accounted for the reduction of gray matter volume in this structure in individuals with MDD, and then demonstrated increased rather than decreased metabolism in subgenual ACG in depressed individuals with MDD (Drevets, 1999). Another study demonstrated that metabolism in rostral anterior cingulate gyrus predicted treatment response in depressed subjects, whereas hypometabolism in this

area predicted poor response to antidepressant treatment; treatment responders had hypermetabolism (Mayberg et al., 1997). A further study demonstrated increased resting blood flow in medial hippocampus, cerebellum, anterior cingulate gyrus, and striatum, and a positive correlation between blood flow in hippocampus and depression severity in female participants, whereas this correlation was reversed in males (Videbech et al., 2002).

Regarding subcortical limbic regions, such as the amygdala, a PET study of patients with familial MDD (Drevets et al., 1992) showed increased resting state blood flow in left amygdala, in addition to left VLPFC, relative to healthy individuals. Other resting-state studies have shown positive correlations between amygdala metabolism, and between amygdala blood flow, and depression severity (Drevets et al., 1992; Abercrombie et al., 1998), and even increased amygdala metabolism in depressed individuals with MDD during sleep (Nofzinger et al., 1999). Subsequent research also demonstrated increased left amygdala metabolism in unmedicated depressed individuals, although in this study, the elevated amygdala metabolism normalized with treatment (Drevets et al., 2002). A more recent SPET study has also shown an *inverse* correlation between blood flow in amygdala and depression severity (Perico et al., 2005). Thus, the role of resting-state amygdala metabolism in depression warrants further investigation.

We next describe studies that have employed PET and SPET to examine abnormalities in metabolism and blood flow, and studies that employed functional Magnetic Resonance Imaging (fMRI) to measure neural activity, during executive control and emotional challenge paradigms in individuals with MDD during depressed episodes.

Studies employing PET and SPET to examine metabolism and blood flow during executive control paradigms in MDD

These studies have mainly demonstrated abnormally reduced metabolism in depressed MDD individuals in different prefrontal cortical regions implicated in cognitive control processes. Using a Stroop divided attention task, which measures the ability to redirect attention toward one and away from another stimulus feature, an early study (George et al., 1997) found decreased blood flow in anterior cingulate gyrus, although increased blood flow in dorsolateral prefrontal cortex, in depressed MDD individuals. Another study, using the Tower of London task, a well-validated task measuring planning and working memory (Elliott *et al.*, 1997) demonstrated attenuation of prefrontal cortical blood flow, as well as significantly reduced blood flow in anterior cingulate gyrus and striatum. The same paradigm (Elliott *et al.*, 1998) was also used to examine neural blood flow to positive or negative feedback. In this study, depressed MDD individuals failed to show blood flow in neural regions implicated in reward mechanisms – medial caudate and ventromedial orbitofrontal cortex.

A SPET study on verbal fluency (Audenaert *et al.*, 2002), measuring working memory, found blunted blood perfusion in ACC and inferior prefrontal cortex in depressed MDD relative to healthy individuals, that was associated with poorer task performance.

Studies employing fMRI to examine neural activity during executive control paradigms in MDD

Here, we describe findings from studies that employed fMRI to measure blood oxygen level-dependent (BOLD) signal change, an indirect measure of neural activity, in MDD individuals during depressed episodes. Many of these studies, similar to studies employing PET and SPET, demonstrated predominantly abnormal reduction in prefrontal cortical activity during executive control tasks in MDD relative to healthy individuals. In one study, for example (Okada *et al.*, 2003), a verbal fluency task was employed to compare neural activity in depressed MDD versus healthy individuals. MDD produced significantly fewer words and had reduced activity in left DLPFC than healthy individuals. In other studies MDD and healthy individuals were matched on task performance, although MDD had abnormal neural activity during the tasks. For example, one study (Barch *et al.*, 2003) assessed working memory performance with an N-back working memory task. There were no significant differences between MDD and healthy individuals on N-back task performance, but healthy individuals had significantly greater activity in bilateral thalamus, right precentral gyrus, and right parietal cortex, relative to depressed MDD individuals.

More recent studies, however, have demonstrated increased rather than decreased activity in prefrontal cortical regions in depressed MDD individuals relative to healthy individuals during executive control tasks. In one study of medication-free depressed individuals (Walsh *et al.*, 2007), N-back task performance (with increasing memory load from 1-, 2-, 3-back) was associated with *increased* load-response activity in frontal and posterior cortical regions in depressed MDD relative to healthy individuals. Similarly, another study employing an N-back task (Matsuo *et al.*, 2007) found in unmedicated depressed MDD individuals significantly increased left DLPFC activity during performance of the 2-back versus 1-back contrast, relative to healthy individuals. Again, in a study employing Tower of London and N-back tasks (Fitzgerald *et al.*, 2008b), although depressed MDD did not differ from healthy individuals on N-back task performance (they did differ on the Tower of London task performance), MDD individuals showed abnormally increased activity in right prefrontal regions during both tasks. Together, these latter studies provide evidence in support of increased rather than reduced recruitment of prefrontal cortical regions by depressed MDD individuals in order to achieve the same or even poorer level of performance as healthy individuals on executive control tasks.

Studies employing fMRI to examine neural activity during emotion challenge paradigms in MDD

The majority of neuroimaging studies examining neural systems supporting emotion processing in depressed MDD individuals have employed fMRI rather than PET and SPET, due to the non-invasive nature and better temporal resolution of fMRI. These studies examining neural responses to emotional stimuli in depressed MDD individuals have provided accumulating evidence for a pattern of significant increases in activity in subcortical limbic regions during processing of (mainly negative) emotional stimuli in depressed MDD versus healthy individuals. For example, one study employing an affective go–no-go task, in which individuals are required to inhibit response to non-salient and attend only to salient emotional words, demonstrated a general attenuation of neural response in ventral portions of ACC to emotional words as well as mood-congruent processing bias in depressed

MDD individuals: an attenuated neural response to happy emotional words and enhanced activity to sad emotional words in rostral anterior cingulate gyrus, medial prefrontal cortex, right anterior temporal cortex, left middle temporal gyrus and bilateral medial frontal gyri (Elliott *et al.*, 2002). Another study (Kumari *et al.*, 2003) of treatment-resistant depressed MDD individuals employed emotional and non-emotional pictures paired with congruent and non-congruent captions to evoke the corresponding affect in participants. Here, increased activity within temporal cortex to negative picture–caption pairs and decreased activity in hippocampus to positive stimuli, and in anterior cingulate regions to both positive and negative stimuli, was demonstrated by depressed MDD relative to healthy individuals.

Studies employing emotional facial expressions have provided compelling evidence for a mood-congruent emotion processing bias in depressed MDD individuals. For example, one study (Lawrence *et al.*, 2004) demonstrated increased activity within parahippocampus/hippocampus to mild sad facial expressions, and increased activity to intense fear facial expressions in dorsomedial prefrontal gyrus in depressed MDD relative to healthy individuals. Another study (Surguladze *et al.*, 2005) demonstrated a dissociation in neural activity to happy and sad facial expressions: healthy individuals demonstrated linear increases in activity in bilateral fusiform gyri and right putamen to expressions of increasing degree of happiness (neutral to mild happy to intense happy facial expressions), while depressed individuals demonstrated linear increases in activity in left putamen, left parahippocampal gyrus/amygdala, and right fusiform gyrus to expressions of increasing degree of sadness – from neutral to mild sad to intense sad facial expressions (Figures 10.1–10.4). Similarly, in other studies, in response to sad faces, depressed MDD individuals demonstrated increased activity in left amygdala, ventral striatum, frontoparietal cortex and decreased activity in prefrontal cortex (Fu *et al.*, 2004).

In further studies (Keedwell *et al.*, 2005b), focussing on examination of neural activity to presentations of happy faces during happy mood induction, depressed MDD individuals showed increased activity within the dorsomedial prefrontal cortex, that positively correlated with severity of anhedonia, while activity within the striatum negatively correlated with

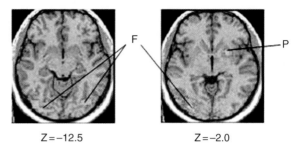

Z=−12.5   Z=−2.0

Figure 10.1 Between-group differences in trends in neural response to happy expressions of increasing intensity of emotion. Two brain slices are depicted at 12.5 and 2 mm below the transcallosal plane, demonstrating significant between-group differences in neural response to expressions of increasing intensity of happiness. Increases in neural response were demonstrated in healthy individuals within right and left fusiform gyri (BA 19) and the right putamen, but decreases in these regions were demonstrated in depressed individuals. The right and the left sides of each brain slice are displayed on the right and left sides of each image, respectively. P, putamen; F, fusiform gyrus; BA, Brodmann area. From Surguladze *et al.* (2005). Copyright 2009, with kind permission from Elsevier Ltd.

anhedonia severity. Another study examined neural activity to positive, negative and neutral words in depressed MDD and healthy individuals (Epstein *et al.*, 2006), and demonstrated abnormally reduced activity in bilateral ventral striatum to positive stimuli, that was associated with decreased interest/pleasure measures. Additionally, one study (Siegle *et al.*, 2002) demonstrated sustained amygdala activity to negatively valenced words which was replicated in a later study (Siegle *et al.*, 2007). One study that specifically examined neural activity during performance of a reward task in depressed MDD individuals (Knutson *et al.*, 2008) showed that although MDD individuals did not differ from healthy individuals in ventral striatal activity, they showed increased dorsal ACG activity during anticipation of gains, suggestive of increased conflict, in addition to showing reduced discrimination of gain versus non-gain outcomes. Together, these findings indicate patterns of abnormal activity in neural regions implicated in emotion and reward processing, and, specifically, increasingly consistent evidence for a mood-congruent emotion processing bias: reduced activity to positive, and increased activity to negative, emotional stimuli in amygdala and striatal regions, in depressed MDD individuals.

We next turn to neuroimaging studies that examined neural activity in MDD individuals after treatment and during remission.

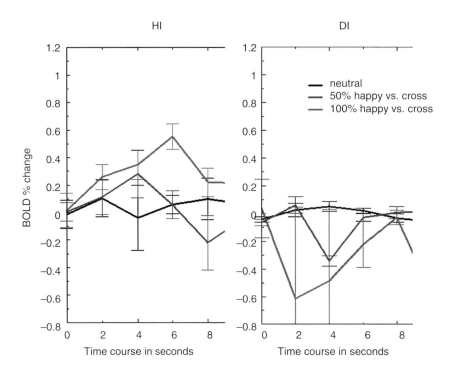

Figure 10.2 Time series of percent change in blood oxygenation level-dependent (BOLD) signal to neutral and both intensities of happy expression in the right fusiform gyrus. The figure represents the time course of BOLD signal change in right fusiform gyrus – average for 16 depressed (DI) and 14 healthy (HI) individuals. From Surguladze *et al.* (2005). Copyright 2009, with kind permission from Elsevier Ltd.

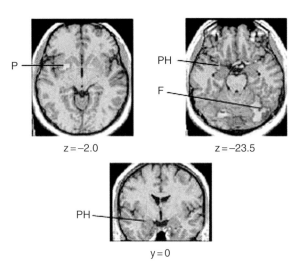

Figure 10.3 Between-group differences in trends in neural response to sad expressions of increasing intensity of emotion. Two brain slices depicted at 2 and 23.5 mm below the transcallosal plane and the slice in coronal plane (*y* = 0) demonstrate significant between-group differences in neural response to expressions of increasing intensity of sadness. Decreases in neural response were demonstrated in healthy individuals within the right fusiform gyrus (BA 37), left parahippocampal/amygdalar region, and left putamen, but increases within these regions were demonstrated in depressed individuals. The right and the left sides of each brain slice are displayed on the right and left sides of each image, respectively. P, putamen; PH, parahippocampal/amygdalar region; F, fusiform gyrus; BA, Brodmann area. From Surguladze *et al.* (2005). Copyright 2009, with kind permission from Elsevier Ltd.

Studies examining changes in neural activity after treatment and recovery from depressed episode in MDD

Here, we describe findings from studies employing PET, SPET and fMRI to examine neural activity in MDD individuals after treatment, and in remitted individuals with a history of MDD.

Successful treatment has been found to reverse patterns of abnormal neural activity in MDD individuals. For example, studies have provided evidence of an imbalance in limbic–cortical pathways in depressed individuals with MDD, and showed reduced blood flow in DLPFC and increased blood flow in rostral ACG that reversed during remission (Mayberg *et al.*, 1999, 2005). Similarly, in an fMRI study (Sheline *et al.*, 2001), abnormally elevated activity within the amygdala to masked fearful facial expressions reduced with antidepressant treatment. Another study (Davidson *et al.*, 2003) demonstrated an effect of treatment in a study employing emotionally negative, positive and neutral stimuli from the IAPS. At baseline, depressed MDD individuals showed reduced activity in left insula and left ACG relative to healthy individuals. After treatment with venlafaxine, the pattern of reduced activity in insula and ACC reversed.

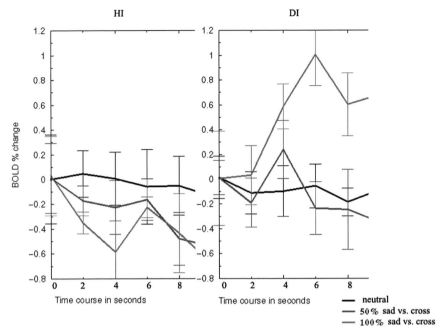

Figure 10.4 Time series of percent change in blood oxygenation level-dependent (BOLD) signal to neutral and both intensities of sad expression in the left parahippocampal/amygdalar region. The figure represents the time course of BOLD signal change in left parahippocampus/amygdala – average for 16 depressed and 14 healthy individuals. HI, healthy individuals; DI, depressed individuals. From Surguladze *et al.* (2005). Copyright 2009, with kind permission from Elsevier Ltd.

Furthermore, depressed MDD individuals with greater ACC activity at baseline to negative versus neutral stimuli showed the most robust treatment response. This finding replicated an earlier report showing that greater pregenual ACC activity at baseline predicted better response to antidepressant treatment in depressed MDD individuals (Mayberg *et al.*, 1997).

Studies employing facial expressions have also shown an amelioration of baseline patterns of abnormal activity after antidepressant (selective serotonin reuptake inhibitor, SSRI) treatment. Here, in response to happy faces (Fu *et al.*, 2007), depressed MDD individuals demonstrated attenuated extrastriate cortical activity that subsequently increased following antidepressant treatment, while symptomatic improvement was associated with greater overall capacity in the hippocampal and extrastriate regions. In contrast, abnormal patterns of increased activity in subcortical and frontal cortical regions to sad facial expression normalized after SSRI treatment in these depressed MDD individuals (Fu *et al.*, 2004). Similarly, in a recent study, subgenual cingulate and extrastriate cortical activity to sad facial expressions was reduced, while extrastriate activity to happy facial expression increased, after antidepressant treatment (Keedwell *et al.*, 2009). Interestingly, in one study (Canli *et al.*, 2005), amygdala activity to either positive or negative facial expressions predicted illness outcome: greater activity in amygdala at baseline predicted lower depression score 8 months later. Recent research on functional connectivity sheds more light on cortico-striatal relationships associated with the treatment response: in a study measuring BOLD response to sad facial expressions, Chen *et al.* (2008) demonstrated treatment-related increased coupling of BOLD response between left amygdala and right middle prefrontal cortex, inferior frontal gyrus, pregenual anterior cingulate, anterior mid cingulate, insula, thalamus, caudate, and putamen. This is in line with the connectivity studies based on resting state low-frequency BOLD-weighted temporal fluctuations (LFBF) described below (Anand *et al.*, 2007).

Studies involving *psychological treatment* have also demonstrated changes in neural activity following remission. Thus, in a PET study employing either paroxetine treatment or interpersonal therapy showed that the decrease in Hamilton depression rating scale was associated in both treatment groups with decreases in normalized PFC and left ACG metabolism, and increases in normalized left temporal lobe metabolism (Brody *et al.*, 2001). A SPET study (Martin *et al.*, 2001) analogously used interpersonal therapy vs. venlafaxine and found that both treatments demonstrated increased basal ganglia blood flow, although there were differences as well: in addition to basal ganglia, clinical improvement in venlafaxine group was associated with right posterior temporal activation, while the IPT group had limbic right posterior cingulate activation.

Broad replication of these results has been reported in a study of CBT vs. venlafaxine (Kennedy *et al.*, 2007). This study showed that response to either treatment modality was associated with decreased glucose metabolism bilaterally in the orbitofrontal cortex and left medial prefrontal cortex, along with increased metabolism in the right occipital-temporal cortex. Changes in metabolism in the anterior and posterior parts of the subgenual cingulate cortex and the caudate differentiated CBT and venlafaxine responders.

A more recent fMRI study examining the effect of CBT showed that pretreatment, MDD individuals had elevated amygdala-hippocampal activity to sad faces, that normalized following 16 sessions of CBT (Fu *et al.*, 2008b). Interestingly, baseline dorsal anterior cingulate activity in depressed MDD individuals showed a significant relationship with subsequent clinical response. Another study demonstrated that more sustained amygdala activity to negative emotional words was associated with better response to CBT in depressed MDD individuals (Siegle *et al.*, 2006).

Regarding neuroimaging studies of remitted individuals with a history of MDD, findings indicate some similarity in neural activity between depressed and remitted individuals with MDD that would indicate persistent abnormalities in neural activity in MDD. For example, one study demonstrated that left amygdala metabolism did not differ between individuals in depressed episode and in remission (Drevets *et al.*, 1992) that motivated the authors to suggest that elevated metabolism in left amygdala may be a trait biomarker in individuals vulnerable to MDD. In a PET study using sad mood induction in remitted MDD, acutely depressed MDD and healthy individuals (Liotti *et al.*, 2002), regional cerebral blood flow (rCBF) in remitted MDD individuals mirrored that of acutely depressed MDD individuals: rCBF was abnormally decreased in medial orbitofrontal cortex in both MDD groups, but unchanged in healthy individuals. In addition, the sad mood provocation paradigm was associated with a pattern of reduced rCBF in pregenual anterior cingulate gyrus that was unique to remitted MDD individuals. The authors proposed that these findings indicated a pattern of rCBF that conferred vulnerability to MDD.

Together, these studies provide converging findings indicating an amelioration of abnormal patterns of pretreatment, baseline neural activity in depressed MDD individuals after pharmacologic and psychological treatments. They also suggest that baseline activity in rostral ACG and amygdala may serve to predict subsequent response to treatment in this population. They also indicate shared patterns of abnormal rCBF in depressed and remitted MDD individuals in amygdala and orbitofrontal cortex at rest and during emotion challenge, which may represent vulnerability to MDD.

It is known that despite progress in pharmacotherapy and advances in psychotherapeutic approaches, up to 20% of patients with major depression fail to respond to traditional methods of therapy, and must undergo treatment with multiple agents and/or electroconvulsive therapy (Fava, 2003). One of the methods offering a promise in managing treatment-resistant depression (TRD) is deep brain stimulation (DBS) – a procedure that involves the direct implantation of stimulation electrodes in localized brain regions with the aim of modifying local and connected brain activity through ongoing, usually high-frequency, stimulation. Although DBS is an invasive procedure with potentially serious side effects, it has advantages over other psychosurgical methods since the implants are minimally destructive of brain tissue (for a review see Fitzgerald, 2008). The pioneering study of 6 patients with TRD (Mayberg *et al.*, 2005) and a subsequent study involving an additional 14 patients (Lozano *et al.*, 2008) reported the results of chronic DBS of subgenual cingulate white matter bilaterally. The stimulation site was chosen according to findings (Mayberg *et al.*, 1999) of involvement of the subgenual cingulate in both acute sadness and antidepressant treatment effects. The results showed that at 12 months from the start of DBS, 55% of patients were responders (50% reduction of Hamilton Rating Scale for Depression, HRSD-17) and 35% achieved or were within 1 point of remission (scoring 8 or less on the HRSD-17 scale).

The effects of DBS on brain functioning were explored with neuroimaging techniques. Whereas the original PET regional blood flow study (Mayberg et al., 2005) showed a decrease in blood flow in the subgenual cingulate gyrus, the subsequent ^{18}F-fluorodeoxyglucose PET study (Lozano et al., 2008) found focal increases in metabolism in the immediate vicinity of the stimulating electrode with decreases in metabolism in the adjacent caudal subcallosal gray matter. Apart from these local changes DBS produced decreases in metabolism in orbital, medial frontal cortex and insula and increases in lateral prefrontal, parietal, mid- and posterior cingulate cortices. The authors hypothesized that DBS disrupted pathological activity in the circuits underlying depression which helped to normalize cerebral function. Another study employing DBS (Schlaepfer et al., 2008) targeted the nucleus accumbens based on the evidence of dysfunction of reward system in depression. One-week stimulation in 3 patients showed a decrease in depression scores (HRSD-24) as well as changes in glucose metabolism in the cortical–limbic networks (measured by PET): increases in metabolism were observed in the nucleus accumbens, amygdala, dorsolateral, and dorsomedial prefrontal cortices; decreases in metabolism were observed in medial prefrontal cortex and caudate.

We next examine findings from neuroimaging studies that employed pharmacologic challenge paradigms to examine the extent to which dysfunction in neural systems implicated in executive control and emotion processing may be associated with deficits in specific neurotransmitters.

Neuroimaging studies combined with pharmacologic challenge paradigms

There is ample evidence that MDD is associated with decreased serotonin metabolism (for review see Booij et al., 2002). Acute tryptophan depletion (ATD) experiments have been shown to induce depressive symptoms in individuals at risk for depression or remitted individuals with a history of MDD, thereby revealing a trait abnormality associated with MDD. In combination with neuroimaging, ATD therefore provides an opportunity to study the neural correlates of this trait abnormality. A PET study examining regional cerebral glucose utilization (rCMRGlu) demonstrated that ATD in individuals with a history of MDD induced a relapse of depression, which was associated with increased glucose utilization in orbitofrontal cortex, medial thalamus, anterior and posterior cingulate cortices, and ventral striatum (Neumeister et al., 2004). These results provide experimental support for previous studies that implicated the above prefrontal cortico-striatal neural systems in MDD and highlight that abnormalities in these neural systems may represent trait-like, vulnerability markers of MDD.

Other studies examined the potential role of other neurotransmitters in MDD. In an fMRI study, oral dextroamphetamine sulphate was administered to stimulate dopaminergic reward systems (Tremblay et al., 2005). Individuals with MDD experienced hypersensitivity to the rewarding effects of dextroamphetamine, although activity was reduced in reward processing neural regions such as orbitofrontal cortex, caudate and putamen. These findings were interpreted as evidence for deficient dopamine-mediated reward processing in MDD. A recent PET fluorodeoxyglucose study (Hasler et al., 2008) employed a catecholamine depletion (CD) paradigm. Glucose metabolism was increased in remitted MDD subjects, but decreased or remained unchanged in healthy individuals in ventromedial frontal polar cortex, midcingulate and subgenual ACG, temporopolar cortex, ventral striatum, and thalamus – regions comprising a limbic–cortical–striatal–pallidal–thalamic network implicated in MDD. Metabolic changes induced by CD in the left ventromedial frontal polar cortex correlated positively with depressive symptoms, whereas changes in the anteroventral striatum were correlated with anhedonic symptoms. Thus, the study highlighted the close association between decreased catecholaminergic neurotransmission, depression and elevated activity in limbic–cortical–striatal–pallidal–thalamic neural system.

Together, these findings indicate that abnormalities in serotonergic and catecholaminergic transmission may together underlie the dysfunction in prefrontal cortical and subcortical limbic neural systems supporting executive control and emotion processing that have been increasingly reported in depressed – and even remitted – individuals with a history of MDD.

We now turn to the emerging studies focusing on examination of neural systems supporting executive control and emotion processing in child and adolescent and in late-life MDD, providing a lifespan perspective to neuroimaging studies of the illness.

Child and adolescent MDD

There have been few neuroimaging studies of child and adolescent MDD. PET and SPET are considered inappropriate for use with children and adolescents because they require exposure to radiation. Therefore, studies to date have employed fMRI. One study (Thomas *et al.*, 2001) reported a blunted amygdala response to fearful facial expressions in children with depression, and exaggerated response in children with anxiety. In contrast, another, larger study (Roberson-Nay *et al.*, 2006) found elevated amygdala activity in adolescents with MDD during incidental memory encoding of faces.

Exploring the functioning of reward-related systems in children and adolescents with MDD, another study (Forbes *et al.*, 2006) reported blunted activity in ACC, bilateral caudate, and inferior orbito-frontal cortex bilaterally during both anticipation and outcome phases of reward processing, together with increased amygdala activity in the outcome phase. These findings were interpreted as indicating a generally diminished responsiveness to reward in childhood onset MDD.

This small number of studies in child and adolescent MDD provides parallel findings to those in adult MDD, namely, reduced activity in emotion and reward processing neural regions during positive emotion and reward processing paradigms, although to date findings have been less consistent regarding the role of the amygdala in response to negative emotional stimuli. Clearly, further studies examining neural activity during emotion processing and cognitive control are needed in this vulnerable population of children and adolescents with MDD.

Functional neuroimaging studies of MDD in late-life depression

Late-life depression (LLD) has been variably defined as depression that starts between 50 and 65 years of life (for a review, see Vaishnavi and Taylor, 2006). LLD is often under-recognized, and there is surprisingly little research on neural abnormalities accompanying this condition. One of the reasons for this lack of research is a high heterogeneity of this sample with regard to psychiatric and general medical comorbidity, which complicates the examination of the mood disorder itself. Therefore, researchers need to take into account any age-related changes in brain structure and function, e.g. the selective aging in prefrontal cortex (Raz *et al.*, 1997). On the other hand, there may be abnormalities in neural systems that are specific to LLD. For example, there are indications of high rates of "silent strokes" in individuals with LLD that support a "vascular depression" hypothesis for the illness (Alexopoulos *et al.*, 1997). The age-related specificity of brain abnormalities in LLD is further supported by findings of significantly more deep white matter hyperintensities and periventricular hyperintensities in individuals with the first onset of major depression over age 50 years compared with those individuals with earlier age of onset (Hickie *et al.*, 1995; Salloway *et al.*, 1996). Recent volumetric studies have been able to detect subtler abnormalities in cerebral cortex in patients with LLD, e.g. bilateral gray matter and white matter volume reductions in the anterior cingulate gyrus and medial orbitofrontal cortex (Ballmaier *et al.*, 2004).

We focus here on the limited number of functional neuroimaging studies that have examined relatively homogenous samples of elderly individuals with MDD. These studies point to several characteristics of LLD that are analogous to mid-life MDD, as well as to some features that might be specific for LLD.

Resting state SPET studies showed reductions in temporal lobe perfusion in individuals with LLD compared with early-life depressed MDD and healthy individuals (Ebmeier *et al.*, 1998). Another well-documented finding is prefrontal hypoperfusion (Navarro *et al.*, 2004), accompanied by striatal hyperperfusion (Alexopoulos, 2002). Importantly, perfusion deficits in "vascular depression" may persist even after remission, when compared with non-late-life MDD individuals in remission (Kimura *et al.*, 2003).

Functional MRI studies have examined neural activity associated with performance of executive control and emotion processing in LLD, similar to the studies in younger individuals. One study on sequence learning (Aizenstein *et al.*, 2005) showed that depressed LDD individuals relative to healthy, age-matched individuals showed diminished activity in dorsolateral PFC bilaterally and increased activity in right caudate and putamen, supporting the fronto-striatal dysfunction hypothesis. A study examining neural systems supporting emotion processing in individuals with LLD (Brassen *et al.*, 2008) demonstrated that these individuals showed decreased activity to negative compared with positive word stimuli in ventromedial prefrontal cortex. This finding was consistent with findings from a previous study of mid-life MDD (Keedwell *et al.*, 2005a), and also correlated with the severity of depression and resolved following clinical improvement.

These findings therefore suggest that LLD, like mid-life adult MDD and child and adolescent MDD, is associated with a dissociation between functional abnormalities in neural systems supporting positive and negative emotion processing, and, like mid-life MDD, may also be associated with decreased activity in prefrontal cortical regions subserving executive control. Further neuroimaging studies are needed in this population.

We next describe findings from the very small number of neuroimaging studies that have examined neural activity in individuals at familial risk of MDD.

Individuals at familial risk of MDD

There have been few reports on neuroimaging studies of people at risk for depression.

One study of young offspring of individuals with a history of MDD (Mannie *et al.*, 2008) showed that in an emotional word-counting Stroop task, adults at familial risk of MDD had less activity in the affective subdivision of the ACC, compared with healthy individuals with no familial risk of MDD. This was partially explained by the lack of difference between neural activity in this region to neutral and emotional words in individuals at risk. This finding was consistent with findings of an earlier study (Elliott *et al.*, 2002) that showed a general attenuation of ACC response to emotional words in depressed individuals with MDD.

There is also evidence concurrent with the findings of abnormal activity of amygdala in adult MDD. In another recent study (Monk *et al.*, 2008), high-risk child and adolescent offspring of parents with MDD demonstrated greater amygdala and ventral striatal (NAcc) activity to fearful faces and lower NAcc activity to happy faces. These findings provide evidence that the previously observed dissociation between amygdala and striatal activity to happy and sad emotional facial expressions in depressed individuals with MDD may also represent a vulnerability marker for MDD in familial at-risk but otherwise healthy individuals.

These preliminary findings in individuals at familial at risk of developing MDD suggest converging patterns of abnormality in neural systems supporting

emotion processing in depressed individuals with MDD and those individuals at risk for the illness. This is an exciting area of research and further studies in this field will have the potential to yield important findings that will ultimately help to identify biomarkers of MDD.

Novel neuroimaging techniques in MDD

New methods are now emerging in fMRI studies to examine resting state-related neural activity, measuring the correlation of low-frequency BOLD-weighted temporal fluctuations (LFBF) in steady-state fMRI data as a measure of connectivity between different neural regions (Biswal *et al.*, 1995). One study (Anand *et al.*, 2005a) found that, in a standard task exposing subjects to emotional pictures, depressed MDD individuals showed increased activity in amygdala, striatum, insula, ACG and anteromedial prefrontal cortex, but *decreased* resting state LFBF correlations between cortical and limbic sites compared with healthy individuals. In a subsequent study the authors examined an effect of 6-weeks treatment with an SSRI antidepressant sertraline (Anand *et al.*, 2005b). The LFBF-based connectivity in this study was measured during the presentation of emotionally positive, negative and neutral pictures from IAPS. The results demonstrated that the treatment was associated with the increased connectivity during processing of pleasant and neutral but not negative pictures. A more recent study by the same group (Anand *et al.*, 2007), employing both the activation task to emotionally negative pictures and the resting state LFBF as a measure of connectivity, demonstrated a decrease in previously elevated subcortical limbic activity to negative emotional pictures that was paralleled by an *increase* in LFBF connectivity between pregenual ACC and these subcortical limbic regions. A recent report (Greicius *et al.*, 2007) has shown that resting-state connectivity within a brain "default network", including medial prefrontal cortex and postcingulate gyrus, and that may be implicated in self-referential processing, is increased in depressed MDD individuals.

Another novel technique is a method to examine regional homogeneity (ReHo; Zang *et al.*, 2004). This method is based on measuring the similarity of time series of a given voxel to those of its nearest voxels, and eventually reflecting the temporal homogeneity of regional BOLD signal, which can reflect the temporal homogeneity of neural activity. One study (Yao *et al.*, 2008) found a diffuse ReHo decrease in depressed individuals with MDD during resting state, which was mainly distributed over frontal cortices, subcortical limbic regions and basal ganglia. Importantly, correlational analysis with Hamilton Depression rating score for depression severity showed that several dimensions of depression were significantly and positively associated with ReHo in various limbic and cortical regions, e.g. the severity of hopelessness correlated with ReHo in right ventral anterior cingulate gyrus. This was consistent with previous studies that implicated functional abnormalities in subgenual cingulate cortex in depressed MDD individuals (Drevets *et al.*, 1997).

One new analytical approach to fMRI data utilizes a support vector machine pattern classification method that allows quantification of brain activity patterns in terms of sensitivity and specificity to depression (Fu *et al.*, 2008a). Thus, in a sad facial emotional expression processing task, 84% sensitivity and 89% specificity was achieved in discriminating between depressed MDD and healthy individuals, corresponding to an accuracy of 86% ($p < 0.0001$). This pattern classification method of fMRI data therefore provides for a highly valid test, comparable to other clinical procedures, and may potentially be used for diagnostic purposes. For example, electrocardiogram (ECG) treadmill testing of risk of cardiac disease has a sensitivity of only 67% and specificity of 70%.

Toward a neural model of MDD

The above findings have allowed the development of neural models of MDD that can be used as frameworks for examining in greater detail function within neural systems supporting different executive control and emotion processes to further facilitate identification of biomarkers of the illness. One model (Mayberg, 1997; Mayberg *et al.*, 1999, 2005) proposed an imbalance in limbic–cortical pathways with reduced activity in dorsal lateral prefrontal cortex and increased activity in subgenual anterior cingulate gyrus, which reverses in remitted states.

This is broadly supported by another model (Phillips *et al.*, 2003b) that postulated increased activity within regions important for the identification

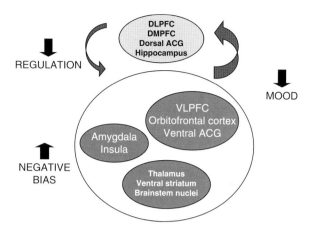

Figure 10.5 Schematic model for the neural basis of the observed deficits in emotion perception and behavior, and the relationship between these and the symptoms of patients with major depression. Volume reductions within the amygdala and other components of the ventral neural system (depicted in dark gray), together with increased rather than decreased activity within these regions during illness, may result in a restricted emotional range, biased toward the predominant role of the amygdala in the perception of negative rather than positive emotions. Structural and functional impairments within regions of the dorsal system (depicted in pale gray), associated with impairments in executive function and effortful regulation of emotional behavior (reduced size of the curved arrow representing the regulation of the ventral by the dorsal system), may perpetuate these phenomena, resulting in depressed mood and anhedonia. DLPFC, dorsolateral prefrontal cortex; DMPFC, dorsomedial prefrontal cortex; ACG, anterior cingulate gyrus; VLPFC, ventrolateral prefrontal cortex. From Phillips *et al.* (2003b). Copyright 2009, with kind permission from Elsevier Ltd.

of emotional stimuli and generation of emotional behavior, including the subgenual cingulate gyrus, ventrolateral prefrontal cortex, amygdala, anterior insula, ventral striatum, and thalamus, and decreased activity within regions implicated in the effortful regulation of emotional behavior, including dorsomedial and dorsolateral prefrontal cortices (Figure 10.5).

Similarly, Drevets and colleagues (1992, 1997, 2008) have proposed that the pattern of brain metabolic abnormalities in depression is characterized by increased glucose metabolism in regions of dorsal and ventromedial prefrontal, frontal polar cortices, pre- and subgenual ACC, posterior cingulate, hippocampus, amygdala and parahippocampal gyrus, ventromedial striatum, and medial thalamus. The metabolism in these regions is normalized with remission.

Recent studies provide evidence for involvement of "default mode network" malfunctioning in depression. This network includes regions of ventromedial prefrontal cortex, posterior cingulate gyrus and inferolateral parietal cortices. Anterior parts of this network are implicated in self-referential processing (Gusnard et al., 2001), and tend to deactivate during performance of cognitive tasks, as cognitive resources are redirected (Raichle et al., 2001; McKiernan et al., 2003). The normal decrease in VMPFC activation during demanding tasks may indicate intact emotional gating (Pochon et al., 2002), and conversely, lack of this deactivation may indicate impaired gating – as reported in a study on working memory (N-back) task (Rose et al., 2006). An fMRI study specifically focusing on resting state activity within the default mode network (Greicius et al., 2007) demonstrated that depressed MDD individuals showed *increased* network functional connectivity in the subgenual cingulate gyrus, the thalamus, the orbitofrontal cortex, and the precuneus.

This is in line with the recent conceptualizations. Gotlib and Hamilton (2008) and Drevets et al. (2008) highlight the closeness of the default network to a "visceromotor system" that modulates introspective functions and visceral reactions to emotional stimuli and is overactive during the depressed state of MDD.

A recent meta-analysis (Fitzgerald et al., 2008a) comprising a large number of neuroimaging studies of resting state, emotional activation and effects of treatment, concluded that since there is limited overlap between the areas found across imaging methods, "pathophysiology as potentially identified with these techniques appears complex and not reducible to simple models or understandable with single imaging methods." Amongst the areas strongly supported by the meta-analysis was the network involving dorsal/pregenual anterior cingulate, bilateral middle frontal gyrus (DLPFC), insula and superior temporal gyrus. This network was characterized by reduced activity in resting state, which normalized with treatment, and relative lack of activation in response to emotionally negative stimuli. Another network, comprising cortico-subcortical limbic structures of medial and inferior frontal cortex, basal ganglia (caudate or putamen) and (less consistently) amygdala and thalamus has been found to be hyperactive in the depressed state and hyper-responsive to both negative and positive stimuli which then normalized following treatment. The meta-analysis did not find either over- or under-activity in subgenual ACC cortex, but demonstrated a reduction in its activity with SSRI antidepressant treatment.

Summary and conclusion

We have described findings from a wide range of different functional neuroimaging studies that have provided converging findings that have contributed to a better understanding of the neural mechanisms underlying MDD, and in turn may begin to help identify potential biomarkers of MDD. There is now increasingly compelling evidence that MDD is associated with dysfunction within different neural systems during rest, during executive control and during emotion processing. Findings from these studies indicate that patterns of increased activity within and functional connectivity between different components of neural systems implicated in emotion and reward processing, and most consistently to negative emotional stimuli, characterize the depressed episode of MDD. Conversely, decreased connectivity between different prefrontal cortical regions implicated in executive control, although inconsistent findings of both decreases and increases in activity within these regions during performance of such tasks are evident in depressed individuals with MDD. These abnormalities ameliorate in part with successful treatment for MDD, although some findings suggest residual abnormalities in these neural systems in remitted individuals with MDD. Abnormalities in both serotonergic and catecholaminergic neurotransmitter systems may underlie the patterns of dysfunction observed macroscopically in MDD. Emerging findings from the relatively small number of studies that have examined activity in these neural systems in children and adolescent with MDD, and in LLD, are beginning to show that similar patterns of dysfunction in these neural systems may characterize MDD at both ends of the lifespan. Furthermore, dysfunction in subcortical limbic regions supporting emotion and reward processing, and in prefrontal cortical regions supporting executive control may also characterize individuals at familial risk of developing MDD. New technologies for investigating connectivity between different regions in these neural systems both at rest and during performance of executive control and emotion processing tasks are promising techniques for more in-depth study of these neural systems, and the extent to which abnormalities in these neural systems may represent illness biomarkers, in MDD.

Box 10.1. Most significant findings of functional neuroimaging studies of major depression

- Depressive episode: resting state
  Reduced metabolism in lateral prefrontal regions
  Increased metabolism in subgenual ACC (especially in treatment responders)
  Increased metabolism in amygdala
- Depressive episode: cognitive tasks
  Increased BOLD signal in dorsolateral prefrontal cortex
- Depressive episode: emotion processing abnormalities that reverse with treatment
  Decreased BOLD signal in ACC and dorsal prefrontal cortex
  Mood-congruent bias of BOLD signal in amygdala, ventral striatum, hippocampus, extrastriate visual cortex
  Reduced connectivity between cortical and limbic structures
- Remitted individuals
  Reduced blood flow in ventral orbitofrontal cortex during sad mood induction
  Increased blood flow in amygdala at rest
- Individuals at familial risk: emotion processing
  Low reactivity of ACC
  Increased amygdala and nucleus accumbens activity to negative signals, decreased nucleus accumbens activity to positive signals
- Children and adolescents with MDD
  Blunted response in orbitofrontal cortex and ACC to reward
  Increased or decreased amygdala to emotional signals
- Late-life depression
  Prefrontal hypoperfusion in resting state
  Reduced prefrontal BOLD signal in cognitive tasks
  Mood-congruent dissociation in ventromedial prefrontal cortex BOLD response to emotional signals, that reverses after treatment

References

Abercrombie H C, Schaefer S M, Larson C L, *et al.* 1998. Metabolic rate in the right amygdala predicts negative affect in depressed patients. *Neuroreport* **9**, 3301–7.

Aizenstein H J, Butters M A, Figurski J L, Stenger V A, Reynolds C F, III and Carter C S. 2005. Prefrontal and striatal activation during sequence learning in geriatric depression. *Biol Psychiatry* **58**, 290–6.

Alexopoulos G S. 2002. Frontostriatal and limbic dysfunction in late-life depression. *Am J Geriatr. Psychiatry* **10**, 687–95.

Alexopoulos G S, Meyers B S, Young R C, Campbell S, Silbersweig D and Charlson M. 1997. "Vascular depression" hypothesis. *Arch Gen Psychiatry* **54**, 915–22.

Anand A, Li Y, Wang Y, *et al.* 2005a. Activity and connectivity of brain mood regulating circuit in depression: A functional magnetic resonance study. *Biol Psychiatry* **57**, 1079–88.

Anand A, Li Y, Wang Y, *et al.* 2005b. Antidepressant effect on connectivity of the mood-regulating circuit: An fMRI study. *Neuropsychopharmacology* **30**, 1334–44.

Anand A, Li Y, Wang Y, Gardner K and Lowe M J. 2007. Reciprocal effects of antidepressant treatment on activity and connectivity of the mood regulating circuit: An fMRI study. *J Neuropsychiatry Clin Neurosci* **19**, 274–82.

Audenaert K, Goethals I, Van Laere K, *et al.* 2002. SPECT neuropsychological activation procedure with the Verbal Fluency Test in attempted suicide patients. *Nucl Med Commun* **23**, 907–16.

Austin M-P, Ross M, Murray C, O'Carroll R E, Ebmeier K P and Goodwin G M. 1992. Cognitive functions in major depression. *J Affect Disord* **25**, 21–30.

Ballmaier M, Toga A W, Blanton R E, *et al.* 2004. Anterior cingulate, gyrus rectus, and orbitofrontal abnormalities in elderly depressed patients: An MRI-based parcellation of the prefrontal cortex. *Am J Psychiatry* **161**, 99–108.

Barch D M, Sheline Y I, Csernansky J G and Snyder A Z. 2003. Working memory and prefrontal cortex dysfunction: Specificity to schizophrenia compared with major depression. *Biol Psychiatry* **53**, 376–84.

Baxter L R, Schwartz J M, Phelps M E, *et al.* 1989. Reduction of prefrontal cortex glucose metabolism common to three types of depression. *Arch Gen Psychiatry* **46**, 243–50.

Baxter L R, Phelps M E, Mazziotta J C, *et al.* 1985. Cerebral metabolic rates for glucose in mood disorders. *Arch Gen Psychiatry* **42**, 441–7.

Beats B C, Sahakian B J and Levy R. 1996. Cognitive performance in tests sensitive to frontal lobe dysfunction in the elderly depressed. *Psychol Med* **26**, 591–603.

Beck A T, Rush A J, Shaw B F and Emery G. 1979. *Cognitive Therapy of Depression.* New York, NY: Guilford.

Bhagwagar Z, Cowen P J, Goodwin G M and Harmer C J. 2004. Normalization of enhanced fear recognition by acute SSRI treatment in subjects with a previous history of depression. *Am J Psychiatry* **161**, 166–8.

Biswal B, Yetkin F Z, Haughton V and Hyde J S. 1995. Functional connectivity in the motor cortex of resting human brain using echo-planar MRI. *Magn Res Med* **34**, 537–41.

Biver F, Goldman S, Delvenne V, *et al.* 1994. Frontal and parietal metabolic disturbances in unipolar depression. *Biol Psychiatry* **36**, 381–8.

Booij L, Van der D W, Benkelfat C, *et al.* 2002. Predictors of mood response to acute tryptophan depletion. A reanalysis. *Neuropsychopharmacology* **27**, 852–61.

Bouhuys A L, Geerts E and Gordijn M C M. 1999. Depressed patients' perceptions of facial emotions in depressed and remitted states are associated with relapse: A longitudinal study. *J Nerv Mental Dis* **187**, 595–602.

Brassen S, Kalisch R, Weber-Fahr W, Braus D F and Buchel C. 2008. Ventromedial prefrontal cortex processing during emotional evaluation in late-life depression: A longitudinal functional magnetic resonance imaging study. *Biol Psychiatry* **64**, 349–55.

Brody A L, Saxena S, Stoessel P, *et al.* 2001. Regional brain metabolic changes in patients with major depression treated with either paroxetine or interpersonal therapy: Preliminary findings. *Arch Gen Psychiatry* **58**, 631–40.

Calder A J, Lawrence A D and Young A W. 2001. Neuropsychology of fear and loathing. *Nat Rev Neurosci* **2**, 352–63.

Canli T, Cooney R E, Goldin P, *et al.* 2005. Amygdala reactivity to emotional faces predicts improvement in major depression. *Neuroreport* **16**, 1267–70.

Charney D S and Babich K S. 2002. Foundation for the NIMH strategic plan for mood disorders research. *Biol Psychiatry* **52**, 455–6.

Chen C H, Suckling J, Ooi C, *et al.* 2008. Functional coupling of the amygdala in depressed patients treated with antidepressant medication. *Neuropsychopharmacology* **33**, 1909–18.

Dalla B G, Parlato V, Iavarone A and Boller F. 1995. Anosognosia, intrusions and "frontal" functions in Alzheimer's disease and depression. *Neuropsychologia* **33**, 247–59.

Davidson R J, Irwin W, Anderle M J and Kalin N H. 2003. The neural substrates of affective processing in depressed patients treated with venlafaxine. *Am J Psychiatry* **160**, 64–75.

Drevets W C. 1999. Prefrontal cortical–amygdalar metabolism in major depression. *Ann N Y Acad Sci* **877**, 614–37.

Drevets W C, Bogers W and Raichle M E. 2002. Functional anatomical correlates of antidepressant drug treatment assessed using PET measures of regional glucose metabolism. *Eur Neuropsychopharmacol* **12**, 527–44.

Drevets W C, Price J L and Furey M L. 2008. Brain structural and functional abnormalities in mood disorders: Implications for neurocircuitry models of depression. *Brain Struct Funct* **213**, 93–118.

Drevets W C, Price J L, Simpson J R, Jr, *et al.* 1997. Subgenual prefrontal cortex abnormalities in mood disorders. *Nature* **386**, 824–7.

Drevets W C, Videen T O, Price J L, Preskorn S H, Carmichael S T and Raichle M E. 1992. A functional anatomical study of unipolar depression. *J Neurosci* **12**, 3628–41.

Ebmeier K P, Glabus M F, Prentice N, Ryman A and Goodwin G M. 1998. A voxel-based analysis of cerebral perfusion in dementia and depression of old age. *Neuroimage* **7**, 199–208.

Elliott R, Baker S C, Rogers R D, *et al.* 1997. Prefrontal dysfunction in depressed patients performing a complex planning task: A study using positron emission tomography. *Psychol Med* **27**, 931–42.

Elliott R, Sahakian B J, Michael A, Paykel E S and Dolan R J. 1998. Abnormal neural response to feedback on planning and guessing tasks in patients with unipolar depression. *Psychol Med* **28**, 559–71.

Elliott R, Rubinsztein J S, Sahakian B J and Dolan R J. 2002. The neural basis of mood-congruent processing biases in depression. *Arch Gen Psychiatry* **59**, 597–604.

Epstein J, Pan H, Kocsis J H, *et al.* 2006. Lack of ventral striatal response to positive stimuli in depressed versus normal subjects. *Am J Psychiatry* **163**, 1784–90.

Fava M. 2003. Diagnosis and definition of treatment-resistant depression. *Biol Psychiatry* **53**, 649–59.

Fitzgerald P. 2008. Brain stimulation techniques for the treatment of depression and other psychiatric disorders. *Austral Psychiatry* **16**, 183–90.

Fitzgerald P B, Laird A R, Maller J and Daskalakis Z J. 2008a. A meta-analytic study of changes in brain activation in depression. *Hum Brain Mapp* **29**, 683–95.

Fitzgerald P B, Srithiran A, Benitez J, *et al.* 2008b. An fMRI study of prefrontal brain activation during multiple tasks in patients with major depressive disorder. *Hum Brain Mapp* **29**, 490–501.

Forbes E E, Christopher M J, Siegle G J, *et al.* 2006. Reward-related decision-making in pediatric major depressive disorder: An fMRI study. *J Child Psychol Psychiatry* **47**, 1031–40.

Fu C H, Mourao-Miranda J, Costafreda S G, *et al.* 2008a. Pattern classification of sad facial processing: Toward the development of neurobiological markers in depression. *Biol Psychiatry* **63**, 656–62.

Fu C H, Williams S C, Cleare A J, *et al.* 2004. Attenuation of the neural response to sad faces in major depression by antidepressant treatment: A prospective, event-related functional magnetic resonance imaging study. *Arch Gen Psychiatry* **61**, 877–89.

Fu C H Y, Williams S C R, Brammer M J, *et al.* 2007. Neural responses to happy facial expressions in major depression following antidepressant treatment. *Am J Psychiatry* **164**, 599–607.

Fu C H Y, Williams S C R, Cleare A J, *et al.* 2008b. Neural responses to sad facial expressions in major depression following cognitive behavioral therapy. *Biol Psychiatry* **64**, 505–12.

George M S, Ketter T A, Parekh P I, Rosinsky N, Ring H A and Pazzaglia P J. 1997. Blunted left cingulate activation in mood disorder subjects during a response interference task (the Stroop). *J Neuropsychiatry Clin Neurosci* **9**, 55–63.

Gonul A S, Kula M, Bilgin A G, Tutus A and Oguz A. 2004. The regional cerebral blood flow changes in major depressive disorder with and without psychotic features. *Prog Neuropsychopharmacol Biol Psychiatry* **28**, 1015–21.

Gotlib I H and Hamilton J P. 2008. Neuroimaging and depression: Current status and unresolved issues. *Curr Dir Psychol Sci* **17**, 159–63.

Gotlib I H and Whiffen V E. 1989. Depression and marital functioning: An examination of specificity of gender differences. *J Abnorm Psychol* **98**, 23–30.

Greicius M D, Flores B H, Menon V, *et al.* 2007. Resting-state functional connectivity in major depression: Abnormally increased contributions from subgenual cingulate cortex and thalamus. *Biol Psychiatry* **62**, 429–37.

Gur R C, Erwin R J, Gur R E, Zwil A S, Heimberg C and Kraemer H C. 1992. Facial emotion discrimination: II. Behavioral findings in depression. *Psychiatry Res* **42**, 241–51.

Gusnard D A, Akbudak E, Shulman G L and Raichle M E. 2001. Medial prefrontal cortex and self-referential mental activity: Relation to a default mode of brain function. *Proc Natl Acad Sci U S A* **98**, 4259–64.

Hariri A R, Tessitore A, Mattay V S, Fera F and Weinberger D R. 2002. The amygdala response to emotional stimuli: A comparison of faces and scenes. *Neuroimage* **17**, 317–23.

Hasler G, Drevets W C, Gould T D, Gottesman I I and Manji H K. 2006. Toward constructing an endophenotype strategy for bipolar disorders. *Biol Psychiatry* **60**, 93–105.

Hasler G, Drevets W C, Manji H K and Charney D S. 2004. Discovering endophenotypes for major depression. *Neuropsychopharmacology* **29**, 1765–81.

Hasler G, Fromm S, Carlson P J, *et al.* 2008. Neural response to catecholamine depletion in unmedicated subjects with major depressive disorder in remission and healthy subjects. *Arch Gen Psychiatry* **65**, 521–31.

Haxby J V, Hoffman E A and Gobbini M I. 2000. The distributed human neural system for face perception. *Trends Cognit Sci* **4**, 223–33.

Hickie I, Scott E, Mitchell P, Wilhelm K, Austin M P and Bennett B. 1995. Subcortical hyperintensities on magnetic resonance imaging: Clinical correlates and prognostic significance in patients with severe depression. *Biol Psychiatry* **37**, 151–60.

Keedwell P, Drapier D, Surguladze S, Giampietro V, Brammer M and Phillips M. 2009. Neural markers of symptomatic improvement during antidepressant therapy in severe depression: subgenual cingulate and visual cortical responses to sad, but not happy, facial stimuli are correlated with changes in symptom score. *J Psychopharmacol* **23**, 775–88.

Keedwell P A, Andrew C, Williams S C, Brammer M J and Phillips M L. 2005a. A double dissociation of ventromedial prefrontal cortical responses to sad and happy stimuli in depressed and healthy individuals. *Biol Psychiatry* **58**, 495–503.

Keedwell P A, Andrew C, Williams S C, Brammer M J and Phillips M L. 2005b. The neural correlates of anhedonia in major depressive disorder. *Biol Psychiatry* **58**, 843–53.

Kennedy S H, Konarski J Z, Segal Z V, *et al.* 2007. Differences in brain glucose metabolism between responders to CBT and venlafaxine in a 16-week randomized controlled trial. *Am J Psychiatry* **164**, 778–88.

Kessler R C, Berglund P, Demler O, *et al.* 2003. The epidemiology of major depressive disorder: Results from the National Comorbidity Survey Replication (NCS-R). *JAMA* **289**, 3095–105.

Kimbrell T A, Ketter T A, George M S, *et al.* 2002. Regional cerebral glucose utilization in patients with a range of severities of unipolar depression. *Biol Psychiatry* **51**, 237–52.

Kimura M, Shimoda K, Mizumura S, *et al.* 2003. Regional cerebral blood flow in vascular depression assessed by ^{123}I-IMP SPECT. *J Nippon Med Sch* **70**, 321–6.

Knutson B, Bhanji J P, Cooney R E, Atlas L Y and Gotlib I H. 2008. Neural responses to monetary incentives in major depression. *Biol Psychiatry* **63**, 686–92.

Koschack J, Hoschel K and Irle E. 2003. Differential impairments of facial affect priming in subjects with acute or partially remitted major depressive episodes. *J NervMental Dis* **191**, 175–81.

Kraemer H C, Gullion C M, Rush A J, Frank E and Kupfer D J. 1994. Can state and trait variables be disentangled? A methodological framework for psychiatric disorders. *Psychiatry Res* **52**, 55–69.

Kraemer H C, Schultz S K and Arndt S. 2002. Biomarkers in psychiatry: methodological issues. *Am J Geriatr Psychiatry* **10**, 653–9.

Kumari V, Mitterschiffthaler M T, Teasdale J D, *et al.* 2003. Neural abnormalities during cognitive generation of affect in treatment-resistant depression. *Biol Psychiatry* **54**, 777–91.

Lang P J, Bradley M M and Cuthbert B N. 2001. *International Affective Picture System (IAPS): Instruction Manual and Affective Ratings.* Technical Report A-5 The Center for Research in Psychophysiology, University of Florida.

Lawrence N S, Williams A M, Surguladze S A, *et al.* 2004. Subcortical and ventral prefrontal cortical neural responses to facial expressions distinguish patients with bipolar disorder and major depression. *Biol Psychiatry* **55**, 578–87.

Libet J and Lewinson P. 1973. Concept of social skills with special reference to the behavior of depressed persons. *J Consult Clin Psychol* **40**, 304–13.

Liotti M, Mayberg H S, McGinnis S, Brannan S L and Jerabek P. 2002. Unmasking disease-specific cerebral blood flow abnormalities: Mood challenge in patients with remitted unipolar depression. *Am J Psychiatry* **159**, 1830–40.

Lozano A M, Mayberg H S, Giacobbe P, Hamani C, Craddock R C and Kennedy S H. 2008. Subcallosal cingulate gyrus deep brain stimulation for treatment-resistant depression. *Biol Psychiatry* **64**, 461–7.

Mannie Z N, Norbury R, Murphy S E, Inkster B, Harmer C J and Cowen P J. 2008. Affective modulation of anterior cingulate cortex in young people at increased familial risk of depression. *Br J Psychiatry* **192**, 356–61.

Martin S D, Martin E, Rai S S, Richardson M A and Royall R. 2001. Brain blood flow changes in depressed patients treated with interpersonal psychotherapy or venlafaxine hydrochloride: Preliminary findings. *Arch Gen Psychiatry* **58**, 641–8.

Martinot J L, Hardy P, Feline A, *et al.* 1990. Left prefrontal glucose hypometabolism in the depressed state: A confirmation. *Am J Psychiatry* **147**, 1313–7.

Masurier M L, Cowen P J and Harmer C J. 2007. Emotional bias and waking salivary cortisol in relatives of patients with major depression. *Psychol Med* **37**, 403–10.

Matsuo K, Glahn D C, Peluso M A, *et al.* 2007. Prefrontal hyperactivation during working memory task in untreated individuals with major depressive disorder. *Mol Psychiatry* **12**, 158–66.

Mayberg H S. 1997. Limbic–cortical dysregulation: A proposed model of depression. *J Neuropsychiatry Clin Neurosci* **9**, 471–81.

Mayberg H S, Brannan S K, Mahurin R K, *et al.* 1997. Cingulate function in depression: A potential predictor of treatment response. *Neuroreport* **8**, 1057–61.

Mayberg H S, Liotti M, Brannan S K, McGinnis B S, Mahurin R K and Jerabek P A. 1999. Reciprocal limbic–cortical function and negative mood: Converging PET findings in depression and normal sadness. *Am J Psychiatry* **156**, 675–82.

Mayberg H S, Lozano A M, Voon V, *et al.* 2005. Deep brain stimulation for treatment-resistant depression. *Neuron* **45**, 651–60.

McKiernan K A, Kaufman J N, Kucera-Thompson J and Binder J R. 2003. A parametric manipulation of factors affecting task-induced deactivation in functional neuroimaging. *J Cognit Neurosci* **15**, 394–408.

Monchi O, Petrides M, Petre V, Worsley K and Dagher A. 2001. Wisconsin Card Sorting revisited: Distinct neural circuits participating in different stages of the task identified by event-related functional magnetic resonance imaging. *J Neurosci* **21**, 7733–41.

Monk C S, Klein R G, Telzer E H, *et al.* 2008. Amygdala and nucleus accumbens activation to emotional facial expressions in children and adolescents at risk for major depression. *Am J Psychiatry* **165**, 90–8.

Moreaud O, Naegele B, Chabannes J P, Roulin J L, Garbolino B and Pellat J. 1996. Frontal lobe dysfunction and depression: Relation with the endogenous nature of the depression. *Encephale* **22**, 47–51.

Mueller T I, Leon A C, Keller M B, *et al.* 1999. Recurrence after recovery from major depressive disorder during 15 years of observational follow-up. *Am J Psychiatry* **156**, 1000–6.

Navarro V, Gasto C, Lomena F, *et al.* 2004. Prognostic value of frontal functional neuroimaging in late-onset severe major depression. *Br J Psychiatry* **184**, 306–11.

Neumeister A, Nugent A C, Waldeck T, *et al.* 2004. Neural and behavioral responses to tryptophan depletion in unmedicated patients with remitted major depressive disorder and controls. *Arch Gen Psychiatry* **61**, 765–73.

Nofzinger E A, Nichols T E, Meltzer C C, *et al.* 1999. Changes in forebrain function from waking to REM sleep in depression: Preliminary analyses of [18F]FDG PET studies. *Psychiatry Res* **91**, 59–78.

Okada G, Okamoto Y, Morinobu S, Yamawaki S and Yokota N. 2003. Attenuated left prefrontal activation during a verbal fluency task in patients with depression. *Neuropsychobiology* **47**, 21–6.

Perico C A M, Skaf C R, Yamada A, *et al.* 2005. Relationship between regional cerebral blood flow and separate symptom clusters of major depression: A single photon emission computed tomography study using statistical parametric mapping. *Neurosci Lett* **384**, 265–70.

Persad S and Polivy J. 1993. Differences between depressed and nondepressed individuals in the recognition of and response to facial cues. *J Abnorm Psychol* **102**, 358–68.

Phillips M L, Drevets W C, Rauch S L and Lane R. 2003a. Neurobiology of emotion perception I: The neural basis of normal emotion perception. *Biol Psychiatry* **54**, 504–14.

Phillips M L, Drevets W C, Rauch S L and Lane R. 2003b. Neurobiology of emotion perception II: Implications for major psychiatric disorders. *Biol Psychiatry* **54**, 515–28.

Phillips M L and Frank E. 2006. Redefining bipolar disorder: Toward DSM-V. *Am J Psychiatry* **163**, 1135–6.

Phillips M L, Ladouceur C D and Drevets W C. 2008. A neural model of voluntary and automatic emotion regulation: Implications for understanding the pathophysiology and neurodevelopment of bipolar disorder. *Mol Psychiatry* **13**, 833–57.

Phillips M L, Young A W, Senior C, *et al.* 1997. A specific neural substrate for perceiving facial expressions of disgust. *Nature* **389**, 495–8.

Pochon J B, Levy R, Fossati P, *et al.* 2002. The neural system that bridges reward and cognition in humans: An fMRI study. *Proc Natl Acad Sci U S A* **99**, 5669–74.

Raichle M E, MacLeod A M, Snyder A Z, Powers W J, Gusnard D A and Shulman G L. 2001. Inaugural Article: A default mode of brain function. *Proc Natl Acad Sci U S A* **98**, 676–82.

Raz N, Gunning F M, Head D, *et al.* 1997. Selective aging of the human cerebral cortex observed in vivo: Differential vulnerability of the prefrontal gray matter. *Cerebral Cortex* **7**, 268–82.

Roberson-Nay R, McClure E B, Monk C S, *et al.* 2006. Increased amygdala activity during successful memory encoding in adolescent major depressive disorder: An fMRI study. *Biol Psychiatry* **60**, 966–73.

Rose E J, Simonotto E and Ebmeier K P. 2006. Limbic over-activity in depression during preserved performance on the n-back task. *Neuroimage* **29**, 203–15.

Salloway S, Malloy P, Kohn R, *et al.* 1996. MRI and neuropsychological differences in early- and late-life-onset geriatric depression. *Neurology* **46**, 1567–74.

Schlaepfer T E, Cohen M X, Frick C, *et al.* 2008. Deep brain stimulation to reward circuitry alleviates anhedonia in refractory major depression. *Neuropsychopharmacology* **33**, 368–77.

Sheline Y I, Barch D M, Donnelly J M, Ollinger J M, Snyder A Z and Mintun M A. 2001. Increased amygdala response to masked emotional faces in depressed subjects resolves with antidepressant treatment: An fMRI study. *Biol Psychiatry* **50**, 651–8.

Siegle G J, Steinhauer S R, Thase M E, Stenger V A and Carter C S. 2002. Can't shake that feeling: Event-related fMRI assessment of sustained amygdala activity in response to emotional information in depressed individuals. *Biol Psychiatry* **51**, 693–707.

Siegle G J, Carter C S and Thase M E. 2006. Use of fMRI to predict recovery from unipolar depression with cognitive behavior therapy. *Am J Psychiatry* **163**, 735–8.

Siegle G J, Thompson W, Carter C S, Steinhauer S R and Thase M E. 2007. Increased amygdala and decreased dorsolateral prefrontal BOLD responses in unipolar depression: Related and independent features. *Biol Psychiatry* **61**, 198–209.

Solomon D A, Keller M B, Leon A C, *et al.* 1997. Recovery from major depression. A 10-year prospective follow-up across multiple episodes. *Arch Gen Psychiatry* **54**, 1001–06.

Sprengelmeyer R, Rausch M, Eysel U T and Przuntek H. 1998. Neural structures associated with recognition of facial expressions of basic emotions. *Proc R Soc Lond B Biol Sci* **265**, 1927–31.

Stuss D T and Levine B. 2002. Adult clinical neuropsychology: Lessons from studies of the frontal lobes. *Annu Rev Psychol* **53**, 401–33.

Surguladze S A, Brammer M J, Keedwell P, *et al.* 2005. A differential pattern of neural response toward sad versus happy facial expressions in major depressive disorder. *Biol Psychiatry* **57**, 201–09.

Surguladze S A, Brammer M J, Young A W, *et al.* 2003. A preferential increase in the extrastriate response to signals of danger. *Neuroimage* **19**, 1317–28.

Surguladze S A, Young A W, Senior C, Brebion G, Travis M J and Phillips M L. 2004. Recognition accuracy and response bias to happy and sad facial expressions in patients with major depression. *Neuropsychology* **18**, 212–8.

Suslow T, Junghanns K and Arolt V. 2001. Detection of facial expressions of emotions in depression. *Percept Motor Skills* **92**, 857–68.

Teasdale J D. 1988. Cognitive vulnerability to persistent depression. *Cogn Emot* **2**, 247–74.

Thomas K M, Drevets W C, Dahl R E, *et al.* 2001. Amygdala response to fearful faces in anxious and depressed children. *Arch Gen Psychiatry* **58**, 1057–63.

Tremblay L K, Naranjo C A, Graham S J, *et al.* 2005. Functional neuroanatomical substrates of altered reward processing in major depressive disorder revealed by a dopaminergic probe. *Arch Gen Psychiatry* **62**, 1228–36.

Üstün B T and Chatterji S. 2001. Global burden of depressive disorders and future projections. In Dawson A and Tylee A (Eds.) *Depression: Social and Economic Timebomb*. London: BMJ, pp. 31–43.

Vaishnavi S and Taylor W D. 2006. Neuroimaging in late-life depression. *Int Rev Psychiatry* **18**, 443–51.

Veiel H O F. 1997. A preliminary profile of neuropsychological deficits associated with major depression. *J Clin Exp Neuropsychol* **19**, 587–603.

Videbech P, Ravnkilde B, Pedersen T H, *et al.* 2002. The Danish PET/depression project: Clinical symptoms and cerebral blood flow. A regions-of-interest analysis. *Acta Psychiatr Scand* **106**, 35–44.

Walsh N D, Williams S C R, Brammer M J, *et al.* 2007. A longitudinal functional magnetic resonance imaging study of verbal working memory in depression after antidepressant therapy. *Biol Psychiatry* **62**, 1236–43.

World Health Organization. 1999. *The World Health Report 1999: Making a Difference*. Geneva: World Health Organization.

Yao Z, Wang L, Lu Q, Liu H and Teng G. 2008. Regional homogeneity in depression and its relationship with separate depressive symptom clusters: A resting-state fMRI study. *J Affect Disord* **115**, 430–8.

Zakzanis K K, Leach L and Kaplan E. 1998. On the nature and pattern of neurocognitive function in major depressive disorder. *Neuropsychiatry, Neuropsychol Behav Neurol* **11**, 111–9.

Zang Y, Jiang T, Lu Y, He Y and Tian L. 2004. Regional homogeneity approach to fMRI data analysis. *NeuroImage* **22**, 394–400.

Zola-Morgan S, Squire L R, varez-Royo P and Clower R P. 1991. Independence of memory functions and emotional behavior: Separate contributions of the hippocampal formation and the amygdala. *Hippocampus* **1**, 207–20.

Molecular imaging of major depression

Julia Sacher and Gwenn S. Smith

Introduction

The initial publications of monoamine receptor binding in the living human brain in the mid 1980s and the progress in neurochemical brain imaging since that time have had a profound influence on our ability to test hypotheses generated from clinical observations, preclinical and post-mortem data regarding the neurochemistry of neuropsychiatric disorders in the living human brain (Wagner *et al.*, 1983; Wong *et al.*, 1984; Arnett *et al.*, 1986). Progress in radiotracer chemistry and instrumentation over the past 20 years has enabled us to test mechanistic hypotheses about pathophysiology, as well as to understand the mechanism of action of psychotropic medications.

The primary focus of radiochemistry development for Positron Emission Tomography (PET) and Single Photon Emission Computed Tomography (SPECT) has been dopamine and serotonin neurotransmission (including imaging of neurotransmitter metabolism/synthesis, transporters and receptors). Major advances have been made in areas including cholinergic (muscarinic and nicotinic), glutamatergic (Brown *et al.*, 2008), and opiate systems (Hashimoto *et al.*, 2008; Hirvonen *et al.*, 2009; Reid *et al.*, 2008; Sorger *et al.*, 2008). More recently, the focus of radiotracer development has broadened to include molecular targets such as signal transduction, inflammation and aspects of neuropathology such as amyloid deposition (Vasdev *et al.*, 2008; Fujita *et al.*, 2008; Suhara *et al.*, 2008). Other more challenging targets of interest for which radiotracers continue to be in development include receptors and transporters for norepinephrine, corticotrophin-releasing factor and the hypothalamo-pituitary–adrenal (HPA) axis and neurogenesis (Schou *et al.*, 2007; Steiniger *et al.*, 2008; Sullivan *et al.*, 2007). Table 11.1 lists the radiotracers in current use for animal and human studies. With respect to instrumentation, the resolution of PET and SPECT scanners has improved considerably over the years. Over the past 10 years, dual-modality scanners such as PET/CT and PET/MR scanners have been developed (for a review, see Myers and Hume, 2002; Riemann *et al.*, 2008; Rowland and Cherry, 2008; Heiss, 2009).

PET and SPECT imaging measures of glucose metabolism, cerebral blood flow and perfusion have provided a fundamental understanding of the neural circuitry associated with affective states in normal control subjects, as well as differences between non-depressed and control subjects, differences between patients who respond to treatment compared to non-responders, and the effects of antidepressant interventions including pharmacologic, non-pharmacologic, and somatic treatments (as reviewed by Mayberg, 2003; Ressler and Mayberg, 2007). The ultimate goal of this work has been to identify the functional circuitry which determines what treatment modality will be indicated for a given patient, which intervention will be indicated for treatment-resistant patients, and how the neuroimaging data could be used to predict recurrence (Mayberg, 2003; Agid *et al.*, 2007). Having identified the functional circuitry implicated in treatment response, we can begin to evaluate specific neurochemical mechanisms using neurochemical brain imaging. A summary of the neurochemical mechanisms that can be measured in vivo with PET and SPECT is shown in Box 11.1.

This chapter will review the PET and SPECT neurochemical brain imaging studies to understand the neurochemical mechanisms underling depression and the response to treatment. A section describing clinical and methodological considerations will be

Table 11.1 Overview of radiotracers in current use for animal and human in vivo PET and SPECT studies

Neurotransmitter site	Radiotracer	Reference*
Dopamine		
Metabolism	L-[18F]-6-fluoroDOPA, L-[β-11 C]DOPA	Garnett *et al.*, 1983; Hartvig *et al.*, 1991
Transporter	[11C]-D-threo-methylphenidate, [18F]-FP-CIT, [11C]-WIN 35,428, [18F]-FECNT, [123I]-betaCIT	Volkow *et al.*, 1995; Chaly *et al.*, 1996; Frost *et al.*, 1993; Davis *et al.*, 2003; Laruelle *et al.*, 1994
Monoamine oxidase inhibitor (A and B)	[11C]-clorgyline, [11C]l-deprenyl, [11C]-harmine	Fowler *et al.*, 1987; Ginovart *et al.*, 2006
Vesicular monoamine transporter (type 2)	[11C]-(+) dihydrotetrabenazine	Frey *et al.*, 1996
D1 Receptor	[11C]-SCH23390, [11C]-NNC112	Suhara *et al.*, 1991; Halldin *et al.,* 1998
D2 Receptor: antagonists	[18F]-*N*-methylspiroperidol, 3-*N*-[11C]-n-methyl-spiperone, 3-(2″-[18F]fluoroethyl)spiperone, [11C]-Raclopride, [18F]-Fallypride, [11C]-FLB 457, [123I]-IBZM, [123I]-Epidepride, [123I]-IBF	Arnett *et al.*, 1986; Wagner *et al.*, 1983; Satyamurthy *et al.*, 1990; Farde *et al.*, 1985; Mukherjee *et al.*, 2002; Halldin *et al.*, 1995; Kung *et al.*, 1990; Kessler *et al.*, 1992; Brücke *et al.*, 1993
D2 Receptor: Agonists	(–)-*N*-[11C]Propyl-Norapomorphine, [11C]-(+)-PHNO	Hwang *et al.*, 2000; Willeit *et al.*, 2006
D3 Receptor**		Leopoldo *et al.*, 2002
D4 Receptor**		Huang *et al.*, 2001
Serotonin		
Metabolism	[11C]-alpha-methyltryptophan	Okazawa *et al.*, 2000
Transporter	[11C]-McN5652, [11C]-DASB, [123I]-β-CIT, [123I]-ADAM	Szabo *et al.*, 1995; Houle *et al.*, 2000; Pirker *et al.*, 2000; Erlandsson *et al.*, 2005
5-HT1A receptor: antagonists	[11C]-carbonyl-WAY100635, *p*-[18F]-MPPF	Farde *et al.*, 1998; Shiue *et al.*, 1997b
5-HT1A receptor: Agonists	[11C]-CUMI-101	Milak *et al.*, 2008
5-HT1B receptor	[11C]-AZ10419369	Pierson *et al.*, 2008
5-HT2A receptor	[18F]-altanserin, [18F]-setoperone, [11C]-MDL100907	Smith *et al.*, 1998; Blin *et al.*, 1990; Ito *et al.*, 1998
5-HT4	[11C]-SB207145, [123I]SB 207710	Marner *et al.*, 2007; Pike *et al.*, 2003
5-HT6	[11C]GSK-215083	Parker *et al.*, 2008
Norepinephrine		
Transporter	(*S,S*)-[18F]FMeNER-D2, (*S, S*)-[11C]MRB	Takano *et al.*, 2008; Ding *et al.*, 2006
Acetylcholine		
Vesicular transporter	[123I]-iodovescamicol	Kuhl *et al.*, 1994
Muscarinic receptors	[11C]-benztropine, [11C]-NMPB, [18F]-FTZP, [123I]-QNB, [123I]4-iododexetimide, [123I]4-iodolevetimide	Dewey *et al.*, 1990; Suhara *et al.*, 1993; Podruchny *et al.*, 2003; Eckelman *et al.*, 1984; Muller-Gartner *et al.*, 1992

Table 11.1 (cont.)

Neurotransmitter site	Radiotracer	Reference*
Nicotinic receptors	[11C]-nicotine, 2-[18F]-F-A85380, [18F]-FPH	Nordberg et al., 1995; Horti et al., 2000; Villemagne et al., 1997
Acetylcholinesterase	[11C]-PMP, [11C]-physostigmine	Koeppe et al., 1999; Pappata et al., 1996
Glutamate		
NMDA receptor	[11C]-ketamine, [18F]FTCP, [18F]methyl-MK-801	Shiue et al., 1997; Ferrarese et al., 1991; Blin et al., 1991
Metabotropic glutamate subtype 5 (mGluR5)	[18F]-SP203	Brown et al., 2008
Benzodiazepine receptor		
Central	[11C]-flumazenil, [123I]-iomazenil	Koeppe et al., 1991; Zoghbi et al., 1992
Peripheral	[11C]-PK11195, [11C]DAA1106	Junck et al., 1989, Yasuno et al., 2008
Opiate	[11C]-carfentanil, [11C]-methyl-naltrindole	Frost et al., 1985; Smith et al., 1999
Neuropeptides		
Corticotrophin releasing factor receptor	[18F]-FBPPA, [11C]R121920, [11C]DMP696	Martarello et al., 2001; Sullivan et al., 2007
Substance P (NK-1)	[18F]-SPA-RQ,	Hargreaves et al., 2002
Arachidonic acid metabolism	[11C]-arachidonic acid	Giovacchini et al., 2002
Phosphodiesterase IV inhibitor	[11C]-rolipram	DaSilva et al., 2002
Alzheimer pathology	[18F]FDDNP	Shoghi-Jadid et al., 2002
Amyloid deposition	[11C]-6-OH-BTA-1, [11C]-SB-13	Mathis et al., 2003; Verhoeff et al., 2004

* If available, studies utilizing human subjects are cited.
**Still in development.

Box 11.1. Molecular brain imaging in affective disorders

Mechanistic Studies
- **Cerebral Metabolism/Blood Flow**
  - Cognitive Activation
  - Pharmacologic Activation
- **Neurotransmitter Synthesis/Vesicular Storage**
- **Neurotransmitter Transporter/Receptor Binding**
- **Endogenous Neurotransmitter Activity**
  - Neurotransmitter Concentrations
  - Neurotransmitter Interactions

presented first, followed by sections summarizing the findings for the serotonin and dopamine systems, as well as other neurochemical and molecular targets. While the majority of studies have been performed in mid-life unipolar depressed patients, the available data on depression subtypes (bipolar disorders and geriatric depression) will be reviewed as well. The neuroimaging data will be reviewed with a particular emphasis on those highly informative studies that have also integrated symptom measures and genotyping with the neurochemical measures to elucidate the variability observed in the neurochemical imaging data.

Clinical and methodological considerations

The clinical and methodological aspects involved in the design, analysis and interpretation of neurochemical imaging studies will be reviewed. While the majority of studies have examined patients and demographically matched controls in a cross-sectional manner, more recent studies have used within-subjects designs to evaluate state- or treatment-dependent effects. The repeated study of patients during the course of treatment provides invaluable information to understanding trait- versus state-related effects, as well as to evaluating the neurochemical substrates of treatment response and treatment resistance.

Clinical considerations
Medication status and treatment

Issues such as prior medication exposure, duration of unmedicated interval for the current episode, and treatment response history may introduce variability into the results obtained. The majority of neurochemical imaging studies were conducted in patients who have never been treated, or who have undergone a medication-free interval. The selection of such patients represents a challenge to patient recruitment, but also has limited the ability to conduct neurochemical imaging studies in severely symptomatic patients or subgroups of patients (e.g. mania, psychotic depression). More information regarding the sensitivity of neurochemical brain imaging measures to psychotropic drug exposure might enable the data obtained in currently treated patients to be interpreted. In the studies involving repeated imaging before and during treatment, the primary consideration is whether the treatment interval is sufficient to observe a consistent response (either response or non-response), and whether the duration between last medication dose and time of scan was controlled.

Psychiatric and medical comorbidity

Another major issue in the design and interpretation of neurochemical brain imaging studies in psychiatric patients is psychiatric and medical comorbidity, particularly in the elderly. Given the high comorbidity of depression with anxiety disorders and addictive disorders, for example, study samples that exclude such individuals may not be representative of the population. At the same time, such comorbid diagnoses may contribute variance into the results and should be considered in data analyses. Medical comorbidity is a major issue in studies of geriatric patients. Conditions such as cerebrovascular disease or diabetes are commonly observed in the elderly. There is no correct approach to addressing these issues. The decision involves either enrolling a highly selected sample of patients, or excluding the patients who are often those who present challenges in clinical management and may have more severe neurochemical deficits. These considerations have limited our ability to study treatment-resistant patients for whom in-vivo neurochemical information could inform clinical management.

Patient characterization, phenomenology and genotyping

Some of the most informative neurochemical imaging studies have explained the variability obtained within groups based upon correlations with affective or cognitive symptoms or particular genotypes. There are numerous examples of studies reviewed in this chapter that have found no between-group differences, but relationships in the patient group between the neuroimaging measures and symptoms or genotypes. The primary limiting factor for this type of investigation is sample size. Most neurochemical imaging studies have relatively limited sample sizes, while studies to evaluate the functional correlates of genetic polymorphisms require larger sample sizes. The pre-selection of patients to enroll in neuroimaging studies based on genotype is a potential approach that could be implemented. In addition, issues such as population stratification and control for multiple comparisons should be addressed. While such strategies are complicated to implement and may require a multi-center approach, the available data suggest that such integrative approaches have yielded highly informative data.

Methodological considerations
Radiotracer properties

After radiochemical synthesis procedures have been developed for a particular target, rodent and non-human primate studies are typically conducted to determine the time course of binding in the brain. Then, the binding profile of the radiotracer is characterized by "blocking" studies (measuring the magnitude occupancy of an unlabelled compound, either the same compound or a similar compound to the labeled agent) for the target of interest, in addition to other sites for which the radiotracer may have a higher affinity.

Several considerations for determining the suitability of a radiotracer for PET or SPECT include the following: (1) how selective is the binding of the radiotracer to the target of interest, (2) how high are the ratios of specific to non-specific binding (typically ratios greater than two are considered acceptable), (3) are the kinetics of the radiotracer such that the radiotracer reaches equilibrium and washes out within several half lives of the radiotracer and in a reasonable amount of time so that the patients can tolerate the scanning duration, and (4) do radiolabeled metabolites of the radiotracer enter the brain and are the metabolites found in high enough amounts to hinder quantification of specific binding?

Acute and chronic treatment

When performing neuroreceptor studies prior to and following treatment, the primary considerations include the effects of the intervention (1) on ligand delivery (particularly with respect to high-affinity ligands), (2) on the rate of metabolism of the radiotracer, and (3) on endogenous neurotransmitter concentrations (if the radiotracer is sensitive to alterations in neurotransmitter concentrations). The ability to interpret the data obtained is largely determined by the degree to which the radiotracer has been characterized in terms of its binding profile and sensitivity to its endogenous competitor. Regarding the design of intervention paradigms, the pharmacologic profile of the intervention agent must be considered, in addition to the time course of the acute (minutes to hours) or chronic (weeks) neuropharmacological effects. In this context, the incorporation of plasma levels of the intervention agents and neuroendocrine measures may enhance the interpretation of the neuroimaging data. Measures of the effects of the interventions on cognition and mood and correlating the neuroimaging data with relevant genotyping may provide useful information with respect to interpretation of between-subject variability of the neuroimaging data.

Instrumentation and study design

In the evaluation of the PET/SPECT studies, there are many issues concerning the design of the imaging protocol and image analysis that may affect the results

obtained and their interpretation. Regarding the conduct of the PET studies, there is potential variability introduced by (1) the specific PET scanner used (which would affect the spatial resolution); (2) the data acquisition mode (two-dimensional versus three-dimensional); and (3) whether the study was quantitative (were venous or arterial blood samples obtained to measure radioactivity/metabolite concentrations), or was a reference region approach used.

Image processing

The two challenging issues are corrections for partial volume effects (imaging of reduced brain tissue in a region of interest due to cerebral atrophy or imaging of a small gray matter structure surrounded by white matter or cerebrospinal fluid) and correction for head movement during the scans. Correction methods for both issues have been proposed and implemented (Rousset *et al.*, 2008; Shidahara *et al.*, 2009; Montgomery *et al.*, 2006; Rahmim *et al.*, 2008). Partial volume effects can result in a signal loss and can be observed as spillover of radioactivity between regions. This phenomenon occurs when the size of the region is similar or smaller than the point spread function, being attributed to the limited spatial resolution of the scanner. Head movement can occur, especially given the long scan protocols for neurochemical radiotracers (60 min or longer), and may be a more critical issue when studying symptomatic rather than treated patients.

Data analysis

Regarding the analysis of the PET data, the considerations in evaluating neurochemical imaging studies include: (1) whether the data are analyzed using a region of interest (ROI) approach or a voxel-wise approach (e.g. statistical parametric mapping, SPM), (2) whether structural brain scans are used for anatomical definition and correction for the effects of cerebral atrophy, (3) whether the tracer kinetic model has been validated; and (4) the statistical procedures used (e.g. analysis of variance, principal component analysis).

The impact of mood disorders

Major Depressive Disorder (MDD, also known as unipolar depression) is the most common psychiatric disorder and is defined as a period of at least two weeks of sustained depressed mood and/or anhedonia (Kessler *et al.*, 2005; First *et al.*, 1995). Other symptoms include loss of appetite, disturbed sleep pattern, loss of energy, irritability, problems with concentration and memory, feelings of worthlessness, and suicidal thoughts (First *et al.*, 1995). The lifetime prevalence for MDD is as high as 20% in the general population worldwide, with a female to male ratio about 5:2 (Weissman *et al.*, 1996).

Bipolar disorder (BD) has a lifetime prevalence of 1–2.4% for subthreshold BD in the United States and ranks sixth as a burden of disease worldwide (Merikangas *et al.*, 2007; Murray, 1996). BD is characterized by the presence of one or more episodes of mania or, if milder, hypomania. Manic episodes commonly alternate with depressive episodes or symptoms, or mixed episodes in which features of both mania and depression are present at the same time. Psychotic major depression (PMD) is a type of depression that can include symptoms such as paranoia, higher levels of anxiety, as well as higher scores of depressed mood, motor retardation, and cognitive disturbance. Thus, clinical course and treatment for PMD differ from those of non-psychotic major depressive disorder, as reviewed by Keller *et al.* (2007). PMD is estimated to affect about 0.4% of the population (Ohayon and Schatzberg, 2002). The prevalence of geriatric depression requiring clinical attention is 13.5% (Beekman *et al.*, 1999), and more than 50% have a chronic course (Beekman *et al.*, 2002; Cole *et al.*, 1999). Cognitive impairment, attention deficits, decreased learning ability, memory loss, and problems in executive function are frequent (Abas *et al.*, 1990; Alexopoulos *et al.*, 2000), and associated with disability and poor treatment outcome (Alexopoulos *et al.*, 1996, 2000; Simpson *et al.*, 1997). Geriatric depression is also associated with a dramatic increase in the rate of completed suicide and with greater mortality in the medically ill elderly (Conwell *et al.*, 1996; Bruce and Leaf, 1989).

Converging clinical, biochemical, neuroimaging, and post-mortem data suggest that MDD, as well as other affective disorders, is unlikely to be an illness of one brain region or a single neurotransmitter system, but a complex disease affecting integrated pathways linking specific cortical, subcortical, and limbic sites and their related neurotransmitter and molecular mediators (Castren, 2004; Krishnan and Nestler, 2008; Ressler and Mayberg, 2007; Smith *et al.*, 2007). In the following section, we will review the studies on neurochemical imaging in depressive illness. While the majority of studies have focused on unipolar depression, we will discuss the available data on other depression subtypes.

Neurochemical imaging in mood disorders

Serotonin system

Serotonin dysfunction in MDD is supported by numerous observations. These findings include reduced cerebrospinal fluid (CSF) concentrations of the serotonin metabolite 5-hydroxyindolacetic acid in medication-free depressed patients; decreased serotonin concentrations in post-mortem brain tissue in depressed and suicidal patients; recurrence of depression after tryptophan depletion in remitted, medication-free patients; and a decrease in serotonin uptake, transporter and receptor binding sites in platelets and the brains of drug-free depressed patients (as reviewed by Mann, 1999; Owens and Nemeroff, 1994; Stockmeier, 2003). In addition, pharmacologic intervention studies have shown a blunted neuroendocrine response to acute pharmacologic interventions of the serotonin system and alterations in mood in depressed patients by pharmacologic manipulations of serotonin system (improvement in mood with increased serotonin and worsening of mood with reduced serotonin concentrations, as reviewed by Kilts, 1994; Maes and Meltzer, 1995; Owens and Nemeroff, 1994; Nobler *et al.*, 1999a, 1999b; Mann, 1999).

With advances in radiotracer chemistry, in-vivo imaging studies have evaluated components of the serotonin system including serotonin synthesis, serotonin transporter, 5-HT1A and 5-HT2A receptors. The majority of these studies have been conducted in mid-life unipolar, depressed patients). Radiotracers for other serotonin receptor sites are being evaluated (5-HT1b (Pierson *et al.*, 2008), 5-HT4 (Comley, *et al.*, 2006), 5-HT6 (Parker *et al.*, 2008); see Table 11.1). Several studies provide evidence for reduced serotonin synthesis in depression. Agren *et al.* (1991) reported lower uptake of [11C]-5-hydroxytryptophan, a radiolabeled precursor for serotonin synthesis, in depressed patients. Serotonin synthesis as measured by trapping of the radiotracer alpha-[11C]-methyl-L-tryptophan was shown to be reduced in anterior cingulate gyrus (bilaterally in females, left hemisphere in males) and left medial temporal cortex in unmedicated depressed patients (Rosa-Neto *et al.*, 2004). These findings suggest that the transporter and receptor alterations observed are related to reduced pre-synaptic serotonin function.

Serotonin transporter (5-HTT)

The human 5-HTT is a 630 amino acid-long receptor that spans the lipid bilayer 12 times with cytoplasmic NH_2 and COOH termini (Blakely et al., 1998). The 5-HTT is particularly relevant to understanding the functional neuroanatomy of depression given its localization in cortical, striatal, and limbic areas (Varnas et al., 2004). Post-mortem autoradiographic studies (Cortes et al., 1988; Hall et al., 1998) have shown that the serotonergic system is hetero-geneously distributed throughout the human brain, with the majority of 5-HT neurons located in the raphe nuclei in the brainstem, as well as in the locus coeruleus, substantia nigra, and some areas of the thalamus and hypothalamus. Intermediate densities of 5-HTT are found in the basal ganglia, various parts of the amygdala and hypothalamus, and in substruc-tures of the pons and medulla oblongata located out-side the raphe nuclei. The lowest density of 5-HTT was measured in the cerebellum, as well as in cortical structures and in most areas of the amygdala (Cortes et al., 1988; Hall et al., 1998). Thus, the localization of the serotonin transmitter suggests that it has a poten-tially important modulatory role with respect to areas implicated in depression.

Two PET radiotracers have been most commonly used to image 5-HTT. The initial human studies were performed with [11C](+)McN5652 (trans-1,2,3,5,6,10-β-hexahydro-6-[4-(methylthio)phenyl]-pyrrolo-[2,1–1]-isoquinoline) (Suehiro et al., 1993). This radiotracer shows good brain uptake and high selectivity for 5-HTT relative to other monoamine transporters (Ikoma et al., 2002; Kung et al., 1999; Parsey et al., 2000; Shank et al., 1988). Due to a low ratio of specific to free and non-specific binding, and modest reversibility of binding during the time frame of the PET scan, measurement of cortical 5-HTT binding with [11C](+)McN5652 is limited (Buck et al., 2000; Frankle et al., 2005; Ikoma et al., 2002; Parsey et al., 2000). At the present time, the PET radiotracer [11C]-DASB (3-amino-4-(2-dimethylaminomethylphenylsulfanyl)-benzonitrile) is the most commonly used radiotracer for 5-HTT. [11C]-DASB is highly selective, shows good brain uptake with an adequate ratio of specific binding relative to non-specific binding with high test–retest reliability of regional 5-HTT binding (Ginovart et al., 2001; Wilson et al., 2002; Frankle et al., 2006). SPECT studies for 5-HTT have been performed using the

radiotracers [123I]-CIT ([123I]-methyl 3-(4-iodophenyl) tropane-2-carboxylate (Kugaya et al., 2003; Pirker et al., 2000; Willeit et al., 2000), and [123I]-ADAM (2-((2-((dimethylamino)methyl)phenyl)thio)-5-iodo-phenylamine (Catafau et al., 2006; Erlandsson et al., 2005; Sacher et al., 2007). [123I]-ADAM is more selective for 5-HTT compared to [123I]-CIT (that also binds to the dopamine transporter).

PET and SPECT studies have evaluated 5-HTT binding in mid-life unipolar and bipolar patients (e.g. Malison et al., 1998; Meyer et al., 2001b; Szabo et al., 2002). Increased 5-HTT (Cannon et al., 2006, 2007), decreased 5-HTT (Malison et al., 1998; Newberg et al., 2005; Parsey et al., 2006a; Reimold et al., 2008; Oquendo et al., 2007), or no difference in unmedicated, recovered or remitted patients (Bhagwagar et al., 2007; Meyer et al., 2004) has been reported. Reduced 5-HTT has been associated with anxiety symptoms in depressed patients (Reimold et al., 2008). It has been suggested that the discrep-ancy between studies may be related to differences between studies in the inclusion of patients with comorbid psychiatric diagnoses, such as post-traumatic stress disorder (PTSD), generalized anxiety dis-order (GAD), binge eating disorder, and simple phobia (Meyer, 2007). The studies that have excluded patients with comorbid Axis I illness have shown increased 5-HTT binding (Ichimiya et al., 2002), whereas the studies that included patients with other Axis I disorders showed lower 5-HTT binding (Parsey et al., 2006a). Higher 5-HTT binding is associated with greater pessimistic thinking as indicated by scores on the dysfunctional attitudes scale (Meyer et al., 2004). Similarly, higher thalamic 5-HTT is asso-ciated with greater neuroticism in young control sub-jects (Takano et al., 2007). Two [11C](+)McN5652 PET studies have reported that higher baseline 5-HTT binding predicted remission to acute fluoxetine treatment, as well as remission at one year (Kugaya et al., 2004; Miller et al., 2008). While the direction of the results across studies is different, the regions implicated are remarkably consistent (e.g. cingulate gyrus, frontal cortex, insula, thalamus and striatum). The factors that may contribute to differences across studies include differences in the radiotracers used ([11C]-DASB versus [11C]-McN5652) and sample characteristics, including comorbid psychiatric diag-noses and duration of medication-free interval.

The serotonin transporter represents the primary target for selective serotonin reuptake inhibitors

In Vivo Serotonin Transporter Binding in the Human

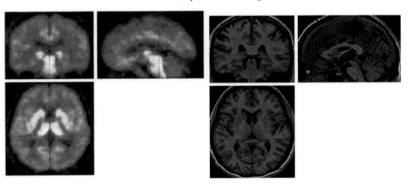

PET Scan of [11C]-DASB

Figure 11.1 A parametric [11C]-DASB PET image of a representative elderly depressed patient (female aged 68 years) co-registered to an MR scan.

(SSRIs), the class of antidepressants most widely prescribed for MDD. SSRIs bind to 5-HTT, thereby blocking serotonin reuptake from the synaptic cleft and subsequently raising extracellular serotonin. Occupancy by SSRIs has been evaluated in controls and depressed patients (Klein *et al.*, 2006, 2007; Meyer *et al.*, 2001b; Parsey *et al.*, 2006a). Studies in controls treated acutely with fluoxetine or depressed patients treated for four weeks with either paroxetine or citalopram have reported significant 5-HTT occupancy in caudate, putamen, thalamus, in addition to prefrontal and anterior cingulate cortices. The magnitude occupancy for these SSRIs was similar (ranging from 65 to 87% across regions; Meyer *et al.*, 2001b). These studies in both controls and depressed patients all demonstrated relatively high brain 5-HTT occupancy even at low plasma concentrations. The studies in patients did not show a correlation between 5-HTT occupancy and improvement in depressive symptoms. A recent study in elderly depressives, who were treated for 8–10 weeks with citalopram to establish treatment response, showed a similar magnitude of striatal and thalamic occupancy, as well as similar relationship between brain occupancy and plasma concentrations to that observed in younger depressed patients also treated with the SSRI citalopram (Smith *et al.*, 2008). A representative [11C]-DASB parametric image from elderly depressed patients is shown in Figure 11.1. In this study of elderly depressed patients, voxel-wise analysis of the 5-HTT data showed that there was a remarkable degree of similarity between regions of 5-HTT occupancy that were correlated with improvement in depressive symptoms and regions of cerebral metabolic decrease (e.g. anterior cingulate gyrus, middle frontal gyrus, precuneus, parahippocampal gyrus) and increase (inferior parietal lobule, cuneus) by citalopram. These data suggest that a serotonergic mechanism may underlie observations of altered cerebral blood flow and metabolism associated with the antidepressant response and that voxel-wise analyses of the neurochemical imaging data may be informative for detecting changes in brain regions with lower concentrations of the transporters and receptors of interest.

In summary, while the data concerning 5-HTT binding in the baseline, unmedicated state in unipolar and bipolar depressed patients are controversial, there is consistency between studies with respect to the brain regions implicated, occupancy by antidepressant medications, as well as the predictive value of baseline 5-HTT binding with respect to treatment outcome and remission. The available data suggest that the correlation of 5-HTT binding with behavioral measures such as pessimistic thinking may explain the variability in patients. While the studies in control subjects have been largely negative with respect to finding an association between 5-HTT binding and genetic polymorphisms for the 5-HTT promoter (Shioe *et al.*, 2003; Willeit *et al.*, 2001), such associations might be informative to study in depressed patients, as the *s* allele has been related to lower serotonin concentrations and slower speed of response relative to the *l* allele (e.g. Lesch *et al.*, 1996; Yu *et al.*, 2002, as reviewed in Smith *et al.*, 2004). As the 5-HTT promoter is a functional polymorphism, the evaluation of the genotype relative to

The Cerebral Metabolic Response to Citalopram Differs as a Function of 5HTTLPR Polymorphisms

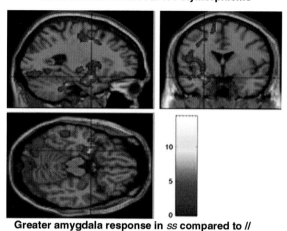

Greater amygdala response in *ss* compared to *ll*

Figure 11.2 The cerebral metabolic response to acute citalopram administration (40 mg, IV) as a function of 5-HTT transporter promoter polymorphisms. Greater left hemisphere response (including the amygdala) associated with the *ss* versus *ll* genotypes in normal control subjects (Smith *et al.*, 2004).

functional serotonin measures may be more revealing. For example (as shown in Figure 11.2), the cerebral metabolic response to citalopram in normal controls with at least one *s* allele showed a blunted response in the right hemisphere and an increased response in the left hemisphere (including the amygdala) relative to subjects with the *ll* genotype, which was similar to the pattern observed in patients with depression (Smith *et al.*, 2004). These PET findings of an increased amygdala response associated with the *s* allele were similar to the results of fMRI studies (Hariri *et al.*, 2003).

Serotonin receptors: overview

With respect to the localization of serotonin receptors, high to intermediate concentrations have been observed throughout the cerebral cortex, amygdala and hippocampus (Hoyer *et al.*, 1986a, 1986b; Varnas *et al.*, 2004; Mengod *et al.*, 1990). Of the 14 serotonin receptor subtypes identified to date, the serotonin 5-HT2A receptor and 5-HT1A subtypes have a more widespread distribution, relatively greater density and better described neurophysiologic roles in the cerebral cortex (frontal, temporal, parietal, cingulate and occipital cortices) and limbic system (hippocampus, entorhinal cortex; Peroutka, 1994; Schotte *et al.*, 1983; Biegon *et al.*, 1986; Pazos *et al.*, 1987). High densities of 5-HT1C (now called 5-HT2C) receptors are found in the substantia nigra, globus pallidus and

choroid plexus (Pazos *et al.*, 1987). 5-HT3 receptors are found in the hippocampus, entorhinal cortex and amygdala (Abi-Dargham *et al.*, 1993).

5-HT1A receptors are located in the soma and dendrites of serotonergic neurons, where they mostly act as autoreceptors (Sotelo *et al.*, 1990). When located in the terminal fields of the serotonergic system such as target neurons in cortical and subcortical regions, they are predominantly post-synaptic receptors (Pazos *et al.*, 1987). Thus, 5-HT1A receptor activation could lead to increased transmission of serotonin when mostly pre-synaptic autoreceptors are involved, whereas a decreased function of the target neurons could subsequently decrease 5-HT1A transmission effects (Blier *et al.*, 1990).

Post-mortem studies have demonstrated alterations in 5-HT1A and 5-HT2A receptors in depression and suicide. These data provided a rationale for neuroimaging studies (e.g. Arango *et al.*, 2002; Mann *et al.*, 2000; Schatzberg, 2002). Alterations of 5HT2A receptors in depression have been reported in several autoradiographic studies (reviewed in detail by Arango *et al.*, 1997; Stockmeier, 2003). Whereas the findings have been controversial to some extent, there is fairly consistent evidence that 5-HT2A receptors are upregulated in the dorsal prefrontal cortex in suicide victims (Arango *et al.*, 1997; Stockmeier, 2003).

Post-mortem data on the 5-HT1A receptors in prefrontal cortex and hippocampus of suicide victims have yielded conflicting results, as some studies report an increase whereas other studies did not detect any significant changes (reviewed in detail by Stockmeier, 2003; e.g. Arango *et al.*, 1995; Stockmeier *et al.*, 1996; Francis *et al.*, 1993). However, several studies suggest reduced receptor function, as depressed subjects show blunted thermic and endocrine responses to 5-HT1A receptor agonist challenge (as reviewed by Drevets *et al.*, 1999). A positive post-mortem study detected a significant decrease in mRNA in the hippocampus of MDD patients who died of suicide (Lopez *et al.*, 1998). Bowden *et al.* (1989) found a decrease in temporal polar and posterior venterolateral prefrontal cortex in MDD and bipolar patients who died of natural causes.

Given the strength of the evidence for a role of the 5-HT1A and 5-HT2A receptor in a variety of neuropsychiatric conditions, as well as the neuroanatomic distribution and neurophysiologic role, radiotracer development has focused on these sites. Thus, the best-validated radiotracers are available for the

5-HT1A and 5-HT2A receptors. The following section provides a summary of the literature.

Serotonin receptors 5-HT1A

11C-[Carbonyl]-WAY-100635 and [18F]-MPPF have been shown to be suitable radiotracers for the 5-HT1A receptors in vivo (Pike *et al.*, 1996; Shiue *et al.*, 1997a). Binding potential values of seven or more are observed in medial temporal structures, where the highest concentration of receptors have been reported (Pike *et al.*, 1996). Data from imaging studies in depressed patients for the 5-HT1A receptor have either shown decreased (Drevets *et al.*, 1999; Sargent *et al.*, 2000; Hirvonen *et al.*, 2008, 2009) or increased (Parsey *et al.*, 2006a) binding. In the study by Parsey *et al.* (2006a), antidepressant-naive subjects and subjects homozygous for the functional 5-HT1A G(-1019) allele of the promoter polymorphism demonstrated higher 5-HT1A binding. A correlation between higher baseline 5-HT1A binding and poorer treatment response has been reported (Parsey *et al.*, 2006b; Moses-Kolko *et al.*, 2007). No alterations of 5-HT1A binding following SSRI treatment has been observed in humans (Sargent *et al.*, 2000, Moses-Kolko *et al.*, 2008), a finding that is in contrast to animal studies showing a functional 5-HT1A response (Cowen, 1996) induced by SSRI treatment. One of the explanations for the lack of an observed effect is that the 5-HT1A antagonist radiotracer binds to low-affinity sites, whereas the changes with treatment may be observed in high-affinity sites. To test this hypothesis, a promising 5-HT1A agonist radiotracer has been developed (Milak *et al.*, 2008). In addition, several promising radiotracers have been developed for the 5-HT1B receptor, which may represent a novel pharmacologic mechanism, as well as a tool for measuring endogenous serotonin concentrations (Pierson *et al.*, 2008).

5-HT1A receptor binding has also been studied in bipolar disorder (as reviewed by Drevets *et al.*, 2000), post-partum depression (Moses-Kolko *et al.*, 2008), and geriatric depression (Meltzer *et al.*, 2004). In all three studies, a significant decrease in receptor availability has been reported for geriatric depressed patients in the dorsal raphe (Meltzer *et al.*, 2004), and for patients with bipolar disorder in midbrain raphe, as well as in limbic and neocortical areas in the mesiotemporal, occipital, and parietal cortex (Drevets *et al.*, 2000; Meltzer *et al.*, 2004). In depressed patients with post-partum onset the decrease in 5-HT1A receptor binding has been detected in anterior cingulate and mesiotemporal cortex (Moses-Kolko *et al.*, 2008).

Several studies have correlated behavioral variables and genetic polymorphisms with 5-HT1A binding. A significant negative correlation between lifetime aggression and 5-HT1A binding was observed in the anterior cingulate, amygdala, dorsal raphe, and medial and orbital prefrontal cortices in healthy controls (Parsey *et al.*, 2002). Anxiety symptoms were positively correlated with 5-HT1A binding in dorsolateral prefrontal cortex, anterior cingulate cortex, parietal cortex, and occipital cortex in control subjects (Tauscher *et al.*, 2001). These observations suggest that behavioral variables such as aggression and anxiety may explain some of the between-subject variability in 5-HT1A binding studies. With respect to genetic studies, lower 5-HT1A receptor binding was associated with the *s* genotype of the 5-HTTLPR rather than the *l* genotype in the absence of an association with 5-HT1A genotypes (David *et al.*, 2005). The study cited above by Parsey *et al.* (2006a) demonstrated an association between 5-HT1A binding and receptor polymorphisms in depressed patients but not in controls. These observations support further studies of the relationship between serotonin genetic polymorphisms and receptor binding measures in controls and MDD patients.

In summary, the 5-HT1A site is the best-studied serotonin receptor site with respect to studies in patients, as well as correlations with behavioral and genetic measures. The baseline comparisons between patients and controls are controversial, but may be explained by some of the associations with behavioral variables and genotypes. While a treatment effect has not been detected with the existing antagonist radiotracers, the development of 5-HT1A agonist, as well as 5-HT1B radiotracers, may be informative with respect to testing the hypothesis of 5-HT1 receptor desensitization as the mechanism of action of SSRIs (Milak *et al.*, 2008; Pierson *et al.*, 2008).

Serotonin receptors 5-HT2A

There are several radiotracers for the 5-HT2A receptor that have suitable imaging properties and are in routine use, including [18F]-Altanserin (Leysen, 1990; Smith *et al.*, 1999), [18F]-Setoperone (Blin *et al.*, 1990), and [(11)C]MDL 100907 (Lundkvist *et al.*, 1996). With respect to differences between depressed patients and controls, the results are controversial. Both focal (right posterolateral orbitofrontal cortex and anterior insular cortex) and global reductions in cortical 5-HT2A binding have been reported (Biver et al., 1997; Messa et al., 2003; Yatham et al., 2000). Reduced prefrontal cortical 5-HT2A binding was observed in suicide attempters compared to control subjects (Van Heeringen et al., 2003). In contrast, two studies showed results (increases) consistent with the post-mortem data. An increase in prefrontal cortical 5-HT2A receptor binding was observed in a subgroup of patients with severe depression and high levels of dysfunctional (more pessimistic) attitudes, but was not observed in the total group of patients (Meyer et al., 1999b). A [18F]-Altanserin PET study identified a positive correlation between 5-HT2A receptor binding and personality risk factors for affective disorders, such as neuroticism, in control subjects (Frokjaer et al., 2008). These observations indicate that in both controls and patients, differences in 5-HT2A receptors emerge when symptoms and personality variables are considered. Recovered, non-medicated patients with a history of recurrent unipolar depression were also shown to have increased 5-HT2A receptor binding in extensive parts of the cortex (Bhagwagar et al., 2006). A study in late-life depressed patients showed no difference in cortical 5-HT2A receptor binding (Meltzer et al., 1999).

The effects of antidepressant treatment on the 5-HT2A receptor are controversial. Meyer et al. (2001b) reported a decrease in 5-HT2A receptor availability after six weeks of paroxetine treatment only in younger depressed patients (under the age of 30). Several earlier studies reported increased cortical binding to the 5-HT2A receptor with antidepressant treatment in depressed patients (Moresco et al., 2000; Massou et al., 1997), but one study reported a decrease (Yatham et al., 1999). The main reason for the discrepancy between studies may be that in the Yatham et al. (1999) study, desipramine was administered, which binds directly to the 5-HT2A receptors, whereas SSRIs were used in the other studies. The effects of electroconvulsive treatment on 5-HT2A receptor availability have been evaluated in non-human primates (Strome et al., 2005). The study demonstrated acute decreases in 5-HT2A receptor availability that persisted for one week and returned to baseline levels two weeks later.

In summary, neurochemical imaging studies demonstrate increased 5-HT2A binding in frontal and other cortical regions in depressed patients, as well as associations with depression-related personality traits in controls. As is the case with the 5-HTT, the

differences emerge when behavioral variables are taken into account. The effects of antidepressant medication are controversial. Future studies of the 5-HT2A receptor should focus on the evaluation of association between 5-HT2A binding and behavioral variables such as treatment response, as well as an evaluation of genetic polymorphisms (e.g. Nomura and Nomura, 2006) that might explain some of the variability between subjects.

Monoamine oxidase A (MAO-A) and vesicular monoamine transporter (VMAT)

Monoamine oxidase A (MAO-A) is a mitochondrial enzyme that breaks down serotonin, norepinephrine and dopamine, and is present throughout the human brain. [11C]-harmine is a selective, reversible PET radiotracer for MAO-A that is preferable to [11C]-clorgyline that binds irreversibly and may be influenced by changes in blood flow (ligand delivery; Ginovart et al., 2006). [11C]-harmine shows high affinity ($K_i = 2$ nM) with high brain uptake in humans, with the greatest uptake in regions with the highest MAO-A density, and the metabolites of harmine have been shown to be polar and not to cross the blood–brain barrier (Tweedie and Burke, 1987).

Specific binding of [11C]-harmine can be fully displaced by MAO-inhibitors in animal models (Bergstrom et al., 1997a). In humans, MAO-inhibitors at clinically tolerable doses can displace 80% of specific binding (Bergstrom et al., 1997a, 1997b; Ginovart et al., 2006). Recently, a significant increase in MAO-A binding has been shown in depressed patients versus healthy controls (Meyer et al., 2006). Radiotracers for the potentially important target, MAO-B, are available (e.g. Fowler et al., 1987) but have not been applied to the study of mood disorders.

The vesicular monoamine transporter (VMAT) accumulates catecholamines, serotonin and tyramine, and the distribution of VMAT parallels that of the plasma membrane dopamine transporter (DAT) in normal subjects. As reviewed in detail by Efange (2000), the radiotracers [11C]TBZOH and [11C]MTBZ have been used successfully with PET to detect changes in VMAT2 density in neuropathology. In a study of asymptomatic, treated bipolar patients with a previous history of manic and psychotic symptoms, an increase in VMAT2 binding in the striatum and thalamus was observed and the regional binding was positively correlated with performance of tasks of executive function (Zubieta *et al.*, 2001b). The patients were medicated at the time of scanning (all with mood stabilizers and some with antipsychotics); however, the radiotracer for VMAT2 has been shown to be insensitive to medication exposure with a variety of classes of psychotropic drugs. These studies provide some evidence for a role of dopamine in the mechanism of action of sodium valproate treatment, for increased VMAT2 binding in bipolar disorders as a trait marker of monoaminergic dysfunction and for an association between VMAT2 binding and executive function.

Dopamine system

The role of the dopamine system in depression has been reviewed in detail (Brown and Gershon, 1993; Nestler and Carlezon, 2006). There are several lines of evidence to support dopamine dysfunction in depression, including: improvement in depressive symptoms with dopamine agonists, the induction of a depressive relapse by pharmacologic depletion of dopamine and low cerebrospinal fluid homovanillic acid levels in depressed patients compared to controls. The limited post-mortem data available do not show differences in D1 and D2 receptors in depressed suicides (Bowden *et al.*, 1997, Allard and Norlén, 2001). In the next section, the available neuroimaging data on the dopamine system in MDD will be reviewed.

With respect to the localization of dopamine receptors in the human brain, intermediate levels of D1 receptors are found diffusely in the cerebral cortex, amygdala and hippocampus, and much lower densities of D2 receptors (slightly higher in temporal and frontal cortices) have been observed (Camps *et al.*, 1989; Cortes *et al.*, 1988). D1 and D2 receptors are in highest concentration in the basal ganglia, whereas D3 receptors are found in areas associated with the limbic system (such as nucleus accumbens, hippocampus). D4 and D5 mRNA are found in greater density in frontal cortex and hippocampus, respectively, and to a much lesser extent in basal ganglia (Van Tol *et al.*, 1991; Sokoloff *et al.*, 1990; Meador-Woodruff *et al.*, 1989). Dopamine transporters are located in high concentrations in the striatum and to a lesser extent in motor, premotor, anterior cingulate, prefrontal, entorhinal/perirhinal, insular, and visual cortices and amygdala (Ciliax *et al.*, 1999). The dopamine system has been the major focus of radiochemistry development, and numerous radiotracers are available for dopamine synthesis and metabolism, dopamine transporter, D1 and D2/D3 receptors (Volkow *et al.*, 1996).

The available imaging data suggest modest decreases or no change in dopamine metabolism, dopamine transporter and D1 and D2 receptor binding (Agren and Reibring, 1994; Meyer *et al.*, 2001a; Suhara *et al.*, 1992). Dopamine transporter binding was reduced in MDD relative to controls (Meyer *et al.*, 2001a). Several studies of striatal D2 receptor availability have shown no differences between patients and controls, even in medication-naive patients (Klimke *et al.*, 1999; Parsey *et al.*, 2001; Hirvonen *et al.*, 2008, 2009). Greater psychomotor slowing has been associated with increased striatal D2 receptor binding, indicating that perhaps differences may be observed in subgroups of depressed patients (Meyer *et al.*, 2006). Pearlson and colleagues demonstrated that D2 binding was increased in patients with schizophrenia and bipolar disorder with psychotic features, but not in bipolar patients without psychotic features (Pearlson *et al.*, 1995). These findings indicated that increased D2 binding was associated with psychosis, but not bipolar disorder. A preliminary study using a high-affinity radiotracer to bind to extrastriatal D2 receptors also observed no difference in D2 receptors in patients relative to controls (Montgomery *et al.*, 2006). With respect to the D1 receptor, decreased binding was observed in the left middle caudate in one report (Cannon *et al.*, 2009). In addition, no differences in amphetamine-induced striatal dopamine release have been observed (Anand *et al.*, 2000; Parsey *et al.*, 2001). Thus, these studies do not provide compelling evidence of striatal D2 dopamine dysfunction in depressed patients, although there is preliminary support for a role of the D1 receptor.

The effects of antidepressant treatment on striatal D2 receptor availability have been studied. The effects of acute and chronic SSRI treatment on striatal D2 receptor availability is modest (Smith *et al.*, 2009; Tiihonen *et al.*, 1996). There is some controversial evidence of changes in striatal D2 binding after total sleep deprivation (TSD) and antidepressant treatment (Ebert *et al.*, 1994; Klimke *et al.*, 1999). Several studies in control subjects have shown that acute prefrontal repetitive transcranial magnetic stimulation (rTMS) increases extracellular dopamine concentrations as measure by decreased D2 receptor availability using PET and SPECT methods (Strafella *et al.*, 2003; Pogarell *et al.*, 2007). The evaluation of this paradigm in MDD patients and the correlation with alterations in depressive symptoms might be revealing.

With respect to bipolar disorders and mood stabilizers, Yatham *et al.* (2002a) studied medication-naive manic patients with [18F]FluoroDOPA. While uptake did not differ between the patients and controls at baseline, treatment with sodium valproate resulted in a decrease in uptake. In contrast, a study of the striatal D2 receptor showed no effect of disease or treatment (Yatham *et al.*, 2002b).

In summary, in contrast to the evidence from pharmacologic and CSF studies that suggest decreased dopamine function and a role of dopamine augmentation in MDD, neurochemical imaging studies do not support a role of the dopamine system in MDD. The evidence of elevated D4 receptor mRNA in the amygdala from a post-mortem study supports the study of the dopamine system in limbic regions (Xiang *et al.*, 2008). Future studies might examine changes in extracellular dopamine concentrations in extrastriatal brain regions, particularly cortical and limbic regions, using high affinity D2 radiotracers and D1 radiotracers when such materials are validated (e.g. Riccardi *et al.*, 2006).

Other neurotransmitters and neuromodulators and molecular targets

The serotonin and dopamine systems have been the major focus of in-vivo neurochemical imaging studies in depression, as well as other conditions including schizophrenia and anxiety disorders. In this section, we will review the available neurochemical imaging data for other neurotransmitter systems, as well as highlighting active areas of radiotracer development for other potentially important neurochemical targets. Many of the mechanisms potentially involved in the pathophysiology of depression have been suggested by recent augmentation studies that show improvement in depressive symptoms by such pharmacologic agents as muscarinic and NMDA antagonists in treatment-resistant patients.

Noradrenergic system

Radiotracer development for the norepinephrine transporter as well as β-adrenergic receptors (β-AR) has been challenging due to the lack of pharmacologically selective agents, and the low signal to noise levels of binding in brain regions due to relatively high levels of non-specific binding (as reviewed by Schou *et al.*, 2007; Ding *et al.*, 2006). Given the role of the norepinephrine transporter in the mechanism of

action of antidepressant agents, a suitable radiotracer would permit drug occupancy studies, as well as studies of pathophysiology. The β-AR is a potentially relevant receptor site because, when stimulated by norepinephrine, the receptor inhibits CRH release and suppresses the stress response of the HPA axis.

Acetylcholine

The role of the cholinergic system in the pathophysiology of MDD has been implicated by the demonstration of centrally active cholinomimetic drugs rapidly inducing depressed mood (as reviewed by Dilsaver, 1986), as well as muscarinic antagonists having a rapid antidepressant effect (Furey and Drevets, 2006). Nicotinic antagonists may also have an antidepressant effect (George *et al.*, 2008). Given the role of nicotine in depression and neurodegenerative diseases such as Alzheimer's and Parkinson's disease, [11C]-nicotine was used for brain imaging of nicotinic receptors. As reviewed by Heiss and Herholz (2006), high binding density was found in pons, cerebellum, occipital cortex, and white matter. However, the tracer has limitations with regards to high non-specific binding and a rapid washout phase. More specific ligands, such as epibatidine and derivatives labeled with 11C or 18F, showed high uptake in thalamus and hypothalamus or midbrain, intermediate uptake in the neocortex and hippocampus, and low uptake in the cerebellum (Villemagne *et al.*, 1997). For other aspects of the cholinergic system, radiotracers have been developed for the vesicular acetylcholine transporter, acetylcholinesterase, and muscarinic receptors. With the exception of the radiotracer [18F]FP-FTZP that is selective for the M2 muscarinic receptor subtypes, the other muscarinic radiotracers are not subtype-selective (Eckelman, 2001). One study using [18F]FP-FTZP observed reduced muscarinic receptor binding in the anterior cingulate gyrus in bipolar depressed patients relative to MDD patients and controls (Cannon *et al.*, 2006). The reduction in receptor binding was negatively correlated with depressive symptoms. The further investigation of muscarinic and nicotinic mechanism in depression would be of mechanistic and therapeutic relevance.

Opiates

The difficulties inherent in radiotracer development for the opiate system have been reviewed (Frost,

2001). Radiotracers have been used in humans for the mu and delta receptor subtypes. [11C]-carfentanil has demonstrated sensitivity to alterations in opiate concentrations (Zubieta et al., 2001a). In a mood induction study using [11C]-carfentanil, the effects of endogenous opioid neurotransmission on mu-opioid receptors differed in depressed patients relative to controls (Zubieta et al., 2003).

HPA axis

The HPA axis is highly relevant to the pathophysiology of mood disorders. Consistent findings show abnormalities in the HPA axis and maladaptive responses to stress to have a central role in the pathophysiology of mood disorders (as reviewed by Holsboer, 2000). To evaluate the HPA axis directly, radiotracer development has focused on the CRF receptor (e.g. Steiniger et al., 2008; Sullivan et al., 2007). However, a radiotracer with suitable properties is not yet available.

Peripheral and central benzodiazepine receptors

For the GABA/benzodiazepine receptor, [11C]-flumazenil, which binds to the antagonist site, and the partial agonist [123I]-iomazenil are the most commonly used radiotracers. The relationship of low occipital GABA levels determined by MR spectroscopy and [123I]-iomazenil binding in depressed patients was evaluated by Kugaya et al. (2003). The investigators observed low GABA levels in this sample replicating earlier findings, but did not observe a difference in [123I]-iomazenil receptor binding or a correlation between the neuroimaging data and GABA levels. Electroconvulsive therapy (ECT) treatment using bitemporal electrode placement, was associated with increased cortical [123I]-iomazenil binding in all regions except temporal cortex (Mervaala et al., 2001). To evaluate theories about the role of neuroinflammation in depression (Raison et al., 2006), peripheral benzodiazepine (PBR) radiotracers can be applied that bind with high affinity to translocator protein (TSPO). TSPO is upregulated in activated microglia and represents a marker of neuroinflammation. A number of radiotracers have been developed and evaluated in human subjects (as reviewed by Chauveau et al., 2008, Fujita et al., 2008), but not yet in depressed patients.

Glutamate

The recent evidence for the antidepressant effects of the N-methyl-D-aspartate (NMDA) antagonist, ketamine, and the genetic data implicating glutamate

receptor polymorphisms in the response to SSRIs has stimulated research to evaluate the role of glutamate in depression (as reviewed by Matthew et al., 2008). Several radiotracers have been evaluated for the NMDA receptor (Blin et al., 1991; Ferrarese et al., 1991; Shiue et al., 1997a) and do not have suitable imaging properties for human studies. The recent emphasis and greatest success for glutamate radiotracer development has been the metabotropic glutamate subtype 5 (MgluR5) receptor (Brown et al., 2008). Such radiotracers could be extremely informative with respect to understanding the possible glutamatergic basis of cerebral hypermetabolism in depression, as well as the role of serotonin modulation of glutamate in the effects of antidepressants (Smith et al., 2008; Marek and Aghajanian, 1998).

Other mechanisms

In addition to neuropeptides associated with the HPA axis, the role of Substance P, the endogenous substrate for the neurokinin 1 (NK-1) receptor, in affective disorders is supported based on the regional localization of the receptors in cortical and limbic regions associated with affective processing and stress, as well as preclinical evidence for antidepressant and anxiolytic effects (as reviewed by Matthew et al., 2008). Both NK-1 and NK-2 trails have shown weak or mixed results with respect to efficacy (Keller et al., 2007; as reviewed by Matthew et al., 2008). Radiotracers for NK-1 receptors are available (Syvanen et al., 2007; Yasuno et al., 2007).

The role of second messengers in the mechanism of action of antidepressant and mood stabilizing agents has been described (Zarate et al., 2006). There are several well-established radiotracers for second messengers that have not yet been investigated in either unipolar or bipolar depressed patients. [11C]-rolipram is a phosphodiesterase (PDE) 4 inhibitor that has been developed as a PET radiotracer, and in unlabelled form has shown promise as an antidepressant drug with anti-inflammatory properties. A second agent is [11C]-arachidonic acid, which has been studied extensively in animal and humans by Rappoport and colleagues (Rappoport, 2008; Pifferi et al., 2008). A radiotracer for cyclic adenosine monophosphate (cAMP; Vasdev et al., 2008) has also been evaluated. These radiotracers could provide unique evidence for a role of second messengers in the mechanisms of action of antidepressants and mood stabilizers as well as the pathophysiology of depression.

183

The most exciting observation in antidepressant physiology has been the observation that antidepressants, such as the SSRIs, and mood stabilizers (lithium, sodium valproate) increase the expression of trophic factors (e.g. brain-derived neurotrophic factor; Duman *et al.*, 1997). While volumetric changes in structural brain imaging have been interpreted as suggestive of neurogenesis, the development of mechanistically selective neuroimaging methods to evaluate such changes in the human brain would be extremely important. The possibility that commonly prescribed psychotropic medications may induce neuronal plasticity has significant implications for the treatment of psychiatric and neurodegenerative diseases.

Conclusions

Neurochemical imaging research in mood disorders has primarily focused on imaging aspects of serotonin and dopamine neurotransmission in the unmedicated state, as well as evaluating the effects of antidepressant treatment. While variable results have been reported, the studies that have incorporated genotyping or behavioral measures have begun to help us interpret the between-subject variability observed. While such integrative research is limited by the small sample sizes of neurochemical imaging studies, such data are invaluable. The rapid scientific development in the areas of pharmacogenetics of antidepressant response and gene expression profiling in affective disorders will have a major influence on the identification of new therapies and neuroimaging targets in the future (Kato and Serretti, 2010; Psychiatric GWAS Consortium Steering Committee, 2009).

There are many critical areas of study that are needed to advance the field of the neurobiology of affective disorders. Studies that involve imaging of comorbidities such as substance abuse or psychiatric disorders such as anxiety disorders are critical to understanding whether the effects of the comorbid disorders are merely additive, or whether there are distinct pathophysiological consequences. A second critical area is the study of affective disorder comorbidity with medical (e.g. cardiovascular disease, diabetes) and neurodegenerative disorders (e.g. Alzheimer's disease, movement disorders), as well as the impact of affective symptoms on individuals at "high risk" for these disorders, such as mild cognitive impairment and gene carriers for conditions such as Huntington's

disease. Longitudinal investigations of disease course have not yet been a major focus of study, but could be very informative in evaluating the effects of repeated episodes on neurochemical function, particularly as many patients become less responsive to treatment with repeated episodes.

With respect to mechanisms of drug action, most studies have focused on evaluating antidepressant effects and measuring occupancy at the initial target sites of action (such as SSRI occupancy of the 5-HTT). Much more work is needed, as driven by preclinical research, to understand the secondary drug effects that may be better linked to treatment response. In this regard, studies examining dynamic changes in neurotransmitter concentrations are potentially informative.

The demonstration that endogenous neurotransmitter concentrations could be measured in vivo by combining neurotransmitter receptor binding measures with acute pharmacologic interventions was an exciting development in neuroimaging methodology in the previous decade (Dewey *et al.*, 1993; Volkow *et al.*, 1994; Smith *et al.*, 1997). The impetus for the development of these methods was the observation that dynamic aspects of neurotransmitter function would be more revealing of pathophysiology and treatment response than static aspects of receptor or transporter binding. This approach can be applied to investigating the changes in a single neurotransmitter system or interactions between neuroanatomically and functionally linked systems. The majority of studies have focused on the dopamine system and modulation of dopamine by neurotransmitter systems (acetylcholine, glutamate, serotonin) and pharmacologic agents that have recently been shown to be effective as antidepressant agents (e.g. scopolamine and ketamine; Furey and Drevets, 2006; Matthew *et al.*, 2008). Such dynamic neurotransmitter paradigms have been applied to depression to a limited extent to examine dopamine concentrations (Anand *et al.*, 2000; Parsey *et al.*, 2001). Methodology development is in progress to extend this approach to other neurotransmitter systems (e.g. sertonin, acetylcholine, and opiates) as well as applications to affective disorders. Figure 11.3 is an example of the effects of acute citalopram on 5-HT2A receptor availability. Citalopram reduced 5-HT2A receptor availability in the cortex consistent with an increase in endogenous serotonin competing for binding to the 5-HT2A receptor and lower receptor availability. The ability

The Effect of Acute Citalopram on Serotonin Receptor Availability

Baseline

Post-Treatment

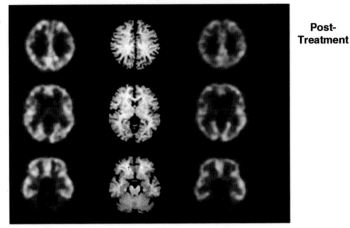

[18F]-Altanserin Distribution Volume Ratio Images

Figure 11.3 The changes in 5-HT2A receptor availability by acute citalopram administration (40 mg, IV) measured by [18F]-altanserin PET studies. Lower cortical binding after citalopram administration is associated with greater competition between higher serotonin concentrations and the radiotracer for binding to the 5-HT2A site.

to evaluate neurotransmitter function and interactions in vivo is a potentially informative approach to understanding the neurobiology of affective disorders that also provides an opportunity to conduct translational studies in mice and rodents for which in-vivo microdialysis methods provide similar dynamic information.

With respect to pharmacologic agents for mood disorders, the mood stabilizers remain an understudied class of medications for which neurochemical imaging methods could be extremely informative. Psychotherapy and somatic treatments (including ECT, deep brain stimulation and rTMS) are also largely understudied with respect to neurochemical brain imaging. The initial studies to evaluate changes in neural circuitry have been highly informative with respect to identifying the pathways involved (as reviewed by Ressler and Mayberg, 2007). The exciting developments of pharmacologic and somatic approaches to treating treatment-resistant patients represent unique opportunities to apply neurochemical imaging methods to understand the neurobiology of treatment resistance and the mechanism of action of these promising treatments. The goal of the chapter was to provide a critical overview of neurochemical imaging research in affective disorders. The findings in many areas are controversial, but highlight the potential of the neuroimaging approaches. The advances in radiotracer chemistry, PET/SPECT instrumentation and small animal PET imaging will enable us to make considerable progress with respect to translational research in affective disorders, drug discovery and human mechanistic studies.

Acknowledgments

Supported in part by National Institute of Health: MH01621, MH49936, MH57078, MH 64823. Clifford I. Workman, BSc is gratefully acknowledged for his input into the chapter.

References

Abas M A, Sahakian B J and Levy R. 1990. Neuropsychological deficits and CT scan changes in elderly depressives. *Psychol Med* **20**, 507–20.

Abi-Dargham A, Laruelle M, Lipska B, *et al.* 1993. Serotonin 5-HT3 receptors in schizophrenia: A postmortem study of the amygdala. *Brain Res* **616**, 53–7.

Agid Y, Buzsáki G, Diamond D M, *et al.* 2007. How can drug discovery for psychiatric disorders be improved? *Nat Rev Drug Discov* **6**, 189–201.

Agren H and Reibring L. 1994. PET studies of presynaptic monoamine metabolism in depressed patients and healthy volunteers. *Pharmacopsychiatry* **27**, 2–6.

Agren H, Reibring L, Hartvig P, *et al.* 1991. Low brain uptake of L-[11C]5-hydroxytryptophan in major depression: A positron emission tomography study on patients and healthy volunteers. *Acta Psychiatr Scand* **83**, 449–55.

Alexopoulos G S, Meyers B S, Young R C, *et al.* 2000. Executive dysfunction and long-term outcomes of geriatric depression. *Arch Gen Psychiatry* **57**, 285–90.

Alexopoulos G S, Vrontou C, Kakuma T, *et al.* 1996. Disability in geriatric depression. *Am J Psychiatry* **153**, 877–85.

Allard P and Norlen M. 2001. Caudate nucleus dopamine D(2) receptors in depressed suicide victims. *Neuropsychobiology* **44**, 70–3.

Anand A, Verhoeff P, Seneca N, *et al.* 2000. Brain SPECT imaging of amphetamine-induced dopamine release in euthymic bipolar disorder patients. *Am J Psychiatry* **157**, 1108–14.

Arango V, Underwood M D, Gubbi A V and Mann J J. 1995. Localized alterations in pre- and postsynaptic serotonin binding sites in the ventrolateral prefrontal cortex of suicide victims. *Brain Res* **688**, 121–33.

Arango V, Underwood M D and Mann J J. 2002. Serotonin brain circuits involved in major depression and suicide. *Progr Brain Res* **136**, 443–53.

Arango V, Underwood M D and Mann J J. 1997. Postmortem findings in suicide victims. Implications for in vivo imaging studies. *Ann N Y Acad Sci* **836**, 269–87.

Arnett C D, Wolf A P, Shiue C Y, *et al.* 1986. Improved delineation of human dopamine receptors using [18F]-*N*-methylspiroperidol and PET. *J Nucl Med* **27**, 1878–82.

Beekman A T, Copeland J R and Prince M J. 1999. Review of community prevalence of depression in later life. *Br J Psychiatry* **174**, 307–11.

Beekman A T, Geerlings S W, Deeg D J, *et al.* 2002. The natural history of late-life depression: A 6-year prospective study in the community. *Arch Gen Psychiatry* **59**, 605–11.

Bergstrom M, Westerberg G, Kihlberg T and Langstrom B. 1997a. Synthesis of some 11C-labelled MAO-A inhibitors and their in vivo uptake kinetics in rhesus monkey brain. *Nucl Med Biol* **24**, 381–8.

Bergstrom M, Westerberg G and Langstrom B. 1997b. 11C-harmine as a tracer for monoamine oxidase A (MAO-A): In vitro and in vivo studies. *Nucl Med Biol* **24**, 287–93.

Bhagwagar Z, Hinz R, Taylor M, Fancy S, Cowen P and Grasby P. 2006. Increased 5-HT(2A) receptor binding in euthymic, medication-free patients recovered from depression: A positron emission study with [(11)C]MDL 100,907. *Am J Psychiatry* **163**, 1580–7.

Bhagwagar Z, Murthy N, Selvaraj S, *et al.* 2007. 5-HTT binding in recovered depressed patients and healthy volunteers: A positron emission tomography study with [11C]DASB. *Am J Psychiatry* **164**, 1858–65.

Biegon A, Kargman S, Snyder L and McEwen B S. 1986. Characterization and localization ofserotonin receptors in human brain postmortem. *Brain Res* **363**, 91–8.

Biver F, Wikler D, Lotstra F, Damhaut P, Goldman S and Mendlewicz J. 1997. Serotonin 5-HT2 receptor imaging in major depression: Focal changes in orbito-insular cortex. *Br J Psychiatry* **171**, 444–8.

Blakely R D, Ramamoorthy S, Schroeter S, *et al.* 1998. Regulated phosphorylation and trafficking of antidepressant-sensitive serotonin transporter proteins. *Biol Psychiatry* **44**, 169–78.

Blier P, de Montigny C and Chaput Y. 1990. A role for the serotonin system in the mechanism of action of antidepressant treatments: Preclinical evidence. *J Clin Psychiatry* **51** (Suppl), 14–20; discussion 21.

Blin J, Denis A, Yamaguchi T, Crouzel C, MacKenzie E T and Baron J C. 1991. PET studies of [18F]methyl-MK-801, a potential NMDA receptor complex radioligand. *Neurosci Lett* **121**, 183–6.

Blin J, Sette G, Fiorelli M, *et al.* 1990. A method for the in vivo investigation of the serotonergic 5-HT2 receptors in the human cerebral cortex using positron emission tomography and 18F-labeled setoperone. *J Neurochem* **54**, 1744–54.

Bowden C, Theodorou A E, Cheetham S C, *et al.* 1997. Dopamine D1 and D2 receptor binding sites in brain samples from depressed suicides and controls. *Brain Res* **752**, 227–33.

Bowden C L, Seleshi E and Javors M A. 1989. Mania associated with high percentage of inhibition of monoamine oxidase. *Am J Psychiatry* **146**, 121.

Brown A K, Kimura Y, Zoghbi S S, *et al.* 2008. Metabotropic glutamate subtype 5 receptors are quantified in the human brain with a novel radioligand for PET. *J Nucl Med* **49**, 2042–8.

Brown A S and Gershon S. 1993. Dopamine and depression. *J Neural Transm* **91**, 75–109.

Bruce M L and Leaf P J. 1989. Psychiatric disorders and 15-month mortality in a community sample of older adults. *Am J Public Hlth* **79**, 727–30.

Brücke T, Kornhuber J, Angelberger P, Asenbaum S, Frassine H, and Podreka I. 1993. SPECT imaging of dopamine and serotosin transporters with [123I]beta-CIT. Binding kinetics in the human brain. *J Neurol Transm Gen Sect* **94**, 137–46.

Buck A, Gucker P M, Schonbachler R D, *et al.* 2000. Evaluation of serotonergic transporters using PET and [11C](+)McN-5652: Assessment of methods. *J Cerebr Blood Flow Metab* **20**, 253–62.

Camps M, Cortés R, Gueye B, Probst A and Palacios J M. 1989. Dopamine receptors in human brain: Autoradiographic distribution of D2 sites. *Neuroscience* **28**, 275–90.

Cannon D M, Ichise M, Fromm S J, *et al.* 2006. Serotonin transporter binding in bipolar disorder assessed using [11C]DASB and positron emission tomography. *Biol Psychiatry* **60**, 207–17.

Cannon D M, Ichise M, Rollis D, *et al.* 2007. Elevated serotonin transporter binding in major depressive disorder assessed using positron emission tomography and [11C]DASB; comparison with bipolar disorder. *Biol Psychiatry* **62**, 870–7.

Cannon D M, Klaver J M, Peck S A, Rallis-Voak D, Erickson K and Drevets W C. 2009. Dopamine type-1 receptor binding in major depressive disorder assessed using positron emission tomography and [11C]NNC-112. *Neuropsychopharmacology*, **5**, 1277–87.

Carson R E, Kiesewetter D O, Jagoda E, Der M G, Herscovitch P and Eckelman W C. 1998. Muscarinic cholinergic receptor measurements with [18F]FP-TZTP: Control and competition studies. *J Cereb Blood Flow Metab* **18**, 1130–42.

Caspi A, Sugden K, Moffitt T E, *et al.* 2003. Influence of life stress on depression: Moderation by a polymorphism in the 5-HTT gene. *Science* **301**, 386–9.

Castren E. 2004. Neurotrophins as mediators of drug effects on mood, addiction, and neuroprotection. *Mol Neurobiol* **29**, 289–302.

Catafau A M, Perez V, Plaza P, *et al.* 2006. Serotonin transporter occupancy induced by paroxetine in patients with major depression disorder: A 123I-ADAM SPECT study. *Psychopharmacology (Berl)* **189**, 145–53.

Chaly T, Dhawan V, Kazumata K, *et al.* 1996. Radiosynthesis of [18F] N-3-fluoropropyl-2-beta-carbomethoxy-3-beta-(4-iodophenyl) nortropane and the first human study with positron emission tomography. *Nucl Med Biol* **23**, 999–1004.

Chauveau F, Boutin H, Van Camp N, Dollé F and Tavitian B. 2008. Nuclear imaging of neuroinflammation: A comprehensive review of [(11C)PK11195 challengers. *Eur J Nucl Med Mol Imaging* **35**, 2304–19.

Ciliax B J, Drash G W, Staley J K, *et al.* 1999. Immunocytochemical localization of the dopamine transporter in human brain. *J Comp Neurol* **409**, 38–56.

Cole M G, Bellavance F and Mansour A. 1999. Prognosis of depression in elderly community and primary care populations: A systematic review and meta-analysis. *Am J Psychiatry* **156**, 1182–9.

Comley R, Parker C, Wishart M, Martarello L, Jakobsen S and Gunn R. 2006. In vivo evaluation and quantification of the 5-HT4 receptor PET ligand [11C]SB-207145. *Neuroimage* **31**, T23.

Conwell Y, Duberstein P R, Cox C, Herrmann J H, Forbes N T and Caine E D. 1996. Relationships of age and axis I diagnoses in victims of completed suicide: A psychological autopsy study. *Am J Psychiatry* **153**, 1001–08.

Cortes R, Soriano E, Pazos A, Probst A and Palacios J M. 1988. Autoradiography of antidepressant binding sites in the human brain: Localization using [3H]imipramine and [3H]paroxetine. *Neuroscience* **27**, 473–96.

Cowen P J. 1996. Advances in psychopharmacology: Mood disorders and dementia. *Br Med Bull* **52**, 539–55.

DaSilva J N, Lourenco C M, Meyer J H, Hussey D, Potter W Z and Houle S. 2002. Imaging cAMP-specific phosphodiesterase-4 in human brain with R-[(11C] rolipram and positron emission tomography. *Eur J Nucl Med Mol Imag* **29**, 1680–3.

David S P, Murthy N V, Rabiner E A, *et al.* 2005. A functional genetic variation of the serotonin (5-HT) transporter affects 5-HT1A receptor binding in humans. *J Neurosci* **25**, 2586–90.

Davis M R, Votaw J R, Bremner J D, *et al.* 2003. Initial human PET imaging studies with the dopamine transporter ligand 18F-FECNT. *J Nucl Med* **44**, 855–61.

Dewey S L, MacGregor R R, Brodie J D, *et al.* 1990. Mapping muscarinic receptors in human and baboon brain using [N-11C-methyl]-benztropine. *Synapse* **5**, 213–23.

Dewey S L, Smith G, Logan J, Brodie J D, Fowler J S and Wolf A P. 1993. Striatal binding of the PET ligand 11C-raclopride is altered by drugs that modify synaptic dopamine levels. *Synapse* **13**, 350–6.

Dilsaver S C. 1986. Cholinergic mechanisms in depression. *Brain Res* **396**, 285–316.

Ding Y S, Lin K S and Logan J. 2006. PET imaging of norepinephrine transporters. *Curr Pharm Des* **12**, 3831–45.

Drevets W C, Frank E, Price J C, *et al.* 1999. PET imaging of serotonin 1A receptor binding in depression. *Biol Psychiatry* **46**, 1375–87.

Drevets W C, Frank E, Price J C, Kupfer D J, Greer P J and Mathis C. 2000. Serotonin type-1A receptor imaging in depression. *Nucl Med Biol* **27**, 499–507.

Duman R S, Heninger G R and Nestler E J. 1997. A molecular and cellular theory of depression. *Arch Gen Psychiatry* **54**, 597–606.

Ebert D, Feistel H, Kaschka W, Barocka A and Pirner A. 1994. Single photon emission computerized tomography assessment of cerebral dopamine D2 receptor blockade in depression before and after sleep deprivation – Preliminary results. *Biol Psychiatry* **35**, 880–5.

Eckelman W C. 2001. Radiolabeled muscarinic radioligands for in vivo studies. *Nucl Med Biol* **28**, 485–91.

Eckelman W C, Reba R C, Rzeszotarski W J, *et al.* 1984. External imaging of cerebral muscarinic acetylcholine receptors. *Science* **223**, 291–3.

Efange S M. 2000. In vivo imaging of the vesicular acetylcholine transporter and the vesicular monoamine transporter. *Faseb J* **14**, 2401–13.

Erlandsson K, Sivananthan T, Lui D, *et al.* 2005. Measuring SSRI occupancy of SERT using the novel tracer [123I] ADAM: A SPECT validation study. *Eur J Nucl Med Mol Imaging* **32**, 1329–36.

Farde L, Ehrin E, Eriksson L, *et al.* 1985. Substituted benzamides as ligands for visualization of dopamine receptor binding in the human brain by positron emission tomography. *Proc Natl Acad Sci USA* **82**, 3863–7.

Farde L, Ito H, Swahn C G, Pike V W and Halldin C. 1998. Quantitative analyses of carbonyl-carbon-11-WAY-100635 binding to central 5-hydroxytryptamine-1A receptors in man. *J Nucl Med* **39**, 1965–71.

Ferrarese C, Guidotti A, Costa E, *et al.* 1991. In vivo study of NMDA-sensitive glutamate receptor by fluorothienylcyclohexylpiperidine, a possible ligand for positron emission tomography. *Neuropharmacology* **30**, 899–905.

First M, Spitzer R, Williams J and Gibbon M. 1995. *Structured Clinical Interview for DSM-IV-Non-Patient Edition* (SCID-NP, Version 1.0)., Washington, D.C.: American Psychiatric Press.

Fowler J S, MacGregor R R, Wolf A P, *et al.* 1987. Mapping human brain monoamine oxidase A and B with 11C-labeled suicide inactivators and PET. *Science* **235**, 481–5.

Francis P T, Pangalos M N, Stephens P H, *et al.* 1993. Antemortem measurements of neurotransmission: Possible implications for pharmacotherapy of Alzheimer's disease and depression. *J Neurol Neurosurg Psychiatry* **56**, 80–4.

Frankle W G, Lombardo I, New A S, *et al.* 2005. Brain serotonin transporter distribution in subjects with impulsive aggressivity: A positron emission study with [11C]McN 5652. *Am J Psychiatry* **162**, 915–23.

Frankle W G, Slifstein M, Gunn R N, *et al.* 2006. Estimation of serotonin transporter parameters with 11C-DASB in healthy humans: Reproducibility and comparison of methods. *J Nucl Med* **47**, 815–26.

Frey K A, Koeppe R A, Kilbourn M R, *et al.* 1996. Presynaptic monoaminergic vesicles in Parkinson's disease and normal aging. *Ann Neurol* **40**, 873–84.

Frokjaer V G, Mortensen E L, Nielsen F A, *et al.* 2008. Frontolimbic serotonin 2A receptor binding in healthy subjects is associated with personality risk factors for affective disorder. *Biol Psychiatry* **63**, 569–76.

Frost J J. 2001. PET imaging of the opioid receptor: The early years. *Nucl Med Biol* **28**, 509–13.

Frost J J, Rosier A J, Reich S G, *et al.* 1993. Positron emission tomographic imaging of the dopamine transporter with 11C-WIN 35,428 reveals marked declines in mild Parkinson's disease. *Ann Neurol* **34**, 423–31.

Frost J J, Wagner H N Jr, Dannals R F, *et al.* 1985. Imaging opiate receptors in the human brain by positron tomography. *J Comp Assist Tomog* **9**, 231–6.

Fujita M, Imaizumi M, Zoghbi S S, *et al.* 2008. Kinetic analysis in healthy humans of a novel positron emission tomography radioligand to image the peripheral benzodiazepine receptor, a potential biomarker for inflammation. *Neuroimage* **40**, 43–52.

Furey M L and Drevets W C. 2006. Antidepressant efficacy of the antimuscarinic drug scopolamine: A randomized, placebo-controlled clinical trial. *Arch Gen Psychiatry* **63**, 1121–9.

Garnett E S, Firnau G and Nahmias C. 1983. Dopamine visualized in the basal ganglia of living man. *Nature* **305**, 137–8.

George T P, Sacco K A, Vessicchio J C, Weinberger A H and Shytle R D. 2008. Nicotinic antagonist augmentation of selective serotonin reuptake inhibitor-refractory major depressive disorder: A preliminary study. *J Clin Psychopharmacol* **28**, 340–4.

Ginovart N, Meyer J H, Boovariwala A *et al.* 2006. Positron emission tomography quantification of [11C]-harmine binding to monoamine oxidase-A in the human brain. *J Cereb Blood Flow Metab* **26**, 330–44.

Ginovart N, Wilson A A, Meyer J H, Hussey D and Houle S. 2001. Positron emission tomography quantification of [(11)C]-DASB binding to the human serotonin transporter: Modeling strategies. *J Cereb Blood Flow Metab* **21**, 1342–53.

Giovacchini G, Chang M C, Channing M A, *et al.* 2002. Brain incorporation of [11C]arachidonic acid in young healthy humans measured with positron emission tomography. *J Cereb Blood Flow Metab* **22**, 1453–62.

Hall H, Halldin C, Farde L and Sedvall G. 1998. Whole hemisphere autoradiography of the postmortem human brain. *Nucl Med Biol* **25**, 715–9.

Halldin C, Farde L, Hogberg T, *et al.* 1995. Carbon-11-FLB 457: A radioligand for extrastriatal D2 dopamine receptors. *J Nucl Med* **36**, 1275–81.

Halldin C, Foged C, Chou Y H, *et al.* 1998. Carbon-11-NNC 112: A radioligand for PET examination of striatal and neocortical D1-dopamine receptors. *J Nucl Med* **39**, 2061–8.

Hargreaves R. 2002. Imaging substance P receptors (NK1) in the living human brain using positron emission tomography. *J Clin Psychiatry* **63**, 18–24.

Hariri A R, Mattay V S, Tessitore A, *et al.* 2002. Serotonin transporter genetic variation and the response of the human amygdala. *Science* **297**, 400–3.

Hartvig P, Agren H, Reibring L, *et al.* 1991. Brain kinetics of L-[beta-11C]dopa in humans studied by positron emission tomography. *J Neural Transm Gen Sect* **86**, 25–41.

Hashimoto K, Nishiyama S, Ohba H, *et al.* 2008. [11C] CHIBA-1001 as a novel PET ligand for alpha7 nicotinic receptors in the brain: A PET study in conscious monkeys. *PLoS ONE* **3**, e3231.

Heiss W D. 2009. The potential of PET/MR for brain imaging. *Eur J Nucl Med Mol Imaging* **36**(Suppl 1), S105–12.

Heiss W D and Herholz K. 2006. Brain receptor imaging. *J Nucl Med* **47**, 302–12.

Henriksson M M, Marttunen M J, Isometsa E T, *et al.* 1995. Mental disorders in elderly suicide. *Int Psychogeriatr* **7**, 275–86.

Hirvonen J, Aalto S, Hagelberg N, *et al.* 2009. Measurement of central micro-opioid receptor binding in vivo with PET and [(11)C]carfentanil: A test–retest study in healthy subjects. *Eur J Nucl Med Mol Imaging* **36**, 275–86.

Hirvonen J, Karlsson H, Kajander J, *et al.* 2008. Striatal dopamine D2 receptors in medication-naïve patients with major depressive disorder as assessed with [11C] raclopride PET. *Psychopharmacology (Berl)* **197**, 581–90.

Holsboer F. 2000. The corticosteroid receptor hypothesis of depression. *Neuropsychopharmacology* **23**, 477–501.

Horti A G, Chefer S I, Mukhin A G, *et al.* 2000. 6-[18F] fluoro-A-85380, a novel radioligand for in vivo imaging of central nicotinic acetylcholine receptors. *Life Sci* **67**, 463–9.

Houle S, Ginovart N, Hussey D, Meyer J H and Wilson A A. 2000. Imaging the serotonin transporter with positron emission tomography: Initial human studies with [11C] DAPP and [11C]DASB. *Eur J Nucl Med* **27**, 1719–22.

Hoyer D, Pazos A, Probst A and Palacios J M. 1986a. Serotonin receptors in the human brain. I. Characterization and autoradiographic localization of 5-HT1A recognition sites. Apparent absence of 5-HT1B recognition sites. *Brain Res* **376**, 85–96.

Hoyer D, Pazos A, Probst A and Palacios J M. 1986b. Serotonin receptors in the human brain. II. Characterization and autoradiographic localization of 5-HT1C and 5-HT2 recognition sites. *Brain Res* **376**, 97–107.

Huang Y, Kegeles L S, Bae S, *et al.* 2001. Synthesis of potent and selective dopamine D(4) antagonists as candidate radioligands. *Bioorg Med Chem Lett* **11**, 1375–7.

Hwang D R, Kegeles L S and Laruelle M. 2000. (–)-*N*-[(11)C] propyl-norapomorphine: A positron-labeled dopamine agonist for PET imaging of D(2) receptors. *Nucl Med Biol* **27**, 533–9.

Ichimiya T, Suhara T, Sudo Y, *et al.* 2002. Serotonin transporter binding in patients with mood disorders: A PET study with [11C](+)McN5652. *Biol Psychiatry* **51**, 715–22.

Ikoma Y, Suhara T, Toyama H, *et al.* 2002. Quantitative analysis for estimating binding potential of the brain serotonin transporter with [11 C]McN5652. *J Cereb Blood Flow Metab* **22**, 490–501.

Ito H, Nyberg S, Halldin C, Lundkvist C and Farde L. 1998. PET imaging of central 5-HT2A receptors with carbon-11-MDL 100,907. *J Nucl Med* **39**, 208–14.

Junck L, Olson J M, Ciliax B J, *et al.* 1989. PET imaging of human gliomas with ligands for the peripheral benzodiazepine binding site. *Ann Neurol* **26**, 752–8.

Kapur S and Mann J J. 1992. Role of the dopaminergic system in depression. *Biol Psychiatry* **32**, 1–17.

Kato M and Serretti A. 2010. Review and meta-analysis of antidepressant pharmacogenetic findings in major depressive disorder. *Mol Psychiatry* **15**, 473–500.

Keller J, Schatzberg A F and Maj M. 2007. Current issues in the classification of psychotic major depression. *Schizophr Bull* **33**, 877–85.

Kessler R C, Chiu W T, Demler O, Merikangas K R and Walters E E. 2005. Prevalence, severity, and comorbidity of 12-month DSM-IV disorders in the national comorbidity survey replication. *Arch Gen Psychiatry* **62**, 617–27.

Kessler R M, Mason N S, Votaw J R, *et al.* 1992. Visualization of extrastriatal dopamine D2 receptors in the human brain. *Eur J Pharmacol* **223**, 105–7.

Kilts C D. 1994. Recent pharmacologic advances in antidepressant therapy. *Am J Med* **97**, 3S–12S.

Klein N, Sacher J, Geiss-Granadia T, *et al.* 2006. In vivo imaging of serotonin transporter occupancy by means of SPECT and [123I]ADAM in healthy subjects administered different doses of escitalopram or citalopram. *Psychopharmacology (Berl)* **188**, 263–72.

Klein N, Sacher J, Geiss-Granadia T, *et al.* 2007. Higher serotonin transporter occupancy after multiple dose administration of escitalopram compared to citalopram: An [123I]ADAM SPECT study. *Psychopharmacology (Berl)* **191**, 333–9.

Klimek V, Schenck J E, Han H, Stockmeier C A and Ordway G A. 2002. Dopaminergic abnormalities in amygdaloid nuclei in major depression: A postmortem study. *Biol Psychiatry* **52**, 740–8.

Klimke A, Larisch R, Janz A, Vosberg H, Muller-Gartner H W and Gaebel W. 1999. Dopamine D2 receptor binding before and after treatment of major depression measured by [123I]IBZM SPECT. *Psychiatry Res* **90**, 91–101.

Koeppe R A, Frey K A, Snyder S E, Meyer P, Kilbourn M R and Kuhl D E. 1999. Kinetic modeling of *N*-[11C] methylpiperidin-4-yl propionate: Alternatives for analysis of an irreversible positron emission tomography trace for measurement of acetylcholinesterase activity in human brain. *J Cereb Blood Flow Metab* **19**, 1150–63.

Koeppe R A, Holthoff V A, Frey K A, Kilbourn M R and Kuhl D E. 1991. Compartmental analysis of [11C] flumazenil kinetics for the estimation of ligand transport rate and receptor distribution using positron emission tomography. *J Cereb Blood Flow Metab* **11**, 735–44.

Krishnan V and Nestler E J. 2008. The molecular neurobiology of depression. *Nature* **455**, 894–902.

Kugaya A, Sanacora G, Staley J K, *et al.* 2004. Brain serotonin transporter availability predicts treatment response to selective serotonin reuptake inhibitors. *Biol Psychiatry* **56**, 497–502.

Kugaya A, Seneca N M, Snyder P J, *et al.* 2003. Changes in human in vivo serotonin and dopamine transporter availabilities during chronic antidepressant administration. *Neuropsychopharmacology* **28**, 413–20.

Kuhl D E, Koeppe R A, Fessler J A, *et al.* 1994. In vivo mapping of cholinergic neurons in the human brain using SPECT and IBVM. *J Nucl Med* **35**, 405–10.

Kung H F, Alavi A, Chang W, *et al.* 1990. In vivo SPECT imaging of CNS D-2 dopamine receptors: Initial studies with iodine-123-IBZM in humans. *J Nucl Med* **31**, 573–9.

Kung M P, Hou C, Oya S, Mu M, Acton P D and Kung H F. 1999. Characterization of [(123)I]IDAM as a novel single-photon emission tomography tracer for serotonin transporters. *Eur J Nucl Med* **26**, 844–53.

Laruelle M, van Dyck C, Abi-Dargham A, *et al.* 1994. Compartmental modeling of iodine-123-iodobenzofuran binding to dopamine D2 receptors in healthy subjects. *J Nucl Med* **35**, 743–54.

Leopoldo M, Berardi F, Colabufo N A, *et al.* 2002. Structure–affinity relationship study on *N*-[4-(4-arylpiperazin-1-yl)butyl]arylcarboxamides as potent and selective dopamine D(3) receptor ligands. *J Med Chem* **45**, 5727–35.

Lesch K P, Bengel D, Heils A, *et al.* 1996. Association of anxiety-related traits with a polymorphism in the serotonin transporter gene regulatory region. *Science* **274**, 1527–31.

Leysen J E. 1990. Gaps and peculiarities in 5-HT2 receptor studies. *Neuropsychopharmacology* **3**, 361–9.

Lopez J F, Chalmers D T, Little K Y and Watson S J. 1998. A.E. Bennett research award. Regulation of serotonin1A, glucocorticoid, and mineralocorticoid receptor in rat and human hippocampus: Implications for the neurobiology of depression. *Biol Psychiatry* **43**, 547–73.

Lu B and Gottschalk W. 2000. Modulation of hippocampal synaptic transmission and plasticity by neurotrophins. *Progr Brain Res* **128**, 231–41.

Lundkvist C, Halldin C, Ginovart N, *et al.* 1996. [11C] MDL 100907, a radioligand for selective imaging of 5-HT(2A) receptors with positron emission tomography. *Life Sci* **58**, PL 187–92.

Maes M and Meltzer H. 1995. The serotonin hypothesis of major depression. In Bloom Kupfer F (ed.) *Psychopharmacology: The Fourth Generation of Progress.* New York, NY: Raven Press, pp. 933–44.

Malison R T, Price L H, Berman R, *et al.* 1998. Reduced brain serotonin transporter availability in major depression as measured by [123I]-2 beta-carbomethoxy-3 beta-(4-iodophenyl)tropane and single photon emission computed tomography. *Biol Psychiatry* **44**, 1090–8.

Mann J J. 1999. Role of the serotonergic system in the pathogenesis of major depression and suicidal behavior. *Neuropsychopharmacology* **21**, 99S–105S.

Mann J J, Huang Y Y, Underwood M D, *et al.* 2000. A serotonin transporter gene promoter polymorphism (5-HTTLPR) and prefrontal cortical binding in major depression and suicide. *Arch Gen Psychiatry* **57**, 729–38.

Marek G J and Aghajanian G K. 1998. The electrophysiology of prefrontal serotonin systems: Therapeutic implications for mood and psychosis. *Biol Psychiatry* **44**, 1118–27.

Marner L, Gillings N, Gunn R, *et al.* 2007. Quantification of 11C-SB207145-PET for 5-HT4 receptors in the human brain: Preliminary results. *J Nucl Med Meeting Abstracts* **48**, 159P.

Martarello L, Kilts C D, Ely T, *et al.* 2001. Synthesis and characterization of fluorinated and iodinated pyrrolopyrimidines as PET/SPECT ligands for the CRF1 receptor. *Nucl Med Biol* **28**, 187–95.

Massou J M, Trichard C, Attar-Levy D, *et al.* 1997. Frontal 5-HT2A receptors studied in depressive patients during chronic treatment by selective serotonin reuptake inhibitors. *Psychopharmacology* **133**, 99–101.

Mathew S J, Manji H K and Charney D S. 2008. Novel drugs and therapeutic targets for severe mood disorders. *Neuropsychopharmacology* **33**, 2080–92.

Mathis C A, Wang Y, Holt D P, Huang G F, Debnath M L and Klunk W E. 2003. Synthesis and evaluation of (11)C-labeled 6-substituted 2-arylbenzothiazoles as amyloid imaging agents. *J Med Chem* **46**, 2740–54.

Mayberg H S. 2003. Modulating dysfunctional limbic-cortical circuits in depression: Towards development of brain-based algorithms for diagnosis and optimised treatment. *Br Med Bull* **65**, 193–207.

Meador-Woodruff J H, Mansour A, Bunzow J R, Van Tol H H, Watson S J Jr and Civelli O. 1989. Distribution of D2 dopamine receptor mRNA in rat brain. *Proc Natl Acad Sci USA* **86**, 7625–8.

Meltzer C C, Price J C, Mathis C A, *et al.* 1999. PET imaging of serotonin type 2A receptors in late-life neuropsychiatric disorders. *Am J Psychiatry* **156**, 1871–8.

Meltzer C C, Price J C, Mathis C A, *et al.* 2004. Serotonin 1A receptor binding and treatment response in late-life depression. *Neuropsychopharmacology* **29**, 2258–65.

Meltzer C C, Smith G, DeKosky S T, *et al.* 1998. Serotonin in aging, late-life depression, and alzheimer's disease: The emerging role of functional imaging. *Neuropsychopharmacology* **18**, 407–30.

Mengod G, Pompeiano M, Martínez-Mir M I and Palacios J M. 1990. Localization of the mRNA for the 5-HT2 receptor by in situ hybridization histochemistry. Correlation with the distribution of receptor sites. *Brain Res* **524**, 139–43.

Merikangas K R, Akiskal H S, Angst J, *et al.* 2007. Lifetime and 12-month prevalence of bipolar spectrum disorder in the national comorbidity survey replication. *Arch Gen Psychiatry* **64**, 543–52.

Mervaala E, Könönen M, Föhr J, *et al.* 2001. SPECT and neuropsychological performance in severe depression treated with ECT. *J Affect Disord* **66**, 47–58.

Messa C, Colombo C, Moresco R M, *et al.* 2003. 5-HT (2A) receptor binding is reduced in drug-naive and unchanged in SSRI-responder depressed patients compared to healthy controls: A PET study. *Psychopharmacology* **167**, 72–8.

Meyer J H. 2007. Imaging the serotonin transporter during major depressive disorder and antidepressant treatment. *J Psychiatry Neurosci* **32**, 86–102.

Meyer J H, Cho R, Kennedy S and Kapur S. 1999a. The effects of single dose nefazodone and paroxetine upon 5-HT2A binding potential in humans using [18F]-setoperone PET. *Psychopharmacology* **144**, 279–81.

Meyer J H, Ginovart N, Boovariwala A, *et al.* 2006. Elevated monoamine oxidase a levels in the brain: An explanation for the monoamine imbalance of major depression. *Arch Gen Psychiatry* **63**, 1209–16.

Meyer J H, Houle S, Sagrati S, *et al.* 2004. Brain serotonin transporter binding potential measured with carbon 11-labeled DASB positron emission tomography: Effects of major depressive episodes and severity of dysfunctional attitudes. *Arch Gen Psychiatry* **61**, 1271–9.

Meyer J H, Kapur S, Houle S, *et al.* 1999b. Prefrontal cortex 5-HT2 receptors in depression: An [18F]setoperone PET imaging study. *Am J Psychiatry* **156**, 1029–34.

Meyer J H, Kruger S, Wilson A A, *et al.* 2001a. Lower dopamine transporter binding potential in striatum during depression. *Neuroreport* **12**, 4121–5.

Meyer J H, McMain S, Kennedy S H, *et al.* 2003. Dysfunctional attitudes and 5-HT2 receptors during depression and self-harm. *Am J Psychiatry* **160**, 90–9.

Meyer J H, Wilson A A, Ginovart N, *et al.* 2001b. Occupancy of serotonin transporters by paroxetine and citalopram during treatment of depression: A [(11)C] DASB PET imaging study. *Am J Psychiatry* **158**, 1843–9.

Milak M S, Severance A J, Ogden R T, *et al.* 2008. Modeling considerations for 11C-CUMI-101, an agonist radiotracer for imaging serotonin 1A receptor in vivo with PET. *J Nucl Med* **49**, 587–96.

Miller J M, Oquendo M A, Ogden R T, Mann J J and Parsey R V. 2008. Serotonin transporter binding as a possible predictor of one-year remission in major depressive disorder. *J Psychiatric Res* **42**, 1137–44.

Montgomery A J, Thielemans K, Mehta M A, Turkheimer F, Mustafovic S and Grasby P M. 2006. Correction of head movement on PET studies: Comparison of methods. *J Nucl Med* **47**, 1936–44.

Moresco R M, Colombo C, Fazio F, *et al.* 2000. Effects of fluvoxamine treatment on the in vivo binding of [F-18] FESP in drug naive depressed patients: A PET study. *Neuroimage* **12**, 452–65.

Moses-Kolko E L, Wisner K L, Price J C, *et al.* 2008. Serotonin 1A receptor reductions in postpartum depression: A positron emission tomography study. *Fertil Steril* **89**, 685–92.

Mukherjee J, Christian B T, Dunigan K A, *et al.* 2002. Brain imaging of 18F-fallypride in normal volunteers: Blood analysis, distribution, test–retest studies, and preliminary assessment of sensitivity to aging effects on dopamine D-2/D-3 receptors. *Synapse* **46**, 170–88.

Muller-Gartner H W, Wilson A A, Dannals R F, Wagner H N Jr and Frost J J. 1992. Imaging muscarinic cholinergic receptors in human brain in vivo with Spect, [123I]4-iododexetimide, and [123I] 4-iodolevetimide. *J Cereb Blood Flow Metab* **12**, 562–70.

Mullins D, Adham N, Hesk D, *et al.* 2008. Identification and characterization of pseudoirreversible nonpeptide antagonists of the neuropeptide Y Y(5) receptor and development of a novel Y(5)-selective radioligand. *Eur J Pharmacol* **601**, 1–7.

Murray C. 1996. *Rethinking DALYs. The Global Burden of Disease: A Comprehensive Assessment of Mortality and Disability from Diseases, Injuries, and Risk Factors in 1990 and Projected to 2020*. Boston, MA: Harvard School of Public Health.

Myers R and Hume S. 2002. Small animal PET. *Eur Neuropsychopharmacol* **12**, 545–55.

Nestler E J and Carlezon W A Jr. 2006. The mesolimbic dopamine reward circuit in depression. *Biol Psychiatry* **59**, 1151–9.

Newberg A B, Amsterdam J D, Wintering N, *et al.* 2005. 123I-ADAM binding to serotonin transporters in patients with major depression and healthy controls: A preliminary study. *J Nucl Med* **46**, 973–7.

Nobler M S, Mann J J and Sackeim H A. 1999a. Serotonin, cerebral blood flow, and cerebral metabolic rate in geriatric major depression and normal aging. *Brain Res* **30**, 250–63.

Nobler M S, Pelton G H and Sackeim H A. 1999b. Cerebral blood flow and metabolism in late-life depression and dementia. *J Geriatric Psychiatry Neurol* **12**, 118–27.

Nomura M and Nomura Y. 2006. Psychological, neuroimaging, and biochemical studies on functional association between impulsive behavior and the 5-HT2A receptor gene polymorphism in humans. *Ann N Y Acad Sci* **1086**, 134–43.

Nordberg A, Lundqvist H, Hartvig P, Lilja A and Langstrom B. 1995. Kinetic analysis of regional (S) (–)11C-nicotine binding in normal and Alzheimer brains – in vivo assessment using positron emission tomography. *Alzheimer Dis Assoc Disord* **9**, 21–7.

Ohayon M M and Schatzberg A F. 2002. Prevalence of depressive episodes with psychotic features in the general population. *Am J Psychiatry* **159**, 1855–61.

Okazawa H, Leyton M, Benkelfat C, Mzengeza S and Diksic M. 2000. Statistical mapping analysis of serotonin synthesis images generated in healthy volunteers using positron-emission tomography and alpha-[11C]methyl-L-tryptophan. *J Psychiatry Neurosci* **5**, 359–70.

Oquendo M A, Hastings R S, Huang Y Y, *et al.* 2007. Brain serotonin transporter binding in depressed patients with bipolar disorder using positron emission tomography. *Arch Gen Psychiatry* **64**, 201–08.

Owens M J and Nemeroff C B. 1994. Role of serotonin in the pathophysiology of depression: Focus on the serotonin transporter. *Clin Chem* **40**, 288–95.

Pappata S, Tavitian B, Traykov L, *et al.* 1996. In vivo imaging of human cerebral acetylcholinesterase. *J Neurochem* **67**, 876–9.

Parker C A, Cunningham V J, Martarello L, *et al.* 2008. Evaluation of the novel 5-HT6 receptor radioligand, [11C]GSK-215083 in human. *Neuroimage* **41**, T20.

Parsey R V, Hastings R S, Oquendo M A, *et al.* 2006a. Lower serotonin transporter binding potential in the human brain during major depressive episodes. *Am J Psychiatry* **163**, 52–8.

Parsey R V, Kegeles L S, Hwang D R, *et al.* 2000. In vivo quantification of brain serotonin transporters in humans using [11C]McN 5652. *J Nucl Med* **41**, 1465–77.

Parsey R V, Kent J M, Oquendo M A, *et al.* 2006b. Acute occupancy of brain serotonin transporter by sertraline as measured by [11C]DASB and positron emission tomography. *Biol Psychiatry* **59**, 821–8.

Parsey R V, Oquendo M A, Ogden R T, *et al.* 2006c. Altered serotonin 1A binding in major depression: A [carbonyl-C-11]WAY100635 positron emission tomography study. *Biol Psychiatry* **59**, 106–13.

Parsey R V, Oquendo M A, Simpson N R, *et al.* 2002. Effects of sex, age, and aggressive traits in man on brain serotonin 5-HT1A receptor binding potential measured by PET using [C-11]WAY-100635. *Brain Res* **954**, 173–82.

Parsey R V, Oquendo M A, Zea-Ponce Y, *et al.* 2001. Dopamine D(2) receptor availability and amphetamine-induced dopamine release in unipolar depression. *Biol Psychiatry* **50**, 313–22.

Pazos A, Probst A and Palacios J M. 1987. Serotonin receptors in the human brain – III. Autoradiographic mapping of serotonin-1 receptors. *Neuroscience* **21**, 97–122.

Pearlson G D, Wong D F, Tune L E, *et al.* 1995. In vivo D2 dopamine receptor density in psychotic and nonpsychotic patients with bipolar disorder. *Arch Gen Psychiatry* **52**, 471–7.

Peroutka S J. 1995. 5-HT receptors: Past, present and future. *Trends Neurosci* **18**, 68–9.

Pierson M E, Andersson J, Nyberg S, *et al.* 2008. [11C] AZ10419369: A selective 5-HT1B receptor radioligand suitable for positron emission tomography (PET). Characterization in the primate brain. *Neuroimage* **41**, 1075–85.

Pifferi F, Tremblay S, Plourde M, Tremblay-Mercier J, Bentourkia M and Cunnane S C. 2008. Ketones and brain function: Possible link to polyunsaturated fatty acids and availability of a new brain PET tracer, 11C-acetoacetate. *Epilepsia* **49** (Suppl 8), 76–9.

Pike V W, Halldin C, Nobuhara K, *et al.* 2003. Radioiodinated SB 207710 as a radioligand in vivo: Imaging of brain 5-HT4 receptors with SPET. *Eur J Nucl Med Mol Imaging* **30**, 1520–8.

Pike V W, McCarron J A, Lammertsma A A, *et al.* 1996. Exquisite delineation of 5-HT1A receptors in human brain with PET and [carbonyl-11 C]WAY-100635. *Eur J Pharmacol* **301**, R5–7.

Pirker W, Asenbaum S, Hauk M, *et al.* 2000. Imaging serotonin and dopamine transporters with 123I-beta-CIT SPECT: Binding kinetics and effects of normal aging. *J Nucl Med* **41**, 36–44.

Podruchny T A, Connolly C, Bokde A, *et al.* 2003. In vivo muscarinic 2 receptor imaging in cognitively normal young and older volunteers. *Synapse* **48**, 39–44.

Pogarell O, Koch W, Pöpperl G, *et al.* 2007. Acute prefrontal rTMS increases striatal dopamine to a similar degree as D-amphetamine. *Psychiatry Res* **156**, 251–5.

Price J C, Kelley D E, Ryan C M, *et al.* 2002. Evidence of increased serotonin-1A receptor binding in type 2 diabetes: A positron emission tomography study. *Brain Res* **927**, 97–103.

Psychiatric GWAS Consortium Steering Committee. 2009. A framework for interpreting genome-wide association studies of psychiatric disorders. *Mol Psychiatry* **14**, 10–7.

Rahmim A, Dinelle K, Cheng J C, *et al.* 2008. Accurate event-driven motion compensation in high-resolution

PET incorporating scattered and random events. *IEEE Trans Med Imaging* **27**, 1018–33.

Raison C L, Capuron L and Miller A H. 2006. Cytokines sing the blues: Inflammation and the pathogenesis of depression. *Trends Immunol* **27**, 24–31.

Rapoport S I. 2008. Brain arachidonic and docosahexaenoic acid cascades are selectively altered by drugs, diet and disease. *Prostagland Leukot Essen Fatty Acids* **79**, 153–6.

Rausch J L, Stahl S M and Hauger R L. 1990. Cortisol and growth hormone responses to the 5-HT1A agonist gepirone in depressed patients. *Biol Psychiatry* **28**, 73–8.

Reid A E, Ding Y S, Eckelman W C, *et al.* 2008. Comparison of the pharmacokinetics of different analogs of 11C-labeled TZTP for imaging muscarinic M2 receptors with PET. *Nucl Med Biol* **35**, 287–98.

Reimold M, Batra A, Knobel A, *et al.* 2008. Anxiety is associated with reduced central serotonin transporter availability in unmedicated patients with unipolar major depression: A [11C]DASB PET study. *Mol Psychiatry* **13**, 606–13, 557.

Ressler K J and Mayberg H S. 2007. Targeting abnormal neural circuits in mood and anxiety disorders: From the laboratory to the clinic. *Nature Neurosci* **10**, 1116–24.

Riccardi P, Li R, Ansari M S, *et al.* 2006. Amphetamine-induced displacement of [18F] fallypride in striatum and extrastriatal regions in humans. *Neuropsychopharmacology* **31**, 1016–26.

Riemann B, Schafers K P, Schober O and Schafers M. 2008. Small animal PET in preclinical studies: Opportunities and challenges. *Q J Nucl Med Mol Imaging* **52**, 215–21.

Rosa-Neto P, Diksic M, Okazawa H, *et al.* 2004. Measurement of brain regional alpha-[11C]methyl-L-tryptophan trapping as a measure of serotonin synthesis in medication-free patients with major depression. *Arch Gen Psychiatry* **61**, 556–63.

Rousset O G, Collins D L, Rahmim A and Wong D F. 2008. Design and implementation of an automated partial volume correction in PET: Application to dopamine receptor quantification in the normal human striatum. *J Nucl Med* **49**, 1097–106.

Rowland D J and Cherry S R. 2008. Small-animal preclinical nuclear medicine instrumentation and methodology. *Semin Nucl Med* **38**, 209–22.

Sacher J, Asenbaum S, Klein N, *et al.* 2007. Binding kinetics of 123I[ADAM] in healthy controls: A selective SERT radioligand. *Int J Neuropsychopharmacol* **10**, 211–8.

Sargent P A, Kjaer K H, Bench C J, *et al.* 2000. Brain serotonin1A receptor binding measured by positron emission tomography with [11C]WAY-100635: Effects of depression and antidepressant treatment. *Arch Gen Psychiatry* **57**, 174–80.

Satyamurthy N, Barrio J R, Bida G T, Huang S C, Mazziotta J C and Phelps M E. 1990. 3-(2'-[18F] fluoroethyl)spiperone, a potent dopamine antagonist: synthesis, structural analysis and in-vivo utilization in humans. *Int J Radiat App Instrument – Part A, Appl Radiat Isotopes* **41**, 113–29.

Saudou F and Hen R. 1994. 5-Hydroxytryptamine receptor subtypes in vertebrates and invertebrates. *Neurochem Int* **25**, 503–32.

Schatzberg A F. 2002. Brain imaging in affective disorders: More questions about causes versus effects. *Am J Psychiatry* **159**, 1807–8.

Schotte A, Maloteaux J M and Laduron P M. 1983. Characterization and regional distribution of serotonin S2-receptors in human brain. *Brain Res* **276**, 231–5.

Schou M, Pike V W and Halldin C. 2007. Development of radioligands for imaging of brain norepinephrine transporters in vivo with positron emission tomography. *Curr Top Med Chem* **7**, 1806–16.

Sen S, Nesse R M, Stoltenberg S F, *et al.* 2003. A BDNF coding variant is associated with the NEO personality inventory domain neuroticism, a risk factor for depression. *Neuropsychopharmacology* **28**, 397–401.

Shank R P, Vaught J L, Pelley K A, Setler P E, McComsey D F and Maryanoff B E. 1988. McN-5652: A highly potent inhibitor of serotonin uptake. *J Pharmacol Exp Therap* **247**, 1032–8.

Shidahara M, Tsoumpas C, Hammers A, *et al.* 2009. Functional and structural synergy for resolution recovery and partial volume correction in brain PET. *Neuroimage* **44**, 340–8.

Shioe K, Ichimiya T, Suhara T, *et al.* 2003. No association between genotype of the promoter region of serotonin transporter gene and serotonin transporter binding in human brain measured by PET. *Synapse* **48**, 184–8.

Shiue C Y, Shiue G G, Mozley P D, *et al.* 1997a. P-[18F]-MPPF: A potential radioligand for PET studies of 5-HT1A receptors in humans. *Synapse* **25**, 147–54.

Shiue C Y, Vallabhahosula S, Wolf A P, *et al.* 1997b. Carbon-11 labelled ketamine-synthesis, distribution in mice and PET studies in baboons. *Nucl Med Biol* **24**, 145–50.

Shoghi-Jadid K, Small G W, Agdeppa E D, *et al.* 2002. Localization of neurofibrillary tangles and beta-amyloid plaques in the brains of living patients with Alzheimer disease. *Am J Geriat Psychiatry* **10**, 24–35.

Simpson S, Talbot P R, Snowden J S and Neary D. 1997. Subcortical vascular disease in elderly patients with treatment resistant depression. *J Neurol Neurosurg Psychiatry* **62**, 196–7.

Smith G, Dewey S L, Brodie J D, *et al.* 1997. Serotonergic modulation of dopamine measured with [11C]raclopride and PET in normal human subjects. *Am J Psychiatry* **154**, 490–6.

Smith G, Kahn A, Hanratty K, *et al.* 2008. Serotonin transporter occupancy by citalopram treatment in geriatric depression. *Neuroimage* **41**, T168.

Smith G, Kramer E, Hermann C, *et al.* 2009a. Serotonin modulation of cerebral glucose metabolism in geriatric depression. *Biol Psychiatry* **66**, 259–66.

Smith G, Kramer E, Hermann C, *et al.* 2009b. The functional neuroanatomy of geriatric depression. *Int J Geriatric Psychiatry* **24**, 798–808.

Smith G, Lotrich F, Malhotra A, *et al.* 2004. The effect of serotonin transporter polymorphisms on serotonin function. *Neuropsychopharmacology* **29**, 2226–34.

Smith G, Price J C, Lopresti B J, *et al.* 1998. Test–retest variability of serotonin 5-HT2A receptor binding measured with positron emission tomography and [18F] altanserin in the human brain. *Synapse* **30**, 380–92.

Smith G S, Gunning-Dixon F M, Lotrich F E, Taylor W D and Evans J D. 2007. Translational research in late-life mood disorders: implications for future intervention and prevention research. *Neuropsychopharmacology* **32**, 1857–75.

Smith G S, Ma Y, Dhawan V, Chaly T and Eidelberg D. 2009. Selective serotonin reuptake inhibitor (SSRI) modulation of striatal dopamine measured with [11C]-raclopride and positron emission tomography. *Synapse* **63**, 1–6.

Smith J S, Zubieta J K, Price J C, *et al.* 1999. Quantification of delta-opioid receptors in human brain with N1'-([11C]methyl) naltrindole and positron emission tomography. *J Cereb Blood Flow Metab* **19**, 956–66.

Smolka M N, Schumann G, Wrase J, *et al.* 2005. Catechol-O-methyltransferase val158met genotype affects processing of emotional stimuli in the amygdala and prefrontal cortex. *J Neurosci* **25**, 836–42.

Sokoloff P, Giros B, Martres M P, Bouthenet M L and Schwartz J C. 1990. Molecular cloning and characterization of a novel dopamine receptor (D3) as a target for neuroleptics. *Nature* **347**, 146–51.

Sorger D, Scheunemann M, Grossmann U, *et al.* 2008. A new 18F-labeled fluoroacetylmorpholino derivative of vesamicol for neuroimaging of the vesicular acetylcholine transporter. *Nucl Med Biol* **35**, 185–95.

Sotelo C, Cholley B, El Mestikawy S, Gozlan H and Hamon M. 1990. Direct immunohistochemical evidence of the existence of 5-HT1A autoreceptors on serotoninergic neurons in the midbrain raphe nuclei. *Eur J Neurosci* **2**, 1144–54.

Staley J K, van Dyck C H, Weinzimmer D, *et al.* 2005. 123I-5-IA-85380 SPECT measurement of nicotinic acetylcholine receptors in human brain by the constant infusion paradigm: Feasibility and reproducibility. *J Nucl Med* **46**, 1466–72.

Steiniger B, Kniess T, Bergmann R, Pietzsch J and Wuest F R. 2008. Radiolabeled glucocorticoids as molecular probes for imaging brain glucocorticoid receptors by means of positron emission tomography (PET). *Mini Rev Med Chem* **8**, 728–39.

Stephenson K A, van Oosten E M, Wilson A A, Meyer J H, Houle S and Vasdev N. 2008. Synthesis and preliminary evaluation of [(18)F]-fluoro-(2S)-exaprolol for imaging cerebral beta-adrenergic receptors with PET. *Neurochem Int* **53**, 173–9.

Stockmeier C A. 2003. Involvement of serotonin in depression: Evidence from postmortem and imaging studies of serotonin receptors and the serotonin transporter. *J Psychiatric Res* **37**, 357–73.

Stockmeier C A, Shapiro L A, Haycock J W, Thompson P A and Lowy M T. 1996. Quantitative subregional distribution of serotonin1A receptors and serotonin transporters in the human dorsal raphe. *Brain Res* **727**, 1–12.

Strafella A P, Paus T, Fraraccio M and Dagher A. 2003. Striatal dopamine release induced by repetitive transcranial magnetic stimulation of the human motor cortex. *Brain* **126**, 2609–15.

Strome E M, Clark C M, Zis A P and Doudet D J. 2005. Electroconvulsive shock decreases binding to 5-HT2 receptors in nonhuman primates: An in vivo positron emission tomography study with [18F]setoperone. *Biol Psychiatry* **57**, 1004–10.

Suehiro M, Scheffel U, Dannals R F, Ravert H T, Ricaurte G A and Wagner N H Jr. 1993. A PET radiotracer for studying serotonin uptake sites: Carbon-11-McN-5652Z. *J Nucl Med* **34**, 120–7.

Suhara T, Fukuda H, Inoue O, *et al.* 1991. Age-related changes in human D1 dopamine receptors measured by positron emission tomography. *Psychopharmacology* **103**, 41–5.

Suhara T, Higuchi M and Miyoshi M. 2008. Neuroimaging in dementia: In vivo amyloid imaging. *Tohoku J Exp Med* **215**, 119–24.

Suhara T, Inoue O, Kobayashi K, Suzuki K and Tateno Y. 1993. Age-related changes in human muscarinic acetylcholine receptors measured by positron emission tomography. *Neurosci Lett* **149**, 225–8.

Suhara T, Nakayama K, Inoue O, *et al.* 1992. D1 dopamine receptor binding in mood disorders measured by positron emission tomography. *Psychopharmacology* **106**, 14–8.

Sullivan G M, Parsey R V, Kumar J S, *et al.* 2007. PET imaging of CRF1 with [11C]R121920 and [11C] DMP696: Is the target of sufficient density? *Nucl Med Biol* **34**, 353–61.

Syvanen S, Eriksson J, Genchel T, Lindhe O, Antoni G and Langstrom B. 2007. Synthesis of two potential NK1-receptor ligands using [1–11C]ethyl iodide and [1–11C] propyl iodide and initial PET-imaging. *BMC Med Imaging* 7, 6.

Szabo Z, Kao P F, Scheffel U, *et al.* 1995. Positron emission tomography imaging of serotonin transporters in the human brain using [11C](+)McN5652. *Synapse* **20**, 37–43.

Szabo Z, McCann U D, Wilson A A, *et al.* 2002. Comparison of (+)-(11)C-McN5652 and (11)C-DASB as serotonin transporter radioligands under various experimental conditions. *J Nucl Med* **43**, 678–92.

Takano A, Arakawa R, Hayashi M, Takahashi H, Ito H and Suhara T. 2007. Relationship between neuroticism personality trait and serotonin transporter binding. *Biol Psychiatry* **62**, 588–92.

Takano A, Gulyas B, Varrone A, *et al.* 2008. Imaging the norepinephrine transporter with positron emission tomography: Initial human studies with (S,S)-[(18)F]FMeNER-D (2). *Eur J Nucl Med Mol Imaging* **35**, 153–7.

Tauscher J, Bagby R M, Javanmard M, Christensen B K, Kasper S and Kapur S. 2001. Inverse relationship between serotonin 5-HT(1A) receptor binding and anxiety: A [(11C)]WAY-100635 PET investigation in healthy volunteers. *Am J Psychiatry* **158**, 1326–8.

Tiihonen J, Kuoppamäki M, Någren K, *et al.* 1996. Serotonergic modulation of striatal D2 dopamine receptor binding in humans measured with positron emission tomography. *Psychopharmacology (Berl)* **126**, 277–80.

Tweedie D J and Burke M D. 1987. Metabolism of the beta-carbolines, harmine and harmol, by liver microsomes from phenobarbitone- or 3-methylcholanthrene-treated mice. Identification and quantitation of two novel harmine metabolites. *Drug Metab Disposition: Biol Fate Chem* **15**, 74–81.

van Heeringen C, Audenaert K, Van Laere K, *et al.* 2003. Prefrontal 5-HT2a receptor binding index, hopelessness and personality characteristics in attempted suicide. *J Affect Disord* **74**, 149–58.

Van Tol H H, Bunzow J R, Guan H C, *et al.* 1991. Cloning of the gene for a human dopamine D4 receptor with high affinity for the antipsychotic clozapine. *Nature* **350**, 610–4.

Varnas K, Halldin C and Hall H. 2004. Autoradiographic distribution of serotonin transporters and receptor subtypes in human brain. *Human Brain Mapp* **22**, 246–60.

Vasdev N, LaRonde F J, Woodgett J R, *et al.* 2008. Rationally designed PKA inhibitors for positron emission tomography: Synthesis and cerebral biodistribution of N-(2-(4-bromocinnamylamino)ethyl)-N-[11C]methyl-isoquinoline-5-sulfonamide. *Bioorg Med Chem* **16**, 5277–84.

Verhoeff N P, Wilson A A, Takeshita S, *et al.* 2004. In-vivo imaging of alzheimer disease beta-amyloid with [11C]SB-13 PET. *Am J Geriatr Psychiatry* **12**, 584–95.

Villemagne V L, Horti A, Scheffel U, *et al.* 1997. Imaging nicotinic acetylcholine receptors with fluorine-18-FPH, an epibatidine analog. *J Nucl Med* **38**, 1737–41.

Volkow N D, Ding Y S, Fowler J S, *et al.* 1995. A new PET ligand for the dopamine transporter: Studies in the human brain. *J Nucl Med* **36**, 2162–8.

Volkow N D, Fowler J S, Gatley S J, *et al.* 1996. PET evaluation of the dopamine system of the human brain. *J Nucl Med* **37**, 1242–56.

Volkow N D, Wang G J, Fowler J S, *et al.* 1994. Imaging endogenous dopamine competition with [11C]raclopride in the human brain. *Synapse* **16**, 255–62.

Wagner N H Jr, Burns H D, Dannals R F, *et al.* 1983. Imaging dopamine receptors in the human brain by positron tomography. *Science* **221**, 1264–6.

Weissman M M, Bland R C, Canino G J, *et al.* 1996. Cross-national epidemiology of major depression and bipolar disorder. *JAMA* **276**, 293–9.

Willeit M, Ginovart N, Kapur S, *et al.* 2006. High-affinity states of human brain dopamine D2/3 receptors imaged by the agonist [11C]-(+)-PHNO. *Biol Psychiatry* **59**, 389–94.

Willeit M, Praschak-Rieder N, Neumeister A, *et al.* 2000. [123I]-beta-CIT SPECT imaging shows reduced brain serotonin transporter availability in drug-free depressed patients with seasonal affective disorder. *Biol Psychiatry* **47**, 482–9.

Willeit M, Stastny J, Pirker W, *et al.* 2001. No evidence for in vivo regulation of midbrain serotonin transporter availability by serotonin transporter promoter gene polymorphism. *Biol Psychiatry* **50**, 8–12.

Wilson A A, Garcia A, Parkes J, *et al.* 2008. Radiosynthesis and initial evaluation of [18F]-FEPPA for PET imaging of peripheral benzodiazepine receptors. *Nucl Med Biol* **35**, 305–14.

Wilson A A, Ginovart N, Hussey D, Meyer J and Houle S. 2002. In vitro and in vivo characterisation of [11C]-DASB: A probe for in vivo measurements of the serotonin transporter by positron emission tomography. *Nucl Med Biol* **29**, 509–15.

Wong D F, Tauscher J and Grunder G. 2009. The role of imaging in proof of concept for CNS drug discovery and development. *Neuropsychopharmacology* **34**, 187–203.

Wong D F, Wagner N H Jr, Dannals R F, *et al.* 1984. Effects of age on dopamine and serotonin receptors measured by positron tomography in the living human brain. *Science* **226**, 1393–6.

Xiang L, Szebeni K, Szebeni A, *et al.* 2008. Dopamine receptor gene expression in human amygdaloid nuclei: Elevated D4 receptor mRNA in major depression. *Brain Res* **1207**, 214–24.

Yasuno F, Ota M, Kosaka J, *et al.* 2008. Increased binding of peripheral benzodiazepine receptor in Alzheimer's disease measured by positron emission tomography with [11C]DAA1106. *Biol Psychiatry* **64**, 835–41.

Yasuno F, Sanabria S M, Burns D, *et al.* 2007. PET imaging of neurokinin-1 receptors with [(18)F]SPA-RQ in human subjects: Assessment of reference tissue models and their test–retest reproducibility. *Synapse* **61**, 242–51.

Yatham L N, Liddle P F, Dennie J, *et al.* 1999. Decrease in brain serotonin 2 receptor binding in patients with major depression following desipramine treatment: A positron emission tomography study with fluorine-18-labeled setoperone. *Arch Gen Psychiatry* **56**, 705–11.

Yatham L N, Liddle P F, Lam R W, *et al.* 2002b. PET study of the effects of valproate on dopamine D(2) receptors in neuroleptic- and mood-stabilizer-naive patients with nonpsychotic mania. *Am J Psychiatry* **159**, 1718–23.

Yatham L N, Liddle P F, Shiah I S, *et al.* 2000. Brain serotonin 2 receptors in major depression: A positron emission tomography study. *Arch Gen Psychiatry* **57**, 850–8.

Yatham L N, Liddle P F, Shiah I S, *et al.* 2002a. PET study of [(18)F]6-fluoro-L-dopa uptake in neuroleptic- and mood-stabilizer-naive first-episode nonpsychotic mania: Effects of treatment with divalproex sodium. *Am J Psychiatry* **159**, 768–74.

Yu Y W, Tsai S J, Chen T J, Lin C H and Hong C J. 2002. Association study of the serotonin transporter promoter polymorphism and symptomatology and antidepressant response in major depressive disorders. *Mol Psychiatry* **7**, 1115–9.

Zarate C A Jr, Singh J and Manji H K. 2006. Cellular plasticity cascades: Targets for the development of novel therapeutics for bipolar disorder. *Biol Psychiatry* **59**, 1006–20.

Zoghbi S S, Baldwin R M, Seibyl J P, *et al.* 1992. Pharmacokinetics of the SPECT benzodiazepine receptor radioligand [123I]iomazenil in human and non-human primates. *Int J Radiat Applic Instrum – Part B, Nucl Med Biol* **19**, 881–8.

Zubieta J K, Ketter T A, Bueller J A, *et al.* 2003. Regulation of human affective responses by anterior cingulate and limbic mu-opioid neurotransmission. *Arch Gen Psychiatry* **60**, 1145–53.

Zubieta J K, Smith Y R, Bueller J A, *et al.* 2001a. Regional mu opioid receptor regulation of sensory and affective dimensions of pain. *Science (New York, NY)* **293**, 311–5.

Zubieta J K, Taylor S F, Huguelet P, Koeppe R A, Kilbourn M R and Frey K A. 2001b. Vesicular monoamine transporter concentrations in bipolar disorder type I, schizophrenia, and healthy subjects. *Biol Psychiatry* **49**, 110–6.

Chapter 12

Neuroimaging of mood disorders: commentary

Paul E. Holtzheimer III and Helen S. Mayberg

Introduction

Over the past several decades, intensive effort has been devoted to the neurobiological investigation of mood disorders, with the goal of improving the prevention and management of these conditions through biologically based interventions. This work has been revolutionized by the advance of neuroimaging methods that allow highly detailed study of the structure and function of the brain in normal and pathological states. The six chapters in this section provide a comprehensive review of the field, highlighting how this larger body of work has contributed to, and largely defined, how we conceptualize the structural and functional neuroanatomy of mood disorders.

In this chapter, we will summarize and synthesize these various findings in an attempt to highlight what has been learned and where future research might be directed. First, the clear variance between study findings will be addressed. This variability is at times striking and potentially argues for a rather skeptical view of the field. However, there are also many reasons for optimism going forward, despite this variability (and possibly because of it). At the very least, it appears that a highly consistent network of brain regions involved in mood regulation is emerging, even if the varied interactions among these regions remain poorly understood. Utilizing this neural network framework – along with continued developments in neuroimaging methods and data analysis – provides a convenient starting point for future mood disorders imaging research.

Interpreting variability: reasons for skepticism

Even a casual reading of the previous chapters will reveal an uneasy reality: despite some degree of agreement, there exists great variability in the structural and functional mood disorders imaging literature that defies simple explanation. The most critical response to these inconsistencies would be to dismiss the findings as irrelevant until greater consistency can be achieved. However, a better understanding of the potential sources of variability in neuroimaging may help reframe this potentially pessimistic state-of-the-art as a reason for optimism.

Challenges inherent to neuroimaging methods

Inherent to all imaging modalities are issues that affect the acquisition and interpretation of data. Obvious concerns are spatial and temporal resolution. Many earlier structural (e.g. computed tomography [CT]) and functional (positron emission tomography [PET], single photon emission computed tomography [SPECT]) approaches were notably limited in both spatial and temporal resolution. This continues to be an issue with many contemporary methods, including magnetic resonance spectroscopy (MRS) (where voxel size is often on the order of centimeters instead of millimeters), structural magnetic resonance imaging (MRI) (where even a 1 mm^3 voxel may not be fine enough to detect subtle structural differences, e.g. in smaller nuclei within the thalamus and amygdala), and DTI (where the voxel size can be thousands of times larger than the individual white matter axons being imaged – a consideration critical to the interpretation of white matter tractography studies using DTI-based methods). In many cases, greater spatial and temporal resolutions are theoretically possible but practically limited by feasibility (e.g. time needed motionless in the scanner) and safety (e.g. field strength of the MRI magnet or total dose of radiation for PET/SPECT studies). These pragmatic issues often lead investigators to choose to optimize one type of resolution (and how much of the brain can be imaged at one time) at the expense of the other.

Functional imaging studies must take into account additional concerns. Much of the functional imaging data in mood disorders relies on studies conducted with subjects "at rest". Given that the human brain is rarely, if ever, truly "at rest", this introduces the confound of what being "at rest" means for a particular individual at a particular time. Important questions must then be addressed, such as: should subjects have eyes open or closed? What instructions should be given prior to the task? And how does one ensure a subject doesn't fall asleep? Theoretically, the "noise" of the resting state can be reduced by using task-based functional studies. However, these studies must deal with other limitations. During fMRI studies, for example, excessive subject motion can degrade the data to the point of being unusable; therefore, tasks must be carefully selected to limit the amount of motion (especially head motion) needed for performance. Additionally, analysis of task-activated data must take into account differences in performance across subjects, validity of the task for assessing the neurological process under investigation, and the potential variance in time course for the brain activity needed to perform the task and the actual monitored behavior (e.g. the activity time needed for the motor cortex to control finger movement versus the time needed to monitor finger movement).

Finally, interpretation of imaging data must keep in mind the relationship between the data collected and the biological process being studied. In all cases, the signal detected in an imaging scan is a proxy for the process of interest. For example, DTI measures the diffusion of water within each voxel – this information is used as a proxy for white matter integrity based on the presumption that water should diffuse in a spatially coherent way in organized white matter. However, in regions where multiple white matter tracts cross (e.g. in ventral and medial prefrontal areas of particular interest in psychiatry), each tract may be highly organized, but the apparent diffusion of water within the voxel (which would contain multiple crossing fibers) may not reflect this. For this specific example, methods have been developed to begin to address this concern (Behrens *et al.*, 2007), although difficulties remain.

During functional imaging, common proxies of neuronal activity include glucose utilization, blood flow, and the ratio of oxygenated to deoxygenated hemoglobin. With these measures, one must be cognizant of time course (e.g. between increased neuronal activity and increased glucose uptake or blood flow) and conditions that may affect the presumed relationship (e.g. diabetes, hypertension, vascular disease and certain medications). Also, it is relevant to consider what activity might actually mean: for an excitatory neuron, activity means release of neurotransmitters that induce firing in the post-synaptically connected cell; for an inhibitory neuron, the opposite occurs. Ultimately, it must be recognized that imaging data are more or less indirect measures of the biological processes of interest – influenced by a multitude of factors, many of which are not understood.

Challenges inherent to the study of neuropsychiatric disorders

In addition to the methodological imaging issues discussed above, certain difficulties are inherent to the study of mood disorders. These primarily include diagnostic complexity, treatment variability, and etiologic variability including complicated gene–environment interactions.

By definition, mood disorders are syndromal conditions diagnosed by mostly subjective symptoms. Using DSM-IV criteria, it is possible for patients with highly variable symptomatic presentations to meet criteria for the same mood episode; it is unknown whether these different presentations result from different alterations of neural function, although previous attempts to subtype mood episodes based on symptomatic presentation (e.g. anxious vs. non-anxious, melancholic vs. atypical) have not proven to have much neurobiological or clinical relevance. The course of mood disorder is also highly inconsistent across patients, and it is again unknown whether this variance has biological meaning. For example, some bipolar I disorder patients have a single manic episode early in life, followed by recurrent severe depressive episodes; others may continue to have manic episodes intermixed with depressive and mixed episodes throughout their course of illness. As the chapters on bipolar disorder highlight, many of these imaging studies have included subjects with bipolar I and bipolar II disorders, occasionally in different phases of the illness at the time of scanning. Finally, it is unknown what impact successive mood episodes have on the brain; there is some suggestion from both the bipolar and unipolar data that being ill may be toxic in a real anatomical sense (Sheline *et al.*, 2003; Farrow *et al.*, 2005).

In addition to variability in presentation of a mood disorder, a number of subject-level characteristics may influence the results of imaging studies. As reviewed in the previous chapters, these include, but are likely not limited to, age of the subject (e.g. child, young adult, older adult), gender, age of onset (e.g. childhood, adulthood, later life), and genetic predisposition. Also, there is etiological variability: many cases of depression arise following a significant psychosocial stressor, while others emerge *de novo*. As mood disorders are probably best conceptualized as the result of complex gene–environment interactions, it becomes of concern to what degree genetics and previous experience (and the interaction of these) may influence the imaging data collected. At the extreme, it may be that imaging results are specific to certain subjects (age, gender, age of onset), with a specific genotype, with a specific environmental history, presenting with a coherent and consistent phenomenology.

In addition to this phenomenological heterogeneity, the majority of mood disorder patients receive at least some form of treatment before ever presenting for a research study. This treatment can vary according to treatment provider, patient concerns, financial issues, etc. As discussed throughout this book, current and prior treatment may impact the neuroimaging data collected – potentially independent of effects on the underlying mood disorder. Therefore, simply including "medication-free" subjects may not adequately address this concern: first, the brain may not return to its "pre-medication" state even a few weeks off of a psychotropic medication due to plastic changes (e.g. downregulation of postsynaptic receptors) that may have occurred; second, previous medications may have specific effects on structural and functional neuroanatomy that may depend on duration of treatment and the presence of other medications – both of which are difficult to accurately document historically; and third, as suggested in earlier chapters, medication effects may be independent of time since treatment. Focusing study on never-treated subjects has its own disadvantages: many subjects with bipolar disorder present with a major depressive episode; patients with more severe illness will likely remain medication-free for a shorter time compared to patients with less severe illness;

patients may opt against treatment for subtle reasons that may relate to potentially neurobiologically important differences in personality and coping style.

If, at the end of the day, all of these potential sources of variability have a significant impact on structural and functional neuroimaging findings, then we will have reached a nearly impossible situation: the ideal study must then include subjects essentially identical – including same symptomatic presentation, age of onset, and identical treatment history. Fortunately, we do not believe this to be the case. Despite the limitations described above – as well as numerous others that arise in specific imaging studies – it is still possible to draw some important conclusions from these data to justify optimism for the field going forward.

Consistency despite variability: reasons for optimism

When reviewing the mood disorders neuroimaging literature to date, one can appreciate a consistent set of brain regions (including gray and white matter components) as critical to normal and abnormal mood regulation. These include:

- dorsolateral prefrontal (Brodmann Areas 9/46);
- Ventrolateral prefrontal (Brodmann Areas 45/47);
- dorsomedial prefrontal (Brodmann Areas 9/10);
- ventromedial prefrontal, including paracingulate regions (Brodmann Area 10/32);
- orbitofrontal (Brodmann Area 11);
- anterior cingulate, especially perigenual (Brodmann Area 24a/b) and subgenual (Brodmann Area 24a/25) portions;
- amygdala;
- hippocampus;
- thalamus, especially anterior and mediodorsal portions;
- basal ganglia, especially caudate, putamen and ventral striatum; and
- less consistently, portions of the parietal lobe, occipital lobe, hypothalamus, brainstem and cerebellum have been identified.

Regardless of the direction of abnormality (smaller vs. larger; more vs. less active; type of neurochemical disturbance), these regions are frequently identified in structural and functional imaging studies in depression and bipolar disorder. This has led to the

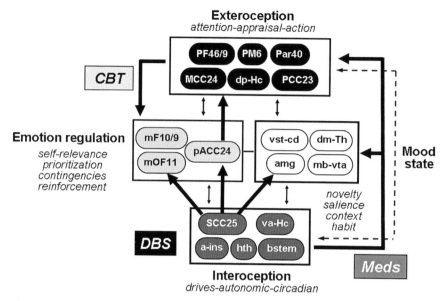

Figure 12.1 A proposed mood regulation model showing brain regions implicated in mood disorders based on neuroimaging data. PF46/9, dorsolateral prefrontal cortex; PM6, premotor area; Par40, dorsal parietal cortex; MCC24, midcingulate cortex/Brodmann Area 24; dp-hc, dorsal portion of the hippocampus; PCC23, posterior cingulate cortex; mF10/9, medial frontal cortex; mOF11, medial orbitofrontal cortex; pACC24, pregenual anterior cingulate cortex/Brodmann Area 24; vst-cd, ventral striatum–caudate; dm-Th, dorsomedial thalamus; amg, amygdala; mb-vta, midbrain/ventral tegmental area; SCC25, subcallosal cingulate cortex/Brodmann Area 25; va-Hc, ventral area of the hippocampus; a-ins, anterior insula; hth, hypothalamus; bstem, brainstem nuclei; CBT, cognitive behavioral therapy; DBS, deep brain stimulation of Brodmann area 25; Meds, antidepressant medications.

conceptualization of a mood regulation neural network (Mayberg, 2003; Phillips *et al.*, 2003); one example is shown in Figure 12.1. It is hypothesized that abnormal function within this network leads to mood disturbance; this might result from dysfunction of a critical node (e.g. left prefrontal cortex following a stroke (Robinson *et al.*, 1983)), dysfunction of multiple nodes, or disturbed communication between nodes resulting from white matter disruption. Despite the variability seen throughout the chapters in this book, we posit that the consistent identification of this similar group of brain regions validates a role for these regions in the pathophysiology of mood disorders.

Within this neural network framework, another way to understand neuroimaging variability emerges: the impact of the brain's attempt to compensate for abnormality. In the face of dysfunction, one would expect the brain – as a dynamic homeostatic system – to try to overcome this dysfunction. Therefore, the brain's state at time of scanning likely reflects not only the neuropathology of the underlying disruption, but also this attempt at compensation (Figure 12.2). By including this notion of compensatory response into

the interpretation of imaging findings, a rational explanation for certain differences (e.g. variable findings in first-episode vs. recurrent episode patients, or in patients with different ages of onset) can be postulated, akin to theories implicating sustained allostatic load in models of metabolic stress and addiction (McEwen, 1998; Koob and Le Moal, 2001).

A more dynamic, neural network approach to mood disorders research also argues against the univariate analytic approaches most often used in neuroimaging studies. Univariate approaches to data analysis necessarily treat each variable (e.g. each voxel or brain region) independently, potentially losing critical information about how variables may be interacting and interdependent. By contrast, multivariate analytic methods treat several variables simultaneously to potentially identify meaningful *patterns* of variance. So, by example, the isolated activity of the dorsolateral prefrontal cortex in depressed vs. control subjects may be less relevant than a pattern of activity across the prefrontal cortex, perigenual cingulate and amygdala. Multivariate approaches to seemingly inconsistent neuroimaging data sets may help identify coherence not detected through standard univariate

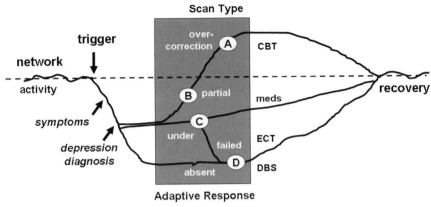

Figure 12.2 Potential time course of neural network changes during a depressive episode and recovery emphasizing the possible role of compensatory response. Functional abnormalities can be seen as resulting from the combined effect of a triggering event (e.g. stressor), the brain's immediate response, and subsequent intrinsic adaptive or maladaptive responses. Different compensatory responses (over-correction [A], partial correction [B], under-correction [C]; or absent/failed correction [D]) may lead to different brain states – and possibly the need for different types of treatment. CBT, cognitive behavioral therapy; meds, antidepressant medications; ECT, electroconvulsive therapy; DBS, deep brain stimulation.

analyses and provide the basis for more complex hypothesis development and testing. The application of multivariate analyses to mood disorders neuroimaging data is on the rise (Seminowicz *et al.*, 2004; Fu *et al.*, 2008; Craddock *et al.*, 2009; James *et al.*, 2009).

Future directions

The consistency across imaging studies in location of abnormality, if not always direction, provides a useful starting point for future investigation. We suggest two primary goals for a mood disorders imaging research agenda: (1) increasing the signal-to-noise ratio for structural and functional imaging studies through technological developments, large-scale multi-center trials and novel analytic methods; and (2) shifting from hypothesis-free to hypothesis-guided investigations based within developing neural network models.

Decreasing noise, increasing signal

A major aim in neuroimaging research is, and will continue to be, limiting the variability in findings due to noise inherent to the methods. Much of this will come from further technological and methodological advances, such as safe and well-tolerated higher intensity scanners (e.g. >9 Tesla MRI) and novel data analytic techniques. These technological developments will also improve the ability of investigators to pool data acquired on different scanners with varied acquisition parameters – a critically important step required for large-scale, multi-center studies that

will mitigate the noise from phenomenological and clinical heterogeneity through recruitment of greater numbers of subjects.

For functional imaging studies, one of the greatest sources of variability is difference in the task paradigm used: therefore, more consistency in task among studies – or at least in domains assessed – would be of benefit. An important intermediate goal for the mood disorders functional imaging community could be to review, agree upon and standardize a set of tasks relevant to the study of depression and bipolar disorder, a strategy similar to those being tested in the schizophrenia and Alzheimer's Dementia research communities (Cho *et al.*, 2005; Jack *et al.*, 2008).

Novel approaches to data analysis will likely play a critically important role in improving signal detection in neuroimaging studies of depression and bipolar disorder. As discussed above, multivariate analytic techniques provide opportunities for identifying relevant patterns of activity or structural changes that may distinguish mood disorder patients from controls, or potentially subgroups of mood disorder patients from each other. Combining different types of data may also be useful. For example, DTI tractography might be used to help define regions of interest (ROIs) for functional imaging analyses, especially those focused on functional connectivity. Joint independent component analysis (ICA), a multivariate technique designed to identify shared variance patterns among two diverse data sets (Calhoun *et al.*, 2006), might be applied to identify shared structural and functional brain abnormalities.

Model-based, hypothesis-driven research

Although hypotheses are often stated for neuroimaging studies in depression or bipolar disorder, the individual study often fits only loosely within a model or paradigm for brain dysfunction in mood disorders. As the neural network involved in mood regulation becomes better understood, it would seem reasonable to begin framing hypotheses within this framework; this allows both a stronger, more generalized basis for the hypothesis and a more direct test of the model itself. For example, using a putative neural network model derived from neuroimaging data, it was hypothesized that focal stimulation of the white matter adjacent to Brodmann Area 25 in the subgenual cingulate cortex could effect functional changes throughout the network leading to clinical improvement in patients with severe, treatment-resistant depression. This hypothesis was supported in a small, proof-of-concept study (Mayberg *et al.*, 2005; Lozano *et al.*, 2008). Similar model-based, hypothesis-driven investigations should become a focus of research going forward.

Conclusion

The field of mood disorders neuroimaging is vibrant, productive and at times chaotic. Over the past nearly 30 years, we have seen an explosion of structural and functional data that has dramatically changed how we think about the neurobiology of depression and bipolar disorder. Along with genetic, metabolic, neuroendocrinological and neuroimmunological studies, neuroimaging findings have helped establish mood disorders as physiological disorders of the brain. This has likely played a pivotal role in the slow but steady destigmatization of mood disorders among the lay public, non-psychiatric clinicians, and other neuroscientists.

The results of neuroimaging studies to date have not always been consistent. Significant variability is often more the rule than the exception. Much of this variability is likely due to methodological limitations inherent to the field, as well as clinical and phenomenological heterogeneity among mood disorder patients. However, in spite of this variability, some important trends are emerging: most specifically, a consistent set of brain regions involved in normal and abnormal mood regulation has been identified that can be organized into a putative mood regulation neural network.

As the field continues to progress, technological developments will continue to help decrease or at least explain some of the residual variability. Large-scale trials and novel approaches to data analysis will further improve our ability to confidently identify meaningful structural and functional abnormalities that characterize mood disorder patients as well as patient subgroups. We are also at a stage where the neural network that has emerged can be used to develop more relevant model-based hypotheses to guide future investigations.

So, notwithstanding the many inconsistencies and limitations of mood disorders neuroimaging results thus far, there are more reasons for optimism than pessimism. The field is strong and getting stronger through multidisciplinary contributions from biomedical engineering, imaging physics, biostatistics, cognitive neuroscience and neuropsychiatry. Sooner rather than later, it is expected that neuroimaging findings will be able to play a vital role in diagnosis, treatment planning, and treatment development. And, these results will continue to define and at times redefine how we conceptualize these serious disorders of mood, thought and behavior.

Box 12.1. Overview of mood disorders neuroimaging data

- Significant variability exists in the published literature; potential sources include:
  Noise inherent to current neuroimaging methods
  Methodological variability between studies
  Biological heterogeneity of the underlying disorders
- Despite this variability, a highly reliable network of brain regions has been implicated in the pathophysiology of mood disorders
- Future directions include:
  Continued improvement of imaging technologies
  Multi-modal imaging (e.g. combination of structural and functional imaging methods)
  Large, multi-site neuroimaging studies
  Shifting from univariate to multivariate analytic methods
  Shifting from hypothesis-free to hypothesis-driven investigations; i.e. increasing power by focusing on the more limited network of brain regions consistently implicated in these disorders

References

Behrens T E, Berg H J, Jbabdi S, *et al.* 2007. Probabilistic diffusion tractography with multiple fibre orientations: What can we gain? *Neuroimage* **34**, 144–55.

Calhoun V, Adali T, Liu J, *et al.* 2006. A feature-based approach to combine functional MRI, structural MRI and EEG brain imaging data. *Conf Proc IEEE Eng Med Biol Soc* **1**, 3672–5.

Cho R Y, Ford J M, Krystal J H, *et al.* 2005. Functional neuroimaging and electrophysiology biomarkers for clinical trials for cognition in schizophrenia. *Schizophr Bull* **31**, 865–9.

Craddock R C, Holtzheimer P E, Hu X P, *et al.* 2009. Disease state prediction from resting state functional connectivity. *Magn Reson Med* **62**, 1619–28.

Farrow T F, Whitford T J, Williams L M, *et al.* 2005. Diagnosis-related regional gray matter loss over two years in first episode schizophrenia and bipolar disorder. *Biol Psychiatry* **58**, 713–23.

Fu C H, Mourao-Miranda J, Costafreda S G, *et al.* 2008. Pattern classification of sad facial processing: Toward the development of neurobiological markers in depression. *Biol Psychiatry* **63**, 656–62.

Jack C R Jr, Bernstein M A, Fox N C, *et al.* 2008. The Alzheimer's Disease Neuroimaging Initiative (ADNI): MRI methods. *J Magn Reson Imaging* **27**, 685–91.

James G A, Kelley M E, Craddock R C, *et al.* 2009. Exploratory structural equation modeling of resting-state fMRI: Applicability of group models to individual subjects. *Neuroimage* **45**, 778–87.

Koob G F and Le Moal M. 2001. Drug addiction, dysregulation of reward, and allostasis. *Neuropsychopharmacology* **24**, 97–129.

Lozano A M, Mayberg H S, Giacobbe P, *et al.* 2008. Subcallosal cingulate gyrus deep brain stimulation for treatment-resistant depression. *Biol Psychiatry* **64**, 461–7.

Mayberg H S. 2003. Modulating dysfunctional limbic-cortical circuits in depression: Towards development of brain-based algorithms for diagnosis and optimised treatment. *Br Med Bull* **65**, 193–207.

Mayberg H S, Lozano A M, Voon V, *et al.* 2005. Deep brain stimulation for treatment-resistant depression. *Neuron* **45**, 651–60.

McEwen B S. 1998. Stress, adaptation, and disease. Allostasis and allostatic load. *Ann N Y Acad Sci* **840**, 33–44.

Phillips M L, Drevets W C, Rauch S L, *et al.* 2003. Neurobiology of emotion perception II: Implications for major psychiatric disorders. *Biol Psychiatry* **54**, 515–28.

Robinson R G, Starr L B, Kubos K L, *et al.* 1983. A two-year longitudinal study of post-stroke mood disorders: Findings during the initial evaluation. *Stroke* **14**, 736–41.

Seminowicz D A, Mayberg H S, McIntosh A R, *et al.* 2004. Limbic–frontal circuitry in major depression: A path modeling metanalysis. *Neuroimage* **22**, 409–18.

Sheline Y I, Gado M H, Kraemer H C, *et al.* 2003. Untreated depression and hippocampal volume loss. *Am J Psychiatry* **160**, 1516–8.

Structural imaging of post-traumatic stress disorder

Mark W. Gilbertson

Post-traumatic stress disorder (PTSD) includes a constellation of disabling behavioral and emotional symptoms that occur in a proportion of individuals exposed to severe psychological trauma. PTSD can be a chronic and debilitating condition in which intrusive memories, hypervigilence, heightened physiological reactivity to reminders of the traumatic event, and avoidance can lead to significant social and occupational impairment. Understanding the neurobiology of this disorder has not only served as validation of PTSD as a diagnostic entity, but may ultimately be critical to the development of more effective therapeutic interventions.

Neuroimaging studies of structural brain abnormalities in PTSD have largely emerged in the context of two principal lines of evidence in the literature. First, early animal research provided compelling evidence that exposure to severe and chronic stress, a process that may be mediated by the neurotoxic impact of elevated corticosteroids, can damage the hippocampal formation, namely, CA3 neuronal cell loss, diminished neuronal regeneration, atrophy of dendritic branching, and reduced levels of brain-derived neurotrophic factor (Gould et al., 1997; Margarinos et al., 1996; McEwen, 1995; Sapolsky et al., 1990; Smith et al., 1995; Uno et al., 1989). As a result, the initial neuroanatomical investigations of PTSD centered largely upon the morphology of the hippocampus. Second, an improved understanding in recent years of the neurocircuitry underlying conditioned fear acquisition and extinction in animals has identified a number of specific brain regions of interest (Herry et al., 2008; Maren, 2005) that are potentially relevant to an understanding of the symptomatology of PTSD (Rauch et al., 2006). In this regard, the literature has not only identified the hippocampus as an important component of the fear circuit, but dominant roles also appear to be played by other brain regions, principally the amygdala and medial prefrontal cortex (mPFC). Structural neuroimaging findings pertaining to specific brain regions in adults with PTSD are reviewed below, followed by a discussion of findings relevant to pediatric studies of PTSD.

Adult neuroimaging studies

Hippocampus

The pioneering studies of hippocampal volume in PTSD (Bremner et al., 1995, 1997; Gurvits et al., 1996; Stein et al., 1997) all found significant reductions in hippocampal volume among PTSD patients relative to both non-traumatized and traumatized controls without PTSD, lending support to the notion that, as with animals, severe stress may also damage the hippocampus in humans. These early studies employed structural MRIs in chronic populations of PTSD patients, namely, combat veterans and adult survivors of childhood abuse, and diminutions in hippocampal size ranged from 5 to 26%. Since that time, over 20 published studies examining hippocampal volume have now appeared in the literature, the clear majority of which provide empirical support for smaller hippocampal volume in PTSD (Bonne et al., 2008; Bossini et al., 2008; Bremner et al., 2003; Chen et al., 2006; Emdad et al., 2006; Gilbertson et al., 2002; Hedges et al., 2003; Kasai et al., 2008; Letizia et al., 2008; Lindauer et al., 2004; Nakano et al., 2002; Pavić et al., 2007; Shin et al., 2004; Villarreal et al., 2002a; Vythilingam et al., 2005; Wignall et al., 2004; Winter et al., 2004). In addition to combat veterans and adult survivors of abuse, smaller hippocampal volumes have also been demonstrated in firefighters, policemen, cancer and burn patients, and mixed trauma groups (e.g. rape, physical assaults, traffic, and occupational accidents) with PTSD. It should be noted, however, that a number of studies have failed to find significant differences in hippocampal volume, most consistently and notably among pediatric PTSD samples (Carrion et al., 2001; De Bellis et al., 1999, 2001, 2002a), suggesting the possible impact of neuromaturational factors (see the section on pediatric neuroimaging below). Interestingly, a few studies of elderly PTSD patients (Freeman et al., 2006; Golier et al.; 2005) have also failed to show significantly smaller hippocampal volume compared with traumatized controls, perhaps representing a confounding impact of aging on the measurement of hippocampal differences or reflecting the overall neurological robustness and resilience of those individuals (regardless of PTSD) who survive into older age. In general, adult PTSD studies that have failed to find smaller hippocampal volumes have largely employed subject populations with less severe or less chronic illness (Bonne et al., 2001; Fennema-Notestine et al., 2002; Jatzko et al., 2006; Pederson et al., 2004; Yamasue et al., 2003; Yehuda et al., 2007). Empirical findings have suggested that severity of illness is an important factor in determining effect size of hippocampal differences in PTSD (Gilbertson et al., 2002; Karl et al., 2006). However, at least one study employing patients with recent onset and less severe PTSD (Wignall et al., 2004) has reported smaller hippocampi. Additionally, although Yehuda et al. (2007) failed to find significant overall group differences between their PTSD and non-PTSD samples, they did report that individuals within the PTSD group who developed PTSD following their first traumatic exposure (versus those who did not) did demonstrate smaller hippocampal volumes (perhaps suggesting that hippocampal volume represents a PTSD-related resilience factor).

Meta-analyses of the available literature regarding hippocampal volume in PTSD (Karl et al., 2006; Kitayama et al., 2005; Smith, 2005; Woon et al., 2008) have all supported the presence of bilateral hippocampal diminution in adult PTSD. In a highly controlled meta-analysis reported by Smith (2005) that encompassed 215 PTSD subjects and 325 control subjects, adult patients with PTSD demonstrated on average a 6.9% smaller left hippocampal volume and a 6.6% smaller right hippocampal volume compared with control subjects. MRI hippocampal volume studies have employed a diverse set of methodologies, including differences in slice thickness, scanner resolution, anatomical boundary definitions, and a variety of other acquisition parameters. In a large-scale meta-analysis, Karl et al. (2006) reported that MRI studies employing high spatial resolution and whole-brain volume correction were more likely to find significant hippocampal differences when comparing PTSD patients to trauma-exposed controls. However, other meta-analyses have not found methodological differences in general to constitute a significant moderator variable in PTSD hippocampal studies (Kitayama et al., 2005; Smith, 2005), and the fact that hippocampal differences have emerged regardless of methodological differences likely argues for the robust nature of the findings.

A number of sample-related factors have also been examined with regard to volumetric differences of the hippocampus in PTSD. Although individual studies have shown variations in identifying right, left, or bilateral hippocampal volume diminutions, current meta-analyses have consistently concluded that smaller hippocampal volume in PTSD is best characterized as bilateral with no significant differences in right versus left volumes. Likewise, the majority of meta-analyses have not provided strong evidence for a gender effect; that is, male and female PTSD patients do not appear to differ significantly in effect size for hippocampal volume differences. However, many studies may lack sufficient statistical power to discern subtle gender differences, and one meta-analytic study (Karl et al., 2006) found evidence for samples containing more males to show larger effect sizes, with the effect being more pronounced in the right hemisphere.

It should be noted that a number of unresolved issues persist regarding the interpretation of hippocampal volume differences that have been observed in PTSD. Psychiatric comorbidity is a common confounding factor in PTSD research, particularly with regard to the co-existing conditions of alcohol abuse and depression. It is important to note that both depression and alcohol abuse have been independently associated with reduced hippocampal volume (Bremner et al., 2000; Laakso et al., 2000). As a result, many volumetric studies of the hippocampus in PTSD have been confounded by the comorbid presence of alcohol abuse and depression, or both.

More recently, however, a number of studies have attempted to control for the impact of these comorbid conditions, and have concluded that hippocampal volume differences in PTSD do not appear to be accounted for merely by histories of alcohol abuse or depression (Bonne *et al.*, 2008; Emdad *et al.*, 2006; Gilbertson *et al.*, 2002; Hedges *et al.*, 2003; Letizia *et al.*, 2008; Lindauer *et al.*, 2004; Pavić *et al.*, 2007). In contrast, at least one recent, well-controlled study (Woodward *et al.*, 2006a) has reported that hippocampal volume differences were only apparent in PTSD patients with comorbid alcoholism (versus PTSD patients without comorbid alcoholism). Further work is required to more fully elucidate the potential impact of comorbid disorders.

A second unresolved issue concerns the origin of hippocampal volume differences in PTSD. It has often been reasonably assumed that smaller hippocampal volume results from trauma-related neurotoxic processes analogous to those documented in animal studies. However, an alternative literature also exists to support the idea that pre-existing genetic variations in hippocampus size can impact subsequent fear-related behavior in animals (Crusio *et al.*, 1989; Schwegler *et al.*, 1983). These competing literatures lay the foundation for an obvious "chicken or egg" problem, namely, is smaller hippocampal size in PTSD a result of trauma exposure, or does it exist as a pre-trauma risk factor that increases the likelihood of developing PTSD once exposed to a traumatic stressor? In an effort to address this issue, Gilbertson *et al.* (2002) studied identical twin brothers discordant for combat service in Vietnam in which some index combat twins developed chronic PTSD whereas other combat exposed twins did not. As expected, combat veterans with PTSD had smaller hippocampi than combat veterans who never developed PTSD. Of greater interest, however, was the finding that the identical twin brothers of combat veterans with PTSD, who themselves had neither combat experience nor PTSD, nonetheless had hippocampal volumes comparable to their PTSD brothers, and smaller than combat veterans without PTSD (and their brothers). This study provided the first evidence in humans that hippocampal volume may serve as a predisposing risk factor rather than as a neurotoxic product of trauma exposure. However, other neuroimaging evidence is not fully consistent with a "risk factor only" interpretation. A number of meta-analyses (Karl *et al.*, 2006; Smith, 2005) have

demonstrated that while PTSD patients show smaller hippocampi relative to traumatized controls, this difference is smaller than that observed in the comparison between PTSD patients and non-traumatized controls. That is, traumatized individuals without PTSD may also demonstrate some degree of hippocampal diminution, which suggests either the presence of a trauma-induced atrophy or that hippocampal volume may also represent a risk factor for trauma exposure itself. Furthermore, Bonne *et al.* (2001), in one of the few longitudinal studies of hippocampal volume in PTSD to be published, failed to find volume differences, pre-existing or otherwise, in traumatized individuals who eventually developed PTSD-related symptoms. However, as previously noted, patients with PTSD in this study demonstrated only mild, recent-onset symptomatology (as well as being followed for only a brief time period). To the degree that hippocampal volume differences exist, they may potentially represent both a predisposing factor as well as a neurotoxic product of trauma, and resolution of this issue must await further longitudinal studies.

Finally, studies employing an alternative structural imaging methodology, magnetic resonance spectroscopic imaging (MRSI), have also reported deficits in the integrity of the hippocampus in PTSD. MRSI quantifies the concentration of *N*-acetylaspartate (NAA), a putative marker of neuronal density. Numerous studies have now demonstrated a significant reduction of NAA, namely, loss of neuronal density, in the hippocampus of individuals diagnosed with PTSD (Freeman *et al.*, 1998; Ham *et al.*, 2007; Li *et al.*, 2006; Mahmutyazicioğlu *et al.*, 2005; Mohanakrishnan Menon *et al.*, 2003, 2004; Schuff *et al.*, 2001, 2008; Villarreal *et al.*, 2002b). At least one study (Freeman *et al.*, 2006) failed to find significant PTSD-related reductions in NAA concentration, albeit in an elderly population of patients, a finding that mirrors previously discussed MRI findings. Also similar to MRI findings, mixed patterns of left, right, or bilateral hippocampal differences have been reported by individual MRSI studies. In an effort to examine the impact of alcohol abuse, a recent MRSI study (Schuff *et al.*, 2008) carefully controlled for presence and absence of comorbid alcoholism, and concluded that hippocampal NAA reduction in PTSD cannot be explained by alcohol abuse/dependence as a confounding factor. It has furthermore been suggested that MRSI may represent a more sensitive measure of hippocampal integrity than structural MRI. In support of this proposition, Schuff et al. (2008) have found hippocampal NAA concentration reductions in PTSD samples in which MRI hippocampal volumetric measures did not reach significance.

Amygdala

Far fewer structural imaging studies examining amygdala volume in PTSD have been published, and many have been reported as control measures in the context of hippocampal volume studies. One study (Matsuoka et al., 2003) has reported reduced left amygdala volume in cancer survivors with traumatic intrusive recollections, although only a very small percentage of the subjects in this sample were actually diagnosed with PTSD. However, the majority of MRI imaging studies have failed to find significant PTSD-related volumetric differences in the amygdala (Bonne et al., 2001; Bremner et al., 1997; De Bellis et al., 1999, 2001, 2002a; Fennema-Notestine et al., 2002; Gilbertson et al., 2002; Gurvits et al., 1996; Lindauer et al., 2004; Wignall et al., 2004). As such, structural findings are in contrast to functional neuroimaging studies that have consistently demonstrated increased activation of the amygdala in adult patients with PTSD (Hull, 2002; Pitman et al., 2001), and which are reviewed fully elsewhere in this volume. Available meta-analyses regarding MRI volumetric studies of the amygdala and PTSD (Karl et al., 2006; Woon et al., 2008) have also failed to find strong or consistent evidence for volumetric differences in PTSD. However, Karl et al. (2006) did note some evidence for a significant but small reduction in left amygdala volume in PTSD patients. The reported effect sizes were small (0.13–0.14) but suggestive of amygdala asymmetry in PTSD.

Frontal lobe

A growing literature in PTSD neuroimaging studies has reported significant volume reductions in frontal regions of the brain, especially medial prefrontal cortex (mPFC). Although reduced orbitofrontal cortex (Hakamata et al., 2007) and cortical thinning in bilateral superior and middle frontal gyri (Geuze et al., 2008) have also been reported, a focal area of interest has been the anterior cingulate cortex (ACC), an area thought to exert significant top-down inhibition (along with the hippocampus) of the amygdala (Rauch et al., 2003). A number of

structural MRI studies have now documented reduced ACC volume in PTSD (Araki et al., 2005; Chen et al., 2006; Kasai et al., 2008; Kitayama et al. 2006; Rauch et al., 2003; Woodward et al., 2006b; Yamasue et al., 2003). A meta-analysis of this literature (Karl et al., 2006) has supported the conclusion of reduced ACC volume with moderate effect sizes. A few studies (Corbo et al., 2005; Hakamata et al., 2007) have failed to find clear ACC volume differences in more acute PTSD; however, one of these studies (Corbo et al., 2005) nonetheless reported significant differences in the "shape" of the ACC even in the absence of actual volume differences. Although structural findings to date appear largely consistent in identifying smaller ACC volume, little consensus has yet emerged regarding laterality or regional specificity within the ACC. Individual studies, as with hippocampal studies cited previously, have varied in their report of bilateral (Kasai et al., 2008; Rauch et al., 2003), left (Chen et al., 2006; Yamasue et al., 2003), and right (Kitayama et al., 2006) ACC reductions. Likewise, some studies have reported ACC reductions in only the pregenual region of the ACC (as well as closely associated subcallosal cortex) (Kasai et al., 2008), whereas others have reported differences in both pregenual and dorsal ACC (Kitayama et al., 2006; Woodward et al., 2006b). In contrast to previously reported findings in the hippocampus, a study of combat-discordant twins has suggested that reduction in pregenual ACC may represent an acquired sign in PTSD, namely, trauma-induced reduction only seen in combat veterans with PTSD, as opposed to a pre-existing vulnerability (Kasai et al., 2008).

Other structural imaging methodologies have provided additional evidence for the relevance of ACC alterations in PTSD. As with the hippocampus, recent MRSI studies of the ACC have reported diminished neuronal density, namely, reduced NAA, in PTSD patients (Ham et al., 2007; Mahmutyazicioğlu et al., 2005; Schuff et al., 2008). Furthermore, a relatively new methodology, diffusion tensor imaging (DTI), has been employed recently to explore the existence of white matter abnormalities in medial frontal cortex in PTSD. DTI provides a measure of the integrity of specific white matter tracts in the brain by examining the movement of water molecules as a function of the degree of density and coherence of local tissue components. A number of initial DTI studies have provided evidence for aberrant white matter integrity in the cingulum bundle, a major neuronal tract connecting the ACC with the amygdala (Abe *et al.*, 2006; Kim *et al.*, 2005, 2006).

Other brain regions

Although the majority of adult neuroimaging reports have centered on the hippocampus, medial prefrontal cortex, and amygdala, structural studies have examined potential abnormalities in other brain regions as well. Some of these regions have served as control sites for previously described studies, and most lack a sufficient database from which to draw firm conclusions. For example, the caudate nucleus has been employed as a control region in hippocampal studies (Bremner *et al.*, 1995, 1997) and has not been found to show volumetric changes associated with PTSD. Likewise, the cerebellar vermis has not been shown to differ in patients with PTSD (Levitt *et al.*, 2006). In contrast, the cavum septum pelucidum (CSP), a small cerebrospinal fluid filled cleft in the anterior portion of the septo-callosal junction, has been found to exist with greater frequency in individuals diagnosed with PTSD (May *et al.*, 2004; Myslobodsky *et al.*, 1995). Neurodevelopmental abnormalities in the region of the callosal–fornix–hippocampus circuitry are thought to lead to the persistence of CSP, which normally resolves shortly following birth. In addition, the corpus callosum has been implicated by a small number of studies as a site of reduced volume in adult PTSD especially in the midbody subregion (Kitayama *et al.*, 2007; Villarreal *et al.*, 2004). Similarly, a few studies have found reduced volume of the insula in PTSD (Corbo *et al.*, 2005; Kasai *et al.*, 2008). Finally, some limited evidence suggests general cortical white matter atrophy or lesions to be associated with PTSD in adults (Canive *et al.*, 1997; Villarreal *et al.*, 2002a).

Pediatric neuroimaging studies

To date, only a small number of investigators have published findings regarding structural brain differences in children and adolescents diagnosed with PTSD. Existing studies involving children have revealed a pattern of structural brain deficits that is largely inconsistent with findings reported in the adult PTSD literature. Most notable in this regard is the failure to replicate reduced hippocampal volume (Carrion *et al.*, 2001; De Bellis *et al.*, 1999, 2001, 2002a; Tupler *et al.*, 2006). To some degree, this failure appears to reflect the fact that total intracranial

and/or cerebral volume in children with PTSD (unlike adults) has often been found to be smaller relative to non-PTSD control subjects (Carrion *et al.*, 2001; De Bellis *et al.*, 1999, 2002a). As a result, even in those pediatric studies in which smaller hippocampal volume was found, this difference became non-significant when controlling for overall brain volume (Carrion *et al.*, 2001). Tupler and De Bellis (2006) pooled subjects from a number of their previous studies and found that hippocampal volume in children and adolescents with PTSD was actually larger than in control subjects when adjusting for overall brain volume (i.e. less relative volume reduction in the hippocampus than in the brain as a whole). A meta-analysis of 105 children with PTSD versus 160 controls (Woon *et al.*, 2008) concluded that studies of hippocampal volume in pediatric PTSD samples have failed to show significant reductions. Nonetheless, some controversy may still remain in that at least one recent longitudinal study (Carrion *et al.*, 2007) has reported a relative volume loss bilaterally in the hippocampus of abused children followed over a 12–18-month period, especially in those children with higher PTSD symptoms and cortisol levels at baseline. However, the general consensus in failing to find hippocampal diminution in children with PTSD has led to speculations that active neurodevelopmental plasticity and rapid limbic growth in childhood may mask hippocampal atrophy, or that the neurotoxic nature of glucocorticoid exposure associated with trauma may have a more generalized impact (i.e. whole-brain) in childhood, rather than the more localized impact (i.e. hippocampus) of adulthood. Resolution of these questions awaits further research.

In addition to findings demonstrating reduced overall intracranial brain volume in children and adolescents with PTSD, a number of studies have identified specific brain regions that appear altered in volume even after controlling for overall brain size. While specific studies of ACC analogous to those reported in adults have not yet been published, a few studies have identified volumetric differences in prefrontal cortex in pediatric PTSD samples (Carrion *et al.*, 2001; De Bellis *et al.*, 2002a, 2003; Richert *et al.*, 2006). These findings have suggested reduced volume of overall prefrontal cortex (De Bellis *et al.*, 2002a) and dorsal PFC (Richert *et al.*, 2006), larger middle-inferior and ventral PFC (Richert *et al.*, 2006), increased prefrontal lobe and lateral ventricle CSF (De Bellis *et al.*, 2003), and a loss of the normal right > left asymmetry of the frontal lobes (Carrion *et al.*, 2001). In addition to frontal lobe alterations, several studies have consistently reported loss of volume and white matter integrity of the corpus callosum, especially medial and posterior regions, in children with PTSD (De Bellis *et al.*, 1999, 2002a, 2003; Jackowski *et al.*, 2008). As such, these findings appear consistent with the limited reports of corpus callosum reduction in adults with PTSD as previously described. Finally, De Bellis and colleagues (De Bellis *et al.*, 2002b, 2006; Thomas *et al.*, 2004) have also reported a number of isolated findings in children with PTSD, including: larger pituitary volumes in pubertal/postpubertal children (but not prepubertal children), larger superior temporal gyrus volume (especially right hemisphere), and smaller total cerebellum volumes.

Summary

Structural neuroimaging studies have revealed a relatively consistent pattern of volumetric reductions in both the hippocampus and anterior cingulate cortex of adults diagnosed with chronic PTSD. As such, these findings are consistent with a model of PTSD that posits a reduced capacity of hippocampus/ACC to inhibit amygdala-based fear responses, likely reflecting a failure of these brain regions to effectively utilize cues in the environment to signal safety (hippocampus) and to adaptively maintain extinction of conditioned emotional responses (ACC) once traumatic experiences are no longer relevant. As further studies using new imaging technologies such as DTI are completed, findings may extend PTSD-related structural abnormalities of the hippocampus and ACC to the associated white matter tracts relevant to their interconnections (including amygdala) in the broader neural circuitry of fear conditioning and extinction. At this time, only limited data exist to implicate structural alterations in other brain regions (e.g. corpus callosum) and the relevance of these potential brain sites awaits further study. Pediatric studies of PTSD have not fully replicated findings reported in the adult literature, and suggest that the neuroanatomical correlates of PTSD may manifest in a more generalized manner (e.g. reduced total brain volume) in children and adolescents who are traumatized. Further research will be required to advance our understanding of the impact of developmental factors and brain maturation on the expression of PTSD-related brain

abnormalities. Additional longitudinal investigations are also needed to more fully elucidate the source of specific volumetric reductions in PTSD, namely, pre-existing vulnerability traits versus the toxic impact of traumatic exposure itself (or perhaps both). As these issues move toward resolution, neuroimaging studies in PTSD will not only continue to contribute to our understanding of the neuropathology of this psychiatric condition, but more importantly, may offer directions for more effective prevention and treatment.

> **Box 13.1. Summary of structural neuroimaging findings in post-traumatic stress disorder (PTSD)**
>
> - Diminished volumes of the hippocampus and anterior cingulate cortex represent the most frequently replicated findings in patients with PTSD, especially those with chronic and severe disorder.
> - Most studies suggest that observed volumetric reductions in PTSD can not be fully explained by comorbid conditions such as substance abuse and depression.
> - Evidence exists to support both neurotoxicity and pre-existing vulnerability as etiological models of brain volume reductions in PTSD.
> - Structural findings are consistent with a model of PTSD that suggests a reduced capacity of hippocampus/ACC to inhibit amygdala-based fear responses.
> - Pediatric studies of PTSD have not fully replicated findings reported in the adult literature and suggest that trauma in children may have a more generalized impact on the brain.

References

Abe O, Yamasue H, Kasai K, *et al.* 2006. Voxel-based diffusion tensor analysis reveals aberrant anterior cingulum integrity in posttraumatic stress disorder due to terrorism. *Psychiatry Res Neuroimag* **146**, 231–42.

Araki T, Kasai K, Yamasue H, *et al.* 2005. Association between lower P300 amplitude and smaller anterior cingulated cortex volume in patients with posttraumatic stress disorder: a study of victims of Tokyo subway sarin attack. *NeuroImage* **25**, 43–50.

Bonne O, Brandes D, Gilboa A, *et al.* 2001. Longitudinal MRI study of *hippocampal* volume in trauma survivors with PTSD. *Am J Psychiatry* **158**, 1248–51.

Bonne O, Vythilingam M, Inagaki M, *et al.* 2008. Reduced posterior hippocampal volume in posttraumatic stress disorder. *J Clin Psychiatry* **69**, 1087–91.

Bossini L, Tavanti M, Calossi S, *et al.* 2008. Magnetic resonance imaging volumes of the hippocampus in drug-naïve patients with post-traumatic stress disorder without comorbidity conditions. *J Psychiatric Res* **42**, 752–62.

Bremner J A, Narayan M, Anderson E R. 2000. Hippocampal volume reduction in major depression. *Am J Psychiatry* **157**, 115–27.

Bremner J A, Randall P, Scott T M, *et al.* 1995. MRI-based measurements of hippocampal volume in combat-related posttraumatic stress disorder. *Am J Psychiatry* **152**, 973–8.

Bremner J D, Randall P, Vermetten E, *et al.* 1997. Magnetic resonance imaging-based measurement of hippocampal volume in posttraumatic stress disorder related to childhood physical and sexual abuse – A preliminary report. *Biol Psychiatry* **41**, 23–32.

Bremner J D, Vythilingam M, Vermetten E, *et al.* 2003. MRI and PET study of deficits in hippocampal structure and function in women with childhood sexual abuse and posttraumatic stress disorder. *Am J Psychiatry* **160**, 924–32.

Canive J M, Lewine J D, Orrison W W, *et al.* 1997. MRI reveals gross structural abnormalities in PTSD. *Ann N Y Acad Sci* **821**, 512–5.

Carrion V G, Weems C F, Eliez S, *et al.* 2001. Attenuation of frontal asymmetry in pediatric posttraumatic stress disorder. *Biol Psychiatry* **50**, 943–51.

Carrion V G, Weems C F and Reiss A L. 2007. Stress predicts brain changes in children: A pilot longitudinal study on youth stress, posttraumatic stress disorder, and the hippocampus. *Pediatrics* **119**, 509–16.

Chen S, Xia W, Li L, *et al.* 2006. Gray matter density reduction in the insula in fire survivors with posttraumatic stress disorder: A voxel-based morphometric study. *Psychiatry Res Neuroimag* **146**, 65–72.

Corbo V, Clément M H, Armony J L, *et al.* 2005. Size versus shape differences: Contrasting voxel-based and volumetric analyses of the anterior cingulate cortex in individuals with acute posttraumatic stress disorder. *Biol Psychiatry* **58**, 119–24.

Crusio W E, Schwegler H and Van Abeelen J H F. 1989. Behavioral responses to novelty and structural variation of the hippocampus in mice. II. Multivariate genetic analysis. *Behav Brain Res* **32**, 81–8.

De Bellis M D, Hall J, Boring A M, *et al.* 2001. A pilot longitudinal study of hippocampal volumes in pediatric maltreatment-related posttraumatic stress disorder. *Biol Psychiatry* **50**, 305–09.

De Bellis M D and Keshavan M S. 2003. Sex differences in brain maturation in maltreatment-related pediatric posttraumatic stress disorder. *Neurosci Biobehav Rev* **27**, 103–17.

De Bellis M D, Keshavan M S, Clark D B, *et al.* 1999. Developmental traumatology part II: Brain development. *Biol Psychiatry* **45**, 1271–84.

De Bellis M D, Keshavan M S, Frustaci K, *et al.* 2002b. Superior temporal gyrus volumes in maltreated children and adolescents with PTSD. *Biol Psychiatry* **51**, 544–52.

De Bellis M D, Keshavan M S, Shifflett H, *et al.* 2002a. Brain structures in pediatric maltreatment-related posttraumatic stress disorder: A sociodemographically matched study. *Biol Psychiatry* **52**, 1066–78.

De Bellis M D and Kuchibhatla M. 2006. Cerebellar volumes in pediatric maltreatment-related posttraumatic stress disorder. *Biol Psychiatry* **60**, 697–703.

Emdad R, Bonekamp D, Sondergaard H P, *et al.* 2006. Morphometric and psychometric comparisons between non-substance-abusing patients with posttraumatic stress disorder and normal controls. *Psychother Psychosom* **75**, 122–32.

Fennema-Notestine C, Stein M B, Kennedy C M, *et al.* 2002. Brain morphometry in female victims of intimate partner violence with and without posttraumatic stress disorder. *Biol Psychiatry* **51**, 1089–101.

Freeman T W, Cardwell D, Karson C N and Komoroski R A. 1998. In vivo proton magnetic resonance spectroscopy of the medial temporal lobes of subjects with combat-related posttraumatic stress disorder. *Magn Reson Med* **40**, 66–71.

Freeman T, Kimbrell T, Booe L, *et al.* 2006. Evidence of resilience: Neuroimaging in former prisoners of war. *Psychiatry Res Neuroimag* **146**, 59–64.

Geuze E, Westenberg H G M, Heinecke A, *et al.* 2008. Thinner prefrontal cortex in veterans with posttraumatic stress disorder. *NeuroImage* **41**, 675–81.

Gilbertson M W, Shenton M E, Ciszewski A, *et al.* 2002. Smaller hippocampal volume predicts pathologic vulnerability to psychological trauma. *Nature Neurosci* **5**, 1242–7.

Golier J A, Yehuda R, DeSanti S, *et al.* 2005. Absence of hippocampal volume differences in survivors of the Nazi Holocaust with and without posttraumatic stress disorder. *Psychiatry Res Neuroimag* **139**, 53–64.

Gould E, McEwen B S, Tanapat P, *et al.* 1997. Neurogenesis in the dentate gyrus of the adult tree shrew is regulated by psychosocial stress and NMDA receptor activation. *J Neurosci* **17**, 2492–8.

Gurvits T V, Shenton M E, Hokama H, *et al.* 1996. Magnetic resonance imaging study of hippocampal volume in chronic, combat-related posttraumatic stress disorder. *Biol Psychiatry* **40**, 1091–9.

Hakamata Y, Matsuoka Y, Inagaki M, *et al.* 2007. Structure of orbitofrontal cortex and its longitudinal course in

211

cancer-related post-traumatic stress disorder. *Neurosci Res* **59**, 383–9.

Ham B J, Chey J, Yoon S J, *et al.* 2007. Decreased N-acetyl-aspartate levels in anterior cingulate and hippocampus in subjects with post-traumatic stress disorder: A proton magnetic resonance spectroscopy study. *Eur J Neurosci* **25**, 324–9.

Hedges D W, Allen A, Tate D F, *et al.* 2003. Reduced hippocampal volume in alcohol and substance naïve Vietnam combat veterans with posttraumatic stress disorder. *Cognit Behav Neurol* **16**, 219–24.

Herry C, Ciocchi S, Senn V, *et al.* 2008. Switching on and off fear by distinct neuronal circuits. *Nature* **454**, 589–90.

Hull A M. 2002. Neuroimaging findings in post-traumatic stress disorder. *Br J Psychiatry* **181**, 102–10.

Jackowski A P, Douglas-Palumberi H, Jackowski M, *et al.* 2008. Corpus callosum in maltreated children with posttraumatic stress disorder: A diffusion tensor imaging study. *Psychiatry Res Neuroimag* **162**, 256–61.

Jatzko A, Rothenhöfer S, Schmitt A, *et al.* 2006. Hippocampal volume in chronic posttraumatic stress disorder (PTSD): MRI study using two different evaluation methods. *J Affect Disord* **94**, 121–6.

Karl A, Schaefer M, Malta L S, *et al.* 2006. A meta-analysis of structural brain abnormalities in PTSD. *Neurosci Biobehav Rev* **30**, 1004–31.

Kasai K, Yamasue H, Gilbertson M W, *et al.* 2008. Evidence for acquired pregenual anterior cingulate gray matter loss from a twin study of combat-related posttraumatic stress disorder. *Biol Psychiatry* **63**, 550–6.

Kim M J, Lyoo I K, Kim S J, *et al.* 2005. Disrupted white matter tract integrity of anterior cingulate in trauma survivors. *Neuroreport* **16**, 1049–53.

Kim S J, Jeong D U, Sim M E, *et al.* 2006. Asymmetrically altered integrity of cingulum bundle in posttraumatic stress disorder. *Neuropsychobiology* **54**, 120–5.

Kitayama N, Brummer M, Hertz L, *et al.* 2007. Morphologic alterations in the corpus callosum in abuse-related posttraumatic stress disorder: A preliminary study. *J Nerv Mental Disord* **195**, 1027–9.

Kitayama N, Quinn S and Bremner J D. 2006. Smaller volume of anterior cingulate cortex in abuse-related posttraumatic stress disorder. *J Affect Disord* **90**, 171–4.

Kitayama N, Vaccarino V, Kutner M, *et al.* 2005. Magnetic resonance imaging (MRI) measurement of hippocampal volume in posttraumatic stress disorder: A meta-analysis. *J Affect Disord* **88**, 79–86.

Laakso M P, Vaurio O, Savolainen L, *et al.* 2000. A volumetric MRI study of the hippocampus in type 1 and 2 alcoholism. *Behav Brain Res* **109**, 177–86.

Letizia B, Maricla T, Sara C, *et al.* 2008. Magnetic resonance imaging volumes of the hippocampus in drug-naïve patients with post-traumatic stress disorder without comorbidity conditions. *J Psychiatric Res* **42**, 752–62.

Levitt J J, Chen Q C, May F S, *et al.* 2006. Volume of cerebellar vermis in monozygotic twins discordant for combat exposure: Lack of relationship to posttraumatic stress disorder. *Psychiatry Res Neuroimag* **148**, 143–9.

Li L, Chen S, Liu J, *et al.* 2006. Magnetic resonance imaging and magnetic resonance spectroscopy study of deficits in hippocampal structure in fire victims with recent-onset posttraumatic stress disorder. *Can J Psychiatry* **51**, 431–7.

Lindauer R J L, Vlieger E J, Jalink M, *et al.* 2004. Smaller hippocampal volume in Dutch police officers with posttraumatic stress disorder. *Biol Psychiatry* **56**, 356–63.

Mahmutyazicioğlu K, Konuk N, Ozdemir H, *et al.* 2005. Evaluation of the hippocampus and the anterior cingulate gyrus by proton MR spectroscopy in patients with post-traumatic stress disorder. *Diagn Interven Radiol* **11**, 125–9.

Maren, S. 2005. Building and burying fear memories in the brain. *Neuroscientist* **11**, 89–99.

Margarinos A M, McEwen B S, Flugge G and Fuchs E. 1996. Chronic psychosocial stress causes apical dendritic atrophy of hippocampal CA3 pyramidal neurons in subordinate tree shrews. *J Neurosci* **16**, 3534–40.

Matsuoka Y, Yamawaki S, Inagaki M, *et al.* 2003. A volumetric study of amygdala in cancer survivors with instrusive recollections. *Biol Psychiatry* **54**, 736–43.

May F S, Chen Q C, Gilbertson M W, *et al.* 2004. Cavum septum pellucidum in monozygotic twins discordant for combat exposure: Relationship to posttraumatic stress disorder. *Biol Psychiatry* **55**, 656–8.

McEwen B S. 1995. Stressful experience, brain, and emotions: developmental, genetic, and hormonal influences. In Gazzaniga M S (ed.) *The Cognitive Neurosciences*. Cambridge, MA: MIT Press, pp. 1117–35.

Mohanakrishnan Menon P, Nasrallah H A, Lyons J A, *et al.* 2003. Single-voxel proton MR spectroscopy of right versus left hippocampi in PTSD. *Psychiatry Res Neuroimag* **123**, 101–08.

Mohanakrishnan Menon P, Nasrallah H A, Reeves R R and Ali J A. 2004. Hippocampal dysfunction in gulf war syndrome: A proton MR spectroscopy study. *Brain Res* **1009**, 189–94.

Myslobodsky M S, Glicksohn J, Singer J, *et al.* 1995. Changes of brain anatomy in patients with posttraumatic stress disorder: A pilot magnetic resonance imaging study. *Psychiatry Res* **58**, 259–64.

Nakano T, Wenner M, Inagaki M, *et al.* 2002. Relationship between distressing cancer-related recollections and hippocampal volume in cancer survivors. *Am J Psychiatry* **159**, 2087–93.

Pavić L, Gregurek R, Radoš M, *et al.* 2007. Smaller right hippocampus in war veterans with posttraumatic stress disorder. *Psychiatry Res Neuroimag* **154**, 191–8.

Pederson C L, Maurer S H, Kaminski P L, *et al.* 2004. Hippocampal volume and memory performance in a community-based sample of women with posttraumatic stress disorder secondary to child abuse. *J Traumat Stress* **17**, 37–40.

Pitman R K, Shin L M and Rauch S L. 2001. Investigating the pathogenesis of posttraumatic stress disorder with neuroimaging. *J Clin Psychiatry* **62**, 47–54.

Rauch S L, Shin L M and Phelps E A. 2006. Neurocircuitry models of posttraumatic stress disorder and extinction: Human neuroimaging research – Past, present, and future. *Biol Psychiatry* **60**, 376–82.

Rauch S L, Shin L M, Segal E, *et al.* 2003. Selectively reduced regional cortical volumes in post-traumatic stress disorder. *NeuroReport* **14**, 913–6.

Richert K A, Carrion V G, Karchemskiy A and Reiss A L. 2006. Regional differences of the prefrontal cortex in pediatric PTSD: An MRI study. *Depress Anxiety* **23**, 17–25.

Sapolsky R M, Uno H, Rebert C S and Finch C E. 1990. Hippocampal damage associated with prolonged glucocorticoid exposure in primates. *J Neurosci* **10**, 2897–902.

Schuff N, Neylan T C, Fox-Bosetti S, *et al.* 2008. Abnormal N-acetylaspartate in hippocampus and anterior cingulate in posttraumatic stress disorder. *Psychiatry Res* **162**, 147–57.

Schuff N, Neylan T C, Lenoci M A, *et al.* 2001. Decreased hippocampal N-acetylaspartate in the absence of atrophy in posttraumatic stress disorder. *Biol Psychiatry* **50**, 952–9.

Schwegler H and Lipp H P. 1983. Hereditary covariations of neuronal circuitry and behavior: Correlations between the proportions of hippocampal synaptic fields in the regio inferior and two-way avoidance in mice and rats. *Behav Brain Res* **7**, 1–38.

Shin L M, Shin P S, Heckers S, *et al.* 2004. Hippocampal function in posttraumatic stress disorder. *Hippocampus* **14**, 292–300.

Smith M A, Makino S, Kvetnansky R and Post R M. 1995. Stress and glucocorticoids affect the expression of brain-derived neurotrophic factor and neurotorphin-3 mRNAs in the hippocampus. *J Neurosci* **15**, 1768–77.

Smith M E. 2005. Bilateral hippocampal volume reduction in adults with post-traumatic stress disorder: A meta-analysis of structural MRI studies. *Hippocampus* **15**, 798–807.

Stein M B, Koverola C, Hanna C, *et al.* 1997. Hippocampal volume in women victimized by childhood sexual abuse. *Psychol Med* **27**, 951–9.

Thomas L A and De Bellis M D. 2004. Pituitary volumes in pediatric maltreatment-related posttraumatic stress disorder. *Biol Psychiatry* **55**, 752–8.

Tupler L A and De Bellis M D. 2006. Segmented hippocampal volume in children and adolescents with posttraumatic stress disorder. *Biol Psychiatry* **59**, 523–9.

Villarreal G, Hamilton D A, Graham D P, *et al.* 2004. Reduced area of the corpus callosum in posttraumatic stress disorder. *Psychiatry Res Neuroimag* **131**, 227–35.

Villarreal G, Hamilton D A, Petropoulos H, *et al.* 2002a. Reduced hippocampal volume and total white matter volume in posttraumatic stress disorder. *Biol Psychiatry* **52**, 119–25.

Villarreal G, Petropoulos H, Hamilton D A, *et al.* 2002b. Proton magnetic resonance spectroscopy of the hippocampus and occipital white matter in PTSD: Preliminary results. *Can J Psychiatry* **47**, 666–70.

Vythilingam M, Luckenbaugh D A, Lam T, *et al.* 2005. Smaller head of the hippocampus in Gulf War-related posttraumatic stress disorder. *Psychiatry Res Neuroimag* **139**, 89–99.

Wignall E L, Dickson J M, Vaughn P, *et al.* 2004. Smaller hippocampal volume in patients with recent-onset posttraumatic stress disorder. *Biol Psychiatry* **56**, 832–6.

Winter H and Irle E. 2004. Hippocampal volume in adult burn patients with and without posttraumatic stress disorder. *Am J Psychiatry* **16**, 2194–200.

Woodward S H, Kaloupek D G, Streeter C C, *et al.* 2006a. Hippocampal volume, PTSD, and alcoholism in combat veterans. *Am J Psychiatry* **163**, 674–81.

Woodward S H, Kaloupek D G, Streeter C C, *et al.* 2006b. Decreased anterior cingulate volume in combat-related PTSD. *Biol Psychiatry* **59**, 582–7.

Woon F L and Hedges D W. 2008. Hippocampal and amygdala volumes in children and adults with childhood maltreatment-related posttraumatic stress disorder: A meta-analysis. *Hippocampus* **18**, 729–36.

Uno H, Tarara R, Else J G, *et al.* 1989. Hippocampal damage associated with prolonged and fetal stress in primates. *J Neurosci* **9**, 1705–11.

Yamasue H, Kasai K, Iwanami A, *et al.* 2003. Voxel-based analysis of MRI reveals anterior cingulate gray-matter volume reduction in posttraumatic stress disorder due to terrorism. *Proc Natl Acad Sci* **100**, 9039–43.

Yehuda R, Golier J A, Tischler L, *et al.* 2007. Hippocampal volume in aging combat veterans with and without post-traumatic stress disorder: Relation to risk and resilience factors. *J Psychiatric Res* **41**, 435–45.

Chapter 14

Functional imaging of post-traumatic stress disorder

Lisa M. Shin, Kathryn Handwerger Brohawn, Danielle L. Pfaff and Roger K. Pitman

Introduction

Post-traumatic stress disorder (PTSD) is an anxiety disorder that can develop in individuals who (1) are exposed to an event or events that involve the threat of death or serious injury, and (2) react with intense fear, helplessness or horror (APA, 2000). Individuals with PTSD re-experience the traumatic event in various ways, including nightmares, intrusive recollections, and flashbacks. In addition, patients may attempt to avoid thoughts or reminders of the trauma and may experience a restricted range of affect, especially positive affect. Finally, patients with PTSD report hyperarousal symptoms, such as hypervigilance, exaggerated startle, and difficulty concentrating (APA, 2000).

In this chapter, we will summarize a neurocircuitry model of PTSD and briefly describe the techniques that have been used to study brain function in this disorder. We will then review the findings of relevant functional neuroimaging studies. Given that current neurocircuitry models focus on the amygdala, medial prefrontal cortex, and hippocampus, this review will include studies that have reported significant findings in those brain regions. (For other recent reviews, see Francati et al., 2007; Lanius et al., 2006; Rauch et al., 2006.) Lastly, we will summarize the findings and suggest directions for future research.

Neurocircuitry model of PTSD

Several brain structures have been of interest in functional neuroimaging studies of PTSD. First is the amygdala, because it is involved in the assessment of potential threat or ambiguity in the environment (Davis and Whalen, 2001; Whalen, 1998) and it plays a critical role in fear conditioning (LeDoux, 2000) and

the encoding of emotional memories (McGaugh, 2004; Dolcos et al., 2004). The medial prefrontal cortex (mPFC), including rostral anterior cingulate cortex (rACC), subcallosal gyrus, and medial frontal gyrus, is relevant to PTSD because these brain regions are involved in the inhibition of emotional information during task performance (Bishop et al., 2004; Whalen et al., 1998), as well as in extinction and the retention of extinction memories (Milad and Quirk, 2002; Morgan et al., 1993; Quirk et al., 2000), which appear to be deficient in PTSD (Orr et al., 2000). Finally, the hippocampus is relevant to PTSD because it is involved in the encoding of both neutral and emotional memories (Eichenbaum, 2000; McGaugh, 2004; Dolcos et al., 2004), and in memory for context during fear conditioning and extinction (Sanders et al., 2003; Maren and Holt, 2000; Corcoran and Maren, 2001).

According to neurocircuitry models of PTSD (Rauch et al., 1998, 2006), the amygdala is hyperresponsive, which may account for exaggerated fear responses and the indelible quality of traumatic memories. Furthermore, the mPFC (including the rACC) is hyporesponsive, and fails to inhibit the amygdala. This may underlie deficits in extinction and in inhibiting attention to trauma-related stimuli. Abnormal hippocampal function may be associated with declarative memory impairments, deficits in identifying safe contexts, and impaired regulation of the hypothalamic–pituitary–adrenal (HPA) axis in PTSD. (See also models described by Layton and Krikorian, 2002; Elzinga and Bremner, 2002; Hamner et al., 1999.)

Tasks, stimuli, and techniques

Several different types of tasks have been developed for use in functional neuroimaging studies of PTSD.

Some employ personalized stimuli that cue subjects to recall traumatic as well as other events from their own lives. A technique that is frequently used to accomplish this goal is script-driven imagery, which was developed by Peter Lang and colleagues (1983) and later adapted to the study of PTSD by Roger Pitman and Scott Orr (Pitman *et al.*, 1987). In script-driven imagery, participants write narratives of their own traumatic and other personal events. Later, on the basis of these narratives, "scripts" are composed in the second person, present tense and audiotaped for playback in the scanner. During script-driven imagery scans, participants are asked to recall and imagine the event being described.

Although script-driven imagery is quite effective at provoking symptomatic or emotional states, a disadvantage of this technique is that, because they are personalized, the stimuli vary widely across subjects. In order to decrease variability and increase experimental control, some researchers have designed sets of "standardized" trauma-related stimuli that are tailored to an entire group of trauma survivors as a whole. Such stimuli include photographs, words, sounds, or smells that are relevant to a particular type of trauma, e.g. combat. Some studies require participants simply to attend to these stimuli, whereas others require them to perform a cognitive task involving them.

In order to determine whether functional abnormalities in PTSD are specific to the processing of trauma-related information, some researchers have implemented emotional stimuli that are unrelated to the traumatic event, including imagery scripts of other life events, generally negative and/or positive photographs, and facial expressions. Several studies have even used neutral stimuli, such as neutral words or auditory tones, in cognitive tasks designed to activate specific brain regions of interest.

Researchers have also examined brain activity of PTSD patients at rest. However, interpreting the findings of resting state studies is often difficult given that participants do not perform any specific task in the scanner. Nevertheless, resting state findings can be illuminating especially if they are correlated with symptom severity or treatment response.

A few research groups have attempted to study the relationship between functional neuroimaging measures and treatment response in PTSD. In some studies, researchers scan patients before and after treatment to determine whether changes in brain function are associated with symptomatic improvement. In other studies, functional imaging measures obtained before treatment are used to predict clinical response.

Researchers studying brain function in PTSD have implemented a wide variety of imaging techniques, including positron emission tomography (PET), single photon emission computed tomography (SPECT), and functional magnetic resonance imaging (fMRI). Furthermore, among researchers using PET, some have implemented oxygen-15 labeled water or carbon dioxide to measure regional cerebral blood flow (rCBF), whereas others have used ^{18}F-fluorodeoxyglucose (FDG) to measure regional cerebral metabolic rate for glucose (rCMRglu).

In the following review, we present the results of functional neuroimaging studies that have yielded findings relevant to the amygdala, medial prefrontal cortex, and hippocampus in PTSD. We have organized the studies according to both the type of stimuli and the type of imaging technique used.

Amygdala

Script-driven imagery

PET

Several PET oxygen-15 studies have used script-driven imagery to study individuals with PTSD. Rauch and colleagues (1996) demonstrated amygdala activation in individuals with PTSD during imagery of traumatic as compared to neutral scripts, although there was no non-PTSD comparison group. Shin and colleagues (2004a) found greater amygdala activation in the traumatic vs. neutral contrast in male Vietnam combat veterans with versus without PTSD. Female nurses with PTSD who served in Vietnam did not exhibit exaggerated amygdala activation relative to female nurse veterans without PTSD. However, both male and female participants with PTSD showed positive correlations between amygdala blood flow and PTSD symptom severity. Osuch and colleagues (2008) scanned individuals 10–29 days after experiencing motor vehicle accidents and then assessed their PTSD symptoms 3 months later. Compared to healthy, trauma-unexposed comparison subjects, accident survivors showed less amygdala activation in response to traumatic versus neutral imagery scripts. This would seem to contradict findings of exaggerated amygdala activation in PTSD. However, follow-up assessments revealed that only 4 of the 22 accident survivors developed the disorder. That most

215

of the accident survivors did not develop PTSD suggests that resilience may be characterized by less amygdala responsivity. Britton and colleagues (2005) also reported diminished amygdala activation during traumatic imagery in trauma-exposed individuals without PTSD.

Using functional connectivity methods, Gilboa and colleagues (2004) demonstrated a positive relationship between amygdala, anterior cingulate, subcallosal cortex, and visual cortex in their PTSD group. In contrast, Shin and colleagues (2004a) found a negative correlation between blood flow changes in the amygdala and those in medial prefrontal cortex in PTSD. In a resilient group of accident survivors, Osuch and colleagues (2008) found a positive correlation between activation in the amygdala and rostral anterior cingulate cortex during traumatic vs. neutral script-driven imagery.

fMRI

Piefke and colleagues (2007) studied accident survivors with acute PTSD using fMRI and script-driven imagery. They found amygdala activation during the traumatic condition compared to both a baseline and a negative, non-traumatic condition. However, interpretation of these findings is limited by the lack of a non-PTSD comparison group.

Trauma-related stimuli
PET

Shin and colleagues (1997) reported amygdala activation during visual mental imagery of standardized combat-related photographs in combat veterans with PTSD, but not in combat veterans without PTSD. Pissiota and colleagues (2002) found amygdala activation in response to combat sounds versus white noise in veterans with PTSD; this amygdala activation was positively correlated with subjective ratings of distress. Vermetten and colleagues (2007) presented a combat-related smell (diesel fuel) to combat veterans with versus without PTSD during PET scanning. The PTSD group exhibited greater amygdala activation, distress, and symptom severity in response to the diesel smell than the combat veterans without PTSD.

SPECT

Liberzon and colleagues (1999) presented combat sounds and white noise in separate conditions to combat veterans with versus without PTSD, as well

as to healthy combat-unexposed participants. They found greater amygdala activation in the combat sounds versus white noise contrast in combat veterans with PTSD relative to the other groups.

fMRI

Two recent fMRI studies have reported exaggerated amygdala activation during the presentation of trauma-related photographs to participants with PTSD. Hendler and colleagues (2003) presented combat-related and neutral photographs at varying recognition thresholds to combat veterans with versus without PTSD. They found that the PTSD group had greater amygdala responses to both combat-related and neutral photographs regardless of the recognition threshold. Morey and colleagues (2009) presented combat veterans with task-irrelevant combat-related photographs or neutral photographs while they performed a neutral working memory task in the fMRI scanner. Combat veterans with PTSD showed greater amygdala activation in response to the combat-related versus neutral photographs, whereas the combat veterans without PTSD did not show this effect.

Two fMRI studies have reported amygdala hyper-responsivity to trauma-related words in PTSD. Protopopescu and colleagues (2005) presented trauma-related, panic-related, positive, and neutral words to individuals with PTSD and trauma-unexposed healthy individuals. Relative to the comparison group, the PTSD group showed greater amygdala responses to the trauma-related words versus neutral words. In addition, amygdala activation was positively correlated with PTSD symptom severity. Furthermore, amygdala activation in the trauma vs. neutral word comparison habituated over time in the PTSD group. Driessen and colleagues (2004) presented participants with words that would cue them to recall specific personal traumatic and non-traumatic events. Women with PTSD and borderline personality disorder showed exaggerated amygdala/uncus activation in response to traumatic vs. non-traumatic word cues, whereas women with borderline personality disorder alone did not.

Trauma-unrelated emotional stimuli
PET

Researchers recently have become interested in implementing Pavlovian fear conditioning paradigms during neuroimaging to study amygdala function in patients with this disorder (Rauch *et al.*, 2006). In the first study of its type, Bremner and colleagues (2005) scanned subjects during a fear conditioning phase, which consisted of presenting a specific visual stimulus (blue square) along with a mild electric shock to the forearm. They found that abuse survivors with PTSD showed greater amygdala responses during fear conditioning than healthy control subjects without abuse histories.

fMRI

Exaggerated amygdala activation in PTSD has also been found in response to some types of trauma-unrelated emotional material, such as facial expressions. Rauch and colleagues (2000) presented participants with fearful and happy facial expressions that were "backwardly masked" by neutral facial expressions such that participants did not report seeing the emotional expressions. Relative to the trauma-exposed comparison group, the PTSD group exhibited greater amygdala responses to the masked fearful versus masked happy faces. Furthermore, amygdala responses in the PTSD group were positively correlated with PTSD symptom severity, but not with depression severity. Similarly, Armony and colleagues (2005) reported a positive correlation between amygdala responses to masked fearful faces and PTSD symptom severity. Bryant *et al.* (2008b) found greater amygdala responses to masked fearful versus neutral expressions in a PTSD group than in a trauma-unexposed comparison group. Furthermore, in the PTSD group, amygdala responses were negatively correlated with responses in the rostral anterior cingulate cortex. Using unmasked, i.e. overtly presented, fearful and happy facial expressions, Shin and colleagues (2005) demonstrated exaggerated amygdala responses in individuals with PTSD compared to trauma-exposed individuals without PTSD. (See Figure 14.1.) Furthermore, in the PTSD group, amygdala activation was negatively correlated with activation in medial prefrontal cortex. This study also reported a trend for less habituation to the fearful vs. happy faces in the PTSD group compared to the control group. In a similar study using overtly presented fearful and neutral facial expressions, Williams *et al.* (2006) also reported greater amygdala activation in the PTSD group compared to a trauma-unexposed comparison group. Positive correlations were found in the PTSD group between right amygdala and left anterior cingulate cortex,

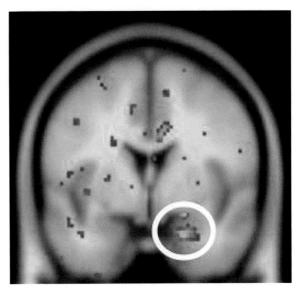

Figure 14.1 Right amygdala activation in response to Fearful vs. Happy facial expressions (*x, y, z*: +22, +2, −14 and +22, 0, −26) that was greater in the PTSD group than in the trauma-exposed control group.

although exactly which portion of the anterior cingulate was correlated with the amygdala was unclear. Dickie and colleagues (2008) showed facial expressions to participants with PTSD during fMRI scanning and afterwards tested their recognition memory for the faces. Although there was no control group, PTSD symptom severity scores were positively correlated with left amygdala activation. In a different memory paradigm that manipulated emotional context, Whalley *et al.* (2009) presented participants with neutral stimuli superimposed upon negative or positive photographs. Later during fMRI, participants' recognition memory for the neutral stimuli was tested. The PTSD group showed greater amygdala/ventral striatum activation associated with the correct recollection of the neutral stimuli.

Neutral stimuli or rest
PET

A study by Semple and colleagues (2000) employed a neutral auditory continuous performance task during PET scanning. Veterans with PTSD and comorbid substance abuse had higher amygdala blood flow compared to a healthy trauma-unexposed comparison group. Shin and colleagues (2004b) studied firefighters with versus without PTSD using a word-stem completion recall task during scanning. Collapsing across deep and shallow recall conditions, the PTSD group had greater rCBF in the amygdala and hippocampus than the non-PTSD group. In contrast, in a resilient group of motor vehicle accident survivors, Osuch *et al.* (2008) found lower blood flow in the amygdala at rest.

SPECT

Chung and colleagues (2006) reported greater amygdala perfusion at rest in a PTSD group compared to a trauma-unexposed healthy control group. However, other resting-state SPECT studies have not revealed exaggerated amygdala activation in PTSD (Bonne *et al.*, 2003; Mirzaei *et al.*, 2001; Pavic *et al.*, 2003; Sachinvala *et al.*, 2000).

fMRI

Bryant and colleagues (2005) used an auditory oddball paradigm and found enhanced amygdala responses to targets in a PTSD group relative to a trauma-unexposed healthy comparison group.

Association with treatment response
SPECT

In a group of patients with subthreshold PTSD, Peres *et al.* (2007) found that amygdala responses to traumatic imagery scripts decreased following exposure and cognitive restructuring therapy.

fMRI

Two recent studies have reported a relationship between amygdala function and clinical response to cognitive-behavioral therapy. Felmingham and colleagues (2007) presented fearful and neutral facial expressions to participants with PTSD both before and after cognitive behavioral therapy. Decreases in amygdala responses were associated with symptomatic improvement. Using a different design, Bryant and colleagues (2008a) found that greater pretreatment amygdala activation to masked fearful vs. neutral faces was associated with a poorer response to cognitive-behavioral therapy.

Summary and comments

Overall, amygdala activation appears to be exaggerated in PTSD, especially in studies involving the use of fearful facial expressions. Additionally, several studies have reported positive correlations between amygdala activation and PTSD symptom severity,

suggesting that amygdala responses are related to the clinical presentation of the disorder. However, not all studies have found this pattern of results (e.g. Bremner *et al.*, 1999a, 1999b; Britton *et al.*, 2005; Lanius *et al.*, 2001, 2002; Shin *et al.*, 1999). There may be multiple reasons for the lack of amygdala activation, particularly in studies that implement PET or SPECT imaging. These techniques have poorer temporal resolution because they require a block design in which blood flow within a condition is typically averaged over a long period of time (from 1 min with PET ^{15}O to 40 min with PET-FDG). Amygdala responses can habituate during this period (Breiter *et al.*, 1996), even in PTSD (Shin *et al.*, 2005; Protopopescu *et al.*, 2005). Averaging blood flow or glucose metabolic rate over several minutes reduces the likelihood of detecting amygdala activation both within and between groups. The lack of amygdala hyper-responsivity in some studies of PTSD also may be due to the use of an imagery task. Amygdala responses to internally generated stimuli appear to be smaller than those in response to externally presented stimuli (Reiman *et al.*, 1997).

Medial prefrontal cortex/rostral anterior cingulate cortex
Script-driven imagery
PET

Studies implementing script-driven imagery have typically reported less activation or even *de*activation in mPFC regions in PTSD during traumatic versus neutral imagery scripts. Bremner and colleagues (1999a) reported deactivation of subcallosal gyrus and a failure to activate the rACC in childhood sexual abuse survivors with PTSD compared to those without PTSD. Shin *et al.* (1999) found relatively less rACC activation in childhood sexual abuse survivors with PTSD compared to those without. (See Figure 14.2.) Using similar techniques, Shin and colleagues (2004a) found less activation in medial frontal gyrus, just anterior to the rACC, in male combat veterans and female nurse veterans with PTSD compared to those without PTSD. In addition, within the PTSD group, rCBF in medial frontal gyrus was negatively correlated with both PTSD symptom severity and rCBF in the amygdala. Similarly, Britton *et al.* (2005) reported lower rACC activation in combat veterans with PTSD than in veterans without PTSD and healthy

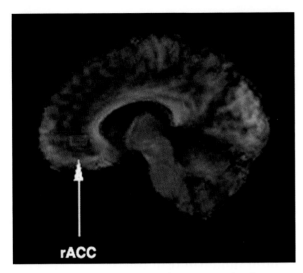

rACC

Figure 14.2 Activation in the rostral anterior cingulate (x, y, z: +7, +38, 0) in the Traumatic vs. Neutral contrast that was lower in women with PTSD than in women without PTSD.

non-combat control subjects. In the PTSD group, dorsomedial prefrontal cortex activation was negatively correlated with PTSD symptom severity.

SPECT

In a study of police officers with versus without PTSD, Lindauer and colleagues (2004) reported lower activation in medial frontal gyrus in response to traumatic versus neutral script-driven imagery in officers with PTSD.

fMRI

In the first fMRI study to implement script-driven imagery in the study of PTSD, Lanius *et al.* (2001) reported significantly diminished activation in the rACC and medial frontal gyrus in the traumatic vs. baseline imagery condition. Diminished ACC responses have also been reported during script-driven imagery involving sad and anxious mood states (Lanius *et al.*, 2003), suggesting that decreased ACC responses are not specific to reminders of trauma. In contrast, this group found that a subgroup of PTSD patients who dissociated, rather than re-experienced, during traumatic imagery showed an opposite pattern of greater activation in the rACC and medial frontal gyrus (Lanius *et al.*, 2002, 2005). This group also found that patients with PTSD and comorbid MDD had greater rACC activation than patients with PTSD alone, although both groups showed less rACC activation than trauma-exposed control

subjects. Hopper and colleagues (2007) recently reported a negative correlation between rACC activation and self-reported re-experiencing during traumatic scripts in PTSD. Frewen *et al.* (2008) reported a negative correlation between activation in the ACC during traumatic script-driven imagery and degree of emotional awareness in PTSD. In contrast, the control group showed a positive correlation between these two variables. In a study of acute accident-related PTSD, Piefke and colleagues (2007) reported rACC activation during traumatic scripts vs. baseline. However, whether this activation deviated from normal is unknown because this study lacked a control group.

Trauma-related stimuli
PET

Bremner and colleagues (1999b) found less activation in the rACC and deactivation in subgenual cortex in response to trauma-related audiovisual stimuli in combat veterans with PTSD. Also using trauma-related visual stimuli, Shin and colleagues (1997) found less blood flow in rACC during the perception of trauma-related vs. neutral photographs, yet greater blood flow in subgenual ACC during visual mental imagery of those photographs. Bremner and colleagues (2004) used an emotional Stroop task, which involved naming the ink color of trauma-related words, to study brain activation in a group of sexual abuse survivors with versus without PTSD. In the trauma-related vs. the neutral comparison, the PTSD group showed significantly less activation in the rACC than the group without PTSD.

SPECT

Two SPECT studies seem to have yielded findings in the mPFC that are different from the findings of other types of studies. Liberzon and colleagues (1999) found equivalent ACC activation in veterans with PTSD, veterans without PTSD, and non-veteran healthy controls during the presentation of combat sounds versus white noise. A different study that employed standardized combat sounds revealed greater medial prefrontal cortex reactivity in veterans with PTSD than in combat and healthy controls (Zubieta *et al.*, 1999).

fMRI

Yang *et al.* (2004) assessed neural correlates of the imagery and perception of earthquake-related pictures in adolescent earthquake survivors. Results revealed that participants without PTSD activated the rACC, whereas those with PTSD did not. Hou and colleagues (2007) found decreased anterior cingulate activation in response to trauma-related pictures vs. neutral pictures in a group of survivors of a coal mining accident with PTSD compared to those without PTSD. In contrast, Morey and colleagues (2009) reported a significant positive correlation between PTSD symptom severity and rACC activation to combat-related vs. neutral photographs. However, this study lacked a comparison group without PTSD. Using an emotional Stroop task with trauma-related words, Shin et al. (2001) reported a failure to activate the rACC in combat veterans with PTSD relative to combat veterans without PTSD. The PTSD group instead showed greater activation of the dorsal ACC (dACC).

Trauma-unrelated emotional stimuli
PET
Studies employing trauma-unrelated emotional stimuli have also reported relatively diminished activation in the rACC in PTSD. Phan and colleagues (2006) presented aversive and neutral photographs to subjects during PET scanning and found deactivation in the ventral mPFC in a PTSD group compared to healthy comparison group. Using emotional word stimuli, Bremner and colleagues (2003b) found blood flow decreases in the rACC and subcallosal cortex during the retrieval of deeply encoded negative vs. neutral words in women with PTSD compared to healthy women without PTSD. In a fear-conditioning and extinction paradigm, Bremner and colleagues (2005) reported decreased activity in the rACC and subcallosal cortex during extinction in women with PTSD relative to trauma-unexposed controls.

fMRI
Using emotional facial expression stimuli, Shin et al. (2005) reported diminished responses to fearful vs. happy expressions in the rACC, dorsal mPFC, and ventral mPFC in men with PTSD compared to trauma-exposed men without PTSD. In addition, rACC activation was negatively correlated with PTSD symptom severity. Relatively diminished rACC activation in response to fearful vs. neutral faces in PTSD has also been reported by Williams and colleagues (2006). Similarly, Kim and colleagues (2008) found diminished rACC activation in response to fearful vs. neutral faces in a PTSD relative to a trauma-

unexposed control group. Rostral ACC activation was negatively correlated with PTSD symptom severity. Dickie et al. (2008) found a negative correlation between symptom severity and ventral mPFC activity in response to subsequently forgotten faces in PTSD. In contrast to the previous studies, Bryant and colleagues (2008b) reported greater ventral mPFC activation during the unconscious processing of fearful vs. neutral faces in PTSD compared to trauma-unexposed control subjects. Using a very different task involving decision-making, Sailer et al. (2008) found diminished activation in medial frontal gyrus and nucleus accumbens in response to gain feedback.

Neutral stimuli or rest
PET
Semple et al. (2000) reported diminished blood flow in the ACC/medial frontal gyrus both at rest and during an auditory continuous performance task in patients with PTSD and histories of substance abuse relative to healthy trauma-unexposed subjects. In a group of resilient motor vehicle accident survivors, most of whom did not develop PTSD, Osuch and colleagues (2008) found greater blood flow at rest in the rACC.

Only three PET studies have utilized FDG to study rCMRglu in PTSD. Molina and colleagues (2010) reported diminished activity in the ACC and medial frontal gyrus in veterans with PTSD relative to those without the disorder. Bremner et al. (1997) found no rCMRglu differences in the ACC between veterans with PTSD and trauma-unexposed healthy individuals. Finally, Shin and colleagues (2009) reported greater rCMRglu in the dACC and midcingulate cortex in combat veterans with PTSD and their identical co-twins compared to combat veterans without PTSD and their identical co-twins. (See Figure 14.3.) This finding suggests that hypermetabolism in this region is a familial risk factor for developing PTSD after trauma exposure, rather than an acquired characteristic of PTSD.

SPECT
Again, SPECT studies have yielded different findings with regard to the ACC in PTSD. Sachinvala and colleagues (2000) found enhanced perfusion at rest in the ACC in individuals with PTSD relative to healthy controls. Chung et al. (2006) reported greater rCBF

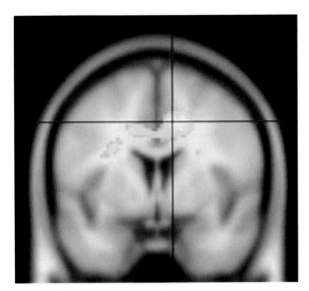

Figure 14.3 Greater glucose metabolism at rest in the dorsal anterior cingulate/midcingulate cortex (x, y, z: +10, +2, +42) in Vietnam veterans with PTSD and their identical co-twins compared to Vietnam veterans without PTSD and their identical co-twins.

in subgenual cingulate cortex at rest in car accident survivors relative to trauma unexposed healthy participants. Bonne *et al.* (2003) found no difference in resting ACC perfusion between PTSD, trauma-exposed control, and trauma-unexposed control groups.

fMRI

The finding of diminished rACC responsivity appears to occur less frequently in fMRI studies that implement neutral stimuli. Bryant and colleagues (2005) used fMRI to study brain responses to an auditory oddball paradigm in individuals with PTSD compared to trauma-unexposed healthy control subjects. The PTSD group showed enhanced rACC and dACC activation (relative to healthy controls) in response to oddball targets versus non-targets. In a study by Shin *et al.* (2007), PTSD and non-PTSD groups did not differ with regard to rACC activation during a neutral Stroop task, although there were trends for greater dACC activation in PTSD. In a group of children with posttraumatic stress symptoms relative to healthy children, Carrion *et al.* (2008) found greater activation in the dACC and rACC during a Go–NoGo task. Finally, in a study of verbal working memory, Moores and colleagues (2008) found diminished ACC activation during working memory updating in a PTSD group relative to a healthy comparison group.

Association with treatment response
PET

Several studies have documented a relationship between activity in the anterior cingulate and improvement following various methods of treatment. In an early case report, Fernandez *et al.* (2001) found that successful treatment of PTSD with fluoxetine was associated with increased activation in ventral prefrontal cortex.

SPECT

Seedat and colleagues (2004) examined brain activation in patients with PTSD both before and after 8 weeks of treatment with citalopram. Perfusion increases in mPFC (left paracingulate gyrus) in response to treatment were correlated with symptomatic improvement. Peres and colleagues (2007) reported a significant increase in left anterior cingulate activity in response to traumatic scripts following exposure-based and restructuring psychotherapy. Similarly, Levin *et al.* (1999) noted increases in ACC activation in a single patient treated with EMDR. Lansing and colleagues (2005) found increased activation with EMDR treatment in medial frontal gyrus/rACC.

fMRI

Felmingham and colleagues (2007) assessed brain activation to fearful vs. neutral faces both before and 6 months following cognitive behavioral therapy in individuals with PTSD. They found significantly increased rACC activation following treatment. In contrast, Bryant *et al.* (2008a) assessed brain responses to masked fearful versus neutral facial expressions in patients with PTSD before undergoing cognitive behavioral treatment. Pretreatment rACC responses were positively correlated with post-treatment PTSD symptom severity scores. Individuals who did not respond well to the CBT displayed significantly greater pretreatment rACC than those who did respond. The researchers speculated that this counterintuitive finding was due to the rapid presentation of fear stimuli, which differed from the types of stimulus presentations used in previous studies.

Summary and comments

Relatively diminished activation of the mPFC, including the rACC, subcallosal gyrus, and medial frontal gyrus, is one of the most robust, although not universal, findings in functional neuroimaging studies of

PTSD. Diminished activation in the mPFC appears to be more commonly found in studies that use trauma-related or emotional stimuli, although it has occurred in some tasks implementing neutral stimuli as well. Overall, mPFC activation appears to correlate negatively with PTSD symptom severity and to increase with successful treatment.

It is important to note that most findings of diminished mPFC activation in PTSD have occurred in rostral or ventral portions of the ACC or the medial frontal gyrus. In fact, several of the reviewed studies suggest that the dorsal portions of the ACC actually may be *hyper-responsive* in PTSD (Bremner *et al.*, 2005; Bryant *et al.*, 2005; Shin *et al.*, 2001, 2007). Thus, when interpreting functional neuroimaging findings within the ACC in PTSD, determining the *location* of the effects, e.g. rostral vs. dorsal, appears to be critical.

Although not reviewed here, some studies have reported decreased volumes of the ACC in PTSD (Rauch *et al.*, 2003; Yamasue *et al.*, 2003; Woodward *et al.*, 2006). Whether diminished volumes can explain diminished function of the ACC is not currently clear, but future studies should evaluate this issue.

Hippocampus
Script-driven imagery
PET

Bremner and colleagues (1999a) used PET and script-driven imagery to study rCBF in childhood sexual abuse survivors. Relative to survivors without PTSD, those with PTSD exhibited rCBF decreases in the hippocampus in the traumatic versus neutral script contrast. Recently, Osuch *et al.* (2008) reported a similar finding of decreased hippocampal blood flow during traumatic vs. neutral imagery in recent motor vehicle accident survivors compared to healthy trauma-unexposed comparison subjects. These researchers also found a significant negative correlation between PTSD symptom severity and right hippocampal blood flow changes. However, as noted previously, only a small percentage of these subjects ended up meeting diagnostic criteria for PTSD. In contrast, Osuch and colleagues (2001) reported a positive correlation between flashback intensity during script-driven imagery and blood flow in the left perihippocampal region, among other areas.

SPECT

In a study implementing SPECT and script-driven imagery before and after treatment with exposure/cognitive restructuring, Peres and colleagues (2007) reported increased left hippocampal activity to traumatic scripts following psychotherapy in a group of individuals with PTSD. Waitlist control subjects showed no rCBF changes over time.

Trauma-related stimuli
fMRI

Using fMRI and a verbal declarative memory task, Thomaes *et al.* (2009) assessed hippocampal function in female childhood abuse survivors with "complex" PTSD versus healthy comparison subjects. During scanning, subjects were presented with abuse-related and neutral words that they encoded either deeply or shallowly. Subjects were also scanned a few minutes later during a recognition test. The PTSD group showed greater activation than controls in the left parahippocampal gyrus during the deep encoding of negative words vs. baseline. The PTSD group also showed greater left hippocampal and parahippocampal activation during the correct recognition of trauma-related words. Thus, it appears that hippocampal activation is not always diminished in PTSD, and that the use of trauma-related stimuli may be more likely to reveal exaggerated hippocampal and parahippocampal activation in PTSD.

Trauma-unrelated emotional stimuli
PET

Bremner *et al.* (2003b) presented childhood sexual abuse survivors with PTSD and healthy trauma-unexposed comparison subjects with neutral and emotional word pairs. Subjects were then scanned during the recollection of the word pairs. Relative to the comparison group, the PTSD group showed greater blood flow decreases in the left hippocampus during the retrieval of the emotional versus neutral word pairs.

Neutral stimuli or rest
PET

Bremner *et al.* (2003b) reported no differences in hippocampal activity between a PTSD and healthy control group during retrieval of neutral word pairs. However, in a separate study, these investigators

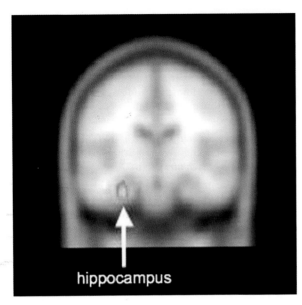

Figure 14.4 Left hippocampal activation (x, y, z: −28, −16, −24) in the deep vs. shallow comparison that was lower in firefighters with PTSD than in firefighters without PTSD.

(Bremner *et al.*, 2003a) found relatively diminished left hippocampal activation in a PTSD versus control group during the encoding of neutral verbal passages. The finding remained even when hippocampal volumes were statistically controlled. In a word-stem cued recall study by Shin and colleagues (2004b), subjects saw neutral words and encoded them either deeply or shallowly before scanning. Subjects were then scanned during recall, and hippocampal blood flow was compared between the deeply encoded and shallowly encoded word conditions. Firefighters with PTSD showed less hippocampal activation than firefighters without PTSD. (See Figure 14.4.) However, this finding was driven by enhanced hippocampal activity in the shallow condition in the PTSD group. In fact, collapsing across conditions revealed that the PTSD group had higher hippocampal blood flow than the non-PTSD group. Other studies have reported evidence for greater hippocampal activity in PTSD during a continuous performance task (Semple *et al.*, 2000), and at rest (Sachinvala *et al.*, 2000). However, Molina and colleagues (2010) reported lower rCMRglu in the hippocampus at rest in combat veterans with PTSD relative to those without PTSD.

fMRI

A number of recent fMRI studies have examined hippocampal activation in tasks involving neutral stimuli. Astur and colleagues (2006) found reduced hippocampal activation during a virtual Morris Water Maze task in a PTSD group relative to a healthy control group. In addition, PTSD symptom severity was negatively correlated with hippocampal activation. Moores *et al.* (2008) found diminished hippocampal activation during working memory updating in PTSD relative to a healthy comparison group. Geuze and colleagues (2008) scanned veterans with versus without PTSD while they encoded and retrieved neutral word-pair associates. In the PTSD group, parahippocampal activation was relatively greater during encoding and relatively less during retrieval. Similar findings were reported by Werner and colleagues (2009), who found greater hippocampal activation during the encoding of paired associates, i.e., face–profession name pairs, and less parahippocampal activation during their retrieval.

Summary and comments

Several studies have reported diminished hippocampal activation in PTSD, especially in those studies that implemented tasks with neutral stimuli. Interestingly, the one study that used trauma-related material in the context of a memory task showed enhanced hippocampal activation in PTSD (Thomaes *et al.*, 2009). Additional studies of this type are needed to more completely characterize hippocampal function in this disorder.

Although not reviewed in the text above, several studies have reported decreased hippocampal volumes in PTSD (Bremner *et al.*, 1995; Gurvits *et al.*, 1996, Karl *et al.*, 2006). Although some functional neuroimaging studies controlled for hippocampal volumes in their analyses (Bremner *et al.*, 2003a, Shin *et al.*, 2004b), additional research is needed to determine the effect of possible volumetric loss on measures of hippocampal function in PTSD.

Future directions

Functional neuroimaging studies of PTSD first appeared in the literature in the early 1990s. Since that time, the field has progressed rapidly, and research has yielded an enormous amount of information concerning the functional neurocircuitry of this disorder. However, many issues remain incompletely investigated, and further research will be required. For example, whether patients with acute PTSD show functional abnormalities similar to those found in the much more frequently studied chronic form of the disorder has not been established; future research might directly compare neuroimaging measures in these two groups. In addition, the extent to which functional abnormalities seen in PTSD are specific to that disorder has not been fully determined. Although the functional neurocircuitry of PTSD does appear to be distinct from that of obsessive–compulsive disorder, how much it differs from panic and social anxiety disorder requires further research. Finally, whether the functional abnormalities described herein represent acquired signs of PTSD or whether they are risk factors for its development after the occurrence of psychological trauma has scarcely been investigated. Future studies utilizing twin and longitudinal designs will be needed to adequately address this issue. If functional neuroimaging abnormalities are determined to be risk factors, then additional research might investigate whether these abnormalities represent endophenotypes for specific genetic polymorphisms (Binder *et al.*, 2008; Koenen *et al.*, 2005; Lee *et al.*, 2005).

Box 14.1.   Summary Box

Amygdala activation is exaggerated in PTSD and correlates positively with symptom severity.

Activation in rostral portions of the medial prefrontal cortex is diminished and correlates inversely with symptom severity.

These results support a neurocircuitry model in which a hyporesponsive medial prefrontal cortex fails to inhibit the amygdala.

This dysfunction may result in failure to inhibit attention to trauma-related stimuli and deficits in the extinction of fear responses.

Functional abnormalities in medial prefrontal regions normalize with successful treatment.

References

APA. 2000. *Diagnostic and Statistical Manual of Mental Disorders, Fourth Edition, Text-Revision*. Washington, DC: American Psychiatric Press.

Armony J L, Corbo V, Clement M H and Brunet A. 2005. Amygdala response in patients with acute PTSD to masked and unmasked emotional facial expressions. *Am J Psychiatry* **162**, 1961–3.

Astur R S, St Germain S A, Tolin D, Ford J, Russell D and Stevens M. 2006. Hippocampus function predicts severity of post-traumatic stress disorder. *Cyberpsychol Behav* **9**, 234–40.

Binder E B, Bradley R G, Liu W, *et al.* 2008. Association of FKBP5 polymorphisms and childhood abuse with risk of posttraumatic stress disorder symptoms in adults. *JAMA* **299**, 1291–305.

Bishop S, Duncan J, Brett M and Lawrence A D. 2004. Prefrontal cortical function and anxiety: Controlling attention to threat-related stimuli. *Nat Neurosci* **7**, 184–8.

Bonne O, Gilboa A, Louzoun Y, *et al.* 2003. Resting regional cerebral perfusion in recent posttraumatic stress disorder. *Biol Psychiatry* **54**, 1077–86.

Breiter H C, Etcoff N L, Whalen P J, *et al.* 1996. Response and habituation of the human amygdala during visual processing of facial expression. *Neuron* **17**, 875–87.

Bremner J D, Innis R B, Ng C K, *et al.* 1997. Positron emission tomography measurement of cerebral metabolic correlates of yohimbine administration in combat-related posttraumatic stress disorder. *Arch Gen Psychiatry* **54**, 246–54.

Bremner J D, Narayan M, Staib L H, Southwick S M, McGlashan T and Charney D S. 1999a. Neural correlates of memories of childhood sexual abuse in women with and without posttraumatic stress disorder. *Am J Psychiatry* **156**, 1787–95.

Bremner J D, Randall P, Scott T M, *et al.* 1995. MRI-based measurement of hippocampal volume in patients with combat-related posttraumatic stress disorder. *Am J Psychiatry* **152**, 973–81.

Bremner J D, Staib L H, Kaloupek D, Southwick S M, Soufer R and Charney D S. 1999b. Neural correlates of exposure to traumatic pictures and sound in Vietnam combat veterans with and without posttraumatic stress disorder: A positron emission tomography study. *Biol Psychiatry* **45**, 806–16.

Bremner J D, Vermetten E, Schmahl C, *et al.* 2005. Positron emission tomographic imaging of neural correlates of a fear acquisition and extinction paradigm in women with childhood sexual-abuse-related post-traumatic stress disorder. *Psychol Med* **35**, 791–806.

Bremner J D, Vermetten E, Vythilingam M, *et al.* 2004. Neural correlates of the classic color and emotional stroop in women with abuse-related posttraumatic stress disorder. *Biol Psychiatry* **55**, 612–20.

Bremner J D, Vythilingam M, Vermetten E, *et al.* 2003a. MRI and PET study of deficits in hippocampal structure and function in women with childhood sexual abuse and posttraumatic stress disorder. *Am J Psychiatry* **160**, 924–32.

Bremner J D, Vythilingam M, Vermetten E, *et al.* 2003b. Neural correlates of declarative memory for emotionally valenced words in women with posttraumatic stress disorder related to early childhood sexual abuse. *Biol Psychiatry* **53**, 879–89.

Britton J C, Phan K L, Taylor S F, Fig L M and Liberzon I. 2005. Corticolimbic blood flow in posttraumatic stress disorder during script-driven imagery. *Biol Psychiatry* **57**, 832–40.

Bryant R A, Felmingham K L, Kemp A H, *et al.* 2005. Neural networks of information processing in posttraumatic stress disorder: A functional magnetic resonance imaging study. *Biol Psychiatry* **58**, 111–8.

Bryant R A, Felmingham K, Kemp A, Das P, Hughes G, Peduto A and Williams L. 2008a. Amygdala and ventral anterior cingulate activation predicts treatment response to cognitive behaviour therapy for post-traumatic stress disorder. *Psychol Med* **38**, 555–61.

Bryant R A, Kemp A H, Felmingham K L, *et al.* 2008b. Enhanced amygdala and medial prefrontal activation during nonconscious processing of fear in posttraumatic stress disorder: An fMRI study. *Hum Brain Mapp* **29**, 517–23.

Carrion V G, Garrett A, Menon V, Weems C F and Reiss A L. 2008. Posttraumatic stress symptoms and brain function during a response-inhibition task: An fMRI study in youth. *Depress Anxiety* **25**, 514–26.

Chung Y A, Kim S H, Chung S K, *et al.* 2006. Alterations in cerebral perfusion in posttraumatic stress disorder patients without re-exposure to accident-related stimuli. *Clin Neurophysiol* **117**, 637–42.

Corcoran K A and Maren S. 2001. Hippocampal inactivation disrupts contextual retrieval of fear memory after extinction. *J Neurosci* **21**, 1720–6.

Davis M and Whalen P J. 2001. The amygdala: Vigilance and emotion. *Mol Psychiatry* **6**, 13–34.

Dickie E W, Brunet A, Akerib V and Armony J L. 2008. An fMRI investigation of memory encoding in PTSD: Influence of symptom severity. *Neuropsychologia* **46**, 1522–31.

Dolcos F, LaBar K S and Cabeza R. 2004. Interaction between the amygdala and the medial temporal lobe memory system predicts better memory for emotional events. *Neuron* **42**, 855–63.

Driessen M, Beblo T, Mertens M, *et al.* 2004. Posttraumatic stress disorder and fMRI activation patterns of traumatic memory in patients with borderline personality disorder. *Biol Psychiatry* **55**, 603–11.

Eichenbaum H. 2000. A cortical–hippocampal system for declarative memory. *Nat Rev Neurosci* **1**, 41–50.

Elzinga B M and Bremner J D. 2002. Are the neural substrates of memory the final common pathway in posttraumatic stress disorder (PTSD)? *J Affect Disord* **70**, 1–17.

Felmingham K, Kemp A, Williams L, *et al.* 2007. Changes in anterior cingulate and amygdala after cognitive behavior therapy of posttraumatic stress disorder. *Psychol Sci* **18**, 127–9.

Fernandez M, Pissiota A, Frans O, von Knorring L, Fischer H and Fredrikson M. 2001. Brain function in a patient with torture related post-traumatic stress disorder before and after fluoxetine treatment: A positron emission tomography provocation study. *Neurosci Lett* **297**, 101–04.

Francati V, Vermetten E and Bremner J D. 2007. Functional neuroimaging studies in posttraumatic stress disorder: Review of current methods and findings. *Depress Anxiety* **24**, 202–18.

Frewen P, Lane R D, Neufeld R W, Densmore M, Stevens T and Lanius R. 2008. Neural correlates of levels of emotional awareness during trauma script-imagery in posttraumatic stress disorder. *Psychosom Med* **70**, 27–31.

Geuze E, Vermetten E, Ruf M, de Kloet C S and Westenberg H G. 2008. Neural correlates of associative learning and memory in veterans with posttraumatic stress disorder. *J Psychiatr Res* **42**, 659–69.

Gilboa A, Shalev A Y, Laor L, *et al.* 2004. Functional connectivity of the prefrontal cortex and the amygdala in posttraumatic stress disorder. *Biol Psychiatry* **55**, 263–72.

Gurvits T V, Shenton M E, Hokama H, *et al.* 1996. Magnetic resonance imaging study of hippocampal volume in chronic, combat-related posttraumatic stress disorder. *Biol Psychiatry* **40**, 1091–9.

Hamner M B, Lorberbaum J P and George M S. 1999. Potential role of the anterior cingulate cortex in PTSD: Review and hypothesis. *Depress Anxiety* **9**, 1–14.

Hendler T, Rotshtein P, Yeshurun Y, *et al.* 2003. Sensing the invisible: Differential sensitivity of visual cortex and amygdala to traumatic context. *Neuroimage* **19**, 587–600.

Hopper J W, Frewen P A, van der Kolk B A and Lanius R A. 2007. Neural correlates of reexperiencing, avoidance, and dissociation in PTSD: Symptom dimensions and emotion dysregulation in responses to script-driven trauma imagery. *J Trauma Stress* **20**, 713–25.

Hou C, Liu J, Wang K, *et al.* 2007. Brain responses to symptom provocation and trauma-related short-term memory recall in coal mining accident survivors with acute severe PTSD. *Brain Res* **1144**, 165–74.

Karl A, Schaefer M, Malta L S, Dorfel D, Rohleder N and Werner A. 2006. A meta-analysis of structural brain abnormalities in PTSD. *Neurosci Biobehav Rev* **30**, 1004–31.

Kim M J, Chey J, Chung A, *et al.* 2008. Diminished rostral anterior cingulate activity in response to threat-related events in posttraumatic stress disorder. *J Psychiatr Res* **42**, 268–77.

Koenen K C, Saxe G, Purcell S, *et al.* 2005. Polymorphisms in FKBP5 are associated with peritraumatic dissociation in medically injured children. *Mol Psychiatry* **10**, 1058–9.

225

Lang P J, Levin D N, Miller G A and Kozak M J. 1983. Fear behavior, fear imagery, and the psychophysiology of emotion: The problem of affective response integration. *J Abnorm Psychol* **92**, 276–306.

Lanius R, Williamson P, Boksman K, *et al.* 2002. Brain activation during script-driven imagery induced dissociative responses in PTSD: A functional magnetic resonance imaging investigation. *Biol Psychiatry* **52**, 305.

Lanius R A, Bluhm R, Lanius U and Pain C. 2006. A review of neuroimaging studies in PTSD: Heterogeneity of response to symptom provocation. *J Psychiatr Res* **40**, 709–29.

Lanius R A, Williamson P C, Bluhm R L, *et al.* 2005. Functional connectivity of dissociative responses in posttraumatic stress disorder: A functional magnetic resonance imaging investigation. *Biol Psychiatry* **57**, 873–84.

Lanius R A, Williamson P C, Densmore M, *et al.* 2001. Neural correlates of traumatic memories in posttraumatic stress disorder: A functional MRI investigation. *Am J Psychiatry* **158**, 1920–2.

Lanius R A, Williamson P C, Hopper J, *et al.* 2003. Recall of emotional states in posttraumatic stress disorder: An fMRI investigation. *Biol Psychiatry* **53**, 204–10.

Lansing K, Amen D G, Hanks C and Rudy L. 2005. High-resolution brain SPECT imaging and eye movement desensitization and reprocessing in police officers with PTSD. *J Neuropsychiatry Clin Neurosci* **17**, 526–32.

Layton B and Krikorian R. 2002. Memory mechanisms in posttraumatic stress disorder. *J Neuropsychiatry Clin Neurosci* **14**, 254–61.

LeDoux J E. 2000. Emotion circuits in the brain. *Annu Rev Neurosci* **23**, 155–84.

Lee H J, Lee M S, Kang R H, *et al.* 2005. Influence of the serotonin transporter promoter gene polymorphism on susceptibility to posttraumatic stress disorder. *Depress Anxiety* **21**, 135–9.

Levin P, Lazrove S. and van der Kolk B. 1999. What psychological testing and neuroimaging tell us about the treatment of Posttraumatic Stress Disorder by Eye Movement Desensitization and Reprocessing. *J Anxiety Disord* **13**, 159–72.

Liberzon I, Taylor S F, Amdur R, *et al.* 1999. Brain activation in PTSD in response to trauma-related stimuli. *Biol Psychiatry* **45**, 817–26.

Lindauer R J, Booij J, Habraken J B, *et al.* 2004. Cerebral blood flow changes during script-driven imagery in police officers with posttraumatic stress disorder. *Biol Psychiatry* **56**, 853–61.

Maren S and Holt W. 2000. The hippocampus and contextual memory retrieval in Pavlovian conditioning. *Behav Brain Res* **110**, 97–108.

McGaugh J L. 2004. The amygdala modulates the consolidation of memories of emotionally arousing experiences. *Annu Rev Neurosci* **27**, 1–28.

Milad M R and Quirk G J. 2002. Neurons in medial prefrontal cortex signal memory for fear extinction. *Nature* **420**, 70–4.

Mirzaei S, Knoll P, Keck A, *et al.* 2001. Regional cerebral blood flow in patients suffering from post-traumatic stress disorder. *Neuropsychobiology* **43**, 260–4.

Molina M E, Isoardi R, Prado M N and Bentolila S. 2010. Basal cerebral glucose distribution in long-term post-traumatic stress disorder. *World J Biol Psychiatry* **11**, 493–501.

Moores K A, Clark C R, McFarlane A C, Brown G C, Puce A and Taylor D J. 2008. Abnormal recruitment of working memory updating networks during maintenance of trauma-neutral information in post-traumatic stress disorder. *Psychiatry Res* **163**, 156–70.

Morey R A, Dolcos F, Petty C M, *et al.* 2008. The role of trauma-related distractors on neural systems for working memory and emotion processing in posttraumatic stress disorder. *J Psychiatr Res* **43**, 809–17.

Morgan M A, Romanski L M and LeDoux J E. 1993. Extinction of emotional learning: Contribution of medial prefrontal cortex. *Neurosci Lett* **163**, 109–13.

Orr S P, Metzger L J, Lasko N B, *et al.* 2000. De novo conditioning in trauma-exposed individuals with and without posttraumatic stress disorder. *J Abnorm Psychol* **109**, 290–8.

Osuch E A, Benson B, Geraci M, *et al.* 2001. Regional cerebral blood flow correlated with flashback intensity in patients with posttraumatic stress disorder. *Biol Psychiatry* **50**, 246–53.

Osuch E A, Willis M W, Bluhm R, Ursano R J and Drevets W C. 2008. Neurophysiological responses to traumatic reminders in the acute aftermath of serious motor vehicle collisions using [^{15}O]-H$_2$O positron emission tomography. *Biol Psychiatry* **64**, 327–35.

Pavic L, Gregurek R, Petrovic R, *et al.* 2003. Alterations in brain activation in posttraumatic stress disorder patients with severe hyperarousal symptoms and impulsive aggressiveness. *Eur Arch Psychiatry Clin Neurosci* **253**, 80–3.

Peres J F, Newberg A B, Mercante J P, *et al.* 2007. Cerebral blood flow changes during retrieval of traumatic memories before and after psychotherapy: A SPECT study. *Psychol Med* **37**, 1481–91.

Phan K L, Britton J C, Taylor S F, Fig L M and Liberzon I. 2006. Corticolimbic blood flow during nontraumatic emotional processing in posttraumatic stress disorder. *Arch Gen Psychiatry* **63**, 184–92.

Piefke M, Pestinger M, Arin T, *et al.* 2007. The neurofunctional mechanisms of traumatic and non-traumatic memory in patients with acute PTSD following accident trauma. *Neurocase* 13, 342–57.

Pissiota A, Frans O, Fernandez M, von Knorring L, Fischer H and Fredrikson M. 2002. Neurofunctional correlates of posttraumatic stress disorder: A PET symptom provocation study. *Eur Arch Psychiatry Clin Neurosci* 252, 68–75.

Pitman R K, Orr S P, Forgue D F, de Jong J B and Claiborn J M. 1987. Psychophysiologic assessment of posttraumatic stress disorder imagery in Vietnam combat veterans. *Arch Gen Psychiatry* 44, 970–5.

Protopopescu X, Pan H, Tuescher O, *et al.* 2005. Differential time courses and specificity of amygdala activity in posttraumatic stress disorder subjects and normal control subjects. *Biol Psychiatry* 57, 464–73.

Quirk G J, Russo G K, Barron J L and Lebron K. 2000. The role of ventromedial prefrontal cortex in the recovery of extinguished fear. *J Neurosci* 20, 6225–31.

Rauch S L, Shin L M and Phelps E A. 2006. Neurocircuitry models of posttraumatic stress disorder and extinction: Human neuroimaging research – Past, present, and future. *Biol Psychiatry* 60, 376–82.

Rauch S L, Shin L M, Segal E, *et al.* 2003. Selectively reduced regional cortical volumes in post-traumatic stress disorder. *Neuroreport* 14, 913–6.

Rauch S L, Shin L M, Whalen P J and Pitman R K. 1998. Neuroimaging and the neuroanatomy of PTSD. *CNS Spectrums* 3 (Suppl 2), 30–41.

Rauch S L, van der Kolk B A, Fisler R E, *et al.* 1996. A symptom provocation study of posttraumatic stress disorder using positron emission tomography and script-driven imagery. *Arch Gen Psychiatry* 53, 380–7.

Rauch S L, Whalen P J, Shin L M, *et al.* 2000. Exaggerated amygdala response to masked facial stimuli in posttraumatic stress disorder: A functional MRI study. *Biol Psychiatry* 47, 769–76.

Reiman E M, Lane R D, Ahern G L, *et al.* 1997. Neuroanatomical correlates of externally and internally generated human emotion. *Am J Psychiatry* 154, 918–25.

Sachinvala N, Kling A, Suffin S, Lake R and Cohen M. 2000. Increased regional cerebral perfusion by 99mTc hexamethyl propylene amine oxime single photon emission computed tomography in post-traumatic stress disorder. *Mil Med* 165, 473–9.

Sailer U, Robinson S, Fischmeister F P, *et al.* 2008. Altered reward processing in the nucleus accumbens and mesial prefrontal cortex of patients with posttraumatic stress disorder. *Neuropsychologia* 46, 2836–44.

Sanders M, Wiltgen B and Fanselow M. 2003. The place of the hippocampus in fear conditioing. *Eur J Pharmacol* 463, 217–23.

Seedat S, Warwick J, van Heerden B, *et al.* 2004. Single photon emission computed tomography in posttraumatic stress disorder before and after treatment with a selective serotonin reuptake inhibitor. *J Affect Disord* 80, 45–53.

Semple W E, Goyer P F, McCormick R, *et al.* 2000. Higher brain blood flow at amygdala and lower frontal cortex blood flow in PTSD patients with comorbid cocaine and alcohol abuse compared with normals. *Psychiatry* 63, 65–74.

Shin L M, Bush G, Whalen P J, *et al.* 2007. Dorsal anterior cingulate function in posttraumatic stress disorder. *J Trauma Stress* 20, 701–12.

Shin L M, Kosslyn S M, McNally R J, *et al.* 1997. Visual imagery and perception in posttraumatic stress disorder. A positron emission tomographic investigation. *Arch Gen Psychiatry* 54, 233–41.

Shin L M, Lasko N B, Macklin M L, *et al.* 2009. Resting metabolic activity in the cingulate cortex and vulnerability to posttraumatic stress disorder. *Arch Gen Psychiatry* 66, 1099–107.

Shin L M, McNally R J, Kosslyn S M, *et al.* 1999. Regional cerebral blood flow during script-driven imagery in childhood sexual abuse-related PTSD: A PET investigation. *Am J Psychiatry* 156, 575–84.

Shin L M, Orr S P, Carson M A, *et al.* 2004a. Regional cerebral blood flow in amygdala and medial prefrontal cortex during traumatic imagery in male and female Vietnam veterans with PTSD. *Arch Gen Psychiatry* 61, 168–76.

Shin L M, Shin P S, Heckers S, *et al.* 2004b. Hippocampal function in posttraumatic stress disorder. *Hippocampus* 14, 292–300.

Shin L M, Whalen P J, Pitman R K, *et al.* 2001. An fMRI study of anterior cingulate function in posttraumatic stress disorder. *Biol Psychiatry* 50, 932–42.

Shin L M, Wright C I, Cannistraro P A, *et al.* 2005. A functional magnetic resonance imaging study of amygdala and medial prefrontal cortex responses to overtly presented fearful faces in posttraumatic stress disorder. *Arch Gen Psychiatry* 62, 273–81.

Thomaes K, Dorrepaal E, Draijer N P, *et al.* 2009. Increased activation of the left hippocampus region in Complex PTSD during encoding and recognition of emotional words: A pilot study. *Psychiatry Res* 171, 44–53.

Vermetten E, Schmahl C, Southwick S M and Bremner J D. 2007. Positron tomography emission study of olfactory induced emotional recall in veterans with and without combat-related posttraumatic stress disorder. *Psychopharmacol Bull* 40, 8–30.

Werner N S, Meindl T, Engel R R, *et al.* 2009. Hippocampal function during associative learning in patients with posttraumatic stress disorder. *J Psychiatr Res* 43, 309–18.

227

Whalen P J. 1998. Fear, vigilance, and ambiguity: Initial neuroimaging studies of the human amygdala. *Curr Dir Psychol Sci* **6**, 178–88.

Whalen P J, Bush G, McNally R J, *et al.* 1998. The emotional counting Stroop paradigm: A functional magnetic resonance imaging probe of the anterior cingulate affective division. *Biol Psychiatry* **44**, 1219–28.

Whalley M G, Rugg M D, Smith A P, Dolan R J and Brewin C R. 2009. Incidental retrieval of emotional contexts in post-traumatic stress disorder and depression: An fMRI study. *Brain Cogn* **69**, 98–107.

Williams L M, Kemp A H, Felmingham K, *et al.* 2006. Trauma modulates amygdala and medial prefrontal responses to consciously attended fear. *Neuroimage* **29**, 347–57.

Woodward S H, Kaloupek D G, Streeter C C, Martinez C, Schaer M and Eliez S. 2006. Decreased anterior cingulate volume in combat-related PTSD. *Biol Psychiatry* **59**, 582–7.

Yamasue H, Kasai K, Iwanami A, *et al.* 2003. Voxel-based analysis of MRI reveals anterior cingulate gray-matter volume reduction in posttraumatic stress disorder due to terrorism. *Proc Natl Acad Sci U S A* **100**, 9039–43.

Yang P, Wu M T, Hsu C C and Ker J H. 2004. Evidence of early neurobiological alternations in adolescents with posttraumatic stress disorder: A functional MRI study. *Neurosci Lett* **370**, 13–8.

Zubieta J K, Chinitz J A, Lombardi U, Fig L M, Cameron O G and Liberzon I. 1999. Medial frontal cortex involvement in PTSD symptoms: A SPECT study. *J Psychiatr Res* **33**, 259–64.

Chapter 15

Molecular imaging of post-traumatic stress disorder

J. Douglas Bremner

Synopsis

Recent advances in brain imaging have permitted an examination of alterations in brain function in patients with post-traumatic stress disorder (PTSD). These studies have been informed by research in the field of neuroscience showing that stress is associated with changes in brain areas involved in the stress response including the amygdala, hippocampus, and prefrontal cortex. Neurochemical/receptor studies in patients with PTSD have replicated findings in animal studies by finding alterations in the hippocampus and frontal cortex. Brain regions implicated in PTSD also play an important role in memory function, highlighting the important interplay between memory and the traumatic stress response. Abnormalities in these brain areas are hypothesized to underlie symptoms of PTSD and other stress-related psychiatric disorders. This chapter reviews findings from neurochemical and neuroreceptor brain imaging measured with positron emission tomography (PET), single photon emission computed tomography (SPECT) and magnetic resonance spectroscopy (MRS). The studies show alterations in neurochemical and neuroreceptor function in brain areas implicated in the stress response and previous functional and structural imaging studies in PTSD, including the hippocampus and prefrontal cortex.

Neural circuits of PTSD

PTSD is characterized by specific symptoms, including intrusive thoughts, hyperarousal, flashbacks, nightmares and sleep disturbances, changes in memory and concentration, and startle responses. Symptoms of PTSD are hypothesized to represent the behavioral manifestation of stress-induced changes in the brain. Stress results in acute and chronic changes in neurochemical systems and specific brain regions, which result in long-term changes in brain "circuits" involved in the stress response (Pitman, 2001; Bremner, 2002; Vermetten and Bremner, 2002a, 2002b). Brain regions that are felt to play an important role in PTSD include the hippocampus, amygdala, and medial prefrontal cortex (Francati et al., 2007; Bremner et al., 2008).

The hippocampus, which is involved in verbal declarative memory, is very sensitive to the effects of stress. Stress in animals has been associated with damage to neurons in the CA3 region of the hippocampus (which may be mediated by hypercortisolemia, decreased brain derived neurotrophic factor, and/or elevated glutamate levels) and inhibition of neurogenesis (Sapolsky et al., 1990; McEwen et al., 1992; Nibuya et al., 1995; Magarinos et al., 1996; Sapolsky, 1996; Gould et al., 1998).

In addition to the hippocampus, other brain structures have been implicated in a neural circuitry of stress including the amygdala and prefrontal cortex. The amygdala is involved in memory for the emotional valence of events, and plays a critical role in the acquisition of fear responses (Davis, 1992). The medial prefrontal cortex includes the anterior cingulate gyrus (Brodmann's area (BA) 32) and subcallosal gyrus (BA 25) as well as the orbitofrontal cortex. Lesion studies demonstrated that the medial prefrontal cortex modulates emotional responsiveness through inhibition of amygdala function (Morgan et al., 1993). Studies show that neurons of the medial prefrontal cortex play an active role in inhibition of fear responses that are mediated by the amygdala (Milad and Quirk, 2002; Milad et al., 2006). Conditioned fear responses are extinguished following

Understanding Neuropsychiatric Disorders, ed. M. E. Shenton and B. I. Turetsky. Published by Cambridge University Press.
© Cambridge University Press 2011.

repeated exposure to the conditioned stimulus (in the absence of the unconditioned aversive, e.g. electric shock stimulus). This inhibition appears to be mediated by medial prefrontal cortical inhibition of amygdala responsiveness. Animal studies also have shown that early stress is associated with a decrease in branching of neurons in the medial prefrontal cortex (Radley *et al.*, 2004). The insula also plays a critical role in integrating the physiological stress response.

Neurochemical brain systems involved in the stress response are also affected by PTSD. These include norepinephrine, the hypothalamic–pituitary–adrenal (HPA) axis, serotonin, opiate and benzodiazepine systems (Vermetten and Bremner, 2002a). In animal studies, chronic stress is associated with changes in benzodiazepine, serotonin, and opiate receptor binding in brain areas outlined above, including hippocampus and frontal cortex (Vermetten and Bremner, 2002a; Bremner, 2004).

Neurochemical and neuroreceptor imaging techniques

Brain chemicals and receptors can be measured with the brain imaging techniques of positron emission tomography (PET), single photon emission computed tomography (SPECT), and magnetic resonance spectroscopy (MRS) (Bremner, 2005).

PET is a type of tomographic imaging that detects positron-emitting substances which are typically made on-site in a cyclotron. PET can be used to measure the concentration of neuroreceptors, in addition to providing assessments of brain blood flow and metabolism, or function (reviewed in another chapter). PET imaging is based on the principles of radioactivity. Radioactive substances are those that are unstable because they have too many positive or negative charges. An atom wants to have an equal balance of negative and positive charges. If it does not, it will change by releasing a negative or positive charge, what is known as *radioactivity*. Imaging devices such as PET cameras can measure these charges when they are let go. If this process is multiplied millions of times, the camera can get a picture of where in the body all of these radioactive atoms are located, and reconstruct a picture of the physiological process of interest. The radioactive substances used in PET can be prepared in an on-site cyclotron, attached to a compound that binds to neuroreceptors, and injected immediately into the patient for imaging.

Neuroreceptors can also be measured with single photon emission computed tomography (SPECT). SPECT differs from PET in that a single photon is emitted from the radionuclide of interest which is detected by the crystals of the camera. SPECT cameras typically use sodium iodide (NaI) crystals, which are optimized for the 140 KeV energy of the typical radiopharmaceutical [Tc-99m] HMPOA (as opposed to the 511 KeV energy of [F-18] FDG). SPECT tracers have much longer half lives than PET tracers which makes them easier to work with for radiochemists. The most common isotope used for neuroreceptor imaging with SPECT is I-123, which has an energy of 159 KeV and a half-life of 13 hours, as opposed to, for instance, C-11, with an energy of 511 KeV and a half-life of 20 minutes.

Radiopharmaceuticals can be labeled with ^{99m}Tc or ^{123}I for SPECT imaging or ^{18}F or ^{11}C for PET imaging of neuroreceptors. Radiopharmaceuticals applied to the study of PTSD to date have involved imaging of benzodiazepine, nicotinic, opiate, and serotonin receptors.

Using magnetic resonance imaging (MRI), it is possible to measure the physical properties, or spectra, of individual chemicals in the brain. Measuring the spectra of the chemicals in a particular region of the brain provides an estimate of the concentration of specific chemicals in that area. One example of this that has been applied to the study of PTSD is the measurement of a chemical called *N*-acetylaspartate (NAA). NAA is an amino acid, the presence of which is felt to correlate with the integrity or health of neurons, which are the basic cells of the brain. Decreases in NAA are felt to represent a loss of neurons or changes in the integrity of neurons that indicate abnormalities. Most studies have looked at the ratio of NAA to creatine (Cr), another chemical not felt to be affected by neuropsychiatric disorders, that acts as a kind of control. Choline (Cho) is another chemical that can be measured with MRS and is felt to be related to glia function or integrity.

Brain imaging studies are consistent with dysfunction of the hippocampus and anterior cingulate in PTSD (Bremner, 2007). Several studies have looked specifically at neurochemical alterations in the hippocampus, and some have also looked at the anterior cingulate, most using NAA as a marker of neuronal integrity (Table 15.1). In an initial pilot study, Schuff *et al.* (1997) measured the ratio of NAA to Cr plus Cho in seven Vietnam veterans with combat-related PTSD

Table 15.1 Published neurochemical and receptor studies in PTSD – methods

Authors	Study population	Sample size	Control group	Sample size	Imaging methods tracer	Receptor/ neurochemical	Finding
Schuff et al., 1997	Vietnam combat-related PTSD	6M/1F	Healthy non-deployed controls	6M/1F	MRS NAA/Cr+Cho	Neuronal integrity	Decreased r. hippocampal
Freeman et al., 1998	Vietnam combat-related PTSD	21M	Veterans without PTSD	8M	MRS NAA/Cr	Neuronal integrity	Decreased hippocampal
De Bellis et al., 2000	Children with maltreatment PTSD	6M/5F	Healthy non-traumatized children	6M/5F	MRS NAA/Cr	Neuronal integrity	Decreased ant. cingulate
Bremner et al., 2000	Vietnam combat-related PTSD	13 M	Healthy non-deployed controls	13M	SPECT/[I-123] iomazenil	Benzodiazepine receptor binding	Decreased prefrontal (9)
Schuff et al., 2001	Vietnam combat-related PTSD	18M	Healthy non deployed controls	19M	MRS NAA	Neuronal integrity	Decreased hipppocampal
Villareal et al., 2002	Mixed PTSD sample	2M/7F	Healthy controls	5M	MRS NAA	Neuronal integrity	Decreased left hippocampal
Lim et al., 2003	Fire victims with PTSD	10M/6F	Healthy controls	6M/2F	MRS NAA	Neuronal integrity	Decreased basal ganglia
Mohanakrishnan Menon et al., 2003	Combat-related PTSD	12M/1F	Veterans without PTSD	6M/1F	MRS NAA/Cr	Neuronal integrity	Decreased L. hippocampal
Fujita et al., 2004	Gulf War combat-related PTSD	19M	Healthy non-deployed controls	19M	SPECT/[I-123] iomazenil	Benzodiazepine receptor binding	No differences; correlation with childhood trauma in r. sup. temp. gyrus
Bonne et al., 2005	Mixed PTSD sample	2M/10F	Healthy non-traumatized controls	1M/10F	PET/[F-18]FC-WAY	Serotonin 5-HT1A receptor binding	No differences
Kimbrell et al., 2005	Veterans with PTSD	68M	Veterans without PTSD	21M	MRS NAA/Cr	Neuronal integrity	No differences; decreased L. hippocampal in non-combat v combat PTSD

Table 15.1 (cont.)

Authors	Study population	Sample size	Control group	Sample size	Imaging methods tracer	Receptor/ neurochemical	Finding
Mahmutyazicioglu et al., 2005	Mixed PTSD sample	7M/3F	Healthy non-PTSD	3M/3F	MRS NAA/Cr	Neuronal integrity	Decreased bilateral hippocampus, anterior cingulate
Seedat et al., 2005	Intimate partner violence PTSD	7F	Violence without PTSD/Healthy	9F/11F	MRS NAA/Cr	Neuronal integrity	No change in ant. cingulate
Freeman et al., 2006	POWs with PTSD	10M	Non-PTSD POWs/ Healthy subject	10M/6M	MRS NAA/Cr	Neuronal integrity	No change in hippocampus
Li et al., 2006	Fire victims with PTSD	4M/8F	Fire victims without PTSD	4M/8F	MRS NAA/Cr	Neuronal integrity	Decreased L. hippocampal
Liberzon et al., 2007	Vietnam combat-related PTSD	16M	Vietnam combat vets without PTSD/HS	14M/15M	PET [C-11]carfentinil	Mu opiate receptor binding	Lower ant. cingulate
Geuze et al., 2008	Dutch veterans with PTSD	9M	Dutch veterans without PTSD	7M	PET [C-11]iomazenil	Benzodiazepine receptor binding	Global reduction; cortex, hippocampus, thalamus
Czermak et al., 2008	Mixed PTSD sample	3M/7F	Healthy controls	3M/7F	SPECT/[I-123]5-IA	Beta2 nicotinic acetylcholine receptor	Increased mesiotemporal (hippocampus) in non-smokers, correlation of re-experiencing with thalamus
Schuff et al., 2008	Veterans with PTSD	50M/5F	Veterans without PTSD	41M/7F	MRS NAA/Cr	Neuronal integrity	Decreased bilateral hippocampus, R. anterior cingulate

and seven healthy non-deployed controls. They found a decrease in right hippocampal NAA/Cr+Cho. Freeman *et al.* (1998) looked at 21 men with Vietnam combat-related PTSD and 8 male veterans without PTSD. They found decreased bilateral hippocampal NAA/Cr. They also found a reduction in left mesiotemporal Cho/Cr. De Bellis *et al.* (2000) studied six boys and five girls with maltreatment-related PTSD and pair-matched healthy, non-traumatized children. They found a reduction in anterior cingulate NAA/Cr. Schuff *et al.* (2001) replicated their pilot study in a group of 18 men with Vietnam combat-related PTSD and 19 male healthy non-deployed veterans showing a decrease in bilateral hippocampal NAA. In a mixed PTSD sample of two men and seven women, Villareal *et al.* (2002) found decreased NAA in the left hippocampus compared to five healthy controls, with no change in occipital NAA/Cr. Lim *et al.* (2003) compared 16 Chinese persons with fire-related PTSD to 8 healthy controls and found a decrease in NAA in the basal ganglia (the hippocampus was not assessed). Mohanakrishnan Menon *et al.* (2003) studied 13 patients with combat-related PTSD and 7 non-PTSD veterans and found decreased left hippocampal NAA/Cr. Kimbrell *et al.* (2005) looked at 68 male veterans with PTSD and 21 male veterans without PTSD and found no differences between the groups in hippocampal NAA/Cr. Patients with non-combat-related PTSD had lower left hippocampal NAA/Cr concentrations than patients with combat-related PTSD. In another study (Mahmutyazicioglu *et al.*, 2005) decreased bilateral hippocampal NAA/Cr was found in a mixed sample of 10 Turkish PTSD patients compared to 6 healthy controls. Hippocampal Cho/Cr was increased.

Seedat *et al.* (2005) found no difference in anterior cingulate NAA/Cr (hippocampus was not examined) between women with intimate partner violence with ($N = 7$) and without ($N = 9$) PTSD, or between 11 healthy women. They did, however, find elevations in choline (Cho/Cr), which they interpreted as possibly being related to proliferation of glia. Freeman *et al.* (2006) found no differences in hippocampal NAA/Cr or Cho/Cr in repatriated prisoners of war with ($N = 10$) and without ($N = 10$) PTSD or healthy subjects ($N = 6$). Li *et al.* (2006) examined 12 patients with fire-related PTSD and matched fire victims without PTSD and showed a decrease in left hippocampal NAA/Cr. Finally, Schuff *et al.* (2008) studied 55 veterans with PTSD

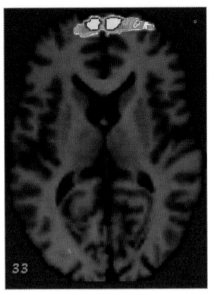

Figure 15.1 Statistical parametric map showing areas of greater decrease (yellow) in benzodiazepine receptor binding in Vietnam combat-related PTSD. Decreases in binding were seen in anterior medial prefrontal cortex.

and 48 veterans without PTSD and showed decreased bilateral hippocampal NAA/Cr and right anterior cingulate NAA/Cr in PTSD. In summary, the finding of decreased hippocampal NAA is a well-replicated finding. These studies indicate that a loss of hippocampal neuronal integrity is associated with PTSD. Some studies are also consistent with altered neuronal integrity in the anterior cingulate.

Studies have begun to use PET and SPECT to measure neuroreceptors in PTSD. Bremner *et al.* (2000) studied 13 male patients with Vietnam combat-related PTSD and 13 healthy non-veteran controls using SPECT [I-123]iomazenil for measurement of brain benzodiazepine receptor binding. They found a reduction in quantitative measures of receptor binding in the anterior prefrontal cortex (Brodmann's Area 9). Fujita *et al.* (2004) studied 19 males with Gulf War-related PTSD and 19 healthy non-deployed veterans using SPECT [I-123]iomazenil. There were no regional or global differences in binding concentrations between groups; there was a correlation between binding in the superior temporal gyrus and childhood trauma exposure. Geuze *et al.* (2008) used PET [C-11]iomazenil to compare benzodiazepine binding in nine Dutch military peacekeeper

233

veterans with PTSD to seven veterans without PTSD. There were global reductions in binding, with the greatest reduction in anterior cingulate, prefrontal and other cortical areas, thalamus and hippocampus. In summary, two-thirds of studies have found reductions in medial prefrontal benzodiazepine receptor binding, with one study showing decreased hippocampal binding as well.

Bonne *et al.* (2005) studied serotonin 5-HT1A receptor binding using [F-18]FC-WAY in 12 patients with PTSD from mixed causes and 11 healthy non-traumatized controls. There were no differences in binding between the groups.

Liberzon and colleagues (2007) used PET and [C-11]carfentinil to measure mu opiate receptor binding in Vietnam combat veterans with ($N = 16$) and without ($N = 14$) PTSD and healthy subjects without combat exposure ($N = 15$). The authors found a reduction in anterior cingulate binding in the PTSD patients compared to the other groups. Both combat groups compared to non-combat had lower binding in amygdala, insular and prefrontal cortex, and nucleus accumbens.

Czermak *et al.* (2008) used SPECT and the marker of the beta2 nicotinic acetylcholine receptor [I-123] 5–IA, in 10 patients with mixed PTSD and 10 healthy controls. PTSD patients showed an increase in mesiotemporal (i.e. hippocampal) binding when the subgroup of non-smokers were compared. Re-experiencing symptom severity in the group as a whole correlated with binding in the thalamus.

Discussion

Neurochemical and neuroreceptor brain imaging studies performed to date are consistent with functional and structural brain imaging studies (reviewed in other chapters) that have implicated the hippocampus and medial prefrontal cortex/anterior cingulate in PTSD. Decreased NAA in these regions indicates a loss of neuronal integrity, either a loss of neurons or neuronal branching. Additionally, since benzodiazepine receptors are ubiquitous on all neurons, the loss of benzodiazepine receptors in these regions could be due to either a decrease in neuronal integrity, and/or a loss of the receptor itself. Decreased opiate binding in anterior cingulate and increased nicotinic binding in the hippocampus indicate involvement of these neurochemical systems in symptoms of PTSD.

Box 15.1. Summary of Findings

- Replicated finding of reduced *N*-acetyl-aspartate (NAA) in hippocampus shows loss of neuronal integrity.
- Replicated finding of reduced NAA in anterior cingulate shows loss of neuronal integrity.
- Possible changes in choline in hippocampus and anterior cingulate of uncertain significance.
- Replicated finding of decreased benzodiazepine receptor binding in frontal cortex.
- Single study of increased nicotinic acetylcholine receptor binding in hippocampus.
- Single study of reduced mu opiate receptor binding in anterior cingulate.
- No change in serotonin 5-HT1A binding in single study performed to date.
- No information on effects of treatment on neurochemical or neuroreceptor binding.

References

Bonne O, Bain E, Neumeister A, *et al.* 2005. No change in serotonin type 1A receptor binding in patients with posttraumatic stress disorder. *Am J Psychiatry* **162**, 383–5.

Bremner J D. 2002. *Does Stress Damage the Brain? Understanding Trauma-Related Disorders from a Mind–Body Perspective.* New York, NY: W.W. Norton.

Bremner J D. 2004. Does stress damage the brain: Understanding trauma related disorders from a mind body perspective. *Dir Psychiatry* **24**, 167–76.

Bremner J D. 2005. *Brain Imaging Handbook.* New York, NY: W.W. Norton.

Bremner J D. 2007. Functional neuroimaging in posttraumatic stress disorder. *Exp Rev Neurotherapy* **7**, 393–405.

Bremner J D, Elzinga B, Schmahl C and Vermetten E. 2008. Structural and functional plasticity of the human brain in posttraumatic stress disorder. *Prog Brain Res* **167**, 171–86.

Bremner J D, Innis R B, White T, *et al.* 2000. SPECT [I-123]iomazenil measurement of the benzodiazepine receptor in panic disorder. *Biol Psychiatry* **47**, 96–106.

Czermak C, Staley J K, Kasserman S, *et al.* 2008. beta2 Nicotinic acetylcholine receptor availability in post-traumatic stress disorder. *Int J Neuropsychopharmacol* **11**, 419–24.

Davis M. 1992. The role of the amygdala in fear and anxiety. *Annu Rev Neurosci* **15**, 353–75.

De Bellis M D, Keshavan M S, Spencer S and Hall J. 2000. *N*-acetylaspartate concentration in the anterior cingulate of maltreated children and adolescents with PTSD. *Am J Psychiatry* **157**, 1175–7.

Francati V, Vermetten E and Bremner J D. 2007. Functional neuroimaging studies in posttraumatic stress disorder:

Review of current methods and findings. *Depress Anxiety* **24**, 202–18.

Freeman T, Kimbrell T, Booe L, *et al.* 2006. Evidence of resilience: Neuroimaging in former prisoners of war. *Psychiatry Res* **146**, 59–64.

Freeman T W, Cardwell D, Karson C N and Komoroski R A. 1998. In vivo proton magnetic resonance spectroscopy of the medial temporal lobes of subjects with combat-related posttraumatic stress disorder. *Magn Reson Med* **40**, 66–71.

Fujita M, Southwick S M, Denucci C C, *et al.* 2004. Central type benzodiazepine receptors in Gulf War veterans with posttraumatic stress disorder. *Biol Psychiatry* **56**, 95–100.

Geuze E, van Berckel B N, Lammertsma A A, *et al.* 2008. Reduced GABAA benzodiazepine receptor binding in veterans with post-traumatic stress disorder. *Mol Psychiatry* **13**, 74–83, 73.

Gould E, Tanapat P, McEwen B S, Flugge G and Fuchs E. 1998. Proliferation of granule cell precursors in the dentate gyrus of adult monkeys is diminished by stress. *Proc Natl Acad Sci USA* **95**, 3168–71.

Kimbrell T, Leulf C, Cardwell D, Komoroski R A and Freeman T W. 2005. Relationship of in vivo medial temporal lobe magnetic resonance spectroscopy to documented combat exposure in veterans with chronic posttraumatic stress disorder. *Psychiatry Res* **140**, 91–4.

Li L, Chen S, Liu J, Zhang J, He Z and Lin X. 2006. Magnetic resonance imaging and magnetic resonance spectroscopy study of deficits in hippocampal structure in fire victims with recent-onset posttraumatic stress disorder. *Can J Psychiatry* **51**, 431–7.

Liberzon I, Taylor S F, Phan K L, *et al.* 2007. Altered central micro-opioid receptor binding after psychological trauma. *Biol Psychiatry* **61**, 1030–8.

Lim M K, Suh C H, Kim H J, *et al.* 2003. Fire-related post-traumatic stress disorder: Brain 1H-MR spectroscopic findings. *Korean J Radiol* **4**, 79–84.

Magarinos A M, McEwen B S, Flugge G and Fluchs E. 1996. Chronic psychosocial stress causes apical dendritic atrophy of hippocampal CA3 pyramidal neurons in subordinate tree shrews. *J Neurosci* **16**, 3534–40.

Mahmutyazicioglu K, Konuk N, Ozdemir H, Atasoy N, Atik L and Gundogdu S. 2005. Evaluation of the hippocampus and the anterior cingulate gyrus by proton MR spectroscopy in patients with post-traumatic stress disorder. *Diagn Interv Radiol* **11**, 125–9.

McEwen B S, Angulo J, Cameron H, *et al.* 1992. Paradoxical effects of adrenal steroids on the brain: Protection versus degeneration. *Biol Psychiatry* **31**, 177–99.

Milad M R and Quirk G J. 2002. Neurons in medial prefrontal cortex signal memory for fear extinction. *Nature* **420**, 70–3.

Milad M R, Rauch S L, Pitman R K and Quirk G J. 2006. Fear extinction in rats: Implications for human brain imaging and anxiety disorders. *Biol Psychol* **73**, 61–71.

Mohanakrishnan Menon P, Nasrallah H A, Lyons J A, Scott M F and Liberto V. 2003. Single-voxel proton MR spectroscopy of right versus left hippocampi in PTSD. *Psychiatry Res* **123**, 101–08.

Morgan C A, Romanski L M and LeDoux J E. 1993. Extinction of emotional learning: Contribution of medial prefrontal cortex. *Neurosci Lett* **163**, 109–13.

Nibuya M, Morinobu S and Duman R S. 1995. Regulation of BDNF and trkB mRNA in rat brain by chronic electroconvulsive seizure and antidepressant drug treatments. *J Neurosci* **15**, 7539–47.

Pitman R K. 2001. Investigating the pathogenesis of posttraumatic stress disorder with neuroimaging. *J Clin Psychiatry* **62**, 47–54.

Radley J J, Sisti H M, Hao J, *et al.* 2004. Chronic behavioral stress induces apical dendritic reorganization in pyramidal neurons of the medial prefrontal cortex. *Neuroscience* **125**, 1–6.

Sapolsky R M. 1996. Why stress is bad for your brain. *Science* **273**, 749–50.

Sapolsky R M, Uno H, Rebert C S and Finch C E. 1990. Hippocampal damage associated with prolonged glucocorticoid exposure in primates. *J Neurosci* **10**, 2897–902.

Schuff N, Marmar C R, Weiss D S, *et al.* 1997. Reduced hippocampal volume and *N*-acetyl aspartate in posttraumatic stress disorder. *Ann N Y Acad Sci* **821**, 516–20.

Schuff N, Neylan T C, Fox-Bosetti S, *et al.* 2008. Abnormal *N*-acetylaspartate in hippocampus and anterior cingulate in posttraumatic stress disorder. *Psychiatry Res* **162**, 147–57.

Schuff N, Neylan T C, Lenoci M A, *et al.* 2001. Decreased hippocampal *N*-acetylaspartate in the absence of atrophy in posttraumatic stress disorder. *Biol Psychiatry* **50**, 952–9.

Seedat S, Videen J S, Kennedy C M and Stein M B. 2005. Single voxel proton magnetic resonance spectroscopy in women with and without intimate partner violence-related posttraumatic stress disorder. *Psychiatry Res* **139**, 249–58.

Vermetten E and Bremner J D. 2002a. Circuits and systems in stress. I. Preclinical studies. *Depress Anxiety* **15**, 126–47.

Vermetten E and Bremner J D. 2002b. Circuits and systems in stress. II. Applications to neurobiology and treatment of PTSD. *Depress Anxiety* **16**, 14–38.

Villarreal G, Hamilton D A, Petropoulos H, *et al.* 2002. Reduced hippocampal volume and total white matter in posttraumatic stress disorder. *Biol Psychiatry* **52**, 119–25.

Structural imaging of obsessive–compulsive disorder

Andrew R. Gilbert, Alison M. Gilbert, Jorge R. C. de Almeida and Philip R. Szeszko

Introduction

Obsessive–compulsive disorder (OCD) is a psychiatric disorder with a substantial prevalence in adulthood (2–3%) and in childhood and adolescence (1–2%), characterized by anxiety-producing obsessions (intrusive, unwanted thoughts or images) and anxiety-neutralizing compulsions (repetitive behaviors). OCD causes significant psychosocial impairment, and in 1996 was recognized by the World Health Organization as one of the top 10 leading causes of years lived with a disability (Murray and Lopez, 1996). With approximately 40% of pediatric OCD patients reporting continued symptoms into adulthood, OCD has a substantial chronic course, contributing to social, academic, occupational and neurocognitive problems across the lifespan (Stewart et al., 2004).

In this chapter we present findings from structural neuroimaging studies of OCD in both pediatric and adult populations. We first briefly discuss neurobiological models of OCD, and next review the structural neuroimaging literature with a focus on regions strongly implicated in the pathophysiology of OCD, including the orbitofrontal cortex, anterior cingulate, basal ganglia, and thalamus. We also discuss the potential role of other brain regions in the pathogenesis of OCD. Neuroimaging evidence that OCD involves a disruption in the brain white matter is reviewed with emphasis placed on results from diffusion tensor imaging (DTI) studies. We finally discuss future directions in structural neuroimaging research in OCD.

Neurobiological models

Although the pathophysiology of OCD remains to be fully elucidated, neuroscientific studies over the past several decades have greatly contributed to our understanding of the neural mechanisms underlying the disorder. The parallel frontal–striatal circuits described by Alexander and colleagues (Alexander et al., 1986, 1990) are frequently integrated into mechanistic neuroanatomical explanations of OCD. For example, several researchers have described an imbalance in systems regarding direct versus indirect basal ganglia pathways in patients with OCD (Baxter et al., 1996; Saxena et al., 2001). These pathways include the orbitofrontal cortex basal ganglia circuit (Saxena et al., 1998; Modell et al., 1989), as well as abnormalities in the striatum (Schwartz, 1998) that alter connectivity between the orbitofrontal cortex and thalamus (Modell et al., 1989). Others have proposed abnormal basal ganglia effects upon both motor and cognitive regulation in OCD (Graybiel and Rauch, 2000). These elegant models are supported by both structural and functional abnormalities in the orbitofrontal cortex, caudate, and thalamus, three regions that are consistently abnormal in patients with OCD compared to healthy controls.

Recent advances in neuroscience have enhanced our understanding of frontal striatal circuitry, which coupled with the growth in neuroimaging studies of OCD have led to broader models of OCD pathophysiology that include the anterior cingulate, hippocampus, parietal lobe and amygdala (Menzies et al., 2008a). Recent functional and structural neuroimaging studies have supported abnormalities in other cortico-striatal–thalamic (CST) circuits, including more lateral frontal systems, and components of disgust and emotion processing systems, such as the insula and amygdala (Menzies et al., 2008a; Valente et al., 2005; Phillips et al., 2000; Aouizerate et al., 2004). Moreover, cognitive deficits in individuals with OCD further support this

Understanding Neuropsychiatric Disorders, ed. M. E. Shenton and B. I. Turetsky. Published by Cambridge University Press.

broad model of cortical dysfunction. For example, abnormalities in response inhibition, set shifting, working memory and planning have all been reported in patients with OCD, and are related to neural regions including the anterior cingulate, dorsolateral prefrontal cortex, insula, temporal and parietal lobes, and the cerebellum (Rauch *et al.*, 2007; Burdick *et al.*, 2008; van den Heuvel *et al.*, 2005; Chamberlain *et al.*, 2005; van der Wee *et al.*, 2003; Christian *et al.*, 2008).

Structural neuroimaging techniques

There has been a substantial increase in the number of structural neuroimaging studies investigating the neurobiology of OCD over the past decade. These studies have identified abnormalities in CST neural systems, especially in the orbitofrontal cortex and have informed many of the dominant neurobiological models of OCD (Baxter *et al.*, 1996; Saxena *et al.*, 1998, 2001; Rauch and Jenike, 1993; Modell *et al.*, 1989). Some of the first studies used computerized tomography (CT), a series of X-rays of limited resolution. The emergence of magnetic resonance (MR) imaging techniques advanced the field by providing higher-resolution images without the potential risk of ionizing radiation. Early MR imaging studies utilized manual tracing techniques to measure specific regions-of-interest (ROIs). Although manual tracing of ROIs has continued and remains the "gold standard" for brain mensuration, more advanced techniques have permitted automated brain measurements to be computed using voxel-wise analysis. Other sophisticated algorithms have permitted investigators to investigate gray matter thickness in OCD across the cortical surface (Narayan *et al.*, 2008; Shin *et al.*, 2007). Because accumulating evidence does not support gross neuroanatomical abnormalities in OCD, structural neuroimaging studies can greatly contribute to our understanding of the more subtle aberrant neural patterns that likely contribute to the disorder.

Orbitofrontal cortex

The orbitofrontal cortex is located in the ventral portion of the prefrontal cortex and has reciprocal projections to and from all sensory modalities (Rolls, 2004). The orbitofrontal cortex plays an important role in human emotion as well as learning the reward and punishment value of sensory stimuli (Hornak *et al.*, 2003; Rolls, 2004), and therefore, has direct relevance to the phenomenology of OCD. Several studies investigating the orbitofrontal cortex in adults with OCD reported less volume in patients compared to healthy controls (Szeszko *et al.*, 1999; Choi *et al.*, 2004; Kang *et al.*, 2004; Atmaca *et al.*, 2006, 2007; Pujol *et al.*, 2004) and that orbitofrontal volume correlates with symptom severity (Kang *et al.*, 2004; Atmaca *et al.*, 2007). In contrast, other studies reported more gray matter in this region in patients compared to healthy controls (Valente *et al.*, 2005; Christian *et al.*, 2008; Kim *et al.*, 2001).

Some data suggest that treatment and/or treatment course may be an important consideration in OCD structural neuroimaging studies investigating orbitofrontal cortex volume. For example, treatment of patients with OCD with selective serotonin reuptake inhibitors (SSRIs) has been linked to changes in brain structure (Gilbert *et al.*, 2000; Szeszko *et al.*, 2004a). In a study investigating the relationship between orbitofrontal cortex volume and treatment response, Atmaca and colleagues (2006) reported that lower orbitofrontal volumes were found in treatment-naive patients compared to treatment-responders and healthy controls. Interestingly, treatment-refractory patients had decreased orbitofrontal volumes compared to treatment-responders. Patients in the study by Kim *et al.* (2001), which identified greater orbitofrontal gray matter density in OCD, included patients who remained psychotropic drug-free for at least 4 weeks. In another study, which compared results obtained using regional volumetry and a voxel-wise analysis, Szeszko *et al.* (2008) reported that psychotropic drug-naive pediatric patients with OCD had more gray matter in the orbitofrontal cortex using both methods compared to healthy controls.

Anterior cingulate cortex

The anterior cingulate cortex is located on the medial surface of the cingulate gyrus and wraps around the anterior portion of the corpus callosum (Barbas, 1992; Vogt *et al.*, 1995). The anterior cingulate is considered an integrative center for cognitive–behavioral and emotional–autonomic, motor neural networks (Bush *et al.*, 2000; Vogt *et al.*, 1992). Several neuroimaging studies of OCD have examined structural alterations in the anterior cingulate, a region that has been linked to difficulties with set-shifting, decision-making and both action and error-monitoring in this

237

disorder (Ursu *et al.*, 2003; Fitzgerald *et al.*, 2005; Maltby *et al.*, 2005). In this regard, a recent meta-analysis combining both adult and pediatric studies reported an overall reduction in anterior cingulate volume in OCD subjects compared to controls (Rotge *et al.*, 2009a). When looking at individual adult studies, however, clear differences in anterior cingulate volumes between patients with OCD and controls were not particularly pronounced. Other studies did not identify significant structural alterations in the anterior cingulate in patients with OCD versus controls (Kang *et al.*, 2004; Grachev *et al.*, 1998). Interestingly, studies in pediatric OCD reported consistent findings of more anterior cingulate gray matter in psychotropic drug-naive patients compared to healthy controls (Rosenberg *et al.*, 1998; Szeszko *et al.*, 2004b, 2008). In contrast, however, another pediatric OCD study reported less anterior cingulate volume in patients compared to controls (Carmona *et al.*, 2007).

Basal ganglia

The basal ganglia refers to a collection of subcortical nuclei that includes the caudate nucleus, putamen, globus pallidus, subthalamic nucleus, and substantia nigra. These structures are involved in multiple segregated parallel loops that regulate cortical activity (Alexander *et al.*, 1986, 1990; Graybiel, 2000). Components of the basal ganglia are implicated in the processing of movement, learning, motivation, and reward (Delgado, 2007; Packard and Knowlton, 2002; Robbins and Everett, 1992) and have been consistently implicated in both adult and pediatric neuroimaging studies of OCD (see Figure 16.1). The basal ganglia include brain regions implicated in tic disorders and other movement disorders and, thus, may play a role in the repetitive behaviors characteristic of OCD. Furthermore, it may be noteworthy that effective deep brain stimulation treatment of OCD specifically targets the anterior limb of the internal capsule, a region linking cortical, thalamic, and basal ganglia structures (Greenberg *et al.*, 2006).

Investigation of basal ganglia volumes from early structural neuroimaging studies of OCD using CT prompted initial interest in the CST pathway. One early study of male adolescents with OCD found decreased caudate volumes in patients compared to controls (Luxenberg *et al.*, 1988). Another study (Stein *et al.*, 1993) found no group differences in

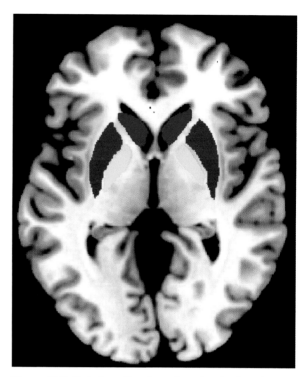

Figure 16.1 Illustration of basal ganglia regions implicated in the neurobiology of OCD (blue, caudate nucleus; red, putamen; yellow, globus pallidus).

caudate or lenticular nucleus volumes in adult OCD patients compared to controls, although CT revealed greater ventricular size in patients with OCD with high versus low neurological soft signs. While these early studies brought interest to a potential role for the CST pathway in the pathophysiology of OCD, methodological limitations of CT limited findings and their interpretation.

Although the striatum (caudate and putamen) is viewed as a key component of the circuitry implicated in OCD, MR imaging ROI studies of the striatum have provided mixed results. Larger (Scarone *et al.*, 1992), smaller (Robinson *et al.*, 1995) and normal (Kang *et al.*, 2004; Atmaca *et al.*, 2006, 2007; Riffkin *et al.*, 2005; Garber *et al.*, 1989; Aylward *et al.*, 1996; Jenike *et al.*, 1996; Kellner *et al.*, 1991) caudate gray matter volumes have been reported in adult OCD patients relative to controls. Results from a study of adult OCD and trichotillomania revealed no significant differences in caudate volume among groups of patients with OCD, trichotillomania and healthy controls (Stein *et al.*, 1997). Smaller caudate volumes in subjects were associated with difficulties in visual-spatial processing on the Rey–Osterreith test (copy dysfunction) and executive control (Stroop Task), lower intellectual functioning and neurological soft signs (i.e. abnormal fine motor coordination, involuntary and mirror movements and visuospatial function). Although caudate volume was related to possible neuropsychological deficits, it was not associated with symptom severity. An explanation for inconsistent findings across studies is the potential for abnormalities to be localized to specific areas of the caudate nucleus in OCD. In this regard, it is noteworthy that Pujol *et al.* (2004) reported that portions of the ventral striatum, including the ventral putamen, were larger in adult OCD patients compared to healthy controls, supporting the possibility of altered motor related circuitry possibly associated with implicit learning difficulties in OCD. Other issues regarding discrepant findings may be related to variation in morphologic delineation criteria including the choice of anatomical landmarks, resolution of images and potential moderators, including different symptom dimensions and sex.

Similar to results from adult studies, basal ganglia findings in pediatric OCD have been mixed. Rosenberg and colleagues (1997a) reported smaller striatal volumes in OCD subjects compared to healthy controls; striatal volumes were inversely correlated with symptom severity but not illness duration. No differences were reported between groups in prefrontal, lateral ventricular or intracranial volumes. In a different cohort of pediatric OCD patients, Szeszko *et al.* (2004b) reported smaller globus pallidus volumes in patients compared to controls, but without associated group differences in volumes of the caudate nucleus or putamen. There were positive correlations between the total globus pallidus and anterior cingulate volumes in the healthy volunteers, but not in the patients with OCD. A voxel-based morphometry study of psychotropic drug-naive children and adolescents with OCD found more gray matter in the putamen compared to healthy control subjects (Szeszko *et al.*, 2008), which was supported by findings using manual volumetry.

Motivated by interest in potential associations between OCD symptoms and streptococcal infections in children and adolescents, Giedd and colleagues studied pediatric OCD subjects with streptococcal infections and healthy controls (Giedd *et al.*, 2000). The group with potential streptococcus-associated OCD and/or tics had larger volumes of the caudate, putamen, and globus pallidus. Peterson and colleagues (2000) examined the relationship between streptococcal infections and gray matter in a group of children and adolescents with OCD, tic disorders, or attention deficit hyperactivity disorder (ADHD) and healthy controls. Interestingly, the subjects with attention deficit hyperactivity disorder or OCD had associations between larger basal ganglia volumes and higher antistreptococcal antibodies. These findings suggest that associations between streptococcal infections and neuropsychiatric disorders may not be specific to OCD and tic disorders and could include other disorders, such as ADHD. However, these findings continue to implicate the basal ganglia in the pathophysiology of OCD and offer one possible mechanism through which structural alterations may occur.

Thalamus

The thalamus is a subcortical structure involved in the relay of information from multiple brain regions to the cortex. It is involved in the regulation of perception, attention and conscious awareness (Jones, 2002). The thalamus has been considered integral to neurobiological models of OCD and several structural neuroimaging studies have implicated this region in the pathophysiology of the disorder. Several adult studies reported larger thalamic volumes in patients with OCD (Atmaca *et al.*, 2007; Kim *et al.*, 2001), both with and without comorbid MDD (Christian *et al.*, 2008) compared to healthy controls. In contrast, however, several studies did not find evidence for thalamic abnormalities in OCD (Kang *et al.*, 2004; Jenike *et al.*, 1996; Kwon *et al.*, 2003). Of particular interest, however, is that a recent meta-analysis reported that thalamic volume was positively associated with OCD symptom severity (Rotge *et al.*, 2009a), consistent with the hypothesis that greater thalamic volume may be pathological in OCD. Along similar lines, Christian *et al.* (2008) reported that among OCD patients without comorbid major depression, more right thalamic gray matter correlated significantly with worse motor functioning. One study reported that thalamic volume was significantly inversely correlated with orbital frontal volumes in patients with OCD, but not among healthy subjects (Rotge *et al.*, 2009b), suggesting that these brain regions may comprise a common neurobiological process in OCD.

There is some evidence that treatment status may be an important consideration in studies investigating thalamic volume in OCD. In the study by Christian and colleagues (2008), which demonstrated larger thalamic volume in patients, patients were still moderately ill as reflected by their Yale Brown Obsessive–Compulsive Scale scores, despite having been treated for their OCD. More direct evidence comes from Atmaca and colleagues (2006), who demonstrated that patients with first-episode OCD had larger bilateral thalamic volumes compared to treatment-responders and healthy controls. Furthermore, treatment-refractory OCD patients demonstrated larger bilateral thalamic volumes compared to treatment responders (Atmaca et al., 2006).

Studies in children and adolescents have also reported larger thalamic volumes in OCD subjects compared to healthy controls. A study of psychotropic drug-naive pediatric OCD patients reported significantly greater thalamic volume compared to healthy controls (Gilbert et al., 2000). Interestingly, the thalamic volumes reduced to levels similar to the healthy comparison group following treatment with the serotonin reuptake inhibitor, paroxetine. The thalamic gray matter reduction was associated with a decrease in OCD symptoms. Of particular interest is that thalamus changes in a pediatric OCD cohort were not evident following non-pharmacologic intervention using cognitive behavioral therapy (Rosenberg et al., 2001).

Other brain regions

While CST networks are most commonly associated with OCD, investigators have also explored the possible role of limbic regions, which are typically associated with fear and anxiety, in the neurobiology of OCD. Several structural neuroimaging studies reported less gray matter in the amygdala (Szeszko et al., 1999; Atmaca et al., 2008) and hippocampus (Atmaca et al., 2008; Hong et al., 2007; Kwon et al., 2003) in adult patients with OCD compared to healthy controls, although Kwon et al. (2003) reported larger amygdala volume in patients. Studies have also found that OCD patients exhibit less hemispheric asymmetry in amygdala and hippocampal volumes compared to healthy controls (Szeszko et al., 1999). In one study, symptom severity was correlated with left hippocampal volume, but not correlated with amygdala volume (Atmaca et al.,

2008). This study also reported that illness duration was negatively associated with both left amygdala and bilateral hippocampal volumes. Alterations in amygdala volume have been reported in a treatment study of pediatric OCD that found significant asymmetry of the amygdala prior to the initiation of treatment (Szeszko et al., 2004a). Following a 16-week course of paroxetine, the pediatric patients with OCD demonstrated a reduction in left amygdala volume. Interestingly, amygdala volume correlated significantly with higher paroxetine dosage at the time of the follow-up scan and total cumulative paroxetine exposure between the two scans.

Voxel-based morphometry studies of OCD have reported gray matter alterations (both increases and decreases) in the insula (Valente et al., 2005; Kim et al., 2001; Pujol et al., 2004), a region associated with disgust, an emotion related to contamination/washing symptoms in OCD patients (Phillips et al., 2000). These same voxel-based morphometry studies also revealed parietal and cerebellar gray matter volume alterations in OCD patients compared to healthy controls. Another study of adult OCD found significantly less gray matter in several dorsal cortical regions (BA6, 8, 9, and 46) and significantly greater gray matter in the midbrain of patients compared to healthy controls (Gilbert et al., 2008). The gray matter differences were correlated with OCD symptom severity. Several recent studies have reported smaller pituitary volumes in both adult (Atmaca et al., 2009; Jung et al., 2009) and pediatric (MacMaster et al., 2006) OCD subjects compared to healthy controls, implicating a potential role of stress in mediating these structural volumes across the age span.

White matter

Despite its relevance to CST models of the disorder, the brain white matter has not been well investigated in OCD. There is now increasing evidence, however, that the brain white matter may be abnormal in OCD and that these abnormalities play an important role in phenomenology. Of particular note is that Stewart and colleagues (2007) reported that variation in several single nucleotide polymorphisms (SNPs) in oligodendrocyte lineage transcription factor 2 was associated with a diagnosis of OCD. Along these lines, several studies used regional volumetry or voxel-based morphometry to assess white matter integrity in patients with OCD. Corpus callosum volumes were reportedly larger in patients with OCD compared to healthy controls (Rosenberg *et al.*, 1997b). Using this same sample, this group also reported lower genu signal intensity in patients with OCD, which may have reflected greater myelinization of the region.

Duran *et al.* (2009) reported significant global white matter reductions in OCD patients compared to controls. Although regional specificity was not evident, these authors reported positive correlations of OCD severity with the anterior limb of the internal capsule. Decreased prefrontal white matter volume was reported in patients with OCD compared to healthy controls (Van den Heuvel *et al.*, 2009; Carmona *et al.*, 2007). In a study investigating white matter in treatment-naive patients, Atmaca *et al.* (2007) reported greater white matter volume in treatment-naive adult patients with OCD compared to healthy volunteers.

Recently, investigators have used DTI to investigate the potential role of white matter abnormalities in the pathogenesis of OCD. This neuroimaging technique permits quantification of water diffusion and can be used to assess white matter integrity via measures such as fractional anisotropy (FA). In one of the first studies to apply this technique to the study of OCD, Szeszko and colleagues (2005) reported lower FA in the cingulate, parietal and occipital regions in patients compared to healthy volunteers. In a partial replication, Cannistraro *et al.* (2007) reported lower FA in the right cingulum of patients with OCD compared to healthy volunteers, but also identified several areas where there was higher FA in patients, including the left cingulum and anterior limb of the internal capsule. Another study reported higher FA in the bilateral semiovale center in patients compared to healthy volunteers (Nakamae *et al.*, 2008). In two DTI studies that assessed the functional significance of white matter abnormalities in OCD, lower FA in the corpus callosum (Saito *et al.*, 2008) and parietal lobe (Szeszko *et al.*, 2005) white matter was associated with greater symptom severity. There is also increasing attention being paid to the possibility of using the brain white matter as an endophenotype in OCD studies. In this regard, Menzies *et al.* (2008b) reported that patients and their first-degree relatives had lower FA in a large region of right inferior parietal white matter and increased FA in a right medial frontal region compared to healthy controls.

Several studies reported changes in white matter integrity in OCD following pharmacologic intervention. In a study assessing white matter in drug-naive patients, Yoo and colleagues (2007) reported higher FA in the corpus callosum, internal capsule, and white matter superiolateral to the right caudate. FA increases were mostly no longer evident following 12 weeks of citalopram treatment, suggesting that the observed abnormalities may be altered by pharmacologic intervention. In another study, treatment-naive children and adolescents with OCD had less right parietal white matter, but this deficit normalized to levels comparable to healthy volunteers following 6 months of treatment (Lazaro *et al.*, 2009). These studies point to the intriguing possibility that medications used to treat OCD may ameliorate some brain white matter structural abnormalities in the disorder, but more research is clearly needed in this area.

Conclusions

Several decades of structural neuroimaging studies in pediatric and adult OCD have supported an evolving, broad model of CST pathology underlying the development and expression of the disorder. Both gray and white matter abnormalities in OCD contribute to this substantially prevalent and potentially disabling condition. Consistent findings of gray matter differences between patients with OCD (both pediatric and adult) and healthy controls in orbitofrontal cortex, basal ganglia, thalamus and anterior cingulate support core abnormalities in CST systems implicated in both cognitive and emotional processing. A growing literature that includes abnormalities in other brain regions in OCD has broadened this neurobiological model; this growth has contributed to a greater understanding of brain–behavior relationships in the disorder. Treatment status and the potential influence of psychotropic medications on brain structure appear to be an important consideration in the interpretation of results from OCD structural neuroimaging studies.

Future directions

Growth in our understanding of neurobiological mechanisms in OCD will likely parallel continued growth in MR imaging and other neuroimaging technologies. The use of a higher magnetic field strength may permit the detection of more subtle structural differences between patients with OCD and healthy controls as well as the potential resolution of the internal architecture of key CST structures that have particular significance for neurobiological models of

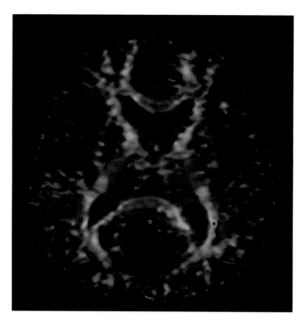

Figure 16.2 Illustration of a colormap from diffusion tensor imaging demonstrating white matter tracts and their directionality (green, anterior/posterior; blue/purple, superior/inferior; red, right/left).

the disorder. Moreover, coupling structural brain imaging with comprehensive neuropsychological examinations will provide important information regarding structure–function relations in OCD. Replication of findings in structural neuroimaging studies should also be an important goal of future research. Multi-site neuroimaging studies will be important in this regard, as studies with small sample sizes may contribute to discrepant findings and disease heterogeneity (i.e. subtypes) can be examined more comprehensively. MR imaging studies linking brain morphology with genetics studies will provide valuable information regarding the potential functional significance of genetic findings. Another important consideration in future structural neuroimaging studies of patients with OCD should be their treatment status as several studies have documented changes in brain structure following pharmacologic intervention consistent with the functional neuroimaging literature. MR imaging done in the context of controlled treatment trials in OCD could be useful in this regard. Furthermore, the use of colormaps (see Figure 16.2) in future DTI studies of OCD will facilitate the identification of specific white matter tracts to inform neurobiological models of the disorder. Finally, to better understand the abnormal neural systems

underlying the pathophysiology of OCD, future studies should include the use of more sophisticated neuroimaging analyses that allow for the investigation of anatomical connectivity.

Acknowledgments

This work was supported in part by grants from the National Center for Research Resources to Dr. Gilbert (05 KL2 RR024154–03) and the National Institute of Mental Health to Dr. Szeszko (MH01990).

Box 16.1. Structural neuroimaging in OCD

- Gray matter volume differences between patients with OCD and healthy controls are consistently found in the following components of cortico-striatal–thalamic pathways:
  Orbitofrontal cortex
  Basal ganglia
  Thalamus
  Anterior cingulate.
- The direction (smaller versus larger) of between-group gray matter differences in structural neuroimaging studies may be related to the following variables:
  Methodological approach (automated vs. manual assessment of brain regions)
  Treatment status (especially serotonin reuptake inhibitors)
  Age (child vs. adult).
- A disruption in the brain white matter may also contribute to the neurobiology of OCD, although the regional localization of abnormalities has not always been consistent.
- Structural neuroimaging studies suggest that the neurobiology of OCD is associated with more widespread neural system dysfunction rather than gross abnormalities in one or two brain regions.
- Heterogeneous findings in structural imaging studies of OCD may reflect and/or explain the clinical heterogeneity of the disorder.
- Future structural neuroimaging studies in OCD could benefit from investigating brain abnormalities in relationship to symptom subtypes and genetic polymorphisms.

References

Alexander G E, Crutcher M D and DeLong M R. 1990. Basal ganglia–thalamocortical circuits: parallel substrates for motor, oculomotor, "prefrontal" and "limbic" functions. *Prog Brain Res* **85**, 119–46.

Alexander G E, DeLong M R and Strick P L. 1986. Parallel organization of functionally segregated circuits linking basal ganglia and cortex. *Annu Rev Neurosci* **9**, 357–81.

Aouizerate B, Guehl D, Cuny E, *et al.* 2004. Pathophysiology of obsessive–compulsive disorder: A necessary link between phenomenology, neuropsychology, imagery and physiology. *Prog Neurobiol* **72**, 195–221.

Atmaca M, Yildirim B H, Ozdemir B H, Aydin B A, Tezcan A E and Ozler A S. 2006. Volumetric MRI assessment of brain regions in patients with refractory obsessive–compulsive disorder. *Prog Neuropsychopharmacol Biol Psychiatry* **30**, 1051–7.

Atmaca M, Yildirim H, Ozdemir H, *et al.* 2008. Hippocampus and amygdalar volumes in patients with refractory obsessive–compulsive disorder. *Prog Neuropsychopharmacol Biol Psychiatry* **32**, 1283–6.

Atmaca M, Yildirim H, Ozdemir H, Tezcan E and Poyraz A K. 2007. Volumetric MRI study of key brain regions implicated in obsessive–compulsive disorder. *Prog Neuropsychopharmacol Biol Psychiatry* **31**, 46–52.

Atmaca M, Yildirim H, Ozler S, Koc M, Kara B and Sec S. 2009. Smaller pituitary volume in adult patients with obsessive–compulsive disorder. *Psychiatry Clin Neurosci* **63**, 516–20.

Aylward E H, Harris G J, Hoehn-Saric R, Barta P E, Machlin S R and Pearlson G D. 1996. Normal caudate nucleus in obsessive–compulsive disorder assessed by quantitative neuroimaging. *Arch Gen Psychiatry* **53**, 577–84.

Barbas H. 1992. Architecture and cortical connections of the prefrontal cortex in the rhesus monkey. *Adv Neurol* **57**, 91–115.

Baxter L R Jr, Saxena S, Brody A L, *et al.* 1996. Brain mediation of obsessive–compulsive disorder symptoms: Evidence from functional brain imaging studies in the human and nonhuman primate. *Semin Clin Neuropsychiatry* **1**, 32–47.

Burdick K E, Robinson D G, Malhotra A K and Szeszko P R. 2008. Neurocognitive profile analysis in obsessive–compulsive disorder. *J Int Neuropsychol Soc* **14**, 640–5.

Bush G, Luu P and Posner M I. 2000. Cognitive and emotional influences in anterior cingulate cortex. *Trends Cogn Sci* **4**, 215–22.

Cannistraro P A, Makris N, Howard J D, *et al.* 2007. A diffusion tensor imaging study of white matter in obsessive–compulsive disorder. *Depress Anxiety* **24**, 440–6.

Carmona S, Bassas N, Rovira M, *et al.* 2007. Pediatric OCD structural brain deficits in conflict monitoring circuits: A voxel-based morphometry study. *Neurosci Lett* **421**, 218–23.

Chamberlain S R, Blackwell A D, Fineberg N A, Robbins T W and Sahakian B J. 2005. The neuropsychology of obsessive compulsive disorder: the importance of failures in cognitive and behavioural inhibition as candidate endophenotypic markers. *Neurosci Biobehav Rev* **29**, 399–419.

Choi J S, Kang D H, Kim J J, *et al.* 2004. Left anterior subregion of orbitofrontal cortex volume reduction and impaired organizational strategies in obsessive–compulsive disorder. *J Psychiatr Res* **38**, 193–9.

Christian C J, Lencz T, Robinson D G, *et al.* 2008. Gray matter structural alterations in obsessive–compulsive disorder: Relationship to neuropsychological functions. *Psychiatry Res* **164**, 123–31.

Delgado M R. 2007. Reward-related responses in the human striatum. *Ann NY Acad Sci* **1104**, 70–88. Epub 2007 Mar 7.

Duran F L, Hoexter M Q, Valente A A Jr, Miguel E C and Busatto G F. 2009. Association between symptom severity and internal capsule volume in obsessive–compulsive disorder. *Neurosci Lett* **452**, 68–71. Epub 2009 Jan 9.

Fitzgerald K D, Welsh R C, Gehring W J, *et al.* 2005. Error related hyperactivity of the anterior cingulate cortex in obsessive–compulsive disorder. *Biol Psychiatry* **57**, 287–94.

Garber H J, Ananth J V, Chiu L C, Griswold V J and Oldendorf W H. 1989. Nuclear magnetic resonance study of obsessive–compulsive disorder. *Am J Psychiatry* **146**, 1001–05.

Giedd J N, Rapoport J L, Garvey M A, Perlmutter S and Swedo S E. 2000. MRI assessment of children with obsessive–compulsive disorder or tics associated with streptococcal infection. *Am J Psychiatry* **157**, 281–3.

Gilbert A R, Mataix-Cols D, Almeida J R, *et al.* 2008. Brain structure and symptom dimension relationships in obsessive–compulsive disorder: A voxel-based morphometry study. *J Affect Disord* **109**, 117–26.

Gilbert A R, Moore G J, Keshavan M S, *et al.* 2000. Decrease in thalamic volumes of pediatric patients with obsessive–compulsive disorder who are taking paroxetine. *Arch Gen Psychiatry* **57**, 449–56.

Grachev I D, Breiter H C, Rauch S L, *et al.* 1998. Structural abnormalities of frontal neocortex in obsessive–compulsive disorder. *Arch Gen Psychiatry* **55**, 181–2.

Graybiel A M. 2000. The basal ganglia. *Curr Biol* **10**, R509–11.

Graybiel A M and Rauch S L. 2000. Toward a neurobiology of obsessive–compulsive disorder. *Neuron* **28**, 343–7.

243

Greenberg B D, Malone D A, Friehs G M, *et al.* 2006. Three-year outcomes in deep brain stimulation for highly resistant obsessive–compulsive disorder. *Neuropsychopharmacology* **31**, 2384–93.

Hong S B, Shin Y W, Kim S H, *et al.* 2007. Hippocampal shape deformity analysis in obsessive–compulsive disorder. *Eur Arch Psychiatry Clin Neurosci* **257**, 185–90.

Hornak J, Bramham J, Rolls E T, *et al.* 2003. Changes in emotion after circumscribed surgical lesions of the orbitofrontal and cingulate cortices. *Brain* **126**, 1691–712. Epub 2003 Jun 4.

Jenike M A, Breiter H C, Baer L, *et al.* 1996. Cerebral structural abnormalities in obsessive–compulsive disorder. A quantitative morphometric magnetic resonance imaging study. *Arch Gen Psychiatry* **53**, 625–32.

Jones E G. 2002. Thalamic organization and function after Cajal. *Prog Brain Res* **136**, 333–57.

Jung M H, Huh M J, Kang D H, *et al.* 2009. Volumetric differences in the pituitary between drug-naive and medicated male patients with obsessive–compulsive disorder. *Prog Neuropsychopharmacol Biol Psychiatry* **33**, 605–09.

Kang D H, Kim J J, Choi J S, *et al.* 2004. Volumetric investigation of the frontal–subcortical circuitry in patients with obsessive–compulsive disorder. *J Neuropsychiatry Clin Neurosci* **16**, 342–9.

Kellner C H, Jolley R R, Holgate R C, *et al.* 1991. Brain MRI in obsessive–compulsive disorder. *Psychiatry Res* **36**, 45–9.

Kim J J, Lee M C, Kim J, *et al.* 2001. Grey matter in obsessive–compulsive disorder: Statistical parametric mapping of segmented magnetic resonance images. *Br J Psychiatry* **179**, 330–4.

Kwon J S, Shin Y W, Kim C W, *et al.* 2003. Similarity and disparity of obsessive–compulsive disorder and schizophrenia in MR volumetric abnormalities of the hippocampus–amygdala complex. *J Neurol Neurosurg Psychiatry* **74**, 962–4.

Lazaro L, Bargalló N, Castro-Fornieles J, *et al.* 2009. Brain changes in children and adolescents with obsessive–compulsive disorder before and after treatment: A voxel-based morphometric MRI study. *Psychiatry Res* **172**, 140–6. Epub 2009 Mar 24.

Luxenberg J S, Swedo S E, Flament M F, Friedland R P, Rapoport J and Rapoport S I. 1988. Neuroanatomical abnormalities in obsessive–compulsive disorder detected with quantitative X-ray computed tomography. *Am J Psychiatry* **145**, 1089–93.

MacMaster F P, Russell A, Mirza Y, *et al.* 2006. Pituitary volume in pediatric obsessive–compulsive disorder. *Biol Psychiatry* **59**, 252–7.

Maltby N, Tolin D F, Worhunsky P, O'Keefe T M and Kiehl K A. 2005. Dysfunctional action monitoring hyperactivates frontal–striatal circuits in obsessive–compulsive disorder: An event-related fMRI study. *Neuroimage* **24**, 495–503.

Menzies L, Chamberlain S R, Laird A R, Thelen S M, Sahakian B J and Bullmore E T. 2008a. Integrating evidence from neuroimaging and neuropsychological studies of obsessive–compulsive disorder: The orbitofronto-striatal model revisited. *Neurosci Biobehav Rev* **32**, 525–49.

Menzies L, Williams G B, Chamberlain S R, *et al.* 2008b. White matter abnormalities in patients with obsessive–compulsive disorder and their first-degree relatives. *Am J Psychiatry* **165**, 1308–15. Epub 2008 Jun 2.

Modell J G, Mountz J M, Curtis G C and Greden J F. 1989. Neurophysiologic dysfunction in basal ganglia/limbic striatal and thalamocortical circuits as a pathogenetic mechanism of obsessive compulsive disorder. *J Neuropsychiatry Clin Neurosci* **1**, 27–36.

Murray C J L and Lopez A D. 1996. *The Global Burden of Disease.* Boston, MA: Harvard School of Public Health.

Nakamae T, Narumoto J, Shibata K, *et al.* 2008. Alteration of fractional anisotropy and apparent diffusion coefficient in obsessive–compulsive disorder: A diffusion tensor imaging study. *Prog Neuropsychopharmacol Biol Psychiatry* **32**, 1221–6. Epub 2008 Mar 25.

Narayan V M, Narr K L, Phillips O R, Thompson P M, Toga A W and Szeszko P R. 2008. Greater regional cortical gray matter thickness in obsessive–compulsive disorder. *Neuroreport* **19**, 1551–5.

Packard M G and Knowlton B J. 2002. Learning and memory functions of the basal ganglia. *Annu Rev Neurosci* **25**, 563–93.

Peterson B S, Leckman J F, Tucker D, *et al.* 2000. Preliminary findings of antistreptococcal antibody titers and basal ganglia volumes in tic, obsessive–compulsive, and attention deficit/hyperactivity disorders. *Arch Gen Psychiatry* **57**, 364–72.

Phillips M L, Marks I M, Senior C, *et al.* 2000. A differential neural response in obsessive–compulsive disorder patients with washing compared with checking symptoms to disgust. *Psychol Med* **30**, 1037–50.

Pujol J, Soriano-Mas C, Alonso P, *et al.* 2004. Mapping structural brain alterations in obsessive–compulsive disorder. *Arch Gen Psychiatry* **61**, 720–30.

Rauch S L and Jenike M A. 1993. Neurobiological models of obsessive–compulsive disorder. *Psychosomatics* **34**, 20–32.

Rauch S L, Wedig M M, Wright C I, *et al.* 2007. Functional magnetic resonance imaging study of regional brain activation during implicit sequence learning in obsessive–compulsive disorder. *Biol Psychiatry* **61**, 330–6.

Riffkin J, Yucel M, Maruff P, *et al.* 2005. Manual and automated MRI study of anterior cingulate and orbito-frontal cortices, and caudate nucleus in obsessive–compulsive disorder: Comparison with healthy controls and patients with schizophrenia. *Psychiatry Res* **138**, 99–113.

Robbins T W and Everitt B J. 1992. Functions of dopamine in the dorsal and ventral striatum. *Sem Neurosci* **4**, 119–27.

Robinson D, Wu H, Munne R A, *et al.* 1995. Reduced caudate nucleus volume in obsessive–compulsive disorder. *Arch Gen Psychiatry* **52**, 393–8.

Rolls E T. 2004. The functions of the orbitofrontal cortex. *Brain Cogn* **55**, 11–29.

Rosenberg D R, Benazon N R, Gilbert A, Sullivan A and Moore G J. 2001. Thalamic volume in pediatric obsessive–compulsive disorder patients before and after cognitive behavioral therapy. *Biol Psychiatry* **50**, 312.

Rosenberg D and Keshavan M. 1998. Toward a neurodevelopmental model of obsessive–compulsive disorder. *Biol Psychiatry* **43**, 623–40.

Rosenberg D R, Keshavan M S, Dick E L, Bagwell W W, MacMaster F P and Birmaher B. 1997a. Corpus callosal morphology in treatment-naive pediatric obsessive compulsive disorder. *Prog Neuropsychopharmacol Biol Psychiatry* **21**, 1269–83.

Rosenberg D R, Keshavan M S, O'Hearn K, *et al.* 1997b. Frontostriatal measurement in treatment-naive children with obsessive compulsive disorder. *Arch Gen Psychiatry* **54**, 824–30.

Rotge J Y, Guehl D, Dilharreguy B, *et al.* 2009a. Meta-analysis of brain volume changes in obsessive–compulsive disorder. *Biol Psychiatry* **65**, 75–83.

Rotge J Y, Dilharreguy B, Aouizerate B, *et al.* 2009b. Inverse relationship between thalamic and orbitofrontal volumes in obsessive–compulsive disorder. *Prog Neuropsychopharmacol Biol Psychiatry* **33**, 682–7. Epub 2009 Mar 21.

Saito Y, Nobuhara K, Okugawa G, *et al.* 2008. Corpus callosum in patients with obsessive–compulsive disorder: Diffusion-tensor imaging study. *Radiology* **246**, 536–42. Epub 2008 Jan 7.

Saxena S, Bota R G and Brody A L. 2001. Brain–behavior relationships in obsessive–compulsive disorder. *Semin Clin Neuropsychiatry* **6**, 82–101.

Saxena S, Brody A L, Schwartz J M and Baxter L R. 1998. Neuroimaging and frontal-subcortical circuitry in obsessive–compulsive disorder. *Br J Psychiatry Suppl* **35**, 26–37.

Scarone S, Colombo C, Livian S, *et al.* 1992. Increased right caudate nucleus size in obsessive–compulsive disorder: Detection with magnetic resonance imaging. *Psychiatry Res* **45**, 115–21.

Schwartz J M. 1998. Neuroanatomical aspects of cognitive-behavioural therapy response in obsessive compulsive disorder. An evolving perspective on brain and behaviour. *Br J Psychiatry Suppl* **35**, 38–44.

Shin Y W, Yoo S Y, Lee J K, *et al.* 2007. Cortical thinning in obsessive compulsive disorder. *Hum Brain Mapp* **28**, 1128–35.

Stein D J, Coetzer R, Lee M, Davids B and Bouwer C. 1997. Magnetic resonance brain imaging in women with obsessive–compulsive disorder and trichotillomania. *Psychiatry Res* **74**, 177–82.

Stein D J, Hollander E, Chan S, *et al.* 1993. Computed tomography and neurological soft signs in obsessive–compulsive disorder. *Psychiatry Res* **50**, 143–50.

Stewart S E, Geller D A, Jenike M, *et al.* 2004. Long-term outcome of pediatric obsessive–compulsive disorder: A meta-analysis and qualitative review of the literature. *Acta Psychiatr Scand* **110**, 4–13.

Stewart S E, Platko J, Fagerness J, *et al.* 2007. A genetic family-based association study of OLIG2 in obsessive–compulsive disorder. *Arch Gen Psychiatry* **64**, 209–14.

Szeszko P R, Ardekani B A, Ashtari M, *et al.* 2005. White matter abnormalities in obsessive–compulsive disorder: A diffusion tensor imaging study. *Arch Gen Psychiatry* **62**, 782–90.

Szeszko P R, Christian C, Macmaster F, *et al.* 2008. Gray matter structural alterations in psychotropic drug-naïve pediatric obsessive–compulsive disorder: An optimized voxel-based morphometry study. *Am J Psychiatry* **165**, 1299–307.

Szeszko P R, MacMillan S, McMeniman M, *et al.* 2004a. Amygdala volume reductions in pediatric patients with obsessive–compulsive disorder treated with paroxetine: Preliminary findings. *Neuropsychopharmacology* **29**, 826–32.

Szeszko P R, MacMillan S, McMeniman M, *et al.* 2004b. Brain structural abnormalities in psychotropic drug-naive pediatric patients with obsessive–compulsive disorder. *Am J Psychiatry* **161**, 1049–56.

Szeszko P R, Robinson D, Alvir J M, *et al.* 1999. Orbital frontal and amygdala volume reductions in obsessive–compulsive disorder. *Arch Gen Psychiatry* **56**, 913–9.

Ursu S, Stenger V A, Shear M K, Jones M R and Carter C S. 2003. Overactive action monitoring in obsessive–compulsive disorder: Evidence from functional magnetic resonance imaging. *Psychol Sci* **14**, 347–53.

Valente A A Jr, Miguel E C, Castro C C, *et al.* 2005. Regional gray matter abnormalities in obsessive–compulsive disorder: A voxel-based morphometry study. *Biol Psychiatry* **58**, 479–87.

Van den Heuvel O A, Remijnse P L, Mataix-Cols D, *et al.* 2009. The major symptom dimensions of obsessive–compulsive disorder are mediated by partially distinct neural systems. *Brain* **132**, 853–68. Epub 2008 Oct 24.

Van den Heuvel O A, Veltman D J, Groenewegen H J, *et al.* 2005. Frontal–striatal dysfunction during planning in obsessive–compulsive disorder. *Arch Gen Psychiatry* **62**, 301–09.

Van der Wee N J, Ramsey N F, Jansma J M, *et al.* 2003. Spatial working memory deficits in obsessive compulsive disorder are associated with excessive engagement of the medial frontal cortex. *Neuroimage* **20**, 2271–80.

Vogt B A, Finch D M and Olson C R. 1992. Functional heterogeneity in cingulate cortex: The anterior executive and posterior evaluative regions. *Cereb Cortex* **2**, 435–43.

Vogt B A, Nimchinsky E A, Vogt L J and Hof P R. 1995. Human cingulate cortex: Surface features, flat maps, and cytoarchitecture. *J Comp Neurol* **359**, 490–506.

Yoo S Y, Jang J H, Shin Y W, *et al.* 2007. White matter abnormalities in drug-naïve patients with obsessive–compulsive disorder: A diffusion tensor study before and after citalopram treatment. *Acta Psychiatr Scand* **116**, 211–9.

Functional imaging of obsessive–compulsive disorder

Bon-Mi Gu, Do-Hyung Kang and Jun Soo Kwon

Functional magnetic resonance imaging (fMRI) research in obsessive–compulsive disorder (OCD) has explored a broad range of cognitive functions, in addition to the neural correlates of symptom provocation and symptom improvement after treatment. Additionally, given the heterogeneity of patients with OCD, some fMRI research has examined symptom-specific neural correlates or comparisons of different symptom dimensions in these patients. fMRI research on OCD has also included family members of patients with OCD, and have suggested trait-dependent neural patterns of cognitive dysfunction and genetic susceptibility to OCD.

The current model of OCD pathophysiology involves cortico basal ganglia–thalamo-cortical loop dysfunction, especially including dysfunction in the orbitofrontal cortex (OFC), caudate nucleus, and anterior cingulate cortex (ACC). The major findings in neuroimaging research in OCD suggest hyperactivation in the ventral frontal–striatal areas, such as the OFC, insula, ACC, and caudate head, during symptom provocation or resting states, and generally show normalized activation after symptom improvement. Additionally, various cognitive paradigms have been applied to fMRI research in OCD, and have provided evidence of neural correlates of specific cognitive dysfunction. The overall results of fMRI research in cognitive paradigms indicate reduced brain activation in the dorsolateral prefrontal cortex (dlPFC) or parietal lobes, related to executive function or cognitive flexibility, increased hippocampus activation, as compensation for dysfunction in the basal ganglia during implicit sequence learning, and hyperactivation in ACC, related to error processing.

Symptom provocation studies

Symptom provocation studies using fMRI in OCD have suggested abnormal activation of affected brain areas in patients during symptom exposure. To date, most findings have been of abnormal activation in the insula and ventrolateral prefrontal cortex (vlPFC) during the processing of disgust-evoking pictures (Adler et al., 2000; Breiter and Rauch, 1996; Mataix-Cols et al., 2004; Phillips et al., 2000; Schienle et al., 2005; Shapira et al., 2003), or during the perception of facial expressions of disgust (Cannistraro et al., 2004; Lawrence et al., 2007). The insula, part of the gustatory cortex that processes unpleasant tastes and smells, is known to mediate the disgust response through various paradigms (Phillips et al., 1997, 1998; Sprengelmeyer et al., 1997). The vlPFC brain area is known to be involved in common emotion processes, integrating information from distributed networks during facial expression recognition (Sprengelmeyer et al., 1998), and to play a role in monitoring of internal states (Critchley et al., 2004). Accordingly, abnormal activation in the insula and vlPFC suggests that patients with OCD may be more prone to experiencing disgust and have increased attention to their bodily responses to facial expressions of disgust.

In the first symptom provocation study using fMRI, Breiter and Rauch (1996) reported increased activation in the OFC, insula, ACC, and temporal and striatal areas in medicated patients with OCD. Similar results were reported in unmedicated patients with OCD (Adler et al., 2000); that study showed increased activation in frontal regions, including the OFC and ACC, and in the temporal cortex during symptom

Understanding Neuropsychiatric Disorders, ed. M. E. Shenton and B. I. Turetsky. Published by Cambridge University Press.
© Cambridge University Press 2011.

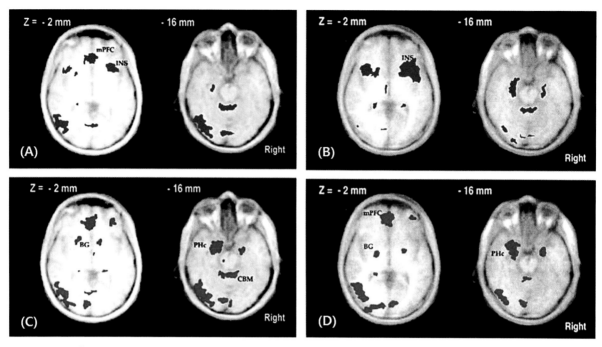

Figure 17.1 Differential brain activation by disgust and threat in healthy volunteers and in patients with OCD. Viewing disgust-inducing pictures versus neutral pictures in healthy volunteers (A) and in patients with OCD (B). Viewing threat-inducing pictures versus neutral pictures in healthy volunteers (C) and in patients with OCD (D). While overall response to threat-inducing pictures was similar between healthy controls and patients with OCD, different brain activation was found during disgust-inducing pictures in several areas, especially in the insula. INS, insula; BG, basal ganglia; mPFC, medial prefrontal cortex; CBM, cerebellum; PHc, parahippocampal region. Adapted with permission (Shapira *et al.*, 2003).

provocation. In that study, provocative stimuli varied widely, based on each subject's symptoms. For example, a patient with an ordering obsession was shown a picture of an overturned suitcase with clothes in disarray, and another patient with a fear of contamination was shown a picture of a dirty paper towel. Another fMRI study attempted to provoke each subject's symptoms using individualized symptom-relevant pictures (Schienle *et al.*, 2005). Schienle and colleagues (2005) used four kinds of stimuli, OCD-irrelevant, disgust-inducing, fear-inducing, and neutral pictures, and OCD-relevant pictures were taken by each patient from their personal environment to specifically trigger their OC symptoms. In the processing of OCD-relevant pictures, as compared to neutral pictures, patients with OCD showed increased activation in the OFC, insula, dlPFC, supramarginal gyrus, left caudate nucleus, and right thalamus, many of which are consistent with previous reports of symptom provocation in OCD. However, even the OCD-irrelevant disgust-inducing, or fear-inducing pictures induced higher activation of the insula in patients with OCD compared to control subjects, suggesting they

had elevated sensitivity for negative cues and were more prone to experience negative somatic states.

However, much of the research reported indicates that the sensitivity to negative stimuli in patients with OCD is restricted to disgust, not fear (Mataix-Cols *et al.*, 2004; Phillips *et al.*, 2000; Shapira *et al.*, 2003). Using disgust-inducing, threat-inducing, and neutral pictures, the neural correlates of disgust and fear have been demonstrated in both patients with OCD and healthy controls. As a result, patients with OCD showed increased activation in the insula during disgust provocation compared to healthy controls, while no difference was observed between the two groups during fear provocation using threat-inducing pictures (Figure 17.1).

In addition to this symptom provocation study, emotional facial recognition tasks also address the differences in fear and disgust information-processing in patients with OCD, as compared to other anxiety disorders. Studies have reported that patients with OCD have deficits when asked to identify facial representations of disgust, as compared to those with other anxiety disorders (Corcoran *et al.*, 2008;

Sprengelmeyer *et al.*, 1997), although an inconsistent report has been published (Parker *et al.*, 2004). With a different response to disgust in OCD compared to other anxiety disorders, the neural response to fear also showed differences between patients with OCD and those with other anxiety disorders (Cannistraro *et al.*, 2004). Contrary to findings of hyperactivity in the amygdala in other mood or anxiety disorders (Rauch *et al.*, 2000; Sheline *et al.*, 2001), patients with OCD demonstrated rather attenuated amygdala responses during the perception of facial emotion expressions of fear compared to healthy controls. The pathophysiology of OCD has been suggested to involve cortico basal ganglia–thalamo-cortical loop dysfunction, including the OFC, insula, ACC, basal ganglia, and thalamus (Saxena *et al.*, 1998; Saxena and Rauch, 2000), and OCD has been suggested to be distinguishable from other anxiety disorders.

Lawrence and colleagues (2007) replicated the finding of the abnormal processing of facial expressions of disgust, but not fear, in OCD using the more sophisticated paradigm of backward masking. In this, they presented photos of fear, disgust, and neutral facial expression just above conscious awareness, masked with neutral facial expression photos. The patients with OCD, especially those with high washing symptoms, showed increased left vlPFC activity with disgust-expression pictures, while they showed no difference with fear-expression pictures, as compared to healthy controls.

Symptom provocation studies have also been used to address the distinct neural correlates of different symptom dimensions. Patients with different symptom dimensions of checking and washing were examined while viewing disgusting pictures (Phillips *et al.*, 2000). Phillips and colleagues (2000) used three kinds of stimuli, neutral, normally disgusting, and washer-relevant pictures (pictures rated as more disgusting by washers than normal controls or checkers) in healthy controls, patients with checking symptom OCD, and those with washing symptom OCD. All three groups showed activation of disgust-related areas, the insular and visual cortical areas, during the normally disgusting picture process. However, washer-relevant pictures induced disgust-related activation only in the washers. This suggested that washers showed different neural responses to washer-relevant stimuli and sensitive emotional responses, unlike the healthy controls and checkers,

who attended more to non-emotive visual details in the washer-relevant stimuli.

While many symptom provocation studies have targeted washing symptoms, other symptom dimensions have also been examined. Mataix-Cols *et al.* (2004) reported distinct neural correlates of washing, checking, and hoarding symptom dimensions in a group of patients with OCD having mixed symptoms. While the subjects were looking at pictures in the fMRI machine, they had to imagine a situation that provoked symptoms, such as with the instructions, "Imagine that you must come into contact with what's shown in the following pictures without washing yourself afterwards" (washing), "Imagine that you are not sure whether you switched off or locked the following objects and it is impossible for you to go back and check" (checking), or "Imagine that the following objects belong to you and that you must throw them away forever" (hoarding). The patients with OCD showed distinct neural activation, according to each symptom provocation, with partially overlapping neural systems. Patients with OCD demonstrated greater activation than healthy controls in the bilateral ventromedial prefrontal (vmPFC) and right caudate nucleus during washing symptom provocation, in motor and attentional function-related areas during checking symptom provocation, and in the left precentral gyrus and right OFC during hoarding symptom provocation. Another study also reported the specific neural basis of hoarding symptoms in a patient displaying hoarding behavior (An *et al.*, 2009). In hoarding-related anxiety provocation, patients with OCD having hoarding symptoms showed increased activation in the bilateral anterior vmPFC, as compared to healthy controls and patients without hoarding symptoms.

fMRI research using cognitive activation paradigms in OCD

Cognitive function in patients with OCD is known to be impaired in several aspects. Deficits in inhibition, cognitive inflexibility, exaggerated error processing, and problems in implicit sequence learning are consistently reported findings regarding cognitive function in OCD. Some of these deficits, such as response inhibition and cognitive inflexibility, have been reported in close relatives of patients with OCD (Bannon *et al.*, 2006; Chamberlain *et al.*, 2006, 2007, 2008), indicating that this cognitive dysfunction could be trait-like in nature, rather than a state-dependent characteristic. Various fMRI paradigms have been used to examine patients with OCD to find neural correlates of cognitive dysfunction or activation to compensate for the deficit.

OCD is characterized by intrusive, unwanted thoughts that cause distress and ritualistic behaviors aimed at reducing these intrusions. Related to these symptoms, deficits in response inhibition and cognitive inflexibility in OCD may constrain patients in rigid conceptual frameworks and disturb them from suppressing their compulsive behaviors. Dysfunction in inhibitory control has long been theorized to be a central feature of OCD (Chamberlain *et al.*, 2005; Rosenberg and Keshavan, 1998; Stein and Ludik, 2000), and various behavioral reports support this postulate (Bannon *et al.*, 2002; Chamberlain *et al.*, 2006; Enright and Beech, 1993; Penades *et al.*, 2007). fMRI studies using a go–no-go paradigm and a stop task, which examine motor inhibitory processes, or the Stroop task, which is related to cognitive inhibition, have been applied in researching inhibition in OCD.

Maltby and colleagues (2005) used a go–no-go task in which participants were instructed to press a button when a go stimulus was presented and to inhibit responding to no-go stimuli as quickly and accurately as possible. The proportion of go to no-go stimuli was 5:1, causing a potent bias toward go stimuli. Under the no-go condition, when the subjects needed strong response inhibition, patients with OCD showed increased activation in the ACC, lateral PFC, lateral OFC, caudate, and thalamus compared to controls. Another study used a go–no-go task (Roth *et al.*, 2007), but the ratio of go to no-go stimuli was 1:1 because of concern for the "oddball" effect of no-go stimuli (Stevens *et al.*, 2000), which has also been reported to be impaired in OCD (Miyata *et al.*, 1998; Morault *et al.*, 1997; Towey *et al.*, 1993). In that study (Roth *et al.*, 2007), while healthy controls showed right hemisphere activation, including the right inferior frontal gyrus, patients with OCD showed more diffuse and bilateral patterns of activation, and less activation in the right inferior and medial frontal areas. The diffuse and bilateral activation in OCD may operate in neural recruitment to compensate for the failure in recruitment of the right inhibitory frontal network during response inhibition. Additionally, symptom scores using Yale–Brown Obsessive Compulsive Scale (Y–BOCS) were negatively correlated with the right OFC and positively correlated with left

thalamus activation during response inhibition, indicating a role of the OFC in suppressing unwanted behaviors and hyperactivation of the thalamus in patients with high OC symptoms (Figure 17.2).

Cognitive inflexibility is frequently reported in patients with OCD (Bannon *et al.*, 2006; Chamberlain *et al.*, 2006; Veale *et al.*, 1996), and among various tasks, reversal learning (Chamberlain *et al.*, 2008; Remijnse *et al.*, 2006) and task-switching paradigms (Gu *et al.*, 2008) have been applied to measure dysfunctional brain activation in OCD. Reversal learning with appropriate behavioral flexibility after negative feedback involves, for example, a previous object that provided a positive answer or reward being changed to a wrong answer, giving negative feedback, so that participants must successfully change their previous favorable choice after the negative feedback. The OFC has long been known to be important in reversal learning (Boulougouris *et al.*, 2007; Dias *et al.*, 1996; Hornak *et al.*, 2004). Using a reversal learning paradigm, Remijnse and colleagues (2006) reported that patients with OCD showed reduced activation in the OFC, dlPFC, anterior PFC, and insula cortex when they successfully adapted their behavior to the negative feedback. Chamberlain and colleagues (2008) also reported reduced activation in the lateral OFC, lateral PFC, and parietal cortices in patients with OCD and their close relatives during reversal learning. These results indicate that dysfunction in the OFC, in addition to the PFC or parietal cortex, is responsible for this deficit in reversal learning and impairs day to day flexibility in patients with OCD.

Gu and colleagues (2008) used a task-switching paradigm to examine cognitive flexibility in OCD, in which subjects had to frequently change the task rules, depending on the presented cue. The task-switching paradigm required the ability to disengage attention from a previous task, resolve interference from previous stimuli or task sets, and update new task sets. Patients with OCD showed increased error rates in switching from a previous task rule, for example, changing the rule from color discrimination to feature discrimination for the stimulus, and decreased brain activation in the dorsal frontal–striatal regions, vmPFC, and right OFC compared to healthy controls. However, the differences in dorsal frontal–striatal regions, including the dlPFC, ACC, and right caudate body, were caused by activation in the healthy controls and inactivation in the patients with OCD, while the ventral frontal areas of OFC and vmPFC differences were due to deactivation in the patients with OCD,

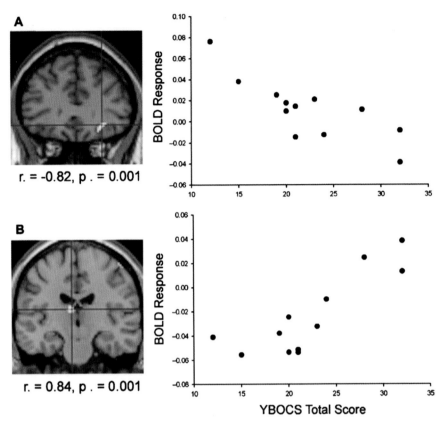

Figure 17.2 Correlations between OCD symptom severity and activation in right orbitofrontal gyrus (A) and left thalamus (B) during response inhibition. Adapted with permission (Roth *et al.*, 2007).

which might suggest an imbalance in the dorsal and ventral frontal regions in these patients (Figure 17.3).

Executive function, such as planning and working memory, has also been examined in patients with OCD using fMRI. Patients with OCD have been reported to perform poorly on spatial working memory tasks, especially as the task becomes more difficult (Purcell *et al.*, 1998a, 1998b). A previous fMRI study also addressed differences in brain activation between patients with OCD and controls, and showed that increased ACC activation was associated with poor performance by patients with OCD (van der Wee *et al.*, 2003). Regarding planning ability, Purcell and colleagues (1998b) reported that patients with OCD were impaired in planning ability, as measured using the Tower of London (ToL) task, and that unaffected relatives of patients with OCD also shared this executive dysfunction (Delorme *et al.*, 2007). Additionally, patients with OCD showed decreased activation in the dlPFC and caudate nucleus during the ToL task, suggesting that the dorsal prefrontal–striatal area is

responsible for the impaired planning capacity in patients with OCD (van den Heuvel *et al.*, 2005).

Another cognitive paradigm applied to OCD is the serial reaction time (SRT) task, which is used to assess implicit information processing and learning. During the SRT task, participants are presented with repeated sequences of visual cues and then the locations of the cues are implicitly predicted and the responses can become faster because of the implicit learning. Striatal dysfunction in OCD has been suggested to underlie the deficit in implicit learning and inability to be aided by implicit learning in improving reaction time (Deckersbach *et al.*, 2002; Rauch, 2003). A PET study showed that patients with OCD exhibited deficient striatal activation and aberrant hippocampal recruitment during implicit sequence learning (Rauch *et al.*, 1997a), and fMRI has shown consistent results (Rauch *et al.*, 2007), with abnormal recruitment of the hippocampus and OFC. Failure in implicit information processing, mediated by striatal areas, is believed to lead to compensatory

251

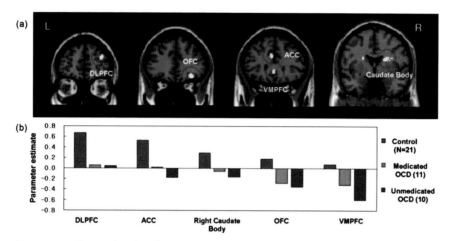

Figure 17.3 The significantly different activation regions during task-switching between patients with OCD and healthy controls. Patients with OCD showed significantly decreased activation in dlPFC, OFC, ACC, vmPFC, and caudate body compared to healthy controls (a). Mean activations for each region of interest shows the inactivation in dorsal frontal–striatal regions and deactivation in ventral frontal regions in the patients with OCD compared to healthy controls (b). dlPFC, dorsolateral prefrontal cortex; OFC, orbitofrontal cortex; ACC, anterior cingulate cortex; vmPFC, ventromedial prefrontal cortex. Adapted with permission (Gu *et al.*, 2008).

involvement of explicit information processing and related brain structures, such as the hippocampus.

Brain activation related to error processing also has been researched in patients with OCD, and excessive error signals generated by the ACC have been suggested to underlie the patients' feeling of being "just not right" and the need for behavioral changes to correct the problem (Pitman, 1987). The ACC is known to be involved in the detection of errors (Gehring *et al.*, 1995; Kiehl *et al.*, 2000; Menon *et al.*, 2001), and both event-related potentials (ERP) and fMRI studies have shown that patients with OCD produce exaggerated error signals in the ACC after errors of commission (Gehring *et al.*, 2000; Johannes *et al.*, 2001; Ursu *et al.*, 2003). However, this hyperactivation in the ACC in patients with OCD has been shown not only during errors of commission, but also during correctly completed, high-conflict trials of a go–no-go task (Maltby *et al.*, 2005) or a continuous performance task (Ursu *et al.*, 2003), suggesting an overactive action-monitoring system in OCD. Additionally, Fitzgerald and colleagues (2005) reported increased error-related activation of the rostral ACC in patients with OCD, and showed a significant correlation between this region and symptom severity in patients.

In summary, various cognitive activation paradigms have been used to examine cognitive deficits in OCD, such as inhibition, cognitive flexibility, implicit learning, executive function, and error processing, and to determine the pathophysiology underlying these

cognitive deficits. Research has also addressed other aspects of cognitive function in OCD, such as the neural correlates of deficits in decision making (Tolin *et al.*, 2009), or different brain activation patterns related to biological motion perception (Jung *et al.*, 2009) related to social functioning (Kim *et al.*, 2005). Recent fMRI research using cognitive activation paradigms has sought to explain the neural correlates of behaviors and cognitive functions of patients with OCD, whether the differential brain activation is primarily caused by the pathophysiology of OCD, especially frontal–striatal dysfunction, or is the result of compensatory activation, rather than the intact recruitment, of corresponding brain areas.

fMRI studies in the family members of patients with OCD

OCD has been suggested to be a heritable neuropsychiatric disorder based on evidence from twin and family studies (Inouye, 1965; Nestadt *et al.*, 2000; Pauls *et al.*, 1995). The level of monozygotic twin concordance has been reported to be between 63 and 87%, and first-degree relatives showed increased rates of OCD (10–22.5%) compared to the normal population risk of 2–3% (Nestadt *et al.*, 2000; Pauls *et al.*, 1995). In an effort to determine objective brain-based measurable traits, or endophenotypes, some fMRI studies have examined brain activation in unaffected close relatives of patients with OCD (Chamberlain *et al.*, 2008), in

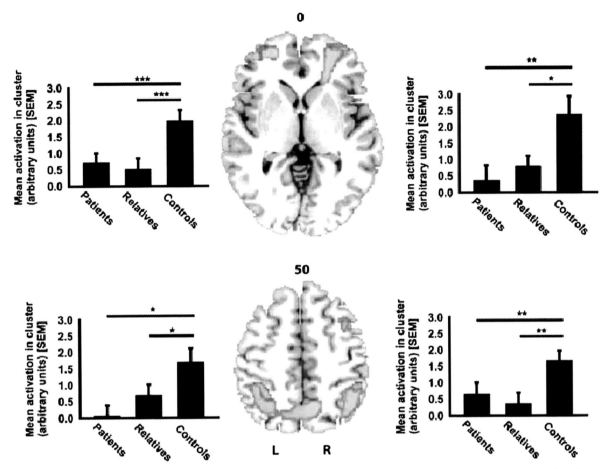

Figure 17.4 Patients with OCD and their unaffected relatives showed underactivation during reversal learning bilaterally in the lateral orbitofrontal cortex (OFC), lateral prefrontal cortex (PFC), and parietal cortices. The images are of representative brain slices showing regions activated during reversal learning across all subjects (yellow area) and regions in which there was a significant effect of group (blue areas). Peripheral graphs indicate mean group activations for each of the four identified clusters where there was a significant effect of group. Top left, left lateral OFC and left lateral PFC, top right, right lateral OFC and right lateral PFC, bottom left, left parietal lobe, bottom right, right parietal lobe. *P<0.05. **P<0.01, ***P<0.001. Adapted with permission (Chamberlain et al., 2008).

addition to behavioral and volumetric markers (Chamberlain et al., 2005; Chamberlain et al., 2007; Menzies et al., 2007).

Using a reversal learning paradigm, Chamberlain and colleagues (2008) reported abnormally reduced activation of the bilateral OFC and inferior parietal lobe in patients with OCD and their unaffected close relatives (Figure 17.4), consistent with other reports of impaired reversal learning and related reduced OFC activation in patients with OCD (Dias et al., 1996; Remijnse et al., 2006). The OFC has an important role in neurobiological models of OCD (Chamberlain et al., 2005; Menzies et al., 2008) and is known to be an important region in behavioral flexibility after negative feedback (Boulougouris et al., 2007;

Dias et al., 1996; Hornak et al., 2004). The result of cognitive inflexibility and related reduced OFC activation in people at increased genetic risk is consistent with the existence of a trait or endophenotype for OCD, even in the absence of chronic treatment or symptom confounds.

In addition to genetic factors, environmental stressors or adverse gene–environment interactions also account for OC symptoms, and the suggested environment risk factors for OCD, for example, streptococcal infection, prenatal problems, psychosocial stress, familial factors, and several life events, such as pregnancy and divorce, may trigger OC symptoms (Alonso et al., 2004; Karno et al., 1988; Miguel et al., 2005). In this regard, discordant OC symptoms have been reported in monozygotic twins, and different brain activation has also been reported (den Braber *et al.*, 2008). The subjects included 17 monozygotic twin pairs, in which one twin with high OC symptoms and the co-twin with low OC symptoms were screened from 419 twin pairs using the Padua Inventory-R (PI-R) as a screening tool for OC behavior (Cath *et al.*, 2008; Sanavio, 1988; van Oppen and Arntz, 1994). During a ToL planning task, twins with OC symptoms showed significantly decreased brain activation in the dlPFC, thalamus pulvina, and inferior parietal cortex compared to the monozygotic twins without OC symptoms. These findings are consistent with previous reports of impaired planning ability in OCD using the ToL task (Purcell *et al.*, 1998a) and decreased dlPFC and caudate nucleus activation related to the ToL task (van den Heuvel *et al.*, 2005). Together, the different brain activation patterns during the planning task in discordant monozygotic twins indicate that neural correlates of OC symptoms may be caused by environmental risk factors or by gene–environment interactions.

fMRI studies related to treatment effects in OCD

The treatment for OCD has long been characterized by a reputation for being highly resistant, but several effective treatments have been recognized recently. According to the effects of pharmacological and/or behavioral treatment, neuroimaging research has addressed changes in brain activation after symptom improvement. Using PET or SPECT studies, reduced glucose metabolism (Baxter *et al.*, 1992; Benkelfat *et al.*, 1990; Swedo *et al.*, 1992) and regional cerebral blood flow in the OFC, caudate nuclei, and thalamus (Kang *et al.*, 2003; Rubin *et al.*, 1995; Saxena *et al.*, 1999, 2002) have been reported after successful treatment. Consistent with this, fMRI has also been used to address the effects of treatment on brain activation during cognitive tasks, such as working memory or the Stroop test, and during symptom provocation (Lazaro *et al.*, 2008; Nabeyama *et al.*, 2008; Nakao *et al.*, 2005b; van der Wee *et al.*, 2007).

Nakao and colleagues (2005b) reported changes in brain activation both during a cognitive task using the Stroop test and during symptom provocation. In that study, symptoms in each patient were provoked through symptom-related word generation, which

had been selected for each patient before the fMRI experiments. After 12 weeks of treatment, pharmacotherapy with fluvoxamine or behavioral therapy, patients with OCD showed mild-to-moderate symptomatic improvement. Related to this improvement, patients with OCD showed decreased activation in the OFC, including the insula, dlPFC, and ACC, following symptom provocation. In contrast, during the Stroop test, patients showed increased activation in broad regions, such as the parietal cortex, cerebellum, dlPFC, and ACC, after treatment. The areas with increased activation are among the prefrontal–subcortical–cerebellar connections believed to play roles in coordinating higher cognitive function (Andreasen *et al.*, 1998; Schmahmann and Pandya, 1997), and among those areas, the ACC has shown decreased activation in patients with OCD in the Stroop test (Nakao *et al.*, 2005a). Accordingly, the increased brain activation related to the Stroop test may reflect changes in cognitive function, such as inhibitory processes, in contrast to decreased brain activation related to the symptom-provocative state in patients with OCD after successful treatment.

Regarding the dissociation between the effects of medication and that of behavioral therapy, Nabeyama and colleagues (2008) examined symptom improvement effects solely induced by behavioral therapy. During the same cognitive task of the Stroop test, patients with OCD showed increased activation in the cerebellum and parietal lobe after treatment, with decreased activation in the OFC, middle frontal gyrus, and temporal regions. While the previous report showed increases in more broad cognitive regions after treatment with applied heterogeneous therapy, including behavioral therapy or pharmacotherapy, behavioral therapy alone primarily increased activation in the posterior brain regions, especially the cerebellum, indicating different effects between behavioral therapy and pharmacotherapy.

Although most neuropsychological studies found no effect of treatment on behavioral performance (Kim *et al.*, 2002; Mataix-Cols *et al.*, 2002; Nielen and Den Boer, 2003), some research has reported limited improvement or even deterioration in neuropsychological performance (Bolton *et al.*, 2000; Sanz *et al.*, 2001). When we consider that treatment using only behavioral therapy improved performance on the Stroop test (Nabeyama *et al.*, 2008), the heterogeneity of treatment, such as intervention with different medications, may have caused the seemingly inconsistent results regarding the treatment effect on performance. Furthermore, the characteristics of the examined cognitive paradigm, the subjects' response to medication, and/or the duration of illness, are other variables that could affect the results of behavioral performance according to treatment.

One study examined changes in brain activation according to the response to pharmacological treatment using fMRI (van der Wee et al., 2007). After 12 weeks of pharmacological treatment, working memory performance and related brain activation were examined in both responders and non-responders. Responders showed significant improvement in performance, as well as overall changes in brain activity related to task difficulty. This result indicates that the working memory deficit and related abnormal brain activation would be, to some extent, state-dependent, as demonstrated by changes in the treatment responders.

Some research on treatment effect has targeted children and adolescents with OCD (Lazaro et al., 2008) because the shorter duration of their disorder would be expected to reduce potential confounding factors, such as prolonged exposure to pharmacological treatment, comorbidity, or chronicity. After 6 months of pharmacological treatment in children and adolescents with OCD, activation in the left insula and putamen during the SRT task decreased significantly compared to the pretreatment state. The SRT task is one of the paradigms measuring ability in implicit serial learning, and implicit serial learning is known to involve the cortico-striatal system (Rauch et al., 1997a, 1997b). The insula and putamen are included in this cortico-striatal system, which is also involved in the pathophysiology of OCD, and the insula is known to play a role in mediating emotional states, including disgust and anxiety.

fMRI research to date regarding treatment effects has generally shown normalized activation compared to the pretreatment state, sometimes with performance improvement. However, the heterogeneity of OCD, with respect to symptom type, duration of illness, and/or comorbidity, may cause inconsistencies in the results, as can the diversity of treatment methods, such as behavioral therapy and pharmacology.

In summary, various approaches of neuroimaging have revealed abnormal brain activations related to symptoms or cognition in patients with OCD. However, there are some discrepancies between findings, which might be caused by the heterogeneous character of OCD, such as the variety of the symptoms and comorbidity, or the diversity of applied cognitive paradigms in neuroimaging research. Future research on symptom-specific neural correlates and related cognitive dysfunctions will bring better understanding to the pathophysiology of OCD. In addition, genetic or family studies will give information regarding traits or state-related characteristics as well as putative vulnerabilities to the disorder. Finally, considering the current model of cortico basal ganglia–thalamo-cortical loop dysfunction of OCD, functional connectivity research that examines the functional relationships between these brain areas will facilitate our understanding of the disorder.

Acknowledgments

This work was supported by the Korea Research Foundation Grant funded by the Korean Government (KRF-2008-313-E00341) and a grant (2009K001270) from the Brain Research Center of the 21st Century Frontier Research Program funded by the Ministry of Science and Technology, Republic of Korea.

Box 17.1. Summary box

The major findings of symptom provocation fMRI research in obsessive–compulsive disorder (OCD) suggest that hyperactivation is found in the ventral frontal–striatal areas of OCD patients, such as in the orbitofrontal cortex (OFC), insula, anterior cingulate cortex (ACC) and caudate head, which generally show normalized activation after symptom improvement. In addition, deficits in cognitive functions, such as those in response inhibition and cognitive flexibility, have been reported in patients with OCD as well as in their genetically close relatives, which implies that these cognitive features are trait-dependent. fMRI research using cognitive paradigms have reported that reduced brain activation in the dorsolateral prefrontal cortex (dlPFC) and parietal lobes are related to cognitive inflexibility and the dysfunction of executive functions. In particular, reduced activation in the lateral OFC, lateral PFC, and parietal cortices during reversal leaning has been reported not only in patients with OCD but also in their genetically close relatives, which sheds some light on the neural correlates of trait-dependent cognitive inflexibility.

255

References

Adler C M, McDonough-Ryan P, Sax K W, Holland S K, Arndt S and Strakowski S M. 2000. fMRI of neuronal activation with symptom provocation in unmedicated patients with obsessive compulsive disorder. *J Psychiatr Res* **34**, 317–24.

Alonso P, Menchon J M, Mataix-Cols D, *et al.* 2004. Perceived parental rearing style in obsessive–compulsive disorder: Relation to symptom dimensions. *Psychiatry Res* **127**, 267–78.

An S K, Mataix-Cols D, Lawrence N S, *et al.* 2009. To discard or not to discard: the neural basis of hoarding symptoms in obsessive–compulsive disorder. *Mol Psychiatry* **14**, 318–31.

Andreasen N C, Paradiso S and O'Leary D S. 1998. "Cognitive dysmetria" as an integrative theory of schizophrenia: A dysfunction in cortical–subcortical–cerebellar circuitry? *Schizophr Bull* **24**, 203–18.

Bannon S, Gonsalvez C J, Croft R J and Boyce P M. 2002. Response inhibition deficits in obsessive–compulsive disorder. *Psychiatry Res* **110**, 165–74.

Bannon S, Gonsalvez C J, Croft R J and Boyce P M. 2006. Executive functions in obsessive–compulsive disorder: State or trait deficits? *Aust N Z J Psychiatry* **40**, 1031–8.

Baxter L R Jr, Schwartz J M, Bergman K S, *et al.* 1992. Caudate glucose metabolic rate changes with both drug and behavior therapy for obsessive–compulsive disorder. *Arch Gen Psychiatry* **49**, 681–9.

Benkelfat C, Nordahl T E, Semple W E, King A C, Murphy D L and Cohen R M. 1990. Local cerebral glucose metabolic rates in obsessive–compulsive disorder. Patients treated with clomipramine. *Arch Gen Psychiatry* **47**, 840–8.

Bolton D, Raven P, Madronal-Luque R and Marks I M. 2000. Neurological and neuropsychological signs in obsessive compulsive disorder: Interaction with behavioural treatment. *Behav Res Ther* **38**, 695–708.

Boulougouris V, Dalley J W and Robbins T W. 2007. Effects of orbitofrontal, infralimbic and prelimbic cortical lesions on serial spatial reversal learning in the rat. *Behav Brain Res* **179**, 219–28.

Breiter H C and Rauch S L. 1996. Functional MRI and the study of OCD: From symptom provocation to cognitive–behavioral probes of cortico-striatal systems and the amygdala. *Neuroimage* **4**, S127–38.

Cannistraro P A, Wright C I, Wedig M M, *et al.* 2004. Amygdala responses to human faces in obsessive-compulsive disorder. *Biol Psychiatry* **56**, 916–20.

Cath D C, van Grootheest D S, Willemsen G, van Oppen P and Boomsma D I. 2008. Environmental factors in obsessive–compulsive behavior: Evidence from discordant and concordant monozygotic twins. *Behav Genet* **38**, 108–20.

Chamberlain S R, Blackwell A D, Fineberg N A, Robbins T W and Sahakian B J. 2005. The neuropsychology of obsessive compulsive disorder: The importance of failures in cognitive and behavioural inhibition as candidate endophenotypic markers. *Neurosci Biobehav Rev* **29**, 399–419.

Chamberlain S R, Fineberg N A, Blackwell A D, Robbins T W and Sahakian B J. 2006. Motor inhibition and cognitive flexibility in obsessive–compulsive disorder and trichotillomania. *Am J Psychiatry* **163**, 1282–4.

Chamberlain S R, Fineberg N A, Menzies L A, *et al.* 2007. Impaired cognitive flexibility and motor inhibition in unaffected first-degree relatives of patients with obsessive–compulsive disorder. *Am J Psychiatry* **164**, 335–8.

Chamberlain S R, Menzies L, Hampshire A, *et al.* 2008. Orbitofrontal dysfunction in patients with obsessive-compulsive disorder and their unaffected relatives. *Science* **321**, 421–2.

Corcoran K M, Woody S R and Tolin D F. 2008. Recognition of facial expressions in obsessive-compulsive disorder. *J Anxiety Disord* **22**, 56–66.

Critchley H D, Wiens S, Rotshtein P, Ohman A and Dolan R J. 2004. Neural systems supporting interoceptive awareness. *Nat Neurosci* **7**, 189–95.

Deckersbach T, Savage C R, Curran T, *et al.* 2002. A study of parallel implicit and explicit information processing in patients with obsessive–compulsive disorder. *Am J Psychiatry* **159**, 1780–2.

Delorme R, Gousse V, Roy I, *et al.* 2007. Shared executive dysfunctions in unaffected relatives of patients with autism and obsessive–compulsive disorder. *Eur Psychiatry* **22**, 32–8.

den Braber A, Ent D, Blokland G A, *et al.* 2008. An fMRI study in monozygotic twins discordant for obsessive-compulsive symptoms. *Biol Psychol* **79**, 91–102.

Dias R, Robbins T W and Roberts A C. 1996. Dissociation in prefrontal cortex of affective and attentional shifts. *Nature* **380**, 69–72.

Enright S J and Beech A R. 1993. Reduced cognitive inhibition in obsessive–compulsive disorder. *Br J Clin Psychol* **32**, 67–74.

Fitzgerald K D, Welsh R C, Gehring W J, *et al.* 2005. Error-related hyperactivity of the anterior cingulate cortex in obsessive–compulsive disorder. *Biol Psychiatry* **57**, 287–94.

Gehring W J, Coles M G, Meyer D E and Donchin E. 1995. A brain potential manifestation of error-related processing. *Electroencephalogr Clin Neurophysiol Suppl* **44**, 261–72.

Gehring W J, Himle J and Nisenson L G. 2000. Action-monitoring dysfunction in obsessive–compulsive disorder. *Psychol Sci* **11**, 1–6.

Gu B M, Park J Y, Kang D H, *et al.* 2008. Neural correlates of cognitive inflexibility during task-switching in obsessive–compulsive disorder. *Brain* **131**, 155–64.

Hornak J, O'Doherty J, Bramham J, *et al.* 2004. Reward-related reversal learning after surgical excisions in orbito-frontal or dorsolateral prefrontal cortex in humans. *J Cogn Neurosci* **16**, 463–78.

Inouye E. 1965. Similar and dissimilar manifestations of obsessive–compulsive neuroses in monozygotic twins. *Am J Psychiatry* **121**, 1171–5.

Johannes S, Wieringa B M, Nager W, *et al.* 2001. Discrepant target detection and action monitoring in obsessive–compulsive disorder. *Psychiatry Res* **108**, 101–10.

Jung W H, Gu B M, Kang D H, *et al.* 2009. BOLD response during visual perception of biological motion in obsessive–compulsive disorder: An fMRI study using the dynamic point-light animation paradigm. *Eur Arch Psychiatry Clin Neurosci* **259**, 46–54.

Kang D H, Kwon J S, Kim J J, *et al.* 2003. Brain glucose metabolic changes associated with neuropsychological improvements after 4 months of treatment in patients with obsessive–compulsive disorder. *Acta Psychiatr Scand* **107**, 291–7.

Karno M, Golding J M, Sorenson S B and Burnam M A. 1988. The epidemiology of obsessive–compulsive disorder in five US communities. *Arch Gen Psychiatry* **45**, 1094–9.

Kiehl K A, Liddle P F and Hopfinger J B. 2000. Error processing and the rostral anterior cingulate: An event-related fMRI study. *Psychophysiology* **37**, 216–23.

Kim J, Doop M L, Blake R and Park S. 2005. Impaired visual recognition of biological motion in schizophrenia. *Schizophr Res* **77**, 299–307.

Kim M S, Park S J, Shin M S and Kwon J S. 2002. Neuropsychological profile in patients with obsessive–compulsive disorder over a period of 4-month treatment. *J Psychiatr Res* **36**, 257–65.

Lawrence N S, An S K, Mataix-Cols D, Ruths F, Speckens A and Phillips M L. 2007. Neural responses to facial expressions of disgust but not fear are modulated by washing symptoms in OCD. *Biol Psychiatry* **61**, 1072–80.

Lazaro L, Caldu X, Junque C, *et al.* 2008. Cerebral activation in children and adolescents with obsessive–compulsive disorder before and after treatment: A functional MRI study. *J Psychiatr Res* **42**, 1051–9.

Maltby N, Tolin D F, Worhunsky P, O'Keefe T M and Kiehl K A. 2005. Dysfunctional action monitoring hyperactivates frontal–striatal circuits in obsessive–compulsive disorder: An event-related fMRI study. *Neuroimage* **24**, 495–503.

Mataix-Cols D, Alonso P, Pifarre J, Menchon J M and Vallejo J. 2002. Neuropsychological performance in medicated vs. unmedicated patients with obsessive–compulsive disorder. *Psychiatry Res* **109**, 255–64.

Mataix-Cols D, Wooderson S, Lawrence N, Brammer M J, Speckens A and Phillips M L. 2004. Distinct neural correlates of washing, checking, and hoarding symptom dimensions in obsessive–compulsive disorder. *Arch Gen Psychiatry* **61**, 564–76.

Menon V, Adleman N E, White C D, Glover G H and Reiss A L. 2001. Error-related brain activation during a Go/NoGo response inhibition task. *Hum Brain Mapp* **12**, 131–43.

Menzies L, Achard S, Chamberlain S R, *et al.* 2007. Neurocognitive endophenotypes of obsessive–compulsive disorder. *Brain* **130**, 3223–36.

Menzies L, Chamberlain S R, Laird A R, Thelen S M, Sahakian B J and Bullmore E T. 2008. Integrating evidence from neuroimaging and neuropsychological studies of obsessive–compulsive disorder: The orbitofronto-striatal model revisited. *Neurosci Biobehav Rev* **32**, 525–49.

Miguel E C, Leckman J F, Rauch S, *et al.* 2005. Obsessive-compulsive disorder phenotypes: Implications for genetic studies. *Mol Psychiatry* **10**, 258–75.

Miyata A, Matsunaga H, Kiriike N, Iwasaki Y, Takei Y and Yamagami S. 1998. Event-related potentials in patients with obsessive–compulsive disorder. *Psychiatry Clin Neurosci* **52**, 513–8.

Morault P M, Bourgeois M, Laville J, Bensch C and Paty J. 1997. Psychophysiological and clinical value of event-related potentials in obsessive–compulsive disorder. *Biol Psychiatry* **42**, 46–56.

Nabeyama M, Nakagawa A, Yoshiura T, *et al.* 2008. Functional MRI study of brain activation alterations in patients with obsessive–compulsive disorder after symptom improvement. *Psychiatry Res* **163**, 236–47.

Nakao T, Nakagawa A, Yoshiura T, *et al.* 2005a. A functional MRI comparison of patients with obsessive–compulsive disorder and normal controls during a Chinese character Stroop task. *Psychiatry Res* **139**, 101–14.

Nakao T, Nakagawa A, Yoshiura T, *et al.* 2005b. Brain activation of patients with obsessive–compulsive disorder during neuropsychological and symptom provocation tasks before and after symptom improvement: A functional magnetic resonance imaging study. *Biol Psychiatry* **57**, 901–10.

Nestadt G, Samuels J, Riddle M, *et al.* 2000. A family study of obsessive–compulsive disorder. *Arch Gen Psychiatry* **57**, 358–63.

Nielen M M and Den Boer J A. 2003. Neuropsychological performance of OCD patients before and after treatment with fluoxetine: Evidence for persistent cognitive deficits. *Psychol Med* **33**, 917–25.

Parker H A, McNally R J, Nakayama K and Wilhelm S. 2004. No disgust recognition deficit in obsessive-compulsive disorder. *J Behav Ther Exp Psychiatry* **35**, 183–92.

Pauls D L, Alsobrook J P 2nd, Goodman W, Rasmussen S and Leckman J F. 1995. A family study of obsessive–compulsive disorder. *Am J Psychiatry* **152**, 76–84.

Penades R, Catalan R, Rubia K, Andres S, Salamero M and Gasto C. 2007. Impaired response inhibition in obsessive compulsive disorder. *Eur Psychiatry* **22**, 404–10.

Phillips M L, Marks I M, Senior C, *et al.* 2000. A differential neural response in obsessive–compulsive disorder patients with washing compared with checking symptoms to disgust. *Psychol Med* **30**, 1037–50.

Phillips M L, Young A W, Scott S K, *et al.* 1998. Neural responses to facial and vocal expressions of fear and disgust. *Proc Biol Sci* **265**, 1809–17.

Phillips M L, Young A W, Senior C, *et al.* 1997. A specific neural substrate for perceiving facial expressions of disgust. *Nature* **389**, 495–8.

Pitman R K. 1987. A cybernetic model of obsessive-compulsive psychopathology. *Compr Psychiatry* **28**, 334–43.

Purcell R, Maruff P, Kyrios M and Pantelis C. 1998a. Cognitive deficits in obsessive–compulsive disorder on tests of frontal–striatal function. *Biol Psychiatry* **43**, 348–57.

Purcell R, Maruff P, Kyrios M and Pantelis C. 1998b. Neuropsychological deficits in obsessive–compulsive disorder: A comparison with unipolar depression, panic disorder, and normal controls. *Arch Gen Psychiatry* **55**, 415–23.

Rauch S L. 2003. Neuroimaging and neurocircuitry models pertaining to the neurosurgical treatment of psychiatric disorders. *Neurosurg Clin N Am* **14**, 213–23, vii–viii.

Rauch S L, Savage C R, Alpert N M, *et al.* 1997a. Probing striatal function in obsessive–compulsive disorder: A PET study of implicit sequence learning. *J Neuropsychiatry Clin Neurosci* **9**, 568–73.

Rauch S L, Wedig M M, Wright C I, *et al.* 2007. Functional magnetic resonance imaging study of regional brain activation during implicit sequence learning in obsessive–compulsive disorder. *Biol Psychiatry* **61**, 330–6.

Rauch S L, Whalen P J, Savage C R, *et al.* 1997b. Striatal recruitment during an implicit sequence learning task as measured by functional magnetic resonance imaging. *Hum Brain Mapp* **5**, 124–32.

Rauch S L, Whalen P J, Shin L M, *et al.* 2000. Exaggerated amygdala response to masked facial stimuli in posttraumatic stress disorder: A functional MRI study. *Biol Psychiatry* **47**, 769–76.

Remijnse P L, Nielen M M, van Balkom A J, *et al.* 2006. Reduced orbitofrontal–striatal activity on a reversal learning task in obsessive–compulsive disorder. *Arch Gen Psychiatry* **63**, 1225–36.

Rosenberg D R and Keshavan M S. 1998. A.E. Bennett Research Award. Toward a neurodevelopmental model of of obsessive–compulsive disorder. *Biol Psychiatry* **43**, 623–40.

Roth R M, Saykin A J, Flashman L A, Pixley H S, West J D and Mamourian A C. 2007. Event-related functional magnetic resonance imaging of response inhibition in obsessive–compulsive disorder. *Biol Psychiatry* **62**, 901–09.

Rubin R T, Ananth J, Villanueva-Meyer J, Trajmar P G and Mena I. 1995. Regional 133xenon cerebral blood flow and cerebral 99mTc-HMPAO uptake in patients with obsessive–compulsive disorder before and during treatment. *Biol Psychiatry* **38**, 429–37.

Sanavio E. 1988. Obsessions and compulsions: The Padua Inventory. *Behav Res Ther* **26**, 169–77.

Sanz M, Molina V, Martin-Loeches M, Calcedo A and Rubia F J. 2001. Auditory P300 event related potential and serotonin reuptake inhibitor treatment in obsessive-compulsive disorder patients. *Psychiatry Res* **101**, 75–81.

Saxena S, Brody A L, Ho M L, *et al.* 2002. Differential cerebral metabolic changes with paroxetine treatment of obsessive–compulsive disorder vs major depression. *Arch Gen Psychiatry* **59**, 250–61.

Saxena S, Brody A L, Maidment K M, *et al.* 1999. Localized orbitofrontal and subcortical metabolic changes and predictors of response to paroxetine treatment in obsessive–compulsive disorder. *Neuropsychopharmacology* **21**, 683–93.

Saxena S, Brody A L, Schwartz J M and Baxter L R. 1998. Neuroimaging and frontal–subcortical circuitry in obsessive–compulsive disorder. *Br J Psychiatry* **35**(Suppl), 26–37.

Saxena S and Rauch S L. 2000. Functional neuroimaging and the neuroanatomy of obsessive–compulsive disorder. *Psychiatr Clin North Am* **23**, 563–86.

Schienle A, Schafer A, Stark R, Walter B and Vaitl D. 2005. Neural responses of OCD patients towards disorder-relevant, generally disgust-inducing and fear-inducing pictures. *Int J Psychophysiol* **57**, 69–77.

Schmahmann J D and Pandya D N. 1997. The cerebrocerebellar system. *Int Rev Neurobiol* **41**, 31–60.

Shapira N A, Liu Y, He A G, *et al.* 2003. Brain activation by disgust-inducing pictures in obsessive–compulsive disorder. *Biol Psychiatry* **54**, 751–6.

Sheline Y I, Barch D M, Donnelly J M, Ollinger J M, Snyder A Z and Mintun M A. 2001. Increased amygdala response to masked emotional faces in depressed subjects resolves with antidepressant treatment: An fMRI study. *Biol Psychiatry* **50**, 651–8.

Sprengelmeyer R, Rausch M, Eysel U T and Przuntek H. 1998. Neural structures associated with recognition of facial expressions of basic emotions. *Proc Biol Sci* **265**, 1927–31.

Sprengelmeyer R, Young A W, Pundt I, *et al.* 1997. Disgust implicated in obsessive–compulsive disorder. *Proc Biol Sci* **264**, 1767–73.

Stein D J and Ludik J. 2000. A neural network of obsessive–compulsive disorder: Modelling cognitive disinhibition and neurotransmitter dysfunction. *Med Hypotheses* **55**, 168–76.

Stevens A A, Skudlarski P, Gatenby J C and Gore J C. 2000. Event-related fMRI of auditory and visual oddball tasks. *Magn Reson Imaging* **18**, 495–502.

Swedo S E, Pietrini P, Leonard H L, *et al.* 1992. Cerebral glucose metabolism in childhood-onset obsessive–compulsive disorder. Revisualization during pharmacotherapy. *Arch Gen Psychiatry* **49**, 690–4.

Tolin D F, Kiehl K A, Worhunsky P, Book G A and Maltby N. 2009. An exploratory study of the neural mechanisms of decision making in compulsive hoarding. *Psychol Med* **39**, 325–36.

Towey J, Bruder G, Tenke C, *et al.* 1993. Event-related potential and clinical correlates of neurodysfunction in obsessive–compulsive disorder. *Psychiatry Res* **49**, 167–81.

Ursu S, Stenger V A, Shear M K, Jones M R and Carter C S. 2003. Overactive action monitoring in obsessive–compulsive disorder: Evidence from functional magnetic resonance imaging. *Psychol Sci* **14**, 347–53.

van den Heuvel O A, Veltman D J, Groenewegen H J, *et al.* 2005. Frontal–striatal dysfunction during planning in obsessive–compulsive disorder. *Arch Gen Psychiatry* **62**, 301–09.

van der Wee N J, Ramsey N F, Jansma J M, *et al.* 2003. Spatial working memory deficits in obsessive compulsive disorder are associated with excessive engagement of the medial frontal cortex. *Neuroimage* **20**, 2271–80.

van der Wee N J, Ramsey N F, van Megen H J, Denys D, Westenberg H G and Kahn R S. 2007. Spatial working memory in obsessive–compulsive disorder improves with clinical response: A functional MRI study. *Eur Neuropsychopharmacol* **17**, 16–23.

van Oppen P and Arntz A. 1994. Cognitive therapy for obsessive–compulsive disorder. *Behav Res Ther* **32**, 79–87.

Veale D M, Sahakian B J, Owen A M and Marks I M. 1996. Specific cognitive deficits in tests sensitive to frontal lobe dysfunction in obsessive–compulsive disorder. *Psychol Med* **26**, 1261–9.

Martijn Figee, Jan Booij and Damiaan Denys

Introduction

Obsessive–compulsive disorder (OCD) is a chronic psychiatric disorder that is characterized by the presence of recurrent and anxiety-provoking thoughts, images or impulses (obsessions), typically followed by repetitive ritualistic behaviors (compulsions) to relieve anxiety. The prevalence of OCD is estimated to be between 1 and 3% (Ruscio et al., 2010; Fullana et al., 2009). Without adequate treatment, obsessions and compulsions can become extremely time-consuming, causing significant impairments in social and occupational functioning. Effective treatment options for OCD are cognitive behavioral therapy, pharmacotherapy or psychosurgical interventions.

Approximately 40–60% of OCD patients respond to pharmacotherapy with drugs that increase intrasynaptic serotonin (Denys 2006; Soomro et al., 2008). Hence, it is often suggested that OCD is related to a dysfunction of brain serotonin systems. Central dopaminergic systems are likely to be involved as well, since patients who do not respond to treatment with serotonin reuptake inhibitors (SRIs) can be successfully augmented with dopamine receptor antagonists (Fineberg et al., 2006; Bloch et al., 2006). Finally, the potential efficacy of glutamate modulating drugs in OCD (Denys, 2006) suggests glutaminergic abnormalities in OCD.

Functional imaging studies indicate involvement of the cortico-striatal–thalamic–cortical circuit in OCD pathophysiology (Saxena and Rauch, 2000; Menzies et al., 2008) and within this circuitry, the neurotransmitters serotonin, dopamine and glutamate are important regulators of neuronal activity. The exact function of these neurotransmitters in OCD is still unclear, however. They may be directly implicated in the pathophysiology of OCD, or only related

to treatment effects. Dysfunctional neurotransmission may be primary, e.g. the result of structural (genetic) defects, or secondary to the illness. Serotonergic, dopaminergic and glutaminergic neurotransmission in OCD has been examined using pharmacological challenge experiments, investigations into metabolites, genetic association studies and animal models. However, these are all indirect measures of neurotransmission, and taken together, they did not reveal consistent results. Neurochemical imaging techniques allow for a more direct examination of neurotransmission systems in OCD patients. Aspects of dopaminergic, serotonergic and glutamatergic systems can be visualized with single photon emission computed tomography (SPECT) and positron emission tomography (PET). In addition, glutaminergic neurotransmission can be measured using ^{1}H magnetic resonance spectroscopy (^{1}H MRS).

SPECT and PET studies may visualize neuroreceptors, but what exactly is being measured with these imaging techniques? SPECT and PET techniques measure binding of radiopharmaceuticals to neurotransmitter transporters or receptors in brain regions of interest, e.g. the serotonin transporter (SERT), the dopamine transporter (DAT), the serotonergic 5-HT$_{2a}$ receptor or the dopaminergic D$_1$ and D$_{2/3}$ receptor. Binding of a specific radiopharmaceutical will occur only if receptors or transporters are available on the surfaces of synaptic membranes. Thus, altered binding reflects altered availability of transporters or receptors. Receptor availability may alter due to up- or downregulation, as a compensatory mechanism in response to neurotransmission. For example, receptors become temporarily unavailable for further stimulation when they are internalized back into the neuronal cell shortly after receptor activation, and

Understanding Neuropsychiatric Disorders, ed. M. E. Shenton and B. I. Turetsky. Published by Cambridge University Press.
© Cambridge University Press 2011.

ת

prolonged activation may decrease the actual number of receptors by lysosomal degradation (Gray and Roth, 2001). SERT and DAT are transporter proteins that are located on membranes of the presynaptic terminals of serotonin- and dopamine-producing neurons, respectively. Because of this localization, decreased availability of SERT may reflect degeneration of serotonergic neurons originating from the raphe nuclei and decreased availability of DAT may have been caused by degeneration of dopaminergic neurons. More specific, degeneration of nigrostriatal or mesocortical neurons is reflected by loss of striatal and cortical DATs, respectively. Finally, availability of receptors and transporters can change in response to short-term alterations in synaptic concentrations of serotonin and dopamine, because of competition with the tracer for binding. For example, lower synaptic serotonin levels means less competition and, thus, more available binding sites for serotonergic radiotracers.

^{1}H MRS is a complementary technique to structural magnetic resonance imaging (MRI), which can graphically visualize a spectrum of magnetic resonances that corresponds to different metabolic compounds in a brain region of choice. It can be used to measure human brain levels of glutamate and its precursor and metabolite glutamine (together: Glx). Glx was found to have a direct relation to glucose metabolism in a combined ^{18}F-fluorodeoxy-glucose PET and ^{1}H MRS study (Pfund et al., 2000), which suggests it is a marker of brain activity.

To explore the role of these neurotransmitters in OCD, we will review all PET and SPECT binding studies on serotonin and dopamine, and all available ^{1}H MRS research into glutamate levels in OCD. We will try to combine these findings into a pathophysiological model for dysfunctional neurotransmission in OCD. Eight studies have investigated serotonergic neurotransmission in OCD, by comparing the availability of SERT or 5-HT$_{2a}$ receptors between patients and healthy controls. In another eight studies, dopaminergic function was examined measuring density of DAT or dopamine D$_1$, D$_{2/3}$ receptors. We will report on combined SERT and DAT studies for each transporter separately. Six studies performed binding scans before and after treatment with SRIs, to study how this affects serotonergic and dopaminergic neurotransmission. Five studies used ^{1}H MRS to estimate brain levels of glutamate in OCD patients and healthy controls, including one study that performed measures

before and after SRI treatment. To the best of our knowledge, no SPECT or PET studies have been performed on imaging of the central glutamatergic system in OCD patients. For a summary of the different studies discussed in this review, see Table 18.1.

Imaging studies on the serotonergic system

Using radiotracers that predominantly bind to SERT in brain areas where this transporter is highly prevalent, e.g. midbrain–pons and thalamic regions, most SERT studies demonstrated decreased SERT availability in OCD, although increased availability was reported in early-onset patients (Pogarell et al., 2003). SERT decreases in thalamic regions were related to OCD severity and duration. Two studies investigated post-synaptic serotonergic 5-HT$_{2a}$ receptors in OCD, showing either increased or decreased availability of the 5-HT$_{2a}$ receptors. Simpson et al. (2003) were the first to study SERT availability in OCD, using PET and ^{11}C-(+)-6β-(4-methylthiophenyl)-1,2,3,5,6α,10β-hexahydropyrrolo[2,1-a]isoquinoline ([^{11}C]McN5652), which is a potent and selective PET tracer for SERT. Comparing 11 OCD patients and 11 age-matched healthy control subjects, they failed to show statistically significant differences in SERT binding within striatal, limbic or cortical areas. This might be partially due to low OCD severity scores in this study (mean Yale–Brown Obsessive Compulsive Scale (Y-BOCS) scores of 20 ± 4 points). Subsequent studies used SPECT imaging to measure uptake of iodine-123-labeled 2β-carbomethoxy-3β-(4-iodophenyl)tropane ([^{123}I]β-CIT). Uptake of this radiotracer reflects predominantly binding to SERT in extrastriatal brain regions. On the other hand, in the striatum, where density of DAT is much higher than that of SERT, it mainly indicates binding to DAT (Laruelle et al., 1993, 1994). The first study using β-CIT found an increase of SERT availability in midbrain–pons, but this was only statistically significant for the early onset patients (<17 years), and it was not correlated with clinical severity measures (Pogarell et al., 2003). The lack of differences in the late-onset OCD group might be explained by older age and more comorbid depression within this group, since these factors are associated with decreased SERT binding (Pirker et al., 2000; Malison et al., 1998). SERT is crucial for maintaining a constant level of intrasynaptic serotonin and, thus, increased SERT may suggest higher levels of intrasynaptic serotonin

Table 18.1 Neurochemical imaging studies in OCD discussed in this chapter

Research group	Imaging method	Patients (controls)	Demographics patient-group	Clinical characteristics	Changes in SERT availability	Correlation with OCD
Simpson et al., 2003	[¹¹C]McN5652 PET	11 (11)	5 female, 6 male mean age 31±12	Heterogeneous Y-BOCS 20±4 Age of onset 17±6 Duration: not reported HAM-D 6±4 drug-free	No differences dorsal caudate, dorsal putamen, ventral striatum, midbrain, thalamus, hippocampus, amygdala and anterior cingulate	No
Pogarell et al., 2003	β-CIT SPECT	9 (10)	4 female, 5 male mean age 34±11	Heterogeneous Y-BOCS 23±8 Age of onset 22±13 Illness duration 12 yrs BDI 16±9 2 drug-free 7 drug-naive	Midbrain–pons ↑	No
van der Wee et al., 2004	β-CIT SPECT	15 (15)	4 female, 11 male mean age 31±9	Heterogeneous Y-BOCS 23±4 10 juvenile onset 5 adult-onset Illness duration 12±7 yrs HAMD 8±4 drug-naive	No differences thalamus, midbrain, pons	No
Stengler-Wenzkle et al., 2004	β-CIT SPECT	10 (7)	6 female, 4 male mean age 29±9	Heterogeneous Y-BOCS 30±3 Age of onset: not reported Illness duration 14 yrs BDI 7 Drug-free	Midbrain/brainstem ↓ Thalamus–hypothalamus ↓ (trend)	No
Hesse et al., 2005	β-CIT SPECT	15 (10)	7 female, 8 male mean age 32±12	Heterogeneous Y-BOCS 25±9 Illness duration 16±9 yrs Age of onset: not reported BDI 7±4 Drug-free	Midbrain/brainstem ↓ Thalamus–hypothalamus ↓	Thalamus–hypothalamus Brainstem (trend)
Hasselbalch et al., 2007	β-CIT SPECT	9 (9)	5 female, 4 male mean age 32 ± 11	Y-BOCS 22 Age of onset 18 Duration 14 yrs HAMD 1 Drug-free	Midbrain–pons ↓	No

Study	Technique	N (N)	Demographics	Clinical	Finding	Region
Zitterl et al., 2007	β-CIT SPECT	24 (24)	11 female, 13 male	OC-checkers Y-BOCS 25±5 Age of onset 22±9 yrs Illness duration 16±11 yrs HAMD 6±3 Drug-free	Thalamus–hypothalamus ↓	Thalamus–hypothalamus
Reimold et al., 2007	[11C]DASB PET	9 (19)	5 male, 4 female mean age 44±9	Y-BOCS 21±8 Illness duration 22±9 Age of onset 22±9 BDI 15±12 2 drug-free 7 drug-naive	Midbrain–thalamus ↓	Thalamus
Adams et al., 2005	[18F]altanserin PET	15 (15)	8 female, 7 male mean age 38	Y-BOCS 30±7 Illness duration16±10 yrs Age of onset 8–48 ys HAMD 6±3 7 drug-free 8 drug-naive	Nucleus caudate ↑	No
Perani et al., 2008	[11C]MDL PET	9 (6)	3 female, 6 male mean age 31±7	Y-BOCS 29±4 Duration 19±9 yrs Age of onset 13±7 Drug-naive	Dorsolateral, frontal polar, and medial frontal cortex, anterior and middle cingulate cortex, parietal and temporal associative cortex ↓	OFC, DLFC, lateral and medial temporal cortex, inferior parietal lobule
Kim et al., 2003	IPT SPECT	15 (9)	4 female, 11 male mean age 29±11	Y-BOCS 30±7 Age of onset 19±10 Duration 9±8 7 MDD 5 tics Drug-free/drug-naive	Striatum ↓	No
Pogarell et al., 2003	β-CIT SPECT	9 (10)	4 female, 5 male mean age 34±11	Y-BOCS 23.0±8.2 Age of onset 22±13 Illness duration 12 yrs BDI 16±9 2 drug-free 7 drug-naive	Striatum ↑ non-significant	No
Van der Wee et al., 2004	β-CIT SPECT	15 (15)	4 female, 11 male mean age 31±9	Y-BOCS 23±4 10 juvenile onset 5 adult-onset Illness duration 12±7 yrs	Left caudate and left putamen ↑ Right caudate and right putamen ↑ non-significant	No

Table 18.1 (cont.)

Research group	Imaging method	Patients (controls)	Demographics patient-group	Clinical characteristics	Changes in SERT availability	Correlation with OCD
				HAMD 8±4 Drug-naive		
Hesse et al., 2005	β-CIT SPECT	15 (10)	7 female, 8 male mean age 32±12	Y-BOCS 25±9 Age of onset: not reported Illness duration 16±9 yrs BDI 7±4 Drug-free	Striatum ↓	No
Denys et al., 2004	IBZM SPECT	10 (10)	7 female, 3 male mean age 36±12	Y-BOCS 26±7 Age of onset 17 Illness duration 16 yrs HAMD 12±5 8 drug-free 2 drug-naive	Left caudatus ↓	No
Schneier et al., 2008	IBZM SPECT	8+8 (7)	OCD: age 33±12 OCD+GSAD: 1 female, 6 male mean age 36±8	OCD: Y-BOCS 23±6 Age of onset 16±8 HAMD 10±6 4 drug-naive 4 drug-free OCD+GSAD: Y-BOCS 21±6 Age of onset 17±14 HAMD 15±4 6 drug-naïve 1 drug-free	OCD: No differences striatum OCD + GSAD: Striatum ↓	No
Perani et al., 2008	[¹¹C]Raclopride PET	9 (9)	3 female, 6 male mean age 31±7	Y-BOCS 29±4 Age of onset 13±7 Illness duration 19±9 No comorbidity Drug-naive	Dorsal caudate and dorsal putamen ↓ Ventral basal ganglia ↓	No
Olver et al., 2008	[¹¹C]-SCH23390 PET	7 (7)	3 female, 4 male mean age 40±14	Y-BOCS 22±8 Illness duration 19±11 HAMD 12±5 5 drug-free 2 drug-naive	Caudate nucleus ↓ and putamen ↓	No

Study	Technique	N	Subjects	Clinical details	Findings	Clinical improvement
Pogarell et al., 2005	β-CIT SPECT	2	Male age 21 and 24	Duration of illness 10 and 8 yrs, Age of onset 11 and 16, Drug-naive, 12 week citalopram 40 mg, Mild response, No Y-BOCS scores	SERT midbrain pons ↓ 38% and 35%, DAT striatum ↑ 34% and 46%	No
Stengler-Wenzke et al., 2006	β-CIT SPECT	5	3 female, 2 male age 29±6	Y-BOCS 32±3, Age of onset 12, Illness duration 16 yrs, Citalopram 60 mg, All responders 57% Y-BOCS↓	SERT midbrain/brainstem ↓, Thalamus ↓	Thalamus
Adams et al., 2005	[18F]altanserin	11	Not reported	Y-BOCS 30, 12–38 wk treatment, Paroxetine (60–80 mg), sertraline (50–150 mg), fluoxetine (60–80 mg), Citalopram (60–80 mg), All responders ↓ 40% Y-BOCS	No sign. 5-HT$_{2A}$ changes in orbito frontal cortex, cerebellum, hippocampus, ventral lateral frontal cortex, insula, lentiform nuclei, anterior cingulate, caudate nuclei, temporal cortex, dorsal lateral prefrontal cortex, thalamus, parietal cortex	No
Moresco et al., 2007	[11C]Raclopride PET	9	2 female, 5 male mean age 29±5	Y-BOCS 30±5, Age of onset n.r., Duration of illness n.r., 12 wk treatment, Fluvoxamine 233±50 mg, 6 responders	D$_{2/3}$ dorsal caudate and putamen ↑ 6.9–9.7%,	No
Kim et al., 2007	IPT SPECT	10	1 female, 9 male mean age 29±11	Illness duration 6±5yrs, Y-BOCS 33±6, 16 wk SRI treatment, 6 fluoxetine 73±5mg, 3 paroxetine 53±6mg, 1 clomipramine 250 mg, All responders 43% Y-BOCS ↓	DAT right BG ↓ 36.7%, left BG ↓ n.s.	Associations with clinical improvement
Zitterl et al., 2008	β-CIT SPECT	24	11 female, 13 male mean age 38±11	OC-checkers, Y-BOCS 25±5, Age of onset 23±10 yrs, Illness duration 16±11 yrs, Drug-free	SERT thalamus–hypothalamus ↓ 47.8%	Negative associations both at baseline and after treatment

Table 18.1 (cont.)

Research group	Imaging method	Patients (controls)	Demographics patient-group	Clinical characteristics	Changes in SERT availability	Correlation with OCD
Rosenberg et al., 2000	¹H MRS 1.5 T	11 (11)	7 female, 4 male mean age 11±3	12 wk treatment Clomipramine 150 mg Y-BOCS ↓ 28% CY-BOCS 30±5 Age of onset 10±2 Illness duration 1±1 yrs HAMD 8±5 12 wks treatment Paroxetine 10–60 mg 9 responders	Left caudate↑ ↓ 23.2% after treatment	Decrease correlated with symptom decrease
Rosenberg et al., 2004	¹H MRS 1.5T	20 (14 C + 14 MDD)	11 female, 9 male mean age 11±3	CY-BOCS 26±5 Illness duration 4±3 HAMD 8±7 Drug-naive	ACC ↓ OCD (15.1%) and MDD (18.7%)	Not analyzed
Whiteside et al., 2006	¹H MRS 1.5 T	15 (15)	6 female, 9 male mean age 41±7	Y-BOCS 24±3 Age of onset 18±8 Illness duration 23±10 HAMD 9±4 Stable on medication	Caudate no sign changes ROF WM ↑	Corr with severity OCD and anxiety and depression (n.s.)
Starck et al., 2008	¹H MRS 1.5 T	8 (12)	3 female, 6 male mean age 33±8	Y-BOCS 23±3 Age of onset 13±4 Illness duration19±8 BDI 16±9 5 SSRI 1 clom + quet + nitraz + alimemazine 2 hypnotics 1 drug-naive	Right caudate no diff ACC no diff occipital cortex ↓	Caudate ↓ Occ ↓ Corr with OCD severity
Yücel et al., 2008	¹H MRS 3 T	20 (26)	10 female, 10 male mean age 34±11	Y-BOCS 20±5 Illness duration 13±11 BDI-II 10±8 12 on medication: 4 fluoxetine 1 fluvoxamine 2 citalopram 1 venlafaxine 4 clomipramine	ACC ↓ females	Corr OCD severity (females)

in the early-onset OCD group. Alternatively, higher SERT might be indicative of an inability to compensate for serotonergic deficits in early-onset patients, which is compatible with research suggesting early-onset OCD is a more severe and SRI-resistant subtype (Rosario-Campos et al., 2001). Three other β-CIT SPECT studies demonstrated decreased SERT availability within midbrain–pons regions. Stengler-Wenzke et al. (2004) found reduced SERT availability in 10 patients compared to 7 controls, Hasselbalch et al. (2007) in 9 patients and 9 controls, and Hesse et al. (2005) comparing 15 patients with 10 controls. In the latter study, SERT reductions were also reported in the thalamus/hypothalamus in correlation with OCD severity and duration, suggesting that SERT alterations in thalamic regions are more strongly related to OCD and occur in the process of illness. Consistent with these results, two studies found reduced SERT in thalamic regions to be strongly correlated with OCD severity. Zitterl et al. (2007) demonstrated reduced SERT in thalamus and hypothalamus, comparing 24 obsessive–compulsive checkers with 24 controls. Decreased thalamic SERT was not only correlated with more severe checking symptoms, but also with shorter illness duration, suggesting that transporter dysfunctions develop early in the course of OCD. Reimold et al. (2007) showed reduced thalamic SERT availability in 9 OCD patients when compared with 19 age-matched controls, using the PET tracer 3-amino-4-(2-dimethylaminomethylphenylsulfanyl)-benzonitrile ([^{11}C]DASB). In contrast, van der Wee et al. (2004) reported no differences in SERT-related β-CIT binding in either midbrain–pons or thalamus between 15 drug-naive OCD patients and 15 controls. This might have been caused by measuring β-CIT uptake after 4 h, since it is uncertain whether this is long enough to visualize SERT optimally (Laruelle et al., 1994; Pirker et al., 2000).

Two groups investigated availability of the 5-HT$_{2a}$ receptor with PET tracers that selectively bind to these receptors. Using [^{18}F]Altanserine PET, Adams et al. (2005) reported increased 5-HT$_{2a}$ receptor availability in both the left and the right caudate nucleus in 15 OCD patients compared to 15 matched controls, which was unrelated to OCD severity. No between-group differences were found in other subcortical or cortical regions. Increased 5-HT$_{2a}$ receptor availability in this study most likely signifies lower concentrations of synaptic serotonin causing more availability of 5-HT$_{2a}$ receptors and upregulation. Since patients in this study were not drug-naive,

upregulation might have occurred secondary to previous SRI treatment. Perani et al. (2008) showed reduced 5-HT$_{2a}$ receptor availability in several cortical brain regions of 9 drug-naive OCD patients compared to 6 matched control subjects, using the radiotracer (R)-(+)-4-(l-hydroxy-1-(2,3-dimethoxyphenyl)methyl)-N-2-(4-fluorophenylethyl)piperidine ([^{11}C]MDL). Reduced 5-HT$_{2a}$ availability in orbitofrontal and dorsolateral frontal cortex was significantly related to OCD severity, but not to disease duration. Decreased 5-HT$_{2a}$ receptor density within these cortical regions could reflect receptor downregulation. Although 5-HT$_{2a}$ receptor upregulation would be expected as a compensation for lower serotonin in OCD, downregulation may indicate further attenuation of serotonergic activity at the post-synaptic level in more severe and untreated OCD patients. Another possible explanation is that OCD is related to a primary dysfunction of cortical 5-HT$_{2a}$ receptors, which might be genetic. Genetic research examining associations between OCD and polymorphisms of the 5-HT$_{2a}$ receptor gene has produced conflicting results (Saiz et al., 2008).

Together, findings from SERT and 5-HT$_{2a}$ imaging studies suggest lower synaptic serotonin in OCD patients, causing presynaptic SERT decreases to compensate for this, and upregulation of post-synaptic striatal 5-HT$_{2a}$ receptors to increase sensitivity for the remaining serotonin. Since specifically decreased thalamic SERT availability was related to illness severity, and to either short or long duration of OCD, this might be an important marker for OCD, but it is still debatable whether the deficit is primary or secondary to the illness. Interestingly, serotonergic deficits were not compensated by SERT decreases in early-onset OCD patients, which might shed some light on the cause of refractoriness to SRIs in this clinical subgroup. In a group of untreated patients, serotonergic neurotransmission was diminished due to a dysfunction of post-synaptic 5-HT$_{2a}$ receptors in cortical brain regions.

Imaging studies on the dopaminergic system

Central dopaminergic neurotransmission in OCD has been imaged with SPECT and PET radiotracers that predominantly bind to striatal DAT, D$_1$ or D$_{2/3}$ receptors. It is not possible to separately visualize D$_2$ and D$_3$ receptors because all available radiotracers bind with equal affinity to both subtypes. Most studies on presynaptic striatal DAT demonstrated increased availability in OCD, whereas one study reported decreased availability. All dopamine D_1 and $D_{2/3}$ binding studies demonstrated decreased striatal availability in OCD. None of these dopaminergic alterations were related to clinical OCD measures. Using SPECT and $[^{123}I]N$-(3-iodopropen-2-yl)-2β-carbomethoxy-3β-(4-chlorophenyl) tropane ($[^{123}I]IPT$), Kim et al. (2003) demonstrated statistically significantly increased DAT availability within the right basal ganglia of 15 OCD patients, compared to 19 age-matched healthy adults. Non-significant increases were shown in the left basal ganglia. Although five OCD patients had a comorbid tic disorder and seven patients had depressive disorder, this did not influence DAT availability. Using β-CIT SPECT, Pogarell et al. (2003) found non-significant increases of striatal DAT availability in 9 predominantly drug-naive OCD patients compared to 10 healthy control subjects that were not properly matched regarding age and gender. Van der Wee et al. (2004) reported increased striatal DAT binding in 15 drug-naive OCD patients, relative to 15 controls. This was statistically significant only for left basal ganglia. Contrasting these previous results, Hesse et al. (2005) found reduced striatal DAT in 15 OCD patients compared to 10 controls. DAT increases in this study may have been overestimated due to age differences between patients and controls.

Using iodine-123-labeled iodobenzamide ($[^{123}I]$ IBZM) SPECT (Figure 18.1), Denys et al. (2004) showed statistically significantly decreased $D_{2/3}$ receptor availability in the left caudate nucleus within a group of 10 OCD patients compared to 10 matched healthy controls. They also demonstrated differences between the left and the right caudate nuclei for $D_{2/3}$ availability and for volume, suggesting laterality in the pathophysiology of OCD. $D_{2/3}$ differences in this study could not be explained by polymorphisms in the dopamine D_2 receptor gene. Schneier et al. (2008) found comparable striatal $D_{2/3}$ decreases in 8 predominantly drug-naive OCD patients compared to 7 control subjects. However, these findings were not statistically significant, possibly owing to the lack of coregistration with MRI for adequate analysis of striatal subregions. The authors did report significantly decreased $D_{2/3}$ availability for a second group of 7 patients with OCD and comorbid generalized social anxiety disorder (GSAD), which is in line with their previous research showing decreased $D_{2/3}$ availability in GSAD patients (Schneier et al., 2000). Using PET imaging and the selective $D_{2/3}$ antagonist $[^{11}C]$

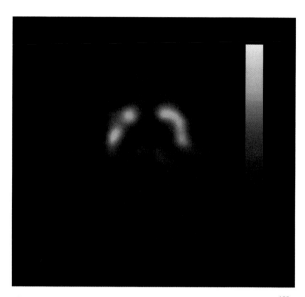

Figure 18.1 Transversal slice at the level of the striatum of an $[^{123}I]$ IBZM SPECT scan (2 h after injection of the radiotracer) performed in a healthy control subject. $[^{123}I]IBZM$ binds in-vivo to dopamine $D_{2/3}$ receptors, especially in the striatum.

raclopride, Perani et al. (2008) demonstrated statistically significantly decreased $D_{2/3}$ binding in dorsal caudate, dorsal putamen and ventral striatum of 9 drug-naive OCD patients compared to 9 controls. $D_{2/3}$ alterations were more prominent in the ventral striatum. Olver et al. (2009) reported reduced availability of dopamine D_1 receptors in caudate nucleus and putamen of 7 OCD patients relative to 7 healthy controls, using PET and the selective D_1 receptor antagonist $[^{11}C]$-SCH23390.

Taken together, findings from DAT, D_1 and $D_{2/3}$ receptor binding studies suggest higher synaptic dopamine levels in the striatum of OCD patients, causing presynaptic DAT elevations for compensatory dopamine reuptake, along with downregulation of post-synaptic D_1 and $D_{2/3}$ receptors to attenuate dopaminergic neurotransmission. Contrary to the serotonergic findings, alterations in dopaminergic neurotransmission were not related to severity, duration or onset of OCD, suggesting that dopaminergic alterations are secondary to the illness.

Serotonergic and dopaminergic changes in response to SRI treatment

At low doses, SRIs already occupy 80% of the SERTs, which will decrease their availability for binding to a SERT tracer. Long-term SRI treatment might cause

SERT downregulation to further increase serotonergic transmission, as has been shown in animals (Benmansour et al., 2002). Accordingly, all studies investigating SRI-induced SERT changes in OCD patients demonstrated decreases of SERT availability (reflecting occupancy of the SERT by the SRI together with a possible downregulation) in midbrain–pons and thalamic regions. Only thalamic SERT occupancy was related to symptom improvement, suggesting this is important for the therapeutic efficacy of SRIs. SERT occupancy was increased following 12 weeks of treatment with citalopram 40 mg in 2 SRIs patients (Pogarell et al., 2005), following one-year treatment with citalopram 60 mg in 5 patients (Stengler-Wenzke et al., 2006), and following 12 weeks of clomipramine 150 mg treatment in 24 obsessive–compulsive checkers (Zitterl et al., 2008). In the latter study, lower baseline SERT was a marker for OCD severity and poor treatment response. The only group investigating 5-HT_{2a} receptor availability after SRI treatment reported no statistically significant alterations following 12–38 weeks of effective treatment with various SRIs in 11 OCD patients (Adams et al., 2005). Measures were performed in the caudate nuclei, where it can be difficult to detect 5-HT_{2a} receptor alterations owing to low 5-HT_{2a} density.

SRIs have been demonstrated to decrease striatal dopamine in animal experiments using $D_{2/3}$ receptor imaging and microdialysis (Dewey et al., 1995). Dopaminergic changes in response to SRI treatment have also been shown in healthy and depressive subjects (Smith et al., 1997; Fowler et al., 1999). Three studies suggest that OCD response to SRI treatment is related to dopaminergic changes. A 12-week treatment period with 40 mg citalopram in 2 drug-naive OCD patients led to a 40% increase in DAT availability in striatum, as measured with β-CIT SPECT (Pogarell et al., 2005). This finding is surprising, since it suggests that OCD treatment with SRIs increases synaptic dopamine levels, although other mechanisms may also be involved (Booij et al., 2007). Treatment response in these two patients was only mild and the exact decreases in Y-BOCS scores were not reported. A SPECT study with [^{123}I]IPT found decreased DAT binding of 37% in the right basal ganglia after a 16-week treatment with SRIs in 10 OCD patients (Kim et al., 2007). Correlation was found between symptom improvement and changes of basal ganglia DAT binding. Moresco et al. (2007) reported a slight but statistically significant increase in striatal [^{11}C]raclopride

binding to $D_{2/3}$ receptors, varying from 6.9 to 9.7%, in 7 drug-naive OCD patients who responded to 12-week treatment with 150–300 mg fluvoxamine. $D_{2/3}$ availability normalized to a level that was previously observed in healthy subjects. No significant correlation was found between clinical measures and baseline $D_{2/3}$ receptor availability, or between Y-BOCS changes and post-treatment receptor availability.

In conclusion, the therapeutic efficacy of SRIs in OCD is related to occupancy of SERT, especially in thalamic regions, but not to changes in 5-HT_{2a} receptors. Moreover, successful SRI treatment in OCD induces decreases of DAT, and elevations of $D_{2/3}$ receptor availability in striatum, indicating normalization of striatal dopaminergic hyperactivity. How serotonin reuptake blocking agents induce dopaminergic changes in OCD treatment is speculative. Dopaminergic and serotonergic neurons are located closely to each other within the striatum. Animal studies suggest that in case of SRI-induced elevation of serotonin, striatal DAT will transport significant amounts of serotonin into dopaminergic terminals (Zhou et al., 2005). Consequently, the competition between dopamine and serotonin for DAT binding will reduce dopaminergic signaling. Additionally, SRIs are able to cause direct dopaminergic alterations independent of changes in synaptic serotonin (Koch et al., 2002). Finally, serotonin has been found to have inhibitory effects on the firing rate of dopaminergic neurons (Dewey et al., 1995; Kapur and Remington, 1996). Of interest, there are some indications that dopaminergic changes are related to higher SRI doses (Koch et al., 2002), and SRI treatment in OCD is only efficacious when using high doses.

Glutaminergic studies

Five studies have used ^{1}H MRS to measure human brain levels of glutamate and its precursor and metabolite glutamine (Glx). The results of these studies suggest elevated caudate Glx levels in OCD, which are normalized in response to SRI treatment. Decreased Glx levels in the anterior cingulate cortex (ACC) were also found; however, this was not illness-specific. Moore et al. (1998) first hypothesized increased caudate Glx in OCD, after having found that paroxetine treatment in a 9-year-old boy with OCD led to a reduction of left caudate Glx. Consistent with this hypothesis, Rosenberg et al. (2000) demonstrated higher Glx levels in the left caudate nucleus of

11 drug-naive OCD children compared to 11 matched healthy children. Glx levels decreased after 12 weeks of treatment with 10–60 mg of paroxetine to levels comparable with those of controls, and these decreases were correlated with improvement of OCD symptoms. In two studies, no caudate Glx abnormalities were found in adult medicated OCD patients. Whiteside et al. (2006) found no differences in caudate Glx between 15 stably SRI-treated patients and 15 controls, while Starck et al. (2008) reported no differences between 8 predominantly medicated patients and 12 controls. These results seem to be in agreement with the pediatric MRS studies, where caudate Glx normalized after SRI treatment. In the Starck study, however, caudate Glx levels were positively correlated with OCD severity. Two studies reported statistically significantly reduced Glx levels in ACC of OCD patients. Rosenberg et al. (2004) showed reduced Glx ACC concentrations in 20 drug-naive children with OCD, compared to 14 matched controls. However, comparable reductions were found in a group of 14 children with major depressive disorder, indicating this finding is not specific to OCD. Yücel et al. (2008) showed reduced ACC Glx in 10 female (mostly medicated) OCD patients compared to healthy females, but no differences for male OCD patients. Again, this suggests that reduced ACC Glx is not specific to OCD.

In summary, OCD may be related to glutaminergic hyperactivity in the caudate nucleus, which can normalize after successful SRI treatment. As a potential marker of brain activity, increased caudate Glx may indicate striatal hyperactivity in OCD. In addition, OCD may be related to reductions of ACC Glx levels; however, this is likely to be less specific for OCD, since it was only found in female OCD patients, and comparable reductions were found in depressed patients.

Conclusion

Results from SPECT and PET binding studies suggest that OCD is related to decreased presynaptic SERT availability in thalamic and midbrain–pons regions, along with increased post-synaptic 5-HT$_{2a}$ receptor availability in cortical areas, indicating diminished serotonergic input into the frontosubcortical circuits. In addition, elevated DAT availability and lower density of dopamine D$_1$ and D$_{2/3}$ receptors in striatum suggest dopaminergic hyperactivity. Whereas only

serotonergic changes are related to OCD course and severity, dopaminergic changes are related to symptom improvement in response to SRI treatment. This suggests that obsessive–compulsive symptoms are primarily caused by a serotonergic deficit, leading to secondary dopaminergic alterations that can be successfully reversed with drugs that increase synaptic serotonin. Serotonergic deficits may cause increased striatal dopamine levels by disinhibiting the dopamine system. Serotonergic projections originating from the brainstem raphe nuclei inhibit the firing of the dopamine cells projecting from the substantia nigra, while in the striatum and cortex they inhibit synaptic release and/or synthesis of dopamine (Kapur and Remington, 1996). Findings from a recent PET study by Wong et al. (2008) suggest dopaminergic hyperactivity in striatum due to serotonin deficits in three patients with Tourette syndrome and comorbid OCD.

^{1}H MRS studies demonstrate striatal glutaminergic hyperactivity in OCD, which is normalized in response to SRI treatment. Both dopamine (through D$_1$ and D$_{2/3}$ receptors) and serotonin (through 5-HT$_{2a}$ receptors) have a modulatory influence on the excitatory activity of glutamate and the inhibitory activity of GABA in the cortico-striatal–thalamic–cortical circuit. Glutamate is an inhibitor of serotonin release and vice versa (Becquet et al., 1990). Decreased serotonergic activity in OCD may therefore lead to increased dopaminergic neurotransmission, through diminished inhibition of GABA interneurons on glutamate projection to the striatum.

How these neurotransmitter changes might be related to the expression of OCD symptoms can only be speculated. Patients with obsessive thoughts are often excessively focused on the potential negative consequences of their own behavior; for example, being constantly worried one might have caused a fire or explosions due to the possibility of not having turned off the gas properly. Compensatory compulsive behaviors, e.g. repetitively checking the gas, may be temporarily rewarding in that they are experienced as reassuring and anxiety-relieving. Several lines of evidence suggest that mesolimbic dopamine neurons are important in detecting potential alerting and rewarding environmental stimuli that can be used for modulation of behavior by reinforcement learning (Schultz, 1998). It can be speculated that dopaminergic hyperactivity in the ventral striatum leads to obsessive awareness of potential alerting events, along with inadequate rewarding of compulsive behaviors. Dopamine-induced reward processing may be enhanced by serotonergic deficits in the raphe nucei as was reported in rats with lesioned midbrain serotonergic neurons (Fletcher *et al.*, 1999). Serotonergic depletion has been demonstrated to cause behaviors that might explain some of the obsessive–compulsive symptoms, such as disinhibition of motor activity, decreased cognitive flexibility and increased focused attention (Olvera-Cortés *et al.*, 2008).

In conclusion, studies that have visualized neurotransmission in OCD clearly indicate abnormalities of serotonin, dopamine and glutamate systems in OCD pathophysiology, but more research is needed to unravel how these abnormalities are related to each other and to the behavioral aspects of OCD.

Box 18.1. Summary Box

- SPECT and PET binding studies on OCD neurotransmission indicate diminished serotonergic input into the frontosubcortical circuits, i.e. decreased availability of serotonin transporter and increased serotonin 5-HT$_{2a}$ receptor availability.
- In addition, elevated availability of dopamine transporter and lower density of dopamine D$_1$ and D$_{2/3}$ receptors in striatum suggest dopaminergic hyperactivity.
- ^{1}H MRS studies demonstrate striatal glutaminergic hyperactivity in OCD.
- Dopaminergic and glutaminergic hyperactivity are normalized in response to SRI treatment of OCD.
- Obsessive–compulsive symptoms might be primarily caused by a serotonergic deficit leading to disinhibition of striatal glutaminergic and dopaminergic activity that can be successfully reversed with drugs that increase synaptic serotonin.

References

Adams K H, Hansen E S, Pinborg L H, *et al.* 2005. Patients with obsessive–compulsive disorder have increased 5-HT2A receptor binding in the caudate nuclei. *Int. J. Neuropsychopharmacol* 8, 391–401.

Becquet D, Faudon M and Hery F. 1990. In vivo evidence for an inhibitory glutamatergic control of serotonin release in the cat caudate nucleus: Involvement of GABA neurons. *Brain Res* 519, 82–8.

Benmansour S, Owens W A, Cecchi M, Morilak D A and Frazer A. 2002. Serotonin clearance in vivo is altered to a greater extent by antidepressant-induced downregulation of the serotonin transporter than by acute blockade of this transporter. *J Neurosci* 22, 6766–72.

Bloch M H, Landeros-Weisenberger A, Kelmendi B, Coric V, Bracken M B and Leckman J F. 2006. A systematic review: Antipsychotic augmentation with treatment refractory obsessive–compulsive disorder. *Mol Psychiatry* 11, 622–32.

Booij J, de Jong J, de Bruin K, Knol R J J, de Win M M and van Eck-Smit B L F. 2007. Quantification of striatal dopamine transporters with [^{123}I] beta-CIT SPECT is influenced by the selective serotonin reuptake inhibitor paroxetine: A double-blind, placebo-controlled, crossover study in healthy controls. *J Nucl Med* 48, 359–66.

Denys D. 2006. Pharmacotherapy of obsessive–compulsive disorder and obsessive–compulsive spectrum disorders. *Psychiatr Clin North Am* 29, 553–84, xi.

Denys D, Klompmakers A A and Westenberg H G. 2004. Synergistic dopamine increase in the rat prefrontal cortex with the combination of quetiapine and fluvoxamine. *Psychopharmacology (Berl)* 176, 195–203.

Dewey S L, Smith G S, Logan J, *et al.* 1995. Serotonergic modulation of striatal dopamine measured with positron emission tomography (PET) and in vivo microdialysis. *J Neurosci* 15, 821–9.

Fineberg N A, Gale T M and Sivakumaran T. 2006. A review of antipsychotics in the treatment of obsessive compulsive disorder. *J Psychopharmacol* 20, 97–103.

Fletcher P J, Korth K M and Chambers J W. 1999. Selective destruction of brain serotonin neurons by 5,7-dihydroxytryptamine increases responding for a conditioned reward. *Psychopharmacology (Berl)* 147, 291–9.

Fowler J S, Wang G J, Volkow N D, *et al.* 1999. PET studies of the effect of the antidepressant drugs nefazodone or paroxetine on [11C]raclopride binding in human brain. *Clin Positron Imaging* 2, 205–09.

Fullana M A, Mataix-Cols D, Caspi A, *et al.* 2009. Obsessions and compulsions in the community: Prevalence, interference, help-seeking, developmental stability, and co-occurring psychiatric conditions. *Am J Psychiatry* 166, 329–36.

Gray J A and Roth B L. 2001. Paradoxical trafficking and regulation of 5-HT(2A) receptors by agonists and antagonists. *Brain Res Bull* 56, 441–51.

Hasselbalch S G, Hansen E S, Jacobsen T B, Pinborg L H, Lønborg J H and Bolwig T G. 2007. Reduced midbrain-pons serotonin transporter binding in patients with obsessive–compulsive disorder. *Acta Psychiatr Scand* 115, 388–94.

Hesse S, Muller U, Lincke T, *et al.* 2005. Serotonin and dopamine transporter imaging in patients with obsessive-compulsive disorder. *Psychiatry Res* 140, 63–72.

Kapur S and Remington G. 1996. Serotonin–dopamine interaction and its relevance to schizophrenia. *Am J Psychiatry* 153, 466–76.

Kim C H, Cheon K A, Koo M S, *et al.* 2007. Dopamine transporter density in the basal ganglia in obsessive–compulsive disorder, measured with [123I]IPT SPECT before and after treatment with serotonin reuptake inhibitors. *Neuropsychobiology* **55**, 156–62.

Kim C H, Koo M S, Cheon K A, Ryu Y H, Lee J D, Lee H S. 2003. Dopamine transporter density of basal ganglia assessed with [123I]IPT SPET in obsessive–compulsive disorder. *Eur J Nucl Med Mol Imaging* **30**, 1637–43.

Koch S, Perry K W, Nelson D L, Conway R G, Threlkeld P G and Bymaster F P. 2002. R-fluoxetine increases extracellular DA, NE, as well as 5-HT in rat prefrontal cortex and hypothalamus: An in vivo microdialysis and receptor binding study. *Neuropsychopharmacology* **27**, 949–59.

Laruelle M, Baldwin R M, Malison R T, *et al.* 1993. SPECT imaging of dopamine and serotonin transporters with [123I]β-CIT: Pharmacological characterization of brain uptake in nonhuman primates. *Synapse* **13**, 295–309.

Laruelle M, Wallace E, Seibyl J P, *et al.* 1994. Graphical, kinetic, and equilibrium analyses of in vivo [123I]β-CIT binding to dopamine transporters in healthy human subjects. *J Cereb Blood Flow Metab* **14**, 982–94.

Malison R T, Price L H, Berman R, *et al.* 1998. Reduced brain serotonin transporter availability in major depression as measured by [123I]-2bcarbomethoxy-3b-(4-iodophenyl)tropane and single photon emission computed tomography. *Biol Psychiatry* **44**, 1090–8.

Menzies L, Chamberlain S R, Laird A R, Thelen S M, Sahakian B J and Bullmore E T. 2008. Integrating evidence from neuroimaging and neuropsychological studies of obsessive compulsive disorder: The orbitofronto-striatal model revisited. *Neurosci Biobehav Rev* **32**, 525–49.

Moore G J, MacMaster F P, Stewart C and Rosenberg D R. 1998. Case study: Caudate glutamatergic changes with paroxetine therapy for paediatric obsessive–compulsive disorder. *J Am Acad Child Adolesc Psychiatry* **37**, 663–7.

Moresco R M, Pietra L, Henin M, *et al.* 2007. Fluvoxamine treatment and D2 receptors: A PET study on OCD drug-naïve patients. *Neuropsychopharmacology* **32**, 197–205.

Olver J S, O'Keefe G, Jones G R, *et al.* 2009. Dopamine D(1) receptor binding in the striatum of patients with obsessive–compulsive disorder. *J Affect Disord* **114**, 321–6.

Olvera-Cortés M E, Anguiano-Rodríguez P, López-Vázquez M A and Alfaro J M. 2008. Serotonin/dopamine interaction in learning. *Prog Brain Res* **172**, 567–602.

Perani D, Garibotto V, Gorini A, *et al.* 2008. In vivo PET study of 5HT(2A) serotonin and D(2) dopamine dysfunction in drug-naïve obsessive–compulsive disorder. *Neuroimage* **42**, 306–14.

Pfund Z, Chugani D C, Juhasz C, *et al.* 2000. Evidence for coupling between glucose metabolism and glutamate cycling using FDG PET and 1H magnetic resonance spectroscopy in patients with epilepsy. *J Cerebr Blood Flow Metab* **20**, 871–8.

Pirker W, Asenbaum S, Hauk M, *et al.* 2000. Imaging serotonin and dopamine transporters with 123I-β-CIT SPECT: Binding kinetics and effects of normal aging. *J Nucl Med* **41**, 36–44.

Pogarell O, Hamann C, Popperl G, *et al.* 2003. Elevated brain serotonin transporter availability in patients with obsessive–compulsive disorder. *Biol Psychiatry* **54**, 1406–13.

Pogarell O, Poepperl G, Mulert C, *et al.* 2005. SERT and DAT availabilities under citalopram treatment in obsessive–compulsive disorder (OCD). *Eur Neuropsychopharmacol* **15**, 521–4.

Reimold M, Smolka M N, Zimmer A, *et al.* 2007. Reduced availability of serotonin transporters in obsessive-compulsive disorder correlates with symptom severity – A [11C]DASB PET study. *J Neural Transm* **114**, 1603–09.

Rosario-Campos M C, Leckman J F, Mercadante M T, *et al.* 2001. Adults with early-onset obsessive–compulsive disorder. *Am J Psychiatry* **158**, 1899–903.

Rosenberg D R, MacMaster F P, Keshavan M S, Fitzgerald K D and Stewart C M. 2000. Decrease in caudate glutamatergic concentrations in paediatric obsessive–compulsive disorder patients taking paroxetine. *J Am Acad Child Adolesc Psychiatry* **39**, 1096–103.

Rosenberg D R, Mirza Y, Russell A, *et al.* 2004. Reduced anterior cingulate glutamatergic concentrations in childhood OCD and major depression versus healthy controls. *J Am Acad Child Adolesc Psychiatry* **43**, 1146–53.

Ruscio A M, Stein D J, Chiu W T and Kessler R C. 2010. The epidemiology of obsessive–compulsive disorder in the National Comorbidity Survey Replication *Mol Psychiatry* **15**, 53–63.

Saiz P A, Garcia-Portilla M P, Arango C, *et al.* 2008. Association study between obsessive–compulsive disorder and serotonergic candidate genes. *Prog Neuropsychopharmacol Biol Psychiatry* **32**, 765–70.

Saxena S and Rauch S L. 2000. Functional neuroimaging and the neuroanatomy of obsessive–compulsive disorder. *Psychiatr Clin North Am* **23**, 563–86.

Schneier F R, Liebowitz M R, Abi-Dargham A, Zea-Ponce Y, Lin S H and Laruelle M. 2000. Low dopamine D(2) receptor binding potential in social phobia. *Am J Psychiatry* **157**, 457–9.

Schneier F R, Martinez D, Abi-Dargham A, *et al.* 2008. Striatal dopamine D(2) receptor availability in OCD with and without comorbid social anxiety disorder: preliminary findings. *Depress Anxiety* **25**, 1–7.

Schultz W. 1998. Predictive reward signal of dopamine neurons. *J Neurophysiol* **80**, 1–27.

Simpson H B, Lombardo I, Slifstein M, *et al.* 2003. Serotonin transporters in obsessive–compulsive disorder: A positron emission tomography study with [11C]McN 5652. *Biol Psychiatry* **54**, 1414–21.

Smith G S, Dewey S L, Brodie J D, *et al.* 1997. Serotonergic modulation of dopamine measured with [11C]raclopride and PET in normal human subjects. *Am J Psychiatry* **154**, 490–6.

Soomro G M, Altman D, Rajagopal S and Oakley-Browne M. 2008. Selective serotonin re-uptake inhibitors (SSRIs) versus placebo for obsessive compulsive disorder (OCD). *Cochrane Database Syst Rev 1*, CD001765.

Starck G, Ljungberg M, Nilsson M, *et al.* 2008. A 1H magnetic resonance spectroscopy study in adults with obsessive compulsive disorder: relationship between metabolite concentrations and symptom severity. *J Neural Transm* **115**, 1051–62.

Stengler-Wenzke K, Müller U, Angermeyer M C, Sabri O and Hesse S. 2004. Reduced serotonin transporter availability in obsessive–compulsive disorder (OCD). *Eur Arch Psychiatry Clin Neurosci* **254**, 252–5.

Stengler-Wenzke K, Müller U, Barthel H, Angermeyer M C, Sabri O and Hesse S. 2006. Serotonin transporter imaging with [123I]beta-CIT SPECT before and after one year of citalopram treatment of obsessive–compulsive disorder. *Neuropsychobiology* **53**, 40–5.

Van der Wee N J, Stevens H, Hardeman J A, *et al.* 2004. Enhanced dopamine transporter density in psychotropic-naïve patients with obsessive–compulsive disorder shown by [123I]{beta}-CIT SPECT. *Am J Psychiatry* **161**, 2201–06.

Whiteside S P, Port J D, Deacon B J and Abramowitz J S. 2006. A magnetic resonance spectroscopy investigation of obsessive–compulsive disorder and anxiety. *Psychiatry Res.* **146**, 137–47.

Wong D F, Brašic J R, Singer H S, *et al.* 2008. Mechanisms of dopaminergic and serotonergic neurotransmission in Tourette Syndrome: Clues from an in vivo neurochemistry study with PET. *Neuropsychopharmacology* **33**, 1239–51.

Yücel M, Wood S J, Wellard R M, *et al.* 2008. Anterior cingulate glutamate–glutamine levels predict symptom severity in women with obsessive–compulsive disorder. *Aust N Z J Psychiatry* **42**, 467–77.

Zhou F M, Liang Y, Salas R, Zhang L, De Biasi M and Dani J A. 2005. Corelease of dopamine and serotonin from striatal dopamine terminals. *Neuron* **46**, 65–74.

Zitterl W, Aigner M, Stompe T, *et al.* 2007. [123I]-beta-CIT SPECT imaging shows reduced thalamus–hypothalamus serotonin transporter availability in 24 drugfree obsessive-compulsive checkers. *Neuropsychopharmacology* **32**, 1661–8.

Zitterl W, Aigner M, Stompe T, *et al.* 2008. Changes in thalamus–hypothalamus serotonin transporter availability during clomipramine administration in patients with obsessive–compulsive disorder. *Neuropsychopharmacology* **33**, 3126–34.

Chapter 19

Structural imaging of other anxiety disorders

José Alexandre de Souza Crippa and Geraldo F. Busatto

Introduction

Compared to the other psychiatric conditions, the diagnostic classification of anxiety disorders was developed relatively late within the history of mental health. This is mainly due to the fact that the various disorders currently referred to as anxious were not even recognized as belonging to the same entity. Until recently, this group of conditions was still thought to be of a purely psychological nature. However, current studies have raised new hypotheses linking biological components to the etiology and to specific symptoms of these disorders.

Besides animal research, earlier post-mortem studies and clinical observations, the research area that has contributed most significantly to bringing new insights into the commonalities and differences among the anxiety disorders and their respective neural circuitries is neuroimaging. Neuroimaging techniques permit the in-vivo evaluation of the human brain, allowing a better understanding of its anatomical, functional and metabolic substrate. Among the various neuroimaging methods used, magnetic resonance (MR) is one of the most frequently employed, mainly because of its high image resolution and the ability to differentiate between different tissues, in addition to being harmless to the patient. MR images can also provide diverse qualitative and quantitative information about the cerebral structure of the patient, allowing the investigation of putative abnormal brain circuits possibly involved in the pathophysiology of psychiatric disorders. Thus, neuroimaging can help elucidate the biological processes that occur in brain regions related to psychological, cognitive and physiological experiences manifested in the different anxiety disorders.

In this chapter, we review the literature which uses MRI for morphometric evaluation of the brain in studies related to anxiety disorders, with an emphasis on panic disorder (PD), generalized anxiety disorder (GAD), social anxiety disorder (SAD), and simple phobias. This review necessarily extends and expands previous reviews that we have written, together with our colleagues, on this same and related topics (Crippa *et al.*, 2004a; Ferrari *et al.*, 2008; Trzesniak *et al.*, 2008).

Structural magnetic resonance (MR) imaging – methods for brain volumetric measurements

One of the most accepted methods used for the investigation of brain morphometry involves the use of regions of interest (ROI). In its most conventional form, an ROI-based approach requires manual delineation of cerebral regions in sequential MRI slices, and the areas obtained in each slice are then summed up to provide a measure of the volume of the brain structure of interest. In order to minimize observer biases, landmarks and rules for manual tracing must be previously defined, and operators must be rigorously trained. This procedure is labor-intensive, thus limiting both the number of brain regions analyzed and the sample size, as well as also requiring investigators to have an a-priori hypothesis regarding specific brain regions (Menzies *et al.*, 2008). Furthermore, ROI-based studies are limited in their treatment of neocortical morphology because of the inherent difficulties in defining structurally complex and variable regions of the human cortex. Thus, the study of neuroanatomy and its relationship to behavior and brain function has received further impetus from the advent of powerful computational tools with which to analyze high-resolution three-dimensional (3D) brain images. The systematic

Understanding Neuropsychiatric Disorders, ed. M. E. Shenton and B. I. Turetsky. Published by Cambridge University Press. © Cambridge University Press 2011.

morphometric evaluation of the brain as a whole has recently become possible with the use of automated techniques such as voxel-by-voxel analysis. Such voxel-wise methods originate from the automated methods developed in the 1990s for the analysis of positron emission tomography (PET) data, most often using a program called Statistical Parametric Mapping (SPM). The application of such methodology to structural MRI, namely voxel-based morphometry (VBM), permits the comparison of the concentration/volume of gray and white matter between groups of interest for each voxel of the cerebral volume after automatic image segmentation, without the need to define ROI regions in advance. Structural MRI scans are spatially normalized to an anatomical template and segmented into gray matter, white matter, and cerebrospinal fluid (CSF) compartments (Ashburner et al., 2000). In optimized versions (OVBM), the VBM methodology allows the creation of study-specific templates that average information from MRI scans acquired with the same equipment and imaging parameters. Processing steps are added to minimize the influence of extracerebral voxels on the routines of spatial normalization and segmentation, and to preserve the volumes of brain structures, which may be considerably deformed during normalization (Good et al., 2001).

In the following sections of this chapter, we present and discuss the findings of MRI studies that have used some of the above morphometric techniques in the investigation of groups of patients with PD, SAD, GAD and phobias.

Neuroanatomic circuits of fear and anxiety

Based on the fear conditioning framework, the anxiety disorders reviewed here are believed to arise from an abnormality in cortical/subcortical interactions, resulting in an inappropriate expression of the fear response (Cammarota et al., 2007). It is well known that the amygdala clearly plays a critical role in the functional neurocircuitry of anxiety disorders. This brain region mediates states of increased arousal as well as the fear response, and its central nucleus serves as the hub both for the integration of information and for the execution of autonomic and behavioral fear. The amygdala is linked to normal fear conditioning and is thought of to be involved in the pathophysiology of different anxiety disorders. Moreover, this brain area is important for other emotional information processing and behavior, such as reward-related processing, encoding of emotionally salient information, risk-taking, processing stimuli of positive valence, and appetitive or aversive olfactory learning (Paulus, 2008). Connections between the amygdala and the sensory thalamus, prefrontal, insular, and somatosensory cortices are also relevant for recognizing threat-related information. For instance, the insular cortex seems to be important for subjective feeling states and interoceptive awareness.

The hippocampus also appears to be important to understanding anxiety disorders and has been suggested to be involved in processing of contextual information. Dysfunction of this brain area has been related to pathological anxiety via overgeneralization, as a consequence of deficient appreciation for the contextual specificity of potentially threatening stimuli.

In addition to the amygdala and hippocampus, a network of other brain structures, including the insula, anterior cingulate gyrus, and medial prefrontal cortex (MPFC), is important for the identification of the emotional significance given to a stimulus, as well as for generating an affective response, and for regulating the affective state. Insula activation is thought to be involved in differential positive versus negative emotion processing, in particular fearful face processing, pain perception, and when individuals are required to make judgments about emotions (Paulus and Stein, 2006; Paulus, 2008). The MPFC cortex and the anterior cingulate gyrus are also important for cognitive and affective aspects of conflict as well as for emotional processing and executive control in response to environmental demands. This neural substrate with executive function seems to modulate the activation of the amygdala and the extended limbic system (Cannistraro et al., 2003).

Panic disorder (PD)

PD is a complex, multi-dimensional psychiatric disorder characterized by the presence of unexpected panic attacks with consequent anticipatory anxiety about experiencing new episodes as well as panic-related phobias (e.g. agoraphobia). The manifestations of PD include a variety of affective, cognitive, behavioral and physiological symptoms. As in the cases of obsessive–compulsive disorder (OCD) and post-traumatic stress disorder (PTSD), PD has been increasingly understood as a disorder with an underlying brain dysfunction. This perspective is supported by the ability to induce panic attacks with pharmacological compounds, by the occurrence of panic symptoms in neurological conditions such as temporal lobe epilepsy, by the response to biological treatment with selective serotonin reuptake inhibitors (SSRIs) and benzodiazepines, and by epidemiological studies showing a higher incidence of PD in first-degree relatives of PD patients (suggestive of genetic vulnerability). The integration of experimental and clinical evidence has provided support for the development of theories concerning the neurobiology of PD.

Deakin and Graeff (1991) proposed that the panic attack corresponds to a spontaneous activation of the fight-or-flight system, while the fear of having new panic attacks (anticipatory anxiety) would inhibit this same system, as observed in the defensive response in the face of distal threat. The increase in the transmission originating from the dorsal raphe nucleus to amygdalar–hippocampal areas would increase anxiety while inhibiting the periaqueductal gray, preventing panic attacks. Conversely, Gorman et al. (2000) established an analogy between PD and conditioned fear. This hypothesis highlights distinct neural substrates involved in aversive conditioning and in the mechanism of fear, and suggests that the central nucleus of the amygdala is the key structure involved in panic attacks, whereas the hippocampus plays an important role in the development of phobic avoidance.

In their anxiety regulation model, Gray and McNaughton (2000) postulate the existence of a "behavioral inhibition system" whose main structure is the septohippocampal system, with inbound and outbound projections – via the parahippocampal cortex – from the Papez circuit, locus coeruleus, raphe nuclei, and prefrontal cortex. The hypothesis is that the hippocampus differentiates between important and meaningless stimuli, thus coordinating different behavioral reactions. Anatomical and functional abnormalities in this system, such as those found in PD, could lead to anomalous defense reactions such as panic attacks and the development of phobic avoidance. Some of these theories suggest that structures located in the temporal lobe are directly or indirectly involved in PD.

Qualitative brain anatomical abnormalities in PD

The qualitative evaluation of MR brain imaging may be a useful technique in the clinical assessment and in research involving PD patients. Pioneer computed

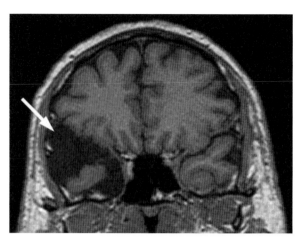

Figure 19.1 Coronal T1-weighted image showing an arachnoid cyst (arrow) in the anterior portion of the temporal pole in a panic disorder patient (56 years old).

tomography (CT) studies provided evidence of brain alterations in PD patients such as regional foci of atrophy, ventricle enlargement, small infarcts (Uhde and Kellner, 1987; Lepola et al., 1990) and enlargement of cortical sulci, predominantly in the prefrontal region and unrelated to the degree of atrophy or the duration of the illness, suggesting that such abnormalities are not progressive (Wurthmann et al., 1997).

Using MR, Ontiveros et al. (1989) found that 43% ($N = 30$) of PD patients who are sensitive to lactate had anatomical abnormalities, mostly in the right temporal lobe, compared to only 10% of healthy controls. The most commonly reported findings were abnormalities in signal intensity and dilation of the temporal horn of the lateral ventricle. The authors also observed that temporal lobe abnormalities were related to severity and duration and early onset of the illness. Thus, these authors suggested that PD may be secondary to temporal lobe dysfunctions and that patients with PD presenting neuroanatomical alterations would have a worse prognosis and require longer pharmacological treatment than those with no such abnormalities. An example of a qualitative brain anatomical abnormality in PD is presented in Figure 19.1.

The above findings were later confirmed in a study involving 31 PD matched to 20 healthy controls. The authors reported a higher frequency of anatomical alterations in patients (40%) – mostly signal abnormalities and asymmetric atrophy in the right temporal lobe – as compared to controls (10%) (Fontaine et al., 1990).

In a sample of 28 patients with electroencephalo-graphic (EEG) alterations, 17 (60.7%) also presented neuroanatomical abnormalities as assessed with MRI, in contrast to 17.9% of patients with normal EEG and only 3.6% of healthy controls. The most commonly found alterations were located in the limbic/septohip-pocampal system. In addition to decreased volume of the right hippocampus, the authors found high rates of cavum septum pellucidum (CSP) in PD patients with EEG abnormalities, which did not occur in patients with a normal EEG (Dantendorfer et al., 1996). The authors argued that CSP may represent a structural abnormality of the septohippocampal system in PD, supporting the hypothesis proposed by Gray and McNaughton (2000). However, definitive conclusions could not be reached, since a high preva-lence of CSP can also be associated with epilepsy (Guru et al., 1998) and schizophrenia (Shenton et al., 2001), among other illnesses. Additionally, the images were analyzed in a qualitative manner and no three-dimensional quantitative method was used. More recently, our group has investigated the preva-lence and size of the CSP in 21 PD patients compared to 21 healthy controls, but no significant differences were detected between groups by manual, ROI-based methods (Crippa et al., 2004b).

Quantitative morphometric MR studies of PD

In the first quantitative MR study of PD, Vythilingam et al. (2000) measured the volume of the temporal lobe, hippocampus and whole brain in 13 PD patients and 14 healthy subjects. The authors found decreased bilateral volume of the temporal lobe in PD patients, although they found no differences in the volume of the hippocampus. Later on, Massana et al. (2003a) evaluated the whole temporal lobe, amygdala and hippocampus of 12 patients with PD compared to 12 healthy controls. This was the first study to deter-mine the volume of the amygdala in PD patients, with the observation of a significant bilateral reduction of this region compared to controls. Later, Uchida et al. (2003), using the same a-priori hypothesis and a manual ROI-based method, detected a reduction of the left temporal lobe in 11 patients with PD com-pared to 11 controls.

The absence of abnormalities of the temporal lobe in the study by Massana et al. (2003a), in contrast to the studies by Uchida et al. (2003) and Vythilingam et al. (2000), may be attributed to a highly conservative

measurement of the ROI employed, which centered only on the medial segment and excluding volumes of the hippocampus and amygdala.

The first study on PD patients using VBM-based methods detected a reduction of gray matter in the left parahippocampal gyrus of PD patients (Massana et al., 2003b). Later, one study (Yoo et al., 2005), using OVBM, demonstrated a bilateral reduction of gray matter in the putamen of 18 patients with PD com-pared to the same number of healthy controls. In this study, the severity of PD symptoms and the duration of the disorder were negatively correlated with the volume of the putamen. Protopopescu et al. (2006), also using OVBM, detected an increased gray mass volume in the brain stem of 10 patients with PD compared to controls, specifically at rostral sites.

More recently, Uchida et al. (2008) assessed gray matter volume in 19 PD patients and 20 healthy vol-unteers using VBM. The authors found a relative increase in gray matter volume in the left insula of PD patients as compared to controls. Increases in the left superior temporal gyrus as well as in the midbrain and pons were also observed in the PD group. Add-itionally, relative gray matter deficits occurred in the right anterior cingulate cortex (Figure 19.2). The authors concluded that insula and anterior cingu-late abnormalities may be relevant to the evaluation process that ascribes negative emotional meaning to potentially distressing cognitive and interoceptive sensory information in PD, and that abnormalities in brainstem structures may be involved in the gener-ation of panic attacks. These results were partially confirmed in a recent study published by Asami and colleagues (2008), in which the anterior cingulate cortex and its subregions were assessed by a combin-ation of ROI and OVBM methods on 26 PD patients and 26 matched healthy controls. Both manual ROI tracing and optimized VBM showed significant volume reduction in the right dorsal anterior cingulate cortex in the PD patients.

The PD and control groups of the above studies were matched for number, age, years of schooling, socioeconomic level and hand dominance. Small samples were investigated in all of these studies, ranging from 10 to 26 patients with PD. However, the studies mainly differed regarding the use of psychotropic medi-cation and presence of comorbidities. The main struc-tural MR studies of PD are presented in Table 19.1.

Diffusion tensor imaging (DTI) is a newly developed MRI technique that allows mapping

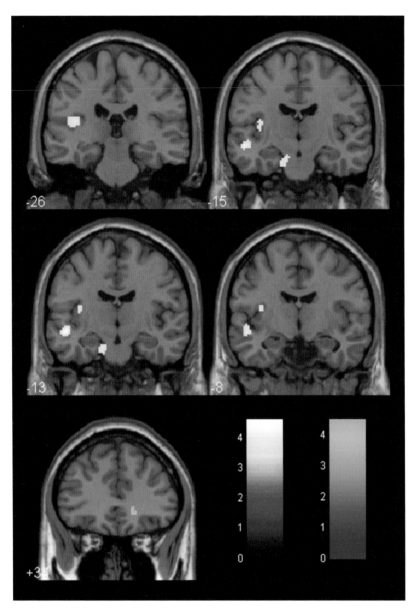

Figure 19.2 Clusters located in brain regions with foci of significantly abnormal gray matter volumes in PD patients (n=19) relative to healthy controls (n=20) are highlighted in yellow (increase) and blue (decrease). Brain regions showing abnormalities in the PD group are labeled with white-printed numbers (1, left insula and claustrum; 2, superior temporal gyrus; 3, midbrain and pons, 4, anterior cingulated gyrus). L, left; R, right. (From the Uchida *et al.*, 2008 study).

anatomical connectivity. It measures the extent of water diffusion in multiple directions and due to the myelination of axons, water diffusion in the direction of neuronal axons is less restricted than in the perpendicular direction. Fractional anisotropy (FA) values obtained from diffusion tensor images represent this level of "anisotropic" water diffusion in white matter regions. Consequently, FA values provide a quantitative indicator of white matter coherence or integrity with lower values signifying

decreased white matter structural connectivity (Basser, 1995). Using this imaging tool, Han *et al.* (2008) evaluated the anterior and posterior cingulate regions of 24 PD patients and the same number of healthy controls. The authors observed that the PD patients presented greater FA values in left anterior and right posterior cingulate regions as compared to the controls. Additionally, the white matter connectivity for these two cingulate regions was also positively correlated with clinical PD severity.

Table 19.1 MR studies in panic disorder

Reference	Subjects (n)	M/F	Age (mean ± SD)	Comorbid agoraphobia	Other comorbidities	Use of medication	Approach	Findings
Vythilingam et al., 2000	13 patients 14 controls	3/1 6/8	38 ± 111 39 ± 9	+	+	Not stated	Manual	- ↓ bilateral temporal lobe
Massana et al., 2003a	12 patients 12 controls	6/6 6/6	26 to 43 years (matched)	+	–	–	Manual	- ↓ bilateral amygdalar volume
Massana et al., 2003b	18 patients 18 controls	11/7 10/8	36.8 ± 11.3	+	–	–	Automated (VBM)	- ↓ GM left parahippocampal gyrus
Uchida et al., 2003	11 patients 11 controls	3/8 5/6	36.86 ± 11.9 34.27 ± 10.2	+	+	+	Manual	- ↓ left temporal lobe - Positive correlation between left hippocampal volume and duration of PD
Crippa et al., 2004	21 patients 21 controls	5/16 5/16	31.1 ± 10.8 38.3 ± 10.0	+	+	+	Manual	- No difference in cavum septum pellucidum
Yoo et al., 2005	18 patients 18 controls	9/9 11/7	33.3 ± 7.1 32.0 ± 5.8	–	–	+ (past)	Automated (OVBM)	- ↓ GM bilateral putamen - Clinical severity was negatively correlated with putamen volume
Protopopescu et al., 2006	10 patients 23 controls	4/6 12/13	35.5 ± 9.7 28.7 ± 7.5	+	+	+ (only one PD)	Automated (OVBM)	- ↑ GM in the midbrain and rostral pons of the brainstem - ↑ ventral hipocampal - ↓ regional prefrontal córtex
Uchida et al., 2008	19 patients 20 controls	3/8 5/6	37.05 ± 9.7 36.45 ± 9.9	+	+	+	Automated (OVBM)	- ↑ left insula - ↑ left superior temporal gyrus - ↑ left parahippocampal gyrus
Asami et al., 2008	26 patients 26 controls	10/16 10/16	19 to 57 years (matched)	+	+	+	Manual *plus* Automated (OVBM)	- ↓ right dorsal ACC (ROI and VBM) - ↓ right rostral ACC (VBM)

↑, increase; ↓, decrease; N, number of participants; F, female; M, male; SD, standard deviation; ACC, anterior cingulate cortex; ROI, region of interest; GM, gray matter; VBM, voxel-based morphometry; OVBM, optimized voxel-based morphometry.

Generalized anxiety disorder (GAD)

GAD is a chronic and recurrent disorder characterized by excessive and uncontrollable worries about a number of events and activities in daily life. Associated symptoms include irritability, restlessness and concentration impairment. Somatic symptoms may include muscle tension, sweating, dry mouth, nausea, and diarrhea. The prevalence of GAD is considered high in the general population and in the primary care setting in particular. GAD symptoms closely resemble those of other anxiety disorders and depression. This has led some investigators to contest it as a distinct diagnostic category.

The neurobiology of GAD seems to involve neurochemical, neuroendocrine, neurophysiological, and genetic factors. For instance, there is evidence of the involvement of the following neurotransmitters and systems in GAD: GABA/benzodiazepine complex, norepinephrine, serotonin (5-HT), cholecystokinin, corticotrophin-releasing factor, hypothalamic–pituitary–adrenal (HPA) axis, and neurosteroids. Furthermore, alterations in the autonomic reactivity have been demonstrated. However, GAD is a relatively new diagnostic category and has gone through major changes in its conceptualization, since the symptoms of this condition closely resemble those of other anxiety disorders and depression. Thus, in spite of the existence of some evidence of a neurobiological foundation for GAD, it is not surprising that there are no consistent neuroanatomical hypotheses specific for this disorder to date. For the same reasons, the number of neuroimaging studies in GAD is also limited, but the literature has increased recently and furthered understanding in regard to the neuroanatomical aspects of this condition.

Neurobiological studies using different investigative techniques (e.g. neurochemistry, physiology, and genetics) in both humans and animals have indicated that, in GAD, there may be abnormalities of some brain regions responsible for emotional processing and social behaviors, such as the amygdala, prefrontal cortex and temporal areas (Jetty *et al.*, 2001). As we previously observed (Ferrari *et al.*, 2008; Crippa *et al.*, 2004b), few studies using structural volumetric MRI have been conducted for this disorder, a fact that prevents definitive conclusions based on brain volumetric data. However, morphometric MRI studies of GAD to date support the hypotheses raised by investigations using other tools, such as functional neuroimaging, which postulate the presence of anatomical abnormalities localized in the amygdala and the temporal lobe, more specifically in the superior temporal gyrus.

The three studies that investigated the volume of brain structures in GAD involved only pediatric samples. De Bellis *et al.* (2000) found greater total and right amygdala volumes in children and adolescents with GAD compared to healthy controls. Later, the same group (De Bellis *et al.*, 2002) reported that children with GAD had a larger volume of the superior temporal gyrus. These studies also investigated other parameters such as intracranial volume, total brain volume, temporal lobe, frontal lobe, thalamus, hippocampus, corpus callosum, and basal ganglia, but no significant differences were found in any of these regions in comparison with healthy controls.

More recently, another morphometric MR study of GAD used the VBM-based approach to compare children with and without anxiety (Milham *et al.*, 2005). The sample of patients with anxiety was heterogeneous, consisting of 9 patients with SAD, 3 with separation anxiety, and 13 with a diagnosis of GAD. Reduction of the volume in the left amygdala was demonstrated in the group of patients with anxiety, although the heterogeneity of anxiety disorders limits the specificity of the findings.

Social anxiety disorder (SAD) and simple phobias

In general, the literature concerning the neural substrates of SAD — also known as social phobia — and specific (or simple) phobias is limited or inconclusive. Similarly, despite some speculation, there are currently no definitive models of the neuroanatomical substrate of phobias. One possibility is that phobias are learned, and thus reflect mostly an example of conditioned fear of a specific stimulus or situation. Conversely, phobias might be the product of dysregulated systems for the detection of threatening stimuli or situations. For example, if humans have a neural network that is specifically designed to assess social signs of threat and another one to evaluate the threat posed by small animals or closed places, these may be the neural substrates underlying the physiopathology of phobias (Rauch and Shin, 2002).

Recent functional neuroimaging studies (Gross-Isseroff *et al.*, 2009; Phan *et al.*, 2009) in patients with SAD suggest that the medial and orbito-prefrontal areas may be involved in the physiopathology of the disorder. However, explicit evidence for this is still lacking. We herein describe a 21-year-old man who developed acute late-onset SAD symptoms after a traumatic brain injury. The patient was involved in a traffic accident at age 17, suffering a contusion on the left frontal lobe with loss of consciousness. He was taken to the local emergency clinic at a municipal hospital, and since no neurological deficits were detected and no particular abnormalities were observed on a brain CT scan, he was discharged. However, a few months after the frontal head trauma, he exhibited excessive shyness and fear of speaking, eating, and writing in front of unfamiliar people, especially women, because of fear of acting in a humiliating way. Exposure to social or performance situations provoked an immediate anxiety response with palpitations, tremors, sweating, and muscle tension, which interfered significantly with the patient's daily routine and social life. After four years of functional disability, he was referred to our social anxiety unit where MR and CT brain scans showed an intradiploic expansive bone formation in the left frontal region, with mass effect and reduction of the frontal horn of the ipsilateral lateral ventricle (Figure 19.3a). Although neuropsychological testing showed no impairments, single-photon emission computed tomography (SPECT) revealed hypoperfusion in blood flow at the medial and orbitofrontal regions (Figure 19.3b). The patient improved after chirurgic resection of the bone lesion and with the use of sertraline at a dosage of 150 mg daily. Although individuals with lesion-induced SAD may be rare, clinicians should be alert to small brain lesions like the one uncovered in this case. However, our interpretation that the expansive lesion located in the frontal brain area, showing the corresponding hypoperfusion on SPECT localized to the orbitofrontal region, is responsible for SAD symptoms, needs to be viewed with caution; other subtle lesions that could not be detected on MRI may exist and the SPECT imaging procedure may be insufficient to detect a small amount of hyper- or hypoperfusion within the orbitofrontal–subcortical circuitry other than the marked hypoperfusion observed in the orbitofrontal area.

No structural neuroimaging studies have been found in the literature involving patients with simple phobia until now, and very few have investigated the volume of brain structures in patients with SAD to date. The first study investigated this issue using

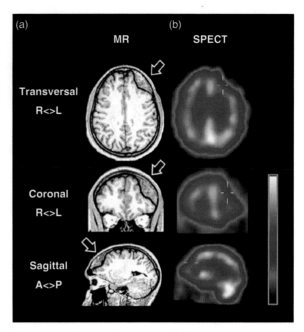

Figure 19.3 (a) Magnetic resonance (MR) scan showing an intradiploic expansive bone formation with mass effect in the left frontal region. (b) Single-photon emission computed tomography (SPECT) revealing hypoperfusion in blood flow in the same region in a patient social anxiety disorder patient (21 years old). (Chaves *et al.*, submitted.)

an ROI-based approach in twenty-two patients and the same number of healthy controls (Potts *et al.*, 1994). The authors did not find differences between groups in volume measures of the total brain, putamen, caudate, or thalamus (Potts *et al.*, 1994). However, they noted that SAD patients had a greater decrease in the volume of the putamen with aging.

The diagnostic frontiers of SAD are still controversial, since it could be described as part of a continuum of severity rather than a disorder based on an arbitrary threshold with qualitative distinctions. Taking this into account, we investigated possible differences among subjects along the social anxiety spectrum using the simulated public speaking test (SPST), an experimental model of human anxiety (Crippa *et al.*, 2008). Afterwards, the anticipatory measures of SPST among groups were correlated with different volume of gray matter regions by MR using the VBM method. We evaluated patients with generalized SAD ($N = 25$), subjects with subclinical SAD (with fear of a social situation without avoidance or impairment; $N = 14$) and healthy controls ($N = 22$). The subjective SPST findings showed that avoidance and functioning impairment were due to a negative

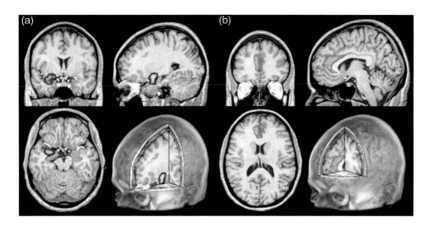

Figure 19.4 (a) Positive correlation between anxiety VAMS scores during public speaking (SPM t map, *p*<0.01, uncorrected) with SVC on right amygdala (highlighted in yellow) in the SAD spectrum (SAD, subclinical SAD and healthy control groups, pooled together) (cluster size = 105; Z = 3.09). (b) Negative correlation between negative self-statement during public speaking (SPM t map, *p*<0.01, uncorrected with SVC) on bilateral anterior cingulate cortex (highlighted in blue) in the SAD group (cluster size = 105; Z = 3.09) (Crippa *et al.*, 2008).

self-evaluation in SPST and not to the level of anxiety experienced. When all groups were pooled together, there was a positive correlation between levels of anxiety experienced and the volume of the right amygdala (Figure 19.4a). The negative self-evaluation of performance in the SPST was associated with a reduction in the volume of the anterior cingulate complex only in the SAD group (Figure 19.4b). These results suggest that the association between anxiety and amygdala volume may be part of a continuum of social anxiety. However, the correlation between self-evaluation of performance with reduced anterior cingulated cortex volume only in the SAD group does not support the idea that this association may be also part of a social anxiety spectrum.

Using DTI, Phan *et al.* (2009) recently observed that SAD patients had significantly lower FA localized to the right uncinate fasciculus white matter, close to the orbitofrontal cortex. The authors suggested that an abnormality in the uncinate fasciculus, the major white matter tract connecting the frontal cortex to the amygdala and other limbic temporal regions, could underlie the aberrant amygdala–prefrontal interactions, resulting in dysfunctional social threat processing in SAD.

Discussion

Given that we have only begun to understand the neural circuitry of anxiety, our current diagnostic system of the anxiety disorders is arguably the most effective tool available for the classification of such conditions. Apart from OCD, the evidence from treatment and neuroimaging studies strongly indicate that the anxiety disorders that are currently classified in separate diagnostic categories may have overlapping pathology, while those that are grouped together within a given category may have very different underlying brain mechanisms. Ongoing efforts in neuroimaging promise to elicit new insights into the commonalities and differences among the anxiety disorders and their respective neural circuitries.

In this chapter, the most consistent finding in quantitative neuroimaging studies of PD was reduced volume of the temporal lobe, although this was not always replicated. The more recent studies implicated other anatomical regions in the pathophysiology of PD, often by means of the VBM technique that allowed the investigation of differences in regional volumes in whole brain. Thus, reductions in anterior cingulate cortex, amygdala and hippocampal region have been described, as well as an increase in gray matter in the insula, superior temporal gyrus and the brainstem structures. In contemporary anatomic models of PD, it is proposed that abnormalities in the insula and anterior cingulate may also be particularly important to the pathophysiology of PD, since these structures participate in the evaluation process of negative emotional meaning to potentially distressing cognitive and interoceptive sensory information. On the other hand, abnormal brain stem structures may be involved in the generation of panic attacks. Brainstem reticular system and mesolimbic dysfunction can account for arousal, anxiety, autonomic, and cardiorespiratory components of PD (Gorman *et al.*, 2000). Recent findings suggestive of a smaller volume of the putamen in patients with PD should also be pointed out, this being an area of the basal ganglia that has also been correlated with the severity of panic symptoms.

Accordingly, due to the nature of the symptoms, subcortical areas such as basal ganglia and limbic system, in addition to the MPFC, have been suggested as being involved in the pathophysiology of PD.

In general, there is some degree of discrepancy between the findings of the various morphometric MRI studies of PD reported to date. Such variability of findings is possibly due to the different techniques of evaluation, the presence of comorbidities among the subjects studied and the small number of participants in the majority of investigations. However, another reason for the discrepant results may also be the multiplicity of brain regions that may be involved in the pathophysiology of PD. In addition, anticipatory anxiety may be related to abnormalities of limbic structures, while phobic avoidance may be related to abnormal activity of the temporal lobe, prefrontal cortical areas, and brainstem (Gorman *et al.*, 2000).

Structural neuroimaging studies of GAD are still in an early phase. The studies reviewed in the present chapter involved highly heterogeneous samples, reflecting the methodological difficulties in conducting studies of this disorder in samples with a precise diagnosis and with no comorbidities. Moreover, these studies were conducted with pediatric samples only, making it difficult to generalize the observed findings to the whole GAD population. However, the detection of a reduction of the amygdala is in agreement with functional imaging studies and with ample theories that relate this region to the mechanisms of recognition and learning in threatening or dangerous situations.

So far, only two structural neuroimaging studies have evaluated the volume of brain structures in patients with SAD. In the first one using a ROI-based approach, the authors found no differences between patients and healthy controls regarding measures of the total brain, putamen, caudate, and thalamus (Potts *et al.*, 1994). In the most recent study in this field conduced by our group (not yet published as a full-length paper), we have also not found differences between SAD patients, subthreshold social phobic subjects and controls, using a VBM-method, although the observed association between anxiety and amygdala volume is suggested as being part of a *continuum* of social anxiety (Crippa *et al.*, 2008). Thus, concurrent with our earlier observations (Ferrari *et al.*, 2008; Crippa *et al.*, 2004b), the present chapter notes the scarce number of morphometric MRI studies on SAD to date. It is surprising that

SAD, one of the most frequent anxiety disorders in the general population, which causes important functional impairments, has not been investigated as often as other anxiety disorders such as OCD and PTSD. In addition, until now no structural neuroimaging paper has been published in samples of subjects with specific phobias. This is especially intriguing considering the relative easiness of recruiting never-medicated SAD and simple phobia patients who are often without significant comorbidities during the initial phases of these conditions. However, DTI methodology has proven to be a useful tool to study these and the other anxiety and psychiatric disorders.

It is important to point out that the inconsistencies in structural imaging findings for the anxiety disorders reviewed in this chapter do not reflect loss of validity of the model of investigation, but may rather reflect confounding factors resulting from the design of the studies. Many studies included subjects with comorbidities such as depression or other anxiety disorders that might have hampered the specificity of the results. Another important point is the inclusion of patients currently or previously taking medications since their use, among other factors, has been shown to affect cerebral morphology of the patients (Ferrari *et al.*, 2008). Differences in age and gender balancing also cause a lack of homogeneity between results across separate studies (Table 19.1).

An additional confounding factor is the presence of patients with different levels and types of symptoms. Regarding PD in particular, previous imaging studies suggested that the different symptomatologic subtypes such as respiratory and non-respiratory (Freire *et al.*, 2009) or lactate responders and non-responders (Maddock *et al.*, 2009) may have distinct neural substrates. In agreement with this, it was suggested that generalized and non-generalized SAD subtypes have distinct neurobiological correlates (Mathew and Ho, 2006). In relation to the subtypes of specific phobia defined by DSM-IV (animal, natural environment, blood/injury, situational), morphological and functional neuroimaging studies among subgroups are still required.

With respect to the methods of MRI analysis, studies with automated analysis methods such as VBM hold the promise of capturing larger numbers of cerebral structures, thus reducing, for example, the difficulty of manual studies in delimiting the anatomical margins of the structure of interest and the problems of the execution and reproducibility of this task. In the selected studies here, analyses by VBM indeed accounted for the observation of changes in other cerebral structures not previously included as a-priori hypotheses in studies that used ROI-based methods. However, the diverse findings obtained in studies using this technique, in addition to sample differences, reveal that VBM still is an evolving method. There are limitations regarding cerebral normalization and smoothing stages that may cause loss of information and degradation of anatomical details across different brain structures (Hulshoff *et al.*, 2001). Thus, it is necessary to determine whether the results obtained with VBM are comparable to those obtained with standard ROI-based morphometry, so that the findings may be better analyzed in the light of these methods, as recently conducted in studies in patients with PD by our group (Uchida *et al.*, 2008) and by Asami *et al.* (2008).

Also with respect to the MRI methodologies, many studies have been carried out using 1.5 T scanners. However, scanners with 3.0 T (or stronger) magnetic fields are increasingly available and may become the standard for research purposes in the next few years. Higher intensity magnets can enhance the signal-to-noise ratio in MRI, improving the distinctions between tissues. The extent to which these differences will impact on research in anxiety disorders should become clearer over the next decade.

It is important to note that the structural neuroimaging findings discussed in the present chapter are not readily reconcilable with previous functional imaging literature on the anxiety disorders evaluated. For instance, in the MR study by Asami *et al.* (2008), in PD patients there was a reduction of the anterior cingulate cortex, whereas previous functional imaging studies demonstrated an increased activity of this region (Javanmard *et al.*, 1999; Bystritsky *et al.*, 2001). Moreover, the decreased activity of the insular cortex in functional imaging studies (e.g. Boshuisen *et al.*, 2002) contrasts with the observed increased volume of this brain region (Uchida *et al.*, 2008). These observations suggest that anatomic findings do not necessarily imply functional changes. In this respect, the structural studies can complement functional ones, especially regarding the delimitation of anatomical changes, the ability to show that increased or reduced tissue volumes are compatible with hyper- and hypometabolism due to compensatory mechanisms.

Finally, it is equally important to make a cautionary note regarding the potential translation of these neuroimaging findings to clinical practice. The majority of neuroimaging studies in psychiatry are research-oriented, and are not designed to have an immediate clinical application. For instance, many neuroimaging findings relate to mean differences in comparisons between groups of patients and controls, and it is difficult to use this information in an individual patient in a clinical setting, especially regarding the anxiety disorders reviewed herein. Nevertheless, neuroimaging studies are increasingly being designed with the aim of translating findings into psychiatric practice, and neuroimaging already plays a major role in the exclusion diagnosis of anxiety disorders due to a general medical condition (see example above; Figure 19.3).

Conclusion

The present chapter indicates that structural neuroimaging methods can be used for a better understanding of the neurobiology of PD, SAD, and other phobic disorders, although they have still been little explored when compared to other anxiety disorders such as OCD and PTSD (Ferrari *et al.*, 2008). Despite a few contradictory findings, mainly due to the variability and limitations of the methodologies used, morphometric abnormalities of some brain structures appear in a more consistent and relatively specific manner in PD. Apparently discrepant results may be due to the different a-priori hypotheses used in studies with ROI, although the findings may indeed reveal distinct brain structures involved in the physiopathology of the same disorder. It will be important for future studies to reproduce prior results and determine which findings are unique to each anxiety disorder. Additionally, it would be important to know whether the brain abnormalities observed in PD and phobias vary progressively during the course of the disorder, as suggested for depression (Frodl *et al.*, 2009) and schizophrenia (Takahashi *et al.*, 2009). Also, it is still not fully understood what the real significance is of the observed qualitative abnormalities in PD. Finally, additional studies will need to establish the extent to which anxiety disorders overlap with comorbid disruptive, mood, anxiety, or psychotic disorders. It is foreseeable that the rapid advancement of neuroimaging techniques, a better sample standardization and greater emphasis on longitudinal studies will permit further clarification of this issue.

Box 19.1. Summary Box

- Structural MRI studies in PD have described reductions of the anterior cingulate cortex, amygdala and hippocampal region, as well as volume increase in the insula, superior temporal gyrus and brain stem structures. These brain regions have been implicated in the neurobiology of fear processes and panic attacks, although their relative contribution to the pathophysiology of PD is still a matter of dispute.
- The observed reduction of the amygdala in GAD is in agreement with the functional imaging studies and with theories linking this region to mechanisms of recognition and learning regarding threatening or dangerous situations. However, structural neuroimaging research in GAD is still in an early phase, and all existing reports have involved pediatric samples only.
- There is a scarce number of morphometric MR studies on SAD and in samples of subjects with specific phobias. However, DTI methodology has proven to be a useful tool to study these and the other anxiety and psychiatric disorders. In addition, the study of SAD as a *continuum* of severity appears to be promising.
- Structural MRI has been increasingly employed with the aim of translating findings into psychiatric practice, and already plays a major role in the exclusion diagnosis of anxiety disorders due to a general medical condition.
- Future investigations about fear mechanisms, PD, GAD, and phobias at the structural, molecular and functional levels should ultimately provide useful insights for a better understanding of the neurobiology of these conditions.

References

Asami T, Hayano F, Nakamura M, *et al.* 2008. Anterior cingulate cortex volume reduction in patients with panic disorder. *Psychiatry Clin Neurosci* **62**, 322–30.

Ashburner J and Friston K J. 2000. Voxel-based morphometry – the methods. *Neuroimage* **11**, 805–21.

Basser P J. 1995. Inferring microstructural features and the physiological state of tissues from diffusion-weighted images. *NMR Biomed* **8**, 333–44.

Boshuisen M L, Ter Horst G J, Paans A M, Reinders A A and den Boer J A. 2002. rCBF differences between panic disorder patients and control subjects during anticipatory anxiety and rest. *Biol Psychiatry* **52**, 126–35.

Bystritsky A, Pontillo D, Powers M, Sabb F W, Craske M G and Bookheimer S Y. 2001. Functional MRI changes during panic anticipation and imagery exposure. *Neuroreport* **21**, 3953–7.

Cammarota M, Bevilaqua L R, Vianna M R, Medina J H and Izquierdo I. 2007. The extinction of conditioned fear: structural and molecular basis and therapeutic use. *Rev Bras Psiquiatr* **29**, 80–5.

Cannistraro P A and Rauch S L. 2003. Neural circuitry of anxiety: Evidence from structural and functional neuroimaging studies. *Psychopharmacol Bull* **37**, 8–25.

Chaves C, Trzesniak C, Derenusson G N, *et al.* Submitted. Late-onset social anxiety disorder after traumatic brain injury.

Crippa J A S, Busatto G and McGuire P K. 2004a. Neuroimagem. In Hetem L A B, Graeff F G (Eds). *Transtornos de Ansiedade*. São Paulo (SP): Atheneu, pp. 133–67.

Crippa J A, Uchida R, Busatto G F, *et al.* 2004b. The size and prevalence of the cavum septum pellucidum are normal in subjects with panic disorder. *Braz J Med Biol Res* **37**, 371–4.

Crippa J A S, Zuardi A W, Busatto Filho, G, *et al.* 2008. Grey matter correlates of cognitive measures of the simulated public speaking test in social anxiety spectrum: a voxel-based study. In 16th European Congress of Psychiatry, 2008, Nice, France. *Eur Psychiatry*, **23**[Abstract].

Dantendorfer K, Prayer D, Kramer J, *et al.* 1996. High frequency of EEG and MRI brain abnormalities in panic disorder. *Psychiatry Res* **68**, 41–53.

De Bellis M D, Casey B J, Dahl R E, *et al.* 2000. A pilot study of amygdala volumes in pediatric generalized anxiety disorder. *Biol Psychiatry* **48**, 51–7.

De Bellis M D, Keshavan M S, Shifflett H, *et al.* 2002. Superior temporal gyrus volumes in pediatric generalized anxiety disorder. *Biol Psychiatry* **51**, 553–62.

Deakin J W F and Graeff F G. 1991. 5-HT and mechanisms of defence. *J Psychopharmacol* **5**, 305–15.

Ferrari M C, Busatto G F, McGuire P K and Crippa J A. 2008. Structural magnetic resonance imaging in anxiety disorders: An update of research findings. *Rev Bras Psiquiatr* **30**, 251–64.

Fontaine R, Breton G, Déry R, Fontaine S and Elie R. 1990. Temporal lobe abnormalities in panic disorder: An MRI study. *Biol Psychiatry* **27**, 304–10.

Freire R C, Lopes F L, Valença A M, *et al.* 2008. Panic disorder respiratory subtype: A comparison between responses to hyperventilation and CO_2 challenge tests. *Psychiatry Res* **157**, 307–10.

Frodl T, Jäger M, Smajstrlova I, *et al.* 2008. Effect of hippocampal and amygdala volumes on clinical outcomes in major depression: A 3-year prospective magnetic resonance imaging study. *J Psychiatry Neurosci* **33**, 423–30.

Good C D, Johnsrude I S, Ashburner J, Henson R N, Friston K J and Frackowiak R S. 2001. A voxel-based morphometric study of ageing in 465 normal adult human brains. *Neuroimage* **14**, 21–36.

Gorman J M, Kent J M, Sullivan G M and Coplan J D. 2000. Neuroanatomical hypothesis of panic disorder, revised. *Am J Psychiatry* **157**, 493–505.

Gray J A and McNaughton N. 2000. *The Neuropsychology of Anxiety. An Enquiry into the Functions of the Septo-Hippocampal System.* 2nd ed. Oxford: Oxford University Press.

Gross-Isseroff R, Kushnir T, Hermesh H, Marom S, Weizman A and Manor D. 2009. Alteration learning in social anxiety disorder: An fMRI study. *World J Biol Psychiatry* **19**, 1–5.

Guru Raj A K, Pratap R C, Jayakumar R and Ariffin W A. 1998. Clinical features and associated radiological abnormalities in 54 patients with cavum septi pellucidi. *Med J Malaysia* **53**, 251–6.

Han D H, Renshaw P F, Dager S R, *et al.* 2008. Altered cingulate white matter connectivity in panic disorder patients. *J Psychiatr Res* **42**, 399–407.

Hulshoff Pol H E, Schnack H G, Mandl R C, *et al.* 2001. Focal gray matter density changes in schizophrenia. *Arch Gen Psychiatry* **58**, 1118–25.

Javanmard M, Shlik J, Kennedy S H, Vaccarino F J, Houle S and Bradwejn J. 1999. Neuroanatomic correlates of CCK-4-induced panic attacks in healthy humans: A comparison of two time points. *Biol Psychiatry* **45**, 872–82.

Jetty P V, Charney D S and Goddard A W. 2001. Neurobiology of generalized anxiety disorder. *Psychiatr Clin North Am* **24**, 75–97.

Lepola U, Nousiainen U, Puranen M, Riekkinen P and Rimón R. 1990. EEG and CT findings in patients with panic disorder. *Biol Psychiatry* **28**, 721–7.

Maddock R J, Buonocore M H, Copeland L E and Richards A L. 2009. Elevated brain lactate responses to neural activation in panic disorder: A dynamic 1H-MRS study. *Mol Psychiatry* **14**, 537–45.

Massana G, Serra-Grabulosa J M, Salgado-Pineda P, *et al.* 2003a. Amygdalar atrophy in panic disorder patients detected by volumetric magnetic resonance imaging. *Neuroimage* **19**, 80–90.

Massana G, Serra-Grabulosa J M, Salgado-Pineda P, *et al.* 2003b. Parahippocampal gray matter density in panic

disorder: A voxel-based morphometric study. *Am J Psychiatry* **160**, 566–8.

Mathew S J and Ho S. 2006. Etiology and neurobiology of social anxiety disorder. *J Clin Psychiatry* **67** (Suppl 12), 9–13.

Menzies L, Chamberlain S R, Laird S M, Thelen S M, Sahakian B J and Bullmore E T. 2008. Integrating evidence from neuroimaging and neuropsychological studies of obsessive–compulsive disorder. *Neurosci Biobehav Rev* **32**, 525–49.

Milham M P, Nugent A C, Drevets W C, *et al.* 2005. Selective reduction in amygdala volume in pediatric anxiety disorders: A voxel-based morphometry investigation. *Biol Psychiatry* **57**, 961–6.

Ontiveros A, Fontaine R, Breton G, Elie R, Fontaine S and Dery R. 1989. Correlation of severity of panic disorder and neuroanatomical changes on magnetic resonance imaging. *J Neuropsychiatry Clin Neurosci* **1**, 404–08.

Paulus M P. 2008. The role of neuroimaging for the diagnosis and treatment of anxiety disorders. *Depress Anxiety* **25**, 348–56.

Paulus M P and Stein M B. 2006. An insular view of anxiety. *Biol Psychiatry* **60**, 383–7.

Phan K L, Orlichenko A, Boyd E, *et al.* 2009. Preliminary evidence of white matter abnormality in the uncinate fasciculus in generalized social anxiety disorder. *Biol Psychiatry* **66**, 691–4.

Potts N L, Davidson J R, Krishnan K R and Doraiswamy P M. 1994. Magnetic resonance imaging in social phobia. *Psychiatry Res* **52**, 35–42.

Protopopescu X, Pan H, Tuescher O, *et al.* 2006. Increased brainstem volume in panic disorder: A voxel-based morphometric study. *Neuroreport* **17**, 361–3.

Rauch S L and Shin L M. 2002. Structural and functional imaging of anxiety and stress disorders. In Davis K L, Dennis Charney D and Coyle J T (Eds). *Neuropsychopharmacology. The Fifth Generation of Progress.* Baltimore, MD: Lippincott Williams and Wilkins, pp. 953–66.

Shenton M E, Dickey C C, Frumin M and McCarley R W. 2001. A review of MRI findings in schizophrenia. *Schizophr Res* **49**, 1–52.

Takahashi T, Wood S J, Yung A R, *et al.* 2009. Progressive gray matter reduction of the superior temporal gyrus during transition to psychosis. *Arch Gen Psychiatry* **66**, 366–76.

Trzesniak C, Araújo D, Crippa J A S. 2008. Magnetic resonance spectroscopy in anxiety disorders. *Acta Neuropsychiatr* **20**, 56–71.

Uchida R R, Del-Ben C M, Busatto G F, *et al.* 2008b. Regional gray matter abnormalities in panic disorder:

A voxel-based morphometry study. *Psychiatry Res* **163**, 21–9.

Uchida R R, Del-Ben C M, Santos A C, *et al.* 2003. Decreased volume of left temporal lobe in panic patients measured through magnetic resonance imaging. *Braz J Med Biol Res* **36**, 925–9.

Uhde T W and Kellner C H. 1987. Cerebral ventricular size in panic disorder. *J Affect Disord* **12**, 175–8.

Vythilingam M, Anderson E R, Goddard A, *et al.* 2000. Temporal lobe volume in panic disorder – a quantitative magnetic resonance imaging study. *Psychiatry Res* **99**, 75–82.

Wurthmann C, Bogerts B, Gregor J, Baumann B, Effenberger O and Döhring W. 1997. Frontal CSF enlargement in panic disorder: A qualitative CT-scan study. *Psychiatry Res* **76**, 83–7.

Yoo H K, Kim M J, Kim S J, *et al.* 2005. Putaminal gray matter volume decrease in panic disorder: An optimized voxel-based morphometry study. *Eur J Neurosci* **22**, 2089–94.

Oliver Tüscher, Daniel J. Zimmerman and David A. Silbersweig

Panic disorder is a common and incapacitating mental disorder (primary as well as comorbid: PD lifetime prevalence 1.6–4.7% and 12-month prevalence in other mental disorders ~69%; Alonso and Lepine, 2007; Kessler *et al.*, 2005). It is characterized by the recurrent, unexpected attacks of multiple somatic (e.g. palpitations, sweating, paresthesias, feeling of shortness of breath or choking) and cognitive fear symptoms (e.g. derealization or depersonalization, fear of losing control or dying), which can occur with or without agoraphobia (fear of experiencing panic in situations from which escape might be difficult). The condition is diagnosed if such panic attacks are followed by persistent concerns about having additional attacks, worry about the implications of the attack or its consequences, and a significant change in the behavior related to the attacks (American Psychiatric Association, 2000).

Brain imaging in panic disorders

Structural and functional neuroimaging studies have contributed enormously to the understanding of the neural substrates of PD. To date, some 200 human neuroimaging studies have been performed using a wide variety of imaging techniques ranging from computed tomography (CT) and structural magnetic resonance imaging (MRI), to positron emission tomography (PET) and single photon emission computed tomography (SPECT), resting state cerebral blood flow (CBF) and receptor binding studies, to functional PET, SPECT and MRI studies using "panicogen" drug challenge (e.g. lactate, CO_2, yohimbine) or cognitive activation paradigms (for reviews see Damsa *et al.*, 2009; Engel *et al.*, 2009; Graeff and Del-Ben, 2008; Rauch *et al.*, 2003). In short, those studies implicated structural as well as functional

alterations in hippocampal and parahippocampal areas (one of the most consistent findings), prefrontal cortex, anterior cingulate gyrus, superior temporal cortex, insula, amygdala, hypothalamus, thalamus and brainstem (mostly interpreted as the periaqueductal gray matter, PAG) of panic patients.

Functional magnetic resonance imaging in panic disorders

There are, however, comparably few functional MRI (fMRI) studies in PD compared to other imaging methods or to other anxiety disorders. Aside from one case report of a spontaneous panic attack in a patient with panic disorder, most fMRI studies have used a panic disorder-related cognitive induction/provocation paradigm.

Along these lines, one of the first fMRI studies on PD used aurally presented (script-driven) imagery exposure that were to specific fearful stimuli of each patient's own fear hierarchy (Bystritsky *et al.*, 2001). Panic patients ($n = 6$, unmedicated for 2 weeks) had increased activity in right inferior frontal cortex, hippocampus and, both, the anterior and posterior cingulate during imagery compared to healthy control subjects. The authors suggested that this pattern of (hyper-)activity indicates an overly active emotional memory system which facilitates encoding and retrieval of fearful or traumatic events leading to recurrent panic attacks (Bystritsky *et al.*, 2001).

Two further studies used threat or panic-related linguistic stimuli to evoke panic disorder-related neural activity. Maddock and colleagues used aurally presented threatening (threat to survival) and neutral words where they asked subjects to silently rate their valence (Maddock *et al.*, 2003). This explicit emotional processing resulted in relative hyperactivity of the left posterior cingulate and left middle/inferior frontal cortex and a more asymmetric activation of the right more than left parahippocampal region in panic patients ($n = 6$, unmedicated for 2 weeks).

In contrast, van den Heuvel and colleagues applied an implicit emotion processing paradigm based on a Stroop color–word paradigm for PD patients, in comparison to obsessive–compulsive disorder (OCD) patients, patients with hypochondriasis, and healthy controls (van den Heuvel et al., 2005). Aside from congruent and incongruent color words, panic- and OCD-related were used. Panic patients ($n = 15$, unmedicated for 4 weeks), compared with control subjects, showed bilaterally increased activation in the anterior prefrontal cortex (PFC), the dorsal cingulate, and inferior parietal cortex and right-sided in the dorso- and ventrolateral PFC, orbitofrontal cortex, thalamus, middle temporal cortex, amygdala, and hippocampus. Similar regions were identified when comparing PD with OCD; however, patients with hypochondriasis compared to healthy controls showed a pattern similar to PD patients but lacking amygdala and ACC hyperactivity. Interestingly, PD patients over-activated a similar fronto-temporo-striatal network in response to OCD-related words as they did to panic-related words, but without the additional amygdala and hypothalamic increase that OCD patients showed to OCD-related words (whereas OCD patients did not show increased activation to panic-related words). In sum, the results intriguingly imply amygdalar and cingulate hyperactivity to panic disorder-specific stimuli (neither OCD nor hypochondriasis patients showed that activity), as well as a tendency for over-generalization to negative/threat-related stimuli in PD (to a lesser extent, this was also true in hypochondriasis).

Of note, although all studies discussed so far used linguistic threat (i.e. preferably left brain-processed) stimuli, all studies showed a relative rightward lateralization of fear/panic-related neural networks. This finding is in line with results of prior PET and SPECT studies, although their results have been questioned as being possible clinching artifacts (for review see Engel et al., 2009; Rauch et al., 2003).

Further corroboration of the importance of (right) amygdalar hyperactivity in PD and panic attacks is presented in a single case study by Pfleiderer et al. (2007). They recently reported a female patient with panic disorder experiencing an (accidental) spontaneous panic attack while taking part in an fMRI auditory habituation paradigm. The panic attack was associated with significantly increased activity in the right amygdala. This is the first report of a spontaneous panic attack within an fMRI setting that supports findings from other neuroimaging techniques (Engel et al., 2009).

Another line of studies used pictures of facial emotion to test for abnormalities in emotion processing in PD.

One other of the first fMRI studies on PD was a study by Thomas et al. (2001) with anxious children (PD, $n = 2$ and/or generalized anxiety disorder, GAD, $n = 11$, mean age around 13 years, all unmedicated; matched depressed children as control group) using a passive facial emotion viewing task (implicit emotion processing). Although only 2 subjects had a diagnosis comparable to adult PD, the results showed that right-sided amygdala hyperactivity is specific to anxiety (compared to healthy and depressed children) and related to the extent of everyday anxiety symptoms. This implies that amygdala hyperactivity might be a trait rather than a state marker of anxiety.

However, comparable to other fMRI studies of facial emotion perception in general and in other psychiatric diseases, amygdala hyperactivity is not always detectable in PD.

Explicit emotion processing in the anterior cingulate and amygdala was tested using facial expression discrimination tasks (subjects were instructed to monitor facial affect and report after scanning) with either fearful and neutral (Pillay et al., 2006), or happy and neutral face presentations (Pillay et al., 2007) in PD patients ($n = 8$, all medicated with either an SSRI and/or a benzodiazepine) and healthy subjects. Compared to control subjects, PD patients showed bilaterally lower activation of the subgenual anterior cingulate cortex (ACC) and the amygdalae but higher activity in more dorsal parts of the anterior cingulate for neutral (Pillay et al., 2006) and even more so for happy faces, as well as increased left amygdala amygdala activity for neutral expressions (Pillay et al., 2007). The authors discussed their findings as a result of attentional processes during cognitive evaluation and a possible reduction in response to acute emotional cues because of a chronic hyperarousal concerning diminished reactivity for fearful faces (Pillay et al., 2006). The ACC increases for happy faces were discussed as a consequence of heightened cognitive demand because of increased conflict monitoring, and their possibly particular emotional relevance as situations absent of threat (Pillay *et al.*, 2007). Aside from confounding factors (medication, small sample size), an additional interpretation of the relatively increased activity in the amygdala for neutral faces could be that it reflects an increase in sensitivity of the amygdala to ambiguity, which biases an organism towards greater sensitivity to negativity (Whalen, 2007).

Further explanation of amygdalar activational differences might come from imaging genetics studies in PD. Domschke *et al.* used an implicit, passive viewing masked facial emotion paradigm (fearful, happy, neutral) to investigate the influence of genetic polymorphisms involved in the serotonin and dopamine metabolism in PD ($n = 20$, 10 medicated with an SSRI, 10 unmedicated) (Domschke *et al.*, 2008). Distinct genetic polymorphisms of the serotonin transporter gene (functional -1019C/G 5-HT1A and 5-HTTLPR) leading to higher concentrations of serotonin in the synaptic cleft resulted in a lower activation of the right prefrontal cortex and increased activity of both amygdalae after presentation of faces with happy emotional expressions (Domschke *et al.*, 2006). In particular, polymorphisms of the serotonin transporter gene are of great interest in PD, since serotonin plays a special role in anxiety, and SSRIs are first-line PD pharmacotherapy (Canli and Lesch, 2007). The same group also reported a role of the functional catechol-*O*-methyltransferase (COMT) val158met polymorphism in the activation of amygdala and prefrontal cortex. In response to fearful faces, increased activation in the right amygdala was observed in PD patients with at least one 158val allele, whereas relatively increased activation of the orbitofrontal and ventromedial prefrontal cortex associated with the 158val allele was shown for the presentation of fearful, angry and happy faces (Domschke *et al.*, 2008). Although findings in both studies were not in line with previous findings of imaging genetics studies of those polymorphisms (Canli and Lesch, 2007; Domschke *et al.*, 2008), genetic characterization to constrain analysis will be of importance in future imaging studies, since those genetic polymorphisms may explain substantial variance in imaging experiments (Meyer-Lindenberg and Weinberger, 2006).

A recent example of a task-wise experimentally refined facial emotion study is that by Chechko *et al.* (2009). The authors used a combination of an explicit facial expression (fearful and happy)

discrimination task with a Stroop emotional-word paradigm by printing either congruently or incongruently the words "fear" or "happy" on the emotional face pictures (Chechko *et al.*, 2009). This task was used first in healthy subjects as an emotional conflict paradigm where it showed reciprocal negative feedback connectivity of the pregenual ACC with the amygdala (Etkin *et al.*, 2006). In PD patients ($n = 18$, all remitted, all medicated with an SSRI), compared to healthy subjects, only previous-trial conflict-related neural activity differed with stronger dorsal anterior cingulate cortex (dACC), temporal, parietal and dorsolateral prefrontal activation during conflict detection after a preceding congruence (Chechko *et al.*, 2009). The context of preceding incongruence lead to diminished dACC and dorsomedial prefrontal cortex activity and increased parahippocampal, amygdala and brainstem (midbrain and dorsal pons) activity in PD patients compared to healthy controls. This pattern of activity with diminished (dorsal) ACC and medial prefrontal cortex activity on one hand and amygdalar hyperactivity on the other resonates with dysfunctional networks in other anxiety disorders, especially PTSD, and in psychiatric disorders in general (Engel *et al.*, 2009; Etkin and Wager, 2007; Rauch *et al.*, 2003). One unique feature of PD might still be the dysfunction of brainstem areas (posterior midbrain and dorsal pons, mostly interpreted as the PAG) which have initially been seen as the key generator region for panic attacks and panic disorder (for review see Del-Ben and Graeff, 2009). Recently, this view has been challenged by an amygdala-centered "fear network" model relying in many ways on the neural basis of classical fear conditioning (Gorman *et al.*, 2000).

Neural substrates of instructed fear in panic disorder

To further discern unique PD-related neural dysfunction in comparison to another major anxiety disorder, and to probe the neural substrates of this fear network, the authors have recently applied an instructed fear paradigm consisting of a Threat and a Safe condition (Tuescher *et al.*, in press) to PD (PD without agoraphobia, $n = 8$, unmedicated), PTSD ($n = 8$, unmedicated) and healthy subjects. In this task, the association of a previously neutral stimulus (visually presented colored squares) with a possible aversive

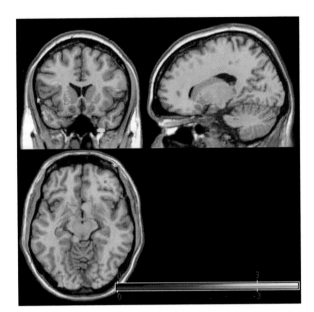

Figure 20.1 Coronal ($y=18$), sagittal ($x=18$) and axial ($z=-11$) sections showing decreased subgenual cingulate (Brodmann area 25), ventral striatum, and extended amygdala activity for the Threat vs. Safe condition in Panic vs. PTSD subjects. Color-coding in the scale represents study-specific t values. (right = right.)

event (electrodermal stimulation) is learned by means of a verbal instruction (Butler *et al.*, 2007; Phelps *et al.*, 2001). Symbolically acquired fear can result in physiological fear responses and functional neuroimaging data comparable to the responses to a conditioned stimulus and its extinction in classical fear conditioning (Butler *et al.*, 2007; Delgado *et al.*, 2008; Phelps *et al.*, 2001). Relative to PTSD and control subjects, PA patients demonstrated significantly less activation to the Threat and increased activity to the Safe condition in the subgenual cingulate (Brodmann Area 25), extending into the ventral striatum and extended amygdala (the bed nucleus of the stria terminalis and its sublenticular extension into the centromedial amygdala; Figure 20.1). PA patients, in contrast to PTSD and control subjects, revealed a marked decrease to the Threat and an increase to the Safe condition over time in midbrain, suggesting abnormal reactivity in this key region for fear expression (Tuescher *et al.*, in press). Importantly, these results extend previous findings of hypoactivation of the cingulate cortex to the subgenual ACC and replicate brainstem dysfunction – in direct contrast to fronto-limbic pathway dysfunction in PTSD. In this experimental context, the increased activity in response to the Safe condition of the subgenual

cingulate, ventral striatum, and extended amygdala might be interpreted as a strong signal for absence of threat (Pillay *et al.*, 2007). It might also be considered in the context of a model that would suggest that in PD, compared with PTSD, the bias is toward internal, viscero-somatic threat, rather than external threat.

Symptom-related neural substrates of instructed fear in panic disorder

In order to test hypotheses concerning fear circuit dysfunction in specific PD symptom domains, the Panic Disorder Severity Scale (PDSS), which assesses symptom status in panic disorder (PD), was entered into a correlational analysis with condition-related blood oxygen level-dependent (BOLD) activity in the instructed fear paradigm (PD without agoraphobia, $n=8$, unmedicated). In PD subjects, the combined frequency and distress severity of panic attacks (PDSS 1 and 2) correlated with increased activity in both, dorsal and extended amygdala, caudal midbrain and pons, and with decreased activity in ventral medial and lateral prefrontal cortex (PFC) in response to the Threat versus Safe condition (Figure 20.2). In turn, the severity of anticipatory anxiety related to panic attacks (PDSS 3) correlated with increased activity in bilateral ventral amygdala, and decreased activity in right lateral orbitofrontal cortex (OFC) and pregenual anterior cingulate cortex in response to the early Threat versus Safe condition (Figure 20.3). The severity of agoraphobic symptoms (PDSS 4) correlated with increased activity in bilateral ventral amygdala, right hippocampus and parahippocampal cortex in response to the early Threat versus Safe condition and with decreased activity in right OFC (Figure 20.4). In summary, symptom severity-dependent neural activity corroborates amygdala hyperactivity and ventral prefrontal hypoactivity in PD in response to cognitively induced threat also representing anticipatory anxiety. With a given symptom, additional brain areas, e.g. hippocampus for agoraphobic symptoms, also respond in a symptom severity-related manner consistent with the function this brain area subserves in that symptom.

Taken together, the fMRI results of cognitively instructed fear in PD presented here support the notion of a dysregulated fear processing neural network in PD while at same time point to the importance of both amygdala and brain stem in PD

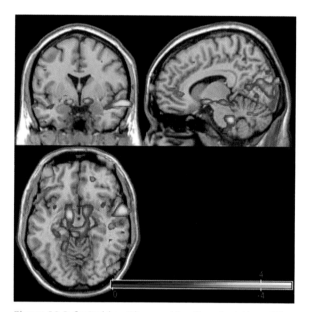

Figure 20.2 Sagittal ($x = 10$), coronal ($y = 0$), and axial ($z = -11$) sections showing that in panic disorder subjects, the combined frequency of and distress severity during panic attacks correlate (PDSS 1 + PDSS 2) with increased activity in both, dorsal and extended amygdala, and caudal midbrain and pons, as well as decreased activity in prefrontal cortex in response to the Threat versus Safe condition. Color-coding in the scale represents study-specific t values. (Right = right.)

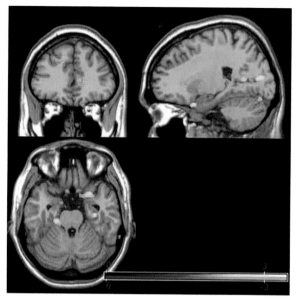

Figure 20.3 Sagittal ($x = -21$), coronal ($y = -2$), and axial ($z = -21$) sections showing that in panic disorder subjects, the severity of anticipatory anxiety related to panic attacks (PDSS 3) correlates with increased activity in bilateral amygdala, and decreased activity in right lateral orbitofrontal cortex and pregenual anterior cingulate cortex in response to the early Threat versus Safe condition. Color-coding in the scale represents study-specific t values. (Right = right.)

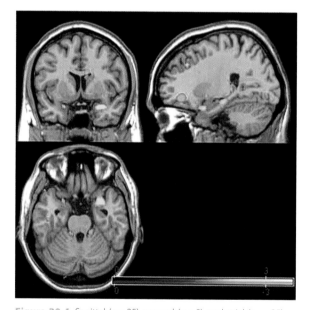

Figure 20.4 Sagittal ($x = 25$), coronal ($y = 8$), and axial ($z = -25$) sections showing that in panic disorder subjects, severity of agoraphobia (PDSS 4) correlates with increased activity in bilateral amygdala, right hippocampus and parahippocampal cortex in response to the early Threat versus Safe condition; correlation with decreased activity occurs in right OFC. Color-coding in the scale represents study-specific t values. (Right = right.)

symptoms. This combined model addresses brain stem functional affiliations, possibly including the PAG with its role in fear expression as well as the ascending reticular activating system, with its role in arousal (the former and latter both affecting autonomic tone). The model also addresses fear perceptual and fear regulating functions associated with the amygdala–hippocampus–ventromedial PFC limbic circuit. Fear perceptual features as anticipatory anxiety, for instance, involve dysfunction of more ventral parts of the amygdala (i.e. the sensory input region) together with prefrontal areas subserving attention, i.e. the pregenual ACC, and evaluation, i.e. ventromedial OFC, of emotionally salient stimuli. Similarly, agoraphobic symptom severity, which can be seen as a form of contextual fear related to an aspect of the environment as a place where a panic attack might have occurred and might occur, is also related to activity in ventral parts of the amygdala in conjunction with the hippocampus. On the other hand, dysregulated fear expression seems to be mediated by dorsal/extended amygdala areas (i.e. the output regions) in concert with brainstem areas as exemplified in comparison to control or PTSD subjects and in correlation with frequency and severity of panic attacks – which can be seen as paroxysmal fear and autonomic activation. Prefrontal cortex hypofunction (mainly ventromedial), however, seems to be common ground for dysregulation of both fear perception and fear expression.

Conclusion

Initial neurocircuitry models of panic disorder have hypothesized that the panic attack itself is generated by certain brainstem areas including the ascending reticular system and respiratory and cardiovascular control centres (for review see Del-Ben and Graeff, 2009). Recent models have proposed a neuronal "fear network" with the amygdala at its center which is controlled by medial prefrontal areas and the hippocampus (Gorman et al., 2000). In this model, amygdala projections to brainstem nuclei might trigger many of the somatic anxiety symptoms during a panic attack. Entero- and exteroceptive awareness are thought be increased by a greater reactivity of the insular cortex and have recently been suggested as the main processing sites for (perceptional and emotional) uncertainty (Simmons et al., 2008). In cognitive symptoms, such as fear expectancies and avoidance, prefrontal cortical areas appear to be involved predominantly.

However, the fMRI studies discussed above as well as panic attacks occurring in an individual with bilateral selective amygdala lesions (Wiest et al., 2006) also suggest that the amygdala is not solely responsible for PD symptoms. A current model of PD might entail amygdalar and brainstem dysfunction on the basis of altered regulation by prefrontal (especially cingulate), hippocampal and insular cortices (Graeff and Del-Ben, 2008; Protopopescu et al., 2006; Tuescher et al., in press). Alternatively, bottom-up limbic and/or brainstem activation is possible. In either case, associated viscero-somatic anxiety, accompanied or driven by autonomic discharge, may result, accounting for the cardinal symptoms of PD. The implementation of new fMRI paradigms targeting discrete symptoms or regions/circuits (Silbersweig and Stern, 1997; Simmons et al., 2008), allowing direct symptom provocation in the scanner (Dieler et al., 2008; Eser et al., 2009; Schunck et al., 2006) and/or direct comparison of disorders in one experimental setting (Stern and Silbersweig, 2001) will help to detail and test such models.

Box 20.1. Summary box

- Functional MRI (fMRI) studies in panic disorder (PD) are infrequent compared with other anxiety disorders and psychiatric conditions, as well as in relation to the prevalence of PD.
- Most fMRI studies in PD are constrained by rather modest sample sizes, medication and genetic effects.
- FMRI studies have highlighted the importance of amygdala, anterior cingulate (ACC) and prefrontal cortex dysfunction in the pathophysiology of PD, features shared by other anxiety disorders.
- Inconsistencies in amygdalar and prefrontal findings might be, in part, due to different task demands, e.g. implicit versus explicit processing of emotional stimuli.
- Brainstem dysfunction has been (re-)established by recent fMRI studies, supported by converging findings using other neuroimaging techniques, and might be a distinguishing characteristic of PD.
- Methodological development (imaging genetics, function or region specific paradigms, data pre- and post-processing inventions) will continue to refine circuit models of PD.
- Further studies comparing PD with other anxiety disorders are needed to discern the unique and overlapping neural network changes in PD.

References

Alonso J and Lepine J P. 2007. Overview of key data from the European Study of the Epidemiology of Mental Disorders (ESEMeD). *J Clin Psychiatry* **68** (Suppl 2), 3–9.

American PsychiatricAssociation. 2000. *Diagnostic and Statistical Manual of Mental Disorders —Text Revision* (4th edition). Philadelphia, PA: APA.

Butler T, Pan H, Tuescher O, et al. 2007. Human fear-related motor neurocircuitry. *Neuroscience* **150**, 1–7.

Bystritsky A, Pontillo D, Powers M, Sabb F W, Craske M G and Bookheimer S Y. 2001. Functional MRI changes during panic anticipation and imagery exposure. *Neuroreport* **12**, 3953–7.

Canli T and Lesch K P. 2007. Long story short: The serotonin transporter in emotion regulation and social cognition. *Nat Neurosci* **10**, 1103–09.

Chechko N, Wehrle R, Erhardt A, Holsboer F, Czisch M and Samann P G. 2009. Unstable prefrontal response to emotional conflict and activation of lower limbic structures and brainstem in remitted panic disorder. *PLoS One* **4**, e5537, 1–11.

Damsa C, Kosel M and Moussally J. 2009. Current status of brain imaging in anxiety disorders. *Curr Opin Psychiatry* **22**, 96–110.

Del-Ben C M and Graeff F G. 2009. Panic disorder: Is the PAG involved? *Neural Plast* 2009, **108135**, 1–9.

Delgado M R, Nearing K I, Ledoux J E and Phelps E A. 2008. Neural circuitry underlying the regulation of conditioned fear and its relation to extinction. *Neuron* **59**, 829–38.

Dieler A C, Samann P G, Leicht G, *et al.* 2008. Independent component analysis applied to pharmacological magnetic resonance imaging (phMRI): New insights into the functional networks underlying panic attacks as induced by CCK-4. *Curr Pharm Des* **14**, 3492–507.

Domschke K, Braun M, Ohrmann P, *et al.* 2006. Association of the functional -1019C/G 5-HT1A polymorphism with prefrontal cortex and amygdala activation measured with 3 T fMRI in panic disorder. *Int J Neuropsychopharmacol* **9**, 349–55.

Domschke K, Ohrmann P, Braun M, *et al.* 2008. Influence of the catechol-O-methyltransferase val158met genotype on amygdala and prefrontal cortex emotional processing in panic disorder. *Psychiatry Res* **163**, 13–20.

Engel K, Bandelow B, Gruber O and Wedekind D. 2009. Neuroimaging in anxiety disorders. *J Neural Transm* **116**, 703–16.

Eser D, Leicht G, Lutz J, *et al.* 2009. Functional neuroanatomy of CCK-4-induced panic attacks in healthy volunteers. *Hum Brain Mapp* **30**, 511–22.

Etkin A, Egner T, Peraza D M, Kandel E R and Hirsch J. 2006. Resolving emotional conflict: A role for the rostral anterior cingulate cortex in modulating activity in the amygdala. *Neuron* **51**, 871–82.

Etkin A and Wager T D. 2007. Functional neuroimaging of anxiety: A meta-analysis of emotional processing in PTSD, social anxiety disorder, and specific phobia. *Am J Psychiatry* **164**, 1476–88.

Gorman J M, Kent J M, Sullivan G M and Coplan J D. 2000. Neuroanatomical hypothesis of panic disorder, revised. *Am J Psychiatry* **157**, 493–505.

Graeff F G and Del-Ben C M. 2008. Neurobiology of panic disorder: From animal models to brain neuroimaging. *Neurosci Biobehav Rev* **32**, 1326–35.

Kessler R C, Berglund P, Demler O, Jin R, Merikangas K R and Walters E E. 2005. Lifetime prevalence and age-of-onset distributions of DSM-IV disorders in the National Comorbidity Survey Replication. *Arch Gen Psychiatry* **62**, 593–602.

Maddock R J, Buonocore M H, Kile S J and Garrett A S. 2003. Brain regions showing increased activation by threat-related words in panic disorder. *Neuroreport* **14**, 325–8.

Meyer-Lindenberg A and Weinberger D R. 2006. Intermediate phenotypes and genetic mechanisms of psychiatric disorders. *Nat Rev Neurosci* **7**, 818–27.

Pfleiderer B, Zinkirciran S, Arolt V, Heindel W, Deckert J, Domschke K. 2007. fMRI amygdala activation during a spontaneous panic attack in a patient with panic disorder. *World J Biol Psychiatry* **8**, 269–72.

Phelps E A, O'Connor K J, Gatenby J C, Gore J C, Grillon C and Davis M. 2001. Activation of the left amygdala to a cognitive representation of fear. *Nat Neurosci* **4**, 437–41.

Pillay S S, Gruber S A, Rogowska J, Simpson N and Yurgelun-Todd D A. 2006. fMRI of fearful facial affect recognition in panic disorder: The cingulate gyrus–amygdala connection. *J Affect Disord* **94**, 173–81.

Pillay S S, Rogowska J, Gruber S A, Simpson N and Yurgelun-Todd D A. 2007. Recognition of happy facial affect in panic disorder: An fMRI study. *J Anxiety Disord* **21**, 381–93.

Protopopescu X, Pan H, Tuescher O, *et al.* 2006. Increased brainstem volume in panic disorder: A voxel-based morphometric study. *Neuroreport* **17**, 361–3.

Rauch S L, Shin L M and Wright C I. 2003. Neuroimaging studies of amygdala function in anxiety disorders. *Ann N Y Acad Sci* **985**, 389–410.

Schunck T, Erb G, Mathis A, *et al.* 2006. Functional magnetic resonance imaging characterization of CCK-4-induced panic attack and subsequent anticipatory anxiety. *Neuroimage* **31**, 1197–208.

Silbersweig D A and Stern E. 1997. Symptom localization in neuropsychiatry. A functional neuroimaging approach. *Ann N Y Acad Sci* **835**, 410–20.

Simmons A, Matthews S C, Paulus M P and Stein M B. 2008. Intolerance of uncertainty correlates with insula activation during affective ambiguity. *Neurosci Lett* **430**, 92–7.

Stern E and Silbersweig D A. 2001. Advances in functional neuroimaging methodology for the study of brain systems underlying human neuropsychological function and dysfunction. *J Clin Exp Neuropsychol* **23**, 3–18.

Tuescher O, Protopopescu X, Pan H, *et al.* in press. Differential activation of the subgenual cingulate and brainstem in Panic Disorder and PTSD.

Thomas K M, Drevets W C, Dahl R E, *et al.* 2001. Amygdala response to fearful faces in anxious and depressed children. *Arch Gen Psychiatry* **58**, 1057–63.

van den Heuvel O A, Veltman D J, Groenewegen H J, *et al.* 2005. Disorder-specific neuroanatomical correlates of attentional bias in obsessive–compulsive disorder, panic disorder, and hypochondriasis. *Arch Gen Psychiatry* **62**, 922–33.

Whalen P J. 2007. The uncertainty of it all. *Trends Cogn Sci* **11**, 499–500.

Wiest G, Lehner-Baumgartner E and Baumgartner C. 2006. Panic attacks in an individual with bilateral selective lesions of the amygdala. *Arch Neurol* **63**, 1798–801.

Molecular imaging of other anxiety disorders

James W. Murrough and Sanjay J. Mathew

Introduction

Neuroimaging research is beginning to define functional anatomical correlates of both normal fear and anxiety as well as the pathological anxiety symptoms found in the anxiety disorders. These studies in humans are guided by molecular biology and behavioral neuroscience research utilizing animal models of fear and anxiety. Anatomical circuits and neurochemicals that may govern normal and abnormal fear and anxiety are beginning to emerge through convergence of both animal and human data. Current research seeks to understand how normal fear systems become dysregulated in clinical anxiety disorders.

This chapter reviews the neurochemical imaging literature in the anxiety disorders, focusing on key findings in post-traumatic stress disorder (PTSD), panic disorder (PD), social anxiety disorder (SAD; also referred to as social phobia) and generalized anxiety disorder (GAD). PTSD develops in a subgroup of individuals who experience a traumatic event (for example, a life-threatening situation), and is characterized by re-experiencing phenomena and intrusive memories related to a traumatic event, hyperarousal (for example, exaggerated startle), and avoidance and emotional numbing. Panic disorder is characterized by the recurrence of discrete panic attacks with the development of anticipatory anxiety and avoidance in between attacks. Panic attacks are the unprovoked, sudden onset of a constellation of psychological and physical symptoms that include intense fear or dread, a feeling of the need to escape, rapid heart beat or palpitations, shortness of breath, dizziness and diaphoresis. Social anxiety disorder consists of excessive embarrassment or humiliation in social situations that leads to behavioral avoidance and occupational or social impairment. Generalized anxiety disorder is characterized by pervasive worry that is excessive and intrusive with accompanying physical symptoms such as muscle tension and fatigue.

Although each of the anxiety disorders has a unique natural history, phenomenology, and symptom profile, they share a common feature of an exaggerated fear response. This observation of an exaggeration of normal fear in anxiety disorders provides the rationale for the application of neurobiological models of fear to the study of the pathophysiology of these disorders. Neuroimaging approaches to the study of anxiety disorders include volumetric magnetic resonance imaging (MRI), functional MRI (fMRI), MR spectroscopic imaging (MRSI), and functional and neuroreceptor studies using positron emission tomography (PET) and single photon emission computed tomography (SPECT). This chapter focuses on neuroreceptor studies of the serotonin (5-HT) system and the gamma-aminobutyric acid (GABA)–benzodiazepine (BZD) system utilizing PET or SPECT, and MRSI studies primarily focusing on the GABA system. A brief review of neuroanatomical and neurochemical aspects of fear and anxiety is presented to provide a neurobiological context for these studies.

Neuroanatomical overview of fear and anxiety

An understanding of neuroanatomical correlates of fear and anxiety-related behaviors that has emerged from preclinical studies provides a structure in which to interpret human neuroimaging studies of anxiety disorders. More than two decades of behavioral neuroscience research has established a set of interconnected brain structures that regulate the expression of fear-related behavior (LeDoux, 2000). Brain

---

Understanding Neuropsychiatric Disorders, ed. M. E. Shenton and B. I. Turetsky. Published by Cambridge University Press.
© Cambridge University Press 2011.

regions that comprise this fear circuitry include the amygdala, the hippocampus, the insula, the orbito-frontal cortex (OFC) and medial prefrontal cortex (mPFC), and related parts of the thalamus, hypothalamus, sensory cortices and brain stem. The amygdala is a critical node in this circuitry and serves to evaluate threat-related sensory information relayed to its lateral nucleus through the anterior thalamus. Output from the central nucleus of the amygdala serves to coordinate threat response through ascending projections to motor cortex, and descending projections to the hypothalamus and brain stem nuclei to modulate endocrine and autonomic responses and arousal/vigilance.

The modulation of emotional behavior in animals and humans is envisioned to depend on functional interactions between the amygdala (and related limbic and paralimbic structures) and regions of the mPFC and OFC (Rauch et al., 2006). These prefrontal structures are thought to represent the significance or salience of a given stimulus to the organisms and interact with the amygdala through dense, reciprocal connections. Regions of the mPFC appear particularly important in reducing fear responses and extinguishing fear-related behaviors that are no longer reinforced (Quirk et al., 2006). PFC regions may serve to suppress amygdala-based fear responses once a threat has passed or the context of the threat has changed. The hippocampus also appears to be important in modulating fear-related behaviors by providing contextual cues through reciprocal connections with the amygdala and through direct modulation of the hypothalamic–pituitary–adrenal (HPA) axis. Dysfunction of the hippocampus has been suggested to contribute to the generalization of fear responses observed in some anxiety disorders.

Neuroimaging studies utilizing fMRI and PET in healthy populations provide evidence for a role for the amygdala, the mPFC, and other regions in emotional behavior in humans that parallels work in animals (Phan et al., 2002). In parallel, neuroimaging studies in anxiety-disorder populations provide evidence of dysfunction in a core system of fear circuitry in humans. In particular, abnormal activation of the amygdala has been demonstrated in many, but not all, neuroimaging studies of anxiety disorders. In PTSD, amygdala hyperactivity has been demonstrated repeatedly during symptom provocation or negative emotional processing (Rauch et al., 2006;

Shin et al., 2004, 2005). Likewise, amygdala hyperactivity has been demonstrated in SAD (Phan et al., 2006; Stein et al., 2002), specific phobia (SP) (Straube et al., 2006), and panic disorder (van den Heuvel et al., 2005). In addition to the amygdala, abnormal insula activity has been observed in multiple neuroimaging studies of anxiety disorders (Paulus and Stein, 2006).

A recent quantitative meta-analysis by Etkin and Wager (2007) compared fMRI and PET studies of PTSD, SAD, SP, and fear conditioning in healthy individuals. In this report, several patterns of activation were found with potential clinical and nosological implications. First, all three anxiety disorders and normal fear activated a set of distinct but overlapping brain regions with two regions being common across all three anxiety disorders: the amygdala and the insula. These findings suggest that PTSD, SAD and SP share a common overactivity of amygdala-based fear circuitry. Second, only patients with PTSD demonstrated regions of hypoactivation compared to healthy controls. These regions included the OFC, regions of mPFC (dorsomedial prefrontal cortex (dmPFC), ventromedial prefrontal cortex (vmPFC), rostral anterior cingulate cortex (rACC), dorsal anterior cingulate cortex (dACC)), midcingulate, anterior hippocampus, and parahippocampal gyrus. All five studies of PTSD demonstrated negative correlations between symptom severity and activity in the mPFC. Hypoactivation of regions of the mPFC in patients with PTSD may reflect a deficit in emotion regulation that is unique to this syndrome among the anxiety disorders.

There have been relatively few neuroimaging studies of GAD relevant to neural circuitry. Three fMRI studies in adolescents with GAD demonstrated both amygdala and vmPFC dysfunction (McClure et al., 2007; Monk et al., 2006, 2008). A recent direct comparison of patients with GAD and SAD revealed distinct neural circuitry abnormalities in the two disorders (Blair et al., 2008). The authors found that SAD was associated with increased responses to fearful facial expressions in the amygdala, consistent with the findings from Etkin and Wager (2007), while GAD was not. In contrast, GAD was associated with increased responses to angry facial expressions in regions of PFC. In both disorders, region-specific patterns of neural responses were associated with severity of anxiety symptoms.

Neurochemical aspects of fear and anxiety relevant to neurochemical imaging of anxiety disorders

The anatomic circuits that underlie fear and anxiety outlined above are modulated by specific neurochemical systems. Among the most closely scrutinized chemical systems include the amino acid neurotransmitters GABA and glutamate, the monoamine neurotransmitters norepinephrine (NE), dopamine (DA), and serotonin (5-HT), the neuropeptides substance P, neuropeptide Y, and corticotropin-releasing hormone (CRH), opioids and cortisol/corticosterone. Stress-related neurochemical alterations have clear adaptive value, for example by increasing the organism's preparedness through increasing attention, vigilance, memory function, as well as peripheral autonomic and endocrine function. However, long-term dysregulation of these systems may underlie a vulnerability to the development of anxiety disorders. Unfortunately, in-vivo imaging methods are currently unavailable for many of the chemical systems identified in preclinical studies of anxiety disorders, for example the noradrenergic system and the HPA axis. However, radioligands are available for the 5-HT$_{1A}$ receptor and the 5-HT reuptake transporter (SERT), for the GABA-BZD receptor, and for the DA transporter (DAT). Additionally, ^{1}H-MRS can estimate steady-state GABA and glutamate concentrations. Below, we provide a partial review of preclinical and human investigations of several neurochemical systems relevant to neurochemical imaging of anxiety disorders: namely the 5-HT, GABA-BZD and DA systems.

Serotonin system

Serotonin is a monoamine neurotransmitter synthesized in brainstem nuclei whose axons project throughout the forebrain to regulate a diverse array of neural functions. Serotonin is also found in the gastrointestinal tract and is known to regulate cardiovascular function. Acute stress increases 5-HT turnover in multiple brain regions including the PFC, nucleus accumbens, amygdala, and lateral hypothalamus (Kent et al., 2002b; Briones-Aranda et al., 2005). Serotonin release may have anxiogenic and anxiolytic effects, depending on the region of the forebrain involved and the receptor subtype activated. Serotonin is thought to act via the amygdala and PFC to enhance defensive responses

to threat on one hand, and act via the dorsal periaqueductal gray (dPAG) to inhibit threat-related behaviors on the other (Graeff, 2002). Anxiogenic effects appear to be mediated via the 5-HT$_{2A}$ receptor, whereas stimulation of 5-HT$_{1A}$ receptors is generally anxiolytic in animals (Graeff, 2004).

There is a ligand available for human in-vivo neurochemical imaging of the 5-HT$_{1A}$ receptor. The behavioral phenotype of 5-HT$_{1A}$ knockout mice includes increases in anxiety-like behaviors (Klemenhagen et al., 2006), whereas in mice overexpressing the 5-HT$_{1A}$ receptor these traits are reduced (Kusserow et al., 2004). Early postnatal shutdown of 5-HT$_{1A}$ receptor expression produces an anxiety phenotype that cannot be rescued with restoration of 5-HT$_{1A}$ receptors (Gross et al., 2002). However, when 5-HT$_{1A}$ receptor expression is reduced in adulthood and then reinstated, the anxiety phenotype is no longer present. These results suggest that altered function of 5-HT$_{1A}$ receptors early in life can produce long-term abnormalities in the regulation of anxiety behaviors.

Another area of investigation has been the SERT, for which an in-vivo radioligand is available for neurochemical imaging in humans. Polymorphisms in the promoter region of the SERT gene, producing a short (s) and long (l) allele, have been linked to behavioral and temperamental traits associated with the development of mood and anxiety disorders (Hariri et al., 2005). Preclinical studies have reported greater anxiety-like behaviors in rodents with altered 5-HT transporters or 5-HT levels (Lesch et al., 1996). Functional MRI studies of healthy volunteers with no psychiatric history showed that carriers of the s allele had higher reactivity in the amygdala to fearful faces (Hariri et al., 2005). Early-life stresses, in combination with the presence of the s allele, confer greater susceptibility to depression or behavioral inhibition in children (Fox et al., 2005), and greater susceptibility to depression in adults (Caspi et al., 2003).

Gamma-aminobutyric acid–benzodiazepine system

γ-Aminobutyric acid is the primary inhibitory neurotransmitter in the brain. GABA exerts an inhibitory influence on neuronal activity via activation of membrane-bound receptors. These receptors include the GABA$_A$ receptor, a fast-acting, ligand-gated chloride channel, and the $GABA_B$ receptor, a slower-acting, G protein-coupled receptor. Agents that are positive allosteric modulators of the $GABA_A$ receptor tend to be anxiolytic, such as benzodiazepines (BZD), barbiturates or ethanol (Kalueff and Nutt, 2007). Benzodiazepine agents bind to distinct BZD sites on $GABA_A$ receptors, potentiating and prolonging the synaptic actions of GABA binding by increasing the frequency of GABA-mediated chloride channel opening (Smith, 2001).

Preclinical investigations have established a primary role for the GABA–BZD system, in particular the α-2 and α-3 subunits, in modulating anxiety (Atack, 2005; Morris et al., 2006). Reduced BZD receptor binding results from acute stress in preclinical models (Kalueff and Nutt, 2007). In humans, pharmacological challenge studies also support a role for GABA–BZD function in anxiety (Nutt and Malizia, 2001). Human anxiety disorders could be related to a down-regulation of BZD receptor binding following exposure to the stress. Other possible explanations are that stress results in changes in receptor affinity, changes in an endogenous BZD ligand (the existence of which is controversial), or stress-related alterations in GABAergic transmission that affect BZD receptor binding. In addition, a preexisting low level of BZD receptor density may be a genetic risk factor for the development of stress-related anxiety disorders (Kalueff and Nutt, 2007).

Dopamine system

Dopamine (DA) is a catecholamine synthesized in a collection of nuclei in the ventral tegmental area (VTA) and substantia nigra (SN) in the brainstem. As with other monoamines, DA regulates diverse neural functions related to mood, cognition, and behavior. In particular, DA appears to play a key role in reward-related behaviors. In animals, acute stress influences DA release and metabolism in a number of specific brain areas important in affective behavior, including the amygdala, the nucleus accumbens and the mPFC. Stress appears to enhance DA release in the mPFC but inhibit DA release in the nucleus accumbens, which may reflect reciprocal interactions between cortical and subcortical DA targets (Ventura et al., 2002).

DA transmission in the mPFC appears to play a critical role in extinction of the conditioned fear in animals. Therefore, reduced prefrontal cortical DA results in the preservation of fear produced by a conditioned stressor, which may have implications for PTSD or other anxiety disorders (Morrow et al., 1999). There is potentially an optimal range for stress-induced DA release in mPFC to facilitate adaptive behavioral responses.

In humans, investigations of serum or cerebrospinal fluid (CSF) levels of DA or its metabolites have failed to demonstrate clear alterations in DA activity. Genetic analyses of polymorphisms of the major DA metabolizing enzyme catechol-O-methyltransferase (COMT) have suggested an association between specific polymorphisms and anxiety disorders, although these findings await replication (Domschke et al., 2007).

Neurochemical imaging findings in specific anxiety disorders
Post-traumatic stress disorder
Serotonin system

A single neuroreceptor PET study of the 5-HT system in patients with PTSD found no evidence for 5-HT dysfunction. Bonne and colleagues employed [^{18}F]-FCWAY to investigate the 5-HT_{1A} receptor in 12 medication-free patients with PTSD (10 females and 2 males) and a matched group of 11 never traumatized, healthy comparison subjects (10 females and one male) (Bonne et al., 2005). The type of trauma in this sample was mixed, with 5 PTSD subjects having suffered prepubertal sexual abuse, 3 having suffered childhood physical or emotional abuse, 2 who had suffered sexual assault as adults, and 2 who had experienced other severe traumatic events as adults. The regions of interest were brain structures with high 5-HT_{1A} receptor density: anterior cingulate cortex (ACC), posterior cingulate cortex, anterior insula, mesiotemporal cortex (hippocampus plus amygdala), anterior temporopolar cortex, and midbrain raphe. No significant differences in 5-HT_{1A} receptor distribution were observed between patients and healthy subjects in any region of interest (ROI). This lack of difference is in contrast to similar studies conducted in patients with panic disorder (Neumeister et al., 2004a) and SAD (Lanzenberger et al., 2007), in which differences in 5-HT_{1A} receptor distribution were found between patients and matched healthy volunteers.

Gamma-aminobutyric acid–benzodiazepine system

Bremner and colleagues investigated the BZD receptor in 13 patients with Vietnam War combat-related PTSD and 13 matched healthy comparison subjects using SPECT imaging of $[^{123}I]$-iomazenil (Bremner et al., 2000a). In the PTSD patients, BZD distribution volume was 41% lower in the prefrontal cortex (Brodmann's area 9) bilaterally relative to comparison subjects. There was no difference in other brain areas including the pons, striatum, thalamus, cerebellum, or midbrain. However, a second study of the BZD receptor in Gulf War-related PTSD failed to replicate the original finding of decreased prefrontal binding. In this second study, Fujita et al. studied 19 veterans with PTSD and 19 age-matched, healthy veterans using $[^{123}I]$-iomazenil SPECT (Fujita et al., 2004). There was no difference in BZD receptor distribution in any region, including the prefrontal cortex. The different findings between these two studies may have been related to differences in the age of the control groups or to differences in the time interval between trauma exposure and scanning.

In a more recent study by Geuze et al., the authors used $[^{11}C]$-flumazenil and PET to investigate the BZD receptor in 9 drug-naive male Dutch veterans with military-related PTSD and 7 male Dutch veterans without PTSD (Geuze et al., 2008). $[^{11}C]$-flumazenil PET is felt to be a more accurate technique for quantifying BZD–GABA$_A$ receptor binding than $[^{123}I]$-iomazenil SPECT. Control veterans without PTSD also met the A1 criterion for PTSD (that is, they had also experienced traumatic events). The authors employed both ROI-based analyses and voxel-wise whole-brain statistical parametric mapping analysis. In this study, veterans with PTSD showed widespread decreases in binding potential throughout the brain including the hippocampus, amygdala, insula, ACC, regions of the PFC, temporal, parietal, and occipital cortices, cerebellum, thalamus, and striatum.

Although not entirely consistent across studies, taken together these findings suggest abnormalities of the GABA–BZD system in PTSD. These findings are also consistent with animal models demonstrating that stress can alter the GABA–BZD system (see above). The observed low GABA–BZD binding in patients with PTSD could reflect a premorbid reduced level of receptor binding sites or decreased receptor binding affinity, or may have resulted from trauma or disease-related reductions in GABA–BZD binding. Of note, Vaiva and colleagues measured serum GABA levels in 108 motor vehicle accident victims immediately after the trauma and then assessed these subjects 6 weeks later for PTSD and found a significant association between low GABA and the eventual development of PTSD (Vaiva et al., 2004).

Panic disorder

Serotonin system

Neumeister and colleagues investigated the 5-HT$_{1A}$ receptor in PD using $[^{18}F]$-FCWAY PET (Neumeister et al., 2004a). The sample in this study consisted of 16 unmedicated patients with PD (10 female, 6 male), 7 of whom also met criteria for MDD, and 15 matched healthy controls (10 female, 5 male). The ROIs examined were similar to those used by Bonne and colleagues (2005) and included the ACC, posterior cingulate cortex, anterior insula, mesiotemporal cortex (hippocampus plus amygdala), anterior temporopolar cortex, and midbrain raphe. In contrast to PTSD, 5-HT$_{1A}$ receptor distribution was lower in the PD group relative to the control group in the ACC, PCC, and raphe. No between-group differences were found in the anterior insula, mesiotemporal cortex, or the anterior temporopolar cortex. Lower 5-HT$_{1A}$ receptor distribution was evident in both the pure PD and the PD plus comorbid depression subgroups relative to the control group and these two PD subgroups did not significantly differ from each other.

Although this finding awaits replication, reduced 5-HT$_{1A}$ binding in PD is consistent with animal studies of the 5-HT$_{1A}$ receptor in anxiety (Graeff, 2004). Reduced density of 5-HT$_{1A}$ receptors may represent a genetic or epigenetic vulnerability of the development of PD and commonly comorbid mood disorders. A polymorphism regulating 5-HT$_{1A}$ receptor transcription was found to be associated with depression and suicide (Lemonde et al., 2003). On the other hand, the finding of reduced 5-HT$_{1A}$ receptor binding may reflect a sequela of the illness or a compensatory process. The specific observation of abnormal 5-HT$_{1A}$ receptor binding in the ACC and PCC has implications for neurocircuitry models of PD given the prominent role of these structures established in human functional neuroimaging investigations (Rauch et al., 2006).

Gamma-aminobutyric acid–benzodiazepine system

Several early studies using SPECT and $[^{123}I]$-iomazenil uptake demonstrated regional alterations in BZD receptor binding in patients with PD (Schlegel et al., 1994; Kaschka et al., 1995; Kuikka et al., 1995). Kaschka et al. compared a group of 9 patients with

PD and depression with a matched control group of 9 dysthymic patients without PD and found bilateral decreases in uptake of [^{123}I]-iomazenil in the inferior frontal and temporal lobes in the PD group relative to the comparison group (Kaschka et al., 1995). Kuikka et al. compared 17 patients with PD with 17 matched healthy control subjects and found reduced uptake in left PFC compared to right PFC in the PD group (Kuikka et al., 1995). The results from these studies, however, may be limited by the use of non-quantitative methods for estimation of BZD receptor binding and other methodological limitations.

Bremner et al. utilized a quantitative method of [^{123}I]-iomazenil SPECT imaging and measurement of radioligand concentration in plasma to better estimate BZD receptor binding in patients with PD ($n = 13$) and healthy controls ($n = 16$) (Bremner et al., 2000b). The authors found decreased BZD receptor binding in left hippocampus and precuneus in PD patients relative to controls. In addition, the authors found decreased BZD receptor binding in PFC (Brodmann's areas 8, 9, and 10) in patients who had a panic attack at the time of the scan compared to patients who did not have a panic attack. The finding of decreased binding in the hippocampus is consistent with preclinical studies showing a decrease in BZD receptor binding in hippocampus with acute and chronic stress.

In addition to SPECT, several groups have investigated the BZD receptor in PD using [^{11}C]-flumazenil PET (Malizia et al., 1998; Cameron et al., 2007; Hasler et al., 2008). Malizia and colleagues found a global reduction in BZD receptor binding with peak reductions in right OFC and insula in PD subjects relative to healthy controls (Malizia et al., 1998). Cameron et al. examined 11 PD patients compared to 21 healthy control subjects and replicated the finding of reduced BZD receptor binding in the insula in the PD group (Cameron et al., 2007). Abnormal GABA function of the insula in PD is interesting in light of the emerging view of the insula in anxiety disorders and may be consistent with some of the symptoms of PD given the involvement of the insula in visceral, somatic, and affective functioning (Paulus and Stein, 2006).

A recent study by Hasler et al. (2008) examined BZD receptor binding with [^{11}C]-flumazenil PET in 15 patients with PD and 18 matched healthy control subjects. In this study, the authors found lower BZD receptor binding in the PD group in multiple brain regions with the largest effect in bilateral dorsal anterolateral PFC (DALPFC). Other brain regions demonstrating reduced binding included right frontal polar cortex, right dorsolateral PFC (DLPFC), bilateral precentral gyrus, right postcentral gyrus, right superior temporal gyrus, ACC, right superior parietal cortex, and left superior occipital gyrus. Unexpectedly, the PD subjects also showed increased binding compared to controls in the hippocampus/parahippocampal gyrus bilaterally and the left DLPFC. In subjects with PD, the severity of panic and anxiety symptoms correlated positively with BZD receptor binding in the DALPFC but negatively with binding in the hippocampus/parahippocampal gyrus.

These results of Hasler et al. are to some extent consistent with those of previous PET [^{11}C]-flumazenil studies in PD. They are also consistent with finding of widespread reductions in GABA–BZD receptor binding in PTSD by Geuze et al. (2008). However, the findings of increased binding in the parahippocampal gyrus/ventral hippocampus by Hasler et al. in PD are in disagreement with those of Cameron et al. (who observed no difference in this area), and Malizia et al. (who found reduced BZD receptor binding in a volume placed over the amygdala and adjacent hippocampus). The results are also in disagreement with those of Bremner et al., who reported decreased BZD binding in the left hippocampus and increased binding in the right dorsolateral PFC with [^{123}I]-iomazenil SPECT (Bremner et al., 2000b). Increased BZD receptor binding in the parahippocampal region conceivably may reflect a compensatory mechanism in PD. The parahippocampal gyrus and anterior ventral hippocampus (containing the subiculum) share extensive anatomical projections with the amygdala and MPFC regions, and participate substantially in the neural circuitry of emotion regulation (Ongur et al., 2003).

In addition to the neuroreceptor studies described above, three studies using ^{1}H-MRS to estimate GABA concentrations have been conducted in PD (Goddard et al., 2001, 2004; Hasler et al., 2009). Goddard and colleagues (2001) estimated total occipital GABA (GABA plus homocarnosine) in 14 unmedicated patients with PD and 14 matched control subjects using ^{1}H-MRS. Patients with PD had a 22% reduction in total occipital cortex GABA concentration compared to controls. This finding adds support to preclinical and human evidence suggesting that deficits in GABA function are associated with PD. In a follow-up study, they examined the response to a BZD challenge (clonazepam administration) in patients with PD (Goddard *et al.*, 2004). They predicted that patients with PD would demonstrate a deficient GABA neuronal response to the challenge. In a repeated measures design, the authors measured occipital cortex GABA responses to acute oral BZD in 10 PD patients and 9 healthy comparison subjects. Panic disorder patients demonstrated a blunted decrease in GABA level to the challenge compared to the healthy controls, who exhibited a significant decrease in occipital GABA. These data may be consistent with a trait-like abnormality in GABA function in patients with PD.

However, in a more recent ^{1}H-MRS study by Hasler *et al.*, the authors examined 17 PD patients and 17 matched controls and found no difference in GABA concentration in PFC (Hasler *et al.*, 2009). In addition, there was no significant difference in glutamate/glutamine (Glx), choline, or *N*-acetyl aspartate concentrations. Of note, the regions of interest (ROI) in the previous studies was the occipital cortex, while the Hasler *et al.* report examined a region of the PFC.

Although there is disagreement among studies of the GABA–BZD system in PD, the preponderance of evidence does suggest an abnormality of this system in the illness. As discussed in relation to the findings of altered GABA–BZD function in PTSD, these findings in humans are consistent with studies of stress in animals (Kalueff and Nutt, 2007). However, it is not known whether altered GABA–BZD function represents a premorbid vulnerability to the disorder or represents a consequence of the disorder.

Social anxiety disorder

Serotonin system

Lanzenberger and collegues investigated the 5-HT$_{1A}$ receptor in 12 medication-free male patients with SAD and 18 healthy male control subjects using [carbonyl-^{11}C]-WAY-100635 PET (Lanzenberger *et al.*, 2007). Major depressive disorder was an exclusion criterion in this study. Regions of interest (ROIs) were defined a priori and included the ACC, OFC, insula, amygdala, hippocampus. The authors found significant 5-HT$_{1A}$ binding reductions in the amygdala (21.4%), the ACC (23.8%), and insula (28.0%). A correlation analysis revealed no significant correlation between state or trait anxiety scores and regional 5-HT$_{1A}$ binding in both groups. The finding of

reduced 5-HT$_{1A}$ binding in the ACC in patients with SAD is consistent with the finding by Neumeister *et al.* (2004b) of reduced 5-HT$_{1A}$ binding in the ACC in patients with PD. This suggests alterations in 5-HT function in limbic and paralimbic areas in patients SAD as well as PD. However, Bonne *et al.* (2005) did not find evidence of altered 5-HT$_{1A}$ function in PTSD.

Kent *et al.* investigated the occupancy of the SERT by paroxetine in 5 patients (3 men, 2 women) with SAD using PET with the [^{11}C]-McN 5652 radioligand (Kent *et al.*, 2002a). Patients were scanned at baseline and then again after 3–6 months of daily paroxetine (20–40 mg/day). Occupancy levels were determined by measuring the decrease in SERT availability between the baseline scan and the treatment scan. Occupancy levels were also compared between different regions (ACC, amygdala, midbrain, thalamus, striatum, and hippocampus). After treatment, large reductions in binding were observed in the midbrain, thalamus, striatum, amygdala, hippocampus, and cingulate cortex. This suggests a marked effect of SERT blockade by paroxetine in patients with SAD, consistent with the therapeutic effects of paroxetine and other selective serotonin reuptake inhibitors (SSRIs) in this disorder.

Van der Wee *et al.* (2008) investigated both the SERT and DAT using ^{123}I-β-CIT SPECT in patients with SAD and healthy controls. ^{123}I-β-CIT can be used to probe both the SERT and DAT because binding of ^{123}I-β-CIT in the striatum primarily reflects DAT density whereas binding in the thalamus and midbrain primary reflects SERT binding (de Win *et al.*, 2005). Average binding ratio for SERT in the left and right thalamus was significantly higher in patients with SAD than in matched healthy controls. No significant differences were found in the midbrain. The average binding ratio for DAT in the striatum was significantly higher in patients than in matched controls. Increased SERT binding may result from increased density of the transporter or else reduced 5-HT concentrations at the transporter, which would decrease competition for the radioligand.

The finding of altered SERT binding in SAD is consistent with a role for abnormal 5-HT function in this disorder, as further suggested by the finding of reduced 5-HT$_{1A}$ receptor binding by Lanzenberger *et al.* (2007). Dysfunction of both 5-HT and DA has been implicated in the pathophysiology of SAD (Mathew *et al.*, 2001). Although these findings await replication, SAD appears to share dysfunction of the 5-HT system in common with PD, but in contrast to PTSD (Bonne *et al.*, 2005; Neumeister *et al.*, 2004a).

Gamma-aminobutyric acid–benzodiazepine system

To date, no neuroreceptor studies of the GABA-BZD system have been conducted in SAD. In a single ^{1}H-MRS study, Pollack *et al.* investigated GABA and glutamate patients with SAD (*N*=10) at baseline compared to a matched group of healthy controls, and changes following 8 weeks of pharmacotherapy with levetiracetam (Pollack *et al.*, 2008). Levetiracetam is an anticonvulsant agent, which may enhance GABAergic activity and has demonstrated anxiolytic effects in animal models of anxiety and in small trials in humans anxiety disorders (Zhang *et al.*, 2005). The authors hypothesized that levels of GABA would be lower and glutamate elevated at baseline compared to healthy controls, and that GABA would increase and glutamate would decrease with treatment. The authors found lower GABA and higher glutamate in the thalamus of patients with SAD compared to controls. There was a significant reduction in thalamic glutamine with levetiracetam treatment but no significant change in GABA.

The finding of reduced GABA in SAD are consistent with the results of Goddard *et al.* (2001) in PD demonstrating a reduction in occipital cortex GABA concentration, but in contrast to those of Hasler *et al.* (2009), who found no difference in GABA in the PFC in patients with PD. However, taken together, the findings of Pollack *et al.* add support to a role for GABA–BZD dysfunction in human anxiety disorders (Geuze *et al.*, 2008; Hasler *et al.*, 2008; Pollack *et al.*, 2008).

Dopamine system

Tiihonen *et al.* (1997a) used [^{123}I]-β-CIT with SPECT to measure DAT binding in 11 patients with SAD and 28 healthy control subjects. The authors found approximately 14% decreased uptake in the striatum of SAD subjects compared to controls. Schneier *et al.* (2000) used the D_2 receptor radiotracer [^{123}I]-iodo-benzamide ([^{123}I]-IBZM) and SPECT to compare D_2 receptor binding in 10 patients with SAD and 10 healthy comparison subjects. The authors found approximately 30% decrease in binding potential in patients with SAD compared to healthy control subjects. In a follow-up study, the same group investigated D_2 binding in patients with OCD with and without comorbid SAD (Schneier *et al.*, 2008). D_2 receptor availability was assessed with [^{123}I]-IBZM SPECT in 7 subjects with OCD comorbid with SAD, 8 with OCD, and 7 matched healthy subjects. There was a mean reduction in striatal [^{123}I]-IBZM binding of 38.7% in the comorbid SAD group compared to healthy controls, but no difference between OCD alone and healthy controls.

As noted above, van der Wee *et al.* (2008) investigated both SERT and DAT binding using SPECT and [^{123}I]-β-CIT in patients with SAD and healthy controls. In contrast to the reports by Tiihonen *et al.* (1997a) and Schneier *et al.* (2000, 2008), van der Wee *et al.* found a significantly higher (25%) average binding ratio for DAT in the striatum in patients compared to matched controls (van der Wee *et al.*, 2008). The reason for the opposite directionality of these findings in SAD is unclear, although these studies are limited by their small sample sizes. Given that altered DAT binding may represent either overactivity or underactivity of the DA system, and the inconsistency of findings, the role of DA in SAD remains unclear.

Generalized anxiety disorder
Serotonin system

Maron and colleagues investigated SERT binding in the midbrain and thalamus in 7 patients with GAD and 7 healthy controls using [^{123}I]-β-CIT SPECT (Maron *et al.*, 2004). The authors found no differences in SERT binding between the patients and controls. Of potential interest was the finding that midbrain SERT binding in patients was significantly and negatively correlated with their anxiety levels measured by a visual analog scale immediately before the scan. However, this study failed to convincingly demonstrate altered 5-HT activity in patients with GAD. This finding is consistent with the lack of difference in 5-HT$_{1A}$ binding in patients with PTSD (Bonne *et al.*, 2005), but in contrast to positive findings in PD (Neumeister *et al.*, 2004a) and SAD (Lanzenberger *et al.*, 2007; van der Wee *et al.*, 2008).

Gamma-aminobutyric acid–benzodiazepine system

Compared to other anxiety disorders, there have been relatively few investigations of the GABA–BZD system in GAD. An early study of the BZD receptor using [^{123}I]-NNC 13–8241 SPECT showed decreased ligand binding in the left temporal pole in 10 female patients with GAD compared to matched healthy control subjects (Tiihonen *et al.*, 1997b). In a second study of 10 unmedicated patients with a mix of anxiety disorders, including 4 with GAD, 5 with PD, and 1 patient with SAD, and matched healthy controls, [^{11}C]-flumazenil PET was used to characterize potential differences in BZD binding (Abadie *et al.*, 1999). The authors found no difference in [^{11}C]-flumazenil binding between the anxiety group and the healthy group in any region. Overall, the role of GABA-BZD in GAD remains to be determined.

Other (non-GABA) proton-magnetic resonance spectroscopy studies

Several studies have utilized ^{1}H-MRS to investigate potential abnormalities in *N*-acetyl-aspartate (NAA), choline (CHO), creatine (CR) or lactate in GAD. An initial study in 15 patients with GAD and 15 matched controls by Mathew *et al.* (2004) demonstrated a 16.5% elevation in NAA in the right DLPFC of patients with GAD. The same group then re-analyzed the data focusing on the centrum semi-ovale as a representative region of cerebral white matter and found decreased concentrations of CHO and CR in GAD patients without a history of early trauma, whereas GAD patients with early trauma were identical to controls (Coplan *et al.*, 2006). This study may have implications for the role of white matter in the pathophysiology of GAD. A recent study of hippocampal NAA in relation to treatment response to the glutamate-modulating agent riluzole found an association between response and increasing NAA levels in patients with GAD (Mathew *et al.*, 2008). Since NAA is taken as a marker of neuronal integrity, an association with response to riluzole is notable. Riluzole is FDA-approved for the treatment of amyotrophic lateral sclerosis, and may possess neurotrophic or neuro-protective properties.

Major depressive disorder with comorbid anxiety disorder

As anxiety disorders are frequently comorbid with mood disorders, investigations of patients with "anxious depression" may be informative in determining specificity of neurochemical abnormalities. Sullivan and colleagues used [^{11}C]-WAY-100635

PET to estimate regional 5-HT$_{1A}$ binding in 28 patients with MDD and comorbid anxiety (Sullivan *et al.*, 2005). Twelve had at least one comorbid anxiety disorder, which included PD ($n = 7$), SAD ($n = 4$), GAD ($n = 2$), or PTSD ($n = 4$). The authors examined correlations between regional 5-HT$_{1A}$ binding and 3 anxiety symtom components referred to as "psychic", "somatic", and "motoric" anxiety. Psycho-metric data from a larger MDD sample ($n = 288$), which included the 28 PET subjects, was used to generate a polychoric correlation matrix of anxiety items from the Hamilton Depression Rating Scale (HDRS) and the Brief Psychiatric Rating Scale (BPRS) for a principal components analysis (PCA). ROIs included OFC, mPFC, ACC, mid cingulate cortex, amygdala, and hippocampus. The authors found that higher psychic and lower somatic anxiety predicted over 50% of the variance in 5-HT$_{1A}$ binding in multiple cortical regions. Psychic anxiety was a positive cor-relate and somatic anxiety was a negative correlate of ligand binding in the four cortical regions examined. There were no correlations between 5-HT$_{1A}$ binding and the three anxiety components in amygdala or hippocampus. They did not find an association between anxiety and 5-HT$_{1A}$ binding in the amyg-dala, hippocampus, or the brainstem. The psychic and somatic anxiety components were not related to depression severity. The authors found lower binding in the subjects with comorbid PD. ANOVAs con-ducted for each ROI individually showed significant main effects of PD diagnosis for all regions except amygdala and occipital cortex.

The finding of reduced 5-HT$_{1A}$ binding in MDD patients with comorbid PD is in line with the findings of Neumeister and colleagues (2004a), described above, in which they report reduced 5-HT$_{1A}$ binding in patients with PD compared to healthy controls. Likewise, the inverse relationship between 5-HT$_{1A}$ binding in the ACC and other cortical regions and somatic anxiety is consistent with 5-HT dysfunction in PD. However, the positive relationship between 5-HT$_{1A}$ binding and psychic anxiety may be some-what unexpected. Psychic anxiety appeared to have opposite relationships with 5-HT$_{1A}$ binding com-pared with somatic/hypochondriacal anxiety and PD in the same cortical regions. The authors speculate whether enhanced neurotransmission at 5-HT$_{1A}$ receptors in cortical regions could result in both anxiogenic and anxiolytic effects depending on the type of anxiety.

- Essential neuroanatomical and neurochemical aspects of fear and anxiety:

  Key brain regions that modulate fear-related behavior – the amygdala, the hippocampus, the insula, the orbitofrontal cortex (OFC) and medial prefrontal cortex (mPFC), and related parts of the thalamus, hypothalamus, sensory cortices and brain stem.

  Key neurochemical modulators of fear circuitry – the amino acid neurotransmitters GABA and glutamate, the monoamine neurotransmitters norepinephrine (NE), dopamine (DA), and serotonin (5-HT), the neuropeptides substance P, neuropeptide Y, and corticotropin-releasing hormone (CRH), opioids and cortisol/corticosterone.

- Summary of neurochemical imaging findings of other anxiety disorders:

  Post-traumatic Stress Disorder – no current evidence for 5-HT dysfunction; some inconsistencies in studies but evidence suggests abnormalities of the GABA–BZD system.

  Panic Disorder – potential dysfunction of 5-HT suggested by single study (lower 5-HT_{1A} receptor distribution in PD in cingulate cortices, and raphe); evidence for regional GABA–BZD abnormalities.

  Social Anxiety Disorder – potential dysfunction of 5-HT suggested by single study (5-HT_{1A} binding reductions in the amygdala, the ACC, and insula); no neuroreceptor studies of the GABA–BZD system to date; a single ^{1}H-MRS study found low GABA and high glutamate; inconsistent findings of altered DAT function.

  Generalized Anxiety Disorder – no current evidence for 5-HT or GABA–BZD dysfunction; ^{1}H-MRS study found decreased concentrations of choline and creatine in GAD patients without a history of early trauma.

- Neurochemical imaging in anxiety disorders – summary:

  Consistent with animal studies, abnormalities of the 5-HT system have been demonstrated in PD and SAD; in contrast, alterations in the 5-HT system have not yet been identified in PTSD or GAD.

  Findings of altered GABA–BZD function have been demonstrated in PD, PTSD and SAD, consistent with preclinical research.

  Caution regarding definitive interpretations is warranted given small sample sizes, varying methodologies and, in some cases, disparate findings between studies.

Conclusions

The neurobiology of anxiety disorders is beginning to be illuminated through complementary human neuroimaging studies and basic and behavior neuroscience investigations in animals. In particular, neurochemical studies utilizing PET or SPECT radioligands and ^{1}H-MRS are starting to characterize abnormalities of the 5-HT, GABA-BZD and DA systems in anxiety disorders, extending preclinical work on the role of these systems in fear and anxiety to humans.

This chapter provided a brief review of neuroanatomical and neurochemical aspects of fear and anxiety, followed by a summary of neurochemical imaging findings in PTSD, PD, SAD and GAD. Consistent with animal studies, abnormalities of the 5-HT system have been demonstrated in PD and SAD. In contrast, alterations in the 5-HT system have not been found in PTSD or GAD. However, as studies have small sample sizes and use varying neuroimaging techniques and heterogeneous clinical samples (with differences across studies in duration of illness, comorbidity, sex distribution, age, etc.), these findings require replication and extension before any definitive conclusions regarding 5-HT function in anxiety disorders can be drawn. Findings of altered GABA–BZD function have been demonstrated in PD, PTSD and SAD, consistent with preclinical research. However, as with the 5-HT system, caution regarding definitive interpretations is warranted given small sample sizes, varying methodologies and, in some cases, disparate findings between studies.

References

Abadie P, Boulenger J P, Benali K, Barre L, Zarifian E and Baron J C. 1999. Relationships between trait and state anxiety and the central benzodiazepine receptor: A PET study. *Eur J Neurosci* **11**, 1470–8.

Atack J R. 2005. The benzodiazepine binding site of GABA (A) receptors as a target for the development of novel anxiolytics. *Exp Opin Investig Drugs* **14**, 601–18.

Blair K, Shaywitz J, Smith B W, *et al*. 2008. Response to emotional expressions in generalized social phobia and generalized anxiety disorder: Evidence for separate disorders. *Am J Psychiatry* **165**, 1193–202.

Bonne O, Bain E, Neumeister A, *et al*. 2005. No change in serotonin type 1A receptor binding in patients with posttraumatic stress disorder. *Am J Psychiatry* **162**, 383–5.

Bremner J D, Innis R B, Southwick S M, Staib L, Zoghbi S and Charney D S. 2000a. Decreased benzodiazepine receptor binding in prefrontal cortex in combat-related posttraumatic stress disorder. *Am J Psychiatry* **157**, 1120–6.

Bremner J D, Innis R B, White T, *et al.* 2000b. SPECT [I-123]iomazenil measurement of the benzodiazepine receptor in panic disorder. *Biol Psychiatry* **47**, 96–106.

Briones-Aranda A, Rocha L and Picazo O. 2005. Influence of forced swimming stress on 5-HT1A receptors and serotonin levels in mouse brain. *Prog Neuropsychopharmacology Biol Psychiatry* **29**, 275–81.

Cameron O G, Huang G C, Nichols T, *et al.* 2007. Reduced gamma-aminobutyric acid(A)–benzodiazepine binding sites in insular cortex of individuals with panic disorder. *Arch Gen Psychiatry* **64**, 793–800.

Caspi A, Sugden K, Moffitt T E, *et al.* 2003. Influence of life stress on depression: moderation by a polymorphism in the 5-HTT gene. *Science (New York, N.Y.)* **301**, 386–9.

Coplan J D, Mathew S J, Mao X, *et al.* 2006. Decreased choline and creatine concentrations in centrum semiovale in patients with generalized anxiety disorder: Relationship to IQ and early trauma. *Psychiatry Res* **147**, 27–39.

de Win M M, Habraken J B, Reneman L, van den Brink W, den Heeten G J and Booij J. 2005. Validation of [(123)I] beta-CIT SPECT to assess serotonin transporters in vivo in humans: A double-blind, placebo-controlled, crossover study with the selective serotonin reuptake inhibitor citalopram. *Neuropsychopharmacology* **30**, 996–1005.

Domschke K, Deckert J, O'Donovan M C and Glatt S J. 2007. Meta-analysis of COMT val158met in panic disorder: ethnic heterogeneity and gender specificity. *Am J Med Genet Part B Neuropsychiatric Genet* **144B**, 667–73.

Etkin A and Wager T D. 2007. Functional neuroimaging of anxiety: A meta-analysis of emotional processing in PTSD, social anxiety disorder, and specific phobia. *Am J Psychiatry* **164**, 1476–88.

Fox N A, Nichols K E, Henderson H A, *et al.* 2005. Evidence for a gene–environment interaction in predicting behavioral inhibition in middle childhood. *Psychol Sci* **16**, 921–6.

Fujita M, Southwick S M, Denucci C C, *et al.* 2004. Central type benzodiazepine receptors in Gulf War veterans with posttraumatic stress disorder. *Biol Psychiatry* **56**, 95–100.

Geuze E, van Berckel B N, Lammertsma A A, *et al.* 2008. Reduced GABAA benzodiazepine receptor binding in veterans with post-traumatic stress disorder. *Mol Psychiatry* **13**, 74–83, 3.

Goddard A W, Mason G F, Almai A, *et al.* 2001. Reductions in occipital cortex GABA levels in panic disorder detected with ^{1}H-magnetic resonance spectroscopy. *Arch Gen Psychiatry* **58**, 556–61.

Goddard A W, Mason G F, Appel M, *et al.* 2004. Impaired GABA neuronal response to acute benzodiazepine administration in panic disorder. *Am J Psychiatry* **161**, 2186–93.

Graeff F G. 2004. Serotonin, the periaqueductal gray and panic. *Neurosci Biobehav Rev* **28**, 239–59.

Graeff F G. 2002. On serotonin and experimental anxiety. *Psychopharmacology* **163**, 467–76.

Gross C, Zhuang X, Stark K, *et al.* 2002. Serotonin1A receptor acts during development to establish normal anxiety-like behaviour in the adult. *Nature* **416**, 396–400.

Hariri A R, Drabant E M, Munoz K E, *et al.* 2005. A susceptibility gene for affective disorders and the response of the human amygdala. *Arch Gen Psychiatry* **62**, 146–52.

Hasler G, Nugent A C, Carlson P J, Carson R E, Geraci M and Drevets W C. 2008. Altered cerebral gamma-aminobutyric acid type A–benzodiazepine receptor binding in panic disorder determined by [11C] flumazenil positron emission tomography. *Arch Gen Psychiatry* **65**, 1166–75.

Hasler G, van der Veen J W, Geraci M, Shen J, Pine D and Drevets W C. 2009. Prefrontal cortical gamma-aminobutyric acid levels in panic disorder determined by proton magnetic resonance spectroscopy. *Biol Psychiatry* **65**, 273–5.

Kalueff A V and Nutt D J. 2007. Role of GABA in anxiety and depression. *Depress Anxiety* **24**, 495–517.

Kaschka W, Feistel H and Ebert D. 1995. Reduced benzodiazepine receptor binding in panic disorders measured by iomazenil SPECT. *J Psychiatric Res* **29**, 427–34.

Kent J M, Coplan J D, Lombardo I, *et al.* 2002a. Occupancy of brain serotonin transporters during treatment with paroxetine in patients with social phobia: A positron emission tomography study with 11C McN 5652. *Psychopharmacology* **164**, 341–8.

Kent J M, Mathew S J and Gorman J M. 2002b. Molecular targets in the treatment of anxiety. *Biol Psychiatry* **52**, 1008–30.

Klemenhagen K C, Gordon J A, David D J, Hen R and Gross C T. 2006. Increased fear response to contextual cues in mice lacking the 5-HT1A receptor. *Neuropsychopharmacology* **31**, 101–11.

Kuikka J T, Pitkanen A, Lepola U, *et al.* 1995. Abnormal regional benzodiazepine receptor uptake in the prefrontal cortex in patients with panic disorder. *Nucl Med Commun* **16**, 273–80.

Kusserow H, Davies B, Hortnagl H, *et al.* 2004. Reduced anxiety-related behaviour in transgenic mice overexpressing serotonin 1A receptors. *Brain Res Mol Brain Res* **129**, 104–16.

Lanzenberger R R, Mitterhauser M, Spindelegger C, *et al.* 2007. Reduced serotonin-1A receptor binding in social anxiety disorder. *Biol Psychiatry* **61**, 1081–9.

LeDoux J E. 2000. Emotion circuits in the brain. *Annu Rev Neurosci* **23**, 155–84.

Lemonde S, Turecki G, Bakish D, *et al.* 2003. Impaired repression at a 5-hydroxytryptamine 1A receptor gene polymorphism associated with major depression and suicide. *J Neurosci* **23**, 8788–99.

Lesch K P, Bengel D, Heils A, *et al.* 1996. Association of anxiety-related traits with a polymorphism in the serotonin transporter gene regulatory region. *Science (New York, N.Y.)* **274**, 1527–31.

Malizia A L, Cunningham V J, Bell C J, Liddle P F, Jones T and Nutt D J. 1998. Decreased brain GABA(A)–benzodiazepine receptor binding in panic disorder: Preliminary results from a quantitative PET study. *Arch Gen Psychiatry* **55**, 715–20.

Maron E, Kuikka J T, Ulst K, Tiihonen J, Vasar V and Shlik J. 2004. SPECT imaging of serotonin transporter binding in patients with generalized anxiety disorder. *Eur Arch Psychiatry Clin Neurosci* **254**, 392–6.

Mathew S J, Coplan J D and Gorman J M. 2001. Neurobiological mechanisms of social anxiety disorder. *Am J Psychiatry* **158**, 1558–67.

Mathew S J, Mao X, Coplan J D, *et al.* 2004. Dorsolateral prefrontal cortical pathology in generalized anxiety disorder: A proton magnetic resonance spectroscopic imaging study. *Am J Psychiatry* **161**, 1119–21.

Mathew S J, Price R B, Mao X, *et al.* 2008. Hippocampal *N*-acetylaspartate concentration and response to riluzole in generalized anxiety disorder. *Biol Psychiatry* **63**, 891–8.

McClure E B, Monk C S, Nelson E E, *et al.* 2007. Abnormal attention modulation of fear circuit function in pediatric generalized anxiety disorder. *Arch Gen Psychiatry* **64**, 97–106.

Monk C S, Nelson E E, McClure E B, *et al.* 2006. Ventrolateral prefrontal cortex activation and attentional bias in response to angry faces in adolescents with generalized anxiety disorder. *Am J Psychiatry* **163**, 1091–7.

Monk C S, Telzer E H, Mogg K, *et al.* 2008. Amygdala and ventrolateral prefrontal cortex activation to masked angry faces in children and adolescents with generalized anxiety disorder. *Arch Gen Psychiatry* **65**, 568–76.

Morris H V, Dawson G R, Reynolds D S, Atack J R and Stephens D N. 2006. Both alpha2 and alpha3 GABAA receptor subtypes mediate the anxiolytic properties of benzodiazepine site ligands in the conditioned emotional response paradigm. *Eur J Neurosci* **23**, 2495–504.

Morrow B A, Elsworth J D, Rasmusson A M and Roth R H. 1999. The role of mesoprefrontal dopamine neurons in the acquisition and expression of conditioned fear in the rat. *Neuroscience* **92**, 553–64.

Neumeister A, Bain E, Nugent A C, *et al.* 2004a. Reduced serotonin type 1A receptor binding in panic disorder. *J Neurosci* **24**, 589–91.

Neumeister A, Nugent A C, Waldeck T, *et al.* 2004b. Neural and behavioral responses to tryptophan depletion in unmedicated patients with remitted major depressive disorder and controls. *Arch Gen Psychiatry* **61**, 765–73.

Nutt D J and Malizia A L. 2001. New insights into the role of the GABA(A)–benzodiazepine receptor in psychiatric disorder. *Br J Psychiatry* **179**, 390–6.

Ongur D, Ferry A T and Price J L. 2003. Architectonic subdivision of the human orbital and medial prefrontal cortex. *J Comp Neurol* **460**, 425–49.

Paulus M P and Stein M B. 2006. An insular view of anxiety. *Biol Psychiatry* **60**, 383–7.

Phan K L, Fitzgerald D A, Nathan P J and Tancer M E. 2006. Association between amygdala hyperactivity to harsh faces and severity of social anxiety in generalized social phobia. *Biol Psychiatry* **59**, 424–9.

Phan K L, Wager T, Taylor S F and Liberzon I. 2002. Functional neuroanatomy of emotion: A meta-analysis of emotion activation studies in PET and fMRI. *Neuroimage* **16**, 331–48.

Pollack M H, Jensen J E, Simon N M, Kaufman R E and Renshaw P F. 2008. High-field MRS study of GABA, glutamate and glutamine in social anxiety disorder: response to treatment with levetiracetam. *Prog Neuropsychopharmacol Biol Psychiatry* **32**, 739–43.

Quirk G J, Garcia R and Gonzalez-Lima F. 2006. Prefrontal mechanisms in extinction of conditioned fear. *Biol Psychiatry* **60**, 337–43.

Rauch S L, Shin L M and Phelps E A. 2006. Neurocircuitry models of posttraumatic stress disorder and extinction: Human neuroimaging research – Past, present, and future. *Biol Psychiatry* **60**, 376–82.

Schlegel S, Steinert H, Bockisch A, Hahn K, Schloesser R and Benkert O. 1994. Decreased benzodiazepine receptor binding in panic disorder measured by IOMAZENIL-SPECT. A preliminary report. *Eur Arch Psychiatry Clin Neurosci* **244**, 49–51.

Schneier F R, Liebowitz M R, Abi-Dargham A, Zea-Ponce Y, Lin S H and Laruelle M. 2000. Low dopamine D(2) receptor binding potential in social phobia. *Am J Psychiatry* **157**, 457–9.

Schneier F R, Martinez D, Abi-Dargham A, *et al.* 2008. Striatal dopamine D(2) receptor availability in OCD with and without comorbid social anxiety disorder: Preliminary findings. *Depress Anxiety* 25, 1–7.

Shin L M, Orr S P, Carson M A, *et al.* 2004. Regional cerebral blood flow in the amygdala and medial prefrontal cortex during traumatic imagery in male and female Vietnam veterans with PTSD. *Arch Gen Psychiatry* 61, 168–76.

Shin L M, Wright C I, Cannistraro P A, *et al.* 2005. A functional magnetic resonance imaging study of amygdala and medial prefrontal cortex responses to overtly presented fearful faces in posttraumatic stress disorder. *Arch Gen Psych* 62, 273–81.

Smith T A. 2001. Type A gamma-aminobutyric acid (GABAA) receptor subunits and benzodiazepine binding: Significance to clinical syndromes and their treatment. *Br J Biomed Sci* 58, 111–21.

Stein M B, Goldin P R, Sareen J, Zorrilla L T and Brown G G. 2002. Increased amygdala activation to angry and contemptuous faces in generalized social phobia. *Arch Gen Psychiatry* 59, 1027–34.

Straube T, Mentzel H J and Miltner W H. 2006. Neural mechanisms of automatic and direct processing of phobogenic stimuli in specific phobia. *Biol Psychiatry* 59, 162–70.

Sullivan G M, Oquendo M A, Simpson N, Van Heertum R L, Mann J J and Parsey R V. 2005. Brain serotonin1A receptor binding in major depression is related to psychic and somatic anxiety. *Biol Psychiatry* 58, 947–54.

Tiihonen J, Kuikka J, Bergstrom K, Lepola U, Koponen H and Leinonen E. 1997a. Dopamine reuptake site densities in patients with social phobia. *Am J Psychiatry* 154, 239–42.

Tiihonen J, Kuikka J, Rasanen P, *et al.* 1997b. Cerebral benzodiazepine receptor binding and distribution in generalized anxiety disorder: A fractal analysis. *Mol Psychiatry* 2, 463–71.

Vaiva G, Thomas P, Ducrocq F, *et al.* 2004. Low posttrauma GABA plasma levels as a predictive factor in the development of acute posttraumatic stress disorder. *Biol Psychiatry* 55, 250–4.

van den Heuvel O A, Veltman D J, Groenewegen H J, *et al.* 2005. Disorder-specific neuroanatomical correlates of attentional bias in obsessive–compulsive disorder, panic disorder, and hypochondriasis. *Arch Gen Psychiatry* 62, 922–33.

van der Wee N J, van Veen J F, Stevens H, van Vliet I M, van Rijk P P and Westenberg H G. 2008. Increased serotonin and dopamine transporter binding in psychotropic medication-naive patients with generalized social anxiety disorder shown by 123I-beta-(4-iodophenyl)-tropane SPECT. *J Nucl Med* 49, 757–63.

Ventura R, Cabib S and Puglisi-Allegra S. 2002. Genetic susceptibility of mesocortical dopamine to stress determines liability to inhibition of mesoaccumbens dopamine and to behavioral "despair" in a mouse model of depression. *Neuroscience* 115, 999–1007.

Zhang W, Connor K M and Davidson J R. 2005. Levetiracetam in social phobia: A placebo controlled pilot study. *J Psychopharmacol (Oxford, England)* 19, 551–3.

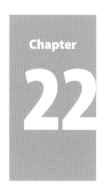

Neuroimaging of anxiety disorders: commentary

Scott L. Rauch

Introduction

In this section, nine chapters summarize brain imaging findings with regard to the structure, funct- ion and chemistry of post-traumatic stress disorder (PTSD) and other anxiety disorders, as well as obsessive–compulsive disorder (OCD). The authors of these reviews have done a marvelous job of captur- ing the tremendous progress that has been made in this field over the last two decades, by succinctly distilling the material into salient points. In many respects, this entire volume is a testament to the progress in psychi- atric neuroscience attributable to the translational tools of neuroimaging. Still, here I wish to underscore the translational potential of neuroimaging, as exem- plified by advances in neuroimaging and the neurocir- cuitry of anxiety disorders. In so doing, I will highlight several themes, spanning the potential contributions of neuroimaging to: diagnosis, pathophysiology, eti- ology, and clinical utility, as well as trends in the evolution of psychiatric neuroimaging as a field.

Diagnosis

Neuroimaging is yet to deliver on the promise of diagnostic value in psychiatry, with very few excep- tions, such as ruling out general medical causes (e.g. tumor, or stroke) of disturbed mental status. Espe- cially with DSM-V looming, there is an amplified yearning in the field for biomarkers of diagnostic specificity and sensitivity sufficient to transform our syndrome-based nosology to one of true pathophysi- ology-based diseases. While we are not yet there, the neuroimaging literature on anxiety disorders aptly illustrates the advances characterized by convergent findings of group differences sufficient to provide heuristic value in shaping circuitry-based models of

disease. We would also wish for data to guide the organization of our diagnostic scheme, in terms of commonalities across the conditions within a category of disorder, as well as distinctions between specific diagnoses. Indeed, what do anxiety disorders have in common, that distinguishes them from other categories of psychiatric conditions, with respect to neural substrates? Leading candidates might include amygdala hyper-responsivity to disorder- specific threat stimuli, as well as hypersensitivity of insular cortex. Conversely, what distinguishes among the anxiety disorders with respect to neural substrates, in a manner that would support their designation as separate, distinct disorders? One important point of differentiation may relate to amygdalar responses to non-specific threat; such probes might cleave the category into those exhibiting hyper-responsivity (e.g. PTSD and panic disorder), those showing no difference from healthy controls (e.g. social and spe- cific phobias), and finally those actually showing blunted amygdalar responses (i.e. OCD). Likewise, the fine mapping of involvement as relates to medial frontal, insular, and hippocampal/parahippocampal cortex could provide the texture necessary to "finger- print" these various disorders. Achieving the ultimate aim of identifying truly pathognomonic characteris- tics of the anxiety disorders may require some com- bination of brain imaging and other indices, such as genetic factors.

Pathophysiology

Beyond diagnosis per se, neuroimaging research is providing clues regarding pathophysiology. This is especially important, because it paves the way toward innovative, new and better treatments. For instance, neuroimaging data can help bridge between animal

Understanding Neuropsychiatric Disorders, ed. M. E. Shenton and B. I. Turetsky. Published by Cambridge University Press.
© Cambridge University Press 2011.

models and human disease. By providing neural validators of animal models to complement crude behavioral indices of validity, we are better equipped to develop more sophisticated animal models of psychiatric diseases. These models then provide a test bed for experimental therapies. One especially compelling example of this relates to the advent of D-cycloserine (DCS) as a pharmacologic augmentation agent in combination with extinction-based behavioral therapies for anxiety disorders. The inspiration for this direction of research came from the use of fear conditioning in animals as a model for anxiety disorders and their treatments; neuroimaging has helped to motivate related hypotheses with regard to neurocircuitry and to test them directly in humans. In addition, as circuitry-based models of disease mature, there will be opportunity to develop more sophisticated circuitry-based therapies via neuromodulation, such as by use of transcranial magnetic stimulation and/or deep brain stimulation. Cell transplantation and targeted genetic therapies may also one day leverage circuitry-based knowledge of neuropsychiatric diseases.

Etiology and pathogenesis

If an understanding of pathophysiology paves the road to better treatments and possibly cures, then knowledge of etiology and pathogenesis provides our most promising path to prevention. Two lines of research have been most fruitful in beginning to shape our understanding of etiology and pathogenesis with respect to anxiety disorders. These entail studies employing: (1) a developmental approach, and (2) genetic methods. In the case of neuroimaging, the advent of methods that obviated exposure to radioactivity were critical to begin gathering developmental data on brain structure, function, and chemistry from an early age. These advances also enabled repeated acquisitions in the same subjects, to plot the trajectories of brain development in healthy subjects, including those at risk for disease, as well as individuals with psychiatric disorders. In particular, in the case of anxiety disorders, there has been interest in the neural substrates of at-risk groups, such as those with behavioral inhibition in childhood, as well as those with high neuroticism in adulthood. Such an approach begins to delineate the backdrop of normal brain development, to characterize biomarkers of high risk, and ultimately to potentially identify

predictors of conversion to full disease. Such would enable the identification of those destined to develop anxiety disorders in advance, thereby providing enriched samples for studies of true prevention strategies.

Studies combining neuroimaging and genetics have begun to elucidate the variance in brain structure and function explained by genotype. Conversely, it is now possible to utilize brain imaging indices as quantitative endophenotypes to guide the analysis of genetic studies. To the degree that contemporary models of anxiety disorders reflect interest in amygdalo-cortical circuitry and monaminergic systems, it is noteworthy that pioneering neuroimaging/genetic studies have largely focused on monoamine oxidase (MAO) and serotonergic reuptake site polymorphisms, as well as differences in amygdala, medial frontal cortex, and hippocampus structure or function. This is a very important area of research, clearly in its infancy.

Clinical utility

As noted above, to date, neuroimaging has very limited clinical utility in psychiatry. Beyond the hope that further research may lead to clinical applications for neuroimaging in psychiatric diagnosis, it is perhaps more likely that neuroimaging indices will become useful in guiding treatment. Several studies have indicated that brain imaging measures can be correlated with, and hence predict, treatment response. If sufficiently refined, one could imagine a scenario whereby neuroimaging tests would be used to evaluate the likelihood of positive/negative responses to various treatments, and thus enable health care providers and patients to prioritize treatment trials in an individualized manner. The predictive power of such methods would need to be high in order to be of true clinical utility; moreover, they would need to be cost-effective.

Evolution of imaging as a field

The studies summarized in this section on anxiety disorders illustrate several important trends in neuroimaging research in general, as well as psychiatric neuroimaging in particular. Over the past 20 years, we have seen a movement toward studies of much larger cohorts of subjects, which helps to mitigate risks of statistical error, by providing greater statistical power and potentially more representative samples. With an accrual of studies using analogous or complementary approaches, meta-analyses have become more common; when done well, such efforts can provide compelling evidence based on convergent findings. Conversely, meta-analysis can help to show inconsistency of findings, that otherwise might be obscured. There are also emerging examples of studies that formally test the reliability of findings, which is an important step toward rigorous methodology in psychiatric neuroimaging.

There is also a movement toward multi-modal imaging, where data gathered across various methods can bring together structural, functional, and chemical indices to provide greater depth, texture, and convergent validity to findings. Likewise, assessment of inter-regional correlations, and methods that enable finer temporal resolution, reflect greater sophistication in assessing the brain basis of healthy functions as well as diseases and their treatments. In this context, there is a growing trend toward appreciating that named gross brain regions are often further divisible into subterritories with distinct anatomic (from connections to cytoarchetectonics) and functional profiles. Prime examples pertinent to anxiety disorders have been the evolution to: (1) subdividing the anterior cingulate cortex (e.g. into dorsal, pregenual, and subgenual subterritories); (2) distinguishing between posteromedial vs. lateral orbitofrontal cortex; (3) distinguishing anterior insula from mid/posterior insula; (4) considering the difference between ventral amygdala and dorsal into extended amygdala; and (5) distinguishing between anterior and posterior hippocampus.

It is noteworthy that the enhanced accessibility and tempered cost of imaging may gradually reduce the threshold for leveraging the power of this technology. However, with progressive focus on lowering health care costs and scrutinizing the cost-efficiency of tests, the clinical utility of neuroimaging tests may be held to an ever-stricter standard in this regard.

Conclusion

Although it has been less than a quarter of a century since the classic pioneering PET studies of anxiety disorders by Baxter, Reiman and others, the field has been revolutionized. Cohesive circuitry models have been posed and refined, informed by animal research, and most directly tested via hypothesis-driven brain imaging studies in humans. Early PET metabolic techniques have been complemented and to some extent eclipsed by PET blood flow, fMRI, and a host of morphometric and neurochemical imaging methods, as well as a dizzying array of innovative paradigms and sophisticated analytic approaches. The centrality of amygdalo-cortical circuitry, including important roles for the insula, medial frontal cortex, and hippocampus, is progressively well established. Still, with each set of findings seems to come a larger number of unanswered questions, and a growing appreciation for the profound complexity of anxiety disorders, especially at the level of their neural substrates. These are tremendously exciting times in this field. Nonetheless, we are yet to deliver on the promise of clinical utility, which should remain a focal point on the horizon to guide us forward into the future. Large-scale studies, with well-established paradigms, together with non-imaging (e.g. genetic) data, and ideally in the context of longitudinal designs, will likely yield the greatest impact in the next few years to come. Currently, there is no better prospect for such work to bear fruit than across the anxiety disorders.

Suggested reading

Baxter L R Jr, Phelps M E, Mazziotta J C, Guze B H, Schwartz J M and Selin C E. 1987. Local cerebral glucose metabolic rates in obsessive–compulsive disorder. A comparison with rates in unipolar depression and in normal controls. *Arch Gen Psychiatry* **44**, 211–8.

Bush G, Luu P and Posner M I. 2000. Cognitive and emotional influences in anterior cingulate cortex. *Trends Cogn Sci* **4**, 215–22.

Cannistraro P A, Wright C I, Wedig M M, *et al.* 2004. Amygdala responses to human faces in obsessive–compulsive disorder. *Biol Psychiatry* **56**, 916–20.

Davis M, Ressler K, Rothbaum B O and Richardson R. 2006. Effects of D-cycloserine on extinction: Translation from preclinical to clinical work. *Biol Psychiatry* **60**, 369–75.

Evans K C, Dougherty D D, Pollack M H and Rauch S L. 2006. Using neuroimaging to predict treatment response in mood and anxiety disorders. *Ann Clin Psychiatry* **18**, 33–42.

Haber S N and Brucker J L. 2009. Cognitive and limbic circuits that are affected by deep brain stimulation. *Front Biosci* **14**, 1823–34.

Hariri A R, Drabant E M and Weinberger D R. 2006. Imaging genetics: Perspectives from studies of genetically driven variation in serotonin function and corticolimbic affective processing. *Biol Psychiatry* **59**, 888–97.

Isacson O and Kordower J H. 2008. Future of cell and gene therapies for Parkinson's disease. *Ann Neurol* **64** (Suppl 2): S122–38.

Kringelbach M L and Rolls E T. 2004. The functional neuroanatomy of the human orbitofrontal cortex: Evidence from neuroimaging and neuropsychology. *Prog Neurobiol* **72**, 341–72.

Paulus M P and Stein M B. 2006. An insular view of anxiety. *Biol Psychiatry* **60**, 383–7.

Rauch S L, Shin L M and Wright C I. 2003. Neuroimaging studies of amygdala function in anxiety disorders. *Ann N Y Acad Sci* **985**, 389–410.

Rauch S L, Shin L M and Phelps E A. 2006. Neurocircuitry models of posttraumatic stress disorder and extinction:

Human neuroimaging research – Past, present, and future. *Biol Psychiatry* **60**, 376–82.

Reiman E M. 1988. The quest to establish the neural substrates of anxiety. *Psychiatr Clin North Am* **11**, 295–307.

Schwartz C E, Wright C I, Shin L M, Kagan J and Rauch S L. 2003. Inhibited and uninhibited infants "grown up": Adult amygdalar response to novelty. *Science* **300**, 1952–3.

Sowell E R, Peterson B S, Thompson P M, Welcome S E, Henkenius A L and Toga A W. 2003. Mapping cortical change across the human life span. *Nat Neurosci* **6**, 309–15.

Structural imaging of Alzheimer's disease

Liana G. Apostolova and Paul M. Thompson

Alzheimer's disease (AD), the most common neuro-degenerative disorder worldwide, is the sixth most common overall cause of death in the USA. It ranks third in health care costs in the USA after heart disease and cancer, and claims an estimated $156 billion USD in direct and indirect costs annually (Wimo *et al.*, 2006). An estimated 13 million elderly will be diagnosed with dementia of the Alzheimer's type (DAT) by the year 2050 in the USA alone (Hebert *et al.*, 2003). As a result of the global aging of the population of all developed countries, the socioeconomic impact of DAT will continue to rise. By the time DAT is clinically diagnosed with current criteria, AD pathology has already spread widely in the brain. To ameliorate the personal and economic impact of DAT, we need to improve on our abilities to diagnose and treat patients as early as possible. This requires improved neuroimaging methods to track pathology in the living brain, and improved computational methods to identify factors that accelerate or resist disease progression.

Mild cognitive impairment (MCI) is an intermediate cognitive state prior to dementia onset, in which people experience some cognitive changes but continue to do well in their daily activities. MCI carries a 4–6-fold increased risk of future diagnosis of dementia. Approximately 10–15% of MCI subjects transition into DAT annually (Petersen, 2007; Petersen *et al.*, 2001), making the MCI state the single most important risk factor of future diagnosis of dementia. A number of pathologic reports have found extensive AD-type pathologic changes in the brains of MCI and cognitively normal elderly (Haroutunian *et al.*, 1998; Price and Morris, 1999), suggesting that there is a long latent pre-dementia stage. Nowadays, the AD research spotlight focuses increasingly on MCI and even

on pre-MCI, as the pre-dementia or pre-symptomatic stages of DAT, respectively, when widespread. This is because widespread neuronal and synaptic loss have usually already occurred by the time dementia can be diagnosed using current criteria.

As treatment is unlikely to reverse all symptoms of full-blown dementia (at the DAT stage), researchers are investigating earlier disease interventions for the pre-DAT stages (Petersen *et al.*, 2005; Salloway *et al.*, 2004). Such a therapeutic intervention is likely to realize the greatest impact (Cummings *et al.*, 2007). Still, a pre-DAT diagnosis is not easy to attain, as all standard diagnostic criteria for AD to date require the presence of a fully developed dementia syndrome. It has been suggested recently to substitute the requirement for functional decline with a positive disease-specific biomarker, which will allow us to make a diagnosis of AD in the pre-DAT stages (Dubois and Albert, 2004; Dubois *et al.*, 2007). This would make it easier to recognize and treat AD earlier then currently feasible. In addition to blood and cerebrospinal fluid markers, neuroimaging has received significant scientific consideration as a promising in-vivo disease-tracking modality that can also provide potential surrogate biomarkers for therapeutic trials. Several non-invasive or mildly invasive neuroimaging techniques such as magnetic resonance imaging (MRI), positron emission tomography (PET) and amyloid imaging have received considerable attention as promising AD biomarkers (de Leon *et al.*, 2007; Dubois *et al.*, 2007).

Most early neuroimaging work in AD and MCI was based on several volumetric methods. The two most widely used methods have been the region-of-interest (ROI) and the voxel-based morphometry techniques (VBM; Ashburner and Friston, 2000). Recent development of several highly advanced computational anatomy techniques has revolutionized the field. This new technology enables us to detect and to visualize discrete changes in cortical and hippocampal integrity and to track the spread of AD pathology throughout the living brain. We can now visualize regionally specific correlations between brain atrophy and important disease-related measures such as neuropsychological tests, age of onset or factors that influence disease progression. In this chapter, we will mostly focus on the new generation of cortical and hippocampal mapping techniques, while reviewing the research findings reported in the literature. We will also discuss strengths and weaknesses of the various analytic approaches.

Computational anatomy approaches for cortical analysis

The computational anatomy field is based on mathematical approaches for modeling anatomical structures in brain images, e.g. by using three-dimensional geometrical surfaces. Computer algorithms can model individual anatomy, and they can also mathematically combine information from many hundreds of subjects in order to examine feature statistics such as cortical gray matter thickness (Bakkour *et al.*, 2009; Dickerson *et al.*, 2009; Lerch *et al.*, 2008; Thompson *et al.*, 2003), fMRI activation (Dickerson and Sperling, 2008), metabolism (Apostolova *et al.*, 2010c), or molecular pathology at the group level (Braskie *et al.*, 2008). Some of the most sophisticated methodologies rely on alignment of cortical features such as gyral/sulcal landmarks identified either by hand or with computer vision approaches followed by statistically guided detection of subtle brain changes associated with prognosis, treatment, or other factors of interest. These 3D cortical statistical maps may also be based on serial scanning of a group of subjects over time (e.g. Gogtay *et al.*, 2004). The resulting animations, or time-lapse maps, can reveal the trajectory of disease, or compare how different drug treatments resist the spread of the disease (Thompson *et al.*, 2004c, 2009).

T1-weighted magnetic resonance imaging (MRI) reveals several characteristic features of DAT-related neurodegeneration. These include progressive enlargement of sulcal and ventricular CSF spaces, and diffuse cortical and white matter atrophy. The sequence of DAT pathologic changes in the human brain follow a characteristic sequence, which is now widely agreed, and relatively well understood. The neurofibrillary

tangles deposit first in the entorhinal cortex and the hippocampus followed by the rest of the limbic system and the rest of the neocortex with a posterior to anterior trajectory; the neuritic plaques also show a posterior to anterior trajectory – plaque deposition typically starts in temporoparietal cortices and spreads to the frontal association cortices (Braak and Braak, 1991). AD is also associated with neuronal shrinkage and death, neuropil loss, and intracortical myelin reduction (Duyckaerts and Dickson, 2003), which are all thought to be responsible for the atrophic changes seen on structural MRI sequences. Prior to assessing the extent and severity of cortical atrophy on an MRI scan, one first has to isolate the cortical gray matter mantle. Many tissue classification methods have been developed to quantify the amount of gray and white matter tissue loss by assigning each image voxel to a specific tissue class. Some of the most recent tissue classifiers rely on sophisticated Bayesian methods accounting for the statistical likelihood of finding each tissue type at each location in a stereotaxic space (Ashburner and Friston, 2000, 2005) to fit statistical models to the MRI signal intensities in a scan, while adjusting for spatial intensity distortions resulting from magnetic field non-uniformities in the scanner (Shattuck *et al.*, 2001; Wells *et al.*, 1996).

The computational anatomy-based cortical thickness approaches are related to the simpler but widely used VBM method. The VBM method computes a local measure of gray matter volume called "gray matter density" (GMD). GMD is the proportion of tissue segmenting as gray matter in a small spherical region (typically of 10–12 mm radius) centered at that point (Thompson *et al.*, 2001; Wright *et al.*, 1995). GMD is easy to measure, as it does not require accurate modeling of the inner and outer cortical surfaces in each scan. The implicit spatial smoothing of the method renders the technique quite robust to image noise. The few shortcomings of technique result from the risk of errors due to misregistration of data into the common space or from potential interactions between diagnosis and registration errors (Bookstein, 2001; Thacker, 2003). The VBM methodology was recently improved and nowadays relies on alignment of brain scans into a common space while adjusting for complex shape differences (Ashburner, 2007; Chiang *et al.*, 2007) resulting in improved power to detect atrophy in multi-subject studies. An entire field of non-linear registration methods has emerged to automatically reshape anatomical scans to match a common brain template, often using fluid transformation models with millions of parameters (see Klein et al., 2009, for a head-to-head comparison of these methods).

These fluid transformations, which align anatomy from one scan to another, may also be used to create detailed maps of atrophy occurring over time within a subject, or in a group of subjects. The resulting approach, called voxel compression mapping (Fox et al., 1999) or tensor-based morphometry (TBM; Lepore et al., 2008; Thompson et al., 2000), can reveal the regions and rates of atrophic changes in 3D throughout the brain. Population studies using TBM have revealed where atrophic rates in elderly subjects are related to genetic risk factors (e.g. the ApoE2 protective gene; Hua et al., 2008), to cardiovascular risk factors such as body mass index (BMI; Raji et al., 2009) and to levels of amyloid pathology measured in spinal CSF (Leow et al., 2009). Current efforts are examining which fluid registration methods have the greatest statistical power to capture disease effects and changes that are correlated with declining cognition (Yanovsky et al., 2009).

Some cortical computational anatomy techniques have evolved feature alignment even further by matching as precisely as possible the ubiquitous cortical anatomical landmarks, such as sulcal lines. This results in further removal of possible confounding variance due to potential mismatch of cortical anatomy across subjects (Thompson et al., 2001). One of these techniques, termed *cortical pattern matching* (Thompson et al., 2004c), is illustrated in Figure 23.1. This method derives a 3D outer surface mesh of each subject's brain onto which any imaging variable of interest (such as cortical thickness, PET, fMRI signals) is then mapped with great anatomical precision after taking full advantage of the detailed morphologic knowledge provided from each subject's sulcal map. As well as matching the entire cortical surface from one subject to another, a higher-order correspondence is also enforced to match a large network of 3D sulcal curves lying in the cortex. This matching is achieved using mathematical methods from differential geometry such as covariant partial differential equations (PDEs) (Joshi et al., 2007; Thompson et al., 2004c), implicit function methods (Leow et al., 2005), harmonic maps (Shi et al., 2007a), diffeomorphic currents (Durrleman et al., 2008), or the Ricci flow method (Wang et al., 2008). The mathematics underlying these methods is often complex, with several new concepts in

mathematics being applied to ensure that the mappings match landmarks precisely while remaining invertible and one-to-one (a property ensured by using "currents"), and with minimal metric distortion (a property enforced using the Ricci flow, which was used to prove Fermat's last theorem; Perelman, 2002).

Because cortical patterns are aligned across subjects, sharp boundaries may emerge in the resulting maps differentiating tissue that is relatively spared (e.g. primary sensorimotor cortex) from other areas that are greatly impaired (e.g. the surrounding association cortices). As well as improving localization of cortical deficits relative to anatomical landmarks, the alignment of cortical features can improve statistical power. These surface-based mapping methods were initially developed to examine cortical gray matter atrophy and its clinical correlates, but they have recently been extended to show that cortical thickness is correlated with functional activation observed with functional MRI (Lu et al., 2009; Rasser et al., 2005) or PET (Apostolova et al., 2010c), and with event-related potential data (Michie et al., 2008), and PET-based measures of amyloid plaque and tangle burden (Braskie et al., 2008).

In AD research, cortical atrophy is a major area of study. The cortical thickness measurement, as a proxy measure for cortical atrophy, can be defined in several different ways, including via the Eikonal equation (Thompson et al., 2005b), which seeks the shortest path joining both the inner and outer cortical sheets, or by line–integral convolution (Aganj et al., 2009), which adjusts the thickness measure for the partial voluming of cortical gray matter voxels with white matter and CSF. One approach we developed for cortical thickness measurement is based on the Eikonal fire equation with fully 3D front propagation (Thompson et al., 2005b). It quantifies the distance of cortical gray matter voxels from the gray/white interface, progressively coding voxels from the inner to the outer cortical surfaces. The method also uses local topological criteria to avoid mis-coding voxels on sulcal banks that are adjacent to each other (Thompson et al., 2005b). The cortical thickness measurements (in millimeters) are plotted at each point on the 3D cortical surface model extracted from the scan. Thickness data across subjects are combined by applying a flow field in spherical coordinates using standard spherical coordinate system as a reference grid onto each subject's cortical surface prior to averaging the data. Additional precision is added from

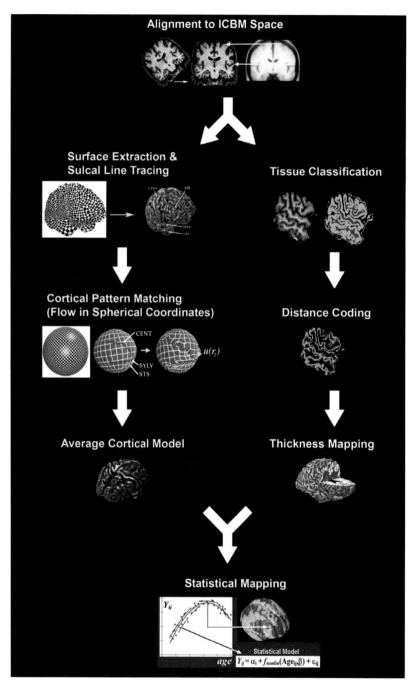

Figure 23.1 Schematic of the cortical pattern matching technique (Thompson *et al.*, 2003). After alignment to a standard coordinate space and removal of the skull and soft tissues, a 3D hemispheric model is derived onto which the sulcal lines are drawn. Sulcal maps are then averaged with the spherical flow model. Each individual's gray matter thickness is estimated using the Eikonal fire equation and mapped onto the 3D hemispheric models prior to group averaging and statistical comparisons.

the information contained in the sulcal/gyral landmarks when averaging data from corresponding cortical regions (Thompson *et al.*, 2004c). This method allows pixel-by-pixel averaging of values of cortical thickness across all subjects and helps to reinforce consistent features, identifying systematic patterns of atrophy. Once each subject's thickness data are aligned to a common space, statistical models are fitted to the thickness measurements at each surface point. The results are displayed in the form of a 3D statistical map, which illustrates the regional significance of the findings.

Regional effects are immensely important for any non-uniform disease process, as is the case in AD. In addition to regional findings, the overall significance of the statistical map can be assessed using formulae for the distribution of features in Gaussian random fields, or by using permutation methods, which randomly assign subjects to groups to find out how likely effects are to occur by accident (Thompson *et al.*, 2004c). These cortical thickness maps have been validated by (1) examining the stability of cortical thickness measures in repeated scans over time (which is around 0.15mm; Sowell *et al.*, 2008), and by (2) showing that the recovered average 3D pattern of thickness agrees well with post-mortem measures derived in independent samples by von Economo (von Economo, 1929). The trajectory of cortical thinning over the human lifespan was recently mapped in 176 subjects aged 7–87, documenting the rapid attrition of cortical gray matter in temporal lobe areas late in life (Sowell *et al.*, 2003a), with some subtle sex differences (Sowell *et al.*, 2007). Such normative data on the expected cortical thickness and its variance at different ages in healthy populations have been useful for detecting characteristic patterns of abnormal cortical thinning in many disorders, including ADHD (Sowell *et al.*, 2003b), schizophrenia (Thompson *et al.*, 2009), bipolar disorder (Bearden *et al.*, 2007), Williams syndrome (Thompson *et al.*, 2005b), Tourette syndrome (Sowell *et al.*, 2008), epilepsy (Lin *et al.*, 2007), HIV/AIDS (Thompson *et al.*, 2005a), and in chronic methamphetamine users (Thompson *et al.*, 2004b).

Sulcal landmarking assures precision, but it comes at a price: it can be quite time-consuming. Several groups are thus attempting to develop a method for automated matching of cortical features by matching mean curvature maps using information theory (Wang *et al.*, 2005), or by attempting to find cortical sulci automatically, using approaches known as graph cuts methods (Shi *et al.*, 2007b) or by fitting geodesic paths between umbilic points on the surface (Liu *et al.*, 2008).

3D surface-based analyses have documented the relentless progression of AD pathology-driven changes from pre-DAT (i.e. the MCI stage) to moderate DAT (Apostolova *et al.*, 2007b; Thompson *et al.*, 2003). The sequence of cortical atrophy follows the expected spread of DAT changes described by Braak and Braak based on sectioning post-mortem brain tissue of DAT patients (Braak and Braak, 1991)

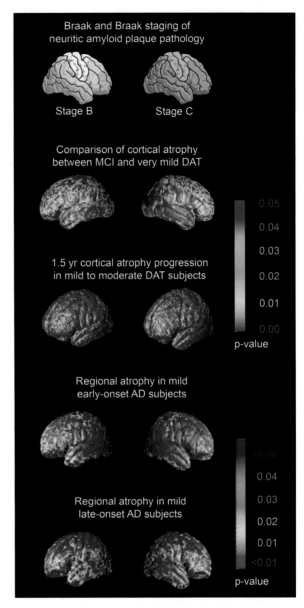

Figure 23.2 Utility of the cortical pattern matching method in structural MRI analyses. Top row: schematic of Braak and Braak amyloid staging. Second row: cross-sectional comparison of MCI vs. very mild DAT patients. Third row: longitudinal study of atrophy progression in DAT subjects (also see 3D animation sequence located at http://www.loni.ucla.edu/~thompson/AD_4D/dynamic.html). Fourth and fifth row: cross-sectional comparison of early vs. late onset DAT.

(see Figure 23.2). Among the many explanations proposed for this sequence are the notion of *retrogenesis* (Reisberg *et al.*, 1999), in which the earliest-developing brain regions (typically primary cortices) are the last to be affected by cortical atrophy in AD.

317

The primary cortices are most heavily myelinated, which may protect them from the burden of AD pathology; by contrast, the high plasticity and metabolic load of the medial temporal lobes may make them more vulnerable to AD-related cell death. Recent time-lapse maps suggest the degenerative sequence is in some respects the opposite of the sequence of cortical maturation in childhood (Gogtay et al., 2004). Cortical development mirrors the evolutionary sequence in which functional areas of the cortex appeared; the primary cortices, which support the most primitive functions, mature earliest in infancy and remain the least vulnerable to AD pathology in later life.

Figure 23.2 shows several useful applications of the cortical pattern matching method that have advanced structural MRI research in AD. Spatially detailed maps have been used to compare the extent of atrophy between subjects with MCI and early DAT (Apostolova et al., 2007b) (Figure 23.2, second row). They have also illustrated the sequence of cortical degeneration in DAT subjects over a 1.5-year period (Thompson et al., 2003) (Figure 23.2, third row). Another application is to show differences between various neurodegenerative disorders, such as between dementia with Lewy bodies, the second most common neurodegenerative dementia in the elderly and DAT (Ballmaier et al., 2004) or between two distinct phenotypes of the same disorder – as in early- and late-onset DAT (Frisoni et al., 2007) (Figure 23.2, fourth and fifth row). In the latter study, age of DAT onset clearly shows a profound effect. Subjects diagnosed with DAT before the age of 65 (early onset Alzheimer's dementia, EOAD) show greater cortical involvement relative to age-matched controls (19.5% atrophy) relative to subjects with age of onset after 65 years (late onset Alzheimer's dementia, LOAD who show 11.9% atrophy relative to age-matched controls) (Frisoni et al., 2007). Such data implicate age as a critical factor in how much gray matter loss is necessary for cognitive decline in different age groups.

Using similar computational anatomy techniques other research groups have reported consistent findings. Lerch et al. (2005) reported 18% thinner cortices in mild to moderate DAT subjects relative to healthy controls in a regional pattern consistent with that depicted in Figure 23.2. In the MCI stage, the differences seemed to localize to the entorhinal and lateral

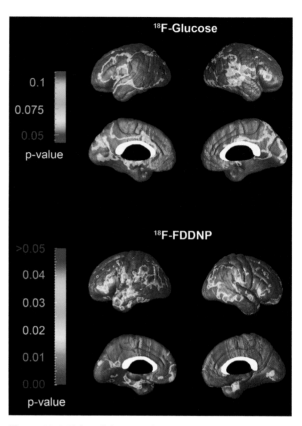

Figure 23.3 Utility of the cortical pattern matching method in functional analyses. Top panel: longitudinal FDG PET metabolic decline in a typical DAT pattern in elderly subjects over 2 years. Bottom panel: significant associations between cognitive performance and [^{18}F]-FDDNP cortical binding.

occipito temporal cortices (Singh et al., 2006). Another research group developed a set of 9 ROIs based on the regions that best differentiated DAT from cognitively normal elderly (Dickerson et al., 2009). These included the medial and inferior temporal, temporopolar, supramarginal and angular, superior and inferior frontal, superior parietal and precuneus regions. They termed the combination of these ROIs "the cortical signature of DAT". Cortical thinning in these predefined regions was robust across four independent DAT samples (Dickerson et al., 2009) and was also present in subjects with questionable DAT who later progressed to mild DAT (Bakkour et al., 2009).

In recent years, we have also used cortical pattern matching to improve the precision of mapping and empower the statistical analyses of functional neuroimaging data of DAT subjects (Figure 23.3). In a longitudinal PET study, cognitively normal subjects who demonstrated cognitive decline over a 2-year period showed 10–15% interim metabolic decline in posterior cortical areas including lateral temporal, parietal and occipital cortices as well as the posterior cingulate and precuneus (Apostolova *et al.*, 2010c) (Figure 23.3, top panel).

Molecular imaging has revolutionized DAT imaging research. Several new compounds capable of selective binding to aberrant intra- and extracellular protein deposits are increasingly pursued for their potential ability to visualize AD pathology in the pre-symptomatic latent disease stages. One recent [18F]-FDDNP study (Braskie *et al.*, 2008) examined the relationship between cognitive performance and amyloid/tau deposition in 10 cognitively normal, 6 MCI and 7 DAT subjects. We reported significant correlations between [18F]-FDDNP binding and mean cognitive performance on a cognitive battery consisting of three episodic memory and three executive tests (calculated as the average Z score from the six individual test Z scores for each subject) (Figure 23.3; bottom panel). Next, we grouped the subjects based on their cognitive performance in four groups – a highly performing cognitively normal group (average Z = 2 corresponding to 2 standard deviations (SD) above age-adjusted norms), a group performing as well as expected for age (averages Z = 0), a group performing on average 2 SD below age-corrected norms (Z = –2) and a cognitively demented group with an average Z score = 4. A time-lapse movie illustrating the progressive [18F]-FDDNP cortical binding with worsening cognition (see Figure 23.4) may be viewed at http://www.loni.ucla.edu/~thompson/FDDNP/video.html. This movie sequence shows a striking resemblance to the previously documented spread of cortical atrophy over 1.5 years in DAT subjects (a cortical atrophy time-lapse movie can be viewed at http://www.loni.ucla.edu/~thompson/AD_4D/dynamic.html) and the Braak and Braak amyloid staging based on pathologic investigation of post-mortem specimens shown in figure 1.1 of Braak and Braak (1991).

Another important utility of the cortical mapping approaches is the exploration of brain–behavior correlations. DAT patients manifest with relentlessly progressive decline across all cognitive domains as well as with neuropsychiatric abnormalities. The human cortex is known for its functional compartmentalization. For instance, the language functions are primarily housed in the perisylvian areas of

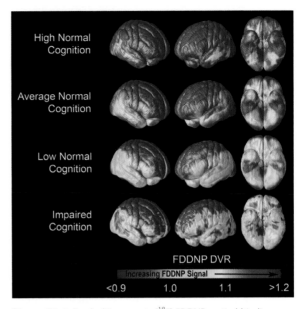

Figure 23.4 Gradual increase in [18F]-FDDNP cortical binding with declining cognitive performance (also see 3D animation sequence located at http://www.loni.ucla.edu/~thompson/FDDNP/video.html).

the left hemisphere in right-handed individuals. AD is one disorder that gives us an exceptional opportunity to study cortical specialization, as it is a disease that results in the progressive breakdown of cognition. For instance, one might expect a strong linkage between declining language performance and cortical atrophy in the perisylvian areas of the left hemisphere as we have previously demonstrated (Apostolova *et al.*, 2008). Global cognitive measures, on the other hand, are expected to map onto both hemispheres. Two recent Mini-Mental Examination (MMSE) cortical pattern matching studies confirm this expectation (Apostolova *et al.*, 2006c; Thompson *et al.*, 2001). Apathy is a behavioral abnormality thought to result from disruption of the connections of or from direct structural damage to the anterior cingulate gyrus. In DAT subjects, apathy maps to the posterior parts of the posterior cingulate gyrus (Apostolova *et al.*, 2007a). These reports could also be credited for demonstrating an important parallel between cognitive decline and structural changes as any disease-modifying therapeutic agent should in addition to cognitive and behavioral improvement also demonstrate an arrest in the spread of brain pathology and the associated cortical atrophy.

319

Computational anatomy approaches for hippocampal analysis

Despite its anatomic complexity, the hippocampus is one of the most researched brain regions in DAT. Historically, DAT hippocampal research has relied on the ROI technique followed by hippocampal volume measurement and between-group statistical comparisons. Innumerable hippocampal volumetric reports have ascertained that AD-type pathology results in progressive hippocampal shrinkage (Jack et al., 2004) which links to memory decline (de Toledo-Morrell et al., 2000; Grundman et al., 2003).

Many techniques focusing on subcortical structures proceed by first extracting the structure of interest from the original scan. The extraction is typically done by having an expert manually trace the outline of the structure on each successive image slice, following a standardized tracing protocol with explicit rules. Although such segmentation can be highly accurate in the hands of the experienced and knowledgeable tracer, it is highly time-consuming. Because it is operator-dependent, it is also prone to human bias. In our experience, tracing one hippocampus on 1-mm thick coronal T1-weighted MRI sections requires approximately 30 min. Such a timeframe makes automated segmentation techniques highly appealing.

Over the last few years, several fully and semi-automated methodologies have been proposed to segment the hippocampus, but none is currently in wide use. Hogan et al. (2000) used a deformable template approach to elastically deform a hippocampal model to match its counterpart in a target scan. This method was successful, but required 10–15 min of user interaction to define both global and hippocampal-specific landmarks. Other closely related atlas-deformation approaches have been published as well (Carmichael et al., 2005; Chupin et al., 2007; Crum et al., 2001; Shen et al., 2002). Another approach called ITK-SNAP (Yushkevich et al., 2006) uses active surface methods implemented in a level-set framework. In ITK-SNAP, the user must first determine an approximate boundary for the structure of interest, and the final segmentation depends to some extent on the starting position of the active surface. Also, the deforming surface is driven by an intensity-based energy minimization functional. This makes it very difficult to segment a structure such as the hippocampus as local intensity information is not sufficient to determine the hippocampal boundary, particularly its junction with the amygdala. The technique proposed by Shen et al. (2002) used an active contour method augmented by a-priori shape information. Nevertheless, that method is still subject to some of the same limitations as ITK-SNAP, requiring some user initialization.

Fully automatic methods do not require any user input, and are usually based on extracting and combining some set of image features to determine the structure boundary. Some commonly used features include image intensity, gradients, curvatures, tissue classifications, local filters, or spectral decompositions (e.g. wavelet analysis). However, determining which features are informative for segmentation, and how to combine them, is difficult without expert knowledge of the problem domain, and without proper features for each different problem, segmentation becomes very challenging. Lao et al. (2006) used a multispectral approach to segment white matter lesions based on co-registered MRI scans with different T1- and T2-dependent contrasts. They used support vector machines (SVMs) to combine the intensity profile of these different scans, and perform multivariate classification in the joint signal space. This will only work if segmentation is possible with only these specific MRI signals, which in general it is not. Powell et al. (2008) also used SVMs and artificial neural networks to segment out the hippocampus. Although they report very good segmentation for their data, their test size was small (5 brains) and they used 25 manually selected features, which means that generalization to other data sets is not guaranteed. Golland et al. (2005) proposed using a large feature pool, and Principal Component Analysis (PCA) to reduce the size of the feature pool, followed by SVM for classification. PCA does not choose features that are necessarily well suited for segmentation, it only chooses features with a large variance. Therefore, the features chosen by PCA are not guaranteed to give good classification results. Another common approach for fully automated segmentation is to nonlinearly transform an atlas, where the hippocampus is already segmented, onto a new brain scan, using deformable registration. Such an approach was proposed by Hammers et al. (2007), but its accuracy depends on the image data used to construct the atlas, as well as the registration model (e.g. octree- or spline-based, elastic, or fluid) and may have difficulty in labeling new scans with image intensities or anatomical shapes that differ substantially from the atlas. A fully automatic extension of the level-set approach was suggested by Pohl *et al.* (2007). In this approach, the traditional signed distance function applied in most level-set implementations is transformed into a probability using the LogOdds space. This can lead to a more natural formulation of the multi-class segmentation problem by incorporating statistical information into the level-set approach. Powell *et al.* (2008) presented several automated segmentation methods using multidimensional registration, and compared template, probability, artificial neural network (ANN) and SVM-based automated segmentation methods. They found that machine learning methods (which is the category in which our method falls) generally outperform template- and probability-based methods, and show promise in becoming as reliable as manual raters while requiring no rater intervention.

Another fully automated approach for subcortical segmentation is FreeSurfer by Fischl *et al.* (2002, 2004). FreeSurfer uses a Markov Random Field to approximate the posterior distribution for anatomical labelings at each voxel in the brain. However, in addition to this, they use a very strong statistical prior distribution based on the knowledge of where structures are in relation to each other. For instance, the amygdala is difficult to distinguish from the hippocampus based on intensity alone. However, they always have the same spatial relationship, with the amygdala immediately anterior to the hippocampus, and this is encoded by the statistical prior in FreeSurfer to separate them correctly. FreeSurfer also makes use of additional statistical priors on the likely location of structures after scans are aligned into a standard stereotaxic space, and their expected intensities based on spatially adaptive fitting of Gaussian mixture models to classify tissues in a training data set. As FreeSurfer is a freely available package over the internet, we have and will continue to compare its segmentation results to ours (Morra *et al.*, 2010). This required us to develop some extensions of the freely available capabilities of FreeSurfer, such as converting its usual outputs – multi-class segmented volumes – into parametric surfaces, allowing us to compare surface-based statistical maps of disease effects, based on the outputs of all segmentation methods.

Our group recently developed a new hippocampal segmentation approach based on a well-established machine learning approach called adaptive boosting,

or AdaBoost. AdaBoost is highly underutilized in medical imaging, although it has generated great interest in the field of pattern recognition and other fields of engineering (see Morra *et al.*, 2009d, for a comparison with other methods). The algorithm requires a small set of manually traced structures of interest to automatically develop and learn a set of classification/segmentation rules for segmenting future images. Using image-based features as input, the AdaBoost determines the combination of classifiers that can determine most accurately which image voxels belong to the structure of interest and which do not (i.e. binary output). As with other adaptive boosting methods, it is not expected that each of the features used has good classification ability in its own right; in fact, any adaptive boosting method uses so-called "weak learners", with individual classification performance only slightly better than chance, and combines them effectively using the boosting strategy.

AdaBoost iteratively selects classifiers from a candidate pool and combines them into a strong learner (Freund and Shapire, 1997). Features that have proven useful in medical image segmentation are those that can be derived from each voxel in all brains such as image intensity, tissue classification maps of gray matter, white matter, and CSF, x, y, and z stereotaxic coordinates after spatial normalization to the standard space (along with combinations of positions such as $x+y$ or $x*z$), curvature filters, gradient filters, mean filters, standard deviation filters, and Haar filters (Viola and Jones, 2004) of sizes varying from $1\times1\times1$ to $7\times7\times7$. Rather than the algorithm developer selecting which features might help to classify the hippocampus, the algorithm itself uses all 20 000 or so possible features and retains only those that reduce the classification error on the training set. Two key features give AdaBoost its power. First, it may be considered a "voting" method, in which each individual feature contributing to the classification may perform very poorly, only slightly better than chance (i.e. random guessing). Second, during training, a successively higher weight is given, at each iteration, to voxels that are incorrectly labeled, resulting in a classifier with extremely high accuracy. A good metric of the benefit of an automated approach is to see how well it agrees with human raters who were not involved with training it. In terms of precision, the agreement in hippocampal volumes between two different human raters was only about 3% higher than the agreement between the

321

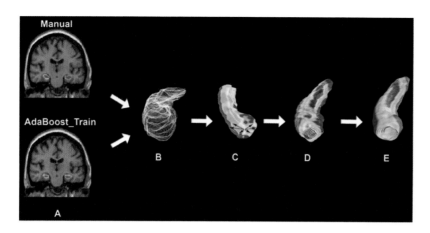

Figure 23.5 Schematic of the hippocampal radial distance technique. After manual or automated hippocampal extraction (A), a 3D hippocampal meshed model is built (B) and the radial distance to each surface point is estimated (C) and mapped onto the surface of each individual (D) prior to group averaging (E) and statistical comparisons.

algorithm and the rater not used to train it, with all values in the 83–89% range (Morra *et al.*, 2008a).

Once the algorithm acquires sufficient segmentation knowledge from the training data set (typically within 48–72 h of intense computation) it can be applied to the full data set. With sufficient computer power, AdaBoost will segment all hippocampal structures from any size data set (tested successfully in over nine hundred subjects from the Alzheimer's Disease Neuroimaging Initiative data set, ADNI) in as little as 1 min. The time required to apply the model to new data sets is substantially less than the time required to train it, and arbitrarily many data sets may be segmented without needing any user interaction.

Undoubtedly, the time saving that such a methodology assures is highly appealing and of critical value for large and very large studies. However, one must bear in mind the implicit limitations of such approaches. Such techniques may not be ideal for small-scale studies, which would benefit much more from the greatest precision possible. Thus, for small data sets, it may be most appropriate to continue to rely on manual segmentation by experienced and highly knowledgeable raters with proven high inter- and intra-rater reliability. Still, for any medium-sized to very large data sets (e.g. more than 50 scans), the AdaBoost technique is invaluable. Another major limitation of AdaBoost lies in its dependency of the quality of the training data set. Any inconsistencies and inaccuracies in the manually traced training data set would degrade the segmentation algorithm underscoring again the extreme importance of having a reliable and well-trained human rater.

Several papers report on the development, validation and robustness of the AdaBoost mapping method (Morra *et al.*, 2008a, 2008b, 2009b, 2009c). The initial validation report specifically shows that the algorithm performance compares as favorably as another human rater to one manual rater's performance (used as the gold standard for hippocampal segmentation; Morra *et al.*, 2008a). Similarly, it compares favorably to the performance of automated hippocampal segmentation Freesurfer technique (Morra *et al.*, 2008a).

Automated segmentation is a noteworthy achievement that assures fast segmentation of the structure of interest, but it is only the first step of the research methodology. It can be followed by the classic simple volumetric analyses where volumes of the structure of interest are determined from the segmentations and used as numerical measures in straightforward statistical data models. The other possibility is to subject the segmented hippocampi to more advanced computational modeling approaches. These techniques can provide 3D visualization and result in better understanding of the regional changes of the hippocampal structure. One such technique – the hippocampal radial distance mapping approach (Thompson *et al.*, 2004a) – fits each hippocampal mesh model with a medial curve composed of the centroid points of each slice and then calculates the distance from the medial core to each hippocampal surface point thus providing a measure sensitive to local atrophy (i.e. the hippocampal radius or thickness; Figure 23.5). After 3D averaging of these shape models, general linear, nonlinear or correlational analyses are employed to show the relationship between hippocampal atrophy (or thinning) and covariates of interest, such as diagnosis, cognitive scores as proxy measures of disease severity, future outcomes (i.e. future conversion to DAT), etc.

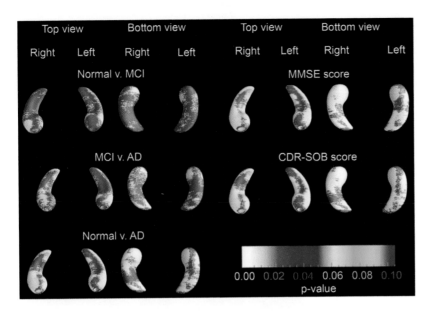

Figure 23.6 Examples of hippocampal radial distance mapping results following automated AdaBoost hippocampal segmentation of the very large ADNI imaging data set. Left panel: cross-sectional between group comparisons. Right panel: cross-sectional analyses of the association between hippocampal radial distance and cognitive measures.

Using the radial distance and other conceptually related approaches, several research groups have demonstrated astounding agreement of the hippocampal 3D generated results with the known progression of AD pathology through the hippocampal structure – first affecting the CA1 and the subiculum (Apostolova *et al.*, 2006b, 2010a, 2010b; Csernansky *et al.*, 2000;, 2005) and later the CA2 and CA3 (Apostolova *et al.*, 2006a, 2010a, 2010b). For a review of these studies please see Apostolova and Thompson (2007, 2008) and Thompson and Apostolova (2007).

Map-based analysis of hippocampal anatomy can now be performed in large populations, due to the development of the automated AdaBoost technique described above. We recently applied the AdaBoost segmentation methodology paired with the radial distance mapping approach in studies of the hippocampal data from the baseline and 1 year follow-up ADNI data set (Morra *et al.*, 2009b, 2009c). The two largest AD-related hippocampal studies to date, conducted with the AdaBoost/radial distance hippocampal approach, agree with the literature. Furthermore, the AdaBoost technique proved very well suited for diagnostic determinations (i.e. differentiating between cognitively normal and MCI or DAT or between MCI and DAT, Figure 23.6, left column) and for demonstrating cognitive correlations between global cognitive measures such as the MMSE and the Clinical Dementia Rating scale (CDR) and hippocampal atrophy (Figure 23.6, right column) (Morra *et al.*, 2008a, 2009a, 2009b). The cognitive models

(where cognitive measures were the predictors and hippocampal radial distance was the dependent variable) were found to have greater statistical power relative to the models using diagnostic group as the predictor variable (Morra *et al.*, 2009a). While true continuous variables (in this case, cognitive scores) generally associate with more statistical power than closely related categorical variables (in this case diagnosis), this finding also demonstrates that a diagnostic "fitting" of subjects in one of three diagnostic labels – even when soundly based on well-established diagnostic criteria – is an oversimplification of the progressive and continuous disease process. In our follow-up paper (Morra *et al.*, 2009c), we searched for associations between the amount of hippocampal atrophy measured with the radial distance method accrued by the ADNI subjects over 12-month period and the associated change in cognition. While all diagnostic groups showed significant change in hippocampal radial distance from baseline to follow-up, of all the clinical covariates tested (conversion from MCI to DAT, MMSE, CDR scores, homocysteine serum level, systolic and diastolic blood pressure, and education) only conversion from MCI to DAT showed significant association with hippocampal atrophy on the right.

Hippocampal atrophy is generally perceived to be a highly desirable disease proxy measure that could prove useful for determination of disease-modifying effects in clinical trials. For decades, DAT clinical trial design has relied solely on cognitive and functional outcome measures. In recent years, there has been increased interest in using various disease biomarkers as surrogate outcome measures, even though none has quite claimed that status yet. The major advantages of these biomarkers would be the ability to rapidly screen potential drug candidates in phase II trials by evaluating their effect on the biomarker instead of relying on very long trial duration to show cognitive or functional benefit. This is expected to lead to faster evaluation of potential compounds and the ability to decrease phase III trial duration and to shrink the sample sizes necessary to detect specific outcomes. A primary prevention phase III DAT trial of a successful compound that reduces DAT incidence rates by 50% (assuming 6% incidence of DAT in the 75–79 years old age group and 12% incidence in the 80–84 years old age group) would need to enroll 5000 subjects and last for 5 years (Thal *et al.*, 1997). All of the above benefits would result in substantial cost savings and would free resources for development of more promising compounds. Furthermore, biomarkers are the only feasible approach for quantifying disease-associated changes in the presymptomatic AD stage (Cummings *et al.*, 2007). The AdaBoost/radial distance technique seems to not only be a fast, high throughput approach very well suited for clinical trials, it also proved to be a sensitive, reliable and robust method for application to medium to very large epidemiological and clinical trial data sets.

Computational anatomy approaches for ventricular analyses

Ventricular enlargement is another consistent finding in DAT. Despite its relative lack of specificity for any single neurodegenerative disorder (i.e. it is readily observed in many neurodegenerative disorders and is not as tightly linked to actual disease pathology as regional hippocampal and cortical atrophy are), it is a well-documented and powerful DAT imaging biomarker (Jack *et al.*, 2004). Similar to the hippocampus, the ventricles may be segmented as an internal cerebral structure and modeled in 3D. Some recently developed automated ventricular segmentation techniques have proved to be immensely useful. The MAFIA approach (multi-atlas fluid image alignment; Figure 23.7), for instance, relies on fluid registration of several (usually four to six) surface-based ventricular models also called atlases (Chou *et al.*, 2008b). These atlases are single-subject 3D parametric meshes

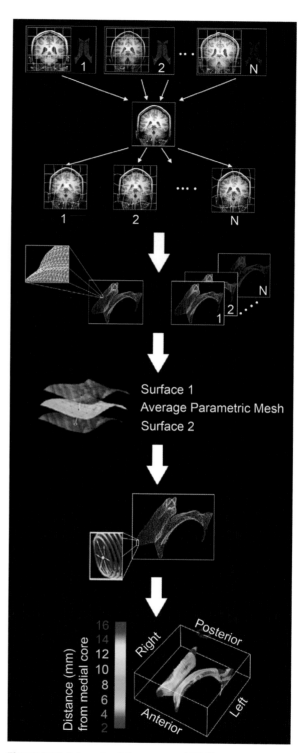

Figure 23.7 Schematic of the automated MAFIA ventricular extraction approach followed by radial distance mapping for ventricular analyses.

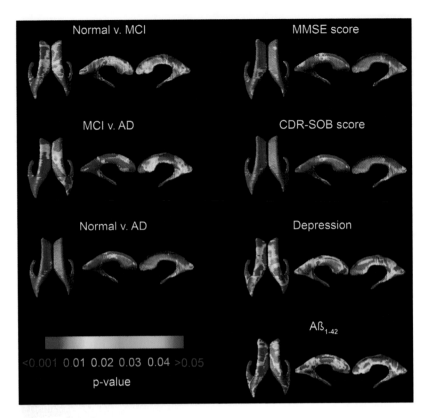

Normal v. MCI

MMSE score

MCI v. AD

CDR-SOB score

Normal v. AD

Depression

$A\beta_{1-42}$

<0.001 0.01 0.02 0.03 0.04 >0.05
p-value

Figure 23.8 Examples of hippocampal radial distance mapping results following the automated MAFIA ventricular segmentation approach of ADNI data. Left panel: cross-sectional between group comparisons. Right panel: cross-sectional analyses of the association between hippocampal radial distance and clinical and laboratory measures known to associate with DAT.

developed from manually drawn ventricular contours by an experienced rater. Using a Navier–Stokes viscous fluid model (Christensen *et al.*, 1996) these atlases are fluidly registered to the lateral ventricles of each study subject (i.e. diffeomorphically propagated to each unlabeled image). Each final individual ventricular model is derived by averaging of all mesh models obtained via fluid registration of the four to six initial atlases (there are four to six ventricular segmentations for each subject that are then averaged into the final 3D model used in further analyses). As is the case with the hippocampus, the automated approach saves time and manual effort and reduces the possibility of subjective bias. This is then followed by the radial distance technique. Averaging of four to six ventricular models for each individual optimizes the extraction and minimizes any potential misregistration bias. Such bias is optimally minimized when no less then four atlases are applied, and the use of multiple atlas results in tangible gains in statistical power for detecting disease effects and gene effects on ventricular expansion (Chou *et al.*, 2007). Using the single-atlas approach, we reported findings that agree with a-priori hypotheses of progressive

ventricular enlargement from cognitively normal elderly to DAT (Carmichael *et al.*, 2007).

Using the MAFIA approach, our group recently mapped the 3D pattern of ventricular differences between AD and cognitively normal subjects and between ApoE4 carriers and non-carriers in a relatively small sample of 17 DAT and 18 cognitively normal subjects (Chou *et al.*, 2008a). AD subjects showed significant posterior and frontal expansions of the lateral ventricle relative to controls while ApoE4 carriers demonstrated mainly frontal horn dilations relative to ApoE4 non-carriers. In one of the largest ventricular mapping studies to date using 80 DAT, 80 MCI and 80 cognitively normal controls from the ADNI data set, ventricular enlargement provided excellent power for discriminating DAT or MCI from cognitively normal subjects (Figure 23.8, left panel) (Chou *et al.*, 2009). CDR and MMSE scores showed the expected strong linkage with ventricular enlargement (Figure 23.8, first and second row of the right panel). The presence of depression likewise showed linkage to ventricular enlargement in the full sample (Figure 23.8, third row of the right panel), which could be partly attributed to its increasing prevalence with disease severity. The authors also investigated the associations between several CSF DAT biomarkers (Amyloid β or $A_{\beta 1-42}$, Tau, phosphorylated tau or pTau, as well as the ratios $A_{\beta 1-42}$/Tau and $A_{\beta 1-42}$/CSF pTau). CSF $A_{\beta 1-42}$ was the only CSF biomarker that showed a significant positive association with ventricular radial distance (Figure 23.8, bottom row of the right panel).

Conclusions

A major advantage of computational anatomy techniques is to track the disease process in 3D, revealing the dynamic sequence in which brain structures are affected. In longitudinal studies, where subjects are scanned repeatedly over time, time-lapse movies can be reconstructed to show the evolution of cortical (Thompson *et al.*, 2004c) and hippocampal atrophy (Apostolova *et al.*, 2010a, 2010b), and plaque and tangle deposition (Braskie *et al.*, 2008). The agreement between these tracking methods with post-mortem pathology suggests that detailed measures of disease progression are obtainable in the living brain, even before cognitive decline is detectable using clinical criteria.

Initial tests of these approaches in clinical trials suggests that differences between comparable medications can be tracked over intervals as short as 3 months, using cortical modeling and successive MRIs (Thompson *et al.*, 2009). For disease biomarkers to be valuable measures in a clinical trial, they must be not only sensitive to subtle changes, but also efficient to measure. As publications emerge from the ADNI initiative (Jack *et al.*, 2008), the most high-throughput methods have been those for automatically segmenting the hippocampus, where close to a thousand scans have been analyzed in a single analysis (Morra *et al.*, 2009c; Schuff *et al.*, 2009). Similar approaches for automated segmentation of the ventricles and caudates have also shown high efficiency and detection sensitivity (Apostolova *et al.*, 2010d; Chou *et al.*, 2008b). Some approaches, such as tensor-based morphometry, are ideal for mapping the profile of atrophy throughout the whole brain in 3D, and are especially suitable for detecting changes in the white matter, which other morphometric approaches may overlook. All of these automated measures show a robust and reliable association with diagnostic categorization and with several measures of disease progression, including CSF-based measures of pathology. Currently, many of these methods are being compared head-to-head in terms of their ability to detect slowing of AD in a clinical trial setting. Ultimately, the approaches used are likely to be those that detect changes over the shortest follow-up intervals, require the smallest sample sizes, and those that are the most efficient to apply.

Box 23.1. Main points

Alzheimer's dementia (AD) is the sixth overall cause of death in the USA, ranking third in health care cost in the US after heart disease and cancer.

By the time AD is diagnosed, pathologic changes such as neuritic plaques, neurofibrillary tangles, synaptic and neuronal loss are widespread.

Substituting the requirement for functional decline with a positive disease-specific biomarker (such as hippocampal atrophy or low cerebrospinal fluid amyloid beta level) will allow us to introduce therapeutic interventions earlier.

Recent advances in computational neuroanatomy have allowed us to visualize highly specific regional atrophic changes in those at risk.

Future implementation of imaging biomarkers as primary or secondary outcome measures in clinical trials will result in cost-effectiveness and efficiency as smaller sample sizes and trial duration will be possible.

References

Aganj I, Sapiro G, Parikshak N, Madsen S K and Thompson P M. 2009. Measurement of cortical thickness from MRI by minimum line integrals on soft-classified tissue. *Hum Brain Mapp* **30**, 3188–99.

Apostolova L G, Akopyan G G, Partiali N, *et al.* 2007a. Structural correlates of apathy in Alzheimer's disease. *Dement Geriatr Cogn Disord* **24**, 91–7.

Apostolova L G, Beyer M K, Green A E, *et al.* 2010d. Hippocampal, caudate and ventricular changes in Parkinson's disease with and without dementia. *Mov Disord* **25**, 687–8.

Apostolova L G, Dinov I D, Dutton R A, *et al.* 2006a. 3D comparison of hippocampal atrophy in amnestic mild cognitive impairment and Alzheimer's disease. *Brain* **129**, 2867–73.

Apostolova L G, Dutton R A, Dinov I D *et al.* 2006b. Conversion of mild cognitive impairment to Alzheimer disease predicted by hippocampal atrophy maps. *Arch Neurol* **63**, 693–9.

Apostolova L G, Lu P, Rogers S, *et al.* 2008. 3D mapping of language networks in clinical and pre-clinical Alzheimer's disease. *Brain Lang* **104**, 33–41.

Apostolova L G, Lu P H, Rogers S, *et al.* 2006c. 3D mapping of mini-mental state examination performance in clinical and preclinical Alzheimer disease. *Alzheimer Dis Assoc Disord* **20**, 224–31.

Apostolova L G, Mosconi L, Thompson P M, *et al.* 2010a. Subregional hippocampal atrophy predicts future decline to Alzheimer's dementia in cognitively normal subjects. *Neurobiol Aging* **31**, 1077–1088.

Apostolova L G, Steiner C A, Akopyan G G, *et al.* 2007b. Three-dimensional gray matter atrophy mapping in mild cognitive impairment and mild Alzheimer disease. *Arch Neurol* **64**, 1489–95.

Apostolova L G and Thompson P M. 2007. Brain mapping as a tool to study neurodegeneration. *Neurotherapeutics* **4**, 387–400.

Apostolova L G and Thompson P M. 2008. Mapping progressive brain structural changes in early Alzheimer's disease and mild cognitive impairment. *Neuropsychologia* **46**, 1597–612.

Apostolova L G, Thompson P M, Green A E, *et al.* 2010b. 3D comparison of low, intermediate and advanced hippocampal atrophy in MCI. *Brain* **31**, 786–97.

Apostolova L G, Thompson P M, Rogers S A, *et al.* 2010c. Surface feature-guided mapping of longitudinal FDG-PET changes in nondemented elderly. *Mol Imag Biol* **12**, 218–24.

Ashburner J. 2007. A fast diffeomorphic image registration algorithm. *Neuroimage* **38**, 95–113.

Ashburner J and Friston K J. 2000. Voxel-based morphometry – The methods. *Neuroimage* **11**, 805–21.

Ashburner J and Friston K J. 2005. Unified segmentation. *Neuroimage* **26**, 839–51.

Bakkour A, Morris J C and Dickerson B C. 2009. The cortical signature of prodromal AD. Regional thinning predicts mild AD dementia. *Neurology* **72**, 1048–55.

Ballmaier M, O'Brien J T, Burton E J, *et al.* 2004. Comparing gray matter loss profiles between dementia with Lewy bodies and Alzheimer's disease using cortical pattern matching: Diagnosis and gender effects. *Neuroimage* **23**, 325–35.

Bearden C E, Thompson P M, Dalwani M, *et al.* 2007. Greater cortical gray matter density in lithium-treated patients with bipolar disorder. *Biol Psychiatry* **62**, 7–16.

Bookstein F L. 2001. "Voxel-based morphometry" should not be used with imperfectly registered images. *Neuroimage* **14**, 1454–62.

Braak H and Braak E. 1991. Neuropathological staging of Alzheimer-related changes. *Acta Neuropathol (Berl)* **82**, 239–59.

Braskie M N, Klunder A D, Hayashi K M, *et al.* 2010. Plaque and tangle imaging and cognition in normal aging and Alzheimer's disease. *Neurobiol Aging* Nov 10. **31**, 1669–78.

Carmichael O T, Aizenstein H A, Davis S W, *et al.* 2005. Atlas-based hippocampus segmentation in Alzheimer's disease and mild cognitive impairment. *Neuroimage* **27**, 979–90.

Carmichael O T, Kuller L H, Lopez O L, *et al.* 2007. Ventricular volume and dementia progression in the Cardiovascular Health Study. *Neurobiol Aging* **28**, 389–97.

Chiang M C, Dutton R A, Hayashi K M, *et al.* 2007. 3D pattern of brain atrophy in HIV/AIDS visualized using tensor-based morphometry. *Neuroimage* **34**, 44–60.

Chou Y, Lepore N, Avedissian C, *et al.* 2009. Mapping correlations between ventricular expansion and CSF amyloid and tau biomarkers in 240 subjects with Alzheimer's disease, mild cognitive impairment and elderly controls. *Neuroimage* **46**, 394–410.

Chou Y, Lepore N, Zubicaray G I, *et al.* 2007. Automated 3D mapping and shape analysis of the lateral ventricles via fluid registration of multiple surface-based atlases. *Proceedings of the 4th IEEE International Symposium on Biomedical Imaging: From Nano to Macro*. Arlington, VA: IEEE Press, 1288–91.

Chou Y, Lepore N, de Zubicaray G I, *et al.* 2008a. Automated ventricular mappping with multi-atlas fluid image allignment reveals genetic effects in Alzheimer's disease. *Neuroimage* **40**, 615–30.

Chou Y Y, Lepore N, de Zubicaray G I, *et al.* 2008b. Automated ventricular mapping with multi-atlas fluid image alignment reveals genetic effects in Alzheimer's disease. *Neuroimage* **40**, 615–30.

Christensen G E, Rabbitt R D and Miller M I. 1996. Deformable templates using large deformation kinematics. *IEEE Trans Image Process* **5**, 1435–47.

Chupin M, Mukuna-Bantumbakulu A R, Hasboun D, *et al.* 2007. Anatomically constrained region deformation for the automated segmentation of the hippocampus and the amygdala: Method and validation on controls and patients with Alzheimer's disease. *Neuroimage* **34**, 996–1019.

Crum W R, Scahill R I and Fox N C. 2001. Automated hippocampal segmentation by regional fluid registration of serial MRI: Validation and application in Alzheimer's disease. *Neuroimage* **13**, 847–55.

Csernansky J G, Wang L, Joshi S, *et al.* 2000. Early DAT is distinguished from aging by high-dimensional mapping of the hippocampus. Dementia of the Alzheimer type. *Neurology* **55**, 1636–43.

Csernansky J G, Wang L, Swank J, *et al.* 2005. Preclinical detection of Alzheimer's disease: Hippocampal shape and volume predict dementia onset in the elderly. *Neuroimage* **25**, 783–92.

Cummings J L, Doody R and Clark C. 2007. Disease-modifying therapies for Alzheimer disease: Challenges to early intervention. *Neurology* 69, 1622–34.

de Leon M J, Mosconi L, Blennow K, *et al.* 2007. Imaging and CSF studies in the preclinical diagnosis of Alzheimer's disease. *Ann N Y Acad Sci* 1097, 114–45.

de Toledo-Morrell L, Dickerson B, Sullivan M P, Spanovic C, Wilson R and Bennett D A. 2000. Hemispheric differences in hippocampal volume predict verbal and spatial memory performance in patients with Alzheimer's disease. *Hippocampus* 10, 136–42.

Dickerson B C, Bakkour A, Salat D H, *et al.* 2009. The cortical signature of Alzheimer's disease: Regionally specific cortical thinning relates to symptom severity in very mild to mild AD dementia and is detectable in asymptomatic amyloid-positive individuals. *Cereb Cortex* 19, 497–510.

Dickerson B C and Sperling R A. 2008. Functional abnormalities of the medial temporal lobe memory system in mild cognitive impairment and Alzheimer's disease: Insights from functional MRI studies. *Neuropsychologia* 46, 1624–35.

Dubois B and Albert M L. 2004. Amnestic MCI or prodromal Alzheimer's disease? *Lancet Neurology* 3, 246–8.

Dubois B, Feldman H H, Jacova C, *et al.* 2007. Research criteria for the diagnosis of Alzheimer's disease: Revising the NINCDS-ADRDA criteria. *Lancet Neurol* 6, 734–46.

Durrleman S, Pennec X, Trouve A, Thompson P and Ayache N. 2008. Inferring brain variability from diffeomorphic deformations of currents: An integrative approach. *Med Image Anal* 12, 626–37.

Duyckaerts C and Dickson D W. 2003. Neuropathology of Alzheimer's disease. In Dickson D W (Ed.) *Neurodegeneration: The Molecular Pathology of Dementia and Movement Disorders.* Basel: ISN Neuropath Press, pp. 47–65.

Fischl B, Salat D H, Busa E, *et al.* 2002. Whole brain segmentation: Automated labeling of neuroanatomical structures in the human brain. *Neuron* 33, 341–55.

Fischl B, Salat D H, van der Kouwe A J, *et al.* 2004. Sequence-independent segmentation of magnetic resonance images. *Neuroimage* 23 (Suppl 1), S69–84.

Fox N C, Warrington E K and Rossor M N. 1999. Serial magnetic resonance imaging of cerebral atrophy in preclinical Alzheimer's disease. *Lancet* 353, 2125.

Freund Y and Shapire R. 1997. A decision-theoretic generalization of online learning and an application to boosting. *J Comp Sys Sci* 55, 119–39.

Frisoni G B, Pievani M, Testa C, *et al.* 2007. The topography of grey matter involvement in early and late onset Alzheimer's disease. *Brain* 130, 720–30.

Gogtay N, Giedd J N, Lusk L, *et al.* 2004. Dynamic mapping of human cortical development during childhood through early adulthood. *Proc Natl Acad Sci U S A* 101, 8174–9.

Golland P, Grimson W E, Shenton M E and Kikinis R. 2005. Detection and analysis of statistical differences in anatomical shape. *Med Image Anal* 9, 69–86.

Grundman M, Jack C R Jr, Petersen R C, *et al.* 2003. Hippocampal volume is associated with memory but not monmemory cognitive performance in patients with mild cognitive impairment. *J Mol Neurosci* 20, 241–8.

Hammers A, Heckemann R, Koepp M J, *et al.* 2007. Automatic detection and quantification of hippocampal atrophy on MRI in temporal lobe epilepsy: A proof-of-principle study. *Neuroimage* 36, 38–47.

Haroutunian V, Perl D P, Purohit D P, *et al.* 1998. Regional distribution of neuritic plaques in the nondemented elderly and subjects with very mild Alzheimer disease. *Arch Neurol* 55, 1185–91.

Hebert L E, Scherr P A, Bienias J L, Bennett D A and Evans D A. 2003. Alzheimer disease in the US population: Prevalence estimates using the 2000 census. *Arch Neurol* 60, 1119–22.

Hogan R E, Mark K E, Wang L, Joshi S, Miller M I and Bucholz R D. 2000. Mesial temporal sclerosis and temporal lobe epilepsy: MR imaging deformation-based segmentation of the hippocampus in five patients. *Radiology* 216, 291–7.

Hua X, Leow A D, Parikshak N, *et al.* 2008. Tensor-based morphometry as a neuroimaging biomarker for Alzheimer's disease: An MRI study of 676 AD, MCI, and normal subjects. *Neuroimage* 43, 458–69.

Jack C R Jr, Bernstein M A, Fox N C, *et al.* 2008. The Alzheimer's Disease Neuroimaging Initiative (ADNI): MRI methods. *J Magn Reson Imaging* 27, 685–91.

Jack C R Jr, Shiung M M, Gunter J L, *et al.* 2004. Comparison of different MRI brain atrophy rate measures with clinical disease progression in AD. *Neurology* 62, 591–600.

Joshi A A, Shattuck D W, Thompson P M and Leahy R M. 2007. Surface-constrained volumetric brain registration using harmonic mappings. *IEEE Trans Med Imaging* 26, 1657–69.

Klein A, Andersson J, Ardekani B A, *et al.* 2009. Evaluation of 14 nonlinear deformation algorithms applied to human brain MRI registration. *Neuroimage* 46, 786–802.

Lao Z, Shen D, Jawad A, *et al.* 2006. Automated segmentation of white matter lesions in 3D brain MRI images, using multivariate pattern classification. In *Proceedings of the 3rd IEEE International Symposium on Biomedical Imaging.* Arlington, VA, IEEE Press, pp. 307–10.

Leow A, Yu C L, Lee S J, *et al.* 2005. Brain structural mapping using a novel hybrid implicit/explicit framework based on the level-set method. *Neuroimage* 24, 910–27.

Leow A D, Yanovsky I, Parikshak N, *et al.* 2009. Alzheimer's Neuroimaging Initiative: A one-year follow-up study correlating degenerative rates, biomarkers and cognition. *Neuroimage* 45, 645–55.

Lepore N, Brun C, Chou Y Y, *et al.* 2008. Generalized tensor-based morphometry of HIV/AIDS using multivariate statistics on deformation tensors. *IEEE Trans Med Imaging* 27, 129–41.

Lerch J P, Pruessner J C, Zijdenbos A, *et al.* 2005. Focal decline of cortical thickness in Alzheimer's disease identified by computational neuroanatomy. *Cereb Cortex* 15, 995–1001.

Lerch J P, Pruessner J, Zijdenbos A P, *et al.* 2008. Automated cortical thickness measurements from MRI can accurately separate Alzheimer's patients from normal elderly controls. *Neurobiol Aging* 29, 23–30.

Lin J J, Salamon N, Lee A D, *et al.* 2007. Reduced neocortical thickness and complexity mapped in mesial temporal lobe epilepsy with hippocampal sclerosis. *Cereb Cortex* 17, 2007–18.

Liu L M, Wang Y L, Thompson P M and Chan T F. 2008. Optimized conformal parameterization of cortical surfaces using shape based matching of landmark curves. *Medical Image Computing and Computer Assisted Intervention, Lecture Notes in Computer Science*, 494–502.

Lu L H, Dapretto M, O'Hare E D, *et al.* 2009. Experience mediates brain function–brain structure correlates in children. *J Neurosci* Feb 24. [Epub ahead of print].

Michie P T, Budd T W, Fulham W R, *et al.* 2008. The potential for new understandings of normal and abnormal cognition by integration of neuroimaging and behavioral data: not an exercise bringing coals to Newcastle. *Brain Imag Behav* published online, December 2008.

Morra J H, Tu Z, Apostolova L G, Green A, Toga A W and Thompson P M. 2010. Comparison of Adaboost and Support Vector Machines for detecting Alzheimer's disease through automated hippocampal segmentation. *IEEE Trans Med Imaging* 29, 30–43.

Morra J H, Tu Z, Apostolova L G, *et al.* 2008a. Validation of a fully automated 3D hippocampal segmentation method using subjects with Alzheimer's disease mild cognitive impairment, and elderly controls. *Neuroimage* 43, 59–68.

Morra J H, Tu Z, Apostolova L G, *et al.* 2009a. Automated 3D mapping of hippocampal atrophy and its clinical correlates in 400 subjects with Alzheimer's disease, mild cognitive impairment and elderly controls. *Hum Brain Mapp* 30, 2766–88.

Morra J H, Tu Z, Apostolova L G, *et al.* 2009b. Automated 3D mapping of hippocampal atrophy and its clinical correlates in 400 subjects with Alzheimer's disease, mild cognitive impairment, and elderly controls.. *Hum Brain Mapp* 30, 2766–88.

Morra J H, Tu Z, Apostolova L G, *et al.* 2009c. Automated mapping of hippocampal atrophy in 1-year repeat MRI data from 490 subjects with Alzheimer's disease, mild cognitive impairment, and elderly controls. *Neuroimage* 45 (1 Suppl), S3–15.

Morra J H, Tu Z, Apostolova L G, Green A E, Toga A W and Thompson P M. 2008b. Automatic subcortical segmentation using a contextual model. *Med Image Comput Comput Assist Interv Int Conf Med Image Comput Comput Assist Interv* 11, 194–201.

Morra J H, Tu Z, Toga A W and Thompson P M. 2009d. Machine learning for brain image segmentation. In Gonzalez F and Romero E (Eds.) *Biomedical Image Analysis and Machine Learning Technologies.* Available from: http://ebook30.com/internet/internet/ 199031/biomedical-image-analysis-and-machine-learning-technologies-applications-and-techniques-premier-reference-source.html

Perelman G. 2002. The entropy formula for the Ricci flow and its geometric applications. arXiv:math. DG/0211159 2002.

Petersen R C. 2007. Mild cognitive impairment. *Contin Lifelong Learning Neurol* 13, 13–36.

Petersen R C, Doody R, Kurz A, *et al.* 2001. Current concepts in mild cognitive impairment. *Arch Neurol* 58, 1985–92.

Petersen R C, Thomas R G, Grundman M, *et al.* 2005. Vitamin E and donepezil for the treatment of mild cognitive impairment. *N Engl J Med* 352, 2379–88.

Pohl K M, Kikinis R and Wells W M. 2007. Active mean fields: Solving the mean field approximation in the level set framework. *Inf Process Med Imaging* 20, 26–37.

Powell S, Magnotta V A, Johnson H, Jammalamadaka V K, Pierson R and Andreasen N C. 2008. Registration and machine learning-based automated segmentation of subcortical and cerebellar brain structures. *Neuroimage* 39, 238–47.

Price J L and Morris J C. 1999. Tangles and plaques in nondemented aging and "preclinical" Alzheimer's disease. *Ann Neurol* 45, 358–68.

Raji C A, Ho A J, Parikshak N, *et al.* 2009. Tensor Based Morphometry of body mass index, insulin and type II diabetes effects on brain structure in the Cardiovascular Health Cognition study. *PNAS* submitted.

Rasser P E, Johnston P, Lagopoulos J, *et al.* 2005. Functional MRI BOLD response to Tower of London performance

329

of first-episode schizophrenia patients using cortical pattern matching. *Neuroimage* **26**, 941–51.

Reisberg B, Franssen E H, Hasan S M, *et al.* 1999. Retrogenesis: Clinical, physiologic, and pathologic mechanisms in brain aging, Alzheimer's and other dementing processes. *Eur Arch Psychiatry Clin Neurosci* **249** (Suppl 3), 28–36.

Salloway S, Ferris S, Kluger A, *et al.* 2004. Efficacy of donepezil in mild cognitive impairment: A randomized placebo-controlled trial. *Neurology* **63**, 651–7.

Schuff N, Woerner N, Boreta L, *et al.* 2009. Progression of hippocampal decline in Alzheimer's disease and mild cognitive impairmant in relation to ApoE status and CSF biomarkers: An MRI study of ADNI. *Brain* **132**, 1067–77.

Shattuck D W, Sandor-Leahy S R, Schaper K A, Rottenberg D A and Leahy R M. 2001. Magnetic resonance image tissue classification using a partial volume model. *Neuroimage* **13**, 856–76.

Shen D, Moffat S, Resnick S M and Davatzikos C. 2002. Measuring size and shape of the hippocampus in MR images using a deformable shape model. *Neuroimage* **15**, 422–34.

Shi Y, Thompson P M, Dinov I, Osher S and Toga A W. 2007a. Direct cortical mapping via solving partial differential equations on implicit surfaces. *Med Image Anal* **11**, 207–23.

Shi Y, Tu Z, Reiss A L, *et al.* 2007b. Joint sulci detection using graphical models and boosted priors. *Inf Process Med Imaging* **20**, 98–109.

Singh V, Chertkow H, Lerch J P, Evans A C, Dorr A E and Kabani N J. 2006. Spatial patterns of cortical thinning in mild cognitive impairment and Alzheimer's disease. *Brain* **129**, 2885–93.

Sowell E R, Kan E, Yoshii J, *et al.* 2008. Thinning of sensorimotor cortices in children with Tourette syndrome. *Nat Neurosci* **11**, 637–9.

Sowell E R, Peterson B S, Kan E, *et al.* 2007. Sex differences in cortical thickness mapped in 176 healthy individuals between 7 and 87 years of age. *Cereb Cortex* **17**, 1550–60.

Sowell E R, Peterson B S, Thompson P M, Welcome S E, Henkenius A L and Toga A W. 2003a. Mapping cortical change across the human life span. *Nat Neurosci* **6**, 309–15.

Sowell E R, Thompson P M, Welcome S E, Henkenius A L, Toga A W and Peterson B S. 2003b. Cortical abnormalities in children and adolescents with attention-deficit hyperactivity disorder. *Lancet* **362**, 1699–707.

Thacker N. 2003. Tutorial: A critical analysis of VBM. Available at: http://www.tina-vision.net/docs/memos/2003-011.pdf. Last updated 08/28/05. Accessed 03/17/07 2003.

Thal L J, Carta A, Doody R, *et al.* 1997. Prevention protocols for Alzheimer disease. Position paper from the International Working Group on Harmonization of Dementia Drug Guidelines. *Alzheimer Dis Assoc Disord* **11** (Suppl 3), 46–9.

Thompson P M and Apostolova L G. 2007. Computational anatomical methods as applied to ageing and dementia. *Br J Radiol* **80** (Spec No 2), S78–91.

Thompson P M, Bartzokis G, Hayashi K M, *et al.* 2009. Time-lapse mapping reveals different disease trajectories in schizophrenia depending on antipsychotic treatment. *Cereb Cortex* **19**, 1107–23.

Thompson P M, Dutton R A, Hayashi K M, *et al.* 2005a. Thinning of the cerebral cortex visualized in HIV/AIDS reflects CD4+ T lymphocyte decline. *Proc Natl Acad Sci U S A* **102**, 15 647–52.

Thompson P M, Giedd J N, Woods R P, MacDonald D, Evans A C and Toga A W. 2000. Growth patterns in the developing brain detected by using continuum mechanical tensor maps. *Nature* **404**, 190–3.

Thompson P M, Hayashi K M, de Zubicaray G, *et al.* 2003. Dynamics of gray matter loss in Alzheimer's disease. *J Neurosci* **23**, 994–1005.

Thompson P M, Hayashi K M, De Zubicaray G I, *et al.* 2004a. Mapping hippocampal and ventricular change in Alzheimer disease. *Neuroimage* **22**, 1754–66.

Thompson P M, Hayashi K M, Simon S L, *et al.* 2004b. Structural abnormalities in the brains of human subjects who use methamphetamine. *J Neurosci* **24**, 6028–36.

Thompson P M, Hayashi K M, Sowell E R, *et al.* 2004c. Mapping cortical change in Alzheimer's disease, brain development, and schizophrenia. *Neuroimage* **23** (Suppl 1), S2–18.

Thompson P M, Lee A D, Dutton R A, *et al.* 2005b. Abnormal cortical complexity and thickness profiles mapped in Williams syndrome. *J Neurosci* **25**, 4146–58.

Thompson P M, Mega M S, Woods R P, *et al.* 2001. Cortical change in Alzheimer's disease detected with a disease-specific population-based brain atlas. *Cereb Cortex* **11**, 1–16.

Viola P and Jones M. 2004. Robust real-time face detection. *Int J Comp Vision* **57**, 137–54.

von Economo C. 1929. *The Cytoarchitectonics of the Human Cerebral Cortex.* London: Oxford Medical Publications.

Wang Y L, Chiang M C and Thompson P M. 2005. *Automated Surface Matching Using Mutual Information Applied to Reimann Surface Structures.* MICCAI. Palm Springs, CA., Berlin: Springer, pp. 666–74.

Wang Y L, Gu X, Chan T F, Thompson P M and Yau S T. 2008. Brain mapping with the Ricci flow conformal parametrization and multivariate statistics on deformation tensors. MICCAI Workshop on

Mathematical Foundations of Computational Anatomy (MFCA), 13 May 2008.

Wells W M III, Grimson W E L, Kikinis R and Jolesz F A. 1996. Adaptive segmentation of MRI data. *Med Imag IEEE Trans* **15**, 429–42.

Wimo A, Jonsson L and Winblad B. 2006. An estimate of the worldwide prevalence and direct costs of dementia in 2003. *Dement Geriatr Cogn Disord* **21**, 175–81.

Wright I C, McGuire P K, Poline J B, *et al.* 1995. A voxel-based method for the statistical analysis of gray and white matter density applied to schizophrenia. *Neuroimage* **2**, 244–52.

Yanovsky I, Leow A D, Osher S J and Thompson P M. 2009. Asymmetric and symmetric unbiased image registration: Statistical assessment of performance. *Med Image Anal* **13**, 679–700.

Yushkevich P A, Piven J, Hazlett H C, *et al.* 2006. User-guided 3D active contour segmentation of anatomical structures: Significantly improved efficiency and reliability. *Neuroimage* **31**, 1116–28.

Chapter 24

Functional imaging of Alzheimer's disease

Vanessa Taler and Andrew J. Saykin

Alzheimer's disease

Background

Alzheimer's disease (AD) is a devastating progressive neurodegenerative disorder that is the most common cause of age-related dementia, accounting for between 60 and 80% of cases of dementia. In 2008, around 5.2 million Americans had AD, with an approximate annual cost of $100 billion. It is estimated that between 11 and 16 million people will be diagnosed with AD in the United States by 2050 (Alzheimer's Association, 2008).

Neuropathological alterations in AD include synaptic loss and cortical atrophy, buildup of beta-amyloid fragments into the "senile" plaques between neurons identified a century ago, and of tau protein into the hallmark neurofibrillary tangles within dead or dying neurons. Cholinergic and glutaminergic pathways are prominently involved in the patho-physiology of AD. While the genetic bases of sporadic late-onset AD are not yet well understood, there are several genetic factors that have been identified as playing a role in the disease. A small number of AD cases ($< 5\%$) are familial in nature and caused by rare mutations in the amyloid precursor protein (APP) or presenilin (PSEN) genes. Presence of the ε4 allele of the apolipoprotein-E (APOE) gene confers increased risk of the more prominent late-onset form of AD, and many studies aiming to identify risk markers for AD focus on these genes.

Declines are observed in a number of cognitive domains in AD, including memory, executive function, and lexical–semantic language abilities, among others. Functional neuroimaging studies examining metabolism, brain activity, and blood flow alterations during cognitive tasks in the early stages of AD have

been performed with the aim of determining the way in which AD neuropathology alters cortical activation patterns, identifying possible markers of imminent development of AD, and examining response to therapeutic interventions.

Early stages of AD

One of the major goals of AD research is to identify as early as possible those individuals who will go on to develop the disease, in order to initiate pharmacological treatment as early in the disease course as possible. In recent decades, it has become clear that a subset of elderly adults exhibit cognitive impairment but do not meet the criteria for full-blown dementia (e.g. Graham et al., 1997; Levy, 1994). In 1999, Petersen and colleagues defined the syndrome of mild cognitive impairment (MCI), where patients exhibit objective and subjective cognitive impairment but not dementia. MCI patients develop AD at a rate of around 10–15% per annum, compared to 1–2% in the general elderly population (Petersen, 2007). However, some MCI patients appear to remain stable or even recover (Winblad et al., 2004); MCI is considered a risk factor for AD rather than a prodromal stage of the disease by some investigators, where others believe it is in fact an early stage of AD (Morris, 2006).

Anatomical brain changes: structural imaging in AD, MCI and cognitive complaints

Volumetric measures of the medial temporal lobe and hippocampus distinguish AD from healthy control subjects with 78–94% sensitivity and 60–100% specificity (Bosscher and Scheltens, 2001). In AD, cortical gray matter changes spread from temporal and limbic to frontal and occipital regions, while sensorimotor regions are relatively spared; some evidence suggests that progression is faster in left than right hemisphere (Thompson *et al.*, 2003). Neuropathological changes are known to occur prior to clinical onset of AD: hippocampal atrophy occurs before dementia onset (Fox *et al.*, 1996; Visser *et al.*, 1999; Jack *et al.*, 1997, 1999), predicts decline to AD (de Leon *et al.*, 1989, 1993), and progresses subsequent to clinically identifiable dementia (Fox *et al.*, 1996). In MCI, recent research has indicated greater rates of atrophy in converters than non-converters in hippocampus, entorhinal cortex, temporal pole, and middle temporal, fusiform, and inferior temporal gyri (Desikan *et al.*, 2008). Analysis of a large cohort of MCI patients ($n = 62$) indicates that degree of neurodegeneration in the medial temporal lobe best predicts conversion to AD within one year; decreased left hippocampal volume was the most robust marker of imminent conversion (Risacher *et al.*, 2009).

An even earlier stage of cognitive decline may be represented by subjects who exhibit marked subjective cognitive complaints but no significant neuropsychological deficits. These subjects have been shown to manifest hippocampal gray matter changes similar to those observed in amnestic MCI (Saykin *et al.*, 2006) (see Figure 24.1). Functional neuroimaging studies in this population are limited, but hold the promise of significant advances in identification and understanding of the earliest stages of cognitive decline and dementia.

Functional neuroimaging in AD patients

Although structural imaging plays a critical role in understanding AD, regions of cortical atrophy are not always in accord with measures of decreased regional cerebral blood flow (Matsuda *et al.*, 2002). Functional neuroimaging studies of AD patients provide a unique opportunity to study in vivo the way in which AD neuropathology influences cortical activation during cognitive processing. We will review findings from various cognitive tasks conducted in three modalities: functional magnetic resonance imaging (fMRI), positron emission tomography (PET) and perfusion single photon emisson computed tomography (SPECT).

Functional magnetic resonance imaging (fMRI)

Functional MRI studies of AD patients performing various cognitive tasks have revealed three distinct patterns of alteration in cortical activation. First, a number of studies have suggested decreased activation in AD relative to healthy elderly. For instance, hippocampal, several studies have reported reduced frontal and temporal activation in AD during visual and verbal encoding (Kato *et al.*, 2001; Small *et al.*, 1999; Rombouts *et al.*, 2000; Sperling *et al.*, 2003) and verbal learning (Schröder *et al.*, 2001). In contrast, other studies have found *increased* activation during cognitive processing in AD compared to healthy elderly, including in lateral temporal areas in a semantic task (Grossman *et al.*, 2003) and in visual areas in a visuospatial task (Kato *et al.*, 2001). Significant correlations have been observed between activation and atrophy in the left inferior frontal gyrus during a semantic task in AD but not in healthy elderly (Johnson *et al.*, 2000). Finally, recent studies suggest that AD and control subjects may engage differing cortical regions during cognitive processing. In semantic and episodic memory tasks, controls have been found to recruit left prefrontal and temporal cortex, while AD patients appear to recruit bilateral dorsolateral prefrontal and posterior cortices (Grady *et al.*, 2003). Activation of prefrontal and posterior regions in AD patients has been correlated with better task performance (Grady *et al.*, 2003). Similar results have been reported for memory encoding and recognition, with AD patients manifesting decreased hippocampal activation and increased parietal and frontal activation relative to control subjects (Pariente *et al.*, 2005).

While the differing findings may reflect differences in clinical assessment of the patient groups, task modalities and demands, and analytic methods (Craig-Schapiro *et al.*, 2009), they may also reflect qualitative differences in processing across groups. The combination of decreased and increased activation in AD patients relative to healthy elderly adults, as well as engagement of differing cortical regions, suggests that increased activation may be due to compensatory activity during cognitive processing (Masdeu *et al.*, 2005). One possibility is that the differing results may reflect qualitative changes as the disease progresses: increases in

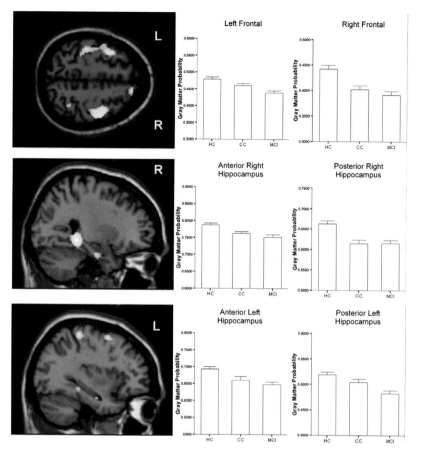

Figure 24.1 Structural changes (with permission from Saykin *et al.*, 2006) Regions showing significant GM atrophy in the MCI and the CC groups compared to HC group. Displayed at the left of each panel are images showing selected regions with group differences in the overall analysis, including bilateral frontal (top), right hippocampus (middle), and left hippocampus (bottom, $p < 0.001$). Also displayed are graphs of group differences in signal intensity from spherical regions of interest in each of the corresponding brain areas.

activity with slight neuronal dysfunction or loss, and subsequent decreases with greater neuronal dysfunction (Masdeu *et al.*, 2005). This will be discussed further in below.

A second issue to consider is the involvement of networks rather than isolated areas. During a verbal learning task, diminished activation has been reported in AD relative to control subjects in a network involving occipital, temporal and frontal cortex (Schröder *et al.*, 2001), suggesting that AD pathology results in altered patterns of cortical activity rather than deficits in any single area. This conclusion is bolstered by the finding that areas not typically thought to be involved in AD pathology, such as sensorimotor areas, have been found to exhibit lower activation in AD than control subjects (Buckner *et al.*, 2000, D'Esposito *et al.*, 2003), likely reflecting disrupted cortical networks. These findings are reviewed in greater detail below.

Positron emission tomography (PET)

Regional cerebral glucose metabolism (CMRgl) can be assessed using ^{18}F-2-deoxy-2-fluoro-D-glucose (FDG-PET) as a marker. Decreased metabolism has been observed in AD in temporoparietal cortex (e.g. Hoffman *et al.*, 2000; Sakamoto *et al.*, 2002), posterior cingulate (e.g. Minoshima *et al.*, 1997; Nestor *et al.*, 2003a), association cortex (Mosconi *et al.*, 2005), hippocampal complex, medial thalamic, and mamillary bodies (e.g. Nestor *et al.*, 2003a; for a review, see Matsuda, 2001). Increased CMRgl has been observed in limbic regions in early-onset relative to late-onset AD (Mosconi *et al.*, 2005). A recent analysis involving a large multi-center cohort (Alzheimer's Disease Neuroimaging Initiative, www.adni-info.org) demonstrated reduced CMRgl bilaterally in posterior cingulate, precuneus, parietotemporal and frontal cortex in AD relative to healthy control subjects; greater disease severity correlated with declines in these regions as well as in left frontal and temporal regions (Langbaum *et al.*, 2009).

Differing patterns of activation during cognitive tasks are also observed in AD patients and cognitively normal subjects. Whole-brain activation deficits have been reported in a visual recognition task (Kessler *et al.*, 1991). In verbal episodic retrieval, reductions in blood flow have been observed in left hippocampus and parietal cortex, and increases have been observed in left prefrontal cortex and cerebellum (Bäckman *et al.*, 1999). In rehearsal of word lists, AD patients exhibited bilateral frontal activation, while in healthy control subjects only the right frontal cortex was activated (Woodard *et al.*, 1998). Reduced activation in AD-affected brain regions and increased frontal activation was observed in episodic (Becker *et al.*, 1996b) and short-term memory (Becker *et al.*, 1996a) tasks. As in the fMRI results discussed above, the combination of reduced and increased activation may reflect impairment and concomitant compensatory processing.

Perfusion single photon emisson computed tomography (SPECT)

Like PET, SPECT is a nuclear imaging technique in which radiolabeled molecules are used to measure regional cerebral blood flow. Researchers should be aware of the importance of correction for atrophy-related partial volume effects in analysis of SPECT measures (Sakamoto *et al.*, 2003); this is also the case for PET. Although SPECT perfusion imaging is significantly less accurate than PET in detecting AD (Silverman, 2004), its lower cost and greater accessibility means that it is still widely used. SPECT studies have indicated several regions of blood flow alterations in AD: temporoparietal association cortices (Julin *et al.*, 1998), posterior cingulate (Kogure *et al.*, 2000; Johnson *et al.*, 1998), and hippocampal–amygdaloid complex (Kogure *et al.*, 2000; Lehtovirta *et al.*, 1996; Johnson *et al.*, 1998; Ohnishi *et al.*, 1995; Julin *et al.*, 1997). Greater hemispheric asymmetry has been observed in women than men with AD (Ott *et al.*, 2000). In general, SPECT results have been consistent with the findings from PET and fMRI in terms of regional involvement.

Functional neuroimaging: early detection of AD

Attempts to delineate the earliest markers of AD using functional neuroimaging have focused on patients exhibiting memory impairment in the absence of dementia (MCI) or significant subjective cognitive complaints, on those with a family history of AD, and on patients known to be at genetic risk, either because they carry an autosomal dominant genetic mutation that is deterministic for AD (PSEN or APP mutation) or because they carry the APOE-ε4 allele, which is the major genetic risk factor for development of sporadic late-onset AD. Here we review findings from studies of these populations using fMRI, PET and SPECT, and discuss the implications for early detection of AD-related alterations in patterns of cortical activation.

Mild cognitive impairment
Functional magnetic resonance imaging (fMRI)

Functional MRI studies have indicated changes in MCI relative to healthy elderly adults (see Figure 24.2). In MCI, decreased activation of medial temporal lobe (Machulda *et al.*, 2003; Petrella *et al.*, 2007) and increased activtion of posteromedial cortex (Petrella *et al.*, 2007) has been observed in memory encoding. Johnson *et al.* reported that healthy elderly but not MCI subjects exhibited dynamic signal attenuation in hippocampal and parahippocampal regions during associative learning (Johnson *et al.*, 2008) and face repetition (Johnson *et al.*, 2004). This reduced signal activation was not associated with gray matter atrophy in the MCI patients (Johnson *et al.*, 2004). In associative encoding, increased hippocampal activation has been reported in MCI relative to healthy elderly (Dickerson *et al.*, 2005). This increased activation was correlated with better memory performance in these patients (Dickerson *et al.*, 2004). These results indicate the existence of a link between these patients' learning difficulties and the medial temporal region, although the precise way in which they are linked remains unclear.

In assessing the various studies reporting reduced or increased activation in MCI of various cortical regions during memory tasks, it is important to distinguish between the encoding and recognition components of memory processing. Studies that have examined these processes separately have indicated differing patterns of activation for the two stages. For instance, Johnson *et al.* (2006a) demonstrated reduced activation in hippocampus in MCI relative to control subjects during encoding, and in posterior cingulate during recognition. Similarly, Trivedi *et al.*

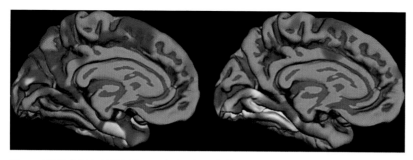

Figure 24.2 fMRI in MCI (with permission from Dickerson and Sperling, 2008) High-quality image (349K) The localization, magnitude, and extent of abnormalities observed in fMRI studies of patients with neurologic diseases depend on both localization and severity of pathology and on functional networks engaged by the particular fMRI task, as well as participant performance on the task. In this illustration, regions of cortical thinning in Alzheimer's disease from structural MRI (left, Dickerson *et al.*, 2007a) are compared with cortical areas activated, as measured with fMRI, in normals during an event-related study of successful learning of new information that was able to later be freely recalled (right, Dickerson *et al.*, 2007b). Analytic tools are emerging that enable the direct investigation of relationships between functional and structural abnormalities in MCI/AD and other disorders.

(2008a) report that, relative to healthy control subjects, MCI patients showed greater hippocampal activation and reduced frontal activation during successful encoding, while during successful recognition, reduced medial temporal activation but greater frontal activation was observed.

As noted for AD patients above, it is important in interpreting these results to consider the degree of impairment exhibited by the MCI patients. An independent components analysis of fMRI activity in mild AD patients, mildly and more severely impaired MCI patients during an associative memory task indicated the presence of multiple memory-related neural networks whose activation varied across participant groups. Activation of hippocampal regions was associated with deactivation of parietal regions across all subjects. Relative to control subjects, less impaired MCI patients showed increased activation of hippocampus, while more impaired MCI patients and AD patients showed decreased hippocampal activation; meanwhile, parietal regions were more deactivated in mild MCI and less deactivated in more impaired MCI and mild AD patients. This reduced deactivation was related to increased activation of attentional networks, suggesting a complex pattern of engagement of memory and attentional regions that evolves over the course of the disease (Celone *et al.*, 2006).

Finally, it should be recalled that a subset of MCI patients may represent relatively cognitively healthy elderly adults who perform poorly on neuropsychological testing at a particular point in time. This is in contrast to the more typical progressive memory loss seen in MCI. The differences between these subgroups may reflect differential regional involvement of medial temporal structures. For example, in a study of face classification in patients with an isolated memory impairment (comparable to MCI), in which patients could be divided into two subgroups, one that showed decreased activation throughout all hippocampal regions relative to healthy elderly adults, similar to AD patients, and another whose dysfunction was limited to the subiculum (Small *et al.*, 1999). These results suggest that all hippocampal regions are involved in early AD, and that age-related (non-AD) memory decline may be related to dysfunction limited to the subiculum.

PET

PET studies have suggested hypometabolism in various brain regions in MCI, including medial temporal, cingular, cingulo-parietal, and prefrontal cortex and precuneus (Devanand *et al.*, 2006; Langbaum *et al.*, 2009; Seo *et al.*, 2009; Nobili *et al.*, 2008); hypometabolism in these regions was correlated with cognitive performance in MCI (Perneczky *et al.*, 2007; Chételat *et al.*, 2003; Nishi *et al.*, 2010). Posterior cingulate, specifically retrosplenial cortex, has been suggested as an important junction between prefrontal areas that play a role in episodic retrieval and memory processing instantiated in the hippocampus (Nestor *et al.*, 2003b). Impairment in functions such as attention and visuospatial functions that are cortically mediated have been found to occur 8–37 months after reductions in cerebral blood flow in temporoparietal regions (for a review, see Wolf *et al.*, 2003).

Several studies have demonstrated that conversion from MCI to probable AD appears to be predicted by declines in regional CMRglc in brain regions associated with AD pathology: temporoparietal (Arnaiz *et al.*, 2001), hippocampus, parahippocampal cortex, and lingual and fusiform gyri (Chételat *et al.*, 2005), and parietal cortex (Mosconi *et al.*, 2004b; Caselli *et al.*, 2008). In a prospective study using generalized estimating equation analyses, Devanand *et al.* (2006) found that a resting PET covariance pattern previously found to discriminate between AD and control subjects was able to predict conversion to AD in an independent sample of MCI patients. Low baseline entorhinal cortex metabolism has been found to predict both conversion from cognitively normal to MCI and subsequent involvement of temporal neocortex (de Leon *et al.*, 2001).

PET imaging can also be used to assess cerebral blood flow during cognitive tasks. In an episodic memory task using semantically related word pairs, MCI patients and healthy control subjects showed differing patterns of activation for retrieval, right frontal and left temporal activation was reduced in MCI patients relative to control subjects, while increased activation was observed in left frontal regions. These results suggest differences in the way in which memories are retrieved by MCI patients and healthy older adults (Moulin *et al.*, 2007).

SPECT

Consistent with the findings in AD as well as the MCI findings from other modalities, SPECT studies of MCI have indicated hypoperfusion in temporoparietal, posterior cingulate, and medial temporal regions, with increasing hypoperfusion as the disease progresses (Kogure *et al.*, 2000; Johnson *et al.*, 1998; Bradley *et al.*, 2002). MRI and/or CT have been reported to better discriminate normal controls from MCI than the widely used measure of cerebellum-to-region of interest ratios, as measured by SPECT (Scheltens *et al.*, 1997). However, more recent research has indicated that conversion from MCI to AD can be predicted by lower perfusion in cingular cortex (Johnson *et al.*, 2007a), and that early-stage AD can be discriminated from other dementia types through automated assessment of perfusion to posterior cingulate gyrus, precuneus and parietal cortices (Waragai *et al.*, 2008). As discussed above, the wide availability and relatively low cost of SPECT relative to PET or fMRI means that it has retained its importance in clinical settings.

APOE-ε4 carriers

fMRI

The majority of fMRI studies of non-demented APOE-ε4 carriers have indicated increased brain activation relative to non-carriers. This increase in activation is not restricted to medial temporal lobe structures, but encompasses large areas of the brain. A study of verbal learning indicated that these tasks result in increased activation of hippocampus, prefrontal and parietal cortex in ε4-carriers relative to non-carriers (Bookheimer *et al.*, 2000), while verbal paired-associate encoding and consolidation appear to result in recruitment of a wide network of right hemisphere structures (Han *et al.*, 2007). Increased activation in parietal cortex has been observed in verbal fluency (Smith *et al.*, 2002) and mental rotation (Yassa *et al.*, 2008), and increased parietal and frontal activation has been observed in working memory tasks (Wishart *et al.*, 2006; Filbey *et al.*, 2006). Increased memory load has been associated with greater activation of dorsolateral prefrontal cortex in homozygous ε4 carriers relative to homozygous ε3 carriers (Petrella *et al.*, 2002). Bondi *et al.* (2005) reported that in a picture learning task, ε4 carriers exhibited increased activation in multiple, widespread brain regions, including hippocampal, parahippocampal, frontal, and parietal cortices. These widespread patterns of increased activation have been interpreted as reflecting compensatory activation (Wierenga and Bondi, 2007) or increased cognitive effort for ε4 carriers relative to non-carriers, and does not appear to reflect task difficulty per se (Burggren *et al.*, 2002).

In contrast, some studies have indicated decreases in activation in ε4 carriers relative to non-carriers, both at rest and during cognitive tasks (for a review, see Scarmeas and Stern (2006)). For instance, decreased hippocampal activation has been observed during episodic encoding for carriers relative to non-carriers (Trivedi *et al.*, 2006, 2008b). In semantic categorization, dose-related decreased activation has been observed in left inferior parietal cortex and bilateral anterior cingulate (Lind *et al.*, 2006b), and parietal activation during categorization predicted subsequent episodic memory performance within the ε4 carriers group (Lind *et al.*, 2006a). Carriers showed decreased response in cingulate cortex and precuneus in episodic face recognition (Xu *et al.*, 2008), and alterations in activation in ventral visual pathways, including medial temporal regions, were observed during visuospatial encoding (Borghesani et al., 2008). In a study of memory function, non-carriers exhibited learning-related increases in activation in bilateral hippocampal, left orbital and middle frontal, and left middle temporal regions, while carriers exhibited a decrease in activation in these regions (Mondadori et al., 2007). Decreased activation was observed in carriers in bilateral mid- and posterior inferotemporal regions relative to non-carriers during visual naming and letter fluency tasks (Smith et al., 1999).

Overall, the varying activation patterns in ε4 carriers compared to non-carriers likely reflect a pattern of impairment and compensatory processing, as for the MCI group discussed above. However, as observed by Scarmeas and Stern (Scarmeas and Stern, 2006), the mixed findings may reflect incipient AD pathology or may simply be due to genetic differences across subjects in terms of brain structure and function.

PET

Although similar patterns of cerebral hypometabolism have been reported in ε4 carriers and non-carriers with AD (bilateral temporal, parietal, posterior cingulate, and prefrontal cortex), more pronounced hypometabolism has been reported in AD patients that carry the ε4 allele, relative to non-carriers, in parietal, temporal, and posterior cingulate cortex (Drzezga et al., 2005), anterior cingulate and frontal cortex (Mosconi et al., 2004c, 2005), association and limbic cortices (Mosconi et al., 2004a). These effects interacted with age: CMRgl decreases were greater with increasing age in ε4 carriers than in non-carriers (Mosconi et al., 2004c), and hypometabolism was more pronounced in the hippocampi and basal frontal cortex in early-onset ε4 carriers than in late-onset carriers and all non-carriers, possibly reflecting reduced tolerance to AD pathophysiology in certain brain regions in carriers (Mosconi et al., 2005). The effects of the ε4 allele on CMRgl were found to be present in very mild but not mild or moderate-to-severe AD, suggesting that this allele plays a role in the development of the disease but not its metabolic progression (Lee et al., 2003). One study has found that dementia severity and ε4 status appear to be independent predictors of the cerebral metabolic pattern in AD patients (Mielke et al., 1998).

Research has also indicated that asymptomatic ε4 carriers exhibit abnormally low CMRgl in Alzheimer's-associated regions, including cingulate and temporal association cortices (Rimajova et al., 2008), precuneus and posterior cingulate, parietotemporal, and frontal cortex (Reiman et al., 1996). This reduction was dose-dependent (Reiman et al., 2005) and occurred as early as 20–39 years of age (Reiman et al., 2004). Left–right parietal asymmetry in CMRgl has also been found to be higher in non-demented ε4 carriers than non-carriers (Small et al., 1995).

Combining functional imaging and genotyping holds considerable promise for identifying patients with early AD (Rapoport, 1997; Small et al., 1996), determining prognosis for patients at risk of developing AD (Drzezga et al., 2005), and testing the efficacy of treatments (Small et al., 1996; Reiman et al., 2001). A recent study found that a combination of FDG-PET findings and APOE genotyping allows classification of MCI subjects into likely converters and non-converters with significantly better sensitivity and specificity than either method alone (Drzezga et al., 2005). In a group of APOE-ε4 carriers with non-symptomatic memory decline (characterized as "pre-MCI" subjects), Caselli et al. (2008) found that lower baseline CMRgl in posterior cingulate, bilateral parietal, and left prefrontal cortex correlated with subsequent verbal memory decline. That is, declines in CMRgl in AD-affected regions prior to onset of cognitive symptoms preceded and predicted verbal memory decline in these patients. APOE-ε4 carriers with MCI showed hypometabolism in temporoparietal and posterior cingulate cortex, and ε4 carriers who went on to develop AD showed additional reductions in anterior cingulate and inferior frontal cortex. CMRgl in these frontal regions has been reported to predict conversion to AD in the ε4 carriers with 100% sensitivity, 90% specificity, and 94% accuracy (Mosconi et al., 2004b).

Consistent with the findings from fMRI studies, functional imaging studies using $H_2^{15}O$ PET have found decreased activation in multiple brain regions during non-verbal memory tasks in healthy young (Scarmeas et al., 2005), older (Scarmeas et al., 2004b), and AD (Scarmeas et al., 2004a) carriers of the ε4 allele, indicating that the effects of the ε4 allele are observable even in college-age carriers.

SPECT

SPECT analyses have indicated that carriers of the ε4 allele exhibit greater hypoperfusion over larger areas of frontal, parietotemporal and occipital cortex

(Sakamoto *et al.*, 2003; Høgh *et al.*, 2001), and greater parietal rCBF asymmetry has been observed in non-carriers relative to carriers (van Dyck *et al.*, 1998). Differences in occipital cortex have been demonstrated to be dose-dependent (Lehtovirta *et al.*, 1996). Perfusion differences became more marked as the disease progressed (Sakamoto *et al.*, 2003; Lehtovirta *et al.*, 1998), even when carriers and non-carriers did not differ in global clinical severity (Lehtovirta *et al.*, 1998). SPECT measures indicated that APOE status interacted with age, with ε4-related differences in frontal association hypoperfusion being most marked in elderly patients (Høgh *et al.*, 2001).

Family history of AD

A family history of AD is an important risk factor for development of AD. Studies of family history have focused on either autosomal dominant genetic mutations that are deterministic for AD (APP, PSEN-1, and PSEN-2), or on the effects of a family history of sporadic AD. We will discuss each of these in turn.

APP and PSEN genes

In subjects carrying a mutation in the PSEN-1 gene, PET and SPECT studies have indicated abnormalities in regions typically affected in sporadic AD: parietal, temporal, anterior frontal and entorhinal cortex, cingulate and hippocampal complex (Mosconi *et al.*, 2006; Fox *et al.*, 1997; Johnson *et al.*, 2001), although two studies report no effect of PSEN mutations on CMRgl in non-demented carriers (Higuchi *et al.*, 1997; Almkvist *et al.*, 2003). Similar alterations have been reported in carriers of the APP mutation (Basun *et al.*, 2008; Julin *et al.*, 1998; Wahlund *et al.*, 1999), although again non-demented carriers appeared to have more or less normal CMRgl (Almkvist *et al.*, 2003). Any observed changes were most marked in carriers with a diagnosis of AD, and similar but less severe patterns have been reported for asymptomatic mutation carriers (for a discussion of the APP mutation, see Rossor *et al.*, 1993, 1996).

Family history of sporadic AD

In fMRI, altered activation patterns in AD-affected brain regions have been observed during cognitive tasks in patients with a family history of AD, independent of APOE status (Bassett *et al.*, 2006), or patients at high risk of AD due to APOE status and family history (Fleisher *et al.*, 2005; Smith *et al.*, 1999,

2005). PET studies have indicated similar results for maternal but not paternal history of AD (Mosconi *et al.*, 2007). In an fMRI study of monozygotic twins where one is affected with AD, the affected twin exhibited greater bilateral parietal involvement than the unaffected twin during visuospatial and verbal working memory tasks, and decreased dorsolateral prefrontal cortex activation was observed during a visuospatial working memory task (Lipton *et al.*, 2003). It should be noted that a first-degree family history of AD appears to influence the expression of APOE-ε4, modulating hippocampal and medial temporal response in encoding (Johnson *et al.*, 2006b), face recognition (Xu *et al.*, 2008), and self-appraisal (Johnson *et al.*, 2007b).

Subjective cognitive complaints

While structural imaging studies have indicated atrophy in areas known to be affected by MCI and AD in older adults with significant subjective cognitive complaints (Saykin *et al.*, 2006; Wang *et al.*, 2006c), very little research has been published to date examining functional imaging measures in these subjects. An early study using FDG-PET indicates that a decline in self-reported use of mnemonics (i.e. a subtype of subjective memory complaint) correlates with decreased frontal lobe function, although no effects were observed on parietal or temporal metabolism (Small *et al.*, 1994). A recent PET study indicated that subjects with significant subjective cognitive complaints had reduced CMRgl in parietotemporal and parahippocampal regions. This effect was found to interact with APOE status: ε4 carriers with cognitive complaints showing the lower CMRgl than either carriers with no cognitive complaints, or non-carriers (Mosconi *et al.*, 2008). Further research is clearly needed in this important area.

Functional connectivity

Researchers have recently begun to focus on the possibility that deficits in AD may be caused by declines in functional connectivity between regions rather than solely to focal neurodegeneration (e.g. Matsuda *et al.*, 2002). Functional connectivity refers to the functional links between brain regions, and is measured by the temporal synchrony and correlations in activation between distinct brain regions (Wang *et al.*, 2007). This connectivity can be assessed during performance of a cognitive task or while at rest, using data from a variety of methodologies including fMRI and PET.

Functional connectivity during cognitive tasks

Changes in functional brain connectivity in AD have also been explored in AD using memory tasks. In a study of short-term verbal memory, Grady *et al.* (2001) found a reduced correlation between activation in prefrontal regions and hippocampus in AD patients relative to control subjects, and suggest that a reduction in integrated activity within a distributed network including these areas may underlie memory breakdowns in AD. Similarly, Lekeu *et al.* (2003) reported a correlation between performance on a free recall task and right frontal regions, while performance on cued recall was correlated with residual parahippocampal activity. These results suggest that impairments in retrieval may be due to a loss of functional connectivity between frontal and parahippocampal regions, and that patients performed this task by retrieving semantic associations in the absence of recollection. In MCI, decreased connectivity has been observed relative to healthy control subjects between fusiform gyrus and visual/medial frontal areas when performing a face-matching task (Bokde *et al.*, 2006), and between the hippocampus and prefrontal, temporal, parietal and cerebellar regions in a memory task (Bai *et al.*, 2009).

Enhanced connectivity has also been reported in at-risk subjects. In an associative memory task (face–name learning), ε4 carriers showed strengthened connectivity of hippocampus to anterior cingulate, inferior parietal/postcentral gyrus region, and caudate nucleus (Bartrés-Faz *et al.*, 2008). The authors interpreted this as reflecting additional activity in cortico-subcortical network. This finding may indicate compensatory increases in those at risk.

Desgranges *et al.* (1998) used PET to assess the relationships between cognitive decline and CMRgl. They found an association between verbal episodic memory impairment and changes in a network including limbic structures, and right parietotemporal and frontal association cortices; between tests of short-term memory and posterior association cortex; and between tests of semantic memory scores correlated with activity in left temporoparietal and frontal association cortices. Such studies of functional anatomic links to cognitive performance are an important extension of research focusing on focal neurodegeneration.

Functional connectivity in the resting state

Interpretation of alterations in functional connectivity associated with performance on cognitive tasks has been complicated by several factors. First, decreased neural metabolism is associated with declines in cognitive performance (Small *et al.*, 2000, 2002; de Leon *et al.*, 2001), meaning that low activation during cognitive tasks in AD could be the cause or the consequence of poor performance (Rombouts and Scheltens, 2005). Second, performance of cognitive tasks can be difficult for AD patients. In addition, there may be compensatory changes during early stages of decline. Therefore, additional alternative approaches to assessing functional brain changes are desirable (Rombouts and Scheltens, 2005).

In order to get around these issues, a number of studies have examined the default resting state network in AD. The default network is a set of functionally intercorrelated regions, including posterior cingulate/precuneus, inferior parietal, left dorsolateral frontal, and left lateral inferior frontal cortex, left inferior temporal gyrus, medial frontal regions, and the right amygdala, that are often deactivated when a subject performs a task that requires attention, relative to when the subject is at rest in the scanner (Shulman *et al.*, 1997).

Decreased resting state connectivity has been observed in AD patients in several regions: between frontal and parietal regions (Horwitz *et al.*, 1987; Wang *et al.*, 2007), between hippocampus and various brain regions including medial prefrontal cortex, ventral anterior cingulate cortex and posterior cingulate cortex (Wang *et al.*, 2006b; Zhou *et al.*, 2008); between cerebellum and cortical, subcortical, and limbic regions, especially frontal cortex (Allen *et al.*, 2007); in the posterior cingulate and hippocampus (Greicius *et al.*, 2004) (see Figure 24.3); and between entorhinal cortex and limbic and paralimbic systems, including the posterior cingulate cortex, anterior cingulate cortex, lingual gyri and left middle temporal gyrus (Hirao *et al.*, 2006). While decreased connectivity has been observed between anterior and posterior regions, studies have indicated *increased* connectivity within lobes, and disruptions are observed in anti-correlated networks (mutually inhibitory connections)

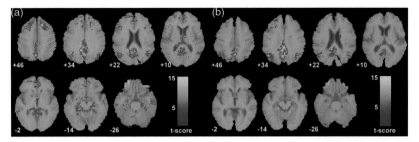

Figure 24.3 Default mode network (with permission from Greicius *et al.*, 2004) Default-mode network in healthy elderly and AD subjects (Washington University data). Axial images showing the default-mode network for the healthy elderly (A) and AD (B) groups. The blue arrows indicate the PCC. The hippocampus and underlying entorhinal cortex (green arrows) were detected bilaterally in healthy elderly subjects (A) but only in the right hemisphere in the AD group (B). Joint height and extent thresholds of $p < 0.0001$ were used to determine significant clusters. The numbers beneath each image refer to the *z* coordinate in Talairach space. *T* score bars are shown at right. Functional images were overlaid on the group-averaged structural image.

(Wang *et al.*, 2007). Some researchers have suggested that AD pathophysiology may be associated with abnormalities in resting-state low-frequency fluctuations (< 0.08 Hz) between posterior cingulate and hippocampus (Greicius *et al.*, 2004), within the hippocampus (Li *et al.*, 2002), and in occipital and temporal lobes and posterior cingulate cortex/precuneus (He *et al.*, 2007). In the latter study, the decrease in functional connectivity was correlated with disease severity as measured by scores on the Mini-Mental State Exam.

An important property of functional networks in healthy subjects is that they are "small-world" networks, characterized by many connections over a short distance in addition to a few long-distance connections in random places (for a recent review and discussion of these networks, see Guye *et al.*, 2008). A loss of small-world properties has been observed in functional networks in AD, with a lower clustering coefficient both overall and within the hippocampi (Supekar *et al.*, 2008). In the latter study, AD and control subjects could be accurately distinguished on the basis of the network clustering coefficient alone, with a sensitivity of 72% and a specificity of 78%. Another study found that AD and control subjects could be discriminated at 83% accuracy based on the correlation and anticorrelation coefficients of intrinsically anticorrelated (i.e. mutually inhibitory) networks, using leave-one-out cross-validation (Wang *et al.*, 2006a). Additionally, a greater persistence of resting fMRI noise has been reported in AD than control subjects in the medial and lateral temporal lobes, insula, dorsal cingulate/medial premotor cortex, and left pre- and post-central gyrus (Maxim *et al.*, 2005), and reduced task-related deactivation of

the default-mode network has been observed in AD patients relative to healthy control subjects during an episodic encoding task (Persson *et al.*, 2008).

Very little research on functional connectivity has been done in MCI, although a recent fMRI study indicates that reduced connectivity is observed in MCI relative to control subjects between both hippocampi and posterior cingulate (Sorg *et al.*, 2007), consistent with the findings in AD.

Neuroimaging of drug effects
A number of studies have explored the effects of cholinergic medications in AD and MCI using fMRI. For example, in AD, cholinesterase inhibitors have been found to improve visuoattentional response in extrastriate and frontoparietal regions in AD (Bentley *et al.*, 2008), and in face recognition in fusiform gyrus (Kircher *et al.*, 2005).

A recent study examining memory encoding and retrieval during face recognition found that acute treatment with galantamine (a single dose) resulted in increased activation during memory retrieval in posterior cingulate, left inferior parietal, and anterior temporal regions in MCI, and increased hippocampal activation during memory encoding in AD. In contrast, more prolonged exposure (5 days) resulted in *decreased* activation in posterior cingulate and prefrontal regions during retrieval in MCI, and in hippocampus during encoding in AD (Goekoop *et al.*, 2006). Seven-day treatment with galantamine resulted in increased hippocampal activation during a spatial navigation task (Grön *et al.*, 2006).

More extended cholinergic treatment (approximately 6 weeks) in MCI has been shown to increase

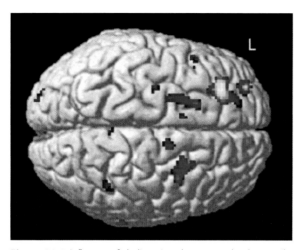

Figure 24.4 Influence of cholinergic enhancement by donepezil on fMRI activation during working memory (from Saykin et al., 2004, with permission). Statistical parametric maps displaying the results of the group × time interaction analysis. This image shows regions that were more activated in patients with MCI than healthy controls at Time 2 (post-medication) compared with Time 1 (baseline).

frontal activation during an n-back working memory task; this activation was correlated with improvement in task performance and baseline hippocampal volume (Saykin *et al.*, 2004) (see Figure 24.4). In another study with 12–24 weeks of donepezil treatment, MCI patients showed increased frontal activation during delayed-response visual memory task, while a placebo group showed decreased frontal activation (Petrella *et al.*, 2009).

In sum, these findings provide evidence for (a) important involvement of cholinergic system in memory function in MCI and AD; (b) different functional status of cholinergic system in these groups; and (c) the sensitivity of fMRI as a biomarker for assessment of pharmacologically induced changes.

Amyloid imaging

A variety of tracers have recently been developed to allow in-vivo imaging of the beta-amyloid (Aβ) deposits that are one of the neuropathological hallmarks of AD. These include [F-18]BAY94–9172, [F-18]AV-45, [F-18]AH110690, and [F-18]FDDNP (for a recent discussion, see Klunk and Mathis, 2008). The most widely used of these agents, however, is Pittsburgh Compound B (PiB), whose use was first reported in 2004 (Klunk *et al.*, 2004). This technique

involves PET imaging with the positron emitter carbon-11. In case studies, a good correspondence has been demonstrated between in-vivo measures of Aβ using PiB and post-mortem measures (Ikonomovic *et al.*, 2008; Bacskai *et al.*, 2007), suggesting that it is a valid marker for these deposits.

Increased PiB uptake, indicating Aβ deposits, has been demonstrated in MCI (e.g. Kemppainen *et al.*, 2007, Pike *et al.*, 2007, Forsberg *et al.*, 2008) (see Figure 24.5), across all subtypes (Wolk *et al.*, 2009), and, interestingly, in some cognitively normal elderly adults (e.g. Aizenstein *et al.*, 2008; Mintun *et al.*, 2006). This uptake is correlated with measures of episodic memory in both cognitively normal and MCI subjects (Pike *et al.*, 2007). A recent study indicated correlations between Aβ deposits, hippocampal atrophy, and measures of episodic memory, suggesting that Aβ-induced hippocampal atrophy may drive episodic memory declines in healthy elderly and MCI (Mormino *et al.*, 2009). Amyloid imaging is clearly an important avenue for future research to expand our understanding of the neural substrates of cognitive impairment in MCI and AD as well as presymptomatic stages of disease.

Conclusions and future directions

Neuroimaging can be expected to take on an increasingly important role in research and patient care for Alzheimer's disease, prodromal states and related neurodegenerative disorders. Until recently, the major role of imaging was to help with a clinical diagnosis of AD by exclusion of other etiologies for cognitive decline. Now, specific patterns of antecedent structural changes and metabolic profiles have been identified on MRI and FDG-PET, with a continuous performance test (CPT) code for differential diagnosis of dementia now being available for PET. Molecular imaging of amyloid deposition as a measure of plaque burden seems poised to become a major surrogate biomarker for disease status in AD. In the near future, preclinical diagnosis of AD by PET and MRI, coupled with lumbar puncture for CSF biomarker studies (e.g. Koivunen *et al.*, 2008), will likely become widespread. Functional MRI including connectivity analyses, ASL perfusion, MRS, and iron detection studies also suggest potential roles for these MR-based modalities that can provide complementary information. However, more research is required, particularly of a longitudinal nature. Although approved pharmacological interventions to

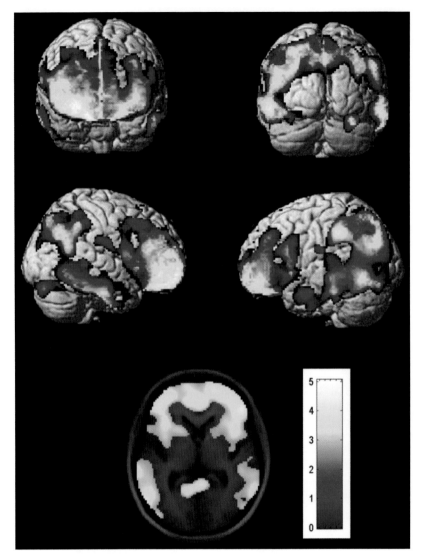

Figure 24.5 PiB (with permission from Kemppainen *et al.*, 2007) Visualization of the results of Statistical Parametric Mapping analysis. The regions with significant increases (corrected *p* value at cluster level < 0.01) in *N*-methyl-[^{11}C]2-(4'-methylaminophenyl)-6-hydroxybenzothiazole [^{11}C]PIB uptake in patients with mild cognitive impairment vs control subjects visualized using surface rendering are shown in two upper rows. The red-yellow scale indicates the level of significance of the differences in [^{11}C]PIB uptake (yellow = most significant difference). The lowest row depicts an axial slice visualizing the increase in the subcortical structures and related color bar indicating *T* values. Image is presented in the neurologic convention (right is right).

date have shown limited disease modification properties, there is a rich drug development pipeline for AD with numerous promising targets. These interventions are likely to have disease-modifying or preventative potential only if administered very early in the course of illness, perhaps a decade or more before an AD diagnosis. Neuroimaging will play an increasing role in early detection (Weiner, 2009), and is likely to take on an equally important role as a biomarker for treatment response (e.g. Dickerson and Sperling, 2005; Saykin *et al.*, 2004; Petrella *et al.*, 2009; Klunk *et al.*, 2004; Klunk and Mathis, 2008). The NIA-sponsored Alzheimer's Disease Neuroimaging Initiative (ADNI)

is assessing the role of many of the imaging methods described in this chapter as biomarkers for early detection and progression in AD. In addition to the US ADNI, parallel efforts have been initiated worldwide including consortia in Europe, Australia, Japan, and most recently China. This is the largest neuroimaging research initiative ever launched and should lead to advances not only in AD but also in the design of clinical trials employing neuroimaging methodology. All of these research efforts can be expected to yield critical new knowledge that will impact the care of patients suffering from this devastating disease.

Patients with Alzheimer's disease (AD) show altered patterns of cortical activation during various tasks that tap cognitive processing, including memory, visuospatial, and semantic processing.

In populations at risk for AD, such as patients with mild cognitive impairment (MCI) or carriers of the ε4 allele of the APOE gene, both increases and decreases in activation have been reported, depending on the task, modality, and region.

These results may reflect qualitative changes in activation as the disease progresses (e.g. increased activation reflects compensatory activation, while decreased activation reflects more impaired processing as the disease progresses).

Changes also likely occur in networks involving topographically distributed cortical regions, both at rest and during cognitive processing.

Neuroimaging biomarkers are likely to prove useful in a number of areas, including imaging of treatment response, and earlier detection of AD.

Exploration of network-level changes in functional connectivity, for example using diffusion tensor imaging (DTI), will add to our current knowledge of activation changes in individual cortical regions.

Amyloid imaging (e.g. PET imaging with Pittsburgh compound B) is an important new direction to expanding our understanding of neurological changes in MCI and AD.

References

Aizenstein H J, Nebes R D, Saxton J A, et al. 2008. Frequent amyloid deposition without significant cognitive impairment among the elderly. *Arch Neurol* **65**, 1509–17.

Allen G, Barnard H, McColl R, Hester A L, Fields J A and Weiner M F. 2007. Reduced hippocampal functional connectivity in Alzheimer disease. *Arch Neurol* **64**, 1482–7.

Almkvist O, Axelman K, Basun H et al. 2003. Clinical findings in nondemented mutation carriers predisposed to Alzheimer's disease: A model of mild cognitive impairment. *Acta Neurol Scand Suppl* **179**, 77–82.

Alzheimer's Association. 2008. Alzheimer's disease facts and figures. *Alzheimer's Dementia* **4**, 110–33.

Arnaiz E, Jelic V, Almkvist O, et al. 2001. Impaired cerebral glucose metabolism and cognitive functioning predict deterioration in mild cognitive impairment. *Neuroreport* **12**, 851–5.

Bäckman L, Andersson J L, Nyberg L, Winblad B, Nordberg A and Almkvist O. 1999. Brain regions associated with episodic retrieval in normal aging and Alzheimer's disease. *Neurology* **52**, 1861–70.

Bacskai B J, Frosch M P, Freeman S H, et al. 2007. Molecular imaging with Pittsburgh Compound B confirmed at autopsy: A case report. *Arch Neurol* **64**, 431–4.

Bai F, Zhang Z, Watson D R, et al. 2009. Abnormal functional connectivity of hippocampus during episodic memory retrieval processing network in amnestic mild cognitive impairment. *Biol Psychiatry* **65**, 951–8.

Bartrés-Faz D, Serra-Grabulosa J M, Sun F T, et al. 2008. Functional connectivity of the hippocampus in elderly with mild memory dysfunction carrying the APOE epsilon4 allele. *Neurobiol Aging* **29**, 1644–53.

Bassett S S, Yousem D M, Cristinzio C, et al. 2006. Familial risk for Alzheimer's disease alters fMRI activation patterns. *Brain* **129**, 1229–39.

Basun H, Bogdanovic N, Ingelsson M, et al. 2008. Clinical and neuropathological features of the arctic APP gene mutation causing early-onset Alzheimer disease. *Arch Neurol* **65**, 499–505.

Becker J T, Mintun M A, Aleva K, Wiseman M B, Nichols T and Dekosky S T. 1996a. Alterations in functional neuroanatomical connectivity in Alzheimer's disease. Positron emission tomography of auditory verbal short-term memory. *Ann N Y Acad Sci* **777**, 239–42.

Becker J T, Mintun M A, Aleva K, Wiseman M B, Nichols T and Dekosky S T. 1996b. Compensatory reallocation of brain resources supporting verbal episodic memory in Alzheimer's disease. *Neurology* **46**, 692–700.

Bentley P, Driver J and Dolan R J 2008. Cholinesterase inhibition modulates visual and attentional brain responses in Alzheimer's disease and health. *Brain* **131**, 409–24.

Bokde A L, Lopez-Bayo P, Meindl T, et al. 2006. Functional connectivity of the fusiform gyrus during a face-matching task in subjects with mild cognitive impairment *Brain* **129**, 1113–24.

Bondi M W, Houston W S, Eyler L T and Brown G G. 2005. fMRI evidence of compensatory mechanisms in older adults at genetic risk for Alzheimer's disease. *Neurology* **64**, 501–8.

Bookheimer S Y, Strojwas M H, Cohen M S, et al. 2000. Patterns of brain activation in people at risk for Alzheimer's disease. *N Engl J Med* **343**, 450–6.

Borghesani P R, Johnson L C, Shelton A L, et al. 2008. Altered medial temporal lobe responses during visuospatial encoding in healthy APOEε4 carriers. *Neurobiol Aging* **29**, 981–91.

Bosscher L and Scheltens P H. 2001. *MRI of the Temporal Lobe. Evidence-Based Dementia.* Oxford: Blackwell.

Bradley K M, O'sullivan V T, Soper N D, et al. 2002. Cerebral perfusion SPECT correlated with Braak pathological stage in Alzheimer's disease. *Brain* **125**, 1772–81.

Buckner R L, Snyder A Z, Sanders A L, Raichle M E and Morris J C. 2000. Functional brain imaging of young, nondemented, and demented older adults. *J Cogn Neurosci* **12** (Suppl. 2), 24–34.

Burggren A C, Small G W, Sabb F W and Bookheimer S. 2002. Specificity of brain activation patterns in people at genetic risk for Alzheimer disease. *Am J Geriatr Psychiatry* **10**, 44–51.

Caselli R J, Chen K, Lee W, Alexander G E and Reiman E M. 2008. Correlating cerebral hypometabolism with future memory decline in subsequent converters to amnestic pre-mild cognitive impairment. *Arch Neurol* **65**, 1231–6.

Celone K A, Calhoun V D, Dickerson B C, *et al.* 2006. Alterations in memory networks in mild cognitive impairment and Alzheimer's disease: An independent component analysis. *J Neurosci* **26**, 10 222–31.

Chételat G, Desgranges B, De La Sayette V, *et al.* 2003. Dissociating atrophy and hypometabolism impact on episodic memory in mild cognitive impairment. *Brain* **126**, 1995–67.

Chételat G, Eustache F, Viader F, *et al.* 2005. FDG-PET measurement is more accurate than neuropsychological assessments to predict global cognitive deterioration in patients with mild cognitive impairment *Neurocase* **11**, 14–25.

Craig-Schapiro R, Fagan A M and Holtzman D M. 2009. Biomarkers of Alzheimer's disease. *Neurobiol Dis* **35**, 128–40.

D'Esposito M, Deouell L Y and Gazzaley A. 2003. Alterations in the BOLD fMRI signal with ageing and disease: A challenge for neuroimaging. *Nat Rev Neurosci* **4**, 863–72.

De Leon M, Golomb J, George A E, *et al.* 1993. The radiologic prediction of Alzheimer disease: The atrophic hippocampal formation. *Am J Neuroradiol* **13**, 897–906.

De Leon M J, Convit A, Wolf O T, *et al.* 2001. Prediction of cognitive decline in normal elderly subjects with 2-[(18)F]fluoro-2-deoxy-d-glucose/positron-emission tomography (FDG/PET). *Proc Natl Acad Sci U S A* **98**, 10 966–71.

De Leon M J, George A E, Stylopoulos L A, Smith G and Miller D C. 1989. Early marker for Alzheimer's disease: The atrophic hippocampus. *Lancet* **2**, 672–3.

Desgranges B, Baron J C, De La Sayette V, *et al.* 1998. The neural substrates of memory systems impairment in Alzheimer's disease. A PET study of resting brain glucose utilization. *Brain* **121**, 611–31.

Desikan R S, Fischl B, Cabral H J, *et al.* 2008. MRI measures of temporoparietal regions show differential rates of atrophy during prodromal AD. *Neurology* **71**, 819–25.

Devanand D P, Habeck C G, Tabert M H, *et al.* 2006. PET network abnormalities and cognitive decline in patients with mild cognitive impairment. *Neuropsychopharmacology* **31**, 1327–34.

Dickerson B C, Bakkour A, Salat D H, *et al.* 2007a. The cortical signature of Alzheimer's disease (AD): A high throughput in vivo MRI-based quantitative biomarker. In *Massachusetts Alzheimer's Disease Research Center 20th Annual Scientific Poster Symposium*, Boston, MA.

Dickerson B C, Miller S L, Greve D N, *et al.* 2007b. Prefrontal–hippocampal–fusiform activity during encoding predicts intraindividual differences in free recall ability: An event-related functional–anatomic MRI study. *Hippocampus* **17**, 1060–70.

Dickerson B C, Salat D H, Bates J F, *et al.* 2004. Medial temporal lobe function and structure in mild cognitive impairment. *Ann Neurol* **56**, 27–35.

Dickerson B C, Salat D H, Greve D N, *et al.* 2005. Increased hippocampal activation in mild cognitive impairment compared to normal aging and AD. *Neurology* **65**, 404–11.

Dickerson B C and Sperling R A. 2005. Neuroimaging biomarkers for clinical trials of disease-modifying therapies in Alzheimer's disease. *NeuroRX* **2**, 348–60.

Drzezga A, Grimmer T, Riemenschneider M, *et al.* 2005. Prediction of individual clinical outcome in MCI by means of genetic assessment and (18)F-FDG PET. *J Nucl Med* **46**, 1625–32.

Filbey F M, Slack K J, Sunderland T P and Cohen R M. 2006. Functional magnetic resonance imaging and magnetoencephalography differences associated with APOEepsilon4 in young healthy adults. *Neuroreport* **17**, 1585–90.

Fleisher A S, Houston W S, Eyler L T, *et al.* 2005. Identification of Alzheimer disease risk by functional magnetic resonance imaging. *Arch Neurol* **62**, 1881–8.

Forsberg A, Engler H, Almkvist O, *et al.* 2008. PET imaging of amyloid deposition in patients with mild cognitive impairment. *Neurobiol Aging* **29**, 1456–65.

Fox N C, Kennedy A M, Harvey R J, *et al.* 1997. Clinicopathological features of familial Alzheimer's disease associated with the M139V mutation in the presenilin 1 gene. Pedigree but not mutation specific age at onset provides evidence for a further genetic factor. *Brain* **120**, 491–501.

Fox N C, Warrington E K, Stevens J M and Rossor M N. 1996. Atrophy of the hippocampal formation in early familial Alzheimer's disease. A longitudinal MRI study of at-risk members of a family with an amyloid precursor protein 717Val-Gly mutation. *Ann N Y Acad Sci* **777**, 226–32.

Goekoop R, Scheltens P, Barkhof F and Rombouts S A. 2006. Cholinergic challenge in Alzheimer patients and mild cognitive impairment differentially affects hippocampal activation – A pharmacological fMRI study. *Brain* **129**, 141–57.

Grady C L, Furey M L, Pietrini P, Horwitz B and Rapoport S I. 2001. Altered brain functional connectivity and impaired short-term memory in Alzheimer's disease. *Brain* **124**, 739–56.

Grady C L, Mcintosh A R, Beig S, Keightley M L, Burlan H and Black S E. 2003. Evidence from functional neuroimaging of a compensatory prefrontal network in Alzheimer's disease. *J Neurosci* **23**, 986–93.

Graham J E, Rockwood K, Beattie B L, *et al.* 1997. Prevalence and severity of cognitive impairment with and without dementia in an elderly population. *Lancet* **349**, 1793–6.

Greicius M D, Srivastava G, Reiss A L and Menon V. 2004. Default-mode network activity distinguishes Alzheimer's disease from healthy aging: Evidence from functional MRI. *Proc Natl Acad Sci U S A* **101**, 4637–42.

Grön G, Brandenburg I, Wunderlich A P and Riepe M W. 2006. Inhibition of hippocampal function in mild cognitive impairment: Targeting the cholinergic hypothesis. *Neurobiol Aging* **27**, 78–87.

Grossman M, Koenig P, Glosser G, *et al.* 2003. Neural basis for semantic memory difficulty in Alzheimer's disease: An fMRI study. *Brain* **126**, 292–311.

Guye M, Bartolomei F and Ranjeva J P. 2008. Imaging structural and functional connectivity: Towards a unified definition of human brain organization? *Curr Opin Neurol* **21**, 393–403.

Han S D, Houston W S, Jak A J, *et al.* 2007. Verbal paired-associate learning by APOE genotype in non-demented older adults: fMRI evidence of a right hemispheric compensatory response. *Neurobiol Aging* **28**, 238–47.

He Y, Wang L, Zang Y, *et al.* 2007. Regional coherence changes in the early stages of Alzheimer's disease: A combined structural and resting-state functional MRI study. *Neuroimage* **35**, 488–500.

Higuchi M, Arai H, Nakagawa T, *et al.* 1997. Regional cerebral glucose utilization is modulated by the dosage of apolipoprotein E type 4 allele and alpha1-antichymotrypsin type A allele in Alzheimer's disease. *Neuroreport* **8**, 2639–43.

Hirao K, Ohnishi T, Matsuda H, *et al.* 2006. Functional interactions between entorhinal cortex and posterior cingulate cortex at the very early stage of Alzheimer's disease using brain perfusion single-photon emission computed tomography. *Nucl Med Commun* **27**, 151–6.

Hoffman J M, Welsh-Bohmer K A, Hanson M, *et al.* 2000. FDG PET imaging in patients with pathologically verified dementia. *J Nucl Med* **41**, 1920–8.

Høgh P, Knudsen G M, Kjaer K H, Jørgensen O S, Paulson O B and Waldemar G. 2001. Single photon emission computed tomography and apolipoprotein E in Alzheimer's disease: Impact of the epsilon4 allele on regional cerebral blood flow. *J Geriatr Psychiatry Neurol* **14**, 42–51.

Horwitz B, Grady C L, Schlageter N L, Duara R and Rapoport S I. 1987. Intercorrelations of regional cerebral glucose metabolic rates in Alzheimer's disease. *Brain Res* **407**, 294–306.

Ikonomovic M D, Klunk W E, Ambrahamson E E, *et al.* 2008. Post-mortem correlates of in vivo PiB-PET amyloid imaging in a typical case of Alzheimer's disease. *Brain* **131**, 1630–45.

Jack C R, Petersen R C, Xu Y C, *et al.* 1999. Prediction of AD with MRI-based hippocampal volume in mild cognitive impairment. *Neurology* **52**, 1397–403.

Jack C R J, Petersen R C, Xu Y C, *et al.* 1997. Medial temporal atrophy on MRI in normal aging and very mild Alzheimer's disease. *Neurology* **49**, 786–94.

Johnson K A, Jones K, Holman B L, *et al.* 1998. Preclinical prediction of Alzheimer's disease using SPECT. *Neurology* **50**, 1563–71.

Johnson K A, Lopera F, Jones K, *et al.* 2001. Presenilin-1-associated abnormalities in regional cerebral perfusion. *Neurology* **56**, 1545–51.

Johnson K A, Moran E K, Becker J A, Blacker D, Fischman A J and Albert M S. 2007a. Single photon emission computed tomography perfusion differences in mild cognitive impairment. *J Neurol Neurosurg Psychiatry* **78**, 240–7.

Johnson S C, Baxter L C, Susskind-Wilder L, Connor D J, Sabbagh M N and Caselli R J. 2004. Hippocampal adaptation to face repetition in healthy elderly and mild cognitive impairment. *Neuropsychologia* **42**, 980–99.

Johnson S C, Ries M L, Hess T M, *et al.* 2007b. Effect of Alzheimer disease risk on brain function during self-appraisal in healthy middle-aged adults. *Arch Gen Psychiatry* **64**, 1163–71.

Johnson S C, Saykin A J, Baxter L C, *et al.* 2000. The relationship between fMRI activation and cerebral atrophy: Comparison of normal aging and Alzheimer disease. *Neuroimage* **11**, 179–87.

Johnson S C, Schmitz T W, Asthana S, Gluck M A and Myers C. 2008. Associative learning over trials activates the hippocampus in healthy elderly but not mild cognitive impairment. *Neuropsychol Dev Cogn B Aging Neuropsychol Cogn* **15**, 129–45.

Johnson S C, Schmitz T W, Moritz C H, *et al.* 2006a. Activation of brain regions vulnerable to Alzheimer's disease: The effect of mild cognitive impairment. *Neurobiol Aging* **27**, 1604–12.

Johnson S C, Schmitz T W, Trivedi M A, *et al.* 2006b. The influence of Alzheimer disease family history and apolipoprotein E epsilon4 on mesial temporal lobe activation. *J Neurosci* **26**, 6069–76.

Julin P, Almkvist O, Basun H, *et al.* 1998. Brain volumes and regional cerebral blood flow in carriers of the

Swedish Alzheimer amyloid protein mutation. *Alzheimer Dis Assoc Disord* **12**, 49–53.

Julin P, Lindqvist J, Svensson L, Slomka P and Wahlund L O. 1997. MRI-guided SPECT measurements of medial temporal lobe blood flow in Alzheimer's disease. *J Nucl Med* **38**, 914–9.

Kato T, Knopman D S and Liu H. 2001. Dissociation of regional activation in mild AD during visual encoding: A functional MRI study. *Neurology* **57**, 812–6.

Kemppainen N M, Aalto S, Wilson I A, *et al.* 2007. PET amyloid ligand [11C]PIB uptake is increased in mild cognitive impairment. *Neurology* **68**, 1603–06.

Kessler J, Herholz K, Grond M and Heiss W D. 1991. Impaired metabolic activation in Alzheimer's disease: A PET study during continuous visual recognition. *Neuropsychologia* **29**, 229–43.

Kircher T T, Erb M, Grodd W and Leube D T. 2005. Cortical activation during cholinesterase-inhibitor treatment in Alzheimer disease: Preliminary findings from a pharmaco-fMRI study. *Am J Geriatr Psychiatry* **13**, 1006–13.

Klunk W E, Engler H, Nordberg A, *et al.* 2004. Imaging brain amyloid in Alzheimer's disease with Pittsburgh Compound-B. *Ann Neurol* **55**, 306–19.

Klunk W E and Mathis C A. 2008. The future of amyloid-beta imaging: A tale of radionuclides and tracer proliferation. *Curr Opin Neurol* **21**, 683–7.

Kogure D, Matsuda H, Ohnishi T, *et al.* 2000. Longitudinal evaluation of early Alzheimer's disease using brain perfusion SPECT. *J Nucl Med* **41**, 1155–62.

Koivunen J, Pirttilä T, Kemppainen N, *et al.* 2008. PET amyloid ligand [11C]PIB uptake and cerebrospinal fluid beta-amyloid in mild cognitive impairment. *Dementia Geriatr Cogn Disord* **26**, 378–83.

Langbaum J B, Chen K, Lee W, *et al.* 2009. Categorical and correlational analyses of baseline fluorodeoxyglucose positron emission tomography images from the Alzheimer's Disease Neuroimaging Initiative (ADNI). *Neuroimage* **45**, 1107–16.

Lee K U, Lee J S, Kim K W, *et al.* 2003. Influence of the apolipoprotein E type 4 allele on cerebral glucose metabolism in Alzheimer's disease patients. *J Neuropsychiatry Clin Neurosci* **15**, 78–83.

Lehtovirta M, Kuikka J, Helisalmi S, *et al.* 1998. Longitudinal SPECT study in Alzheimer's disease: Relation to apolipoprotein E polymorphism. *J Neurol Neurosurg Psychiatry* **64**, 742–6.

Lehtovirta M, Soininen H, Laakso M P, *et al.* 1996. SPECT and MRI analysis in Alzheimer's disease: Relation to apolipoprotein E epsilon 4 allele. *J Neurol Neurosurg Psychiatry* **60**, 644–9.

Lekeu F, Van Der Linden M, Chicherio C, *et al.* 2003. Brain correlates of performance in a free/cued recall task

with semantic encoding in Alzheimer disease. *Alzheimer Dis Assoc Disord* **17**, 35–45.

Levy R. 1994. Aging-associated cognitive decline. *Int Psychogeriatr* **6**, 63–8.

Li S J, Li Z, Wu G, Zhang M J, Franczak M and Antuono P G. 2002. Alzheimer Disease: Evaluation of a functional MR imaging index as a marker. *Radiology* **225**, 253–9.

Lind J, Ingvar M, Persson J, *et al.* 2006a. Parietal cortex activation predicts memory decline in apolipoprotein E-epsilon4 carriers. *Neuroreport* **17**, 1683–6.

Lind J, Persson J, Ingvar M, *et al.* 2006b. Reduced functional brain activity response in cognitively intact apolipoprotein E epsilon4 carriers. *Brain* **129**, 1240–8.

Lipton A M, McColl R, Cullum C M, *et al.* 2003. Differential activation on fMRI of monozygotic twins discordant for AD. *Neurology* **60**, 1713–6.

Machulda M M, Ward H A, Borowski B, *et al.* 2003. Comparison of memory fMRI response among normal, MCI, and Alzheimer's patients. *Neurology* **61**, 500–6.

Masdeu J C, Zubieta J L and Arbizu J. 2005. Neuroimaging as a marker of the onset and progression of Alzheimer's disease. *J Neurol Sci* **236**, 55–64.

Matsuda H. 2001. Cerebral blood flow and metabolic abnormalities in Alzheimer's disease. *Ann Nucl Med* **15**, 85–92.

Matsuda H, Kitayama N, Ohnishi T, *et al.* 2002. Longitudinal evaluation of both morphologic and functional changes in the same individuals with Alzheimer's disease. *J Nucl Med* **43**, 304–11.

Maxim V, Sendur L, Fadili J, *et al.* 2005. Fractional Gaussian noise, functional MRI and Alzheimer's disease. *Neuroimage* **25**, 141–58.

Mielke R, Zerres K, Uhlhaas S, Kessler J and Heiss W D. 1998. Apolipoprotein E polymorphism influences the cerebral metabolic pattern in Alzheimer's disease. *Neurosci Lett* **254**, 49–52.

Minoshima S, Giordani B, Berent S, Frey K A, Foster N L and Kuhl D E. 1997. Metabolic reduction in the posterior cingulate cortex in very early Alzheimer's disease. *Ann Neurol* **42**, 85–94.

Mintun M A, Larossa G N, Sheline Y I, *et al.* 2006. [11C]PIB in a nondemented population: Potential antecedent marker of Alzheimer disease. *Neurology* **67**, 446–52.

Mondadori C R, De Quervain D J, Buchmann A, *et al.* 2007. Better memory and neural efficiency in young apolipoprotein E epsilon4 carriers. *Cerebral Cortex* **17**, 1934–47.

Mormino E C, Kluth J T, Madison C M, *et al.* 2009. Episodic memory loss is related to hippocampal-mediated {beta}-amyloid deposition in elderly subjects. *Brain* **132**, 1310–23.

Morris J C. 2006. Mild cognitive impairment is early-stage Alzheimer disease: Time to revise diagnostic criteria. *Arch Neurol* **63**, 15–6.

Mosconi L, Brys M, Switalski R, *et al.* 2007. Maternal family history of Alzheimer's disease predisposes to reduced brain glucose metabolism. *Proc Natl Acad Sci U S A* **104**, 19 067–72.

Mosconi L, De Santi S, Brys M, *et al.* 2008. Hypometabolism and altered cerebrospinal fluid markers in normal apolipoprotein E E4 carriers with subjective memory complaints. *Biol Psychiatry* **63**, 609–18.

Mosconi L, Herholz K, Prohovnik I, *et al.* 2005. Metabolic interaction between ApoE genotype and onset age in Alzheimer's disease: Implications for brain reserve. *J Neurol Neurosurg Psychiatry* **76**, 15–23.

Mosconi L, Nacmias B, Sorbi S, *et al.* 2004a. Brain metabolic decreases related to the dose of the ApoE e4 allele in Alzheimer's disease. *J Neurol Neurosurg Psychiatry* **75**, 370–6.

Mosconi L, Perani D, Sorbi S, *et al.* 2004b. MCI conversion to dementia and the APOE genotype: A prediction study with FDG-PET. *Neurology* **63**, 2332–40.

Mosconi L, Sorbi S, De Leon M J, *et al.* 2006. Hypometabolism exceeds atrophy in presymptomatic early-onset familial Alzheimer's disease. *J Nucl Med* **47**, 1778–86.

Mosconi L, Sorbi S, Nacmias B, *et al.* 2004c. Age and ApoE genotype interaction in Alzheimer's disease: An FDG-PET study. *Psychiatry Res* **130**, 141–51.

Moulin C J, Laine M, Rinne J O, Kaasinen V S, Hiltunen J and Kangasmäki A. 2007. Brain function during multi-trial learning in mild cognitive impairment: A PET activation study. *Brain Res* **1136**, 132–41.

Nestor P G, Fryer T D, Smielewski P and Hodges J R. 2003a. Limbic hypometabolism in Alzheimer's disease and mild cognitive impairment. *Ann Neurol* **54**, 343–51.

Nestor P G, Fryer T D, Ikeda M and Hodges J R. 2003b. Retrosplenial cortex (BA 29/30) hypometabolism in mild cognitive impairment (prodromal Alzheimer's disease). *Eur J Neurosci* **18**, 2663–7.

Nishi H, Sawamoto N, Namiki C, *et al.* 2010. Correlation between cognitive deficits and glucose hypometabolism in mild cognitive impairment. *J Neuroimaging* **20**, 29–36.

Nobili F, Salmaso D, Morbelli S, *et al.* 2008. Principal component analysis of FDG PET in amnestic MCI. *Eur J Nucl Med Mol Imaging* **35**, 2191–202.

Ohnishi T, Hoshi H, Nagamachi S, *et al.* 1995. High-resolution SPECT to assess hippocampal perfusion in neuropsychiatric diseases. *J Nucl Med* **36**, 1163–9.

Ott B R, Heindel W C, Tan Z and Noto R B. 2000. Lateralized cortical perfusion in women with Alzheimer's disease. *J Gender-Spec Med* **3**, 29–35.

Pariente J, Cole S, Henson R, *et al.* 2005. Alzheimer's patients engage an alternative network during a memory task. *Ann Neurol* **58**, 870–9.

Perneczky R, Hartmann J, Grimmer T, Drzezga A and Kurz A. 2007. Cerebral metabolic correlates of the clinical dementia rating scale in mild cognitive impairment. *J Geriatr Psychiatry Neurol* **20**, 84–8.

Persson J, Lind J, Larsson A, *et al.* 2008. Altered deactivation in individuals with genetic risk for Alzheimer's disease. *Neuropsychologia* **46**, 1679–87.

Petersen R C. 2007. Mild cognitive impairment: Current research and clinical implications. *Semin Neurol* **27**, 22–31.

Petersen R C, Smith G E, Waring S C, Ivnik R J, Tangalos E G and Kokmen E. 1999. Mild cognitive impairment: Clinical characterization and outcome. *Arch Neurol* **56**, 303–08.

Petrella J R, Lustig C, Bucher L A, Jha A P and Doraiswamy P M. 2002. Prefrontal activation patterns in subjects at risk for Alzheimer disease. *Am J Geriatr Psychiatry* **10**, 112–3.

Petrella J R, Prince S E, Krishnan S, Husn H, Kelley L and Doraiswamy P M. 2009. Effects of donepezil on cortical activation in mild cognitive impairment: A pilot double-blind placebo-controlled trial using functional MR imaging. *Am J Neuroradiol* **30**, 411–6.

Petrella J R, Wang L, Krishnan S, *et al.* 2007. Cortical deactivation in mild cognitive impairment: High-field-strength functional MR imaging. *Radiology* **245**, 224–35.

Pike K E, Savage G, Villemagne V L, *et al.* 2007. Beta-amyloid imaging and memory in non-demented individuals: Evidence for preclinical Alzheimer's disease. *Brain* **130**, 2837–44.

Rapoport S I. 1997. Discriminant analysis of brain imaging data identifies subjects with early Alzheimer's disease. *Int Psychogeriatr* **9** (Suppl. 1), 229–35.

Reiman E M, Caselli R J, Chen K, Alexander G E, Bandy D and Frost J. 2001. Declining brain activity in cognitively normal apolipoprotein E epsilon 4 heterozygotes: A foundation for using positron emission tomography to efficiently test treatments to prevent Alzheimer's disease. *Proc Natl Acad Sci U S A* **98**, 3334–9.

Reiman E M, Caselli R J, Yun L S, *et al.* 1996. Preclinical evidence of Alzheimer's disease in persons homozygous for the epsilon 4 allele for apolipoprotein E. *N Engl J Med* **334**, 752–8.

Reiman E M, Chen K, Alexander G E, *et al.* 2004. Functional brain abnormalities in young adults at genetic risk for late-onset Alzheimer's dementia. *Proc Natl Acad Sci U S A* **101**, 284–9.

Reiman E M, Chen K, Alexander G E, *et al.* 2005. Correlations between apolipoprotein E epsilon4 gene dose and brain-imaging measurements of regional hypometabolism. *Proc Natl Acad Sci U S A* **102**, 8299–302.

Rimajova M, Lenzo N P, Wu J S, *et al.* 2008. Fluoro-2-deoxy-D-glucose (FDG)-PET in APOEepsilon4 carriers in the Australian population. *J Alzheimer's Dis* **13**, 137–46.

Risacher S L, Saykin A J, West J D, *et al.* 2009. Baseline MRI predictors of conversion from MCI to probable AD in the ADNI cohort. *Curr Alzheimer Res* **6**, 347–61.

Rombouts S A, Barkhof F, Veltman D J, *et al.* 2000. Functional MR imaging in Alzheimer's disease during memory encoding. *Am J Neuroradiol* **21**, 1869–75.

Rombouts S A and Scheltens P. 2005. Functional connectivity in elderly controls and AD patients using resting-state fMRI: A pilot study. *Curr Alzheimer Res* **2**, 115–6.

Rossor M, Kennedy A M and Frackowiak R S. 1996. Clinical and neuroimaging features of familial Alzheimer's disease. *Ann N Y Acad Sci* **777**, 49–56.

Rossor M, Newman S, Frackowiak R S, Lantos P and Kennedy A M. 1993. Alzheimer's disease families with amyloid precursor protein mutations. *Ann N Y Acad Sci* **695**, 198–202.

Sakamoto S, Ishii K, Sasaki M, *et al.* 2002. Differences in cerebral metabolic impairment between early and late onset types of Alzheimer's disease. *J Neurol Sci* **200**, 27–32.

Sakamoto S, Matsuda H, Asada T, *et al.* 2003. Apolipoprotein E genotype and early Alzheimer's disease: A longitudinal SPECT study. *J Neuroimag* **13**, 113–23.

Saykin A J, Wishart H A, Rabin L A, *et al.* 2004. Cholinergic enhancement of frontal lobe activity in mild cognitive impairment. *Brain* **127**, 1574–83.

Saykin A J, Wishart H A, Rabin L A, *et al.* 2006. Older adults with cognitive complaints show brain atrophy similar to that of amnestic MCI. *Neurology* **67**, 834–42.

Scarmeas N, Anderson K E, Hilton J, *et al.* 2004a. APOE-dependent PET patterns of brain activation in Alzheimer disease. *Neurology* **63**, 913–5.

Scarmeas N, Habeck C, Anderson K E, *et al.* 2004b. Altered PET functional brain responses in cognitively intact elderly persons at risk for Alzheimer disease (carriers of the E4 allele). *Am J Geriatr Psychiatry* **12**, 596–605.

Scarmeas N, Habeck C, Hilton J, *et al.* 2005. APOE related alterations in cerebral activation even at college age. *J Neurol Neurosurg Psychiatry* **76**, 1440–4.

Scarmeas N and Stern Y. 2006. Imaging studies and APOE genotype in persons at risk for Alzheimer's disease. *Curr Psychiatry Rep* **8**, 11–7.

Scheltens P, Launer L J, Barkhof F, Weinstein H C and Jonker C. 1997. The diagnostic value of magnetic resonance imaging and technetium 99m-HMPAO single-photon-emission computed tomography for the diagnosis of Alzheimer disease in a community-dwelling elderly population. *Alzheimer Dis Assoc Disord* **11**, 63–70.

Schröder J, Buchsbaum M S, Shihabuddin L, *et al.* 2001. Patterns of cortical activity and memory performance in Alzheimer's disease. *Biol Psychiatry* **49**, 426–36.

Seo S W, Cho S S, Park A, Chin J and Na D L. 2009. Subcortical vascular versus amnestic mild cognitive impairment: Comparison of cerebral glucose metabolism. *J Neuroimag* **19**, 213–9.

Shulman G L, Fiez J A, Corbetta M, *et al.* 1997. Common blood flow changes across visual tasks: II. Decreases in cerebral cortex. *J Cogn Neurosci* **9**, 648–63.

Silverman D H. 2004. Brain 18F-FDG PET in the diagnosis of neurodegenerative dementias: Comparison with perfusion SPECT and with clinical evaluations lacking nuclear imaging. *J Nucl Med* **45**, 594–607.

Small B J, Mazziotta J C, Collins M T, *et al.* 1995. Apolipoprotein E type 4 allele and cerebral glucose metabolism in relatives at risk for familial Alzheimer disease. *J Am Med Assoc* **273**, 942–7.

Small G W, Komo S, La Rue A, *et al.* 1996. Early detection of Alzheimer's disease by combining apolipoprotein E and neuroimaging. *Ann N Y Acad Sci* **802**, 70–8.

Small G W, Okonek A, Mandelkern M A, *et al.* 1994. Age-associated memory loss: Initial neuropsychological and cerebral metabolic findings of a longitudinal study. *Int Psychogeriatr* **6**, 23–44.

Small S A, Perera G M, Delapaz R, Mayeux R and Stern Y. 1999. Differential regional dysfunction of the hippocampal formation among elderly with memory decline and Alzheimer's disease. *Ann Neurol* **45**, 466–72.

Small S A, Tsai W Y, De La Paz R, Mayeux R and Stern C E. 2002. Imaging hippocampal function across the human life span: Is memory decline normal or not? *Ann Neurol* **51**, 290–5.

Small S A, Wu E X, Bartsch D, *et al.* 2000. Imaging physiologic dysfunction of individual hippocampal subregions in humans and genetically modified mice. *Neuron* **28**, 653–4.

Smith C D, Andersen A H, Kryscio R J, *et al.* 1999. Altered brain activation in cognitively intact individuals at high risk for Alzheimer's disease. *Neurology* **53**, 1391–6.

Smith C D, Andersen A H, Kryscio R J, *et al.* 2002. Women at risk for AD show increased parietal activation during a fluency task. *Neurology* **58**, 1197–202.

Smith C D, Kryscio R J, Schmitt F A, *et al.* 2005. Longitudinal functional alterations in asymptomatic women at risk for Alzheimer's disease. *J Neuroimag* **15**, 271–7.

Sorg C, Riedl V, Mühlau M, *et al.* 2007. Selective changes of resting-state networks in individuals at risk for Alzheimer's disease. *Proc Natl Acad Sci U S A* **104**, 18 760–5.

Sperling R A, Bates J F, Chua E F, *et al.* 2003. fMRI studies of associative encoding in young and elderly controls and mild Alzheimer's disease. *J Neurol Neurosurg Psychiatry* **74**, 44–50.

349

Supekar K, Menon V, Rubin D, Musen M and Greicius M D. 2008. Network analysis of intrinsic functional brain connectivity in Alzheimer's disease. *PLoS Comput Biol* **4**, e1000100.

Thompson P M, Hayashi K M, De Zubicaray G, *et al.* 2003. Dynamics of gray matter loss in Alzheimer's disease. *J Neurosci* **23**, 994–1005.

Trivedi M A, Murphy C M, Goetz C, *et al.* 2008a. fMRI activation changes during successful episodic memory encoding and recognition in amnestic mild cognitive impairment relative to cognitively healthy older adults. *Dementia Geriatr Cogn Disord* **26**, 123–37.

Trivedi M A, Schmitz T W, Ries M L, *et al.* 2006. Reduced hippocampal activation during episodic encoding in middle-aged individuals at genetic risk of Alzheimer's disease: A cross-sectional study. *BMC Med* **4**, 1.

Trivedi M A, Schmitz T W, Ries M L, *et al.* 2008b. fMRI activation during episodic encoding and metacognitive appraisal across the lifespan: Risk factors for Alzheimer's disease. *Neuropsychologia* **46**, 1667–78.

Van Dyck C H, Gelernter J, Macavoy M G, *et al.* 1998. Absence of an apolipoprotein E epsilon4 allele is associated with increased parietal regional cerebral blood flow asymmetry in Alzheimer disease. *Arch Neurol* **55**, 1460–6.

Visser P J, Scheltens P, Verhey F R, *et al.* 1999. Medial temporal lobe atrophy and memory dysfunction as predictors for dementia in subjects with mild cognitive impairment. *J Neurol* **246**, 477–85.

Wahlund L, Basun H, Almkvist O, *et al.* 1999. A follow-up study of the family with the Swedish APP 670/671 Alzheimer's disease mutation. *Dementia Geriatr Cogn Disord* **10**, 526–33.

Wang K, Jiang T, Liang M, *et al.* 2006a. Discriminative analysis of early Alzheimer's disease based on two intrinsically anti-correlated networks with resting-state fMRI. *Med Image Comput ComputAssist Interv* **9**, 340–7.

Wang K, Liang M, Wang L, *et al.* 2007. Altered functional connectivity in early Alzheimer's disease: A resting-state fMRI study. *Hum Brain Mapp* **28**, 967–78.

Wang L, Zang Y, He Y, *et al.* 2006b. Changes in hippocampal connectivity in the early stages of Alzheimer's disease: Evidence from resting state fMRI. *Neuroimage* **31**, 496–504.

Wang P J, Saykin A J, Flashman L A, *et al.* 2006c. Regionally specific atrophy of the corpus callosum in AD, MCI and cognitive complaints. *Neurobiol Aging* **27**, 1613–7.

Waragai M, Mizumura S, Yamada T and Matsuda H. 2008. Differentiation of early-stage Alzheimer's disease from other types of dementia using brain perfusion single photon emission computed tomography with easy z-score imaging system analysis. *Dementia Geriatr Cogn Disord* **26**, 547–55.

Weiner M W. 2009. Imaging and biomarkers will be used for detection and monitoring progression of early Alzheimer's disease. *J Nutr Health Aging* **13**, 332.

Wierenga C E and Bondi M W. 2007. Use of functional magnetic resonance imaging in the early identification of Alzheimer's disease. *Neuropsychol Rev* **17**, 127–43.

Winblad B, Palmer K, Kivipelto M, *et al.* 2004. Mild cognitive impairment – Beyond controversies, towards a consensus: Report of the International Working Group on Mild Cognitive Impairment. *J Int Med* **256**, 240–6.

Wishart H A, Saykin A J, Rabin L A, *et al.* 2006. Increased brain activation during working memory in cognitively intact adults with the APOE epsilon4 allele. *Am J Psychiatry* **163**, 1603–10.

Wolf H, Jelic V, Gertz H J, Nordberg A, Julin P and Wahlund L O. 2003. A critical discussion of the role of neuroimaging in mild cognitive impairment. *Acta Neurol Scand Suppl* **179**, 52–76.

Wolk D A, Price J C, Saxton J A, *et al.* 2009. Amyloid imaging in mild cognitive impairment subtypes. *Ann Neurol* **65**, 557–68.

Woodard J L, Grafton S T, Votaw J R, Green R C, Dobraski M E and Hoffman J M. 1998. Compensatory recruitment of neural resources during overt rehearsal of word lists in Alzheimer's disease. *Neuropsychology* **12**, 491–504.

Xu G, Mclaren D G, Ries M L, *et al.* 2008. The influence of parental history of Alzheimer's disease and apolipoprotein E {varepsilon}4 on the BOLD signal during recognition memory. *Brain* **132**, 383–91.

Yassa M A, Verduzco G, Cristinzio C and Bassett S S. 2008. Altered fMRI activation during mental rotation in those at genetic risk for Alzheimer disease. *Neurology* **70**, 1898–904.

Zhou Y, Dougherty J H J, Hubner K F, Bai B, Cannon R L and Hutson R K. 2008. Abnormal connectivity in the posterior cingulate and hippocampus in early Alzheimer's disease and mild cognitive impairment *Alzheimer's Dementia* **4**, 265–70.

Chapter 25

Molecular imaging of Alzheimer's disease

Norbert Schuff

Abstract

Neurochemical imaging offers an opportunity to study at a molecular level in-vivo the neuronal substrates that underpin Alzheimer's disease (AD) and related disorders, such as mild cognitive impairment (MCI). In particular, proton magnetic resonance spectroscopic imaging (^{1}H MRSI) is unique among diagnostic imaging modalities because the method can measure several different brain metabolites simultaneously, including N-acetylaspartate (NAA), a neuronal integrity marker, and *myo*-inositol (MI), a potential glial marker. The goal of this chapter is to review key findings of ^{1}H MRSI in AD, MCI and aging, and to discuss the potential value of this technology for diagnosis and prognosis of AD as well as for the assessment of therapeutic intervention. Other neurochemical imaging technologies such as direct mapping of neurotransmitter systems using emission tomography (PET) tracers and new trends, such as amyloid PET imaging are also briefly discussed.

Introduction

Alzheimer's disease (AD) is the most common cause of dementia and a growing health problem globally, affecting 20% of the population over 80 years of age (Ferri *et al.*, 2005). Currently, the definite diagnosis of AD can only be made through autopsy to find the pathological hallmarks of the disease: microscopic amyloid plaques and neurofibrillary tangles. Macroscopically, AD is characterized by progressive loss of brain tissue that leads to a rapid decline in cognitive function. The development of markers that can reliably indicate presence of the disease at the earliest possible stage is therefore an important public health goal. In addition to AD, there is nowadays also a particular interest in older individuals who lie cognitively somewhere in the middle between normal and dementia and who fit the concept of mild cognitive impairment (MCI) (Petersen *et al.*, 1999), because this syndrome is thought to be a transitional stage to AD. MCI may define a window for the prediction of AD as well as therapeutic interventions with the prospect of slowing progression or even preventing the disease, though not all patients with MCI go on to develop AD (Panza *et al.*, 2005).

Neurochemical imaging technologies offer an extraordinary opportunity to study in-vivo the neuronal substrates that underpin AD and MCI at a molecular level and therefore hold great promise for the identification of a marker of AD. In particular, magnetic resonance spectroscopy (MRS) is unique among diagnostic imaging modalities because the method can measure several different brain metabolites simultaneously, providing in principle a multivariate spectroscopic profile of a disease. The goal of this chapter is to review key MRS findings in AD and MCI and discuss the potential value of MRS for diagnosis and prognosis of AD as well as for the assessment of therapeutic intervention. Other promising neurochemical imaging modalities that directly probe neurotransmitter systems using radioactive positron emission tomography (PET) tracers are also briefly reviewed and new trends, such as amyloid PET imaging are also discussed.

Magnetic resonance spectroscopy

Magnetic resonance-detectable cerebral metabolites

Magnetic resonance spectroscopy enables non-invasive analysis of the chemical composition of biological tissue, and when combined with magnetic resonance imaging techniques, it provides a readily available

Understanding Neuropsychiatric Disorders, ed. M. E. Shenton and B. I. Turetsky. Published by Cambridge University Press.
© Cambridge University Press 2011.

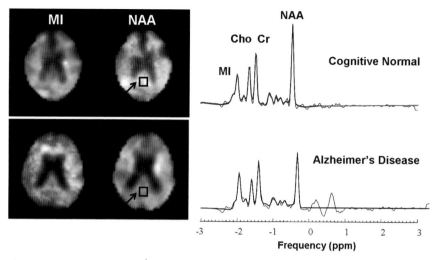

Figure 25.1 Examples of brain ^{1}H MRSI metabolite maps of *N*-acetylaspartate (NAA), a marker of neuronal integrity and *myo*-inositol (MI), a potential glial marker, from a 76-year-old patient with Alzheimer's disease (bottom) and a cognitive normal subject of the same age. The ^{1}H MRSI data were obtained at the standard clinical magnetic field strength of 1.5 T. Also shown are the entire proton magnetic resonance spectra for each subject from a location in the posterior brain (indicated by a black square). They show NAA is lower and MI slightly higher in the AD compared with the control subject. A reduction of the resonance of choline moiety (Cho), presumably reflecting cell membrane breakdown, can also be seen in the AD patient. In contrast, the patient and the control subject have comparable levels of creatine (Cr).

method for mapping abundant (i.e. concentrations in the range of a few millimoles) and small molecules in the human brain. Depending on the nucleus, different metabolic aspects can be assessed, but because of its wide availability on clinical MRI systems, proton magnetic resonance spectroscopic imaging (^{1}H MRSI) is most widely used. ^{1}H MRSI can measure several abundant cerebral metabolites simultaneously, including *N*-acetylaspartate (NAA), a key molecule involved in the metabolism of aspartate (Koller *et al.*, 1984) and excitatory dipeptide *N*-acetyl-aspartyl-glutamate (Birken and Oldendorf, 1989), synthesis of lipid (Urenjak *et al.*, 1993), and regulation of cellular osmosis (Blakely and Coyle, 1988). Using immuno-histochemical techniques, NAA has been shown to be predominantly localized in neurons, axons and dendrites within the central nervous system (Simmons *et al.*, 1991), while it is largely absent in mature glial cells (Urenjak *et al.*, 1993). Animal models of neuronal injury have also been shown to give good correlations between NAA levels (as measured by MRS) and neuronal counts on histology (Guimaraes *et al.*, 1995). NAA is therefore considered a neuron marker and has been studied extensively in AD. In addition to NAA, other prominent spectral features in ^{1}H MRSI are the resonances of the moieties of choline (Cho), creatine (Cr) as well as *myo*-inositol (MI). Cho is mainly composed of cytosolic phosphocholine and glycerophosphocholine, which are the products of membrane breakdown and precursors of choline acetylcholine synthesis. Free choline and acetylcholine, which have very low abundance in brain tissue, make practically no detectable contributions to Cho (Klein, 2000). Cr reflects the sum of phosphocreatine and free creatine. MI is primarily present in glial cells (Glanville *et al.*, 1989), but virtually absent in neuronal cell cultures (Brand *et al.*, 1993). Increased MI levels correlate with glial proliferation in inflammatory processes in the central nervous system (Bitsch *et al.*, 1999) and are possibly an index of glial activation and proliferation in AD. The possibility of measuring neuronal processes selectively through NAA and inflammatory processes through MI has been a major motivation for many researchers to utilize ^{1}H MRSI for studies of dementia.

^{1}H MRSI in AD

Representative ^{1}H MRSI metabolite maps of the brain, showing the distribution of NAA and MI from a cognitive normal individual and a patient diagnosed with AD are depicted in Figure 25.1. Also shown for each subject is an entire ^{1}H MR spectrum from a particular brain location (black square). The spectra indicate lower NAA and slightly higher MI levels in the AD patient compared to the control subject. Reduced NAA levels have been reported consistently by ^{1}H MR spectroscopy studies in various brain regions in AD, but predominantly in gray matter regions in the parietal lobe (Moats *et al.*, 1994; Rose *et al.*, 1999; Shonk *et al.*, 1995; Tedeschi *et al.*, 1996), the temporal lobe (Parnetti *et al.*, 1996; Tedeschi *et al.*, 1996), and the hippocampus (Dixon *et al.*, 2002; Jessen *et al.*, 2001; Schuff *et al.*, 1997). Some of these studies were performed using single-voxel ^{1}H MR spectroscopy, a technical simplification of ^{1}H MRSI that measures metabolites at one location at a time only. Nonetheless, single-voxel and spectroscopic imaging measurements yielded generally similar results. Although these metabolite changes are not specific to AD, several studies have shown that AD is associated with a characteristic regional pattern of reduced NAA concentration that involves predominantly parietal and temporal lobe gray matter, including the hippocampus, while white matter and frontal lobe gray matter regions are typically spared (Schuff *et al.*, 2002; Zhu *et al.*, 2006). This distribution resembles the regional neuropathological involvement in AD. Moreover, it has been shown that the typical distribution of low NAA in AD is different from the patterns of low NAA in other types of dementias. For example, ischemic vascular dementia and frontotemporal dementia both exhibit low NAA, usually in frontal lobe regions and white matter, while the parietal lobe is spared (Capizzano *et al.*, 2000; Ernst *et al.*, 1997; Mihara *et al.*, 2006; Schuff *et al.*, 2003). However, while regional differences between the various dementias may be prominent during the mild stage of each disease, the difference can disappear with increasing dementia severity as the pathology spreads throughout the brain. Several studies using structural MRI and ^{1}H MRSI together also showed that the NAA reduction in AD can occur irrespective of brain atrophy (Pfefferbaum *et al.*, 1999; Schuff *et al.*, 2002), implying that ^{1}H MRSI and structural MRI each provide complementary information. Indeed, NAA measurements can improve the classification between AD patients and cognitively normal elderly subjects over the classification using structural MRI measures, such as hippocampal atrophy, alone (Schuff *et al.*, 1997).

Imaging of MI, which is technically more demanding than imaging of NAA because the signal of MI decays faster than does that of NAA, shows consistently elevated MI levels in AD. Generally, the regional distribution of elevated MI in AD mirrors that of reduced NAA (Zhu *et al.*, 2006). However,

the increase of MI levels does not always correlate with the decrease of NAA levels, despite the observation that MI and NAA alterations occur in the same brain region. In particular, one ^{1}H MRSI study found increased MI levels of white matter in AD in absence of any significant NAA changes (Siger *et al.*, 2009). This result suggests that increased MI may be an even more robust and sensitive indication for AD pathology than NAA, at least with regard to white matter. Studies that used MI and NAA together typically achieved 90% correct classification between AD patients and cognitively normal subjects (Fernandez *et al.*, 2005; Zhu *et al.*, 2006). However, the results should be interpreted with caution, because these studies relied on a clinical determination of AD without confirmation by autopsy. Only few spectroscopy studies with confirmed diagnosis of AD by autopsy have been reported so far (Kantarci *et al.*, 2008; Klunk *et al.*, 1992). These studies revealed correlations between MR metabolites and density of plaques and tangles in the brain tissue, where the strongest correlation was observed for the ratio of NAA to MI.

Reports of altered Cho levels in AD are conflicting. Some studies reported elevated Cho levels (Kantarci *et al.*, 2000; Meyerhoff *et al.*, 1994) in AD, whereas others found normal levels (Parnetti *et al.*, 1997; Schuff *et al.*, 1997). In contrast to Cho, most studies found no significant alterations of Cr levels in AD and Cr is often being used as an internal reference. However, Cr levels between white matter and gray matter differ about twofold, which can mimic metabolite variations in ^{1}H MRSI voxels with heterogeneous tissue compositions. In quantitative studies, ^{1}H MRSI is often used together with structural MRI to account for tissue variations (Schuff *et al.*, 2001).

^{1}H MRSI in MCI

Several MRI studies reported NAA and MI alterations in MCI that resembled the distribution already seen in AD, although the magnitude of the changes are usually lower than those in AD (Ackl *et al.*, 2005; Chantal *et al.*, 2004; Chao *et al.*, 2005; Kantarci *et al.*, 2000, 2002). One ^{1}H MRSI study in particular found substantial NAA reduction in the medial temporal lobe, including the hippocampus, in MCI, whereas atrophy of the hippocampus or cortex in these patients was only minor (Chao *et al.*, 2005). Moreover, in these subjects, the decrease of NAA was more strongly correlated with impaired memory functions than hippocampal atrophy. Observations of abnormal NAA and MI levels in absence of significant brain atrophy even extended to minimally impaired subjects, who show informant-based functional decline that sets them apart from cognitive normal peers, but who are otherwise too minimally impaired to meet MCI criteria (Chao *et al.*, 2010). The alterations of NAA and MI levels in MCI may therefore be sensitive to biochemical changes before tissue loss is measurable. However, whether NAA or MI is a more sensitive marker of early biochemical changes in MCI is still a matter of debate. Several ^{1}H MRSI studies of MCI reported increased MI levels in absence of significant NAA alterations (Catani *et al.*, 2001; Kantarci *et al.*, 2000; Siger *et al.*, 2009), consistent with the idea that increase in MI occurs earlier than the NAA degrees during the progression toward AD. However, not all MCI subjects convert to AD. More prospective ^{1}H MRSI studies that follow-up MCI subjects clinically and confirm AD by autopsy are necessary to compare the sensitivity of MI and NAA to detect early AD pathology.

Box 25.1. ^{1}H MRSI in AD and MCI

- ^{1}H MRSI enables non-invasive mapping of abundant and small molecules in the brain, such as *N*-acetylaspartate (NAA), a marker of neuronal integrity and *myo*-inositol (MI), a potential marker of gliosis.
- In AD, NAA is reduced and MI elevated predominantly in the parietal and temporal lobe regions, including the hippocampus.
- In MCI, the extent of NAA and MCI alterations are between those seen in AD and normal aging.
- NAA and MI alterations can occur even in absence of measurable brain atrophy, implying that they reflect neuronal damage before it can be detected structurally.

Prospective ^{1}H MRSI studies

An important potential application of ^{1}H MRSI is in the prediction of cognitive decline that might lead to the development of AD, since the feasibility of protecting a healthy brain is always greater than trying to repair one that is already damaged. The interest in prospective ^{1}H MRSI studies to predict cognitive decline has been growing in recent years, although such studies are still far fewer in numbers than cross-sectional ^{1}H MRSI studies. In general, NAA levels

decline with progressive cognitive impairment in patients with clinically established AD (Adalsteinsson *et al.*, 2000; Jessen *et al.*, 2001), and recently, a similar pattern of NAA decline has also been reported in MCI (Kantarci *et al.*, 2007). Furthermore, several studies found that MCI patients, who later progressed to AD, have lower NAA levels at baseline than those MCI patients who remain stable (Chao *et al.*, 2005; Metastasio *et al.*, 2006). In particular, NAA/MI ratios have been shown to be an efficient predictor for decline of memory functions (Kantarci *et al.*, 2002), as well as for decline of executive functions (Olson *et al.*, 2008) in MCI. Furthermore, NAA of medial temporal lobe including the hippocampus used together with structural MRI measure of brain atrophy predicted conversion from MCI to AD better than structural MRI alone (Chao *et al.*, 2010). Additional support for the predictive values of NAA and MI comes from a recent prospective ^{1}H MRSI study that followed patients to autopsy (Kantarci *et al.*, 2008). This showed that decreased NAA and increased MI levels were associated with higher neuritic plaque scores and greater likelihood of AD. The NAA/MI ratio proved to be the strongest predictor of pathologic likelihood of AD. Although the odds of developing AD when presenting low NAA and high MI levels have not yet been established, the findings – taken together – suggest that NAA and MI are useful objective measures of cognitive decline and potentially early markers for AD. Interestingly, a recent longitudinal study found Cho/Cr ratios increased in patients with MCI, who progressed to AD (Kantarci *et al.*, 2007), despite conflicting results of Cho alterations in AD from cross-sectional studies. In contrast, Cho/Cr ratios decreased in MCI patients, who remained stable. The findings suggest a possible relationship between the compensatory cholinergic mechanisms of MCI and decreased Cho/Cr ratios.

Box 25.2. Prospective ^{1}H MRSI studies

- The NAA/MI ratio is an efficient predictor for decline of memory functions.
- The NAA/MI ratio is also the strongest predictor of pathologic likelihood of AD, as determined by brain autopsy.
- Low NAA and high MCI levels at baseline are associated with higher rates of conversion to AD.
- The findings suggest that NAA and MI are useful objective measures of cognitive decline and potentially early markers for AD.

Use of ^{1}H MRSI in treatment trials

^{1}H MRSI measurements of NAA seem particularly suited for monitoring the efficiency of potentially neuroprotective pharmacological interventions in AD, because NAA is considered a marker of neuronal integrity. Recent data indicate that NAA levels may show modest short-term improvement after cholinesterase treatment in AD, even in the absence of clinical improvement compared with the placebo group (Krishnan et al., 2003). However, the data were not entirely conclusive in regard to a drug effect, because NAA tended to initially increase in the first half of the trial, consistent with an improvement, but then decreased to levels not different from baseline, implying that treatment was only of temporary use. In another clinical trial involving ^{1}H MRSI, Memantine, an N-methyl-D-aspartate (NMDA) antagonist and approved treatment in the US and Europe of moderate to severe AD, was associated with reduced glutamate levels, consistent with the expected anti-excitotoxic properties of the drug (Glodzik et al., 2008). (The resonances of glutamate and its precursor glutamine are readily detectable at ^{1}H MR spectra at higher magnetic fields and reflect that metabolic pool of this neurotransmitter.) No changes over time were found for NAA either in the treatment or in the placebo group, implying that the measured decrease in glutamate levels in the treatment group was unlikely to be related to neuron loss, but more likely reflected a therapeutic effect. The use of ^{1}H MRSI in clinical trials is only at the beginning, and several technical hurdles to perform spectroscopy studies uniformly at multiple centers must still be overcome.

Other neurochemical imaging modalities

Positron emission tomography of neurotransmitter systems

The development of molecular imaging techniques such as positron emission tomography (PET) using specific radioligands has paved the way for direct measurements of neurotransmitters systems. While almost all neurotransmitters are affected in AD, the disease is especially known for impairment of cholinergic transmission in hippocampal and the basal forebrain (Engelborghs and De Deyn, 1997). PET studies using a substrate for acetylcholinesterase demonstrated in-vivo that the loss of acetylcholinesterase was most profound in the amygdala, followed by the cerebral cortex and the hippocampus (Kuhl et al., 1999; Shinotoh et al., 2003). Investigators have also used PET radioligands to visualize cholinergic nicotinic receptors in AD, which have been found to correlate with cognitive measures of attention (Kadir et al., 2006). An early PET study demonstrated reduced uptake of [^{11}C]-nicotine binding in AD, reflecting losses in high and low affinity nicotinic receptor sites (Nordberg et al., 1990). In addition, significantly lower [^{11}C] nicotine binding was observed in the frontal cortex, temporal cortex, and hippocampus of AD patients compared with controls (Nordberg et al., 1995). The degree of reduction corresponded to the severity of cognitive impairment, but was reversible with administration of tacrine, a cholinesterase inhibitor (Nordberg, 1993). Acetylcholine muscarinic receptors on the other hand, appear to be preserved in AD until more advanced stages of dementia (Wyper et al., 1993).

The central serotonin (5-HT) system, one of the most widely distributed neurotransmitter systems throughout the brain, is thought to play a major role in cognition. The effects of 5-HT are exercised through binding to a variety of membrane-based receptors, but the most extensively studied receptor is 5-HT$_{1A}$. A recent PET study using a selective [^{18}F] molecular imaging probe for 5-HT$_{1A}$ receptors, termed MPPF, showed a striking reduction of MPPF binding in the hippocampus in AD patients compared to cognitive normal controls, consistent with loss of hippocampal neurons (Kepe et al., 2006). MCI patients exhibited intermediate MPPF binding values between AD and controls. Representative MPPF images are shown in Figure 25.2 (top row), depicting regionally diminished signal intensities of MPPF, especially in the hippocampus in an AD patient and less prominent reductions in an MCI patient relative to a cognitively normal subject. Discrepant to this, however, is another [^{18}F] MPPF study that reported a downregulation of hippocampal 5-HT$_{1A}$ binding in patients with mild AD but an upregulation in patients with MCI (Truchot et al., 2007). The discrepancy remains unexplained but the main concerns are the small number of subjects in each study (about 10 patients per group in each study) and the clinical heterogeneity across the sample. Variability between subjects in disease severity and duration as well as comorbidity with other disorders such as depression could influence the results significantly.

Amyloid PET imaging

Another promising development in imaging is the recent discovery of PET tracer compounds that enable detection of amyloid plaques in the living brain, one

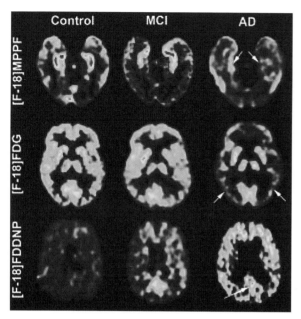

Figure 25.2 Representative examples of brain PET images from a control subject (*Left*), an MCI subject (*Center*), and an AD patient (*Right*): Images of [¹⁸F] MPPF binding (summed 30–60 min) to serotonin (5-HT_{1A}) receptors, are shown at the *Top*. The images from the AD patient show strongly decreased [¹⁸F] MPPF binding in the hippocampus (arrows in *Top*), coinciding with globally decreased cortical metabolism, as reflected by images of deoxy-[¹⁸F]-fluoro-D-glucose (FDG), shown in the *Middle*, and increased cortical binding of [¹⁸F] FDDNP, a molecule that binds to plaques and tangles, shown at the *Bottom*. Reproduced from Kepe *et al.* (2006) with permission from the National Academy of Sciences of the USA.

> **Box 25.3. PET of neurotransmitter systems**
>
> - Developments of specific PET radioligands have paved the way for direct measurements of neurotransmitter systems.
> - Acetylcholine receptors were most profoundly diminished in the amygdala in AD.
> - Cholinergic nicotinic receptors were reduced in the hippocampus and temporal cortex in AD.
> - Serotonin 5-HT$_{1A}$ receptors were reduced in the hippocampus in AD and to a lesser extent also in MCI.

> **Box 25.4. Amyloid PET**
>
> - An [¹¹C] radiotracer-labeled compound (PIB) has been developed, which binds to amyloid-β plaques but not to tangles.
> - Amyloid PET has shown high amyloid load in AD and in MCI.
> - Amyloid PET shows higher amyloid load in MCI patients who convert to AD than in those who remain stable.
> - However, amyloid PET is at its beginning and its diagnostic accuracy still needs to be determined.

of the defining hallmarks of AD, previously only detectable at autopsy. The most extensive experience has been with the amyloid-binding [¹¹C] radiotracer-labeled Pittsburgh compound B (or in short PIB), which binds to amyloid-β plaques but not to tangles. Representative PIB images from a patient with AD and a cognitively normal elderly subject are shown in Figure 25.3 (bottom row), superimposed on

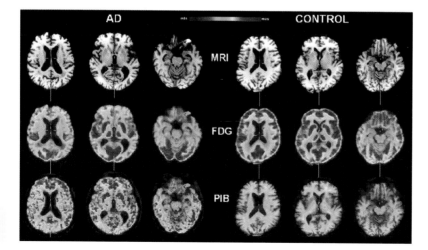

Figure 25.3 Representative brain amyloid PET images (*Bottom*) with the [¹¹C] Pittsburg compound B (PIB) from an AD patient (*Left*) and a control subject (*Right*). The images from the AD patient show highly increased binding of PIB in cortical regions, which coincides with decreased cortical metabolism, as reflected by images of FDG-PET, shown in the *Middle*. The corresponding structural MRI data are shown (*Top*) for anatomical reference. Data made available with permission from the Alzheimer's Disease Neuroimaging Initiative (ADNI).

structural MRI data. Higher PIB binding, reflecting higher amyloid load as represented by warmer colors, is clearly visible in the images of the AD patient. It has been shown that MCI patients can have a PIB uptake similar to that in AD (Forsberg *et al.*, 2008; Kemppainen *et al.*, 2007), suggesting that amyloid deposition occurs early. Furthermore, converters from MCI to AD had a significantly higher uptake of the amyloid tracer in the posterior cingulum than non-converters (Forsberg *et al.*, 2008). However, some MCI patients show no tracer binding at all (Price *et al.*, 2005). Amyloid imaging could therefore become useful for predicting the future disease course in at risk elders. However, because the early amyloid burden spares the hippocampus, which is known to be impacted early in AD (Braak and Braak, 1998), amyloid PET is unlikely to replace the need for imaging the hippocampal formation by other means. It is also not yet known whether amyloid imaging correlates more tightly than structural, functional or neurochemical imaging with cognitive decline. Nonetheless, the development of joint analyses utilizing amyloid PET as well as neurochemical, structural and functional imaging measures together may accomplish greater predictive power than either imaging modality can provide on its own.

Future perspectives

The studies reviewed above indicate that ^{1}H MRSI measures have the potential of offering a relatively direct window into neurochemical alterations in the brain and such measures might indicate neurodegenerative events more accurately than measures derived from peripheral tissue. However, potentially useful biomarkers need to undergo pathological validation in order to be deemed clinically useful. Most ^{1}H MRSI studies of AD lack clinical validation of the cohorts under investigation, a problem that also applies to neurotransmitter studies by PET. Only recently have ^{1}H MRSI measures been subjected to pathological validations in patients who were followed to autopsy (Kantarci *et al.*, 2008). More prospective ^{1}H MRSI studies that include pathological validations are necessary to determine if the metabolite alterations are useful as surrogates for neurodegeneration. This may require many years of data collection.

From a technical perspective, in-vivo ^{1}H MRSI will likely continue to benefit from new developments, such as stronger MRI magnets and refined acquisition methods. MRI scanners operating at a magnetic field strength of 3 Tesla compared to the established strength of 1.5 Tesla are now being more and more integrated into clinical practice, and 7 Tesla magnets are in operation at several research sites worldwide. An increased signal-to-noise ratio at higher field strength and greater spectral dispersion is expected to increase the diagnostic accuracy and test–retest reproducibility of ^{1}H MRSI. Paralleling the development of stronger magnets, new methods are being developed by physicists to simplify ^{1}H MRSI data to allow for more accurate quantification of metabolites such as glutamate, glutamine, and GABA (4-aminobutyric acid, the major inhibitory neurotransmitter in the mammalian brain). Accurate quantification of these metabolites currently suffers from significant spectral overlap with resonances from other metabolites (Kaiser *et al.*, 2008). These metabolites might provide additional diagnostic information in dementia. Furthermore, MRSI studies based on other nuclei, specifically ^{13}C, should become more feasible at higher magnetic fields. ^{13}C MRS measures of the neuronal tricarboxylic acid cycle, glucose oxidation and glutamate neurotransmission – to name a few – may provide additional markers for neurochemical processes in AD (Lin *et al.*, 2003; Ross *et al.*, 2003).

Box 25.5. Future perspectives

- ^{1}H MRSI will benefit from new developments that improve measurement precision, including the detection of additional metabolites, such as glutamate, glutamine, and GABA.
- Development of new PET radioligands will make possible the investigation of more neurotransmitter systems, such as several serotonin receptor subtypes.
- Multi-transmitter PET imaging will provide the possibility to explore how different transmitter systems interact.
- Development of an [^{18}F]-labeled derivative as amyloid tracer will allow for wider distribution and application of amyloid PET.

The work in PET neurotransmitters briefly reviewed above constitutes only a beginning in the exploration of the role of the various neurotransmitter systems in human cognition. For example, several serotonin receptor subtypes other than 5-HT$_{1A}$ have been implicated on cognitive functions from animal models. Future radioligand development will allow for further investigation of the functional role of other serotonergic subtypes in humans. In addition, multi-transmitter system imaging will provide the possibility to explore how different transmitter systems interact.

Amyloid imaging technology holds particular promise for more efficient assessment of pharmacologic interventions that aim to clear amyloid from the brain. However, the diagnostic potential of amyloid imaging will not be fully realized until an effective treatment exists for AD and amyloid load changes over time can be measured. At that time, the ability to identify early and perhaps presymptomatic conditions that might be slowed or even reversed by therapy will become essential. Development of a [^{18}F]-labeled derivative of PIB is also underway, which will allow for wider distribution and application of amyloid imaging.

Summary

Neurochemical imaging modalities provide a powerful tool in studies of Alzheimer's disease and related cognitive disorders, expanding our knowledge of the neuronal underpinning of the disease and potentially aiding development of targets for pharmacological treatment. Present data support the concept that ^{1}H MRSI measures of reduced NAA, a neuronal integrity marker and elevated MI may be valuable in predicting development of dementia and monitoring early disease progression for preventive therapies. However, investigations of ^{1}H MRSI as a marker for differential diagnosis and progression of dementia have been largely limited to clinically confirmed cohorts, and more studies are necessary to validate potential ^{1}H MRSI markers by histopathology at autopsy, a limitation that ^{1}H MRSI currently shares with PET imaging of neurotransmitter systems. Overall, MRS is a promising investigational technique in dementia and related cognitive disorders at this time that provides unique measures of multivariate spectroscopic profiles of the brain. The potential clinical application of ^{1}H MRSI in aging and dementia is expected to grow with technical advances in the field.

Acknowledgments

I am indebted to Dr. Michael W. Weiner, Director of the Center for Imaging of Neurodegenerative iseases (CIND), for his scientific guidance and support. This work was funded in part by support by grants from US Department of Defense, a grant from the Michael J. Fox Foundation for Parkinson's Disease Research, and grant (RR23953) from the National Center for Research Resources of NIH (Dr. Weiner).

References

Ackl N, Ising M, Schreiber Y A, Atiya M, Sonntag A and Auer D P. 2005. Hippocampal metabolic abnormalities in mild cognitive impairment and Alzheimer's disease. *Neurosci Lett* **384**, 23–8.

Adalsteinsson E, Sullivan E V, Kleinhans N, Spielman D M and Pfefferbaum A. 2000. Longitudinal decline of the neuronal marker N-acetyl aspartate in Alzheimer's disease. *Lancet* **355**, 1696–7.

Birken D L and Oldendorf W H. 1989. N-acetyl-L-aspartic acid: A literature review of a compound prominent in 1H-NMR spectroscopic studies of brain. *Neurosci Biobehav Rev* **13**, 23–31.

Bitsch A, Bruhn H, Vougioukas V, et al. 1999. Inflammatory CNS demyelination: Histopathologic correlation with in vivo quantitative proton MR spectroscopy. *Am J Neuroradiol* **20**, 1619–27.

Blakely R D and Coyle J T. 1988. The neurobiology of N-acetylaspartylglutamate. *Int Rev Neurobiol* **30**, 39–100.

Braak H and Braak E. 1998. Evolution of neuronal changes in the course of Alzheimer's disease. *J Neural Transm Suppl* **53**, 127–40.

Brand A, Richter-Landsberg C and Leibfritz D. 1993. Multinuclear NMR studies on the energy metabolism of glial and neuronal cells. *Dev Neurosci* **15**, 289–98.

Capizzano A A, Schuff N, Amend D L, et al. 2000. Subcortical ischemic vascular dementia: Assessment with quantitative MR imaging and 1H MR spectroscopy. *Am J Neuroradiol* **21**, 621–30.

Catani M, Cherubini A, Howard R, et al. 2001. (1)H-MR spectroscopy differentiates mild cognitive impairment from normal brain aging. *Neuroreport* **12**, 2315–7.

Chantal S, Braun C M, Bouchard R W, Labelle M and Boulanger Y. 2004. Similar 1H magnetic resonance spectroscopic metabolic pattern in the medial temporal lobes of patients with mild cognitive impairment and Alzheimer disease. *Brain Res* **1003**, 26–35.

Chao L L, Mueller S G, Buckley S T, et al. 2010. Evidence of neurodegeneration in brains of older adults who do not yet fulfill MCI criteria. *Neurobiol Aging* **31**, 368–77.

Chao L L, Schuff N, Kramer J H, et al. 2005. Reduced medial temporal lobe N-acetylaspartate in cognitively impaired but nondemented patients. *Neurology* **64**, 282–9.

Dixon R M, Bradley K M, Budge M M, Styles P and Smith A D. 2002. Longitudinal quantitative proton magnetic resonance spectroscopy of the hippocampus in Alzheimer's disease. *Brain* **125**, 2332–41.

Engelborghs S and De Deyn P P. 1997. The neurochemistry of Alzheimer's disease. *Acta Neurol Belg* **97**, 67–84.

Ernst T, Chang L, Melchor R and Mehringer C M. 1997. Frontotemporal dementia and early Alzheimer disease: Differentiation with frontal lobe H-1 MR spectroscopy. *Radiology* **203**, 829–36.

Fernandez A, Garcia-Segura J M, Ortiz T, *et al.* 2005. Proton magnetic resonance spectroscopy and magnetoencephalographic estimation of delta dipole density: A combination of techniques that may contribute to the diagnosis of Alzheimer's disease. *Dement Geriatr Cogn Disord* **20**, 169–77.

Ferri C P, Prince M, Brayne C, *et al.* 2005. Global prevalence of dementia: A Delphi consensus study. *Lancet* **366**, 2112–7.

Forsberg A, Engler H, Almkvist O, *et al.* 2008. PET imaging of amyloid deposition in patients with mild cognitive impairment. *Neurobiol Aging* **29**, 1456–65.

Glanville N T, Byers D M, Cook H W, Spence M W and Palmer F B. 1989. Differences in the metabolism of inositol and phosphoinositides by cultured cells of neuronal and glial origin. *Biochim Biophys Acta* **1004**, 169–79.

Glodzik L, King K G, Gonen O, Liu S, De Santi S and de Leon M J. 2008. Memantine decreases hippocampal glutamate levels: A magnetic resonance spectroscopy study. *Prog Neuropsychopharmacol Biol Psychiatry* **32**, 1005–12.

Guimaraes A R, Schwartz P, Prakash M R, *et al.* 1995. Quantitative in vivo 1H nuclear magnetic resonance spectroscopic imaging of neuronal loss in rat brain. *Neuroscience* **69**, 1095–101.

Jessen F, Block W, Traber F, *et al.* 2001. Decrease of *N*-acetylaspartate in the MTL correlates with cognitive decline of AD patients. *Neurology* **57**, 930–2.

Kadir A, Almkvist O, Wall A, Langstrom B and Nordberg A. 2006. PET imaging of cortical 11C-nicotine binding correlates with the cognitive function of attention in Alzheimer's disease. *Psychopharmacology (Berl)* **188**, 509–20.

Kaiser L G, Young K, Meyerhoff D J, Mueller S G and Matson G B. 2008. A detailed analysis of localized J-difference GABA editing: theoretical and experimental study at 4 T. *NMR Biomed* **21**, 22–32.

Kantarci K, Jack C R, Jr., Xu Y C, Campeau N G, O'Brien P C, Smith G E, *et al.* 2000. Regional metabolic patterns in mild cognitive impairment and Alzheimer's disease: A 1H MRS study. *Neurology* 2000; **55**: 210–7.

Kantarci K, Knopman D S, Dickson D W, *et al.* 2008. Alzheimer disease: Postmortem neuropathologic correlates of antemortem 1H MR spectroscopy metabolite measurements. *Radiology* **248**, 210–20.

Kantarci K, Smith G E, Ivnik R J, *et al.* 2002. 1H magnetic resonance spectroscopy, cognitive function, and apolipoprotein E genotype in normal aging, mild cognitive impairment and Alzheimer's disease. *J Int Neuropsychol Soc* **8**, 934–42.

Kantarci K, Weigand S D, Petersen R C, *et al.* 2007. Longitudinal 1H MRS changes in mild cognitive impairment and Alzheimer's disease. *Neurobiol Aging* **28**, 1330–9.

Kemppainen N M, Aalto S, Wilson I A, *et al.* 2007. PET amyloid ligand [11C]PIB uptake is increased in mild cognitive impairment. *Neurology* **68**, 1603–06.

Kepe V, Barrio J R, Huang S C, *et al.* 2006. Serotonin 1A receptors in the living brain of Alzheimer's disease patients. *Proc Natl Acad Sci USA* **103**, 702–07.

Klein J. 2000. Membrane breakdown in acute and chronic neurodegeneration: Focus on choline-containing phospholipids. *J Neural Transm* **107**, 1027–63.

Klunk W E, Panchalingam K, Moossy J, McClure R J and Pettegrew J W. 1992. *N*-acetyl-L-aspartate and other amino acid metabolites in Alzheimer's disease brain: A preliminary proton nuclear magnetic resonance study. *Neurology* **42**, 1578–85.

Koller K J, Zaczek R and Coyle J T. 1984. *N*-acetyl-aspartyl-glutamate: Regional levels in rat brain and the effects of brain lesions as determined by a new HPLC method. *J Neurochem* **43**, 1136–42.

Krishnan K R, Charles H C, Doraiswamy P M, *et al.* 2003. Randomized, placebo-controlled trial of the effects of donepezil on neuronal markers and hippocampal volumes in Alzheimer's disease. *Am J Psychiatry* **160**, 2003–11.

Kuhl D E, Koeppe R A, Minoshima S, *et al.* 1999. In vivo mapping of cerebral acetylcholinesterase activity in aging and Alzheimer's disease. *Neurology* **52**, 691–9.

Lin A P, Shic F, Enriquez C and Ross B D. 2003. Reduced glutamate neurotransmission in patients with Alzheimer's disease – an in vivo (13)C magnetic resonance spectroscopy study. *Magma* **16**, 29–42.

Metastasio A, Rinaldi P, Tarducci R, *et al.* 2006. Conversion of MCI to dementia: Role of proton magnetic resonance spectroscopy. *Neurobiol Aging* **27**, 926–32.

Meyerhoff D J, MacKay S, Constans J M, *et al.* 1994. Axonal injury and membrane alterations in Alzheimer's disease suggested by in vivo proton magnetic resonance spectroscopic imaging. *Ann Neurol* **36**, 40–7.

Mihara M, Hattori N, Abe K, Sakoda S and Sawada T. 2006. Magnetic resonance spectroscopic study of Alzheimer's disease and frontotemporal dementia/Pick complex. *Neuroreport* **17**, 413–6.

Moats R A, Ernst T, Shonk T K and Ross B D. 1994. Abnormal cerebral metabolite concentrations in patients with probable Alzheimer disease. *Magn Reson Med* **32**, 110–5.

Nordberg A. 1993. Clinical studies in Alzheimer patients with positron emission tomography. *Behav Brain Res* **57**, 215–24.

Nordberg A, Hartvig P, Lilja A, *et al*. 1990. Decreased uptake and binding of 11C-nicotine in brain of Alzheimer patients as visualized by positron emission tomography. *J Neural Transm Park Dis Dement Sect* **2**, 215–24.

Nordberg A, Lundqvist H, Hartvig P, Lilja A and Langstrom B. 1995. Kinetic analysis of regional (S)(–)11C-nicotine binding in normal and Alzheimer brains – In vivo assessment using positron emission tomography. *Alzheimer Dis Assoc Disord* **9**, 21–7.

Olson B L, Holshouser B A, Britt W 3rd, *et al*. 2008. Longitudinal metabolic and cognitive changes in mild cognitive impairment patients. *Alzheimer Dis Assoc Disord* **22**, 269–77.

Panza F, D'Introno A, Colacicco A M, *et al*. 2005. Current epidemiology of mild cognitive impairment and other predementia syndromes. *Am J Geriatr Psychiatry* **13**, 633–44.

Parnetti L, Lowenthal D T, Presciutti O, *et al*. 1996. 1H-MRS, MRI-based hippocampal volumetry, and 99mTc-HMPAO-SPECT in normal aging, age-associated memory impairment, and probable Alzheimer's disease. *J Am Geriatr Soc* **44**, 133–8.

Parnetti L, Tarducci R, Presciutti O, *et al*. 1997. Proton magnetic resonance spectroscopy can differentiate Alzheimer's disease from normal aging. *Mech Ageing Dev* **97**, 9–14.

Petersen R C, Smith G E, Waring S C, Ivnik R J, Tangalos E G and Kokmen E. 1999. Mild cognitive impairment: Clinical characterization and outcome. *Arch Neurol* **56**, 303–08.

Pfefferbaum A, Adalsteinsson E, Spielman D, Sullivan E V and Lim K O. 1999. In vivo brain concentrations of N-acetyl compounds, creatine, and choline in Alzheimer disease. *Arch Gen Psychiatry* **56**, 185–92.

Price J C, Klunk W E, Lopresti B J, *et al*. 2005. Kinetic modeling of amyloid binding in humans using PET imaging and Pittsburgh Compound-B. *J Cereb Blood Flow Metab* **25**, 1528–47.

Rose S E, de Zubicaray G I, Wang D, *et al*. 1999. A 1H MRS study of probable Alzheimer's disease and normal aging: Implications for longitudinal monitoring of dementia progression. *Magn Reson Imaging* **17**, 291–9.

Ross B, Lin A, Harris K, Bhattacharya P and Schweinsburg B. 2003. Clinical experience with 13C MRS in vivo. *NMR Biomed* **16**, 358–69.

Schuff N, Amend D, Ezekiel F, *et al*. 1997. Changes of hippocampal N-acetylaspartate and volume in Alzheimer's disease: A proton MR spectroscopic imaging and MRI study. *Neurology* **49**, 1513–21.

Schuff N, Capizzano A A, Du A T, *et al*. 2003. Different patterns of N-acetylaspartate loss in subcortical ischemic vascular dementia and AD. *Neurology* **61**, 358–64.

Schuff N, Capizzano A A, Du A T, *et al*. 2002. Selective reduction of N-acetylaspartate in medial temporal and parietal lobes in AD. *Neurology* **58**, 928–35.

Schuff N, Ezekiel F, Gamst A C, *et al*. 2001. Region and tissue differences of metabolites in normally aged brain using multislice 1H magnetic resonance spectroscopic imaging. *Magn Reson Med* **45**, 899–907.

Shinotoh H, Fukushi K, Nagatsuka S, *et al*. 2003. The amygdala and Alzheimer's disease: Positron emission tomographic study of the cholinergic system. *Ann N Y Acad Sci* **985**, 411–9.

Shonk T K, Moats R A, Gifford P, *et al*. 1995. Probable Alzheimer disease: Diagnosis with proton MR spectroscopy. *Radiology* **195**, 65–72.

Siger M, Schuff N, Zhu X, Miller B L and Weiner M W. 2009. Regional myo-inositol concentration in mild cognitive impairment using 1H magnetic resonance spectroscopic imaging. *Alzheimer Dis Assoc Disord* **23**, 57–62.

Simmons M L, Frondoza C G and Coyle J T. 1991. Immunocytochemical localization of N-acetyl-aspartate with monoclonal antibodies. *Neuroscience* **45**, 37–45.

Tedeschi G, Bertolino A, Lundbom N, *et al*. 1996. Cortical and subcortical chemical pathology in Alzheimer's disease as assessed by multislice proton magnetic resonance spectroscopic imaging. *Neurology* **47**, 696–704.

Truchot L, Costes S N, Zimmer L, *et al*. 2007. Up-regulation of hippocampal serotonin metabolism in mild cognitive impairment. *Neurology* **69**, 1012–7.

Urenjak J, Williams S R, Gadian D G and Noble M. 1993. Proton nuclear magnetic resonance spectroscopy unambiguously identifies different neural cell types. *J Neurosci* **13**, 981–9.

Wyper D J, Brown D, Patterson J, *et al*. 1993. Deficits in iodine-labelled 3-quinuclidinyl benzilate binding in relation to cerebral blood flow in patients with Alzheimer's disease. *Eur J Nucl Med* **20**, 379–86.

Zhu X, Schuff N, Kornak J, *et al*. 2006. Effects of Alzheimer disease on fronto-parietal brain N-acetyl aspartate and myo-inositol using magnetic resonance spectroscopic imaging. *Alzheimer Dis Assoc Disord* **20**, 77–85.

Chapter 26

Neuroimaging of Parkinson's disease

Raúl de la Fuente-Fernández and A. Jon Stoessl

Introduction

Parkinson's disease (PD) is the second most common neurodegenerative disorder after Alzheimer's disease (de Lau and Breteler, 2006). PD is characterized by the progressive loss of dopamine neurons in the substantia nigra pars compacta (SNpc), which leads to striatal dopamine denervation, particularly affecting the dorsolateral part of the putamen (Kish et al., 1988; Fearnley and Lees, 1991). As this part of the putamen is mostly involved in motor performance, motor dysfunction is the chief manifestation of PD. However, it has become increasingly recognized that other brain systems and functions are impaired in PD. Thus, behavior disorders and cognitive dysfunction are often present in PD, and constitute a major source of disability (Dubois and Pillon, 1997; Schrag et al., 2000; Aarsland et al., 2001; Weintraub et al., 2004). The actual prevalence rates of cognitive dysfunction and dementia in PD are difficult to determine, as they will depend upon whether extensive neuropsychological analysis was used or not, as well as several confounding factors (e.g. age, presence of depression). In general, it is accepted that at least some 30% of PD subjects will end up developing dementia (Dubois and Pillon, 1997). The risk of dementia can be up to sixfold higher in PD compared to subjects without PD (Aarsland et al., 2001).

The underlying mechanisms by which these non-motor manifestations of PD actually come into play are still poorly understood. It is well known that the Lewy body, the pathological hallmark of PD (Gibb and Lees, 1988; Fearnley and Lees, 1991) or Lewy neurites, can be present not only in surviving dopamine neurons of the midbrain, but also in the cerebral cortex and other brainstem nuclei (Gibb and

Lees, 1988; Gibb et al., 1989; Kosaka and Iseki, 1996; Del Tredici et al., 2002; Braak et al., 2003). While some subjects with Lewy body pathology develop cognitive impairment as an early or even initial manifestation of disease – a condition named dementia with Lewy bodies (DLB) – most of them initially present with typical motor symptoms and then go on to develop dementia, an entity known as PD dementia (PDD) (Gibb et al., 1989; Del Tredici et al., 2002; Braak et al., 2003). In all likelihood both conditions are nothing more than the two ends of the same spectrum (de la Fuente-Fernández and Calne, 1996).

Pathological observations suggest that PD usually first affects the lower brainstem structures, and then progresses in a caudo-rostral direction to affect midbrain structures (particularly SNpc) and finally the cerebral cortex (Braak et al., 2003). Cases that follow this pattern would ultimately present with clinical features of PDD. However, Lewy body pathology can affect the cerebral cortex from the beginning of illness, which would manifest clinically as DLB (Gibb et al., 1989; Braak et al., 2003). Still, PD subjects without frank dementia, where Lewy body pathology is presumably restricted to the brainstem, most often present with signs of frontal–executive dysfunction (Cools, 2006; Dagher and Nagano-Saito, 2007; Grahn et al., 2008). There is evidence that such frontal dysfunction is likely related, at least in great part, to "deafferentation" caused by striatal dopamine deficiency (Cools, 2006; Grahn et al., 2008). As we will see in this review, recent neuroimaging studies have started to unravel some of the mysteries behind the behavior and cognitive manifestations of PD (Postuma and Dagher, 2006; Nandhagopal et al., 2008).

Topography of dopamine depletion in PD

Most of the burden of Lewy body pathology involves dopamine cells in the ventrolateral tier of SNpc (Fearnley and Lees, 1991), a region that primarily projects to the dorsal striatum (nigrostriatal dopamine pathway), particularly the dorsolateral part of the putamen, but also dorsal parts of the caudate nucleus (Bernheimer *et al.*, 1973; Kish *et al.*, 1988, 1992). Less affected by Lewy body pathology are dopamine cells located in medial and dorsal regions of SNpc, and even less affected are dopamine cells in the ventral tegmental area (VTA). Dopamine cells from the VTA send projections to the ventral striatum and other limbic structures (mesolimbic dopamine pathway). The ventral striatum is a structure that includes the nucleus accumbens as well as the ventral parts of the caudate and putamen. In addition to these dopamine projections to dorsal and ventral striatum, there are also direct dopamine projections from VTA and the medial part of SNpc to the frontal cortex (mesocortical dopamine pathway). There is evidence to suggest that this pathway is also damaged in PD (Javoy-Agid and Agid, 1980; Scatton *et al.*, 1983). Asymmetries in the damage to the different dopaminergic regions may help explain some the variability in motor and cognitive function often encountered in PD (Cheesman *et al.*, 2005; Foster *et al.*, 2008).

Cortico-striatal loops

The basal ganglia consist of several structures involved in a complex functional network. Following an oversimplified model, there are three major anatomical and functional cortico-striatal loops, which are mostly organized in parallel (Alexander *et al.*, 1986; Albin *et al.*, 1989; Middleton and Strick, 2000; Obeso *et al.*, 2000; see Figure 26.1). (1) The motor loop, where several cortical motor regions, particularly the supplementary motor area (SMA), connect with the putamen, which in turn modulates the same cortical motor areas through several relays involving the internal pallidum/substantia nigra pars reticulata (GPi/SNpr) and the ventrolateral nucleus of the thalamus. (2) The cognitive loop, connecting the dorsolateral prefrontal cortex (PFC) to the dorsolateral part of the head of the caudate nucleus, which in turn sends

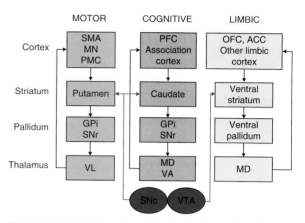

Figure 26.1 Parallel loops involving the basal ganglia and responsible for regulation of motor, cognitive and behavioral function. ACC, anterior cingulate cortex; GPI, internal globus pallidus; M1, motor cortex; MD, medial dorsal nucleus; OFC, orbitofrontal cortex; PFC, prefrontal cortex; PMC, premotor cortex; SNc, substantia nigra pars compacta; SNr, substantia nigra pars reticulata; VA, ventral anterior; VTA, ventral tegmental area. Adapted from Alexander *et al.* (1986).

back modulatory adjustments to the dorsolateral prefrontal PFC through GPi/SNpr and the mediodorsal and ventral anterior thalamic nuclei. (3) The limbic loop, with inputs from the orbitofrontal cortex (OFC) to the ventral caudate nucleus, and from the anterior cingulate cortex (ACC), amygdala and hippocampus to the nucleus accumbens; these two structures of the ventral striatum modulate the corresponding cortical and limbic regions through the ventral pallidum and the mediodorsal nucleus of the thalamus. As mentioned earlier, dopamine inputs originating in SNpc modulate the motor and cognitive loops by acting on dopamine receptors in the dorsal striatum (putamen and caudate), respectively. Dopamine inputs from VTA modulate the limbic loop by acting on dopamine receptors in the ventral striatum.

In-vivo anatomical and functional confirmation of these cortico-striatal loops in humans comes from magnetic resonance imaging techniques (Bestmann *et al.*, 2004; Lehéricy *et al.*, 2004). In addition, in-vivo experiments in humans combining positron emission tomography (PET) and repetitive transcranial magnetic stimulation (rTMS) techniques also support the notion that these cortico-striatal loops are indeed segregated. Thus, while rTMS of the motor cortex induces the release of dopamine in the putamen, rTMS applied to the dorsolateral PFC induces dopamine release in the caudate nucleus (Strafella et al., 2001, 2003b).

It remains unknown whether the mesocortical dopamine pathway modifies the functional interface of these three parallel loops (Cools, 2006). Interestingly, while dopamine D2-type receptors are particularly abundant in the striatum (Cooper et al., 2003), D1-type receptors may predominate in the PFC (Bergson et al., 1995; Williams and Goldman-Rakic, 1995; Sawaguchi, 2000). In addition, there are differences in dopamine handling among the nigrostriatal, mesolimbic and mesocortical pathways (Cooper et al., 2003), which may also explain in part their distinct response to dopaminergic treatment in PD. All these factors should be taken into account when examining the function of the cortico-striatal loops (Kimberg and D'Esposito, 2003; Cools, 2006). In fact, it has long been recognized that dopaminergic treatment can have both positive and negative effects on cognitive function in PD subjects (Gotham et al., 1986, 1988; Owen et al., 1993b; Kulisevsky et al., 1996, Cools et al., 2001b; Lewis et al., 2005). Dopamine replacement therapy can also act as a mood modifier (Black et al., 2005).

Frontal lobe dysfunction in PD

The three major cortico-striatal loops outlined above involve a number of frontal cortical areas, which are functionally (and perhaps structurally) differently impaired at different stages of PD (Lange et al., 1992; Owen et al., 1992, 1993a; Owen, 1997; Fera et al., 2007). In the early stages of PD, frontal lobe dysfunction most likely reflects deafferentation in relation to dopamine deficiency, first in the dorsal striatum and later in the ventral striatum as well. In keeping with this notion, the administration of a dopamine D2 receptor antagonist to healthy volunteers reproduces to a great extent the cognitive deficits often seen in PD subjects (Mehta et al., 1999). In later stages of the disease, however, damage to the mesocortical dopamine pathway, and even direct damage to frontal cortical areas (cortical Lewy body pathology), may contribute to impair normal frontal lobe function. In fact, dementia in PD is related to the loss of dopamine cells in the medial part of SNpc (Rinne et al., 1989), where the mesocortical dopamine pathway originates. There is some indication that frontal lobe dysfunction may predict incident dementia in PD (Woods and Tröster, 2003).

The cortico-striatal motor loop: motor tasks in PD

In keeping with current motor program models of basal ganglia function (Mink, 1996), PET studies measuring cerebral blood flow (CBF) have shown that the basal ganglia and SMA play a major role in motor sequence control (Boecker et al., 1998). As expected, compared to normal controls, PD subjects have less activation in the contralateral putamen and the corresponding frontal motor regions, such as SMA, while performing motor tasks (Playford et al., 1992). Interestingly, a similar covariance pattern was obtained under resting conditions using PET with fluorodeoxyglucose (FDG-PET) (Asanuma et al., 2006). Greater deficits of activation occur in self-initiated movements as compared to externally triggered movements (Jahanshahi et al., 1995). In contrast, PD subjects often show over-activity in cortical areas that are relatively putamen-independent, particularly when performing more complex motor tasks (Samuel et al., 1997a). These activation abnormalities are corrected after normalization of basal ganglia function by either pharmacological (Jenkins et al., 1992; Rascol et al., 1992) or surgical approaches (Grafton et al., 1995; Limousin et al., 1997; Samuel et al., 1997b; Ceballos-Baumann et al., 1999; Fukuda et al., 2001; Strafella et al., 2003a; Asanuma et al., 2006). Functional magnetic resonance (fMRI) studies have in general yielded similar results (Haslinger et al., 2001; Buhmann et al., 2003), although there are some conflicting observations (Sabatini et al., 2000; Peters et al., 2003). It is worth noting that the functional changes observed during performance of motor tasks most likely also reflect some additional frontal lobe abnormalities in relation to attention, planning, and working memory (Owen et al., 1992; Rowe et al., 2002; Dirnberger et al., 2005). Thus, PD subjects performing simple motor tasks also show under-activation of frontal areas not directly involved in the motor loop, such as the PFC and ACC (Playford et al., 1992). Interestingly, compensatory reorganization of the cortical–striatal motor loop has been found during the presymptomatic phase of PD (Buhmann et al., 2005).

The cortico-striatal cognitive loop: cognitive tasks in PD

Normal performance of typical frontal lobe cognitive tasks, such as the Wisconsin Card Sorting Task or the Tower of London planning task, depends upon several frontal executive functions including attention, planning, and cognitive flexibility. Functional neuroimaging studies in healthy human subjects have shown that the dorsal striatum (in particular, the caudate nucleus) and the dorsolateral PFC are activated during task set-shifting (Dagher *et al.*, 1999; Sohn *et al.*, 2000; Monchi *et al.*, 2001; Lewis *et al.*, 2004). In contrast, PD subjects off medication have impaired task set-shifting (Cools *et al.*, 2001a), presumably in relation to deafferentation of the dorsolateral PFC, which is dependent on inputs from the dorsal part of the caudate nucleus (Cools *et al.*, 2001b). In this context, it is worth noting that PD is characterized by substantial dopamine depletion in the most rostrodorsal part of the caudate nucleus (Kish *et al.*, 1988). In fact, after the putamen, the dorsal part of the caudate nucleus is the striatal structure with greater dopamine depletion in PD. As the rostrodorsal part of the caudate is connected with the dorsolateral PFC (Yeterian and Pandya, 1991), impairments in tasks involving attentional set-shifting can be predicted to occur in PD, even in early stages of disease (Owen *et al.*, 1993b; Cools *et al.*, 2001a).

In keeping with these anatomical considerations, and also in keeping with the clinical observations, CBF PET studies have found reduced activation in the basal ganglia of PD subjects during performance of the Tower of London test (Owen *et al.*, 1998; Dagher *et al.*, 2001). In addition, the degree of impairment on executive tasks was found to correlate with dopaminergic hypofunction in the caudate nucleus (Marié *et al.*, 1999; Brück *et al.*, 2001). At the PFC level, however, the results are not so clear-cut and, in fact, there have been some a-priori conflicting observations. As expected, fMRI studies have shown that PD subjects with executive dysfunction do have underactivation of the cognitive loop (caudate and PFC) as compared to PD subjects without dysexecutive dysfunction (Lewis *et al.*, 2003). However, several functional neuroimaging studies, including PET and fMRI, have also shown that, as compared to healthy controls, PD subjects have increased (not decreased) activation in the dorsolateral PFC during performance of PFC-sensitive cognitive tasks (Dagher *et al.*, 2001; Cools *et al.*, 2002b; Mattay *et al.*, 2002). As levodopa administration (i.e. dopamine replacement) normalized these activation pattern abnormalities, the authors proposed that over-activation of the dorsolateral PFC observed in PD subjects could be related to dysfunction in the mesocortical dopamine pathway

(e.g. reduced dopamine levels in PFC) (Cools *et al.*, 2002b; Mattay *et al.*, 2002). Naturally, one cannot be absolutely certain as to whether the normalizing effect of dopamine replacement occurs at the level of the caudate nucleus (normalization of the nigrostriatal dopamine pathway) or at the level of the frontal cortex (normalization of the mesocortical dopamine pathway). Nonetheless, current models of basal ganglia function do suggest that the effect of dopamine replacement in the caudate nucleus should lead to an increase (not a decrease) in PFC activity (Alexander *et al.*, 1986; Albin *et al.*, 1989), which lends support to the notion of a dysfunctional mesocortical dopamine pathway in PD.

More recent fMRI studies in early PD subjects have yielded more detailed information on this issue (Monchi *et al.*, 2004, 2007). It has been shown that, as compared to normal controls, PD subjects have both over-activation in the dorsolateral PFC and under-activation in the ventrolateral PFC during performance of the Wisconsin Card Sorting Task (Monchi *et al.*, 2004). More importantly, using the Montreal Card Sorting Task, the same authors demonstrated that the pattern of activation in PD was dependent upon whether the cognitive task involved the caudate nucleus or not. Only when the task was caudate-dependent did PD subjects show prefrontal under-activation, in both the dorsolateral and ventrolateral PFC (Monchi *et al.*, 2007). In contrast, when the cognitive task was caudate-independent, PD subjects actually showed over-activation, not only in PFC, but also in cortical regions not normally involved in the performance of the task (Monchi *et al.*, 2007). Taken together, these observations suggest that, in addition to dopamine depletion in the caudate nucleus, the mesocortical dopamine pathway most likely also plays a role in the pattern of cognitive dysfunction observed in PD. Nonetheless, changes in the ventral part of the caudate nucleus, which is connected to the ventrolateral PFC (Yeterian and Pandya, 1991), may also contribute to the PD activation pattern.

The cortico-striatal limbic loop: reversal learning tasks and behavior in PD

In contrast to the severely affected dopaminergic projections to the dorsal striatum (caudate and putamen), the dopaminergic projection to the ventral striatum seems to be essentially normal in PD, at least in the early stages of the disease (Kish *et al.*, 1988).

This simple observation has profound implications for understanding why dopamine replacement therapy sometimes leads to behavioral disorders in PD subjects. Nonetheless, a recent PET study suggested that depression, which sometimes precedes PD motor symptoms, may be associated with loss of dopamine terminals in the ventral striatum (Remy et al., 2005).

There is compelling evidence that probabilistic reversal learning tasks are well suited to examine the function of the ventral striatum, in particular the nucleus accumbens (Cools et al., 2007). To perform these tasks, subjects must reject the learned rule in favor of a contradictory rule (Swainson et al., 2000). Hence, probabilistic reversal learning tasks, as is the case for the cognitive tasks used to examine the cortico-striatal cognitive loop, are also dependent on cognitive flexibility. However, they are conceptually different from typical set-shifting tasks such us the Wisconsin Card Sorting Test. Essentially, reversal learning tasks test for balance between "go" and "no-go" signals (Frank et al., 2004). fMRI studies on healthy human volunteers have shown that probabilistic reversal learning tasks activate the ventral striatum and the corresponding ventrolateral PFC (Cools et al., 2002a). This pattern of activation (accumbens–ventrolateral PFC) contrasts with the pattern obtained during performance of set-shifting tasks (caudate–dorsolateral PFC). As expected, PD subjects off medication perform much better on reversal learning tasks than on tasks involving the dorsal striatum circuitry (Swainson et al., 2000) and show normal activation in the nucleus accumbens (Cools et al., 2007). However, dopamine replacement therapy may actually worsen the performance of reversal learning tasks in PD subjects, and this deleterious effect is reversed by levodopa withdrawal (Cools et al., 2001b).

To explain this paradoxical effect (i.e. worsening on dopamine replacement therapy), it has long been proposed that treatment may "over-dose" the essentially normal ventral striatum, and the corresponding limbic loop, in PD subjects (Gotham et al., 1986, 1988; Cools, 2006). Accordingly, while dopamine replacement therapy improves function in circuitries dependent upon structures with major PD-related dopamine depletion (dorsal striatum), the same treatment paradoxically impairs function in areas with no (or only minor) dopamine depletion, such as the ventral striatum (Cools, 2006). Interestingly, the administration of direct dopamine agonists to

healthy human subjects also leads to impairments in reversal-learning performance (Mehta et al., 2001).

It is well known that the mesolimbic dopamine pathway and corresponding cortical frontal areas are involved in reward processing and goal-directed behaviors (Schultz, 2002; Brown and Braver, 2005; Knutson et al., 2005). Hence, functional abnormalities in the limbic loop may also explain why medicated PD subjects sometimes develop a number of behavioral disorders, including impulsivity, compulsive eating and shopping, hypersexuality, drug-seeking behavior, pathological gambling and other risk-taking behaviors (Goodwin et al., 1971; Vogel and Schiffter, 1983; Nausieda, 1985; Lawrence et al., 2003; Nandhagopal et al., 2008). Several experiments have shown that medicated PD subjects may have an impaired capacity to gauge different probability values (Knowlton et al., 1996) as well as the predicted reward value (Schott et al., 2007), and often exhibit abnormal betting strategies (Cools et al., 2003). Thus, while PD subjects off medication tend to avoid negative outcomes, they are particularly sensitive to positive outcomes when on medication (Frank et al., 2004). In other words, dopamine replacement therapy favors "go" signals over "no-go" signals.

These experimental observations set the foundations to explain the behavioral disorders sometimes encountered in PD, and suggested that medicated PD subjects may indeed have greater than normal levels of dopamine in the ventral striatum. A recent PET study has lent support to this prediction (Evans et al., 2006). After levodopa administration, PD subjects with the so-called "dopamine dysregulation syndrome" (i.e. subjects with abusive use of medication) release substantially more dopamine in the ventral striatum than PD subjects without this behavioral disorder. It is assumed that such increased levels of dopamine in the ventral striatum, particularly in the nucleus accumbens, must trigger rewarding signals, which perpetuates the abnormal behavior in question, be it abusive use of anti-PD medication or pathological gambling or sex, to name but a few. In fact, the same (or very similar) mechanism seems to be implicated in addiction to drugs of abuse, where the dopamine reward signal seems to be amplified (Schultz, 2002). There is also evidence to suggest that signals from the caudate nucleus may contribute to modulate these abnormal behaviors (Kaasinen et al., 2001; Tricomi et al., 2004).

Cognition and cortical pathology in PD

In keeping with neuropathological studies, which have demonstrated Lewy bodies and cell loss in medial temporal lobe areas (Braak *et al.*, 2003), high-resolution MRI images have demonstrated hippocampal atrophy in PD (Camicioli *et al.*, 2003; Burton *et al.*, 2004; Nagano-Saito *et al.*, 2005; Summerfield *et al.*, 2005). This hippocampal atrophy, which may precede frank dementia in PD, was correlated with impairments in memory tests. Naturally, frontal lobe dysfunction (see above) or direct Lewy body pathology in the frontal lobe (Braak *et al.*, 2003) may also contribute to memory deficits in PD. In fact, cortical Lewy body pathology is common in paralimbic, temporal and frontal areas of the neocortex in PD subjects with dementia (Kosaka and Iseki, 1996; Braak *et al.*, 2003). On the other hand, while the FDG-PET pattern of glucose metabolism in non-demented PD subjects is characterized by hypometabolism in frontal areas (Huang *et al.*, 2007), visual hallucinations, which are a major clinical criterion for the diagnosis of dementia with Lewy bodies, are associated with relative frontal lobe hypermetabolism and relative hypometabolism in posterior (parieto-occipital) cortical areas (Nagano-Saito *et al.*, 2004). This pattern of posterior hypometabolism may help distinguish dementia related to Lewy body pathology from Alzheimer's disease (Minoshima *et al.*, 2001). In addition, there is pathological (Scatton *et al.*, 1983) and in-vivo PET evidence that other neurotransmitters, particularly cholinergic pathways, are also involved in PD dementia (Bohnen *et al.*, 2003; Hilker *et al.*, 2005). Indeed, cholinergic dysfunction can be even more severe in PD subjects with dementia than in Alzheimer's disease (Bohnen *et al.*, 2003). Finally, in-vivo PET studies are currently investigating whether concomitant amyloid pathology may contribute to dementia in PD subjects, although at this point, it appears that amyloid deposition is associated more with DLB than with PDD (Edison *et al.*, 2008; Gomperts *et al.*, 2008).

References

Aarsland D, Andersen K, Larsen J P, *et al.* 2001. Risk of dementia in Parkinson's disease: a community-based, prospective study. *Neurology* **56**, 730–6.

Albin R L, Young A B and Penney J B. 1989. The functional anatomy of basal ganglia disorders. *Trends Neurosci* **12**, 366–75.

Alexander G E, DeLong, M R, and Strick P L. 1986. Parallel organization of functionally segregated circuits linking basal ganglia and cortex. *Annu Rev Neurosci* **9**, 357–81.

Asanuma K, Tang C, Ma Y, *et al.* 2006. Network modulation in the treatment of Parkinson's disease. *Brain* **129**, 2667–78.

Bergson C, Mrzljak L, Smiley J F, Pappy M, Levenson R, and Goldman-Rakic P S. 1995. Regional, cellular, and subcellular variations in the distribution of D1 and D5 dopamine receptors in primate brain. *J Neurosci* **15**, 7821–36.

Bernheimer H, Birkmayer W, Hornykiewicz O, Jellinger K, and Seitelberger F. 1973. Brain dopamine and the syndromes of Parkinson and Huntington: Clinical, morphological and neurochemical correlations. *J Neurol Sci* **20**, 415–55.

Bestmann S, Baudewig J, Siebner H R, Rothwell J C and Frahm J. 2004. Functional MRI of the immediate impact of transcranial magnetic stimulation on cortical and subcortical motor circuits. *Eur J Neurosci* **19**, 1950–62.

Black K J, Hershey T, Hartlein J M, Carl J L and Perlmutter J S. 2005. Levodopa challenge neuroimaging of levodopa-related mood fluctuations in Parkinson's disease. *Neuropsychopharmacology* **30**, 590–601.

Boecker H, Dagher A, Ceballos-Baumann A O, *et al.* 1998. Role of the human rostral supplementary motor area and the basal ganglia in motor sequence control: investigations with H2 15O PET. *J Neurophysiol* **79**, 1070–80.

Bohnen N I, Kaufer D I, Ivanco L S, *et al.* 2003. Cortical cholinergic function is more severely affected in parkinsonian dementia than in Alzheimer disease: An in vivo positron emission tomographic study. *Arch Neurol* **60**, 1745–8.

Box 26.1. Causes of cognitive impairment in Parkinson's disease

- Cortical Lewy body/Lewy neurite pathology.
- Loss of caudate and cortical dopamine innervation.
- Inverted U-shaped dose–response curve for dopamine in cortex.
  Worsening by dopaminergic therapy on probabilistic reversal learning tasks.
- Altered activity in cortico-striatal–thalamo-cortical loops.
- Cholinergic denervation.
- Concomitant amyloid deposition ± Alzheimer pathology.

Braak H, Del Tredici K, Rüb U, de Vos R A, Jansen Steur E N and Braak E. 2003. Staging of brain pathology related to sporadic Parkinson's disease. *Neurobiol Aging* **24**, 197–211.

Brown J W and Braver T S. 2005. Learned predictions of error likelihood in the anterior cingulate cortex. *Science* **307**, 1118–21.

Brück A, Portin R, Lindell A, *et al.* 2001. Positron emission tomography shows that impaired frontal lobe functioning in Parkinson's disease is related to dopaminergic hypofunction in the caudate nucleus. *Neurosci Lett* **311**, 81–4.

Buhmann C, Binkofski F, Klein C, *et al.* 2005. Motor reorganization in asymptomatic carriers of a single mutant Parkin allele: A human model for presymptomatic parkinsonism. *Brain* **128**, 2281–90.

Buhmann C, Glauche V, Sturenburg H J, Oechsner M, Weiller C and Buchel C. 2003. Pharmacologically modulated fMRI-cortical responsiveness to levodopa in drug-naive hemiparkinsonian patients. *Brain* **126**, 451–61.

Burton E J, McKeith I G, Burn D J, Williams E D and O'Brien J T. 2004. Cerebral atrophy in Parkinson's disease with and without dementia: a comparison with Alzheimer's disease, dementia with Lewy bodies and controls. *Brain* **127**, 791–800.

Camicioli R, Moore M M, Kinney A, Corbridge E, Glassberg K and Kaye J A. 2003. Parkinson's disease is associated with hippocampal atrophy. *Mov Disord* **18**, 784–90.

Ceballos-Baumann A O, Boecker H, Bartenstein P, *et al.* 1999. A positron emission tomographic study of subthalamic nucleus stimulation in Parkinson disease: Enhanced movement-related activity of motor-association cortex and decreased motor cortex resting activity. *Arch Neurol* **56**, 997–1003.

Cheesman A L, Barker R A, Lewis S J, Robbins T W, Owen A M and Brooks D J. 2005. Lateralisation of striatal function: Evidence from 18F-dopa PET in Parkinson's disease. *J Neurol Neurosurg Psychiatry* **76**, 1204–10.

Cools R. 2006. Dopaminergic modulation of cognitive function – implications for L-DOPA treatment in Parkinson's disease. *Neurosci Biobehav Rev* **30**, 1–23.

Cools R, Barker R A, Sahakian B J and Robbins T W. 2001a. Mechanisms of cognitive set flexibility in Parkinson's disease. *Brain* **124**, 2503–12.

Cools R, Barker R A, Sahakian B J and Robbins T W. 2001b. Enhanced or impaired cognitive function in Parkinson's disease as a function of dopaminergic medication and task demands. *Cereb Cortex* **11**, 1136–43.

Cools R, Barker R A, Sahakian B J and Robbins T W. 2003. L-Dopa medication remediates cognitive inflexibility, but increases impulsivity in patients with Parkinson's disease. *Neuropsychologia* **41**, 1431–41.

Cools R, Clark L, Owen A M and Robbins T W. 2002a. Defining the neural mechanisms of probabilistic reversal learning using event-related functional magnetic resonance imaging. *J Neurosci* **22**, 4563–7.

Cools R, Lewis S J, Clark L, Barker R A and Robbins T W. 2007. L-DOPA disrupts activity in the nucleus accumbens during reversal learning in Parkinson's disease. *Neuropsychopharmacology* **32**, 180–9.

Cools R, Stefanova E, Barker R A, Robbins T W and Owen A M. 2002b. Dopaminergic modulation of high-level cognition in Parkinson's disease: The role of the prefrontal cortex revealed by PET. *Brain* **125**, 584–94.

Cooper J R, Bloom F E and Roth R H. 2003. *The Biochemical Basis of Neuropharmacology.* 8th Ed. Oxford: Oxford University Press.

Dagher A and Nagano-Saito A. 2007. Functional and anatomical magnetic resonance imaging in Parkinson's disease. *Mol Imaging Biol* **9**, 234–42.

Dagher A, Owen A M, Boecker H and Brooks D J. 1999. Mapping the network for planning: A correlational PET activation study with the Tower of London task. *Brain* **122**, 1973–87.

Dagher A, Owen A M, Boecker H and Brooks D J. 2001. The role of the striatum and hippocampus in planning: A PET activation study in Parkinson's disease. *Brain* **124**, 1020–32.

de la Fuente-Fernández R and Calne D B. 1996. What do Lewy bodies tell us about dementia and parkinsonism? In Perry R H, McKeith I G, Perry E K (Eds.). *Dementia with Lewy Bodies.* New York, NY: Cambridge University Press, pp. 287–301.

de Lau L M L and Breteler M M B. 2006. Epidemiology of Parkinson's disease. *Lancet Neurol* **5**, 525–35.

Del Tredici K, Rüb U, De Vos R A, Bohl J R and Braak H. 2002. Where does Parkinson disease pathology begin in the brain? *J Neuropathol Exp Neurol* **61**, 413–26.

Dirnberger G, Frith C D and Jahanshahi M. 2005. Executive dysfunction in Parkinson's disease is associated with altered pallidal–frontal processing. *Neuroimage* **25**, 588–99.

Dubois B and Pillon B. 1997. Cognitive deficits in Parkinson's disease. *J Neurol* **244**, 2–8.

Edison P, Rowe C C, Rinne J O, *et al.* 2008. Amyloid load in Parkinson's disease dementia and Lewy body dementia measured with [^{11}C]PIB positron emission tomography. *J Neurol Neurosurg Psychiatry* **79**, 1331–8.

Evans A H, Pavese N, Lawrence A D, *et al.* 2006. Compulsive drug use linked to sensitized ventral striatal dopamine transmission. *Ann Neurol* **59**, 852–8.

Fearnley J M and Lees A J. 1991. Ageing and Parkinson's disease: substantia nigra regional selectivity. *Brain* **114**, 2283–301.

Fera F, Nicoletti G, Cerasa A, *et al.* 2007. Dopaminergic modulation of cognitive interference after pharmacological washout in Parkinson's disease. *Brain Res Bull* **74**, 75–83.

Foster E R, Black K J, Antenor-Dorsey J A, Perlmutter J S and Hershey T. 2008. Motor asymmetry and substantia nigra volume are related to spatial delayed response performance in Parkinson disease. *Brain Cogn* **67**, 1–10.

Frank M J, Seeberger L C and O'Reilly R C. 2004. By carrot or by stick: Cognitive reinforcement learning in parkinsonism. *Science* **306**, 1940–3.

Fukuda M, Mentis M, Ghilardi M F, *et al.* 2001. Functional correlates of pallidal stimulation for Parkinson's disease. *Ann Neurol* **49**, 155–64.

Gibb W R and Lees A J. 1988. The relevance of the Lewy body to the pathogenesis of idiopathic Parkinson's disease. *J Neurol Neurosurg Psychiatry* **51**, 745–52.

Gibb W R, Luthert P J, Janota I and Lantos P L. 1989. Cortical Lewy body dementia: Clinical features and classification. *J Neurol Neurosurg Psychiatry* **52**, 185–92.

Gomperts S N, Rentz D M, Moran E, *et al.* 2008. Imaging amyloid deposition in Lewy body diseases. *Neurology* **71**, 903–10.

Goodwin F K, Murphy D L, Brodie H K and Bunney W E Jr. 1971. Levodopa: Alterations in behavior. *Clin Pharmacol Ther* **12**, 383–96.

Gotham A M, Brown R G and Marsden C D. 1986. Levodopa treatment may benefit or impair "frontal" function in Parkinson's disease. *Lancet* **2**, 970–1.

Gotham A M, Brown R G and Marsden C D. 1988. "Frontal" cognitive function in patients with Parkinson's disease "on" and "off" levodopa. *Brain* **111**, 299–321.

Grafton S T, Waters C, Sutton J, Lew M F and Couldwell W. 1995. Pallidotomy increases activity of motor association cortex in Parkinson's disease: A positron emission tomographic study. *Ann Neurol* **37**, 776–83.

Grahn J A, Parkinson J A and Owen A M. 2008. The cognitive functions of the caudate nucleus. *Prog Neurobiol* **86**, 141–55.

Haslinger B, Erhard P, Kämpfe N, *et al.* 2001. Event-related functional magnetic resonance imaging in Parkinson's disease before and after levodopa. *Brain* **124**, 558–70.

Hilker R, Thomas A V, Klein J C, *et al.* 2005. Dementia in Parkinson disease: Functional imaging of cholinergic and dopaminergic pathways. *Neurology* **65**, 1716–22.

Huang C, Mattis P, Tang C, Perrine K, Carbon M and Eidelberg D. 2007. Metabolic brain networks associated with cognitive function in Parkinson's disease. *Neuroimage* **34**, 714–23.

Jahanshahi M, Jenkins I H, Brown R G, Marsden C D, Passingham R E and Brooks D J. 1995. Self-initiated versus externally triggered movements. I. An investigation using measurement of regional cerebral blood flow with PET and movement-related potentials in normal and Parkinson's disease subjects. *Brain* **118**, 913–33.

Javoy-Agid F and Agid Y. 1980. Is the mesocortical dopaminergic system involved in Parkinson disease? *Neurology* **30**, 1326–30.

Jenkins I H, Fernandez W, Playford E D, *et al.* 1992. Impaired activation of the supplementary motor area in Parkinson's disease is reversed when akinesia is treated with apomorphine. *Ann Neurol* **32**, 749–57.

Kaasinen V, Nurmi E, Bergman J, *et al.* 2001. Personality traits and brain dopaminergic function in Parkinson's disease. *Proc Natl Acad Sci USA* **98**, 13 272–7.

Kimberg D and D'Esposito M. 2003. Cognitive effects of the dopamine agonist pergolide. *Neuropsychologia* **41**, 1020–7.

Kish S J, Shannak K and Hornykiewicz O. 1988. Uneven pattern of dopamine loss in the striatum of patients with idiopathic Parkinson's disease. Pathophysiologic and clinical implications. *N Engl J Med* **318**, 876–80.

Kish S J, Shannak K, Rajput A, Deck J H and Hornykiewicz O. 1992. Aging produces a specific pattern of striatal dopamine loss: Implications for the etiology of idiopathic Parkinson's disease. *J Neurochem* **58**, 642–8.

Knowlton B J, Mangels J A and Squire L R. 1996. A neostriatal habit learning system in humans. *Science* **273**, 1399–402.

Knutson B, Taylor J, Kaufman M, Peterson R and Glover, G. 2005. Distributed neural representation of expected value. *J Neurosci* **25**, 4806–12.

Kosaka K and Iseki E. 1996. Dementia with Lewy bodies. *Curr Opin Neurol* **9**, 271–5.

Kulisevsky J, Avila A, Barbanoj M, *et al.* 1996. Acute effects of levodopa on neuropsychological performance in stable and fluctuating Parkinson's disease patients at different levodopa plasma levels. *Brain* **119**, 2121–32.

Lange K W, Robbins T W, Marsden C D, James M, Owen A M and Paul G M. 1992. L-dopa withdrawal in Parkinson's disease selectively impairs cognitive performance in tests sensitive to frontal lobe dysfunction. *Psychopharmacology (Berl)* **107**, 394–404.

Lawrence A D, Evans A H and Lees A J. 2003. Compulsive use of dopamine replacement therapy in Parkinson's disease: Reward systems gone awry? *Lancet Neurol* **2**, 595–604.

Lehéricy S, Ducros M, Van de Moortele P F, *et al.* 2004. Diffusion tensor fiber tracking shows distinct corticostriatal circuits in humans. *Ann Neurol* **55**, 522–9.

Lewis S J, Dove A, Robbins T W, Barker R A and Owen A M. 2003. Cognitive impairments in early Parkinson's disease are accompanied by reductions in activity in frontostriatal neural circuitry. *J Neurosci* **23**, 6351–6.

Lewis S J, Dove A, Robbins T W, Barker R A and Owen A M. 2004. Striatal contributions to working memory: A functional magnetic resonance imaging study in humans. *Eur J Neurosci* **19**, 755–60.

Lewis S J, Slabosz A, Robbins T W, Barker R A and Owen A M. 2005. Dopaminergic basis for deficits in working memory but not attentional set-shifting in Parkinson's disease. *Neuropsychologia* **43**, 823–32.

Limousin P, Greene J, Pollak P, Rothwell J, Benabid A L and Frackowiak R. 1997. Changes in cerebral activity pattern due to subthalamic nucleus or internal pallidum stimulation in Parkinson's disease. *Ann Neurol* **42**, 283–91.

Marié R M, Barré L, Dupuy B, Viader F, Defer G and Baron J C. 1999. Relationships between striatal dopamine denervation and frontal executive tests in Parkinson's disease. *Neurosci Lett* **260**, 77–80.

Mattay V S, Tessitore A, Callicott J H, *et al.* 2002. Dopaminergic modulation of cortical function in patients with Parkinson's disease. *Ann Neurol* **51**, 156–64.

Mehta M A, Sahakian B J, McKenna P J and Robbins T W. 1999. Systemic sulpiride in young adult volunteers simulates the profile of cognitive deficits in Parkinson's disease. *Psychopharmacology (Berl)* **146**, 162–74.

Mehta M A, Swainson R, Ogilvie A D, Sahakian J and Robbins T W. 2001. Improved short-term spatial memory but impaired reversal learning following the dopamine D2 agonist bromocriptine in human volunteers. *Psychopharmacology (Berl)* **159**, 10–20.

Middleton F A and Strick P L. 2000. Basal ganglia and cerebellar loops: Motor and cognitive circuits. *Brain Res Brain Res Rev* **31**, 236–50.

Mink J W. 1996. The basal ganglia: Focused selection and inhibition of competing motor programs. *Prog Neurobiol* **50**, 381–425.

Minoshima S, Foster N L, Sima A A, Frey K A, Albin R L and Kuhl D E. 2001. Alzheimer's disease versus dementia with Lewy bodies: Cerebral metabolic distinction with autopsy confirmation. *Ann Neurol* **50**, 358–65.

Monchi O, Petrides M, Doyon J, Postuma R B, Worsley K and Dagher A. 2004. Neural bases of set-shifting deficits in Parkinson's disease. *J Neurosci* **24**, 702–10.

Monchi O, Petrides M, Mejia-Constain B and Strafella A P. 2007. Cortical activity in Parkinson's disease during executive processing depends on striatal involvement. *Brain* **130**, 233–44.

Monchi O, Petrides M, Petre V, Worsley K and Dagher A. 2001. Wisconsin Card Sorting revisited: Distinct neural circuits participating in different stages of the task identified by event-related fMRI. *J Neurosci* **21**, 7733–41.

Nagano-Saito A, Washimi Y, Arahata Y, *et al.* 2004. Visual hallucination in Parkinson's disease with FDG PET. *Mov Disord* **19**, 801–06.

Nagano-Saito A, Washimi Y, Arahata Y, *et al.* 2005. Cerebral atrophy and its relation to cognitive impairment in Parkinson disease. *Neurology* **64**, 224–9.

Nandhagopal R, McKeown M J and Stoessl A J. 2008. Functional imaging in Parkinson's disease. *Neurology* **70**, 1478–88.

Nausieda P A. 1985. Sinemet "abusers". *Clin Neuropharmacol* **8**, 318–27.

Obeso J A, Rodríguez-Oroz M C, Rodríguez M, *et al.* 2000. Pathophysiology of the basal ganglia in Parkinson's disease. *Trends Neurosci* **23**, S8–19.

Owen A M. 1997. The functional organization of working memory processes within human lateral frontal cortex: The contribution of functional neuroimaging. *Eur J Neurosci* **9**, 1329–39.

Owen A M, Beksinska M, James M, *et al.* 1993a. Visuospatial memory deficits at different stages of Parkinson's disease. *Neuropsychologia* **31**, 627–44.

Owen A M, Doyon J, Dagher A, Sadikot A and Evans A C. 1998. Abnormal basal ganglia outflow in Parkinson's disease identified with PET. Implications for higher cortical functions. *Brain* **121**, 949–65.

Owen A M, James M, Leigh P N, *et al.* 1992. Fronto-striatal cognitive deficits at different stages of Parkinson's disease. *Brain* **115**, 1727–51.

Owen A M, Roberts A C, Hodges J R, Summers B A, Polkey C E and Robbins T W. 1993b. Contrasting mechanisms of impaired attentional set-shifting in patients with frontal lobe damage or Parkinson's disease. *Brain* **116**, 1159–75.

Peters S, Suchan B, Rusin J, *et al.* 2003. Apomorphine reduces BOLD signal in fMRI during voluntary movement in Parkinsonian patients. *Neuroreport* **14**, 809–12.

Playford E D, Jenkins I H, Passingham R E, Nutt J, Frackowiak R S and Brooks D J. 1992. Impaired mesial frontal and putamen activation in Parkinson's disease: A positron emission tomography study. *Ann Neurol* **32**, 151–61.

Postuma R B and Dagher A. 2006. Basal ganglia functional connectivity based on a meta-analysis of 126 positron emission tomography and functional magnetic resonance imaging publications. *Cereb Cortex* **16**, 1508–21.

Rascol O, Sabatini U, Chollet F, *et al.* 1992. Supplementary and primary sensory motor area activity in Parkinson's disease. Regional cerebral blood flow changes during finger movements and effects of apomorphine. *Arch Neurol* **49**, 144–8.

Remy P, Doder M, Lees A, Turjanski N and Brooks D. 2005. Depression in Parkinson's disease: Loss of dopamine and noradrenaline innervation in the limbic system. *Brain* **128**, 1314–22.

Rinne J O, Rummukainen J, Paljärvi L and Rinne U K. 1989. Dementia in Parkinson's disease is related to neuronal loss in the medial substantia nigra. *Ann Neurol* **26**, 47–50.

Rowe J, Stephan K E, Friston K, Frackowiak R, Lees A and Passingham R. 2002. Attention to action in Parkinson's disease: Impaired effective connectivity among frontal cortical regions. *Brain* **125**, 276–89.

Sabatini U, Boulanouar K, Fabre N, *et al.* 2000. Cortical motor reorganization in akinetic patients with Parkinson's disease: a functional MRI study. *Brain* **123**, 394–403.

Samuel M, Ceballos-Baumann A O, Blin J, *et al.* 1997a. Evidence for lateral premotor and parietal overactivity in Parkinson's disease during sequential and bimanual movements. A PET study. *Brain* **120**, 963–76.

Samuel M, Ceballos-Baumann A O, Turjanski N, *et al.* 1997b. Pallidotomy in Parkinson's disease increases supplementary motor area and prefrontal activation during performance of volitional movements. An H2O PET study. *Brain* **120**, 1301–13.

Sawaguchi T. 2000. The role of D1-dopamine receptors in working memory-guided movements mediated by frontal cortical areas. *Parkinsonism Relat Disord* **7**, 9–19.

Scatton B, Javoy-Agid F, Rouquier L, Dubois B and Agid Y. 1983. Reduction of cortical dopamine, noradrenaline, serotonin and their metabolites in Parkinson's disease. *Brain Res* **275**, 321–8.

Schott B H, Niehaus L, Wittmann B C, *et al.* 2007. Ageing and early-stage Parkinson's disease affect separable neural mechanisms of mesolimbic reward processing. *Brain* **130**, 2412–24.

Schrag A, Jahanshahi M and Quinn N. 2000. What contributes to quality of life in patients with Parkinson's disease? *J Neurol Neurosurg Psychiatry* **69**, 308–12.

Schultz W. 2002. Getting formal with dopamine and reward. *Neuron* **36**, 241–63.

Sohn M H, Ursu S, Anderson J R, Stenger V A and Carter C S. 2000. The role of prefrontal cortex and posterior parietal cortex in task switching. *Proc Natl Acad Sci USA* **97**, 13 448–53.

Strafella A P, Dagher A and Sadikot A. 2003. Cerebral blood flow changes induced by subthalamic stimulation in Parkinson's disease. *Neurology* **60**, 1039–42.

Strafella A P, Paus T, Barrett J and Dagher A. 2001. Repetitive transcranial magnetic stimulation of the human prefrontal cortex induces dopamine release in the caudate nucleus. *J Neurosci* **21**, RC157.

Strafella A P, Paus T, Fraraccio M and Dagher A. 2003. Striatal dopamine release induced by repetitive transcranial magnetic stimulation of the human motor cortex. *Brain* **126**, 2609–15.

Summerfield C, Junqué C, Tolosa E, *et al.* 2005. Structural brain changes in Parkinson disease with dementia: A voxel-based morphometry study. *Arch Neurol* **62**, 281–5.

Swainson R, Rogers R D, Sahakian B J, Summers B A, Polkey C E and Robbins T W. 2000. Probabilistic learning and reversal deficits in patients with Parkinson's disease or frontal or temporal lobe lesions: Possible adverse effects of dopaminergic medication. *Neuropsychologia* **38**, 596–612.

Tricomi E M, Delgado M R and Fiez J A. 2004. Modulation of caudate activity by action contingency. *Neuron* **41**, 281–92.

Vogel H P and Schiffter R. 1983. Hypersexuality – A complication of dopaminergic therapy in Parkinson's disease. *Pharmacopsychiatria* **16**, 107–10.

Weintraub D, Moberg P J, Duda J E, Katz I R and Stern M B. 2004. Effect of psychiatric and other nonmotor symptoms on disability in Parkinson's disease. *J Am Geriatr Soc* **52**, 784–8.

Williams G V and Goldman-Rakic P S. 1995. Modulation of memory fields by dopamine D1 receptors in prefrontal cortex. *Nature* **376**, 572–5.

Woods S P and Tröster A I. 2003. Prodromal frontal/executive dysfunction predicts incident dementia in Parkinson's disease. *J Int Neuropsychol Soc* **9**, 17–24.

Yeterian E H and Pandya D N. 1991. Prefrontostriatal connections in relation to cortical architectonic organization in rhesus monkeys. *J Comp Neurol* **312**, 43–67.

Chapter 27

Neuroimaging of other dementing disorders

William Hu and Murray Grossman

Introduction

Alzheimer's disease (AD) is the most common form of dementing illness in the elderly (Kokmen et al., 1993), but advances in molecular pathology over the past few decades have led to the identification of other common neurodegenerative disorders (Prusiner and Hsiao, 1994; Neary et al., 1998; McKhann et al., 2001; Boeve et al., 2003; Lippa et al., 2007; Murray et al., 2007). Patients with these non-Alzheimer dementia disorders frequently have similar subjective complaints as patients with AD, but atypical features in the evaluation of these cognitively impaired patients should alert the astute physician of an alternative non-AD diagnosis, including behavioral and language variants of frontotemporal dementia (Neary et al., 1998; McKhann et al., 2001), dementia with Lewy bodies (Lippa et al., 2007), vascular dementia, and other forms of less common neurological disorders, including Creutzfeldt–Jakob disease (Prusiner and Hsiao, 1994). The utility of imaging studies has been studied extensively in many of these disorders, and this chapter will focus on the group differences between disorders and highlight the role of structural and functional imaging in non-Alzheimer dementias. Disease-specific features unique to one type or one group of disorders are frequently congruent with the localization model of neurodegenerative disease based on prominent clinical deficits, but the majority of these studies lack the power to determine the positive and negative predictive values of disease-specific features at the group level when used on an individual patient basis, despite variable amount of anecdotal clinical evidence. With a few exceptions, these imaging features – when present – should only be used as supportive evidence to complement clinical impression when present. Unusual imaging features should broaden instead of narrow the clinical differential diagnosis, and additional investigational modalities should be considered to better define the disease process.

Frontotemporal dementia – behavioral variant (bv-FTD)

Frontotemporal dementia is the second most common dementing illness in those under the age of 65 (Knopman et al., 2004). The clinical syndrome of frontotemporal dementia includes behavioral (bv-FTD) and language variants (McKhann et al., 2001), and the two disorders not infrequently share features of the other (Neary et al., 1998). Historically, cases of bv-FTD often carried the clinical diagnosis of Pick's disease (McKhann et al., 2001), although Pick's disease pathology of tau-positive Pick bodies is not universally present in cases of clinically diagnosed Pick's disease. In fact, when multiple clinicopathologic series were examined, Pick's disease with tau-positive Pick bodies only represented a minority of bv-FTD with autopsy confirmation (Hodges et al., 2004; Kertesz et al., 2005; Forman et al., 2006a; Josephs et al., 2006b). About half of the bv-FTD patients have neuritic or intracellular lesions immunoreactive to TAR DNA binding protein of ~43 kDa (TDP-43; Neumann et al., 2006) and these patients are said to have frontotemporal lobar degeneration associated with TDP-43 (FTLD-TDP). The other patients have pathologic changes consistent with Pick's disease (Dickson, 2001), corticobasal degeneration (CBD; Murray et al., 2007), progressive supranuclear palsy (PSP; Dickson, 2008), frontotemporal dementia with parkinsonism linked to chromosome 17 (FTDP-17; van Swieten and Spillantini, 2007), or

---

Understanding Neuropsychiatric Disorders, ed. M. E. Shenton and B. I. Turetsky. Published by Cambridge University Press.
© Cambridge University Press 2011.

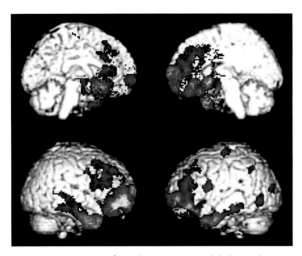

Figure 27.1 Patterns of atrophy in patients with behavioral variant of frontotemporal dementia (bv-FTD).

tangle-predominant dementia (Jellinger and Attems, 2007). The common link among these disorders is the presence of hyperphosphorylated tau in neurofibrillary tangles, and they are grouped together as tauopathies. Patients with clinical bv-FTD can also have pathology in keeping with AD, and they are sometimes considered to have frontal-variant of AD (Johnson *et al.*, 1999; Grossman *et al.*, 2008).

Modern imaging techniques have allowed for structural and functional analysis of patients with bv-FTD. Due to the clinical and pathologic heterogeneity of FTD, information on bv-FTD has come from both studies on clinically diagnosed cases with variable pathologic confirmation and analysis of pathologically confirmed FTLD cases, with bv-FTD the most common clinical diagnosis in most series. Magnetic resonance imaging (MRI) of the brain is the most utilized modality in the clinical evaluation of patients suspected of having bv-FTD, and patients often have frontal and/or temporal atrophy, although more global atrophy may also exist. Voxel-based morphometry (VBM) analysis of patients with clinical bv-FTD generally showed atrophy in the right dorsolateral prefrontal cortex, anterior cingulate cortex, and insula, and additional atrophic regions have been identified in different clinical series, including orbitofrontal and left motor cortices (Rosen *et al.*, 2002a), as well as right posterolateral temporal cortical atrophy (Grossman *et al.*, 2004). Certain behavioral characteristics common in bv-FTD are also associated with patterns of focal brain atrophy,

including disinhibition with orbitofrontal and right medial temporal limbic structure atrophy (Zamboni *et al.*, 2008), apathy with dorsolateral prefrontal atrophy (Zamboni *et al.*, 2008; Massimo and Grossman, 2008), poor emotional comprehension with right amygdala and orbitofrontal atrophy (Rosen *et al.*, 2002b), disagreeableness with left orbitofrontal atrophy (Rankin *et al.*, 2004), and binge eating with right insular circuit atrophy (Woolley *et al.*, 2007). At the same time, frontal atrophy is often found in cognitively normal control subjects, and left frontal lobe atrophy was found to be more associated with bv-FTD than right frontal lobe atrophy in a comparison study between 30 cognitively normal subjects and 16 bv-FTD patients (Chow *et al.*, 2008).

Patterns of brain atrophy in FTLD can also be analyzed according to the subtypes of pathologic disorders giving rise to bv-FTD. As a group, autopsy-confirmed cases of FTLD had more atrophy in frontal lobar regions, anterior cingulate gyri, and the insula compared with autopsy-confirmed cases of AD (Rabinovici *et al.*, 2007). However, no group differences were found between tau-positive and tau-negative (FTLD-TDP) cases of FTLD in two series comparing a total of 16 cases of FTLD-TDP and 15 cases of tauopathies using VBM analysis (Whitwell *et al.*, 2004; Kim *et al.*, 2007). When examined according to the exact pathologic diagnosis rather than presence or absence of tau pathology, each type of TDP-43- or tau-positive pathology was associated with a particular pattern of brain atrophy: FTLD-TDP with atrophy in the bilateral orbitofrontal cortices, posterior superior temporal lobes, and posterior fusiform gyri; Pick's disease with Pick bodies with bilateral dorsolateral prefrontal atrophy; frontotemporal dementia with parkinsonism linked to chromosome 17 (FTDP-17) with atrophy in the right temporal lobe and orbitofrontal cortex, CBD with atrophy in the frontoparietal cortical regions and subcortical nuclei; PSP with atrophy in the brainstem, cortical regions, and the adjacent white matter (Whitwell *et al.*, 2005; Josephs *et al.*, 2008a). Given the multitude of atrophy patterns associated with the pathologic heterogeneity of FTD, it is thus possible that atrophy pattern alone from one time point is insufficient to distinguish FTLD-TDP from tauopathies. In cases with serial volumetric imaging, longitudinal patterns of atrophy can be examined by brain and ventricular boundary-shift integral analysis. Using such analysis in a cohort of 12 patients with FTLD-TDP (10 with bv-FTD) and 10 patients with CBD or PSP (3 with bv-FTD), CBD cases were found to have the highest annual rate of brain atrophy at 2.3% per year, while FTLD-TDP cases had an annual rate of brain atrophy at 1.7% per year (Whitwell *et al.*, 2007b). In contrast, AD cases and control cases had annual rates of brain atrophy at 1.1 and 0.3% per year, respectively. Hence, compared with AD, FTLD case had more frontal or temporal atrophy and faster annual rates of atrophy, and some tau-positive cases (CBD) had significantly faster annual rates of atrophy than other pathologic subtypes of FTLD.

At the individual patient level, imaging studies should aid the clinician in the distinction between FTD and other non-FTD dementing illnesses. Structural imaging could be sensitive early in the disease course, but is insufficiently specific in patients eventually diagnosed with FTD. In one study of serially diagnosed and followed patients with dementia, 40 of 63 FTD patients had more prominent frontal and temporal atrophy out of proportion to generalized atrophy, with positive and negative predictive values of frontotemporal abnormalities in FTD diagnosis at 66 and 69%, respectively (Mendez *et al.*, 2007). The utility of volumetric MRI in distinguishing AD and FTD was addressed in a recent study using 37 clinically diagnosed AD patients and 12 clinically diagnosed FTD patients (8 with bv-FTD). With VBM and high-dimensional pattern classification, the average accuracy in differentiating AD from FTD on an individual patient basis was 84% (Davatzikos *et al.*, 2008).

Box 27.1. Behavioral variant frontotemporal dementia (bv-FTD)

Characterized clinically by change in comportment, apathy, disinhibition, poor planning/judgment.
Atrophy seen in dorsolateral prefrontal cortex, orbitofrontal cortex, anterior cingulated gyrus, insula, posterior temporal lobe.
Reduced cerebral blood flow and cerebral metabolism seen in frontal or frontotemporal regions.

In searching for an imaging biomarker for FTD or FTLD, functional brain imaging studies – including both single-photon emission computed tomography (SPECT) and positron emission tomography (PET) – represented a significant step forward in the clinical diagnosis of bv-FTD. Reduction in frontal cerebral blood flow on SPECT was seen in 80% of

autopsy-confirmed cases of FTLD, and reduction in parietal cerebral blood flow present in 90% of autopsy-confirmed AD cases was found in 28% of autopsy-confirmed FTLD (McNeill *et al.*, 2007). Similar to VBM, patterns of hypoperfusion in FTD may also correspond to behavioral deficits, such as right frontal hypoperfusion with loss of insight, left frontal hypoperfusion with change in hygiene, and left temporal hypoperfusion with compulsion and mental rigidity (McMurtray *et al.*, 2006). In clinically diagnosed patients with FTD, PET using 18-F fluoro-deoxyglucose (FDG-PET) tended to show fronto-temporal hypoperfusion (Ishii *et al.*, 1998b), while parietal–temporal hypoperfusion was more common in AD patients (Minoshima *et al.*, 1997). In patients with autopsy-confirmation, FDG-PET with stereotactic surface projection (SSP) was able to achieve diagnostic accuracy of 89% with significant inter-rater diagnostic agreement (Foster *et al.*, 2007). Importantly, FDG-PET results improved overall clinical diagnostic accuracy from 79 to 90%. A direct comparison of diagnostic accuracy between SPECT/PET imaging and volumetric MRI imaging further showed increased sensitivity and specificity in the diagnosis of FTD (Mendez *et al.*, 2007). Currently, FDG-PET is approved by the Centers for Medicare and Medicaid Services in the US for improving clinical diagnostic accuracy of FTD or AD in cases of atypical dementia, and the utility of FDG-PET scan in distinguishing bv-FTD from AD may be as early as the mild cognitive impairment (MCI) stage, as some patients diagnosed with clinical MCI already demonstrated different patterns of hypoperfusion consistent with either AD or FTD (Mosconi *et al.*, 2008).

Familial FTLD-TDP

A significant proportion of patients with bv-FTD have a family history of dementia, parkinsonian disorder, or amyotrophic lateral sclerosis. Over the past decade, a number of mutations have been identified to be associated with familial FTD that clinically often presents with bv-FTD. This includes mutations in the microtubule-associated protein tau (MAPT) that cause the tauopathy FTDP-17, and mutations in progranulin (PGRN), charged multi-vesicular body protein 2B (CHMP2B), and valosin-containing protein (VCP), all of which cause familial tau-negative FTLD-TDP. Only limited information is available on the imaging findings of these patients, and no systemic characterization of imaging characteristics yet exists for familial FTLD-TDP of known mutations. As a group, patients with PGRN mutations had more severe atrophy affecting the frontal, temporal, and parietal lobes than patients without PGRN mutations (Whitwell *et al.*, 2007a). This widespread pattern of atrophy is possibly associated with the more severe clinical phenotypes in patients with PGRN mutations, some of whom also demonstrated deficits reflecting parietal lobe dysfunction in addition to frontal and temporal lobar dysfunction (Beck *et al.*, 2008; Le Ber *et al.*, 2008; Rohrer *et al.*, 2008). CHMP2B mutations were found in a large Danish pedigree with autosomal dominant FTD linked to chromosome 3 (Skibinski *et al.*, 2005) and a Belgian patient with familial FTD (van der Zee *et al.*, 2008). Imaging studies of affected patients have shown mild to generalized cortical atrophy on CT, and hypoperfusion in the frontal, parietal, and temporal lobes on SPECT (Gydesen *et al.*, 2002; van der Zee *et al.*, 2008). Mutations in VCP lead to a multi-system disorder involving FTD, inclusion body myopathy, and Paget's disease of the bone, and are associated with ubiquitin- and TDP-43-immunoreactive lesions distinct from the typical FTLD (Forman *et al.*, 2006b). Limited imaging data are available on patients with FTD and VCP mutations. Case reports or case series have shown minimal to severe cortical atrophy on CT or MRI (Le Ber *et al.*, 2004; Bersano *et al.*, 2007; Watts *et al.*, 2007; Viassolo *et al.*, 2008), prominent callosal and frontal white matter atrophy on MRI (Krause *et al.*, 2007), and/or mild to severe diffuse frontal lobe hypoperfusion on SPECT (Le Ber *et al.*, 2004; Watts *et al.*, 2007). The mixed imaging findings likely reflect the relatively heterogeneous clinical phenotypes involved with each mutation, but it appears that no imaging abnormality is reliably associated with one particular type of familial FTLD mutation. Radiological evidence of differential gray and white matter involvement may be indicative of underlying disease mechanism by which mutations in these ubiquitous proteins lead to focal frontotemporal dysfunction. In the future, imaging modalities using substrate-specific ligands targeting abnormal proteins should allow for more accurate diagnosis in suspected familial cases and clinically asymptomatic carriers.

Semantic dementia

Semantic dementia (SD) represents a fluent form of primary progressive aphasia (PPA) or language variant-FTD (lv-FTD). It is characterized by marked loss of semantic knowledge in both spontaneous speech and confrontational naming, degraded object knowledge, circumlocution, mildly slowed rate of speech production, and preserved grammar and repetition (Neary *et al.*, 1998). Behaviorally, patients with SD are much more likely to have symptoms reminiscent of bv-FTD than patients with other forms of lv-FTD or AD (Rosen *et al.*, 2006). Subtle behavioral features may also be preferentially associated with SD, such as unusual food preferences rather than general hyperorality seen in bv-FTD (Seeley *et al.*, 2005). In clinico-pathologic series, the most common pathologic diagnosis in SD patients was FTLD-TDP, with AD being the next most common cause and tauopathies only infrequently associated with SD (Forman *et al.*, 2006a; Snowden *et al.*, 2007; Knibb *et al.*, 2006). When FTLD-TDP pathologic pattern was further examined according to microscopic structures immunoreactive to TDP-43 and ubiquitin, SD was found to have mostly abundant dystrophic neurites and rare intracellular lesions (MacKenzie Type II, Sampathu Type I) (Grossman *et al.*, 2007; Snowden *et al.*, 2007). Gross examination of the brain in autopsy-confirmed cases often, but not universally, showed lobar asymmetry corresponding to the clinical aphasic presentation (Snowden *et al.*, 2007).

Early work showed left hemispheric atrophy in small groups of patients clinically diagnosed with SD, especially in the left temporal pole (Mummery *et al.*, 2000). However, bilateral atrophy can also occur in SD, especially later in the disease course (Garrard and Hodges, 2000). Compared to control subjects, SD patients had more atrophy in the anterior inferior temporal gyrus, anterior superior temporal gyrus, posterior amygdala, and ventromedial frontal cortex bilaterally (Rosen *et al.*, 2002b). All these regions except the ventromedial frontal cortex also showed more atrophy in SD when compared with bv-FTD, and these findings have been confirmed in subsequent series of patients using VBM analysis (Gorno-Tempini *et al.*, 2004; Davies *et al.*, 2008). Atrophy in SD likely extends beyond gray matter, as white matter atrophy was also found in SD compared with bv-FTD and control subjects (Chao *et al.*, 2007). One diffusion

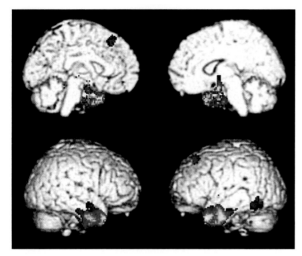

Figure 27.2 Patterns of atrophy in patients with semantic dementia (SD).

Deficits in SD patients have yielded important information on the neurological substrate for single word and sentence comprehension through correlational analysis. Single word meaning impairment correlates with left posterolateral and ventral temporal atrophy in SD (Mummery *et al.*, 2000; Grossman *et al.*, 2004; Bright *et al.*, 2008) and bilateral anterior temporal lobe hypometabolism (Nestor *et al.*, 2006). With disease progression, SD patients can additionally develop difficulties in sentence comprehension, which correlates with atrophy in the posterolateral portion of the left temporal cortex (Grossman and Moore, 2005; Davies *et al.*, 2008). More posterior cortical disease involvement in SD patients can manifest as degraded visual–perceptual feature knowledge of concrete object and actions. This has been correlated with atrophy in the visual association cortex likely reflecting deficits in semantic association (Yi *et al.*, 2007). A neuropsychological correlate of the bilateral temporal involvement in SD is poor comprehension of emotion, especially emotions with negative valence such as sadness. This deficit in SD correlates with atrophy in the right amygdala and right orbitofrontal cortex (Rosen *et al.*, 2002b), and provides further evidence that SD is more than a left-hemispheric degenerative process, and this pattern of bi-temporal degeneration may be associated with the specific pathology morphology of prominent dystrophic neurites.

Progressive non-fluent aphasia

Progressive non-fluent aphasia (PNFA) is a non-fluent form of lv-FTD, characterized by effortful speech, shortened phrase length, and reduced use of grammatical elements (Kartsounis *et al.*, 1991; Grossman *et al.*, 1996a; Turner *et al.*, 1996). Single word comprehension is usually preserved, but comprehension of grammatically complex (Mesulam *et al.*, 2008) sentences is impaired (Turner *et al.*,

tensor imaging (DTI) study revealed disruption of the inferior longitudinal fasciculus connecting the anterior temporal and frontal regions (Borroni *et al.*, 2007). We have performed similar DTI analysis in SD patients, and found abnormalities in the white matter connecting the anterior temporal region to the frontal and parietal integration regions (Asmuth *et al.*, 2008). FDG-PET studies in SD patients have shown dysfunction in the bilateral temporal regions and medial orbitofrontal regions, reflecting results from VBM analysis (Desgranges *et al.*, 2007; Drzezga *et al.*, 2008). The degree of dysfunction on FDG-PET analysis was more severe than the degree of atrophy on VBM analysis, likely reflecting substrate- (FTLD-TDP) or region-specific neuronal dysfunction before the development of lobar atrophy. As some cases of SD also have cerebrospinal fluid (CSF) profiles suggestive of AD (Hu and Grossman, unpublished data) or AD pathology on autopsy (Knibb *et al.*, 2006), amyloid-specific imaging has also been performed in eight clinically diagnosed SD patients (Drzezga *et al.*, 2008). Interestingly, none of these patients demonstrated retention of Pittsburgh Compound B, leading the investigators to the conclusion that SD can be accurately diagnosed clinically. However, as the sensitivity of [11C]-PIB PET in non-AD cases still needs to be confirmed, this small study should be interpreted with caution especially given the common occurrence of AD pathology in autopsy-confirmed series of SD.

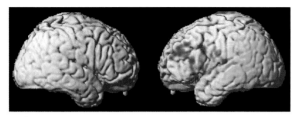

Figure 27.3 Patterns of atrophy in patients with progressive non-fluent aphasia (PNFA) if the underlying pathology is frontotemporal lobar degeneration (red) or Alzheimer's disease (green).

1996). In particular, impairments of verb processing may be more pronounced than noun processing in sentence comprehension (Rhee *et al.*, 2001). Patients with a PNFA-like form of primary progressive aphasia are variably classified as PNFA or non-fluent PPA in published studies, although there is high agreement between cases of PNFA and cases of non-fluent PPA (Clark *et al.*, 2005; Knibb *et al.*, 2006; Mesulam *et al.*, 2008). Patients with PNFA usually do not have prominent behavioral features early in the disease course, although they may demonstrate behavioral abnormalities later in the disease course including hyperorality, disinhibition, or apathy. Pathologically, PNFA is highly associated with tauopathies in most clinicopathologic series, although clinically diagnosed cases of PNFA can also have pathologic changes in keeping with Alzheimer disease or FTLD-TDP (Forman *et al.*, 2006a; Josephs *et al.*, 2006b; Knibb *et al.*, 2006; Mesulam *et al.*, 2008). Dysarthria is more common in the non-fluent form of PPA than fluent forms (Clark *et al.*, 2005). Apraxia of speech (AOS), a disorder of motor speech planning, can be present in PNFA with or without non-verbal oral apraxia (Gorno-Tempini *et al.*, 2004).

Volumetric MRI studies in individual patients with PNFA have shown minimal atrophy, left perisylvian atrophy, or left-hemispheric atrophy (Caselli *et al.*, 1992; Turner *et al.*, 1996; Nestor *et al.*, 2003). A detailed VBM analysis showed significant atrophy in the pars opercularis, triangularis, pars orbitalis of the left inferior frontal gyrus, left precentral gyrus of the insula with extension into the inferior precentral gyrus and middle frontal gyrus, bilateral caudate nuclei, and left putamen (Gorno-Tempini *et al.*, 2004). The atrophy in PNFA is also more severe on a group level compared with other forms of FTD-related disorders (Grossman *et al.*, 2004). While atrophy surrounding the left perisylvian fissure is

insufficient by itself for the diagnosis of PNFA as it can also be seen in AD cases without aphasia (Nestor *et al.*, 2003; Gorno-Tempini *et al.*, 2004), its presence is often considered supporting evidence for PNFA (Mesulam *et al.*, 2008). It is also important to note that while this radiographic change is common in the clinical diagnosis of PNFA, its presence likely only reflects the neuro-anatomical basis of the clinical syndrome and should not be used in the prediction of pathology. In one detailed clinicopathologic series of patients with non-fluent aphasia, three cases of PNFA with asymmetric left frontal atrophy in one series all had AD pathology on autopsy (Knibb *et al.*, 2006). Interestingly, even in cases of PNFA with AD pathology, the degree of asymmetry in AD pathology as might be expected from the lateralized clinical phenotype is minimal despite asymmetric atrophy (Mesulam *et al.*, 2008). This may be in part due to the extensive interhemispheric abnormalities seen on DTI studies of PNFA patients (Asmuth *et al.*, 2008). Alternatively, this has led to speculations that AD changes in these cases of non-FTLD PNFA may represent late-stage changes, although further confirmatory evidence is necessary before the association between AD pathology and PNFA phenotype can be discounted.

AOS has been the subject of a number of clinicopathologic analyses. Whereas PNFA with apraxia of speech is most often associated with tauopathies, PNFA cases without AOS are more likely to have pathologic findings of FTLD-TDP (Josephs *et al.*, 2006a; Snowden *et al.*, 2007). In one of these series of patients with PNFA-related disorder and autopsy-confirmed FTLD, AOS was present in more than half of the cases, and was the dominant clinical feature in 40% (Josephs *et al.*, 2006a). VBM analysis of patients with AOS only showed atrophy predominantly affecting the bilateral superior premotor cortex, with extension into the precentral gyrus and supplemental motor area. In contrast, patients with PNFA plus AOS showed atrophy in the superior premotor cortex, greater involvement of the posterior inferior frontal lobe, but without involvement of the supplemental motor region (Josephs *et al.*, 2006a). All of the AOS cases and PNFA plus AOS cases had tauopathies on pathologic examination, so the distinctions in clinical phenotypes and imaging analysis cannot be explained by differences between tauopathies and FTLD-TDP alone. However, with the majority of AOS cases having pathology of PSP and all cases of PNFA plus AOS having CBD pathology, the observed difference in atrophy may instead reflect the exact pathologic subtype of tauopathy rather than general presence of absence of tau-related changes.

Consistent with the pattern of atrophy seen in volumetric analysis, functional imaging using SPECT and FDG-PET has also shown left-hemispheric hypoperfusion or hypometabolism (Turner *et al.*, 1996; Nestor *et al.*, 2003; Clark *et al.*, 2005). Using the region-of-interest (ROI) method in PET analysis, a group of PNFA cases had general left-hemisphere hypometabolism compared to controls, and more hypometabolism in the left inferior frontal, superior and middle temporal gyri relative to clinically probable AD (Grossman *et al.*, 1996b). Additional areas identified via ROI analysis include bi-frontal and left temporoparietal regions, and left subcortical nuclei (Talbot *et al.*, 1995; Newberg *et al.*, 2000). Using statistical parametric mapping, one subsequent study showed that patients with pure and possibly early PNFA had hypometabolism more restricted to the left anterior insula, and PNFA cases with more cognitive impairment demonstrated more severe patterns of hypometabolism with extension into Broca's area, superior temporal gyrus, inferior frontal gyrus, and dorsomedial frontal region (Nestor *et al.*, 2003). These abnormalities in metabolism were distinct from both cognitively normal control subjects and patients with AD. Specifically, analysis of PNFA cases against AD cases yielded a single focus of hypometabolic cluster in the left frontal operculum (Nestor *et al.*, 2003). On a qualitative level, abnormalities on SPECT and FDG-PET are more pronounced than abnormalities seen in VBM analysis alone.

Clinically characterized by effortful speech, agrammatism, difficulty with comprehension of grammatically complex sentences, with preserved comprehension and object knowledge.

Can be with or without apraxia of speech.

Atrophy in left perisylvian fissure.

Cerebral hypometabolism in left insula and left perisylvian fissure.

Correlational analysis between patterns of brain imaging abnormalities and neuropsychological deficits has been able to confirm the neuro-anatomical basis of many language deficits observed in PNFA.

Early in the disease course of PNFA, patients tend to have greater difficulty understanding grammatically complex sentences compared to grammatically simple sentences (Grossman and Moore, 2005). In healthy seniors, fMRI studies have shown an association between grammatical components of sentence processing and ventral portions of left inferior frontal cortex (Grossman *et al.*, 2002). Difficulties in sentence comprehension by PNFA patients may thus be associated with dysfunction in this region. In a SPECT analysis, hypoperfusion in the lateral superior and inferior portions of the left frontal lobe and left anterior superior temporal lobe was associated with difficulties in understanding sentences containing a grammatically subordinate clause (Grossman *et al.*, 1998). A similar finding has been documented in a VBM analysis relating left inferior frontal and anterior superior cortical atrophy to reduced speech fluency in a semi-structured speech sample (Ash *et al.*, 2009). In a blood oxygen level-dependent (BOLD) fMRI study, PNFA patients were presented with grammatically complex sentences. PNFA patients with grammatical comprehension difficulties showed only limited left inferior frontal recruitment during the task (Cooke *et al.*, 2003). Reduced activity in the left frontal lobe shown on a study of arterial spin labeling in PNFA patients was related to their difficulties in sentence comprehension (Grossman *et al.*, 2001). In comparison, non-aphasic patients showed good activation of the left inferior frontal region in the BOLD fMRI study (Cooke *et al.*, 2003).

The strong association between the clinical phenotype of PNFA and pathologic changes consistent with tauopathies, especially with the concurrent symptoms of AOS and grammatical difficulties, makes PNFA the ideal clinical correlate to pathologic tauopathies. Recognition of the dominant clinical deficits and left perisylvian atrophy or dysfunction will be crucial in the identification of patients with PNFA and highly probable underlying tau-positive pathology, such that PNFA patients could be included in therapeutic trials targeting hyperphosphorylated tau.

Logopenic progressive aphasia

It has long been observed that up to 33% of patients with lv-FTD may have pathology consistent with AD (Hodges *et al.*, 2004). This, along with the clinical observation that some patients with progressive aphasia cannot be easily classified as either SD or PNFA, has led to studies to characterize patients with the clinical syndrome of primary progressive aphasia and pathologic findings of AD. Gorno-Tempini and colleagues have proposed the diagnosis of logopenic progressive aphasia, characterized by slow, effortful speech with word finding pauses, impaired repetition and comprehension for longer sentences but preserved functioning for single words, and preserved grammar (Gorno-Tempini *et al.*, 2004; Gorno-Tempini *et al.*, 2008). Atrophy on MRI and hypoperfusion on SPECT in these patients are evident in the posterior left temporal lobe and inferior parietal lobule, distinct from patterns seen in SD and PNFA. In our experience, many of these clinically diagnosed patients have cerebrospinal fluid profiles consistent with AD (elevated tau level and tau/Aβ42 ratio, 11 out of 15), and this profile has been associated with autopsy confirmation of AD (Bian *et al.*, 2008) and the presence of cerebral amyloid by using PET imaging with amyloid-specific substrate Pittsburgh compound B (PIB-PET) as would be expected in AD (Fagan *et al.*, 2006). Mesulam and colleagues recently characterized patients with primary progressive aphasia according to their clinical and pathologic diagnoses, and found AD to be the most common source of pathology in patients with logopenic aphasia (7 out of 11; Mesulam *et al.*, 2008). Similar to clinically diagnosed LPA patients, progressive aphasic patients with pathologic AD have also been found to have predominantly temporoparietal cortical atrophy (Josephs *et al.*, 2008b). Unlike AD cases with prominent memory impairment, these aphasic AD patients had demonstrated relative sparing of the hippocampal structures. Thus, clinical, imaging, and pathologic data all point to an aphasic disorder with AD pathology unique from aphasic variants of FTLD or amnestic variants of AD, and future studies will be necessary to determine how diagnostic accuracy of LPA is influenced by functional and amyloid-specific imaging studies.

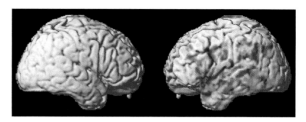

Figure 27.4 Patterns of atrophy in patients with logopenic progressive aphasia (LPA) if the underlying pathology is frontotemporal lobar degeneration (red) or Alzheimer's disease (green).

Frontotemporal dementia with motor neuron disease

A small proportion of patients with behavioral or language-variant FTD can develop symptoms of motor neuron disease (MND) an average of 12–13 months into the disease course (Hu *et al.*, 2009b). The emergence of motor neuron symptoms is nearly universally associated with significantly worse prognosis than FTD without MND (Josephs *et al.*, 2005), although some patients can have less rapid decline than the typical patients with FTD-MND (Hu *et al.*, 2009b). Patients with amyotrophic lateral sclerosis (ALS) can also develop a dementing syndrome indistinguishable from FTD (Phukan *et al.*, 2007). Therefore, FTD, FTD-MND, ALS with dementia (ALS-D), and ALS are thought to represent different stages of a disease spectrum. However, few empirical data exist to determine whether FTD-MND represents secondary motor neuron involvement in susceptible FTD patients or a unique disease entity that simultaneously affects two vulnerable neuronal populations, and whether FTD-MND and ALS-D are more similar to each other on the molecular level than to their constituent disorders. In this section, we will discuss both imaging characteristics that potentially distinguish the combined disorders from FTD or ALS alone, and findings that may support a more continuous nature of the disorder spectrum.

Volumetric imaging studies have echoed pathologic findings (Geser *et al.*, 2008) that ALS is a diffuse

---

Box 27.4. Logopenic progressive aphasia (LPA)

Clinically characterized by word finding pauses, circumlocution, impaired repetition and comprehension of longer sentences, preserved grammar and single word comprehension.
Atrophy in left temporal–parietal region.

Box 27.5. FTD with motor neuron disease (FTD-MND)

Clinically characterized by onset of ALS/MND before or after onset of FTD.
Atrophy seen in motor and pre-motor cortices and frontal lobes.
Less temporal atrophy in FTD-MND than bv-FTD.

disorder that involves extramotor regions during the disease course. VBM analysis of patients with ALS and ALS/FTD showed common areas of atrophy involving motor and pre-motor cortices, bilateral frontal lobes, superior temporal gyri, temporal poles, and left posterior thalamus, but ALS/FTD patients had more significant atrophy in the frontal regions compared with non-demented ALS patients (Chang et al., 2005). Furthermore, in non-demented ALS patients, those with subclinical cognitive impairment had more prominent atrophy in the right frontal, parietal, and limbic regions compared with ALS patients without any cognitive deficits (Murphy et al., 2007). The degree of frontal lobe involvement in ALS thus parallels the extent of clinical cognitive impairment. Interestingly, while one might expect the most severe stage of dementia in ALS to reflect patterns of atrophy seen in FTLD-TDP without motor neuron disease, this has not been found. While patients with autopsy-confirmed FTLD-TDP without motor neuron involvement had atrophy in the frontal and temporal lobes, patients with FTLD-TDP with motor neuron involvement only had prominent atrophy in the frontal lobe. Thus, FTLD disorders involving motor neurons may preferentially affect the frontal regions more than the temporal regions, while FTLD-TDP without motor neuron involvement appears to preferentially affect both the frontal and temporal lobes. In addition, abnormalities on T2-weighted images have been reported in some patients with FTLD-MND, possibly reflecting region-specific myelin loss (Mori et al., 2007). However, due to the relative rarity of FTD-MND or ALS-FTD, findings from small series of patients with both FTD and ALS must be confirmed in larger collaborative studies.

Magnetic resonance spectroscopy (MRS) has been used to identify region-specific neuronal dysfunction, and we have used ^{1}H-MRS to evaluate patients with bv-FTD. When the region of interest analysis was performed on the primary motor cortex, we found half of the patients with bv-FTD to have a decreased N-acetylaspartate peak and an increased choline peak, even though these patients had no clinical evidence of a motor system disorder. As a similar proportion of bv-FTD patients have FTLD-TDP on autopsy, one hypothesis would be that all FTLD-TDP patients presenting with bv-FTD have neuronal loss in the primary motor cortex and possibly subclinical motor neuron disease, and a small proportion

of them would go on to develop clinical ALS. However, the proportion of patients who develop ALS is small, and the interval periods between onset of FTD and MND symptoms in FTD-MND and ALS-D patients form a bimodal rather than continuous distribution. Thus, MRS abnormality may be associated with the underlying pathologic change, but may lack value in predicting which FTD patients would develop ALS. Longitudinal studies in patients studied with spectroscopy are needed to evaluate this hypothesis.

Corticobasal syndrome/corticobasal degeneration

Corticobasal syndrome (CBS) is frequently considered part of the FTD spectrum disorder, as patients with CBS often have frontal cognitive deficits, and corticobasal degeneration (CBD) represents a significant pathologic category in those with bv-FTD and non-fluent lv-FTD. In this chapter, CBS refers to the clinical syndrome that may or may not have pathologic substrate of CBD, and CBD is used strictly to refer to the pathologic substrate that includes features of cortical atrophy, ballooned neurons, and tau-immunoreactive lesions in the neurons and astrocytic plaques (Dickson et al., 2002). No consensus criteria yet exist for the clinical diagnosis of CBS, but experts generally agree that CBS patients have combined deficits reflecting cortical and subcortical (basal ganglia) disease usually in an asymmetric fashion (Boeve et al., 2003; Litvan et al., 2003; Murray et al., 2007). Cortical features common in CBS include apraxia, cortical sensory loss, alien-limb phenomenon, visual–spatial difficulties, and language deficits such as PNFA; subcortical features of CBS can include asymmetric dystonia, rigidity, tremor, and myoclonus (Litvan et al., 2003). Pathology of clinical CBS can include tauopathies such as CBD and PSP, AD, and CJD, and pathology of CBD can give rise to the clinical syndromes of bv-FTD, non-fluent lv-FTD, and CBS (Dickson et al., 2002; Forman et al., 2006a; Murray et al., 2007; Fulbright et al., 2008).

The most remarkable feature in structural imaging of CBS reflects the asymmetric disease involvement. One could frequently detect asymmetric atrophy in the frontal and/or parietal lobes corresponding to the asymmetric clinical abnormalities. VBM analysis of CBS patients showed atrophy in the premotor cortex and subcortical white matter (Soliveri et al., 1999;

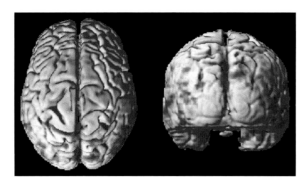

Figure 27.5 Asymmetric pattern of parietal atrophy in patients with corticobasal syndrome (CBS).

Boxer et al., 2006). The imaging asymmetry is highly correlated with the clinical asymmetry at the individual patient level, and is highly dependent on the inclusion or exclusion of patients with speech disorders on the group level (Kitagaki et al., 2000; Josephs et al., 2004; Groschel et al., 2004). In other words, patients diagnosed with CBS with apraxia of speech are likely to have left-hemispheric atrophy (Boxer et al., 2006), while CBS patients without speech disorders are more likely to have right-hemispheric atrophy (Hu and Grossman, unpublished data). Furthermore, T2 signal abnormalities on MRI have been observed in the more atrophic gyri, possibly reflecting gliosis (Soliveri et al., 1999; Hu et al., 2005). While this has been considered as a possible predictor of the underlying disease process, the possible association between this signal abnormality and specific FTLD pathology has since been invalidated, as it has also been shown to be associated with AD pathology. Nevertheless, regardless of the underlying pathology, asymmetric cortical atrophy appears to be common in CBS in our experience, along with possible atrophy in the contralateral dorsomedial frontal cortex (Listerud et al., 2009). This pattern of atrophy appears to extend beyond only those diagnosed clinically with CBS. In autopsy-confirmed cases of CBD, VBM analysis has shown significant cortical atrophy involving the posterior inferior, middle and superior frontal lobes, the superior premotor cortex, the posterior temporal and parietal lobes, insula cortex, supplemental motor area, and subcortical gray matter including the globus pallidus, putamen, and head of the caudate nucleus compared to control subjects (Josephs et al., 2008a). Cortical atrophy was more prominent in those who presented with a cognitive disorder than with an extrapyramidal disorder, and white matter atrophy may be more pronounced in

patients with a clinical parkinsonian disorder. Lastly, atrophy in the middle corpus callosum is common in CBD (Groschel et al., 2004; Josephs et al., 2008b). This has been speculated to be associated with the presence of the alien-limb phenomenon, although the emergence of alien limbs is perhaps more likely due to cortical involvement rather than a disconnection syndrome.

Similar to its utility in differentiating AD from FTD, functional imaging studies have been studied extensively for their potential in differentiating a tauopathy such as CBS from an alpha synucleinopathy such as idiopathic Parkinson's disease (Blin et al., 1992; Eckert et al., 2005). One study using MRS demonstrated a significantly reduced N-acetylaspartate to choline ratio in the parietal cortex contralateral to the most affected side in CBS patients (Tedeschi et al., 1997). In early FDG-PET studies, CBS patients showed diffuse cortical and subcortical hypometabolism, and the brain regions with the most pronounced changes invariably corresponded to the most affected limb sites (Eidelberg et al., 1991; Blin et al., 1992). In addition to severe hypometabolism contralateral to the most affected side, hypometabolism in the ipsilateral side was also seen in the motor and/or premotor cortical region in one study (Lutte et al., 2000). In one large subsequent series, patients with CBS were found to have asymmetric uptake of radiotracers, characterized by hypometabolism in the cortex and basal ganglia contralateral to the most affected limbs, and additionally hypermetabolism in the cortex and basal ganglia ipsilateral to the most affected side (Eckert et al., 2005). This pattern is quite unique from idiopathic Parkinson's disease, which is associated with subcortical gray hypermetabolism and bilateral frontal and/or parietal hypometabolism, and progressive supranuclear palsy, which is associated with hypometaboslim of the brainstem and frontal cortex, plus hypermetabolism of the parietal cortex. PET analysis using fluorodopa also demonstrated more prefrontal involvement and less subcortical hypometabolism in CBS than in idiopathic Parkinson's disease cases (Laureys *et al.*, 1999).

With the variety of unique symptoms that can emerge in the course of CBS, correlational studies have been used to identify anatomical regions responsible for symptoms such as apraxia and alien-limb phenomenon. Atrophy in the temporal cortex of CBS patients accounted for 41% of the variance in cognitive performance, and 33% of the neuropsychiatric symptoms (Groschel *et al.*, 2004). Using 18 patients with CBS, anterior cingulate hypometabolism was associated with poor performance on praxis tasks, and dysfunction in the superior parietal lobule and supplementary motor area identified CBS patients who were unable to correct their praxis errors (Peigneux *et al.*, 2001). This difficulty in self-correction in CBS probably reflects dysfunction in dynamic coding of body position and movements associated with disruption in the frontal–parietal circuits (Buxbaum *et al.*, 2007). CBS patients also have impairments in calculations that require number representation (Halpern *et al.*, 2003). In healthy adults, number representation has been primarily associated with the parietal cortex and prefrontal cortex, and the parietal atrophy in CBS may account for the clinical difficulty in calculation and relative magnitudes (Halpern *et al.*, 2004).

A future direction in the clinical and investigational characterization of CBS involves the use of functional imaging in pathologic prediction. In autopsy-confirmed cases of CBS with either CBD pathology or AD pathology, prominent hypoperfusion in the parietal lobe – similar to that seen in amnestic cases of AD – was more common in AD cases presenting with CBS than CBD cases presenting with CBS (Hu *et al.*, 2009a). While the number of these cases is small, studies such as this suggest that functional imaging along with substrate-specific biomarkers such as cerebrospinal fluid amyloid-beta level (Bian *et al.*, 2008), or amyloid-specific imaging (Rabinovici *et al.*, 2007) can reliably identify CBS cases associated with AD. As tauopathies and AD account for the vast majority of CBS cases, patients with CBS and supporting studies not suggestive of AD can be presumed to have tauopathies with relatively high confidence, and future natural history, correlational, and therapeutic CBS studies should no longer be hampered by the inclusion of a high proportion of AD patients.

Alzheimer's disease with TDP-43 immunoreactivity

No discussion on FTLD-related disorders is complete without discussion of AD cases with TDP-43 copathology. Since the discovery of TDP-43 immunoreactive lesions in ubiquitin-positive, tau-negative cases of FTLD, TDP-43 immunoreactivity has been found in up to 40% of AD cases (Amador-Ortiz and Dickson, 2008; Hu *et al.*, 2008). While the exact pathologic and clinical significance of this copathology remains to be defined, AD patients with TDP-43 copathology were found to have more atrophy in the bilateral hippocampal regions (Josephs *et al.*, 2008c). In turn, this may modify the clinical AD phenotype, or accelerate the overall process of neurodegeneration due to synergistic interaction between the two pathologic processes. In addition, a small proportion of patients with familial FTD have co-existing AD pathology of intermediate severity (Mukherjee *et al.*, 2006), and all these patients with co-existing FTLD and AD pathology may have laboratory evidence in favor of AD pathology, including CSF studies and amyloid-specific imaging. While some patients with clinical features of FTD patients have pathologic evidence of AD without FTLD, it is important to not discount the possibility of AD as a copathology in patients otherwise determined to have FTD.

Dementia with Lewy bodies and Parkinson's disease dementia

Dementia with Lewy bodies (DLB) and Parkinson's disease dementia (PDD) are two dementing illnesses associated with idiopathic Parkinson's disease (PD). DLB is thought to represent the second most common cause of dementia in the elderly, accounting for 10–15% of cases in autopsy series (McKeith *et al.*, 1996). PDD is estimated to occur in up to 41% of patients with PD (Apaydin *et al.*, 2002). DLB and PDD share the clinical features of cognitive and movement disorders, plus pathologic Lewy bodies immunoreactive to alpha-synuclein on autopsy (Colosimo *et al.*, 2003; Noe *et al.*, 2004). DLB and PDD are differentiated clinically by the temporal sequence of symptomatic onset: DLB is diagnosed when dementia occurs before or concurrently with parkinsonism, and PDD is diagnosed when dementia develops in a patient with established PD (McKeith *et al.*, 2005). Subtle clinical and pathologic differences have been reported between DLB and PDD. Clinically, DLB patients are more likely to have visual hallucination than PDD patients (Mosimann *et al.*, 2006), and may have worse levodopa response than PDD patients (Apaydin *et al.*, 2002; Burn *et al.*, 2003; Bonelli *et al.*, 2004). DLB cases on autopsy may have more Lewy body pathology and AD pathology than PDD cases (Harding and Halliday, 2001; Ballard *et al.*, 2006). On cognitive testing, patients with both DLB and PDD commonly present with executive dysfunctions, and DLB patients may have more prominent conceptual and attentional errors than PDD patients (Downes *et al.*, 1998; Aarsland *et al.*, 2003). Investigation into the imaging correlate of clinical features has frequently followed the clinical division differentiating DLB and PDD, and will be reviewed here separately and then jointly.

Mixed results have come from early structural imaging analysis of DLB. Most studies prior to 2000 showed relative preservation of cortical structures compared with control subjects (Barber *et al.*, 2000), although hippocampal atrophy was found in DLB (Hashimoto *et al.*, 1998). Subsequent studies using VBM analysis showed volume loss in the frontal, temporal, and insular cortical regions compared with control subjects, but less medial temporal and hippocampal atrophy compared to AD cases (Burton *et al.*, 2002; Ballmaier *et al.*, 2004; Tam *et al.*, 2005). More subcortical atrophy has also been recently reported in one study (Burton *et al.*, 2004). One recent VBM analysis again showed less cortical atrophy in patients with DLB, with scattered areas of atrophy identified in the hippocampus, parietal lobe, and frontal lobe. More significant atrophy was found in the dorsal midbrain, substantia innominata, and hypothalamus via VBM analysis and region of interest analysis (Whitwell *et al.*, 2007c). The discrepancies in contemporary studies may in part reflect differences in clinical duration and severity, as findings of more significant cortical atrophy in DLB had mean minimental status score in the range of 13–16, compared with 22 out of 30 in the study with relatively prominent subcortical atrophy.

Fewer volumetric studies are available on PDD. One early study reported hippocampal atrophy more prominent than that seen in AD (Laakso *et al.*, 1996), and hippocampal atrophy was correlated with clinical measures of memory impairment (Riekkinen *et al.*, 1998). The first large series of PDD patients were found to have diffuse pattern of cortical volume loss

in the bilateral temporal and occipital lobes, along with right middle and inferior frontal gyri, left inferior and superior parietal lobe, right caudate and putamen, and bilateral thalamus. When compared with other patients with similar symptoms, PDD patients had more atrophy in the left occipital cortex than PD patients without dementia, but less significant atrophy in the bilateral medial temporal structures compared with AD patients (Burton *et al.*, 2004). In a separate study, PDD patients were found to have less atrophy than AD patients in multiple brain regions, including in the amygdala and middle temporal gyrus bilaterally, along with the right insula and post-central gyrus, and left hippocampus and middle occipital gyrus (Beyer *et al.*, 2007).

Two studies referenced above have also directly compared patients with DLB and PDD. In the first, there was no difference in severity of atrophy between DLB patients and PDD patients (Burton *et al.*, 2004), In the second study, DLB patients were found to have more atrophy in the temporal, parietal, and occipital lobes than in PDD (Beyer *et al.*, 2007). The discordant findings again may reflect different clinical disease severity, as DLB patients in the earlier study had more cognitive impairment (mean MMSE 16.5 vs. 19.4) and were younger (mean age 77.9 vs. 73.6 years). Further analysis taking disease severity into account is necessary to determine whether there is any definitive difference in atrophy pattern between DLB and PDD, although consistent findings from available studies seem to point to a diffuse pattern of atrophy for both entities between that of AD and control subjects. Furthermore, no focal atrophy (as may be seen in FTD-related disorders) has been identified to correlate with the clinical or pathologic diagnosis of DLB and PDD.

Functional imaging studies have offered more definitive findings in DLB and PDD. Occipital hypoperfusion has been reliably identified in DLB, with relative preservation of temporal perfusion compared with AD patients (Donnemiller *et al.*, 1997; Ishii *et al.*, 1999; Lobotesis *et al.*, 2001). Similar patterns of hypometablism in the primary visual and/or visual association cortex have also been observed, and the hypometabolism was associated with more severe pathologic changes (Ishii *et al.*, 1998a; Higuchi *et al.*, 2000; Minoshima *et al.*, 2001). PDD patients have also been observed to have more occipital hypoperfusion than AD patients (Vander Borght *et al.*, 1997; Firbank *et al.*, 2003). The decreased occipital perfusion has been correlated with increased fluctuation of consciousness, while decreased posterior cingulate perfusion was associated with hallucination severity in some studies but not in others (O'Brien et al., 2004, 2005; Osaki et al., 2005). When patients were imaged longitudinally, DLB patients were found to have increased perfusion to the putamen which was correlated with worsening of parkinsonism. On the other hand, PDD patients did not demonstrate a significant change in putamenal perfusion compared with control subjects, although striatal perfusion did correlate with worsening parkinsonism on an individual basis (Firbank et al., 2005). Direct comparison of metabolic rates showed that DLB and PDD patients had very similar patterns of hypometabolism, although DLB patients had more metabolic decrease in the anterior cingulate region compared with PDD patients (Yong et al., 2007). These findings in DLB and PDD patients complement patterns of atrophy observed in structural analysis, and the differences in DLB and PDD patients may offer functional support for the observed differences in degree of atrophy between DLB and PDD.

> **Box 27.7. Dementia with Lewy bodies (DLB) and Parkinson's disease dementia (PDD)**
>
> Clinically characterized by concurrent onset of cognitive and parkinsonian symptoms (DLB) or onset of cognitive symptoms in the setting of parkinsonism (PDD).
>
> DLB shows more atrophy in frontal/temporal cortices and subcortical structures than control subjects, but less medial temporal atrophy than AD.
>
> PDD shows more atrophy in frontal/temporal/occipital cortices than control subjects, but less medial temporal atrophy than AD.
>
> Cerebral hypoperfusion and hypometabolism in occipital regions in DLB and PDD.

Substrate-specific imaging has been increasingly used in PD-related disorders to analyze striatal dopamine transporter loss. Iodine I-123-radiolabeled 2β-carbomethoxy-3β-(4-iodophenyl)-N-(3-fluoropropyl) nortropane (^{123}I-FP-CIT) is a ligand with high specificity for the dopamine transporter (Walker et al., 1999). In a clinical cohort, striatal binding of ^{123}I-CIT was significantly decreased in PD compared to control subjects and patients with vascular parkinsonism, drug-induced parkinsonism, or essential tremor (Eerola et al., 2005). Patients with PD, PDD,

and DLB all have reduced ^{123}I-FP-CIT SPECT uptake in the caudate and putamen compared with AD patients and control subjects (Walker et al., 2002; O'Brien et al., 2004). When specific parts of the basal ganglia were analyzed, PDD patients had the most severe loss of dopamine transporter in the caudate and putamen, followed by DLB and PD patients, and PD patients had the largest differential dopamine transporter loss between caudate and posterior putamen. Statistical parametric mapping of ^{123}I-FP-CIT SPECT images confirmed reduced ligand uptake in the bilateral caudate and putamen in DLB and PD patients compared with AD patients and control subjects (Colloby et al., 2004), and the rate of dopamine transporter loss was similar among patients with PD, PDD, and DLB over time (Colloby et al., 2005). In a phase III, multi-center study, ^{123}I-FP-CIT SPECT imaging showed sensitivity of 77.7% and specificity of 90.4% in the diagnosis of DLB (McKeith et al., 2007). Abnormality in dopamine transporter on SPECT has since been introduced as a suggestive feature in the diagnosis of DLB (McKeith et al., 2005).

A similar receptor-specific ligand imaging approach has been used to investigate the density of muscarinic acetylcholine receptors in DLB and PDD, as loss of acetylcholine receptors may reflect cognitive decline. Compared to control subjects, muscarinic receptors were increased in the right occipital lobe in DLB, and bilateral occipital lobes in PDD, possibly corresponding to previous changes in perfusion seen in similar regions (Colloby et al., 2006). In the same study, bilateral frontal and temporal receptor loss was observed in PDD, but not in DLB. While loss of cholinergic neurons may explain the receptor upregulation in the occipital regions, the cause and functional consequence of decreased frontal and temporal receptor density remain unclear. In a clinicopathologic study, increased muscarinic receptor binding in Brodmann area 36 in the temporal lobe was positively correlated with delusions in autopsy-confirmed DLB patients, although PDD patients were not assessed. The conflicting findings between in-vivo imaging and direct pathologic analysis may reflect differences in disease duration or in-vivo specificity of ligand binding, and caution must be exercised in interpreting such imaging results. However, results from studies using dopamine transporter imaging remain encouraging, with potential utility in differentiating parkinsonian disorders associated with alpha-synucleinopathies from those associated instead with tauopathies (Kim *et al.*, 2002; Plotkin *et al.*, 2005).

Vascular dementia

Vascular dementia is a clinically and pathologically heterogeneous entity. Clinically, cognitive impairment and dementia can result from large vessel disease or small vessel disease. Dementia can result from large vessel disease by large territory cortical infarcts or strategically located infarcts, and small vessel disease dementia often stems from lacunar infarcts, accumulation of clinically silent infarcts, or extensive small vessel disease. While a history of multiple clinically apparent infarctions can be useful in the diagnosis of multi-infarct dementia or dementia from large vessel disease, neuroimaging is essential in the diagnosis of small vessel disease. The most commonly used vascular dementia criteria are from the National Institute of Neurological Disorders and Stroke Association Internationale pour la Recherche et l'Enseignement en Neurosciences (NINDS-AIREN), which incorporate the use of neuroimaging as part of the diagnostic algorithm (Roman *et al.*, 1993).

Large vessel disease

1. Topography: radiological lesions associated with dementia include any of the following or combination thereof:
   a. bilateral anterior cerebral artery territory;
   b. posterior cerebral artery territory, including paramedian thalamic infarctions and inferior medial temporal lobe lesions;
   c. cortical association areas, including parietal–temporal regions, temporal–occipital regions, and angular gyrus;
   d. watershed carotid territories in the superior frontal and parietal regions.
2. Severity – in addition to the above, relevant radiological lesions associated with dementia include:
   a. large vessel lesions of the dominant hemisphere.
3. Bilateral large vessel hemispheric strokes.

Small vessel disease

4. Topography: multiple basal ganglia and frontal white matter lacunar infarcts; extensive peri-ventricular white matter lesions; bilateral thalamic infarcts.
5. Severity – leukoencephalopathy involving at least 25% of the total white matter.

While it is commonly accepted that cerebrovascular disease contributes to the development of cognitive impairment and/or dementia either directly or in conjunction with degenerative causes, it remains controversial whether some types of cerebrovascular lesions are more detrimental cognitively than others. Patients often have a combination of large and small vessel disease, along with vascular risk factors shared by cerebrovascular disease and Alzheimer disease. On MRI, large vessel disease is characterized by cortical infarcts in the corresponding vascular or watershed territories. Lacunar infarcts are small, cavitated lesions located in areas commonly associated with unique clinical syndromes in some but can be clinically silent in others, including the thalamus, basal ganglia, internal capsule, thalamus, pons, corona radiata, and centrum semiovale. The cavitary center shares the same imaging intensity as CSF on both CT and MRI, and is more easily visualized on MRI due to improved sensitivity. Population studies have shown increasing prevalence of clinically silent lacunar infarcts with age (Price *et al.*, 1997; Vermeer *et al.*, 2002; DeCarli *et al.*, 2005). White matter hyperintensities (WMH) are also frequent findings in the elderly patients with and without dementia, and are associated with demyelination and gliosis reflecting tissue degeneration of variable severity (Englund, 1998, 2002). Longitudinally, WMH progression is common in the subcortical white matter, and new lacunes frequently also occur in the subcortical white matter, especially in the frontal lobe (Gouw *et al.*, 2008). The exact association between these vascular lesions and dementia requires further clarification, but potential mechanisms include direct causal relationship between cumulative white matter injury and dementia, additive or synergistic effect of vascular lesions with age-related AD pathology, and common risk factors predisposing to vascular and AD pathology.

Analysis of the cerebrovascular contribution to dementia is complicated by the observation that risk factors predisposing individual patients to vascular pathology – hypertension, hyperlipidemia, and diabetes – are the same risk factors that increase the likelihood of and rate of decline in AD (Mielke *et al.*, 2007), and clinically silent infarcts – at times numerous – can be seen in cognitively normal subjects. Similarly, patients with vascular lesions and AD pathology have lower AD pathologic burden for the same degree of clinical impairment compared with those without vascular lesions (Snowdon *et al.*, 1997), but not all radiographical WMH are thought to be pathological in nature (Sze *et al.*, 1986). Various studies have examined patients with different levels of vascular lesions and co-existing AD pathology. At the microvascular level, patients with mild WMH based on neuroimaging have worse performance on memory/language tests than executive control tests, and patients with moderate to severe WMH have the reverse pattern of worse executive functions than memory/language functions (Price *et al.*, 2005). In direct comparison of potential predictors associated with subcortical vascular lesion burden, severity of cognitive impairment is associated with total WMH burden, hippocampal atrophy and cortical atrophy than number of lacunes (Fein *et al.*, 2000; Mungas *et al.*, 2001). Specifically, brain atrophy is correlated with all cognitive domains, WMH is associated with impaired short-term memory/language and mental inflexibility, and strategic infarcts in the thalamus and/or cortical gray matter are associated with poor short-term and working memory but not with mental flexibility (Swartz *et al.*, 2008). Unlike deep white matter lesions, periventricular WMH did not appear to be correlated with cognitive impairment (Delano-Wood *et al.*, 2008). Furthermore, there may exist a threshold beyond which the cumulative WMH becomes clinically significant (Price *et al.*, 2005; Chui *et al.*, 2006; Libon *et al.*, 2008).

When vascular lesions and AD pathology were examined in clinicopathologic series, a slightly different pattern of clinical significance emerges for microinfarcts, periventricular and diffuse white matter demyelination co-existing with AD pathology. One such large clinicopathologic study identified 156 brains with a spectrum of AD pathology, lacunes, and microvascular pathology including cortical microinfarcts, diffuse and focal gliosis, periventricular and deep white matter demyelination without any other form of pathology or copathology such as Lewy bodies (Gold *et al.*, 2007). The presence of clinical dementia was independently correlated with Braak and Braak staging of AD pathology, Aβ deposition stage, cortical microinfarct density, and thalamic and basal ganglion lacunar infarct number. In this study, white matter lacunes, periventricular and

diffuse white matter demyelination scores, and cortical gliosis were not associated with the presence of clinical dementia. The inclusion of both ends of the vascular–degenerative dementia spectrum (high probability AD with mild microvascular lesions, and low probability AD with severe microvascular lesions) and quantitative confirmation of AD and vascular lesions proved powerful in elucidating the interaction between AD and microvascular pathology. Namely, even in cases of severe AD pathology, presence of vascular lesions – both those that would be visible on neuroimaging and those that would be difficult to assess on conventional neuroimaging – still affected the severity of cognitive impairment in patients with clinical dementia. However, this likely does not contradict the previous imaging-based findings, as the contribution of white matter lesions to clinical dementia may only be significant in milder cases of AD (more "pure" vascular dementia) and be diluted in series incorporating cases with moderate to severe AD pathology (Snowdon *et al.*, 1997; Kovari *et al.*, 2007).

When larger cortical infarcts are also analyzed alongside AD pathology and microvascular pathology, yet another pattern of relative contribution has been reported. In a large clinicopathologic study of 153 brains including those with microvascular and macrovascular infarcts, nearly 50% of patients with microvascular infarcts also had macrovascular infarcts, and the presence of macrovascular infarcts did not seem to correlate with severity of AD pathology (Schneider *et al.*, 2007). As expected, the presence of macrovascular infarctions increased the odds of developing clinical dementia, especially multiple, large, and subcortical infarctions. Microscopic infarctions also contributed to dementia independent of macroscopic infarctions and AD pathology. In a follow-up study, the same group reported that the presence of microvascular infarcts increased the risk of dementia fourfold (Schneider *et al.*, 2007). Thus, multiple variants of cerebrovascular lesions may significantly contribute to the development of dementia, with or without the existence of significant AD pathology. Nevertheless, it remains to be determined whether vascular dementia (moderate to severe vascular pathology with mild AD pathology), mixed dementia (moderate to severe vascular and AD pathology), and clinically probable AD (moderate to severe AD pathology, mild vascular pathology) can be reliably distinguished clinically and radiographically. Prospective studies incorporating both detection of AD pathologic substrate (^{11}C-PIB-PET) and white matter lesions/integrity (MRI/DTI) will be necessary to define the vascular–degenerative spectrum.

Creutzfeldt–Jakob disease

Creutzfeldt–Jakob disease (CJD) is a rare neuroinfectious disorder that often enters the differential diagnosis of a patient with dementia, and will only be briefly discussed in this chapter. It is thought to be caused by the incorrectly folded human prion protein. It has a sporadic and familial form. Clinically, CJD is characterized by rapidly progressive dementia associated with myoclonus, ataxia, and seizure, although the combination of these symptoms do not always translate into clinical or pathologic prionopathies (Hu et al., 2006; Geschwind et al., 2008). The first antemortem diagnostic tests for CJD came from cerebrospinal fluid analysis and elecroencephalography (EEG), when it was found that patients with autopsy-confirmed CJD had elevated 14–3–3 protein, a neuronal nuclear protein involved in the stress response, and periodic sharp wave complexes (PSWC). Different cut-off values for CSF 14–3–3 generated diagnostic thresholds of either high sensitivity or high specificity, but CSF 14–3–3 assays are not widely available and could only be performed in limited specialty laboratories in the USA. With increasing clinical recognition of CJD and availability of MRI, it became apparent that many CJD patients had patterns of MRI abnormalities not seen in other neurodegenerative disorders. In sporadic cases of CJD (sCJD), T2 and diffusion weighted imaging (DWI) abnormalities have been observed in the cortical and deep gray matter. Furthermore, the patterns of MRI abnormalities are correlated with the polymorphic codon 129 of prion protein gene: MM1/MV1/MV2 cases had frequent striatal abnormalities, MM2 had rare striatal abnormalities but more frequent cortical abnormalities, VV1 cases had high frequency of cortical abnormalities but also some striatal abnormalities, and VV2 cases had high prevalence of striatum, thalamus, and cortical abnormalities (Parchi et al., 1996). Most patients with PSWC on EEG had MRI DWI abnormalities (Kandiah et al., 2008), and patients with isolated DWI abnormalities in the cortex may be associated with slightly better prognosis than those with affected cortical and striatal regions (Meissner et al., 2008). DWI was associated with

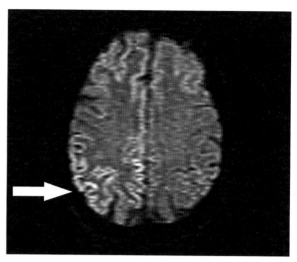

Figure 27.6 DWI abnormalities in the cortical ribbon region of a sporadic Creutzfeldt-Jakob disease (CJD) case. (Image courtesy of Dr. Keith A. Josephs.)

improved clinical diagnostic accuracy of 90.5% compared with other laboratory tests: 57.1% for neuron-specific enolase and 76.2% for 14–3–3 (Satoh et al., 2007).

Box 27.8. Creutzfeldt–Jakob disease (CJD)

Clinically characterized by rapidly progressive dementia, ataxia, myoclonus, with supporting evidence of EEG abnormalities and elevated 14–3–3 in CSF.

DWI abnormalities in cortical regions, thalamus, and/or striatum.

"Pulvinar sign" suggestive but not diagnostic of variant CJD.

In familial CJD, DWI abnormalities in the caudate nucleus are sensitive and highly specific, and FLAIR abnormalities were slightly more sensitive but less specific than DWI findings (Fulbright et al., 2008). In variant CJD (vCJD), DWI abnormalities in the pulvinar nucleus of the thamalus were seen in 32 out of 36 patients which led to the introduction of the "pulvinar sign" in CJD diagnosis (Zeidler et al., 2000). Unlike sCJD, these patients generally do not have EEG abnormalities, and CSF 14–3–3 is only elevated in about half of the cases (Will et al., 2000). Hence, DWI abnormalities significantly improve the diagnostic accuracy of sCJD, and can be crucial in the diagnosis of vCJD, although sCJD cases could also have DWI appearances mimicking those seen in vCJD (Martindale *et al.*, 2003). At the same time, subtle MRI changes associated with CJD can be missed by inexperienced readers, and should be examined with care in patients clinically suspected to having a prionopathy.

Summary

In conclusion, non-AD neurodegenerative disorders frequently give rise to clinical phenotypes distinctly different from clinically probable AD with prominent memory impairment, although structural and functional imaging studies could serve as useful biomarkers in cases lacking collateral history or cases too impaired for objective testing. Common patterns of imaging findings (for example, frontotemporal abnormalities in FTLD, temporoparietal abnormalities in AD) could also be useful in the identification of atypical dementia variants of common pathology, as evidenced by imaging findings in LPA being more similar to AD than FTLD. When used appropriately, volumetric brain analysis of demented patients may be sufficiently sensitive and specific to improve the clinical diagnostic accuracy, although the development of radio-ligands specific for each neuropathologic substrate involved in AD, FTD, and DLB will significantly enhance the clinical diagnosis of neurodegenerative disorders, especially in cases of co-existing pathology. The utility of imaging will likely extend beyond diagnostic aide to involve better understanding of the basic neuropathologic process, and can serve as measurable endpoints to identify therapies of high promise and yield. It is thus of crucial importance for clinicians involved in the care and research of patients suffering from common and unusual dementing illnesses to familiarize themselves with the general patterns and caveats of these degenerative conditions.

References

Aarsland D, Litvan I, Salmon D, *et al.* 2003. Performance on the dementia rating scale in Parkinson's disease with dementia and dementia with Lewy bodies: Comparison with progressive supranuclear palsy and Alzheimer's disease. *J Neurol Neurosurg Psychiatry* **74**, 1215–20.

Amador-Ortiz C and Dickson D W. 2008. Neuropathology of hippocampal sclerosis. *Handb Clin Neurol* **89**, 569–72.

Apaydin H, Ahlskog J E, Parisi J E, *et al.* 2002. Parkinson disease neuropathology: Later-developing dementia and loss of the levodopa response. *Arch Neurol* **59**, 102–12.

Ash S, Moore P, Vesely L, *et al.* 2009. Non-fluent speech in frontotemporal lobar degeneration. *J Neuroling* **22**, 370–83.

Asmuth J, Zhang H, Vesely L, *et al.* 2008. DTI analysis of white matter deficits in frontotemporal lobar dementia. *Neurology* **70**, A452.

Ballard C, Ziabreva I, Perry R, *et al.* 2006. Differences in neuropathologic characteristics across the Lewy body dementia spectrum. *Neurology* **67**, 1931–4.

Ballmaier M, O'Brien J T, Burton E J, *et al.* 2004. Comparing gray matter loss profiles between dementia with Lewy bodies and Alzheimer's disease using cortical pattern matching: diagnosis and gender effects. *Neuroimage* **23**, 325–35.

Barber R, Ballard C, McKeith I G, *et al.* 2000. MRI volumetric study of dementia with Lewy bodies: A comparison with AD and vascular dementia. *Neurology* **54**, 1304–9.

Beck J, Rohrer J D, Campbell T, *et al.* 2008. A distinct clinical, neuropsychological and radiological phenotype is associated with progranulin gene mutations in a large UK series. *Brain* **131**, 706–20.

Bersano A, Del Bo R, Lamperti C, *et al.* 2007. Inclusion body myopathy and frontotemporal dementia caused by a novel VCP mutation. *Neurobiol Aging* **30**, 752–8.

Beyer M K, Larsen J P, Aasrland D, *et al.* 2007. Gray matter atrophy in Parkinson disease with dementia and dementia with Lewy bodies. *Neurology* **69**, 747–54.

Bian H, Van Swieten J C, Leight S, *et al.* 2008. CSF biomarkers in frontotemporal lobar degeneration with known pathology. *Neurology* **70**, 1827–35.

Blin J, Vidailhet M J, Pillon B, *et al.* 1992. Corticobasal degeneration: Decreased and asymmetrical glucose consumption as studied with PET. *Mov Disord* **7**, 348–54.

Boeve B F, Lang A E, Litvan I, *et al.* 2003. Corticobasal degeneration and its relationship to progressive supranuclear palsy and frontotemporal dementia. *Ann Neurol* **54** (Suppl 5), S15–9.

Bonelli S B, Ransmayr G, Steffelbauer M, *et al.* 2004. L-dopa responsiveness in dementia with Lewy bodies, Parkinson disease with and without dementia. *Neurology* **63**, 376–8.

Borroni B, Brambati S M, Agosti C, *et al.* 2007. Evidence of white matter changes on diffusion tensor imaging in frontotemporal dementia. *Arch Neurol* **64**, 246–51.

Boxer A L, Geschwind M D, Belfor N, *et al.* 2006. Patterns of brain atrophy that differentiate corticobasal degeneration syndrome from progressive supranuclear palsy. *Arch Neurol* **63**, 81–6.

Bright P, Moss H E, Stamatakis E A, *et al.* 2008. Longitudinal studies of semantic dementia: The relationship between structural and functional changes over time. *Neuropsychologia* **46**, 2177–88.

Burn D J, Rowan E N, Minett T, *et al.* 2003. Extrapyramidal features in Parkinson's disease with and without dementia and dementia with Lewy bodies: A cross-sectional comparative study. *Mov Disord* **18**, 884–9.

Burton E J, Karas G, Paling S M, *et al.* 2002. Patterns of cerebral atrophy in dementia with Lewy bodies using voxel-based morphometry. *Neuroimage* **17**, 618–30.

Burton E J, McKeith I G, Burn D J, *et al.* 2004. Cerebral atrophy in Parkinson's disease with and without dementia: A comparison with Alzheimer's disease, dementia with Lewy bodies and controls. *Brain* **127**, 791–800.

Buxbaum L J, Kyle K, Grossman M, *et al.* 2007. Left inferior parietal representations for skilled hand-object interactions: Evidence from stroke and corticobasal degeneration. *Cortex* **43**, 411–23.

Caselli R J, Jack C R Jr, Petersen R C, *et al.* 1992. Asymmetric cortical degenerative syndromes: Clinical and radiologic correlations. *Neurology* **42**, 1462–8.

Chang J L, Lomen-Hoerth C, Murphy C J, *et al.* 2005. A voxel-based morphometry study of patterns of brain atrophy in ALS and ALS/FTLD. *Neurology* **65**, 75–80.

Chao L L, Schuff N, Clevenger E M, *et al.* 2007. Patterns of white matter atrophy in frontotemporal lobar degeneration. *Arch Neurol* **64**, 1619–24.

Chow T W, Binns M A, Freedman M, *et al.* 2008. Overlap in frontotemporal atrophy between normal aging and patients with frontotemporal dementias. *Alzheimer Dis Assoc Disord* **22**, 327–35.

Chui H C, Zarow C, Mack W J, *et al.* 2006. Cognitive impact of subcortical vascular and Alzheimer's disease pathology. *Ann Neurol* **60**, 677–87.

Clark D G, Charuvastra A, Miller B L, *et al.* 2005. Fluent versus nonfluent primary progressive aphasia: A comparison of clinical and functional neuroimaging features. *Brain Lang* **94**, 54–60.

Colloby S J, O'Brien J T, Fenwick J D, *et al.* 2004. The application of statistical parametric mapping to 123I-FP-CIT SPECT in dementia with Lewy bodies, Alzheimer's disease and Parkinson's disease. *Neuroimage* **23**, 956–66.

Colloby S J, Pakrasi S, Firbank M J, *et al.* 2006. In vivo SPECT imaging of muscarinic acetylcholine receptors using (R, R) ^{123}I-QNB in dementia with Lewy bodies and Parkinson's disease dementia. *Neuroimage* **33**, 423–9.

Colloby S J, Williams E D, Burn D J, *et al.* 2005. Progression of dopaminergic degeneration in dementia with Lewy bodies and Parkinson's disease with and without dementia assessed using ^{123}I-FP-CIT SPECT. *Eur J Nucl Med Mol Imaging* **32**, 1176–85.

Colosimo C, Hughes A J, Kilford L, *et al.* 2003. Lewy body cortical involvement may not always predict dementia in Parkinson's disease. *J Neurol Neurosurg Psychiatry* **74**, 852–6.

Cooke A, DeVita C, Gee J, *et al.* 2003. Neural basis for sentence comprehension deficits in frontotemporal dementia. *Brain Lang* **85**, 211–21.

Davatzikos C, Resnick S M, Wu X, *et al.* 2008. Individual patient diagnosis of AD and FTD via high-dimensional pattern classification of MRI. *Neuroimage* **41**, 1220–7.

Davies R R, Halliday G M, Xuereb J H, *et al.* 2008. The neural basis of semantic memory: Evidence from semantic dementia. *Neurobiol Aging* **30**, 2043–52.

DeCarli C, Massaro J, Harvey D, *et al.* 2005. Measures of brain morphology and infarction in the Framingham heart study: Establishing what is normal. *Neurobiol Aging* **26**, 491–510.

Delano-Wood L, Abeles N, Sacco J M, *et al.* 2008. Regional white matter pathology in mild cognitive impairment: Differential influence of lesion type on neuropsychological functioning. *Stroke* **39**, 794–9.

Desgranges B, Matuszewski V, Poilino P, *et al.* 2007. Anatomical and functional alterations in semantic dementia: A voxel-based MRI and PET study. *Neurobiol Aging* **28**, 1904–13.

Dickson D W. 2001. Neuropathology of Pick's disease. *Neurology* **56** (11 Suppl 4), S16–20.

Dickson D W. 2008. Neuropathology of progressive supranuclear palsy. *Handb Clin Neurol* **89**, 487–91.

Dickson D W, Bergeron C, Chin S S, *et al.* 2002. Office of Rare Diseases neuropathologic criteria for corticobasal degeneration. *J Neuropathol Exp Neurol* **61**, 935–46.

Donnemiller E, Heilmann J, Wenning G K, *et al.* 1997. Brain perfusion scintigraphy with 99mTc-HMPAO or 99mTc-ECD and 123I-beta-CIT single-photon emission tomography in dementia of the Alzheimer-type and diffuse Lewy body disease. *Eur J Nucl Med* **24**, 320–5.

Downes J J, Priestley N M, Doran M, *et al.* 1998. Intellectual, mnemonic, and frontal functions in dementia with Lewy bodies: A comparison with early and advanced Parkinson's disease. *Behav Neurol* **11**, 173–83.

Drzezga A, Grimmer T, Henriksen G, *et al.* 2008. Imaging of amyloid plaques and cerebral glucose metabolism in semantic dementia and Alzheimer's disease. *Neuroimage* **39**, 619–33.

Eckert T, Barnes A, Dhawan V, *et al.* 2005. FDG PET in the differential diagnosis of parkinsonian disorders. *Neuroimage* **26**, 912–21.

Eerola J, Tienari P J, Kaakkola S, *et al.* 2005. How useful is [123I]beta-CIT SPECT in clinical practice? *J Neurol Neurosurg Psychiatry* **76**, 1211–6.

Eidelberg D, Dhawan V, Moeller J R, *et al*. 1991. The metabolic landscape of cortico-basal ganglionic degeneration: Regional asymmetries studied with positron emission tomography. *J Neurol Neurosurg Psychiatry* **54**, 856–62.

Englund E. 1998. Neuropathology of white matter changes in Alzheimer's disease and vascular dementia. *Dement Geriatr Cogn Disord* **9** (Suppl 1), 6–12.

Englund E. 2002. Neuropathology of white matter lesions in vascular cognitive impairment. *Cerebrovasc Dis* **13** (Suppl 2), 11–5.

Fagan A M, Mintun M A, Mach R H, *et al*. 2006. Inverse relation between in vivo amyloid imaging load and cerebrospinal fluid Abeta42 in humans. *Ann Neurol* **59**, 512–9.

Fein G, Di Sclafani V, Tanabe J, *et al*. 2000. Hippocampal and cortical atrophy predict dementia in subcortical ischemic vascular disease. *Neurology* **55**, 1626–35.

Firbank M J, Burn D J, McKeith I G, *et al*. 2005. Longitudinal study of cerebral blood flow SPECT in Parkinson's disease with dementia, and dementia with Lewy bodies. *Int J Geriatr Psychiatry* **20**, 776–82.

Firbank M J, Colloby S J, Burn D J, *et al*. 2003. Regional cerebral blood flow in Parkinson's disease with and without dementia. *Neuroimage* **20**, 1309–19.

Forman M S, Farmer J, Johnson J K, *et al*. 2006a. Frontotemporal dementia: clinicopathological correlations. *Ann Neurol* **59**, 952–62.

Forman M S, Mackenzie I R, Cairns N J, *et al*. 2006b. Novel ubiquitin neuropathology in frontotemporal dementia with valosin-containing protein gene mutations. *J Neuropathol Exp Neurol* **65**, 571–81.

Foster N L, Heidebrink J L, Clark C M, *et al*. 2007. FDG-PET improves accuracy in distinguishing frontotemporal dementia and Alzheimer's disease. *Brain* **130**, 2616–35.

Fulbright R K, Hoffmann C, Leed H, *et al*. 2008. MR imaging of familial Creutzfeldt-Jakob disease: A blinded and controlled study. *Am J Neuroradiol* **29**, 1638–43.

Garrard P and Hodges J R. 2000. Semantic dementia: Clinical, radiological and pathological perspectives. *J Neurol* **247**, 409–22.

Geschwind M D, Tan K M, Lennon V A, *et al*. 2008. Voltage-gated potassium channel autoimmunity mimicking Creutzfeldt–Jakob disease. *Arch Neurol* **65**, 1341–6.

Geser F, Winton M J, Kwong L K, *et al*. 2008. Pathological TDP-43 in parkinsonism–dementia complex and amyotrophic lateral sclerosis of Guam. *Acta Neuropathol* **115**, 133–45.

Gold G, Giannakopoulos P, Herrmann F R, *et al*. 2007. Identification of Alzheimer and vascular lesion thresholds for mixed dementia. *Brain* **130**, 2830–6.

Gorno-Tempini M L, Brambati S M, Ginex V, *et al*. 2008. The logopenic/phonological variant of primary progressive aphasia. *Neurology* **71**, 1227–34.

Gorno-Tempini M L, Dronkers N F, Rankin K P, *et al*. 2004. Cognition and anatomy in three variants of primary progressive aphasia. *Ann Neurol* **55**, 335–46.

Gouw A A, van der Flier W M, Fazekas F, *et al*. 2008. Progression of white matter hyperintensities and incidence of new lacunes over a 3-year period: The Leukoaraiosis and Disability study. *Stroke* **39**, 1414–20.

Groschel K, Hauser T K, Luft A, *et al*. 2004. Magnetic resonance imaging-based volumetry differentiates progressive supranuclear palsy from corticobasal degeneration. *Neuroimage* **21**, 714–24.

Grossman M, Alsop D, Detre J A, *et al*. 2001. Perfusion fMRI using arterial spin labeling in Alzheimer's disease and frontotemporal dementia: Correlations with language. *Brain Lang* **79**, 94–5.

Grossman M, CookeA, DeVita C, *et al*. 2002. Sentence processing strategies in healthy seniors with poor comprehension: An fMRI study. *Brain Lang* **80**, 296–313.

Grossman M, D'Esposito M, Hughes E, *et al*. 1996a. Language comprehension profiles in Alzheimer's disease, multi-infarct dementia, and frontotemporal degeneration. *Neurology* **47**, 183–9.

Grossman M, McMillan C, Moore P, *et al*. 2004. What's in a name: Voxel-based morphometric analyses of MRI and naming difficulty in Alzheimer's disease, frontotemporal dementia and corticobasal degeneration. *Brain* **127**, 628–49.

Grossman M, Mickanin J, Onishi K, *et al*. 1996b. Progressive nonfluent aphasia: language, cognitive, and PET measures contrasted to probable Alzheimer's disease. *J Cogn Neurosci* **8**, 135–54.

Grossman M and Moore P. 2005. A longitudinal study of sentence comprehension difficulty in primary progressive aphasia. *J Neurol Neurosurg Psychiatry* **76**, 644–9.

Grossman M, Payer F, Onishi K, *et al*. 1998. Language comprehension and regional cerebral defects in frontotemporal degeneration and Alzheimer's disease. *Neurology* **50**, 157–63.

Grossman M, Wood E M, Moore P, *et al*. 2007. TDP-43 pathologic lesions and clinical phenotype in frontotemporal lobar degeneration with ubiquitin-positive inclusions. *Arch Neurol* **64**, 1449–54.

Grossman M, Xie S X, Libon D J, *et al*. 2008. Longitudinal decline in autopsy-defined frontotemporal lobar degeneration. *Neurology* **70**, 2036–45.

Gydesen S, Brown J M, Brun A, *et al*. 2002. Chromosome 3 linked frontotemporal dementia (FTD-3). *Neurology* **59**, 1585–94.

Halpern C, McMillan C, Moore P, *et al.* 2003. Calculation impairment in neurodegenerative diseases. *J Neurol Sci* **208**, 31–8.

Halpern C H, Glosser G, Clark R, *et al.* 2004. Dissociation of numbers and objects in corticobasal degeneration and semantic dementia. *Neurology* **62**, 1163–9.

Harding A J and Halliday G M. 2001. Cortical Lewy body pathology in the diagnosis of dementia. *Acta Neuropathol* **102**, 355–63.

Hashimoto M, Kitagaki H, Imamura T, *et al.* 1998. Medial temporal and whole-brain atrophy in dementia with Lewy bodies: A volumetric MRI study. *Neurology* **51**, 357–62.

Higuchi M, Tashiro M, Arai H, *et al.* 2000. Glucose hypometabolism and neuropathological correlates in brains of dementia with Lewy bodies. *Exp Neurol* **162**, 247–56.

Hodges J R, Davies R R, Xuereb J H, *et al.* 2004. Clinicopathological correlates in frontotemporal dementia. *Ann Neurol* **56**, 399–406.

Hu W T, Josephs K A, Ahlskog J E, *et al.* 2005. MRI correlates of alien leg-like phenomenon in corticobasal degeneration. *Mov Disord* **20**, 870–3.

Hu W T, Josephs K A, Knopman D S, *et al.* 2008. Temporal lobar predominance of TDP-43 neuronal cytoplasmic inclusions in Alzheimer disease. *Acta Neuropathol* **116**, 215–20.

Hu W T, Murray J A, Greenaway M C, *et al.* 2006. Cognitive impairment and celiac disease. *Arch Neurol* **63**, 1440–6.

Hu W T, Rippon G, Boeve F, *et al.* 2009a. Alzheimer disease and corticobasal degeneration presenting as corticobasal syndrome. *Mov Disord* **24**, 1375–9.

Hu W T, Seelaar H, Josephs K A, *et al.* 2009b. Survival profiles of patients with frontotemporal dementia and motor neuron disease. *Arch Neurol* **66**, 1359–64.

Ishii K, Imamura T, Sasaki M, *et al.* 1998a. Regional cerebral glucose metabolism in dementia with Lewy bodies and Alzheimer's disease. *Neurology* **51**, 125–30.

Ishii K, Sakamoto S, Sasaki M, *et al.* 1998b. Cerebral glucose metabolism in patients with frontotemporal dementia. *J Nucl Med* **39**, 1875–8.

Ishii K, Yamaji S, Kitagaki H, *et al.* 1999. Regional cerebral blood flow difference between dementia with Lewy bodies and AD. *Neurology* **53**, 413–6.

Jellinger K A and Attems J. 2007. Neurofibrillary tangle-predominant dementia: Comparison with classical Alzheimer disease. *Acta Neuropathol* **113**, 107–17.

Johnson J K, Head E, Kim R, *et al.* 1999. Clinical and pathological evidence for a frontal variant of Alzheimer disease. *Arch Neurol* **56**, 1233–9.

Josephs K A, Duffy J R, Strand E A, *et al.* 2006a. Clinicopathological and imaging correlates of progressive aphasia and apraxia of speech. *Brain* **129**, 1385–98.

Josephs K A, Knopman D S, Whitwell J L, *et al.* 2005. Survival in two variants of tau-negative frontotemporal lobar degeneration: FTLD-U vs FTLD-MND. *Neurology* **65**, 645–7.

Josephs K A, Petersen R C, Knopman D S, *et al.* 2006b. Clinicopathologic analysis of frontotemporal and corticobasal degenerations and PSP. *Neurology* **66**, 41–8.

Josephs K A, Tang-Wai D F, Edland S D, *et al.* 2004. Correlation between antemortem magnetic resonance imaging findings and pathologically confirmed corticobasal degeneration. *Arch Neurol* **61**, 1881–4.

Josephs K A, Whitwell J L, Dickson D W, *et al.* 2008a. Voxel-based morphometry in autopsy proven PSP and CBD. *Neurobiol Aging* **29**, 280–9.

Josephs K A, Whitwell J L, Duffy J R, *et al.* 2008b. Progressive aphasia secondary to Alzheimer disease vs FTLD pathology. *Neurology* **70**, 25–34.

Josephs K A, Whitwell J L, Knopman D S, *et al.* 2008c. Abnormal TDP-43 immunoreactivity in AD modifies clinicopathologic and radiologic phenotype. *Neurology* **70**, 1850–7.

Kandiah N, Tan K, Pan A B, *et al.* 2008. Creutzfeldt–Jakob disease: Which diffusion-weighted imaging abnormality is associated with periodic EEG complexes? *J Neurol* **255**, 1411–4.

Kartsounis L D, Crellin R F, Crewes H, *et al.* 1991. Primary progressive non-fluent aphasia: A case study. *Cortex* **27**, 121–9.

Kertesz A, McMonagle P, Blair M, *et al.* 2005. The evolution and pathology of frontotemporal dementia. *Brain* **128**, 1996–2005.

Kim E J, Rabinovici G D, Seeley W W, *et al.* 2007. Patterns of MRI atrophy in tau positive and ubiquitin positive frontotemporal lobar degeneration. *J Neurol Neurosurg Psychiatry* **78**, 1375–8.

Kim Y J, Ichise M, Erami S S, *et al.* 2002. Combination of dopamine transporter and D2 receptor SPECT in the diagnostic evaluation of PD, MSA, and PSP. *Mov Disord* **17**, 303–12.

Kitagaki H, Hirono N, Ishii K, *et al.* 2000. Corticobasal degeneration: Evaluation of cortical atrophy by means of hemispheric surface display generated with MR images. *Radiology* **216**, 31–8.

Knibb J A, Xuereb J H, Patterson K, *et al.* 2006. Clinical and pathological characterization of progressive aphasia. *Ann Neurol* **59**, 156–65.

Knopman D S, Petersen R C, Edland S D, *et al.* 2004. The incidence of frontotemporal lobar degeneration in

Rochester, Minnesota, 1990 through 1994. *Neurology* **62**, 506–08.

Kokmen E, Beard C M, O'Brien P C, *et al.* 1993. Is the incidence of dementing illness changing? A 25-year time trend study in Rochester, Minnesota (1960–1984). *Neurology* **43**, 1887–92.

Kovari E, Gold G., Herrmann F R, *et al.* 2007. Cortical microinfarcts and demyelination affect cognition in cases at high risk for dementia. *Neurology* **68**, 927–31.

Krause S, Gohringer T, Walter M C, *et al.* 2007. Brain imaging and neuropsychology in late-onset dementia due to a novel mutation (R93C) of valosin-containing protein. *Clin Neuropathol* **26**, 232–40.

Laakso M P, Partanen K, Riekkinen P, *et al.* 1996. Hippocampal volumes in Alzheimer's disease, Parkinson's disease with and without dementia, and in vascular dementia: An MRI study. *Neurology* **46**, 678–81.

Laureys S, Salmon E, Garraux G, *et al.* 1999. Fluorodopa uptake and glucose metabolism in early stages of corticobasal degeneration. *J Neurol* **246**, 1151–8.

Le Ber I, Camuzat A, Hannequin D, *et al.* 2008. Phenotype variability in progranulin mutation carriers: A clinical, neuropsychological, imaging and genetic study. *Brain* **131**, 732–46.

Le Ber I, Martinez M, Campion D, *et al.* 2004. A non-DM1, non-DM2 multisystem myotonic disorder with frontotemporal dementia: Phenotype and suggestive mapping of the DM3 locus to chromosome 15q21–24. *Brain* **127**, 1979–92.

Libon D J, Price C C, Giovannetti T, *et al.* 2008. Linking MRI hyperintensities with patterns of neuropsychological impairment: Evidence for a threshold effect. *Stroke* **39**, 806–13.

Lippa C F, Duda J E, Grossman M, *et al.* 2007. DLB and PDD boundary issues: Diagnosis, treatment, molecular pathology, and biomarkers. *Neurology* **68**, 812–9.

Listerud J, Anderson C, Moore P, *et al.* 2009. Neuropsychological patterns in MRI-defined subgroups of patients with degenerative dementia. *J Int Neuropsychol Soc,* **15**, 459–70.

Litvan I, Bhatia K P, Burn D J, *et al.* 2003. Movement Disorders Society Scientific Issues Committee report: SIC Task Force appraisal of clinical diagnostic criteria for Parkinsonian disorders. *Mov Disord* **18**, 467–86.

Lobotesis K, Fenwick J D, Phipps A, *et al.* 2001. Occipital hypoperfusion on SPECT in dementia with Lewy bodies but not AD. *Neurology* **56**, 643–9.

Lutte I, Laterre C, Bodart J M, *et al.* 2000. Contribution of PET studies in diagnosis of corticobasal degeneration. *Eur Neurol* **44**, 12–21.

Martindale J, Geschwind M D, De Armond S, *et al.* 2003. Sporadic Creutzfeldt–Jakob disease mimicking variant Creutzfeldt–Jakob disease. *Arch Neurol* **60**, 767–70.

Massimo L and Grossman M. 2008. Patient care and management of frontotemporal lobar degeneration. *Am J Alzh Dis Other Dementias* **23**, 125–31.

McKeith I, O'Brien J, Walker Z, *et al.* 2007. Sensitivity and specificity of dopamine transporter imaging with 123I-FP-CIT SPECT in dementia with Lewy bodies: A phase III, multicentre study. *Lancet Neurol* **6**, 305–13.

McKeith I G, Dickson D W, Lowe J, *et al.* 2005. Diagnosis and management of dementia with Lewy bodies: Third report of the DLB Consortium. *Neurology* **65**, 1863–72.

McKeith I G, Galasko D, Kosaka K, *et al.* 1996. Consensus guidelines for the clinical and pathologic diagnosis of dementia with Lewy bodies (DLB): Report of the consortium on DLB international workshop. *Neurology* **47**, 1113–24.

McKhann G M, Albert M S, Grossman M, *et al.* 2001. Clinical and pathological diagnosis of frontotemporal dementia: Report of the Work Group on Frontotemporal Dementia and Pick's Disease. *Arch Neurol* **58**, 1803–09.

McMurtray A M, Chen A K, Shapira J S, *et al.* 2006. Variations in regional SPECT hypoperfusion and clinical features in frontotemporal dementia. *Neurology* **66**, 517–22.

McNeill R, Sare G M, Manoharan M, *et al.* 2007. Accuracy of single-photon emission computed tomography in differentiating frontotemporal dementia from Alzheimer's disease. *J Neurol Neurosurg Psychiatry* **78**, 350–5.

Meissner B, Kallenberg K, Sanchez-Juanc P, *et al.* 2008. Isolated cortical signal increase on MR imaging as a frequent lesion pattern in sporadic Creutzfeldt–Jakob disease. *Am J Neuroradiol* **29**, 1519–24.

Mendez M F, Shapira J S, McMurtray A, *et al.* 2007. Accuracy of the clinical evaluation for frontotemporal dementia. *Arch Neurol* **64**, 830–5.

Mesulam M, Wicklund A, Johnson N, *et al.* 2008. Alzheimer and frontotemporal pathology in subsets of primary progressive aphasia. *Ann Neurol* **63**, 709–19.

Mielke M M, Rosenberg P B, Tschanz J, *et al.* 2007. Vascular factors predict rate of progression in Alzheimer disease. *Neurology* **69**, 1850–8.

Minoshima S, Foster N L, Sima A A, *et al.* 2001. Alzheimer's disease versus dementia with Lewy bodies: Cerebral metabolic distinction with autopsy confirmation. *Ann Neurol* **50**, 358–65.

Minoshima S, Giordani B, Berent S, *et al.* 1997. Metabolic reduction in the posterior cingulate cortex in very early Alzheimer's disease. *Ann Neurol* **42**, 85–94.

Mori H, Yagishita A, Takeda T, *et al.* 2007. Symmetric temporal abnormalities on MR imaging in amyotrophic lateral sclerosis with dementia. *Am J Neuroradiol* **28**, 1511–6.

Mosconi L, Tsui W H, Herholz K, *et al.* 2008. Multicenter standardized 18F-FDG PET diagnosis of mild cognitive impairment, Alzheimer's disease, and other dementias. *J Nucl Med* **49**, 390–8.

Mosimann U P, Rowan E N, Partington C E, *et al.* 2006. Characteristics of visual hallucinations in Parkinson disease dementia and dementia with Lewy bodies. *Am J Geriatr Psychiatry* **14**, 153–60.

Mukherjee O, Pastor P, Cairns N J, *et al.* 2006. HDDD2 is a familial frontotemporal lobar degeneration with ubiquitin-positive, tau-negative inclusions caused by a missense mutation in the signal peptide of progranulin. *Ann Neurol* **60**, 314–22.

Mummery C J, Patterson K, Price C J, *et al.* 2000. A voxel-based morphometry study of semantic dementia: Relationship between temporal lobe atrophy and semantic memory. *Ann Neurol* **47**, 36–45.

Mungas D, Jagust W J, Reed B R, *et al.* 2001. MRI predictors of cognition in subcortical ischemic vascular disease and Alzheimer's disease. *Neurology* **57**, 2229–35.

Murphy J M, Henry R G, Langmore S, *et al.* 2007. Continuum of frontal lobe impairment in amyotrophic lateral sclerosis. *Arch Neurol* **64**, 530–4.

Murray R, Neumann M, Forman M S, *et al.* 2007. Cognitive and motor assessment in autopsy-proven corticobasal degeneration. *Neurology* **68**, 1274–83.

Neary D, Snowden J S, Gustafson L, *et al.* 1998. Frontotemporal lobar degeneration: a consensus on clinical diagnostic criteria. *Neurology* **51**, 1546–54.

Nestor P J, Fryer T D, Hodges J R, *et al.* 2006. Declarative memory impairments in Alzheimer's disease and semantic dementia. *Neuroimage* **30**, 1010–20.

Nestor P J, Graham N L, Fruer T D, *et al.* 2003. Progressive non-fluent aphasia is associated with hypometabolism centred on the left anterior insula. *Brain* **126**, 2406–18.

Neumann M, Sampathu D M, Kwong L K, *et al.* 2006. Ubiquitinated TDP-43 in frontotemporal lobar degeneration and amyotrophic lateral sclerosis. *Science* **314**, 130–3.

Newberg A B, Mozley P D, Sadek A H, *et al.* 2000. Regional cerebral distribution of [Tc-99m] hexylmethylpropylene amineoxine in patients with progressive aphasia. *J Neuroimaging* **10**, 162–8.

Noe E, Marder K, Bell K L, *et al.* 2004. Comparison of dementia with Lewy bodies to Alzheimer's disease and Parkinson's disease with dementia. *Mov Disord* **19**, 60–7.

O'Brien J T, Colloby S, Fenwick J, *et al.* 2004. Dopamine transporter loss visualized with FP-CIT SPECT in the differential diagnosis of dementia with Lewy bodies. *Arch Neurol* **61**, 919–25.

O'Brien J T, Firbank M J, Mosimann U P, *et al.* 2005. Change in perfusion, hallucinations and fluctuations in consciousness in dementia with Lewy bodies. *Psychiatry Res* **139**, 79–88.

Osaki Y, Morita Y, Fukumoto M, *et al.* 2005. Three-dimensional stereotactic surface projection SPECT analysis in Parkinson's disease with and without dementia. *Mov Disord* **20**, 999–1005.

Parchi P, Castellani R, Capellari S, *et al.* 1996. Molecular basis of phenotypic variability in sporadic Creutzfeldt–Jakob disease. *Ann Neurol* **39**, 767–78.

Peigneux P, Salmon E, Garraux G, *et al.* 2001. Neural and cognitive bases of upper limb apraxia in corticobasal degeneration. *Neurology* **57**, 1259–68.

Phukan J, Pender N P, Hardiman O, *et al.* 2007. Cognitive impairment in amyotrophic lateral sclerosis. *Lancet Neurol* **6**, 994–1003.

Plotkin M, Amthauer H, Klaffke S, *et al.* 2005. Combined 123I-FP-CIT and 123I-IBZM SPECT for the diagnosis of parkinsonian syndromes: Study on 72 patients. *J Neural Transm* **112**, 677–92.

Price C C, Jefferson A L, Merino J G, *et al.* 2005. Subcortical vascular dementia: Integrating neuropsychological and neuroradiologic data. *Neurology* **65**, 376–82.

Price T R, Manolio T A, Kronmal R A, *et al.* 1997. Silent brain infarction on magnetic resonance imaging and neurological abnormalities in community-dwelling older adults. The Cardiovascular Health Study. CHS Collaborative Research Group. *Stroke* **28**, 1158–64.

Prusiner S B and Hsiao K K. 1994. Human prion diseases. *Ann Neurol* **35**, 385–95.

Rabinovici G D, Furst A J, O'Neil J P, *et al.* 2007. 11C-PIB PET imaging in Alzheimer disease and frontotemporal lobar degeneration. *Neurology* **68**, 1205–12.

Rankin K P, Rosen H J, Kramer J H, *et al.* 2004. Right and left medial orbitofrontal volumes show an opposite relationship to agreeableness in FTD. *Dement Geriatr Cogn Disord* **17**, 328–32.

Rhee J, Antiquena P, Grossman M, *et al.* 2001. Verb comprehension in frontotemporal degeneration: The role of grammatical, semantic and executive components. *Neurocase* **7**, 173–84.

Riekkinen P Jr, Kejonen K, Laakso M P, *et al.* 1998. Hippocampal atrophy is related to impaired memory, but not frontal functions in non-demented Parkinson's disease patients. *Neuroreport* **9**, 1507–11.

Rohrer J D, Warren J D, Omar R, *et al.* 2008. Parietal lobe deficits in frontotemporal lobar degeneration caused by a mutation in the progranulin gene. *Arch Neurol* **65**, 506–13.

Roman G C, Tatemichi T K, Erkinjuntti T, *et al.* 1993. Vascular dementia: Diagnostic criteria for research studies. Report of the NINDS-AIREN International Workshop. *Neurology* 43, 250–60.

Rosen H J, Allison S C, Ogar J M, *et al.* 2006. Behavioral features in semantic dementia vs other forms of progressive aphasias. *Neurology* 67, 1752–6.

Rosen H J, Gorno-Tempini M L, Goldman W P, *et al.* 2002a. Patterns of brain atrophy in frontotemporal dementia and semantic dementia. *Neurology* 58, 198–208.

Rosen H J, Perry R J, Murphy J, *et al.* 2002b. Emotion comprehension in the temporal variant of frontotemporal dementia. *Brain* 125, 2286–95.

Satoh K, Shirabe S, Tsujino A, *et al.* 2007. Total tau protein in cerebrospinal fluid and diffusion-weighted MRI as an early diagnostic marker for Creutzfeldt–Jakob disease. *Dement Geriatr Cogn Disord* 24, 207–12.

Schneider J A, Boyle P A, Arvanitakis Z, *et al.* 2007. Subcortical infarcts, Alzheimer's disease pathology, and memory function in older persons. *Ann Neurol* 62, 59–66.

Seeley W W, Bauer A M, Miller B L, *et al.* 2005. The natural history of temporal variant frontotemporal dementia. *Neurology* 64, 1384–90.

Skibinski G, Parkinson N J, Brown J M, *et al.* 2005. Mutations in the endosomal ESCRTIII-complex subunit CHMP2B in frontotemporal dementia. *Nat Genet* 37, 806–08.

Snowden J, Neary D, Mann D, *et al.* 2007. Frontotemporal lobar degeneration: Clinical and pathological relationships. *Acta Neuropathol* 114, 31–8.

Snowdon D A, Greiner L H, Mortimer J A, *et al.* 1997. Brain infarction and the clinical expression of Alzheimer disease. The Nun Study. *JAMA* 277, 813–7.

Soliveri P, Monza D, Paridi D, *et al.* 1999. Cognitive and magnetic resonance imaging aspects of corticobasal degeneration and progressive supranuclear palsy. *Neurology* 53, 502–07.

Swartz R H, Stuss D T, Gao F, *et al.* 2008. Independent cognitive effects of atrophy and diffuse subcortical and thalamico-cortical cerebrovascular disease in dementia. *Stroke* 39, 822–30.

Sze G, De Armond S J, Brandt-Zawadzki M, *et al.* 1986. Foci of MRI signal (pseudo lesions) anterior to the frontal horns: Histologic correlations of a normal finding. *Am J Roentgenol* 147, 331–7.

Talbot P R, Snowden J S, Lloyd J J, *et al.* 1995. The contribution of single photon emission tomography to the clinical differentiation of degenerative cortical brain disorders. *J Neurol* 242, 579–86.

Tam C W, Burton E J, McKeith I G, *et al.* 2005. Temporal lobe atrophy on MRI in Parkinson disease with dementia: A comparison with Alzheimer disease and dementia with Lewy bodies. *Neurology* 64, 861–5.

Tedeschi G, Litvan I, Bonavita S, *et al.* 1997. Proton magnetic resonance spectroscopic imaging in progressive supranuclear palsy, Parkinson's disease and corticobasal degeneration. *Brain* 120, 1541–52.

Turner R S, Kenyon L C, Trojanowski J Q, *et al.* 1996. Clinical, neuroimaging, and pathologic features of progressive nonfluent aphasia. *Ann Neurol* 39, 166–73.

van der Zee J, Urwin H, Engelborghs S, *et al.* 2008. CHMP2B C-truncating mutations in frontotemporal lobar degeneration are associated with an aberrant endosomal phenotype in vitro. *Hum Mol Genet* 17, 313–22.

van Swieten J and Spillantini M G. 2007. Hereditary frontotemporal dementia caused by Tau gene mutations. *Brain Pathol* 17, 63–73.

Vander Borght T, Minoshima S, Giordani B, *et al.* 1997. Cerebral metabolic differences in Parkinson's and Alzheimer's diseases matched for dementia severity. *J Nucl Med* 38, 797–802.

Vermeer S E, Koudstaal P J, Oudkerk M, *et al.* 2002. Prevalence and risk factors of silent brain infarcts in the population-based Rotterdam Scan Study. *Stroke* 33, 21–5.

Viassolo V, Previtali S C, Schiatti E, *et al.* 2008. Inclusion body myopathy, Paget's disease of the bone and frontotemporal dementia: Recurrence of the VCP R155H mutation in an Italian family and implications for genetic counselling. *Clin Genet* 74, 54–60.

Walker Z, Costa D C, Ince P, *et al.* 1999. In-vivo demonstration of dopaminergic degeneration in dementia with Lewy bodies. *Lancet* 354, 646–7.

Walker Z, Costa D C, Walker R W, *et al.* 2002. Differentiation of dementia with Lewy bodies from Alzheimer's disease using a dopaminergic presynaptic ligand. *J Neurol Neurosurg Psychiatry* 73, 134–40.

Watts G D, Thomasova D, Ramdeen S K, *et al.* 2007. Novel VCP mutations in inclusion body myopathy associated with Paget disease of bone and frontotemporal dementia. *Clin Genet* 72, 420–6.

Whitwell J L, Jack C R Jr, Kantacri K, *et al.* 2007a. Voxel-based morphometry in frontotemporal lobar degeneration with ubiquitin-positive inclusions with and without progranulin mutations. *Arch Neurol* 64, 371–6.

Whitwell J L, Jack C R Jr, Parisi J E, *et al.* 2007b. Rates of cerebral atrophy differ in different degenerative pathologies. *Brain* 130, 1148–58.

Whitwell J L, Josephs K A, Rossor M N, *et al.* 2005. Magnetic resonance imaging signatures of tissue pathology in frontotemporal dementia. *Arch Neurol* 62, 1402–08.

Whitwell J L, Warren J D, Josephs K A, *et al.* 2004. Voxel-based morphometry in tau-positive and tau-negative

393

frontotemporal lobar degenerations. *Neurodegener Dis* **1**, 225–30.

Whitwell J L, Weigand S D, Shiung M M, *et al.* 2007c. Focal atrophy in dementia with Lewy bodies on MRI: A distinct pattern from Alzheimer's disease. *Brain* **130**, 708–19.

Will R G, Zeidler M, Stewart G E, *et al.* 2000. Diagnosis of new variant Creutzfeldt–Jakob disease. *Ann Neurol* **47**, 575–82.

Woolley J D, Gorno-Tempini M L, Seeley W W, *et al.* 2007. Binge eating is associated with right orbitofrontal–insular–striatal atrophy in frontotemporal dementia. *Neurology* **69**, 1424–33.

Yi H A, Moore P, Grossman M, *et al.* 2007. Reversal of the concreteness effect for verbs in patients with semantic dementia. *Neuropsychology* **21**, 9–19.

Yong S W, Yoon J K, An Y S, *et al.* 2007. A comparison of cerebral glucose metabolism in Parkinson's disease, Parkinson's disease dementia and dementia with Lewy bodies. *Eur J Neurol* **14**, 1357–62.

Zamboni G, Huey E D, Krueger F, *et al.* 2008. Apathy and disinhibition in frontotemporal dementia: Insights into their neural correlates. *Neurology* **71**, 736–42.

Zeidler M, Sellar R J, Collie D A, *et al.* 2000. The pulvinar sign on magnetic resonance imaging in variant Creutzfeldt–Jakob disease. *Lancet* **355**, 1412–8.

Chapter 28

Neuroimaging of cognitive disorders: commentary

Mony J. de Leon, Henry Rusinek, Wai Tsui, Thomas Wisniewski, Jerzy Wegiel and Ajax George

When my career-long colleagues and I look back, we are struck by the wealth of accumulated knowledge derived from the structural imaging of patients with Alzheimer's disease (AD). While many of these advances were made possible by improvements in imaging hardware, creative image analysis protocols and new software tools, the key to improved understanding of AD was the interdisciplinary interactions across the fields of neuropathology, biology, and neuropsychology. We note also that much of the research reviewed in the previous chapters on AD and non-AD dementias would not have been possible without such interdisciplinary interactions and important advances in neuroimaging techniques that have taken place over the past two decades. In this brief commentary, we offer our highly personal view of three-dimensional tomographic imaging related to AD. We describe important research themes that emerged over the past 30 years and which continue to be successfully employed to understand and to ultimately prevent AD.

Hardware advances

The age of structural imaging in AD began with X-ray computed tomography (CT). In spite of the advances made with CT between 1975 and 1985 (see Figure 28.1), poor soft tissue contrast, beam hardening artifacts, and long acquisition times limited the descriptions of the gross atrophy and limited the systematic search for specific anatomical targets of AD. It was not until about 1979, about 7 years after CT first became available, that we identified cortical atrophy as the second radiological feature of AD that exceeded age effects (de Leon *et al.*, 1979). Ventricular dilatation was the first recognized abnormality of AD (Barron *et al.*, 1976), no doubt having its roots in prior observations made with

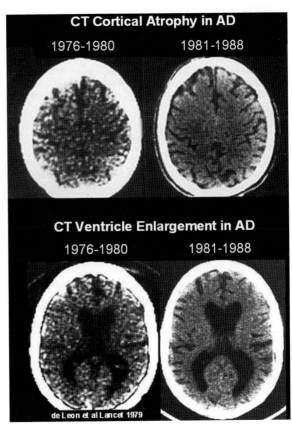

Figure 28.1 CT scans taken with first and second generation commercial CT cameras. Top images demonstrated improvements in imaging cortical atrophy and bottom images the improvements in appreciating ventricle size.

pneumoencephalography. That the CT characterization of excess cortical atrophy in AD was difficult to discern, given the well-known post-mortem "walnut" appearance of the cortical convexities, highlights the initial challenges in using this technology. Still, the semiquantitative methods used to observe the CT detectable

---

Understanding Neuropsychiatric Disorders, ed. M. E. Shenton and B. I. Turetsky. Published by Cambridge University Press.
© Cambridge University Press 2011.

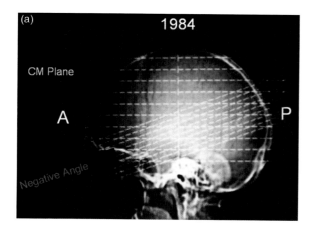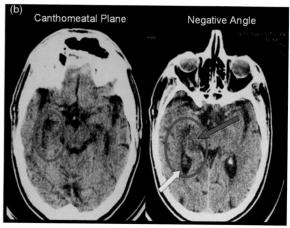

Figure 28.2 (a) Lateral scout view highlighting the cantho-meatal and negative angulation planes. Note the approximate 25° difference between the planes. The negative angulation plane is designed to parallel the long (anterior–posterior) axis of the hippocampus. (b) Axial CT scans at the level of the hippocampus highlighting the cantho-meatal (left) and negative angulation planes (right). The negative angulation plane affords increased visibility for the CSF accumulations in the hippocampal region (arrows).

excess regional cortical atrophy was not very useful in day-to-day clinical work. It was not until the availability of magnetic resonance imaging (MRI) that regional cortical atrophy was readily appreciated visually and quantified. Thus, MRI brought the description of cortical atrophy into the standard clinical use we take for granted today.

Similar technology-driven evolutions occurred both with the appreciation of hippocampal atrophy as an early feature of AD, and for age-related white matter lesions as an indicator of microvascular pathology. In the mid 1980s it was known that hippocampal pathology affected virtually all AD patients and possibly accounted for the memory impairment symptoms. It was also believed that the hippocampus tissue could not be directly studied using CT and the anatomical investigation was off limits. Our CT studies introduced the "negative angulation acquisition plane" to more efficiently reveal and measure temporal horn enlargement and incidentally found evidence for hippocampal atrophy. On CT, we defined hippocampal atrophy as cerebrospinal fluid (CSF) accumulations in the perihippocampal fissures. In 1988, we described the prevalence of hippocampal atrophy in AD (de Leon *et al.*, 1988) (Figure 28.2a and b), and in 1989 we published the first imaging study predicting the transition from mild cognitive impairment (MCI) to AD (de Leon *et al.*, 1989). Later, MRI studies with the capacity to discern the gray matter, white matter and the CSF of the hippocampal region, directly measured (Jack *et al.*, 1989) and post-

mortem validated the hippocampal volume (Bobinski *et al.*, 2000) (Figure 28.3a–c).

The use of CT to detect white matter lesions did not fare as well as either cortical or hippocampal atrophy. CT reports of white matter disease failed to convince readers that white matter pathology was discernable, it was not typically characterized at post-mortem unless correlated with a Binswanger-type profile. The first published clinico-radiological correlations (George *et al.*, 1986a) were not well accepted. To bring the white matter evaluation into routine use required that white matter pathology be sensitively detected, post-mortem verified, and with apparent clinical significance (George *et al.*, 1986b). The solution came with MRI imaging sequences such as long TR dual-echo spin-echo or fluid-attenuated inversion recovery (FLAIR); the latter having the advantage of easily separating white matter lesions (WML) from CSF-like lesions. White matter pathology had bright T2 and FLAIR signals which made for reliable observations. MRI proved to be very sensitive and it allowed the study of WML even in normal aging (Figure 28.4). The increased MRI signals were first referred to as "unidentified bright objects" (UBOs), reflecting their unknown etiology. Here the association between imaging and neuropathology again proved to be invaluable and quite possibly changed the post-mortem exam to include scrutiny of available films. UBOs in elderly populations were soon commonly recognized as common tissue changes,

(a)

CT vs MRI in AD

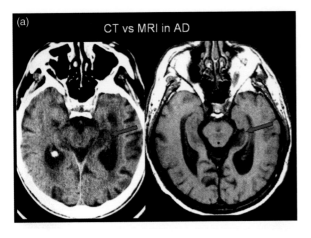

(b)

Longitudinal Hippocampal Atrophy
10-Year decline from NL to AD

NL   MCI   AD

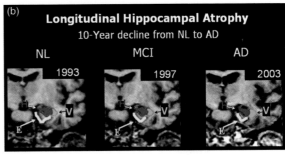

(c)

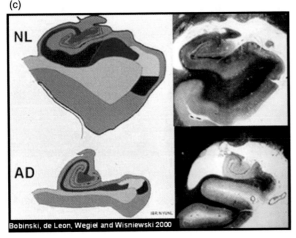

Figure 28.3 (a) Axial CT (left) and MRI (right) scans at the level of the hippocampus with arrow highlighting the hippocampal atrophy as defined by enlarged perihippocampal CSF spaces. (b) MRI scans of a elderly male subject who over the course of 10 years declined from normal cognition to MCI to a dementia diagnosed as AD. The scans highlight in red the hippocampal area, in yellow the entorhinal cortex, and in green the temporal horn of the lateral ventricle. (c) Histololgical validation of the hippocampal volume. Study depicts the regional vulnerability of the hippocampus proper in AD (bottom) vs. control (top). Colors depict the subfields of the hippocampus: central red the dentate gyrus, maroon the CA1, green, yellow and blue the subicular regions.

secondary to microvascular pathology and associated with hypertension and other vascular disease risk factors. Clinically, the UBOs of aging were associated with numerous treatable vascular disease risk factors.

Software advances

Advances in software engineering have further added to our understandings of vulnerable brain tissue and aided in appreciating the progression of AD-related changes. Historically, image registration combined with whole-brain data acquisitions and uniformity corrections led the way in interrogating cross-modality data sets. Structural imaging has been invaluable in

anatomically defining the regional tissue vulnerability and atrophy correction as estimated by FDG-PET (fluorodeoxyglucose positron emission tomography) and amyloid imaging (Li et al., 2008) and other tracers. Notable, and as reviewed by Apostolova and Thompson, are recent studies that show regional hippocampal formation atrophy rates are differentially increased in the presymptomatic phases of AD, thus enabling the detection of possible candidates for primary prevention study (Apostolova et al., 2010; Jack, Jr. et al., 2005; Rusinek et al., 2003). Also contributing to the discovery of brain regions vulnerable in early AD and in other neurodegenerative disorders and enhancing the discovery of functional networks are the voxel-wise image analysis

397

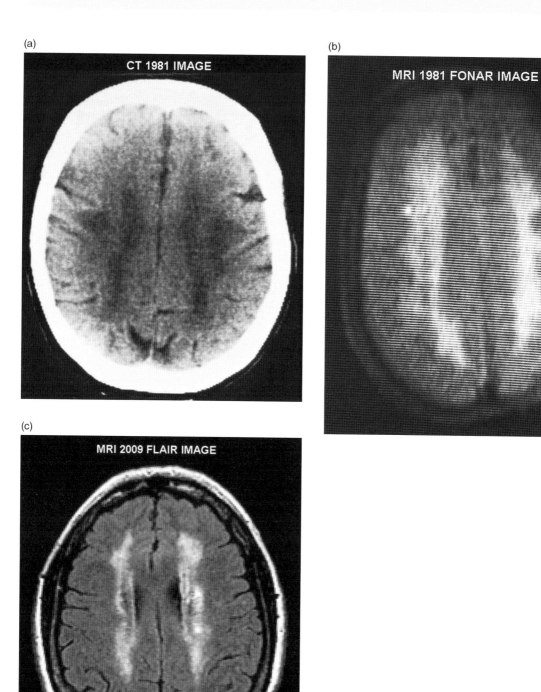

Figure 28.4 (a) WML on 1981 CT. (b) WML on first generation 1981 MRI T2 image. (c) 2009 MRI FLAIR image.

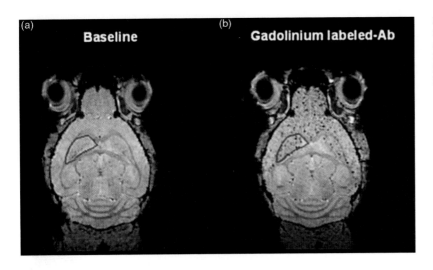

Figure 28.5 MR images from a Tg mouse at baseline and after injecting a gadolinium-labeled amyloid beta. Note the uptake of the tracer in many brain regions. The right hippocampus is outlined in red.

technologies, most notably Statistical Parametric Mapping (SPM) (Friston *et al.* 1995; see Taler and Saykin and de la Fuente-Fernández and Stoessel, this volume).

Pathology correlation and validation

Structural imaging owes a great debt to pathology for the contributions made to understanding the lesions and pathologic anatomy of AD. Over the past 35 years, pioneers such as Blessed, Scheibel, Glenner, Wisniewski, Iqbal, Terry, Braak and others have defined productive pathologic targets for imaging (de Leon, 2006). These studies revealed a topography of affected brain, ranging from the synapses, pyramidal neurons, and interacting glia affected, to the regional distribution and chemistry of the neurofibrillary tangle and the amyloid plaque. This pathological infrastructure continues to be fundamental to launching the structural (and molecular) imaging investigations that target the sites affected in the early stages of disease.

Although MRI imaging has yet to deliver a specific marker of AD pathology, MRI has provided sensitive characterizations of the effects of AD pathology and the promise of new MR contrast agents for identifying amyloid plaque pathology (Poduslo *et al.*, 2002; Sigurdsson *et al.*, 2008) (see Figure 28.5). In the chapters that preceded, we find ample evidence of how novel MRI acquisition modalities and analyses contribute to early diagnosis and to revealing the topography of AD changes. The MR spectroscopy approach is clearly of great interest with respect to improving the staging of brain damage and estimating the risk for the clinical expression of disease and for understanding treatment outcomes (Schuff, this volume). Today, MRI increasingly

contributes to guiding the neuropathology exam rather than exclusively using the post-mortem exam for validation. This new role has been enhanced with high-resolution imaging, an increasing number of novel acquisition protocols tuned to selective pathology, and modeling to describe brain damage (diffusion of water molecules in the white matter, estimations of blood flow based on endogenous oxygen-related tissue contrast, and tracer uptake and clearance).

Yet, an even greater calling is approaching: the revelation of disease mechanism. Here, too, MRI imaging in collaboration with pathology, physiology and biology has begun to make key contributions. Animal models for AD have used fMRI to demonstrate in-vivo the action of soluble β-amyloid (Aβ) in discrete brain areas (Luo *et al.*, 2008), thus enabling the first descriptions of the functional role of Aβ. In another of many examples, human studies show that early in the course of AD there are regional blood flow compensations following cognitive challenge that may underlie cognitive reserve and also identify regions at future risk (Sperling, 2007). These pursuits have moved MR imaging into the role of a primary player for revealing both general brain mechanisms and those that apply to AD and other diseases.

Clinical validation and biomarker correlation

MRI imaging readily lends itself to repeat examinations. It is widely understood that this approach is necessary for revealing correlates of disease progression and for clinical validation. In addition to predicting clinical changes and establishing rates of brain change, longitudinal examinations can also contribute to CSF biomarker development. In particular, several studies have shown that longitudinal measurement of MRI atrophy could statistically contribute to CSF biomarkers that are specific for tauopathy and amyloid pathology to improve the prediction of AD risk (Brys *et al.*, 2009). MRI has also been shown to be useful for correcting the progressive biomarker dilution of brain-derived biomarkers in the increasing CSF spaces characteristic of AD. Specifically, tau and other brain-derived biomarkers measured in the CSF do not show progression effects in spite of an increased topography of affected brain. Studies show that using MRI to correct for the increased CSF volume enables recognition of longitudinal CSF biomarker changes (de Leon *et al.*, 2002).

Standardized image acquisitions and data sharing

Recent large-scale multi-center studies are providing confirmation of MRI results that were previously based on smaller samples of patients. Data sharing is essential to identify clinically valid test measurements that can be collected reliably across sites with different MRI machines, levels of expertise, and time and financial commitment to research questions. In particular, the German Competence Network, the European Union Study and the Alzheimer's Disease Neuroimaging Initiative (ADNI) taking place in North America are good examples of multiple centers collaborating to create large MRI data sets using standardized acquisitions or standardized analyses. While most of the MRI protocols presented in this text were evaluated in single site studies (typically, measures are first studied where they are developed), the future looks bright for successful entry to the public domain of large imaging data sets, such as that provided by ADNI. While shared data sets cannot replace essential site-specific innovations, they will foster standardized and quality-controlled image acquisitions, contribute image analysis solutions for clinical trials and mechanism searches, and improve estimates of risk with translation to community settings.

The past 30 years of imaging in AD have contributed to a remarkable journey marked by a greatly increased understanding of the brain and affording hope to millions of sufferers of neurodegenerative diseases. Without doubt, the future will discover a wealth of new contributions and solutions leading to the prevention of AD. We are grateful to our colleagues at the NIH for their faithful support of this work: Neil Buckholtz, Marcelle Morrison-Bogorod, Tony Phelps, and Richard Hodes. God-speed to the pioneers we lost along the way: Alfred Wolf (PET), David Christman (PET), Jacob Cohen (Biostatistics), and Henryk Wisniewski (Neuropathology).

References

Apostolova L G, Mosconi L, Thompson P, *et al.* 2010. Subregional hippocampal atrophy predicts Alzheimer's dementia in cognitively normal subjects. *Neurobiol Aging* **31**, 1077–88.

Barron S A, Jacobs L and Kinkel W. 1976. Changes in size of normal lateral ventricles during aging determined by computerized tomography. *Neurology* **26**, 1011–3.

Bobinski M, de Leon M J, Wegiel J, *et al.* 2000. The histological validation of post mortem magnetic resonance imaging-determined hippocampal volume in Alzheimer's disease. *Neuroscience* **95**, 721–5.

Brys M, Pirraglia E, Rich K, *et al.* 2009. Prediction and longitudinal study of CSF biomarkers in mild cognitive impairment. *Neurobiol Aging* **30**, 682–90.

de Leon M J. 2006. Hippocampal imaging in the early diagnosis of AD, 1988 to 2006. In Jucker M, Beyreuther K, Haass C, Nitsch R M and Christen Y (Eds.), *Alzheimer: 100 Years and Beyond.* Berlin: Springer.

de Leon M J, Ferris S H, Blau I, *et al.* 1979. Correlations between computerised tomographic changes and behavioral deficits in senile dementia. *Lancet* **20**, 859–60.

de Leon M J, George A E, Stylopoulos L A, Smith G and Miller D C. 1989. Early marker for Alzheimer's disease: The atrophic hippocampus. *Lancet* **2**, 672–3.

de Leon M J, McRae T, Tsai J R, *et al.* 1988. Abnormal cortisol response in Alzheimer's disease linked to hippocampal atrophy. *Lancet* **2**, 391–2.

de Leon M J, Segal C Y, Tarshish C Y, *et al.* 2002. Longitudinal CSF tau load increases in mild cognitive impairment. *Neurosci Lett* **333**, 183–6.

Friston K J, Holmes A P, Worsley K J, *et al.* 1995. Statistical parametric maps in functional imaging: A general linear approach. *Hum Brain Mapp* **2**, 189–210.

George A E, de Leon M J, Gentes C I, *et al.* 1986a. Leukoencephalopathy in normal and pathologic aging: 1. CT of brain lucencies. *Am J Neuroradiol* **7**, 561–6.

George A E, de Leon M J, Kalnin A, Rosner L, Goodgold A and Chase N. 1986b. Leukoencephalopathy in normal and pathologic aging: 2. MRI and brain lucencies. *Am J Neuroradiol* **7**, 567–70.

Jack C R, Twomey C, Zinsmeister A, Sharbrough F, Petersen R and Cascino G. 1989. Anterior temporal lobes and hippocampal formations: Normative volumetric measurements from MR images in young adults. *Radiology* **172**, 549–54.

Jack C R Jr, Shiung M M, Weigand S D, *et al*. 2005. Brain atrophy rates predict subsequent clinical conversion in normal elderly and amnestic MCI. *Neurology* **65**, 1227–31.

Li Y, Rinne J O, Mosconi L, *et al*. 2008. Regional analysis of FDG and PIB-PET images in normal aging, mild cognitive impairment and Alzheimer's disease. *Eur J Nucl Med Mol Imag* **35**, 2169–81.

Luo F, Seifert T R, Edalji R, *et al*. 2008. Non-invasive characterization of [Beta]-Amyloid$_{1-40}$ vasoactivity by functional magnetic resonance imaging in mice. *Neuroscience* **155**, 263–9.

Poduslo J F, Wengenack T M, Curran G L, *et al*. 2002. Molecular targeting of Alzheimer's amyloid plaques for contrast-enhanced magnetic resonance imaging. *Neurobiol Dis* **11**, 315–29.

Rusinek H, De Santi S, Frid D, *et al*. 2003. Regional brain atrophy rate predicts future cognitive decline: 6-year longitudinal MR imaging study of normal aging. *Radiology* **229**, 691–6.

Sigurdsson E M, Wadghiri Y Z, Mosconi L, *et al*. 2008. A non-toxic ligand for voxel-based MRI analysis of plaques in AD transgenic mice. *Neurobiol Aging* **29**, 836–47.

Sperling R A. 2007. Functional MRI studies of associative encoding in normal aging, mild cognitive impairment, and Alzheimer's disease. *Ann NY Acad Sci* **1097**, 146–55.

Substance Abuse

29

Structural imaging of substance abuse

Sandra Chanraud, Anne Lise Pitel and Edith V. Sullivan

The availability of imaging tools has enhanced our appreciation of the effects of chronic and excessive alcohol exposure on the human brain. The specific localization of alcohol effects on the brain could further enhance our understanding of the behavioral, cognitive, and motor impairments associated with alcoholism. Cognitive impairments observed in alcohol dependents can limit a person's ability to sustain sobriety and re-establish normal life function. Indeed, impairment of executive control of behavior may well contribute directly to maintenance of addiction. Thus, assessment and acknowledgment of alcohol dependents' cognitive impairments and their neuroanatomical substrates could inform and direct treatment approaches.

Brain tissue shrinkage, reflected by ventricular and sulcal enlargement, has been reported widely from initial in-vivo imaging studies using computerized tomography (CT) to more recent work using magnetic resonance imaging (MRI) with evidence that these changes are progressive with continued alcohol use, and at least partly reversible with abstinence. In-vivo CT and MRI studies of alcoholism complement post-mortem neuropathological investigations in the search for structural brain abnormalities due to alcoholism, and each type of study has provided focus for the other in targeting structures to investigate (Sheedy *et al.*, 1999; Sullivan *et al.*, 1999).

Careful selection of MR sequence parameters for image data acquisition and semi- or automated methods for image data analysis increase the opportunity for precise identification and quantification of changes in central nervous system morphometry that can then be used to identify subtle changes in the brain. Within specific brain regions, changes in tissue characteristics may also be detectable in a longitudinal assessment. Here, we first review briefly the general principles of brain imaging and of images analyses as they pertain to the characterization of appropriate structural regions. Then, we review the literature on the effects of alcoholism on brain structure as revealed by brain imaging.

Alcoholism: definition and epidemiology

Alcohol use disorders are maladaptive patterns of alcohol consumption that include alcohol abuse and dependence (American Psychiatric Association, 1994) and are associated with domestic violence, economic cost and loss of productivity. According to the DSM IV (First *et al.*, 1998), alcohol abuse is defined as repeated use despite recurrent adverse consequences. It causes clinically significant distress or impairment of social or occupational functioning, as manifested by failure to fulfill major role obligations, repeated exposure hazards, getting into legal difficulties, and developing social and interpersonal problems. Alcohol dependence is considered as alcohol abuse combined with tolerance, withdrawal, and an uncontrollable drive to drink. Alcohol dependents neglect activities, spend inordinate amounts of time drinking or recovering from drinking, and continue consuming alcohol despite alcohol-related physiological or physical problems. According to the National Epidemiologic Survey on Alcohol and Related Conditions (NESARC), a nationwide survey of more than 43 000 adults conducted from 2001 to 2002, 66% of people with alcohol dependence also meet the criteria for alcohol abuse (Hasin *et al.*, 2007). Symptoms of alcohol dependence typically progress from abuse to

Understanding Neuropsychiatric Disorders, ed. M. E. Shenton and B. I. Turetsky. Published by Cambridge University Press.
© Cambridge University Press 2011.

impaired control, to tolerance, and finally, to physio-logical and psychological dependence.

Alcohol dependence is a highly prevalent mental disorder, affecting people of all ages and socioeconomic groups. Alcoholism affects almost three times as many men as women and is particularly common in young adults. Despite its high prevalence, the available data suggest that alcohol dependence and abuse are underdiagnosed. Treatments are available that can assist the patient in attaining abstinence and improve aspects of health that may have been damaged by chronic alcohol intake, but these will likely not reach the patient unless the initial diagnosis is made (Cargiulo, 2007). Only 24.1% of those with alcohol dependence are treated, slightly less than the treatment rate found in 1997 (Hasin *et al.*, 2007). In the year 2000, alcohol consumption was responsible for 85 000 deaths or 3.5% of all deaths in the United States (Cargiulo, 2007). Some of these deaths were attributed to the acute effects of excessive alcohol consumption (injuries and alcohol-related accidents), but many more were attributed to the insidious effects of alcohol abuse and dependence. Indeed, chronic heavy drinking is associated with high risk of developing acute and chronic physical and mental health problems, including cardiovascular disease, central and peripheral neurological impairment, hepatic disease, cancer, fetal alcohol disorders, and psychiatric disorders associated with increased risk of suicide. Significant morbidity and mortality are associated with alcohol dependence, and almost 19 million Americans require treatment for an "alcohol problem". However, only 2.4 million have been diagnosed and just 139 000 receive medication to treat it (To and Vega, 2006). Alcohol treatment usually involves therapy in addition to medication that helps reduce craving. Alcoholism clinicians have access nowadays to a wide range of treatment options for their patients (http://pubs.niaaa.nih.gov/publications/aa49.htm). Some of these treatments, such as 12-step self-help programs (e.g. Alcoholics Anonymous), have been used for decades. Others, including brief intervention (five or fewer standard office visits) and various therapies borrowed from other fields, such as motivational enhancement therapy and couples therapy, are newer concepts that have been shown to be effective in reducing the risk for alcohol-related problems (Cisler *et al.*, 1998; Miller *et al.*, 1999).

Basics of structural and diffusion imaging

Computerized tomography

Originally called computed axial tomography because of its required plane of acquisition, CT scanning is a non-invasive method to image bone and tissue and can provide high-resolution ($\approx$1 mm) information on brain structure in three-dimensional space. Although CT is often used instead of structural MRI in clinical settings because of its lower cost, it poses a risk of radiation because it uses X-rays. The information matrix obtained by CT scanning permits the reconstruction of an image in which skull boundaries, the distribution of cerebrospinal fluid (CSF), and some differentiation between healthy and diseased tissue can be discerned.

However, gray matter and white matter are relatively isointense, rendering CT studies poorly able to distinguish whether expansion of CSF spaces deep in the brain (ventricles) and over its surface (sulci) is due to volume or quality changes in white matter, gray matter, or both. In addition, some of the principal lesion sites associated with Wernicke's encephalopathy, for example, the mammillary bodies are difficult to assess quantitatively on CT scans because they are obscured by artifacts from surrounding bone structures and are not visualized optimally in the axial plane. Although the amount of CSF in the third ventricle has been used as an indirect measure of diencephalic lesions (Shimamura *et al.*, 1988), more direct and quantitative assessment of the tissue itself is essential for determining loci of alcoholism's effect on brain structures. The cerebellum is another site often affected by alcoholism that cannot be optimally viewed with CT. An additional limitation of CT is the exposure of the patient to radiation, which makes it difficult for use in longitudinal studies. The application of nuclear magnetic resonance, which is free of ionizing radiation, has provided opportunities to examine brain structures in living persons repeatedly and to do so with high resolution and improved tissue differentiation.

Magnetic resonance imaging

The nuclei of certain atoms exhibit nuclear magnetic resonance (NMR). That is, when they are exposed to a strong magnetic field, they behave like small, spinning magnets and align themselves within the field. Each type of nucleus spins at its own particular rate (the resonant frequency), which is determined by the strength of the magnetic field. If the nuclei are bombarded with radio waves (energy similar to radio and television signals) at the frequency at which they are spinning, they absorb this energy, and their alignment in the magnetic field is disturbed. When the radio waves are turned off, the transverse vector component produces an oscillating magnetic field, which induces a small current in the receiver coil. This signal is called the free induction decay (FID). In MRI, the static magnetic field can be varied across the body (a field gradient), so that different spatial locations become associated with different precession frequencies. Application of the field gradient destroys the FID signal, but this can be recovered and measured by a refocusing gradient (to create a so-called "gradient echo"), or by a radio frequency pulse (to create a so-called "spin-echo").

The magnetic resonance image is determined primarily by three variables: proton density, T1, and T2. Proton density reflects the number of hydrogen nuclei stimulated. T1 is an exponential time constant that describes the return of the nuclei to equilibrium and realignment with the magnetic field. Higher T1 values mean it takes nuclei longer to return to realignment after perturbation. T2 is the exponential time constant describing signal loss due to interference between hydrogen nuclei. The T1 and T2 tend to reflect proportion of free water to bound water in a tissue; the biological significance of these variables is not yet fully understood.

Proton density, T1, and T2 differ in biological tissues, and this provides the subtle gradations by which details of brain structure can be perceived. A great deal of flexibility is available in designing MRI examinations. In addition to the flexibility in highlighting tissue differences, MRI offers great flexibility in the direction in which the brain is viewed. During scanning, magnetic gradients can be applied in the three (orthogonal) directions, or planes, to provide information about the spatial location of the signals in that plane. This allows the brain and particular structures within it to be viewed, not only from bottom to top (axial), as in conventional CT images, but also from front to back (coronal), from left to right (sagittal), or at any oblique angle to these planes. This flexibility also enables greater accuracy in aligning images with internal landmarks, an essential consideration for ensuring consistency of data

from repeat scans on the same person (Rohlfing et al., 2006).

Diffusion imaging and tracking fibers

Brain functions are emergent properties of interacting brain areas within networks. In contrast with "functional segregation" which aims to localize functions to specific brain areas, "functional integration" describes function in terms of the flow of information between brain areas. The brain is composed of numerous functional networks of interconnected areas, through which information is transferred and transformed. On an anatomical level, functional networks communicate through white matter fibers that are orderly structures.

In the context of diffusion-weighted MRI (Basser, 1995), diffusion describes the stochastic movement of molecules in liquids, called Brownian molecular motion. In unconstrained media, this movement is isotropic, i.e. it can be described by the same Gaussian probability distribution across all spatial directions.

In biological tissue, such as the cerebral white matter, however, the molecular motion of water molecules is restricted by the cellular microstructure. Diffusion barriers, such as the neuronal membrane, myelin sheathes and intra-axonal transport, determine a preferred spatial orientation of the molecular movement. This orientation of diffusion is called anisotropy (Basser, 1995). Diffusion tensor imaging (DTI) is based on this nature of diffusion that can be described mathematically by a tensor and represented as an ellipsoid. The directions of the main axes of the ellipsoid (in the MR scanner's coordinate system) are given by the eigenvectors ($\varepsilon1$, $\varepsilon2$, $\varepsilon3$) with their lengths representing the eigenvalues ($\lambda1$, $\lambda2$, $\lambda3$) of the diffusion tensor. The largest eigenvalue ($\lambda1$) corresponds to the principal eigenvector $\varepsilon1$, which represents the main diffusion direction within the voxel. Commonly used measures of diffusion include fractional anisotropy (FA), which is an estimate of the fraction of the diffusion attributed to anisotropy and ranges between 0 (isotropy) and 1 (diffusion hypothetically only in a single orientation). Another measure that has been used to compare different voxels in terms of diffusion is intervoxel coherence, which quantifies the degree of diffusion collinearity between adjacent voxels (Pfefferbaum et al., 2006a). Measures of diffusivity, such as mean diffusivity (MD) or apparent diffusion coefficient (ADC) and trace of

405

the diffusion tensor (Tr) (all closely related to each other), can also be used to quantify the overall diffusion in a particular voxel or region. However, the ADC does not assess the orientation of molecular movement. Therefore, differences in FA, MD or ADC could reflect differences either in orientation, coherence, or number of fiber tracts.

Methods of brain exploration

A number of studies have tracked anatomical changes in the same group of alcohol dependents over several years, providing *longitudinal* data on the effects of alcohol. *Cross-sectional* studies have investigated anatomical differences between groups of alcohol-dependent subjects and groups of controls of the same age providing data on differences in regional volume or shape.

Studies of changes in brain structure related to alcohol consumption have typically been of two types. Some have been largely quantitative, commonly using measurements calculated from 3D T1-weighted images. Others have been qualitative, comparing high-resolution images of a specific region of interest and neuronal populations.

Generalized differences in cerebral cortical volume were best-appreciated using fully quantitative volumetrics (Chanraud *et al.*, 2007; Cardenas *et al.*, 2007; Rohlfing *et al.*, 2006), whereas more specific damage to small structures, such as the mammillary bodies, or subregions of larger structures, such as the cerebellum and thalamus, can best be appreciated by utilizing a variety of MR sequences and qualitative techniques of measurement (Pearlson and Calhoun, 2007).

Regions of interest

Manual delineation of brain regions of interest (ROI) is the current gold standard for morphometry and anatomical validity. ROI methodology typically involves development of reliable and valid anatomic landmarks, rater training, and inter-rater reliability. Despite its strength, it also has limitations: it is time-consuming and labor-intensive, especially when comparing several brain regions in large groups of subjects. Manually delineated ROIs are also subject to inaccuracy because local individual neuroanatomy can be marked by substantial inter-subject variability, especially in diseased population. The hypothesis-based nature of the ROI method restricts assessment to pre-specified regions. Until recently, most structural MRI brain studies were confined to relatively straightforward ROI-based measurement of brain regions and remains essential for quantification of small structures, such as the mammillary bodies.

Automated data-driven methods

To overcome the laborious nature of manual volumetric methods, automated methods have been developed to determine differences between groups and changes over time in brain structure using hypothesis- and rater-independent approaches. One of the best-established methods is the automated measurement of the whole-brain volume over time, which is already being used as a secondary end point in clinical treatment trials (Kinkingnehun *et al.*, 2008). However, the heuristic value of this method is limited, as only global effects can be recorded without providing information about regionally differentiated effects.

Voxel-based morphometry

Whole-brain analyses such as VBM (Mechelli *et al.*, 2005) has grown in popularity because of its ease of use. VBM and optimized VBM are fully automated measurement methods for examination of structural MR images of the whole brain by voxel-wise comparison of the relative local densities (Sowell *et al.*, 2001) or volumes (Maguire *et al.*, 2000) of brain tissue between two groups of subjects. By giving equal weight to every voxel included in the 3D sampling array, VBM provides an unbiased measure of highly localized regions that might not be examined in hypothesis-based ROI studies, and thus provides a multiple regional comparison. Conceptually, VBM tests for residual tissue density differences remaining after spatial normalization of MRI scans into standardized stereotaxic space. Owing to the nature of this normalization procedure (Ashburner and Friston, 2000), VBM analyses are less sensitive to shape differences and thus may exhibit high reliability at the expense of validity. VBM results can be modulated to account for the variable shape changes in nonlinear normalization and thus preserve the volume of the particular tissue within a voxel. The normalization procedures employed in VBM, although highly reliable because they are automated, make the process less sensitive to group differences in shape or gray–white matter differentiation, and are prone to errors caused by misregistration of anatomical structures.

The method has been updated and optimized (Good et al., 2001) to reduce errors arising from systematic differences in head shape, variations in segmentation, and inconsistent brain stripping as well as errors introduced by spatial normalization. Recently, a VBM study in alcohol dependent subjects, performed using images segmented from non-brain tissue as inputs, resulted in an increased sensitivity for detecting alcohol-related effects (Fein et al., 2006). VBM and ROI methods provide different types of information, and they should therefore be used in tandem, with automated VBM being used to generate hypotheses by identifying areas that can be subsequently be more thoroughly investigated with ROI-based approaches.

Deformation-based morphometry (DBM)

Whereas VBM transforms brain images into a standard space to compensate for global differences but preserves local differences in cortical gray matter distribution, DBM (Gaser et al., 2001) transforms the brain volumes at high resolution to a standard template to eliminate the anatomical differences between the brains. The anatomical information then is not in the MRI images themselves, but in the deformation fields that are required to transform the patient's brain into a standard brain. These deformation fields offer a multivariate vector field of localization information from which regional volume effects can be extrapolated. This method allows searching the entire brain for significant changes, and has been shown to permit longitudinal studies that distinguish between volume differences and volume changes in morphometric analyses of alcohol-dependent subjects (Rohlfing et al., 2006).

Methods of exploration of diffusion-weighted images

Different approaches can be applied to study differences in regional brain anisotropy between subjects. Some studies have used voxel-based approaches (VBA) (Bruno et al., 2008), where data sets from subjects belonging to one diagnostic group have been processed with reference to a specific metric (e.g. FA), normalized to a standard anatomical template, combined and averaged, before being compared to similarly processed data sets from another group. Other studies (Schulte et al., 2005) have used an ROI approach, where ROIs are placed in regions of the brain

thought to be implicated in a particular condition and are compared in terms of an averaged measure of a specific metric between different groups of subjects. Using the multivariate information of diffusion tensors, in-vivo fiber tracking can be performed. This allows reconstructing the fiber tracts originating from selected white matter areas based on individual diffusion-weighted images. Tractography allows segmentation and visualization of putative fiber tracts crossing one or more brain regions, along with measurement of various characteristics over the tract so defined, such as average FA, or average length of the tract. The tract structure can be appreciated and the trajectory can be followed over many slices (Mori and van Zijl, 2002). DTI is well adapted for a general description at a microstructural level of subcortical white matter architecture in the human brain. Unlike anatomical imaging, DTI tractography facilitates the comparison of specific and identified neuronal circuits.

Macrostructural abnormalities in alcoholism

CT findings

The first CT investigations in repeated series from Canada, Sweden, Germany, and England reported convergent findings by showing diffuse abnormalities in the form of ventricular-enlargement and sulcal widening (Carlen et al., 1978; Bergman et al., 1980; Ron et al., 1982; Schroth et al., 1985) in alcoholism. CT studies of healthy subjects spanning the age range demonstrated a considerable shrinkage of tissue complemented with expansion of CSF-filled spaces in the brain associated with aging (Pfefferbaum et al., 1986; Stafford et al., 1988), indicating the need to take normal age-related brain changes into account in investigations of alcoholism and other conditions affecting the brain. Following the method of Pfefferbaum et al. (1986), and later modified (Pfefferbaum et al., 1993) to account for normal variation in intracranial volume (Mathalon et al., 1993), age norms for each CT measure were calculated from healthy subjects and CT measures of alcoholics were then expressed as deviations from age norms. This approach allows determination of the magnitude of tissue shrinkage or sulcal or ventricular expansion for a single individual or a group of patients and to compare different pathological groups with each other.

Several studies of alcoholic patients have reported increases in the size of the lateral ventricles and

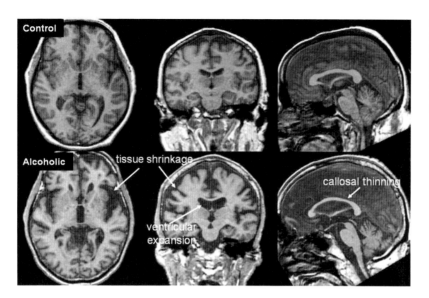

Figure 29.1 MRI scans from a 53-year-old control man (upper) and a 53-year-old alcoholic man (lower) from axial (left), coronal (right) and sagittal (right) views (from Rosenbloom and Pfefferbaum, 2008). Tissue shrinkage, ventricular expansion and corpus callosum thinning are particularly noticeable.

cortical sulci (Lishman *et al.*, 1987; Jernigan *et al.*, 1982). After adjusting for age norms, Pfefferbaum's group found that older alcoholics have more brain shrinkage for their age than do younger alcoholics. The ventricular enlargement revealed in these subjects was related to lifetime alcohol consumption (Pfefferbaum *et al.*, 1988). Not all investigators have been able to demonstrate such a relationship, and some have reported a surprising lack of association between amount of alcohol consumed and amount of cortical shrinkage (for review, see Lishman, 1990).

MRI findings

Since 1981, when Besson *et al.* reported shorter brain T1s in both gray and white matter in intoxicated alcoholics, which lengthened during withdrawal and abstinence (1–6 weeks), several longitudinal studies have reported conflicting results. These studies examined alcoholics at different intervals since last drink, and many had limited control data (Besson *et al.*, 1981, 1989; Schroth *et al.*, 1988; Smith *et al.*, 1985). Chick *et al.* (1989) found longer T1s in the alcoholics measured 2 weeks postwithdrawal, whereas Agartz *et al.* (1991), in a study of comparable design but using a lower field instrument, found no differences in T1 or T2 between alcoholics and controls. Both studies found correlations between volume deficits and T1 (Mander *et al.*, 1989), suggesting that partial voluming (some CSF present in what appears to be a tissue voxel) may contribute to the increased T1 seen in alcoholics.

Cross-sectional MRI studies of chronically alcohol-dependent subjects, without obvious complications from nutritional deficiencies or hepatic disorders, demonstrated cortical and cerebellar shrinkage relative to the controls (Wang *et al.*, 1993; Hayakawa *et al.*, 1992; Shear *et al.*, 1994). Specific brain regions affected by chronic alcohol exposure include cortical gray and white matter (Jernigan *et al.*, 1991; Pfefferbaum *et al.*, 1992), particularly prefrontal areas in older alcoholic individuals (Pfefferbaum *et al.*, 1997; Cardenas *et al.*, 2007), mammillary bodies (Shear *et al.*, 1996; Sullivan *et al.*, 1999), anterior hippocampus (Agartz *et al.*, 1999; Sullivan *et al.*, 1995), thalamus (De Bellis *et al.*, 2005; Sullivan, 2003; Chanraud *et al.*, 2007), pons (Pfefferbaum *et al.*, 2002; Sullivan, 2003; Chanraud *et al.*, 2008), and cerebellum (De Bellis *et al.*, 2005; Sullivan *et al.*, 2000a, 2000c) (Figure 29.1).

MRI: regional specificity
Does brain tissue shrinkage equally involve gray and white matter?

There is pathological evidence showing that alcoholism damages both gray and white matter (Jensen and Pakkenberg, 1993; Kril *et al.*, 1997; Harper, 1998) with the mainstay of cortical loss in the frontal lobes. However, neuropathological studies agree that the reduction in alcoholics' brain weight is largely due to reduction in the white matter volume rather than in the gray matter volume (Harper, 1998). Interestingly, results from a more recent study suggest that some white matter brain regions, e.g. splenium, have greater sensitivity to alcohol-induced damage through different molecular mechanisms (Kashem et al., 2008), due to distinct interaction with the heterogeneous distribution of proteins depending on the nature of the axons. Apparent atrophy of the cerebral cortex, mostly represented by widening of the cortical sulci and narrowing of the gyri in alcoholics, is also reported by the neuropathological studies. This could be explained by white matter shrinkage (Harper, 1998). At a microscopic level, Courville (1955) and later Harper et al. (1987) published quantitative studies documenting neuronal loss in alcoholics. They revealed a reduction of 22% in the number of neurons, and this loss was specifically localized in the superior frontal cortex because no differences were found in other brain regions explored (i.e. motor, cingulate, and inferior temporal cortices). Using a semi-automated procedure to segment brain tissue into gray matter, white matter, and CSF, Pfefferbaum et al. (1992) reported a significant shrinkage of both gray and white matter volume and an increase of CSF-filled spaces. Later, these same investigators studied cortical gray matter volumes extracted from high-resolution T1-weighted MR images in younger and older chronic alcoholics. They found that cortical gray and white matter volumes in prefrontal regions were significantly smaller in younger alcoholics compared with age-matched controls (Pfefferbaum et al., 1997). More recently, VBM studies have confirmed widespread damage in both gray matter and white matter (Jang et al., 2007), with more significant alterations of gray matter in focal regions such as the frontal cortex, the thalamus, the insular cortex, the dorsal hippocampus and the cerebellum and more significant alterations of white matter in periventricular area, pons and cerebellar peduncles (Chanraud et al., 2007; Mechtcheriakov et al., 2007). Gray matter alterations localized to the frontal and temporal lobes have been reported using DBM method (Cardenas et al., 2007). White matter volume deficits in temporal lobe seem to be particularly present in patients with a history of seizure (Sullivan et al., 1996).

Subcortical gray matter

- Striatum

Using a sensitive method of volume estimation for post-mortem specimens, Kril et al. (1997) were unable to show any change in the volumes of the caudate or of

the putamen. By contrast, MRI studies have revealed smaller volumes of caudate and putamen in alcoholics than in controls, regardless of length of sobriety (Jernigan et al., 1991; Sullivan et al., 2005a). In the more recent study, the nucleus accumbens was shown to have greater volume shrinkage in more recent than longer sober alcoholics (Sullivan et al., 2005a).

- Insula

Both shape analysis of the perisylvian region in both hemispheres (Jang et al., 2007; Makris et al., 2008) and VBM studies (Chanraud et al., 2007) have revealed shape or volume differences in the insula of alcoholics compared with controls. Shape deformations revealed by Jang et al. (2007) were localized mainly in the central part of the insula in both hemispheres, with a greater difference in the right than in the left hemisphere. In healthy subjects, the surface of left insula is more convex than the right one. Thus, normal left–right insula asymmetry observed in healthy subjects is reduced in alcoholics.

- Hippocampus

An early experimental rodent model of alcohol toxicity showed that neurons in the hippocampal formation brain region are selectively damaged by alcohol (Walker et al., 1980). However, in humans, glial cell loss (Korbo, 1999) and neuronal dysmorphology (Harding et al., 1997) rather than neuronal loss have been reported in hippocampus. Structural neuroimaging studies have also demonstrated hippocampal volume deficit in alcoholics (Agartz et al., 1999; Laakso et al., 2000; Wilhelm et al., 2008; Sullivan et al., 1995; Kurth et al., 2004). The hippocampal volume shrinkage has been attributed to pathological changes in white matter (decrease in axonal diameter and loss of white matter) (Harding et al., 1997), but the incorporation of newly formed neurons to the dentate gyrus could also be affected by alcohol (He et al., 2005; Nixon and Crews, 2004).

One MRI study measured hippocampus volume in late-onset alcoholics (Type I) and violent, early-onset alcoholics (Type II) compared with non-alcoholic controls (Laakso et al., 2000). The right but not left hippocampus was significantly smaller in both alcoholic groups. Despite the absence of age-related decline in hippocampal volumes in the control subjects, consistent with other reports (Sullivan et al., 2005b), alcoholics with Type I showed a tendency toward decreased volumes with age, confirming earlier

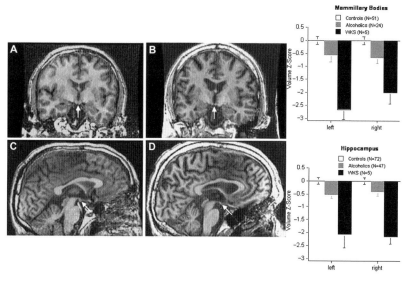

Figure 29.2 T1-weighted Spoiled echo (SPGR) images of a 59-year-old healthy man (left panel) and a 53-year-old man with Korsakoff syndrome (from Rosenbloom and Pfefferbaum, 2008). Note the shrunken mammillary bodies (arrows) in the alcoholic Korsakoff man (B and D) compared with the control (A and C). Mean ± SD of volumes of mammillary bodies and hippocampus are represented in the right side. All volumes are expresses as standardized Z-scores, adjusted for normal variation in intracranial volume and age. The expected value of the controls is 0 (SD = 1) (from Sullivan and Pfefferbaum, 2009).

reports (Sullivan *et al.*, 1995), and also with the duration of alcoholism. A later study reported volume deficits in alcoholics compared with non-alcoholic controls, with left hippocampal volume reduction being slightly greater than on the right (Beresford *et al.*, 2006). Another association was revealed between hippocampal volume and the type of alcoholic beverage consumed, a stronger negative correlation being found in subjects consuming wine and spirits than in subjects consuming beer (Wilhelm *et al.*, 2008). The effects of the different types of alcoholic beverage on hippocampus may be accounted by homocysteine-mediated excitotoxicity. Indeed, homocysteine is a mediator of excitotoxicity and neurotoxicity via overstimulation of N-methyl-D-aspartate (NMDA) receptors (Lipton *et al.*, 1997) and its plasma concentration is dependent on both the type of beverage and amount of alcohol consumed (Bleich *et al.*, 2000). Therefore, these findings suggest that homocysteine-mediated excitotoxicity could be an important pathophysiological mechanism in alcohol-related hippocampus damage. Finally, deficits in alcoholics' hippocampal volume do not seem to be related to seizures (which are usually generalized rather than focal) occurring during first-onset withdrawal (Bleich *et al.*, 2003) or more chronically (Sullivan *et al.*, 1996).

- Mammillary bodies

Atrophic change in the mammillary bodies is a cardinal feature of Wernicke's encephalopathy. Exploration of this brain structure has revealed smaller volumes in amnesic as well as in non-amnesic alcoholics (Sullivan *et al.*, 1999). Therefore, visualizable mammillary body damage does not seem to be necessary for the development of amnesia in alcoholic subjects (Shear *et al.*, 1996).

- Hippocampus vs. mammillary bodies in alcoholics vs. Korsakoff syndrome (KS)

Brain structural volume deficits in the hippocampus and mammillary bodies show a graded effect from uncomplicated alcoholics to alcoholic Korsakoff patients. Sullivan and Pfefferbaum (2009) compared these two groups of alcoholics using manual volumetric quantification of several brain structures. Regional brain volumes were adjusted for normal variation in intracranial volume and age and expressed as standardized Z-scores, where the expected mean of the controls was 0 and standard deviation was 1. Results indicated graded regional brain volume shrinkage, where deficits of uncomplicated alcoholics were significant (generally about 0.5 standard deviation deficit), but less severe than those of KS (about 1–2 standard deviation deficit), notably in the mammillary bodies and hippocampus. Contrary to Squire *et al.* (1990), who reported spared hippocampus but barely detectable mammillary bodies in KS alcoholics, these recent findings suggest that hippocampus volume is as much impaired as mammillary bodies in both uncomplicated and amnesic alcoholics (Figure 29.2), the hippocampus alteration being twice as large as in KS than in uncomplicated alcoholics (Sullivan and Marsh, 2003).

- Brain reward system

Whereas Kril *et al.* (1997) found volume deficits in the amygdala only of alcoholics with KS, Alvarez *et al.* reported a neuronal density reduction in the amygdaloid complex in alcoholics of all ages (Alvarez *et al.*, 1989). Using a modified version of VBM, Fein *et al.* (2006) specifically examined the amygdala in abstinent alcoholics who demonstrate impairment on a simulated gambling task that requires unaltered amygdala and ventromedial prefrontal regions for intact performance. Compared with controls, abstinent alcoholics had significantly less gray matter density in the amygdala. The authors were cautious in attributing this dysmorphology to alcoholism per se, and offered an alternative explanation that the structural abnormality predated alcoholism. Given the amygdala's role in emotional regulation and behavioral control (for review, see McBride, 2002), premorbid deficits in these functions could put individuals at heightened risk for developing alcohol use disorders (Clark *et al.*, 2008; Kamarajan *et al.*, 2006). In additon to being smaller, the amygdala was negatively associated with both alcohol craving and probability of relapse within 6 months following detoxification (Wrase *et al.*, 2008). Another morphometric analysis of brain reward system revealed lower total reward-network volume in alcoholic subjects (Makris *et al.*, 2008). Specifically, notable volume deficits were found in right dorsolateral prefrontal cortex, right anterior insula, and right nucleus accumbens and in left amygdala. Such damage in the brain reward system could predate the onset of alcoholism, result from chronic drinking, or represent an interaction of both possibilities.

- Brainstem

The brainstem is considered critical in development and maintenance of drug dependence (for review, see Koob, 2008). The dorsal and median raphe nuclei, a major source of serotoninergic axons in the brain, have been a focus of investigation ever since the disruptive effects of alcohol on neurotransmission were first described (Balldin *et al.*, 1994). Whereas neuronal counts showed no significant difference in uncomplicated alcoholics, the functionality of these axons was disrupted (Baker *et al.*, 1996). Brain regions that are part of the brainstem have been observed by MRI to be altered in alcoholic men (Sullivan, 2003; Bloomer *et al.*, 2004) and women (Pfefferbaum *et al.*, 2002). More recently, these findings were confirmed

for the pons volume with an ROI approach. Indeed, whereas the midbrain volume did not differ between alcoholics and controls, the volume of the pons was smaller in alcoholics than controls (Chanraud *et al.*, 2008).

- Cerebellum

Neuronal loss occurs in the cerebellum of alcoholics (for review, see Cavanagh *et al.*, 1997). This effect was noted by post-mortem studies of Purkinje cells in the superior vermis (Victor *et al.*, 1959; Torvik and Torp, 1986), in the small rostral and caudate lobes (Phillips *et al.*, 1987), and in the anterior folia of the vermis (Baker *et al.*, 1999). Quantitatively, two large autopsy studies revealed cerebellar atrophy in 26.8–27.6%, of all examined alcoholics (Lindboe and Loberg, 1988; Torvik *et al.*, 1982). Vermal white matter volume is also significantly smaller in alcoholics than non-alcoholic controls (Baker *et al.*, 1999). Different cell types of the cerebellum appear to be differentially susceptible to alcohol-related damage. The Purkinje cells are the most vulnerable and global reductions in Purkinje cell numbers (Phillips *et al.*, 1987), and densities (Andersen 2004; Ferrer *et al.*, 1984; Victor *et al.*, 1959) are commonly observed in the cerebellum of alcoholics.

Cerebellar atrophy as revealed by CT has been reported in a high percentage of alcoholics (Diener *et al.*, 1986; Melgaard and Ahlgren, 1986). More recent MRI studies have revealed gross vermian volume deficit in 33% of chronic alcoholics without KS or Wernicke's encephalopathy (Antunez *et al.*, 1998), both in gray and white matter volumes (Shear *et al.*, 1996; Sullivan, 2003). This is of particular interest given recent data showing the importance of the cerebellum in the organization of higher order cerebral functions (Sullivan *et al.*, 2003; Schmahmann, 2004).

White matter volume

- Corpus callosum

Thinning of the corpus callosum occurs in uncomplicated alcoholics and is more prominent in the anterior rather than posterior regions (Pfefferbaum *et al.*, 1996; Estruch *et al.*, 1997). In addition to macrostructural shrinkage observed in alcoholic women with MRI (Hommer *et al.*, 1996), DTI studies have revealed evidence for microstructural degradation, which is compounded by age (Pfefferbaum and Sullivan, 2005; Pfefferbaum *et al.*,

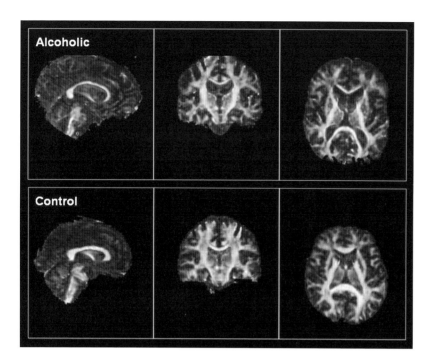

Figure 29.3 Images from sagittal (left), coronal (left) and axial (left) views of a 57-year-old alcoholic man (upper panel) and a 54-year-old control man (lower panel) displaying values for FA and illustrating clearly the white matter architecture of the brain (from Rosenbloom and Pfefferbaum, 2008). Note the robust appearing white matter structures in the control compared with the alcoholic.

2006a). Severe callosal thinning is a marker of Marchiafava–Bignami disease, possibly caused by nutritional deficiency and resulting in severe demyelination and necrosis (Victor *et al.*, 1989). As with Wernicke encephalopathy and Korsakoff syndrome, the reflection of Marchiafava–Bignami disease in alcohol-related callosal damage raises the possibility of a continuum of graded brain dysmorphology associated with chronic alcoholism (Sullivan and Pfefferbaum, 2009).

MR diffusion tensor imaging in alcoholism

Recent developments in neuroimaging have motivated examination of neural circuits. In part, this trend follows system-based hypotheses of mental illnesses proposing that disruption of the circuits (Sullivan *et al.*, 2003; Andreasen *et al.*, 1996) linking "effectively connected" structures produces behavioral manifestations of target disorders. Passingham *et al.* (2002) proposed the concept of a "connectional fingerprint", whereby the function of a cortical area is determined by its extrinsic connections and its intrinsic properties. This conceptualization suggests that functional connectivity has an anatomical basis and that anatomical information is a critical component for distinguishing patterns of brain functional connectivity.

Features of this model can be tested with neuroimaging, and choice of neuroimaging modality determines the level of analysis to test the hypothesis proposed.

When used to study white matter structure (and thus brain *anatomical* connectivity) in alcoholics, DTI has revealed microstructural damage related to alcoholism and in interaction with age in cerebral areas that appear intact from analyses of structural MRI (Pfefferbaum and Sullivan, 2002; Sullivan and Pfefferbaum, 2003) (Figure 29.3). Prior studies have shown widespread FA deficits in both hemispheres (Pfefferbaum *et al.*, 2006b), as well as white matter tract damage in alcoholic subjects in the genu and splenium of the corpus callosum, the centrum semiovale (Pfefferbaum and Sullivan, 2002, 2005; Pfefferbaum *et al.*, 2000), corticopontine bundles (Chanraud *et al.*, 2008), and right frontolimbic connections (Harris *et al.*, 2008).

The association of localized and remote gray matter regional alterations with alterations in brain white matter raises the possibility that damage in alcoholism has a predilection to specific anatomical circuits and thus specific functional networks. Dysfunction of the brain circuitry may account, at least in part, for neuropsychological deficits and their typical pattern in alcohol dependent individuals.

Factors contributing to the heterogeneity of brain damage

Even though ethanol is an agent with apparent direct toxic effects on neurons (Riley and Walker, 1978; McMullen *et al.*, 1984), possibly because of its non-oxidative metabolism to fatty acid ethyl esters within cells (Charness, 1993), the question of its direct, indirect or compounded effects on brain is still a matter of debate. Indeed, the consumption of ethanol is also indirectly associated with a variety of other factors influencing brain morphometry.

Thiamine

A deficiency in the essential nutrient thiamine resulting from chronic alcohol consumption is one factor underlying alcohol-induced brain damage. A reduction in thiamine can interfere with numerous cellular functions, leading to serious brain disorders, including KS subjects. Chronic alcohol consumption can result in thiamine deficiency by causing inadequate nutritional thiamine intake, decreased absorption of thiamine from the gastrointestinal tract, and impaired thiamine utilization in the cells (for review, see Martin *et al.*, 2003). However, people differ in their susceptibility to thiamine deficiency, and different brain regions also may be more or less sensitive to this condition. Various brain regions and even different cell types within one brain region may differ in their sensitivity to alcohol-induced damage as well as in their susceptibility to associated problems, including alcohol-related malnutrition (e.g. thiamine deficiency). For example, human post-mortem studies have found that the anterior superior cerebellar vermis most frequently exhibits alcohol-induced damage (Baker *et al.*, 1999; Victor *et al.*, 1959). Additional studies have found that thiamine deficiency contributes to a reduction in the number and size of a certain cerebellar cell type called Purkinje cells in parts of the cerebellar vermis (Phillips *et al.*, 1987). In-vivo studies mirror post-mortem results, and have found that uncomplicated alcoholics showed the same pattern of focal brain volume deficits as did the KS alcoholics, but in a milder form. When compared with healthy controls, uncomplicated alcoholics had mild to moderate volume deficits and alcoholics with KS had moderate to severe volume deficits in the mammillary bodies, hippocampus, thalamus, cerebellum, and pons (Sullivan and Pfefferbaum, 2009). Thiamine

deficiency seems to contribute to the constellation of cerebral alterations (Butters, 1981). However, the degree of implication of this nutritional deficiency in alcohol-related brain damages is still a matter of debate and is amendable to controlled studies with animal models (Langlais and Zhang, 1997; Pentney and Dlugos, 2000; He *et al.*, 2007; Pfefferbaum *et al.*, 2007).

Aging

Morphological abnormalities in alcoholics are highly similar to brain changes revealed in normal aging (Harper, 1998; Pfefferbaum *et al.*, 2005; Carlen and Wilkinson, 1987). The prominent differences in the frontal lobes and the enlargement of ventricles can be found in alcoholics when compared with healthy subjects, and in normal elderly when compared with younger adults (Pfefferbaum *et al.*, 1997; Sullivan *et al.*, 2000a). Older alcoholics have greater brain dysmorphology than younger ones, and this age-alcoholism interaction is not necessarily related to years of chronic alcoholism. Two hypotheses have been proposed following these findings (see for review Oscar-Berman and Schendan, 2000). The first hypothesis refers to "accelerated aging", whereby alcoholics would show signs of premature aging by precocious onset of neuroanatomical and behavioral changes typically associated with advancing age. The second, "increased vulnerability", differs from the first by the timing of alcohol action. This proposal suggests that an aging brain is more vulnerable to the influences of neurotoxins, including ethanol, than is the brain of a younger person. Thus, only older alcoholics would be more sensitive to the untoward effects of alcoholism and would show more alcohol-related neuroanatomical and neuropsychological abnormalities than younger ones (Pfefferbaum *et al.*, 1998).

Taken together, most of the evidence from neuro-pathological and neuroimaging investigations support the increased vulnerability model (Oscar-Berman and Marinkovic, 2003). Indeed, neuroimaging has highlighted the greater degree of brain alterations in older alcoholics when compared with younger alcoholics in the cerebral cortex (Di Sclafani *et al.*, 1995; Harris *et al.*, 1999, Pfefferbaum *et al.*, 1997), corpus callosum (Pfefferbaum *et al.*, 1996), hippocampus (Laakso *et al.*, 2000; Sullivan *et al.*, 1995), and cerebellum (Harris *et al.*, 1999; Sullivan *et al.*, 2000a). DTI data also provide evidence of such age-related effects on white matter

413

microstructure. In the corpus callosum, findings are in accordance with an interaction between the age and recent drinking history (Pfefferbaum *et al.*, 2006a).

Gender

Neuroimaging studies present some discrepancies regarding gender differences in alcohol-related brain changes. Mann *et al.* (2005a) studied a sample of alcoholic men and women in which women had lower absolute average alcohol consumption in the year before study than men, but equivalent for their weight, and had shorter history of alcohol dependence. Despite the shorter history, women did not differ from men regarding the extent of the brain damage. The authors concluded that reduction of brain volume seemed to develop faster in women, the "telescoping effect", arguing in favor of a greater vulnerability to alcoholism among women than men.

One MRI study reported that although age and alcoholism interacted adversely in both sexes, alcoholic men, but not alcoholic women, had abnormally small cortical white matter and enlarged sulcal volumes compared with same sex healthy comparison groups (Pfefferbaum *et al.*, 2001). By contrast, Hommer *et al.* (2001) reported clear gender differences in the brain structure of alcoholics. In that study, alcoholic men and women had smaller volumes of gray and white matters as well as greater volumes of sulcal and ventricular CSF than non-alcoholic men and women, but these differences were larger for the women than men. Two other studies (Kroft *et al.*, 1991; Pfefferbaum *et al.*, 2002) reported no differences in any brain regions measured (ventricles, corpus callosum, pons and cortical white matter) between alcoholic women and non-alcoholic women of similar ages. Despite lack of abnormalities detectable on a volumetric, macrostructural level, alcoholic women were shown to have white matter microstructural abnormality quantified with a DTI region of interest analysis (Pfefferbaum and Sullivan, 2002). Thus, in some instances, DTI has proved to be a more sensitive measure than MRI in detecting the subtle effects of alcoholism.

Comorbidity

Alcoholism is frequently accompanied by comorbidities of drugs of abuse and psychiatric diseases (Petrakis *et al.*, 2006; Hasin *et al.*, 2007). For example, individuals with schizophrenia are at increased risk

for developing substance abuse disorders (Regier *et al.*, 1990). The tendency among schizophrenic individuals to overvalue alcohol-like rewards and to devalue the potential negative consequences of alcohol abuse may be a contributing factor to their substance abuse risk (Krystal *et al.*, 2006). Alcoholism is also common in subjects with attention deficit/hyperactivity disorder (ADHD), affecting 1 in 5 adults with ADHD (Wilens and Upadhyaya, 2007). The prevalence rates of alcoholism in subjects with bipolar disorder (Vornik and Brown, 2006) and depression (Kessler *et al.*, 1996) are much higher than in the general population. These psychiatric diseases are associated with brain dysmorphology and dysfunction (Malhi and Lagopoulos, 2008), and comorbid association must be taken into account for a more accurate picture of direct and compounded effects of chronic alcoholism (Sullivan *et al.*, 2000b).

Smoking

While smoking rates among non-drinkers are 20–30% in the Western world, rates are up to 80 or 90% among alcohol-dependent subjects. Using high-resolution MRI, Gadzinsky *et al.* (2005b) have observed a different pattern of structure-function relationships in non-smoking alcoholics and in smoking alcoholics. In non-smoking alcoholics, visuospatial learning and memory were positively correlated with temporal white matter and occipital white matter volumes, whereas no significant structure–function relationships were observed in smoking alcoholics. These results suggest that chronic smoking in alcoholics can further disturb brain functional neurocircuitry. Furthermore, chronic smoking associated with alcoholism appears to compound the effects of alcohol-induced neuronal injury and cell membrane dysfunction, inferred from MR spectroscopy, in the frontal lobes and midbrain (Durazzo *et al.*, 2004).

Family history

Results of twin, family, and adoption studies have shown that genes and environment influence vulnerability to alcoholism (Dick and Foroud, 2003; Begleiter and Porjesz, 1999; Schuckit *et al.*, 2004; Whitfield *et al.*, 2004). The Collaborative Studies on Genetics of Alcoholism (COGA) is a multi-site research program that was developed by the National Institute on Alcohol Abuse and Alcoholism (NIAAA) to clarify the relation between genetic contribution to the predisposition for the development of alcoholism and, conversely, alcoholism's effect on gene expression (for reviews, see Porjesz and Rangaswamy, 2007; Bierut et al., 2002; Oscar-Berman and Marinkovic, 2007; Mayfield et al., 2008). Since its inception, multiple members from hundreds of families with a history of alcoholism have been recruited to participate in neuropsychiatric evaluation, genetic screening, and behavioral testing with sensitive and quantitative electrophysiological and neuropsychological examination (Begleiter and Porjesz, 1999). These studies have led to the identification of genes and phenotypes related to alcoholism risk (Edenberg and Foroud, 2006). Offspring from families having a high density of alcoholism differ in both neurophysiological and neuroanatomical characteristics that could not be explained by personal drinking history or particular childhood and adolescent psychopathology and therefore are present before the onset of alcoholism.

Smaller brain volumes were observed in family history positive subjects with high risk for developing alcoholism (e.g. corpus callosum: Venkatasubramanian et al., 2007). More particularly, brain regions within limbic system (hippocampus, amygdala and orbitofrontal cortex) in alcoholics' offspring are smaller than controls at the same age (Benegal et al., 2007; Hill et al., 2001; De Bellis et al., 2000). Such dysmorphology could underlie dysfunctioning in emotional processing and could be involved in the vulnerability to develop alcohol dependence. Because the amygdala tends to increase in volume during childhood and adolescence, smaller volumes observed in high-risk children may indicate a developmental delay that parallels delays seen in visual P300 amplitude (Hill et al., 2001). Curiously, cerebellar volume has been shown to be larger in offspring from alcohol dependent families than in controls age- and sex-matched. This volume difference could be related to less gray matter pruning than normal. Such structural difference in the cerebellum, which plays a role in regulating cognitive functions and has been documented in other genetically related disorders such as autism (Amaral et al., 2008), could also increase the susceptibility for developing alcohol dependence (Hill et al., 2007).

Relations between structural changes and brain functions

A significant percentage of recovering chronic alcoholics exhibit mild to moderate deficits in complex cognitive and motor processes (Oscar-Berman and Marinkovic, 2007; Sullivan et al., 2000d). These functions tend to be impaired but not completely lost. Typically, the processes affected are executive functions (Noel et al., 2001), episodic memory (Pitel et al., 2007), visuospatial abilities (Beatty et al., 1996), and gait and balance (Sullivan et al., 2000c). Although some studies failed to find any relation between brain functions and structural brain data in alcoholics (Demir et al., 2002; Wang et al., 1993), others do provide evidence for such associations (Chick et al., 1989; Fein et al., 2006; Durazzo et al., 2007; Makris et al., 2008; Sullivan and Pfefferbaum, 2001). Performance on a task evaluating global cognitive efficiency (Mini Mental State Examination) have been related to the ventriculocranial ratio (Mochizuki et al., 2005), and more specific cognitive processes have been also associated with abnormalities in more localized brain regions or circuits (Sullivan and Pfefferbaum, 2005).

Executive function deficits in alcoholics were originally examined in relation to prefrontal lobe damage (Nicolas et al., 1993, 1997). Yet, alterations in nodes and connections of the frontocerebellar circuitry seem to be better predictors of executive dysfunctioning than alterations in prefrontal regions (Sullivan et al., 2003). The frontocerebellar circuitry encompasses two loops: a feedback loop involving the thalamus (Haber and McFarland, 2001) and a feedforward loop involving the pons (Schmahmann and Pandya, 1997). When considering this far-reaching multi-modal circuit, executive deficits were found to be related to the gray matter volume in the frontal lobes, cerebellum, pons, and thalamus (Sullivan et al., 2003; Chanraud et al., 2007). Moreover, a tractography study revealed that in alcoholics, the number of white matter fibers reconstructed between the midbrain and the pons correlated with executive performance (Chanraud et al., 2009). Taken together, these findings suggest that, in alcoholics, compromised frontocerebellar circuitry may underlie, at least in part, executive dysfunctions, either by disruption of nodes themselves or by disconnection of circuitry. In addition to the involvement of the frontocerebellar loops, executive functions and attentional processes may be related to the integrity of the corpus callosum (Estruch et al., 1997 Schulte et al., 2004; Pfefferbaum et al., 2000). Such relations were observed with both macrostructural (MRI) and microstructural (DTI) imaging data (Pfefferbaum et al., 2006a; Schulte et al., 2005).

Episodic memory functioning relies on a specific brain network, Papez's circuit, which includes the gray matter structures of the hippocampus, mammillary bodies, thalamus, and cingulate cortex, interconnected by white matter fiber bundles, in particular, the cingulate bundle and the fornix (Papez, 1937). Even though damage to these brain structures and white matter bundles have been reported in alcoholics (see previously in this chapter), little is known about the structural abnormalities underlying episodic memory deficits in alcoholics. Gazdzinski et al. (2005b) have suggested that episodic memory performance is related to white matter in the temporal lobe in alcoholism. However, further investigations are required to specify the relations between episodic memory disorders and Papez's circuit integrity in uncomplicated alcoholics.

Visuospatial abilities are sometimes considered as reflecting the vulnerability of the right hemisphere to alcohol. Although some evidence supports this possibility (Oscar-Berman and Marinkovic, 2003, 2007), other studies found that visuospatial performance was related to white matter volume in the cerebellum (Sullivan, 2003) and microstructural integrity of the splenium (Pfefferbaum et al., 2006a). Concerning motor functions, disorders of control postural, gait and balance as well as ataxia have been related to vermis volume (Sullivan, 2003; Sullivan et al., 2000a, 2006), whereas grip strength has been associated with putamen volume (Sullivan et al., 2005a). These cognitive and motor dysfunctions are most prominently present in alcoholics early in abstinence and during the first weeks of sobriety. Some cognitive and motor recovery may evolve with sustained abstinence from alcohol consumption (Brandt et al., 1983; Fein et al., 1990; Reed et al., 1992; Rourke and Grant, 1999; Rosenbloom et al., 2004; Munro et al., 2000), and it has occasionally been associated with recovery of alcoholism-related structural brain damage (Rosenbloom et al., 2007).

Reversibility of structural brain damage

Potential reversibility of brain damage with abstinence was first investigated in the 1980s with CT scans. The initial seminal report focused on eight alcoholics who were scanned during treatment and then rescanned after a 10- to 14-month interval (Carlen et al., 1978). The four subjects who remained abstinent and improved functionally showed reversal of cerebral shrinkage, whereas the four subjects who continued drinking or demonstrated no functional improvement in the interval showed no change in tissue shrinkage. Subsequent reports of larger samples from this (Carlen et al., 1984) and other laboratories (Ron et al., 1982; Muuronen et al., 1989) confirmed the possibility of reversibility of brain shrinkage in a proportion of abstinent alcoholics. Moreover, analysis showed positive correlations between functional improvement scores on neurological examination and reversible cerebral volume reduction measurements (Carlen et al., 1984). Two years later, a CT study revealed decreased CSF volume and increased cerebral density with maintained abstinence over 4 weeks in alcoholics (Carlen et al., 1986).

Subsequent longitudinal MRI investigations confirmed reduction of ventricular dilatation after several weeks (Schroth et al., 1988; Zipursky et al., 1989) or months (Shear et al., 1994) of drinking cessation. Pfefferbaum et al. (1995) specified the course of the decrease of ventricle volume. MRI data were obtained on a group of alcoholics after an average of 12 days (MRI-1) and 32 days (MRI-2) of sobriety and again 2–12 months after MRI-2 (MRI-3, during which period some maintained abstinence and some relapsed). Results indicated, in abstainers, decline in CSF volume of the lateral ventricles from MRI-1 to MRI-2 and reduction of third ventricular volume from MRI-2 to MRI-3 in abstainers. Therefore, these data suggest that reduction in lateral ventricular volumes occurs early in the course of abstinence and is related to improvement in hematocrit, hemoglobin level and red blood cell count (Pfefferbaum et al., 2004), and that shrinkage in third ventricle volume appears later with continued abstinence (Figure 29.4).

Interestingly, the volume of brain structures belonging to Papez's circuit might be particularly sensitive to abstinence. Indeed, the volume increase of amygdala (Wrase et al., 2008), thalamus (Cardenas et al., 2007), anterior cingulate (Cardenas et al., 2007) and hippocampus (Liu et al., 2000; Wrase et al., 2008) have been described in sober alcoholics. A recent study in rodent models of binge drinking (Nixon, 2006), which focused on the effects of alcohol on structural plasticity in hippocampus during and after intoxication, indicated that adult neurogenesis in the hippocampus is inhibited during alcohol intoxication but returns to normal with cessation of drinking. Whether substantial and functionally viable neurogenesis occurs in the human hippocampus or other brain structures remains however uncertain (Rakic, 2002).

Continued Drinking over 1 Year

Abstinence over 1 Year

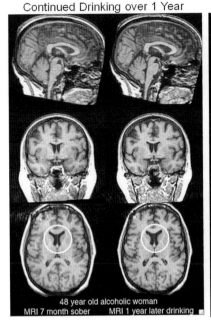
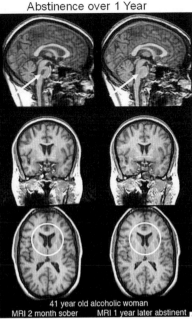

48 year old alcoholic woman
MRI 7 month sober   MRI 1 year later drinking ■

41 year old alcoholic woman
MRI 2 month sober   MRI 1 year later abstinent ▪

Figure 29.4 Here we see the contrast between an alcoholic who continues to drink and one who maintains sobriety (from Rosenbloom and Pfefferbaum, 2008). For both cases, the images to the left were obtained after a period of sobriety and the images to the right were obtained 1 year later. In the lower panel for each woman we see expansion of the lateral ventricles with continued drinking and reduction of the lateral ventricles with continued sobriety. In the upper panel, we see that a lesion in the pons, clearly visible in the first image has resolved after a year of sobriety.

Improvement in abstinent alcoholics was also reported in cerebral cortex (Liu *et al.*, 2000) and temporal and insula cortices (Cardenas *et al.*, 2007), as well as brainstem and cerebellar cortex volume (Liu *et al.*, 2000; Cardenas *et al.*, 2007). The convergence of these findings led Cardenas *et al.* (2007) to suggest that the fronto-ponto-cerebellar circuit, though adversely affected by heavy drinking, is amenable to recovery with abstinence.

In alcoholics with sustained sobriety, several associations between neuropsychological and MRI data have been reported. Lateral ventricular reduction was related to memory improvement (Rosenbloom *et al.*, 2007), third ventricle volume decrease to non-verbal short-term memory improvement (Sullivan *et al.*, 2000c), and fourth ventricle volume decrease to the ataxia improvement (Rosenbloom *et al.*, 2007).

Despite evidence for recovery of brain volume with abstinence, the mechanisms accounting for this recovery remain unclear. The hypothesis of brain rehydration was tested by Schroth *et al.* (1988), who were the first to examine white matter recovery with drinking cessation. No significant increase of T2 values was found, and the authors concluded that alcohol-induced reversible brain effects could not be solely attributed to fluctuation of free water in the brain. The rehydration hypothesis was also considered by Mann *et al.* (1993) but has received little support. Later investigations showed decrease

of white matter in relapsers (Pfefferbaum *et al.*, 1995) and increase in abstainers (Shear *et al.*, 1994), notably in the corpus callosum and subcortical white matter (Cardenas *et al.*, 2007). The mechanism for either volume loss or restoration with abstinence remains controversial but probably involves changes in both myelination and axonal integrity. Wallerian (retrograde) axonal degeneration leads to a permanent reduction in both white and gray matter volume (see Box), explaining why tissue volume recovery appears incomplete with abstinence (for review, see Sullivan and Zahr, 2008). Future longitudinal studies using DTI are required to gain a better understanding of the white matter recovery in sober alcoholics and to specify its role in the cortical volume improvement.

Several factors can predict brain recovery with abstinence. First, the extent of the brain damage may be related to the rapidity of the recovery since smaller brain volumes at baseline were reported to predict faster brain volume gains (Gazdzinski *et al.*, 2005a; Yeh *et al.*, 2007). Gray matter measured at baseline was a better predictor of extent of gray matter recovery than baseline white matter was of its recovery (Cardenas *et al.*, 2007). Second, volume decrease may be associated with interim drinking during the interval of the follow-up (Pfefferbaum *et al.*, 1998), precluding significant volume change (Shear *et al.*, 1994), or even causing decrease of white matter volume (Pfefferbaum *et al.*, 1995) in relapsers.

417

The rapid reversal of brain volume gains in relapsers may be modulated by duration of abstinence and non-abstinence periods, as well as recency of drinking (Gazdzinski et al., 2005a). History of drinking before cessation may also modify brain recovery: the most rapid volume recovery was observed after abstinence in individuals with the greatest drinking severity (Gazdzinski et al., 2005a). Third, concomitant smoking has recently been highlighted as a factor affecting brain damage reversibility (Yeh et al., 2007). Gazdzinsky et al. (2008) found that increase of hippocampus volume correlated with visuospatial memory improvements only in non-smoking alcoholics. These findings suggest, therefore, that chronic cigarette smoking may exacerbate behavioral repercussion of brain volume change. Fourth, alcoholic men and women may also differ regarding brain recovery, improvement being greater and faster in women than in men (Mann et al., 2005a; Schuckit et al., 1995, 1998), but further investigations are required to confirm this conclusion. Finally, investigations regarding neuropsychological recovery suggest a decrease in brain plasticity in aging since older alcoholics have exhibited a slowdown in the course of recovery compared with younger alcoholics (Fein et al., 1990; Munro et al., 2000; Reed et al., 1992; Rourke and Grant, 1999).

The capacity of brain volume to return to normal with drinking cessation is unknown. Short-term abstinence (6 weeks) seems sufficient to induce improvement in brain volume, but not sufficient to return to normal as determined by comparison with control subjects (Mann et al., 2005b). Whether the improvement returned subjects to their own premorbid level cannot be determined; however, three interpretations can be given for these findings. First, extended abstinence longer than the one studied may be required for sober alcoholics to have similar brain volume as control subjects. In that case, a return to normal would imply that there was no pre-existing brain abnormality in alcoholics and that brain damage in alcoholics are entirely the results of the harmful effects of alcohol (possibly compounded by concomitant thiamine deficiency, comorbid diseases, etc.) on the brain. The second explanation is that some brain damage associated with alcoholism, such as neuronal loss (Harper, 2007), may be irreversible, even with extended abstinence. A third explanation is that alcohol-dependent subjects have pre-morbid brain differences from non-dependents that could be considered as a predisposition or risk-factor (Schottenbauer et al., 2007). In that case, even after complete recovery, alcoholics would still have different brain volumes from controls because they started that way. Longer-term longitudinal investigations, including separate samples of offsprings of alcoholic persons, are required to examine these hypotheses.

Interpretation of MRI findings

Even though structural imaging has revealed brain abnormalities in alcohol dependents, what can MRI tell us about the neuropathology of alcoholism? MRI reports must be interpreted with caution because "differences" or "changes" observed do not necessarily reflect a loss of brain tissue. The term "atrophy", for example, describes the end product of a gradual alteration in morphology, followed by a loss of neurons without any products of degradation. The term "degeneration" is used in post-mortem neuropathological studies of alcoholism to describe the result of a more rapid alteration process that affects either the neuron directly or the myelin and that is associated with phagocytosis or gliosis mechanisms resulting in products of degradation (Adams and Victor, 1989). MRI findings likely reflect in part neuropathological processes or outcomes, but whether brain tissue shrinkage reflects fewer neurons, glia, synapses and neuropil remains unknown with current in-vivo structural imaging technology.

Alcohol-related brain changes have the potential of involving cell body death, and loss of axons, dendrites, and synapses, but it is difficult to determine the sequence of events and the causal relationships among these events. Axonal degeneration can precede and sometimes causes neuronal death (for review see Coleman, 2005). Axonal degeneration can be directly triggered by drugs and is a common secondary event in inflammation and myelin disorders (Medana and Esiri, 2003). Lesions affecting the cell body (Figure 29.5A), or affecting the axon (Figure 29.5B), can generate degeneration of the whole axon distal to their sites. It is possible that abnormally low FA in alcohol-dependent subjects reflects alteration of localized white matter fibers and also damage in remote gray matter. More subtle changes in white matter could also result from alcohol's effects on myelin production. Also, programmed axonal self-destruction may be used by unhealthy neurons to eliminate an injured axon or to disconnect it from their post-synaptic targets to conserve resources (Figure 29.5C and D). Finally, a lack of

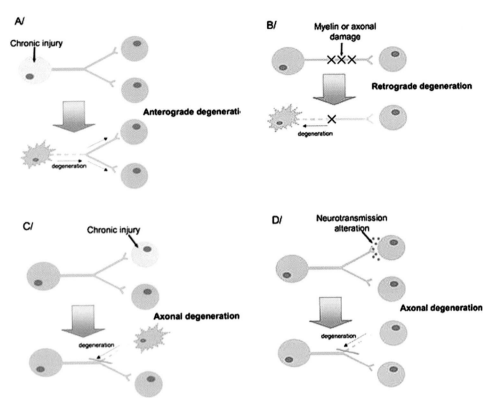

Figure 29.5 Possible mechanisms of neuron damage by: (A) anterograde degeneration due to direct chronic injury of the neuron's cell body; (B) retrograde degeneration due to myelin or axonal damage; (C) axonal degeneration due to chronic injury on post-synaptic neuron; (D) axonal degeneration due to neurotransmission dysfunction.

signals from appropriate target cells can cause the axons to degenerate, as it occurs in culture when the axon of a neuron is locally deprived of brain-derived neurotrophic factor (Figure 29.5C). These potential mechanisms may work independently or in concert to compromise axons either directly or indirectly. Given that axons connect brain regions thus enabling cerebral interneuronal communication, such alterations could also be the substrate of brain dysfunction, characterized by incomplete lesions, disconnection syndrome, and inefficient signal processing.

Conclusion

Alcohol dependence follows a longitudinal course, from initiation to development of dependence, chronic intake, withdrawal, and often relapse. Advances in MRI technologies have enabled exploration of brain changes for each of these steps and, for example, have revealed widespread volume deficits in gray and white matter with a predilection for the prefrontal cortex.

Selective components of function that are impaired in alcohol dependents can persist even after months of sobriety and can linger for years (Rosenbloom et al., 2004). Some impairments have occasionally been related to specific brain abnormalities. The relationships between brain regions and cognitive or motor functions predominantly involve two anatomo-functional circuits (frontocerebellar and Papez circuits) rather than either isolated local brain nodes or global dysmorphology. Variability in the extent and constellation of brain abnormalities and their functional consequences in alcohol-dependent subjects provide clues to alcohol's action on the brain and raise the possibility that individual differences play a major role in alcoholism's detrimental effects. Indeed, individual differences in response to alcohol use and alcohol dependence may reflect variance in patterns of alcohol use (e.g. ventricles (Ding et al., 2004)), nutritional status (e.g. Wernicke–Korsakoff syndrome (Thomson, 2000)), manifestation of withdrawal signs and symptoms (e.g. temporal white matter (Sullivan et al.,

419

Box 29.1.

Brain circuits commonly damaged in alcohol-dependent subjects and related to selective cognitive impairments in these subjects, notably executive functions and episodic memory. Sagittal (top left), coronal (top right) and surface-rendered (bottom left) views of brain regions that are part of the frontocerebellar circuit (in blue) and Papez circuit (in yellow) and their relations with cognitive impairments (bottom right). Alterations within one or both of these circuits (see conclusion) are usually found in alcohol-dependent subjects.

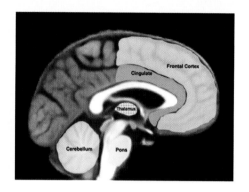 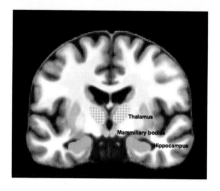

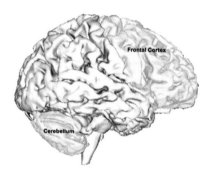

Fronto-cerebellar Circuit	Papez's Circuit
Executive functions	Episodic memory

Main anatomofunctional relationships revealed in alcohol dependent subjects.

1996)), and genetically determined vulnerability (e.g. offspring (Oscar-Berman and Marinkovic, 2007)). Although frontocerebellar and Papez circuits seem to be more particularly altered by alcoholism, damage in both circuits does not necessarily co-occur. Different factors may affect these two circuits, leading to different profiles of brain abnormalities among alcoholics.

Alterations of nodes that are part of frontocerebellar circuit (see Box 29.1, regions highlighted in blue) are related to executive impairments and working memory deficits and are associated with the age at first alcohol intake (Chanraud et al., 2007). Interestingly, parts of this circuit mature late in adolescence (Casey et al., 2008), a time when alcohol use can be heaviest (NESARC), and are particularly sensitive to pathological disruption (Ridler et al., 2006).

Alterations in Papez circuit (see Box 29.1, regions highlighted in yellow) can lead to neurological complications that are related to thiamine deficiency.

Nutritional status may, therefore, interact with alcohol consumption in damaging brain regions within this circuit. Damage to the hippocampus, which is part of this circuit, can differ depending on the nature of the alcohol drunk (Wilhelm et al., 2008). Therefore, drinking history, among multiple other factors, must be taken into account when gauging the neuropathology of alcoholism.

Such factors can be examined with animal models of alcohol dependence and controlled, in terms of alcohol-exposure amount, age at exposure, withdrawal, and nutrition (Crews et al., 2004; Pfefferbaum et al., 2007). In combination with structural imaging, experimental models of alcoholism could be a translational point in identifying mechanisms of alcohol-related brain dysmorphology. Clinically, these neuroimaging tools have unveiled in-vivo characterization of brain tissue abnormalities that predate the development of alcohol dependence and can serve as predisposing factors, those that result from alcohol dependence to help maintain addiction, and those that can manifest neuroplasticity contributing at least some degree of recovery with prolonged sobriety.

Gray matter volume shrinkage of prefrontal cortex, cerebellum (especially anterior vermis), pons, mammillary bodies, hippocampus, and thalamus particularly in older alcoholic individuals.

White matter tract microstructural damage affecting the genu and splenium of the corpus callosum, the centrum semiovale, corticopontine bundles, and frontolimbic connections.

Compounded effects of alcohol with a variety of other factors, including age, gender, nutritional (thiamine) deficiency, drugs of abuse, psychiatric comorbidity, and family history of alcoholism.

Evidence for recovery of brain volume with abstinence, but mechanisms of damage or repair remain elusive.

Impairments involve executive functions, behavioral inhibition, working memory, episodic memory, visuospatial abilities, and gait and balance.

Three major brain circuits are affected and disrupt selective constellations of function.

Frontocerebellar circuit alteration is related to executive dysfunction and postural instability.

Papez's circuit alteration is related to episodic memory impairment.

Ventral–striatal–amygdala circuit alteration is related to difficulties in emotional and affect appreciation and may enable maintenance of alcohol dependence.

Acknowledgments

We thank Adolf Pfefferbaum, MD for inspiration in all aspects of this work and for MR and DT images used in the figures. We also thank Margaret J. Rosenbloom, MA for thoughtful comments on the manuscript. This work was supported by NIH grants AA010723, AA012388, AA017168, AA017923, AA005965.

References

Adams R D and Victor M. 1989. *Principles of Neurology* (4th ed.). New York, NY: McGraw-Hill, Inc.

Agartz I, Momenan R, Rawlings R R, Kerich M J and Hommer D W. 1999. Hippocampal volume in patients with alcohol dependence. *Arch Gen Psychiatry* **56**, 356–63.

Agartz I, Saaf J, Wahlund L O and Wetterberg L. 1991. T1 and T2 relaxation time estimates and brain measures during withdrawal in alcoholic men. *Drug Alcohol Depend* **29**, 157–69.

Alvarez I, Gonzalo L M and Llor J. 1989. Effects of chronic alcoholism on the amygdaloid complex. A study in human and rats. *Histol Histopathol* **4**, 183–92.

Amaral D G, Schumann C M and Nordahl C W. 2008. Neuroanatomy of autism. *Trends Neurosci* **31**, 137–45.

American Psychiatric Association. 1994. *Diagnostic and Statistical Manual of Mental Disorders*. Washington, DC: American Psychiatric Association.

Andersen B B. 2004. Reduction of Purkinje cell volume in cerebellum of alcoholics. *Brain Res* **1007**, 10–8.

Andreasen N C, O'Leary D S, Cizadlo T, *et al.* 1996. Schizophrenia and cognitive dysmetria: A positron-emission tomography study of dysfunctional prefrontal–thalamic–cerebellar circuitry. *Proc Natl Acad Sci USA* **93**, 9985–90.

Antunez E, Estruch R, Cardenal C, Nicolas J M, Fernandez-Sola J and Urbano-Marquez A. 1998. Usefulness of CT and MR imaging in the diagnosis of acute Wernicke's encephalopathy. *Am J Roentgenol* **171**, 1131–7.

Ashburner J and Friston K J. 2000. Voxel-based morphometry – The methods. *Neuroimage* **11**, 805–21.

Baker K G, Halliday G M, Kril J J and Harper C G. 1996. Chronic alcoholics without Wernicke–Korsakoff syndrome or cirrhosis do not lose serotonergic neurons in the dorsal raphe nucleus. *Alcohol Clin Exp Res* **20**, 61–6.

Baker K G, Harding A J, Halliday G M, Kril J J and Harper C G. 1999. Neuronal loss in functional zones of the cerebellum of chronic alcoholics with and without Wernicke's encephalopathy. *Neuroscience* **91**, 429–38.

Balldin J, Berggren U, Engel J and Eriksson M. 1994. Neuroendocrine evidence for reduced serotonergic neurotransmission during heavy drinking. *Alcohol Clin Exp Res* **18**, 822–5.

Basser P J. 1995. Inferring microstructural features and the physiological state of tissues from diffusion-weighted images. *NMR Biomed* **8**, 333–44.

Beatty W W, Hames K A, Blanco C R, Nixon S J and Tivis L J. 1996. Visuospatial perception, construction and memory in alcoholism. *J Stud Alcohol* **57**, 136–43.

Begleiter H and Porjesz B. 1999. What is inherited in the predisposition toward alcoholism? A proposed model. *Alcohol Clin Exp Res* **23**, 1125–35.

Benegal V, Antony G, Venkatasubramanian G and Jayakumar P N. 2007. Gray matter volume abnormalities and externalizing symptoms in subjects at high risk for alcohol dependence. *Addict Biol* **12**, 122–32.

Beresford T P, Arciniegas D B, Alfers J, *et al.* 2006. Hippocampus volume loss due to chronic heavy drinking. *Alcohol Clin Exp Res* **30**, 1866–70.

Bergman H, Borg S, Hindmarsh T, Idestrom C M and Mutzell S. 1980. Computed-tomography of the brain and neuropsychological assessment of alcoholic patients. *Adv Exp Med Biol* **126**, 771–86.

Besson J A, Glen A I, Foreman E I, *et al.* 1981. Nuclear magnetic resonance observations in alcoholic cerebral disorder and the role of vasopressin. *Lancet* **2**, 923–4.

Besson J A, Greentree S G, Foster M A and Rimmington J E. 1989. Effects of ethanol on the NMR characteristics of rat brain. Acute administration, dependency, and long-term effects. *Br J Psychiatry* **155**, 818–21.

Bierut L J, Saccone N L, Rice J P, *et al.* 2002. Defining alcohol-related phenotypes in humans. The Collaborative Study on the Genetics of Alcoholism. *Alcohol Res Health* **26**, 208–13.

Bleich S, Degner D, Kropp S, Ruther E and Kornhuber J. 2000. Red wine, spirits, beer and serum homocysteine. *Lancet* **356**, 512.

Bleich S, Sperling W, Degner D, *et al.* 2003. Lack of association between hippocampal volume reduction and first-onset alcohol withdrawal seizure. A volumetric MRI study. *Alcohol Alcohol* **38**, 40–4.

Bloomer C W, Langleben D D and Meyerhoff D J. 2004. Magnetic resonance detects brainstem changes in chronic, active heavy drinkers. *Psychiatry Res* **132**, 209–18.

Brandt J, Butters N, Ryan C and Bayog R. 1983. Cognitive loss and recovery in long-term alcohol abusers. *Arch Gen Psychiatry* **40**, 435–42.

Bruno S, Cercignani M and Ron M A. 2008. White matter abnormalities in bipolar disorder: A voxel-based diffusion tensor imaging study. *Bipolar Disord* **10**, 460–8.

Butters N. 1981. The Wernicke–Korsakoff syndrome: A review of psychological, neuropathological and etiological factors. *Curr Alcohol* **8**, 205–32.

Cardenas V A, Studholme C, Gazdzinski S, Durazzo T C and Meyerhoff D J. 2007. Deformation-based morphometry of brain changes in alcohol dependence and abstinence. *Neuroimage* **34**, 879–87.

Cargiulo T. 2007. Understanding the health impact of alcohol dependence. *Am J Health Syst Pharm* **64**, S5–11.

Carlen P L, Penn R D, Fornazzari L, Bennett J, Wilkinson D A and Wortzman G. 1986. Computerized tomographic scan assessment of alcoholic brain damage and its potential reversibility. *Alcohol Clin Exp Res* **10**, 226–32.

Carlen P L and Wilkinson D A. 1987. Alcohol-induced brain damage: Confounding variables. *Alcohol Alcohol Suppl* **1**, 37–41.

Carlen P L, Wilkinson D A, Wortzman G and Holgate R. 1984. Partially reversible cerebral atrophy and functional improvement in recently abstinent alcoholics. *Can J Neurol Sci* **11**, 441–6.

Carlen P L, Wortzman G, Holgate R C, Wilkinson D A and Rankin J C. 1978. Reversible cerebral atrophy in recently abstinent chronic alcoholics measured by computed tomography scans. *Science* **200**, 1076–8.

Casey B J, Getz S and Galvan A. 2008. The adolescent brain. *Dev Rev* **28**, 62–77.

Cavanagh J B, Holton J L and Nolan C C. 1997. Selective damage to the cerebellar vermis in chronic alcoholism: A contribution from neurotoxicology to an old problem of selective vulnerability. *Neuropathol Appl Neurobiol* **23**, 355–63.

Chanraud S, Martelli C, Delain F, *et al.* 2007. Brain morphometry and cognitive performance in detoxified alcohol-dependents with preserved psychosocial functioning. *Neuropsychopharmacology* **32**, 429–38.

Chanraud S, Reynaud M, Wessa M, *et al.* 2008. Diffusion tensor tractography in mesencephalic bundles: Relation to mental flexibility in detoxified alcohol-dependent subjects. *Neuropsychopharmacology* **34**, 1223–32.

Charness M E. 1993. Brain lesions in alcoholics. *Alcohol Clin Exp Res* **17**, 2–11.

Chick J D, Smith M A, Engleman H M, *et al.* 1989. Magnetic resonance imaging of the brain in alcoholics: Cerebral atrophy, lifetime alcohol consumption, and cognitive deficits. *Alcohol Clin Exp Res* **13**, 512–8.

Cisler R, Holder H D, Longabaugh R, Stout R L and Zweben A. 1998. Actual and estimated replication costs for alcohol treatment modalities: Case study from Project MATCH. *J Stud Alcohol* **59**, 503–12.

Clark D B, Thatcher D L and Tapert S F. 2008. Alcohol, psychological dysregulation, and adolescent brain development. *Alcohol Clin Exp Res* **32**, 375–85.

Coleman M. 2005. Axon degeneration mechanisms: Commonality amid diversity. *Nat Rev Neurosci* **6**, 889–98.

Courville C. 1955. *Effects of Alcohol on the Nervous System of Man.* Los Angeles, CA: San Lucas Press.

Crews F T, Collins M A, Dlugos C, *et al.* 2004. Alcohol-induced neurodegeneration: When, where and why? *Alcohol Clin Exp Res* **28**, 350–64.

De Bellis M D, Clark D B, Beers S R, *et al.* 2000. Hippocampal volume in adolescent-onset alcohol use disorders. *Am J Psychiatry* **157**, 737–44.

De Bellis M D, Narasimhan A, Thatcher D L, Keshavan M S, Soloff P and Clark D B. 2005. Prefrontal cortex, thalamus, and cerebellar volumes in adolescents and young adults with adolescent-onset alcohol use disorders and comorbid mental disorders. *Alcohol Clin Exp Res* **29**, 1590–600.

Demir B, Ulug B, Lay Ergun E and Erbas B. 2002. Regional cerebral blood flow and neuropsychological functioning in early and late onset alcoholism. *Psychiatry Res* **115**, 115–25.

Di Sclafani V, Ezekiel F, Meyerhoff D J, *et al.* 1995. Brain atrophy and cognitive function in older abstinent alcoholic men. *Alcohol Clin Exp Res* **19**, 1121–6.

Dick D M and Foroud T. 2003. Candidate genes for alcohol dependence: A review of genetic evidence from human studies. *Alcohol Clin Exp Res* **27**, 868–79.

Diener H C, Muller A, Thron A, Poremba M, Dichgans J and Rapp H. 1986. Correlation of clinical signs with CT findings in patients with cerebellar disease. *J Neurol* **233**, 5–12.

Ding J, Eigenbrodt M L, Mosley T H Jr *et al.* 2004. Alcohol intake and cerebral abnormalities on magnetic resonance imaging in a community-based population of middle-aged adults: The Atherosclerosis Risk in Communities (ARIC) study. *Stroke* **35**, 16–21.

Durazzo T C, Cardenas V A, Studholme C, Weiner M W and Meyerhoff D J. 2007. Non-treatment-seeking heavy drinkers: effects of chronic cigarette smoking on brain structure. *Drug Alcohol Depend* **87**, 76–82.

Durazzo T C, Gazdzinski S, Banys P and Meyerhoff D J. 2004. Cigarette smoking exacerbates chronic alcohol-induced brain damage: A preliminary metabolite imaging study. *Alcohol Clin Exp Res* **28**, 1849–60.

Edenberg H J and Foroud T. 2006. The genetics of alcoholism: Identifying specific genes through family studies. *Addict Biol* **11**, 386–96.

Estruch R, Nicolas J M, Salamero M, *et al.* 1997. Atrophy of the corpus callosum in chronic alcoholism. *J Neurol Sci* **146**, 145–51.

Fein G, Bachman L, Fisher S and Davenport L. 1990. Cognitive impairments in abstinent alcoholics. *West J Med* **152**, 531–7.

Fein G, Landman B, Tran H, *et al.* 2006. Brain atrophy in long-term abstinent alcoholics who demonstrate impairment on a simulated gambling task. *Neuroimage* **32**, 1465–71.

Ferrer I, Fabregues I, Pineda M, Gracia I and Ribalta T. 1984. A Golgi study of cerebellar atrophy in human chronic alcoholism. *Neuropathol Appl Neurobiol* **10**, 245–53.

First M B, Spitzer R L, Gibbon M and Williams J B W. 1998. *Structured Clinical Interview for DSM-IV Axis I Disorders (SCID) Version 2.0.* New York, NY: Biometrics Research Department, New York State Psychiatric Institute.

Gaser C, Nenadic I, Buchsbaum B R, Hazlett E A and Buchsbaum M S. 2001. Deformation-based morphometry and its relation to conventional volumetry of brain lateral ventricles in MRI. *Neuroimage* **13**, 1140–5.

Gazdzinski S, Durazzo T C and Meyerhoff D J. 2005a. Temporal dynamics and determinants of whole brain tissue volume changes during recovery from alcohol dependence. *Drug Alcohol Depend* **78**, 263–73.

Gazdzinski S, Durazzo T C, Studholme C, Song E, Banys P and Meyerhoff D J. 2005b. Quantitative brain MRI in alcohol dependence: Preliminary evidence for effects of concurrent chronic cigarette smoking on regional brain volumes. *Alcohol Clin Exp Res* **29**, 1484–95.

Gazdzinski S, Durazzo T C, Yeh P H, Hardin D, Banys P and Meyerhoff D J. 2008. Chronic cigarette smoking modulates injury and short-term recovery of the medial temporal lobe in alcoholics. *Psychiatry Res* **162**, 133–45.

Good C D, Johnsrude I S, Ashburner J, Henson R N, Friston K J and Frackowiak R S. 2001. A voxel-based morphometric study of ageing in 465 normal adult human brains. *Neuroimage* **14**, 21–36.

Haber S and McFarland N R. 2001. The place of the thalamus in frontal cortical–basal ganglia circuits. *Neuroscientist* **7**, 315–24.

Harding A J, Wong A, Svoboda M, Kril J J and Halliday G M. 1997. Chronic alcohol consumption does not cause hippocampal neuron loss in humans. *Hippocampus* **7**, 78–87.

Harper C. 1998. The neuropathology of alcohol-specific brain damage, or does alcohol damage the brain? *J Neuropathol Exp Neurol* **57**, 101–10.

Harper C. 2007. The neurotoxicity of alcohol. *Hum Exp Toxicol* **26**, 251–7.

Harper C G, Kril J J and Daly J M. 1987. The specific gravity of the brains of alcoholic and control patients: A pathological study. *Br J Addict* **82**, 1349–54.

Harris G J, Jaffin S K, Hodge S M, *et al.* 2008. Frontal white matter and cingulum diffusion tensor imaging deficits in alcoholism. *Alcohol Clin Exp Res* **32**, 1001–13.

Harris G J, Oscar-Berman M, Gansler A, *et al.* 1999. Hypoperfusion of the cerebellum and aging effects on cerebral cortex blood flow in abstinent alcoholics: A SPECT study. *Alcohol Clin Exp Res* **23**, 1219–27.

Hasin D S, Stinson F S, Ogburn E and Grant B F. 2007. Prevalence, correlates, disability, and comorbidity of DSM-IV alcohol abuse and dependence in the United States: Results from the National Epidemiologic Survey on Alcohol and Related Conditions. *Arch Gen Psychiatry* **64**, 830–42.

Hayakawa K, Kumagai H, Suzuki Y, *et al.* 1992. MR imaging of chronic alcoholism. *Acta Radiol* **33**, 201–06.

He J, Nixon K, Shetty A K and Crews F T. 2005. Chronic alcohol exposure reduces hippocampal neurogenesis and dendritic growth of newborn neurons. *Eur J Neurosci* **21**, 2711–20.

He X, Sullivan E V, Stankovic R K, Harper C G and Pfefferbaum A. 2007. Interaction of thiamine deficiency and voluntary alcohol consumption disrupts rat corpus callosum ultrastructure. *Neuropsychopharmacology* **32**, 2207–16.

Hill S Y, De Bellis M D, Keshavan M S, et al. 2001. Right amygdala volume in adolescent and young adult offspring from families at high risk for developing alcoholism. Biol Psychiatry 49, 894–905.

Hill S Y, Muddasani S, Prasad K, et al. 2007. Cerebellar volume in offspring from multiplex alcohol dependence families. Biol Psychiatry 61, 41–7.

Hommer D, Momenan R, Kaiser E and Rawlings R. 2001. Evidence for a gender-related effect of alcoholism on brain volumes. Am J Psychiatry 158, 198–204.

Hommer D, Momenan R, Rawlings R, et al. 1996. Decreased corpus callosum size among alcoholic women. Arch Neurol 53, 359–63.

Jang D P, Namkoong K, Kim J J, et al. 2007. The relationship between brain morphometry and neuropsychological performance in alcohol dependence. Neurosci Lett 428, 21–6.

Jensen G B and Pakkenberg B. 1993. Do alcoholics drink their neurons away? Lancet 342, 1201–04.

Jernigan T L, Butters N, Ditraglia G, et al. 1991. Reduced cerebral grey matter observed in alcoholics using magnetic resonance imaging. Alcohol Clin Exp Res 15, 418–27.

Jernigan T L, Zatz L M, Ahumada A J Jr, Pfefferbaum A, Tinklenberg J R and Moses J A Jr. 1982. CT measures of cerebrospinal fluid volume in alcoholics and normal volunteers. Psychiatry Res 7, 9–17.

Kamarajan C, Porjesz B, Jones K, et al. 2006. Event-related oscillations in offspring of alcoholics: Neurocognitive disinhibition as a risk for alcoholism. Biol Psychiatry 59, 625–34.

Kashem M A, Harper C and Matsumoto I. 2008. Differential protein expression in the corpus callosum (genu) of human alcoholics. Neurochem Int 53, 1–11.

Kessler R C, Nelson C B, McGonagle K A, Liu J, Swartz M and Blazer D G. 1996. Comorbidity of DSM-III-R major depressive disorder in the general population: results from the US National Comorbidity Survey. Br J Psychiatry Suppl 17–30.

Kinkingnehun S, Sarazin M, Lehericy S, Guichart-Gomez E, Hergueta T and Dubois B. 2008. VBM anticipates the rate of progression of Alzheimer disease: A 3-year longitudinal study. Neurology 70, 2201–11.

Koob G F. 2008. A role for brain stress systems in addiction. Neuron 59, 11–34.

Korbo L. 1999. Glial cell loss in the hippocampus of alcoholics. Alcohol Clin Exp Res 23, 164–8.

Kril J J, Halliday G M, Svoboda M D and Cartwright H. 1997. The cerebral cortex is damaged in chronic alcoholics. Neuroscience 79, 983–98.

Kroft C L, Gescuk B, Woods B T, et al. 1991. Brain ventricular size in female alcoholics: An MRI study. Alcohol 8, 31–4.

Krystal J H, D'Souza D C, Gallinat J, et al. 2006. The vulnerability to alcohol and substance abuse in individuals diagnosed with schizophrenia. Neurotox Res 10, 235–52.

Kurth C, Wegerer V, Reulbach U, et al. 2004. Analysis of hippocampal atrophy in alcoholic patients by a Kohonen feature map. Neuroreport 15, 367–71.

Laakso M P, Vaurio O, Savolainen L, et al. 2000. A volumetric MRI study of the hippocampus in type 1 and 2 alcoholism. Behav Brain es 109, 177–86.

Langlais P J and Zhang S X. 1997. Cortical and subcortical white matter damage without Wernicke's encephalopathy after recovery from thiamine deficiency in the rat. Alcohol Clin Exp Res 21, 434–43.

Lindboe C F and Loberg E M. 1988. The frequency of brain lesions in alcoholics. Comparison between the 5-year periods 1975–1979 and 1983–1987. J Neurol Sci 88, 107–13.

Lipton S A, Kim W K, Choi Y B, et al. 1997. Neurotoxicity associated with dual actions of homocysteine at the N-methyl-D-aspartate receptor. Proc Natl Acad Sci USA 94, 5923–8.

Lishman W A. 1990. Alcohol and the brain. Br J Psychiatry 156, 635–44.

Lishman W A, Jacobson R R and Acker C. 1987. Brain damage in alcoholism: current concepts. Acta Med Scand Suppl 717, 5–17.

Liu R S, Lemieux L, Shorvon S D, Sisodiya S M and Duncan J S. 2000. Association between brain size and abstinence from alcohol. Lancet 355, 1969–70.

Maguire E A, Gadian D G, Johnsrude I S, et al. 2000. Navigation-related structural change in the hippocampi of taxi drivers. Proc Natl Acad Sci USA 97, 4398–403.

Makris N, Oscar-Berman M, Jaffin S K, et al. 2008. Decreased volume of the brain reward system in alcoholism. Biol Psychiatry 64, 192–202.

Malhi G S and Lagopoulos J. 2008. Making sense of neuroimaging in psychiatry. Acta Psychiatr Scand 117, 100–17.

Mander A J, Young A, Chick J D and Best J J. 1989. The relationship of cerebral atrophy and T1 in alcoholics: An MRI study. Drug Alcohol Depend 24, 57–9.

Mann K, Ackermann K, Croissant B, Mundle G, Nakovics H and Diehl A. 2005a. Neuroimaging of gender differences in alcohol dependence: Are women more vulnerable? Alcohol Clin Exp Res 29, 896–901.

Mann K, Mundle G, Langle G and Petersen D. 1993. The reversibility of alcoholic brain damage is not due to rehydration: A CT study. Addiction 88, 649–53.

Mann K, Schafer D R, Langle G, Ackermann K and Croissant B. 2005b. The long-term course of alcoholism,

5, 10 and 16 years after treatment. *Addiction* **100**, 797–805.

Martin P R, Singleton C K and Hiller-Sturmhofel S. 2003. The role of thiamine deficiency in alcoholic brain disease. *Alcohol Res Health* **27**, 134–42.

Mathalon D H, Sullivan E V, Rawles J M and Pfefferbaum A. 1993. Correction for head size in brain-imaging measurements. *Psychiatry Res* **50**, 121–39.

Mayfield R D, Harris R A and Schuckit M A. 2008. Genetic factors influencing alcohol dependence. *Br J Pharmacol* **154**, 275–87.

McBride W J. 2002. Central nucleus of the amygdala and the effects of alcohol and alcohol-drinking behavior in rodents. *Pharmacol Biochem Behav* **71**, 509–15.

McMullen P A, Saint-Cyr J A and Carlen P L. 1984. Morphological alterations in rat CA1 hippocampal pyramidal cell dendrites resulting from chronic ethanol consumption and withdrawal. *J Comp Neurol* **225**, 111–8.

Mechelli A, Price C J, Friston K J and Ashburner J. 2005. Voxel-based morphometry of the human brain: Methods and applications. *Curr Med Imaging Rev* **1**, 1–9.

Mechtcheriakov S, Brenneis C, Egger K, Koppelstaetter F, Schocke M and Marksteiner J. 2007. A widespread distinct pattern of cerebral atrophy in patients with alcohol addiction revealed by voxel-based morphometry. *J Neurol Neurosurg Psychiatry* **78**, 610–4.

Medana I M and Esiri M M. 2003. Axonal damage: A key predictor of outcome in human CNS diseases. *Brain* **126**, 515–30.

Melgaard B and Ahlgren P. 1986. Ataxia and cerebellar atrophy in chronic alcoholics. *J Neurol* **233**, 13–5.

Miller W R, Meyers R J and Tonigan J S. 1999. Engaging the unmotivated in treatment for alcohol problems: A comparison of three strategies for intervention through family members. *J Consult Clin Psychol* **67**, 688–97.

Mochizuki H, Masaki T, Matsushita S, *et al.* 2005. Cognitive impairment and diffuse white matter atrophy in alcoholics. *Clin Neurophysiol* **116**, 223–8.

Mori S and Van Zijl P C. 2002. Fiber tracking: Principles and strategies – A technical review. *NMR Biomed* **15**, 468–80.

Munro C A, Saxton J and Butters M A. 2000. The neuropsychological consequences of abstinence among older alcoholics: A cross-sectional study. *Alcohol Clin Exp Res* **24**, 1510–6.

Muuronen A, Bergman H, Hindmarsh T and Telakivi T. 1989. Influence of improved drinking habits on brain atrophy and cognitive performance in alcoholic patients: A 5-year follow-up study. *Alcohol Clin Exp Res* **13**, 137–41.

Nicolas J M, Catafau A M, Estruch R, *et al.* 1993. Regional cerebral blood flow-SPECT in chronic alcoholism: Relation to neuropsychological testing. *J Nucl Med* **34**, 1452–9.

Nicolas J M, Estruch R, Salamero M, *et al.* 1997. Brain impairment in well-nourished chronic alcoholics is related to ethanol intake. *Ann Neurol* **41**, 590–8.

Nixon K. 2006. Alcohol and adult neurogenesis: Roles in neurodegeneration and recovery in chronic alcoholism. *Hippocampus* **16**, 287–95.

Nixon K and Crews F T. 2004. Temporally specific burst in cell proliferation increases hippocampal neurogenesis in protracted abstinence from alcohol. *J Neurosci* **24**, 9714–22.

Noel X, Paternot J, Van Der Linden M, *et al.* 2001. Correlation between inhibition, working memory and delimited frontal area blood flow measure by 99mTc-Bicisate SPECT in alcohol-dependent patients. *Alcohol Alcohol* **36**, 556–63.

Oscar-Berman M and Marinkovic K. 2003. Alcoholism and the brain: An overview. *Alcohol Res Health* **27**, 125–33.

Oscar-Berman M and Marinkovic K. 2007. Alcohol: Effects on neurobehavioral functions and the brain. *Neuropsychol Rev* **17**, 239–57.

Oscar-Berman M and Schendan H E. 2000. Asymmetries of brain function in alcoholism: Relationship to aging. In Obler L and Connor L T (Eds.) *Neurobehavior of Language and Cognition: Studies of Normal Aging and Brain Damage.* New York, NY: Kluwer Academic Publishers.

Papez J W. 1937. A proposed mechanism of emotion. *Arch Neurol Psychiatry* **28**, 725–43.

Passingham R E, Stephan K E and Kotter R. 2002. The anatomical basis of functional localization in the cortex. *Nat Rev Neurosci* **3**, 606–16.

Pearlson G D and Calhoun V. 2007. Structural and functional magnetic resonance imaging in psychiatric disorders. *Can J Psychiatry* **52**, 158–66.

Pentney R J and Dlugos C A. 2000. Cerebellar Purkinje neurons with altered terminal dendritic segments are present in all lobules of the cerebellar vermis of ageing, ethanol-treated F344 rats. *Alcohol Alcohol* **35**, 35–43.

Petrakis I L, Poling J, Levinson C, *et al.* 2006. Naltrexone and disulfiram in patients with alcohol dependence and comorbid post-traumatic stress disorder. *Biol Psychiatry* **60**, 777–83.

Pfefferbaum A, Adalsteinsson E, Bell R L and Sullivan E V. 2007. Development and resolution of brain lesions caused by pyrithiamine- and dietary-induced thiamine deficiency and alcohol exposure in the alcohol-preferring rat: A longitudinal magnetic resonance imaging and spectroscopy study. *Neuropsychopharmacology* **32**, 1159–77.

Pfefferbaum A, Adalsteinsson E and Sullivan E V. 2005. Frontal circuitry degradation marks healthy adult aging: Evidence from diffusion tensor imaging. *Neuroimage* **26**, 891–9.

Pfefferbaum A, Adalsteinsson E and Sullivan E V. 2006a. Dysmorphology and microstructural degradation of the corpus callosum: Interaction of age and alcoholism. *Neurobiol Aging* **27**, 994–1009.

Pfefferbaum A, Adalsteinsson E and Sullivan E V. 2006b. Supratentorial profile of white matter microstructural integrity in recovering alcoholic men and women. *Biol Psychiatry* **59**, 364–72.

Pfefferbaum A, Lim K O, Desmond J E and Sullivan E V. 1996. Thinning of the corpus callosum in older alcoholic men: A magnetic resonance imaging study. *Alcohol Clin Exp Res* **20**, 752–7.

Pfefferbaum A, Lim K O, Zipursky R B, *et al.* 1992. Brain gray and white matter volume loss accelerates with aging in chronic alcoholics: A quantitative MRI study. *Alcohol Clin Exp Res* **16**, 1078–89.

Pfefferbaum A, Rosenbloom M, Crusan K and Jernigan T L. 1988. Brain CT changes in alcoholics: Effects of age and alcohol consumption. *Alcohol Clin Exp Res* **12**, 81–7.

Pfefferbaum A, Rosenbloom M, Deshmukh A and Sullivan E. 2001. Sex differences in the effects of alcohol on brain structure. *Am J Psychiatry* **158**, 188–97.

Pfefferbaum A, Rosenbloom M, Serventi K L and Sullivan E V. 2002. Corpus callosum, pons, and cortical white matter in alcoholic women. *Alcohol Clin Exp Res* **26**, 400–06.

Pfefferbaum A, Rosenbloom M J, Serventi K L and Sullivan E V. 2004. Brain volumes, RBC status, and hepatic function in alcoholics after 1 and 4 weeks of sobriety: Predictors of outcome. *Am J Psychiatry* **161**, 1190–6.

Pfefferbaum A and Sullivan E V. 2002. Microstructural but not macrostructural disruption of white matter in women with chronic alcoholism. *Neuroimage* **15**, 708–18.

Pfefferbaum A and Sullivan E V. 2005. Disruption of brain white matter microstructure by excessive intracellular and extracellular fluid in alcoholism: Evidence from diffusion tensor imaging. *Neuropsychopharmacology* **30**, 423–32.

Pfefferbaum A, Sullivan E V, Hedehus M, Adalsteinsson E, Lim K O and Moseley M. 2000. In vivo detection and functional correlates of white matter microstructural disruption in chronic alcoholism. *Alcohol Clin Exp Res* **24**, 1214–21.

Pfefferbaum A, Sullivan E V, Mathalon D H and Lim K O. 1997. Frontal lobe volume loss observed with magnetic resonance imaging in older chronic alcoholics. *Alcohol Clin Exp Res* **21**, 521–9.

Pfefferbaum A, Sullivan E V, Mathalon D H, Shear P K, Rosenbloom M J and Lim K O. 1995. Longitudinal changes in magnetic resonance imaging brain volumes in abstinent and relapsed alcoholics. *Alcohol Clin Exp Res* **19**, 1177–91.

Pfefferbaum A, Sullivan E V, Rosenbloom M J, Mathalon D H and Lim K O. 1998. A controlled study of cortical gray matter and ventricular changes in alcoholic men over a 5-year interval. *Arch Gen Psychiatry* **55**, 905–12.

Pfefferbaum A, Sullivan E V, Rosenbloom M J, Shear P K, Mathalon D H and Lim K O. 1993. Increase in brain cerebrospinal fluid volume is greater in older than in younger alcoholic patients: A replication study and CT/MRI comparison. *Psychiatry Res* **50**, 257–74.

Pfefferbaum A, Zatz L M and Jernigan T L. 1986. Computer-interactive method for quantifying cerebrospinal fluid and tissue in brain CT scans: Effects of aging. *J Comput Assist Tomogr* **10**, 571–8.

Phillips S C, Harper C G and Kril J. 1987. A quantitative histological study of the cerebellar vermis in alcoholic patients. *Brain* **110**, 301–14.

Pitel A L, Beaunieux H, Witkowski T, *et al.* 2007. Genuine episodic memory deficits and executive dysfunctions in alcoholic subjects early in abstinence. *Alcohol Clin Exp Res* **31**, 1169–78.

Porjesz B and Rangaswamy M. 2007. Neurophysiological endophenotypes, CNS disinhibition, and risk for alcohol dependence and related disorders. *Sci World J* **7**, 131–41.

Rakic P. 2002. Neurogenesis in adult primates. *Prog Brain Res* **138**, 3–14.

Reed R J, Grant I and Rourke S B. 1992. Long-term abstinent alcoholics have normal memory. *Alcohol Clin Exp Res* **16**, 677–83.

Regier D A, Farmer M E, Rae D S, *et al.* 1990. Comorbidity of mental disorders with alcohol and other drug abuse. Results from the Epidemiologic Catchment Area (ECA) Study. *JAMA* **264**, 2511–8.

Ridler K, Veijola J M, Tanskanen P, *et al.* 2006. Fronto-cerebellar systems are associated with infant motor and adult executive functions in healthy adults but not in schizophrenia. *Proc Natl Acad Sci USA* **103**, 15 651–6.

Riley J N and Walker D W. 1978. Morphological alterations in hippocampus after long-term alcohol consumption in mice. *Science* **201**, 646–8.

Rohlfing T, Sullivan E V and Pfefferbaum A. 2006. Deformation-based brain morphometry to track the course of alcoholism: Differences between intra-subject and inter-subject analysis. *Psychiatry Res* **146**, 157–70.

Ron M A, Acker W, Shaw G K and Lishman W A. 1982. Computerized tomography of the brain in chronic alcoholism: A survey and follow-up study. *Brain* **105**, 497–514.

Rosenbloom M J and Pfefferbaum A. 2008. Magnetic resonance imaging of the living brain: Evidence for brain degeneration among alcoholics and recovery with abstinence. *Alcohol Res Hlth* **31**, 362–76.

Rosenbloom M J, Pfefferbaum A and Sullivan E V. 2004. Recovery of short-term memory and psychomotor speed but not postural stability with long-term sobriety in alcoholic women. *Neuropsychology* **18**, 589–97.

Rosenbloom M J, Rohlfing T, O'Reilly A W, Sassoon S A, Pfefferbaum A and Sullivan E V. 2007. Improvement in memory and static balance with abstinence in alcoholic men and women: Selective relations with change in brain structure. *Psychiatry Res* **155**, 91–102.

Rourke S B and Grant I. 1999. The interactive effects of age and length of abstinence on the recovery of neuropsychological functioning in chronic male alcoholics: A 2-year follow-up study. *J Int Neuropsychol Soc* **5**, 234–46.

Schmahmann J D. 2004. Disorders of the cerebellum: Ataxia, dysmetria of thought, and the cerebellar cognitive affective syndrome. *J Neuropsychiatry Clin Neurosci* **16**, 367–78.

Schmahmann J D and Pandya D N. 1997. Anatomic organization of the basilar pontine projections from prefrontal cortices in rhesus monkey. *J Neurosci* **17**, 438–58.

Schottenbauer M A, Momenan R, Kerick M and Hommer D W. 2007. Relationships among aging, IQ, and intracranial volume in alcoholics and control subjects. *Neuropsychology* **21**, 337–45.

Schroth G, Naegele T, Klose U, Mann K and Petersen D. 1988. Reversible brain shrinkage in abstinent alcoholics, measured by MRI. *Neuroradiology* **30**, 385–9.

Schroth G, Remmes U and Schupmann A. 1985. Computed tomographic follow-up of brain volume fluctuations before and after alcohol withdrawal treatment. *Rofo* **142**, 363–9.

Schuckit M A, Anthenelli R M, Bucholz K K, Hesselbrock V M and Tipp J. 1995. The time course of development of alcohol-related problems in men and women. *J Stud Alcohol* **56**, 218–25.

Schuckit M A, Daeppen J B, Tipp J E, Hesselbrock M and Bucholz K K. 1998. The clinical course of alcohol-related problems in alcohol dependent and nonalcohol dependent drinking women and men. *J Stud Alcohol* **59**, 581–90.

Schuckit M A, Danko G P and Smith T L. 2004. Patterns of drug-related disorders in a prospective study of men chosen for their family history of alcoholism. *J Stud Alcohol* **65**, 613–20.

Schulte T, Pfefferbaum A and Sullivan E V. 2004. Parallel interhemispheric processing in aging and alcoholism: Relation to corpus callosum size. *Neuropsychologia* **42**, 257–71.

Schulte T, Sullivan E V, Muller-Oehring E M, Adalsteinsson E and Pfefferbaum A. 2005. Corpus callosal microstructural integrity influences interhemispheric processing: A diffusion tensor imaging study. *Cereb Cortex* **15**, 1384–92.

Shear P K, Jernigan T L and Butters N. 1994. Volumetric magnetic resonance imaging quantification of longitudinal brain changes in abstinent alcoholics. *Alcohol Clin Exp Res* **18**, 172–6.

Shear P K, Sullivan E V, Lane B and Pfefferbaum A. 1996. Mammillary body and cerebellar shrinkage in chronic alcoholics with and without amnesia. *Alcohol Clin Exp Res* **20**, 1489–95.

Sheedy D, Lara A, Garrick T and Harper C. 1999. Size of mamillary bodies in health and disease: Useful measurements in neuroradiological diagnosis of Wernicke's encephalopathy. *Alcohol Clin Exp Res* **23**, 1624–8.

Shimamura A P, Jernigan T L and Squire L R. 1988. Korsakoff's syndrome: Radiological (CT) findings and neuropsychological correlates. *J Neurosci* **8**, 4400–10.

Smith M A, Chick J, Kean D M, *et al.* 1985. Brain water in chronic alcoholic patients measured by magnetic resonance imaging. *Lancet* **1**, 1273–4.

Sowell E R, Thompson P M, Mattson S N, *et al.* 2001. Voxel-based morphometric analyses of the brain in children and adolescents prenatally exposed to alcohol. *Neuroreport* **12**, 515–23.

Squire L R, Amaral D G and Press G A. 1990. Magnetic resonance imaging of the hippocampal formation and mammillary nuclei distinguish medial temporal lobe and diencephalic amnesia. *J Neurosci* **10**, 3106–17.

Stafford J L, Albert M S, Naeser M A, Sandor T and Garvey A J. 1988. Age-related differences in computed tomographic scan measurements. *Arch Neurol* **45**, 409–15.

Sullivan E V. 2003. Compromised pontocerebellar and cerebellothalamocortical systems: Speculations on their contributions to cognitive and motor impairment in nonamnesic alcoholism. *Alcohol Clin Exp Res* **27**, 1409–19.

Sullivan E V, Deshmukh A, De Rosa E, Rosenbloom M J and Pfefferbaum A. 2005a. Striatal and forebrain nuclei volumes: Contribution to motor function and working memory deficits in alcoholism. *Biol Psychiatry* **57**, 768–76.

Sullivan E V, Deshmukh A, Desmond J E, Lim K O and Pfefferbaum A. 2000a. Cerebellar volume decline in normal aging, alcoholism, and Korsakoff's syndrome: Relation to ataxia. *Neuropsychology* **14**, 341–52.

Sullivan E V, Deshmukh A, Desmond J E, *et al.* 2000b. Contribution of alcohol abuse to cerebellar volume deficits in men with schizophrenia. *Arch Gen Psychiatry* **57**, 894–902.

Sullivan E V, Harding A J, Pentney R, *et al.* 2003. Disruption of frontocerebellar circuitry and function in alcoholism. *Alcohol Clin Exp Res* **27**, 301–09.

Sullivan E V, Lane B, Deshmukh A, *et al.* 1999. In vivo mammillary body volume deficits in amnesic and nonamnesic alcoholics. *Alcohol Clin Exp Res* **23**, 1629–36.

Sullivan E V and Marsh L. 2003. Hippocampal volume deficits in alcoholic Korsakoff's syndrome. *Neurology* **61**, 1716–9.

Sullivan E V, Marsh L, Mathalon D H, Lim K O and Pfefferbaum A. 1995. Anterior hippocampal volume deficits in nonamnesic, aging chronic alcoholics. *Alcohol Clin Exp Res* **19**, 110–22.

Sullivan E V, Marsh L, Mathalon D H, Lim K O and Pfefferbaum A. 1996. Relationship between alcohol withdrawal seizures and temporal lobe white matter volume deficits. *Alcohol Clin Exp Res* **20**, 348–54.

Sullivan E V, Marsh L, and Pfefferbaum A. 2005b. Preservation of hippocampal volume throughout adulthood in healthy men and women. *Neurobiol Aging* **26**, 1093–8.

Sullivan E V and Pfefferbaum A. 2001. Magnetic resonance relaxometry reveals central pontine abnormalities in clinically asymptomatic alcoholic men. *Alcohol Clin Exp Res* **25**, 1206–12.

Sullivan E V and Pfefferbaum A. 2003. Diffusion tensor imaging in normal aging and neuropsychiatric disorders. *Eur J Radiol* **45**, 244–55.

Sullivan E V and Pfefferbaum A. 2005. Neurocircuitry in alcoholism: A substrate of disruption and repair. *Psychopharmacology (Berl)* **180**, 583–94.

Sullivan E V and Pfefferbaum A. (2009). Neuroimaging of the Wernicke Korsakoff Syndrome. *Alcohol Alcohol* **44**, 155–65.

Sullivan E V, Rose J and Pfefferbaum A. 2006. Effect of vision, touch and stance on cerebellar vermian-related sway and tremor: A quantitative physiological and MRI study. *Cereb Cortex* **16**, 1077–86.

Sullivan E V, Rosenbloom M J, Lim K O and Pfefferbaum A. 2000c. Longitudinal changes in cognition, gait, and balance in abstinent and relapsed alcoholic men: Relationships to changes in brain structure. *Neuropsychology* **14**, 178–88.

Sullivan E V, Rosenbloom M J, and Pfefferbaum A. 2000d. Pattern of motor and cognitive deficits in detoxified alcoholic men. *Alcohol Clin Exp Res* **24**, 611–21.

Sullivan E V and Zahr N M. 2008. Neuroinflammation as a neurotoxic mechanism in alcoholism: Commentary on "Increased MCP-1 and microglia in various regions of human alcoholic brain". *Exp Neurol* **213**, 10–7.

Thomson A D. 2000. Mechanisms of vitamin deficiency in chronic alcohol misusers and the development of the Wernicke–Korsakoff syndrome. *Alcohol Alcohol Suppl* **35**, 2–7.

To S E and Vega C P. 2006. Alcoholism and pathways to recovery: New survey results on views and treatment options. *Med Gen Med* **8**, 2.

Torvik A, Lindboe C F and Rogde S. 1982. Brain lesions in alcoholics. A neuropathological study with clinical correlations. *J Neurol Sci* **56**, 233–48.

Torvik A and Torp S. 1986. The prevalence of alcoholic cerebellar atrophy. A morphometric and histological study of an autopsy material. *J Neurol Sci* **75**, 43–51.

Venkatasubramanian G, Anthony G, Reddy U S, Reddy V V, Jayakumar P N and Benegal V. 2007. Corpus callosum abnormalities associated with greater externalizing behaviors in subjects at high risk for alcohol dependence. *Psychiatry Res* **156**, 209–15.

Victor M, Adams R D and Mancall E L. 1959. A restricted form of cerebellar degeneration occurring in alcohol patients. *Arch Neurol* **1**, 577–688.

Victor M A, Adams R D and Collins G H. 1989. *The Wernicke–Korsakoff syndrome*. Philadelphia, PA: F.A. Davis Company.

Vornik L A and Brown E S. 2006. Management of comorbid bipolar disorder and substance abuse. *J Clin Psychiatry*, **67** (Suppl 7), 24–30.

Walker D W, Barnes D E, Zornetzer S F, Hunter B E and Kubanis P. 1980. Neuronal loss in hippocampus induced by prolonged ethanol consumption in rats. *Science* **209**, 711–3.

Wang G J, Volkow N D, Roque C T, *et al.* 1993. Functional importance of ventricular enlargement and cortical atrophy in healthy subjects and alcoholics as assessed with PET, MR imaging, and neuropsychologic testing. *Radiology* **186**, 59–65.

Whitfield J B, Zhu G, Madden P A, Neale M C, Heath A C and Martin N G. 2004. The genetics of alcohol intake and of alcohol dependence. *Alcohol Clin Exp Res* **28**, 1153–60.

Wilens T E and Upadhyaya H P. 2007. Impact of substance use disorder on ADHD and its treatment. *J Clin Psychiatry* **68**, e20.

Wilhelm J, Frieling H, Hillemacher T, Degner D, Kornhuber J and Bleich S. 2008. Hippocampal volume loss in patients with alcoholism is influenced by the consumed type of alcoholic beverage. *Alcohol Alcohol* **43**, 296–9.

Wrase J, Makris N, Braus D F, *et al.* 2008. Amygdala volume associated with alcohol abuse relapse and craving. *Am J Psychiatry* **165**, 1179–84.

Yeh P H, Gazdzinski S, Durazzo T C, Sjostrand K and Meyerhoff D J. 2007. Hierarchical linear modeling (HLM) of longitudinal brain structural and cognitive changes in alcohol-dependent individuals during sobriety. *Drug Alcohol Depend* **91**, 195–204.

Zipursky R B, Lim K C and Pfefferbaum A. 1989. MRI study of brain changes with short-term abstinence from alcohol. *Alcohol Clin Exp Res* **13**, 664–6.

Chapter 30

Functional imaging of substance abuse

Omar M. Mahmood and Susan F. Tapert

Introduction

Overview of substance abuse

Substance use disorders (SUD; substance abuse or dependence) are prevalent in both adult and adolescent populations. It is estimated that 8% of the US population aged 12 and older currently uses some form of illicit drug, and that this percentage is slightly higher among youths aged 12–17 (9.5%) (Substance Abuse and Mental Health Services Administration (SAMHSA), 2008). The most commonly used substance is alcohol, and the most frequently used illicit drug is cannabis, followed by non-prescribed medications, cocaine, methamphetamines, and hallucinogens. Given their prevalence and deleterious physical, psychosocial, and financial effects, SUDs have become a major focus of research, with a particular recent emphasis on elucidating the mechanisms of addiction-related dysfunction and implications for treatment.

SUDs, as defined in the DSM-IV, include substance dependence and substance abuse. *Substance dependence* refers to recurrent use of a substance resulting in a clinically impairing pattern of repeatedly experiencing at least 3 of the following 7 criteria within a 12-month period: (1) tolerance; (2) use to relieve withdrawal; (3) using larger amounts or for more time than intended; (4) inability to cut down or quit; (5) spending excessive time obtaining, using, or recovering from the substance; (6) giving up important activities due to the substance use; and (7) continued use despite negative consequences, such as in medical or psychological health. *Substance abuse* refers to recurrent use of a substance, also resulting in a clinically impairing pattern, but repeatedly experiencing at least 1 of the following 4 criteria within a 12-month period: (1) an inability to fulfill

major role obligations in a work, school, or home environment; (2) use in physically hazardous situations (e.g. driving while intoxicated); (3) legal problems; or (4) a failure to stop using despite significant social or interpersonal problems caused by the substance abuse (American Psychiatric Association, 1994). Substance abuse is a less severe diagnosis, and can only be met if substance dependence was never present. In 2007, an estimated 22.3 million people in the United States met criteria for substance abuse or dependence according to DSM-IV classifications (SAMHSA, 2008).

Overview of functional magnetic resonance imaging (fMRI)

By detecting changes in arterial blood flow correlated with cognitive functioning, fMRI studies have been particularly useful in identifying patterns of regional brain activity that are specific to SUDs. The signal changes detected and analyzed during an fMRI experiment correspond to blood oxygen level-dependent (BOLD) differences that indicate where neural activity is localized in the brain. Typically, researchers use fMRI to compare differences in activation between substance using and healthy control groups during performance of an identical cognitive task. As we will review here, fMRI studies have found relationships between brain activation patterns and long-term cognitive consequences of using different intoxicating substances. In addition, fMRI has been used to understand the neural substrates of reward systems in substance abusers, and to evaluate susceptibility to relapse and other markers of treatment outcome. What follows is a review of fMRI studies in various SUDs. Unless

Understanding Neuropsychiatric Disorders, ed. M. E. Shenton and B. I. Turetsky. Published by Cambridge University Press.

otherwise noted, all of the studies described include participants with a history of SUD who were abstinent at the time of participation.

> **Box 30.1. Overview of this chapter**
>
> - This chapter will provide a summary of work using fMRI to evaluate (1) cognitive functioning, (2) cue reactivity and reward processing, and (3) neural predictors of treatment outcome in individuals with substance abuse or dependence. Peer-reviewed fMRI studies have now been published on individuals with dependence or abuse of alcohol, cannabis, cocaine, methamphetamine, MDMA, and nicotine.
> - Studies selected for review here include participants who met diagnostic criteria for DSM-IV substance dependence or abuse, or who demonstrated a recurrent and regular pattern of use, utilize BOLD fMRI techniques, and have at least 6 subjects per group. The majority of the studies compared users to a control group of healthy non-users. Participants' duration of abstinence at the time of scanning was characterized. Studies solely designed to examine the acute effects of substances on neural and cognitive functioning were not included in this review.

Alcohol

Alcohol use disorder (AUD; DSM-IV alcohol abuse or dependence) is associated with widespread volume loss in the brain and cortical gray and white matter abnormalities, with particular vulnerability in the prefrontal and frontal regions (Pfefferbaum *et al.*, 1997), as well as impairments in visuospatial functioning, memory, balance, speeded processing, and aspects of executive functioning (Rosenbloom *et al.*, 2007). To probe neural systems subserving these cognitive deficits, Pfefferbaum and colleagues administered a spatial working memory task to adult men with and without AUD in an fMRI paradigm (Pfefferbaum *et al.*, 2001). They found that non-drinking controls exhibited a pattern of brain activation in frontal regions and the dorsal "Where" stream that are typically activated during visuospatial processing tasks, whereas men with AUD exhibited decreased frontal activation and more activation of the ventral "What" stream during performance of the task. As groups did not differ on task accuracy, the authors concluded that the atypical patterns of activation seen in the AUD group suggested the employment of an

inappropriate strategy and functional reorganization of brain systems causing alternative neural pathways to execute the task, because the optimal network had been compromised (Pfefferbaum *et al.*, 2001). Similar results were found when a spatial working memory task was administered during fMRI scanning to young women with a history of AUD and age-matched controls (Tapert *et al.*, 2001). Young women with AUD also demonstrated decreased activation in prefrontal and parietal regions associated with spatial memory functioning, indicating that the adverse impact of alcohol on neural systems may be observable in young adulthood.

In an fMRI study of verbal working memory in chronic alcoholism, individuals with AUD and healthy controls once again demonstrated equivalent performances on the task while exhibiting differences in brain activation (Desmond *et al.*, 2003). While AUD individuals produced a pattern of activation in the left frontal lobe and right cerebellar regions that is expected in verbal working memory processing, they demonstrated greater levels of activation in those regions compared to healthy controls. This finding of increased activation along with more bilateral activation across the brain was suggested to reflect a compensatory response required for individuals with AUD to maintain the same level of performance compared to controls (Desmond *et al.*, 2003).

Adolescents with AUD have been found to exhibit abnormal patterns of brain activation that suggest both reorganization of neural systems and increased compensatory responses as a result of subtle alcohol-related neuronal injury (Tapert *et al.*, 2004b). While performing a spatial working memory task, adolescents with AUD produced an overall pattern of activation that was consistent with expected spatial memory systems. However, this pattern was characterized by less brain response in bilateral cerebellar and left precentral gyrus regions yet more response in bilateral parietal regions than healthy control adolescents evidenced. Further, greater *recent* alcohol use was linked to increased activation, while heavier levels of *lifetime* drinking were linked to particularly low activation in frontal and cerebellar regions. In contrast to these working memory-related differences, adolescents with AUD did not show any divergence in activation from non-drinkers on a simple finger tapping task, suggesting that neural abnormalities may be constrained to cognitive challenges. These findings indicated that even with relatively brief histories of heavy drinking (1–2 years), abnormal brain functioning related to alcohol use is detectable as early as adolescence (Tapert *et al.*, 2004b).

Several fMRI studies have investigated neural response in individuals with AUD when reacting to alcohol-related stimuli. In such studies, the functional brain activity in persons with AUD and healthy controls is compared as the two groups are presented with salient cues (often visual) that are known to elicit craving for alcohol. By studying "cue reactivity" (a conditioned physiological and cognitive response to drug cues) in an fMRI environment, researchers are able to learn more about the neural substrates of reward systems that are thought to maintain addictive behaviors.

The first study of cue reactivity using fMRI and visually presented alcohol stimuli was conducted by George and colleagues (2001). Compared to social drinkers, adults with alcohol dependence exhibited increased activation in the left prefrontal cortex and the anterior thalamus in response to pictures of alcoholic beverages versus non-alcoholic beverages. A similar finding of increased activation in the dorsolateral prefrontal cortex in response to images of alcoholic versus non-alcoholic beverages was found in a pilot study of six adults with AUD, and additional activation was observed in the ventral striatum, anterior cingulate, and orbitofrontal gyrus (Wrase *et al.*, 2002). The authors suggested that in addition to the attention and working memory functioning supported by the prefrontal regions, the reaction to salient alcohol cues elicited activation of the brain's reward system, particularly the anterior cingulate (which is associated with reward-based decision making) and the ventral striatum (which includes the nucleus accumbens, an essential structure in reinforcing pleasurable and rewarding behavior; Wrase *et al.*, 2002). In adolescents and young adults with AUD, many of the same brain systems show increased response to alcohol cues, as compared to healthy controls (Tapert *et al.*, 2003, 2004a). When presented with visual alcohol-related stimuli, adolescents with AUD demonstrated significantly more activation in widespread frontal regions, particularly in the left hemisphere, as well as in a network of areas associated with reward and drug craving (anterior cingulate, subcallosal cortex/nucleus accumbens, and limbic regions; Tapert *et al.*, 2003). Notably, young women with a history of alcohol dependence exhibited a more restricted pattern of activation in left frontal and

limbic regions during visual presentation of alcohol-related words, which may not have elicited as much cue reactivity as pictoral stimuli (Tapert *et al.*, 2004a). In a study that investigated cue reactivity in AUD adults while simultaneously measuring subjective ratings of alcohol craving, the reward pathways seen in previous studies (i.e. anterior cingulate, nucleus accumbens, limbic regions) were again activated in response to visual alcohol cues (Myrick *et al.*, 2004). The authors also found that in addition to the anterior cingulate and nucleus accumbens, real time subjective craving ratings correlated with activation in the left orbitofrontal cortex (Myrick *et al.*, 2004).

In a study of brain response to an olfactory cue (ethanol odor) in alcohol-dependent adults who recently completed detoxification compared to healthy controls, Schneider and colleagues found increased activation in limbic regions (right amygdala/hippocampal area), the superior temporal gyrus, and the cerebellum among alcohol dependent patients (Schneider *et al.*, 2001). Following three weeks of inpatient psychiatric day treatment and cognitive behavioral group therapy focused on alcohol-related problems, alcohol-dependent patients reported significantly reduced craving in response to ethanol odor, and their neural response no longer included increased activation of the limbic regions or the cerebellum. The authors concluded that this change in brain activation following treatment reflected the reduction in craving that is related to emotional reactions supported by the amygdala and learned memory associations supported in part by the cerebellum (Schneider *et al.*, 2001).

Interestingly, fMRI studies can provide unique insights into the effects of treatment for alcohol-related disorders and clinical outcomes for patients. Grüsser and colleagues found that the intensity of brain activation in the anterior cingulate, medial prefrontal cortex and striatum in response to visual alcohol cues predicted subsequent relapse in abstinent AUD individuals (Grüsser *et al.*, 2004). Similar patterns of reward system activation were found in a study that compared activation in adults with and without AUD in response to alcohol versus non-alcohol stimuli and affectively positive versus affectively negative stimuli (Heinz *et al.*, 2007). Although the increased neural response of reward systems to alcohol stimuli did not predict later drinking, greater response in the ventral striatum and thalamus during presentation of non-alcohol affectively positive images was associated with a *lower* relapse risk (Heinz *et al.*, 2007). These clinically useful studies show how fMRI can assess vulnerabilities in patients with AUD, thus helping to optimize interventions.

Studying the neural response to emotional stimuli among AUD individuals provides an understanding of the affective and behavioral dysfunction that is frequently associated with heavy alcohol use. When asked to determine the intensity of various facial expressions, AUD individuals did not differ from healthy controls in accurately decoding emotional intensity (Salloum *et al.*, 2007). However, the alcohol group exhibited less activation than controls in the rostral anterior cingulate cortex when processing negative emotional stimuli (i.e. faces depicting sadness, fear, and disgust). The authors suggested that the observed dysfunction of the affective division of the anterior cingulate reflected the deficits among AUD individuals in integrating emotional and cognitive information that can lead to misinterpretations of social interaction. Gilman and Hommer (2008) presented AUD adults and healthy controls with images designed to arouse positive and negative emotional responses while simultaneously presenting images of alcoholic and non-alcoholic beverages. In the absence of an alcohol cue, AUD individuals showed greater activation to negative images than the control group in the parahippocampal gyrus, lingual gyrus, and the inferior occipital gyrus. When negative images were presented in conjunction with an alcohol cue, AUD individuals exhibited a decrease in activation, particularly in parahippocampal regions, and demonstrated an overall pattern of activity similar to that of controls. The authors concluded that these neural responses underscored the tendency of individuals with AUD to consume alcohol for the effect of blunting the impact of pain or fear emotions.

Cannabis

There is conflicting evidence about whether heavy, chronic use of cannabis is related to structural brain damage (see Quickfall and Crockford, 2006, for a review). Most studies have found no differences between cannabis users and non-users, although some evidence suggests reduced gray matter volumes in parahippocampal regions (Matochik *et al.*, 2005). In functional neuroimaging studies, abstinent cannabis users tend to show global decreases in brain activation compared to control groups, with decreased blood

flow observed in the frontal lobes (Lundqvist *et al.*, 2001), anterior cingulate (Pillay *et al.*, 2004), and the cerebellum (Block *et al.*, 2000). Neuropsychological studies of the residual effects of cannabis have shown deficits in executive functioning (Pope and Yurgelun-Todd, 1996), attention (Solowij *et al.*, 1995), and learning and memory (Solowij and Battisti, 2008) that tend to remit after a month of abstinence in adult users (Pope *et al.*, 2001), but may not in adolescent users (Medina *et al.*, 2007).

Depending on the cognitive task administered, fMRI studies have found that chronic marijuana use is associated with altered brain activation across various neural networks that may be attributable to the widespread distribution of cannabinoid receptors in the brain (Chang and Chronicle, 2007). When heavy cannabis users were compared to controls during performance of a spatial working memory task, they demonstrated increased functional activity in the prefrontal cortex and anterior cingulate (areas associated with spatial working memory), as well as additional activation of the putamen and caudate nucleus (areas thought to have been recruited to compensate for subtle neural deficits) (Kanayama *et al.*, 2004). A similar finding was seen in adolescents, where spatial working memory performance correlated with activation in an expected network supporting spatial perception and working memory (medial prefrontal cortex and bilateral superior parietal regions; Schweinsburg *et al.*, 2008). When compared to non-users, adolescent cannabis users exhibited increased activation in the right superior parietal lobule yet diminished activation in the right dorsolateral prefrontal cortex. Thus, a history of heavy cannabis use during adolescence may have resulted in a reorganization of neural networks characterized by a weakened capacity to rely on executive functioning and a heavier reliance on spatial rehearsal and attentional networks (see Figure 30.1) (Schweinsburg *et al.*, 2008). This compensatory increase of parietal involvement during performance of a spatial working memory task was replicated in another study that also found a positive relationship between adolescent cannabis users' performance and activation in the left temporal lobe, suggesting the employment of a non-optimal verbal strategy that was not seen in non-users (Padula *et al.*, 2007).

Visually tracking and attending to moving stimuli activated a visual attention network (dorsal medial and lateral prefrontal cortex, parietal cortices, and

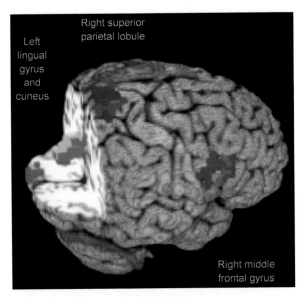

Figure 30.1 Spatial working memory related activation in adolescent cannabis ($n = 15$) users was greater (clusters > 1328 µl, $p < 0.05$) in the right superior parietal lobule (shown here in blue), yet diminished in the right dorsolateral prefrontal regions (shown here in orange), as compared to demographically similar non-users ($n = 17$), suggesting that a history of heavy cannabis use during adolescence may be linked to a reorganization of neural networks characterized by a weakened capacity to rely on executive functioning and heavier reliance on spatial rehearsal and attentional networks (Schweinsburg et al., 2008).

occipital regions) in both cannabis users and non-using controls (Chang et al., 2006). However, among cannabis users, functional activity was relatively weak in these areas, while small regions of activation were observed in frontal, parietal, and temporal cortices that were not present among the controls. The investigators concluded that these differences represented neuroadaptive changes in response to heavy cannabis use (Chang et al., 2006). During performance of an auditory working memory (n-back) task, controls and tobacco-smoking individuals demonstrated a deactivation of the hippocampus across trials that was not exhibited by cannabis users (Jacobsen et al., 2004b). A visual working memory task that required participants to memorize target items (a group of letters) and then decide whether items presented in subsequent trials matched any of the target items elicited a consistent network of activation in cannabis users and non-users (with no differences in the response seen in the anterior cingulate and dorsolateral prefrontal cortex; Jager et al., 2006). However, the authors hypothesized that a greater magnitude of activation observed in the superior parietal regions of cannabis

users' brains suggested that the task demands placed a higher neurophysiological burden on individuals with a history of frequent cannabis use (Jager et al., 2006). A combination of diminished neural function and compensatory hyperactivity during performance of a visual working memory task was observed in an early study by Yurgelun-Todd and colleagues (1999). The authors found that cannabis users exhibited reductions in blood flow to the dorsolateral prefrontal cortex compared to non-users, but increased activation of the anterior cingulate cortex.

Changes in neural processing following long-term, heavy cannabis use have also been found in a number of studies of learning and memory function (Solowij and Battisti, 2008). Nestor and colleagues found that during learning and recall of face–number pairs, cannabis users showed reduced activation in superior and middle frontal regions that suggested an inefficiency in frontally mediated associative learning (Nestor et al., 2008). Although they did not differ in memory performance from the control group, cannabis users exhibited greater activation of the parahippocampal regions that was interpreted as a compensatory shift in neural functioning required to maintain normal memory formation. This finding is in conflict with another study that demonstrated decreased parahippocampal response in cannabis users during a picture-pairing task (Jager et al., 2007). These discrepancies may reflect differences in task demands between the recognition memory paradigm of the picture-pairing task and the memory retrieval required for the picture–number recall task used by Nestor and colleagues.

In a study of verbal memory functioning that examined the interaction between the effects of cannabis use and nicotine withdrawal, adolescent cannabis users and non-users with concomitant tobacco addiction were compared on list-learning abilities and verbal working memory during smoking deprivation and ad-lib smoking conditions (Jacobsen et al., 2007b). When deprived of nicotine, the abstinent cannabis users demonstrated deficits in delayed recall of verbal stimuli that improved when they were allowed to smoke tobacco. In contrast, the control group showed no difference in verbal memory between nicotine withdrawal and ad-lib smoking. During performance of a verbal working memory task in an fMRI environment, nicotine withdrawal elicited increased activation of a network involved in phonological processing and working memory function (inferior parietal cortex, superior temporal gyrus, posterior cingulate gyrus, and the right hippocampus) in cannabis users, but the same effect was not found in the control group. The findings suggested that heavy cannabis use during adolescence may have developmental effects on the neurocircuitry underlying verbal learning and memory that are unmasked in the context of nicotine withdrawal.

Inhibitory processing, a component of executive functioning, has been studied to a limited extent in fMRI investigations of heavy cannabis use. While performing a modified Stroop task that required participants to inhibit the over-learned process of reading a word and instead engage in a less automatic process of identifying the printed (incongruently) color of a word, cannabis users demonstrated less activation of the anterior cingulate but greater activation of mid cingulate regions compared to controls (Gruber and Yurgelun-Todd, 2005). In addition, cannabis users showed more diffuse activity in the bilateral dorsolateral prefrontal cortex compared to the focal, right-sided activation seen in the control group. This failure to strongly activate the anterior cingulate, which is implicated in normal executive functioning, along with the increased and bilateral activity in other cortical regions was interpreted as reflecting neural compensation and the adoption of alternative processing strategies (Gruber and Yurgelun-Todd, 2005). Inhibitory processing in adolescent cannabis users has been studied using a go–no-go task in which participants were asked to respond to most visual stimuli with a button press, and to inhibit their response when presented with a target stimulus (Tapert *et al.*, 2007). Compared to age-matched controls, adolescent users showed substantially greater activation in multiple cortical areas (particularly in dorsolateral prefrontal and parietal), indicating that cannabis users recruited additional neural resources to exert adequate executive control during an inhibition task (see Figure 30.2).

As demonstrated in the studies described, the effects of cannabis use on brain function persist even after periods of abstinence. However, the duration of abstinence may influence the nature of cannabis-related neural changes. Chang and colleagues found that longer periods of abstinence correlated with stronger activation in areas that were diminished in cannabis users, suggesting that with time, abstinent users experience a continued normalization of neural function (Chang *et al.*, 2006).

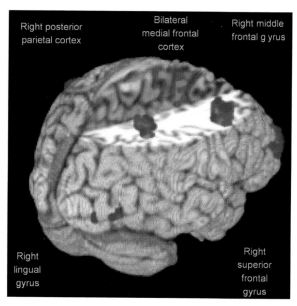

Figure 30.2 Inhibitory processing in adolescent cannabis users was studied using a go–no-go task, in which participants responded to most visual stimuli with a button press, but needed to inhibit responding when presented with a target stimulus. Compared to age-matched controls ($n = 17$), adolescent cannabis users ($n = 16$) showed substantially greater activation (clusters $> 943\ \mu l$, $p < 0.05$) in multiple cortical areas (shown here in blue), including dorsolateral prefrontal and parietal areas, indicating that cannabis users recruited additional neural resources to exert adequate executive control during an inhibition task (Tapert *et al.*, 2007).

Yurgelun-Todd and colleagues observed a similar normalization of cortical activity after 28 days of abstinence (Yurgelun-Todd *et al.*, 1999). Notably, cannabis users still exhibited functional abnormalities, and this persistence of neural response aberrancy has been found in other studies of users with the same duration (~1 month) of abstinence (Padula *et al.*, 2007; Pillay *et al.*, 2008; Schweinsburg *et al.*, 2008; Tapert *et al.*, 2007).

Methamphetamine and cocaine

Methamphetamine and cocaine, the two most commonly used illicit stimulant drugs (SAMHSA, 2008), have been found to cause long-term damage to dopaminergic pathways in the brain (Volkow *et al.*, 1993, 2001). Structural MRI reveals that chronic use of both stimulants is associated with decreased brain volumes in the anterior cingulate cortex as well as the medial temporal lobe region (Franklin *et al.*, 2002; Thompson *et al.*, 2004). In addition, cerebral blood flow abnormalities are detected in widespread cortical areas following a history of protracted stimulant use (Chang *et al.*, 2002; Strickland, 1993). Neuropsychological evidence indicates that stimulant dependent individuals exhibit deficits in executive functioning and learning and memory following 2–5 weeks of abstinence (Beatty *et al.*, 1995; Berry *et al.*, 1993; Scott *et al.*, 2007), with deficits in psychomotor speed and attention persisting even after 1 year of abstinence (Toomey *et al.*, 2003).

A number of neuroimaging studies have focused on the neural substrates of executive dysfunction in stimulant dependence. In a study of response inhibition using a go–no-go task, cocaine users demonstrated poorer inhibitory control compared to non-users (Kaufman *et al.*, 2003). An event-related fMRI study design allowed for analysis of successful inhibition trials, and found cocaine users to show reduced activity in the anterior cingulate cortex and right insula during response inhibition, as compared to non-users. Hypoactivity in the anterior cingulate region as well as right prefrontal cortex was demonstrated during another response inhibition task that also subjected participants to increasing working memory load (Hester and Garavan, 2004). In addition, the authors found that activation of the anterior cingulate remained constant in cocaine users with increasing levels of working memory load, whereas non-users exhibited a greater response in the same region in order to cope with increasing cognitive demand. Similar dysfunction of the frontal–executive systems has been observed in methamphetamine users as well. On a decision-making task, methamphetamine users tended to exhibit more stimulus-driven responses than non-users; and although overall patterns of activation were similar between both groups across various regions of the cortex, dorsolateral prefrontal and orbitofrontal regions were less active among methamphetamine users (Paulus *et al.*, 2002). A subsequent study found that methamphetamine users were less sensitive to the degree of their success or failure on the decision-making test compared to non-users, and this difference in processing information was associated with attenuated activation in the bilateral middle frontal gyrus (Paulus *et al.*, 2003). The authors posited that these findings elucidated the neural substrates of habit-based learning in stimulant dependence, in which users choose responses based on stimulus-driven experiences with little attention to the outcome's success.

Similar to alcohol research, a number of studies have investigated cue reactivity and craving in stimulant-dependent individuals. In one of the first fMRI studies of cue-induced craving in cocaine users, Garavan and colleagues found that users demonstrated an increase in activation across several brain regions (including prefrontal cortex, anterior and posterior cingulate, and bilateral parietal lobes) compared to non-using controls while viewing a film of cocaine cues (Garavan *et al.*, 2000). Exposure to a film of sexually evocative scenes elicited activation of a neural network that overlapped with craving-related activation. However, cocaine users exhibited greater activation in three areas (anterior cingulate, right inferior parietal lobule, and the caudate nucleus) when viewing cocaine cues compared to the sexual stimuli. These findings suggest that cocaine craving is supported by the same neural circuitry that is activated during processing of evocative and rewarding stimuli, and that chronic cocaine abuse may lead to a reorganization of the brain's reward pathways that alters natural emotional drives (Garavan *et al.*, 2000). Subjective reports of cocaine craving amongst users also correlate with this activation of dopaminergic reward pathways in limbic regions, anterior cingulate, and orbitofrontal cortex (Risinger *et al.*, 2005). After visual presentation of cocaine cues replicated the increased anterior cingulate activity seen in other studies, cocaine users who began to experience craving exhibited patterns of activation that mirrored the neural response seen in healthy controls during the viewing of emotionally sad stimuli (Wexler *et al.*, 2001). The investigators posited that, among users, there is a physiologic relationship between reaction to cocaine cues and neural activity associated with dysphoric states.

Given that drug craving is known to increase in times of emotional stress (Jaffe *et al.*, 1989), some researchers have used fMRI to explore the neural substrates of negative emotion in stimulant dependence. Goldstein and colleagues presented cocaine users with verbal drug cues and found that when participants rated the words with more negative emotional valence, they exhibited increased activation of the dorsal anterior cingulate cortex (Goldstein *et al.*, 2007). This may reflect the intrusive and negative nature of the cue-related thoughts that users encounter when experiencing craving. A similar hyperactivation of the dorsal anterior cingulate during exposure to pictures of fearful and angry faces was found in methamphetamine users when compared to non-using controls (Payer *et al.*, 2007). The authors suggested that these results indicated an over-sensitivity to negative cues that could underlie the socio-emotional disturbances frequently seen in stimulant-dependent individuals. In contrast to these findings, Sinha and colleagues found that guided imagery and recall of stressful situations in cocaine users was associated with decreased activation of the anterior cingulate cortex and parahippocampal regions as well as increased activation in the caudate nucleus and putamen, compared to non-using controls (Sinha *et al.*, 2005). This pattern of activation in cocaine-dependent individuals was interpreted as a failure to exert cognitive control and regulation of emotion during stressful experiences and a reliance upon automatic, habit-based compulsions supported by the dorsal striatum that may explain the potential for relapse behaviors during emotional stress.

To determine whether fMRI patterns of activation could predict relapse among methamphetamine users, Paulus and colleagues administered a two-choice decision-making task to recently abstinent users who were subsequently interviewed about relapse behavior one year later (Paulus *et al.*, 2005). The initial neural response patterns in the posterior cingulate, right insular, and temporal cortex correctly predicted individuals who relapsed and those who did not relapse. Methamphetamine users who relapsed exhibited decreased activation in a network of structures implicated in decision-making processes (insula, dorsolateral prefrontal, parietal, and temporal cortices). In contrast, when cocaine dependent individuals were exposed to drug cues in an fMRI study after a 2-week inpatient detoxification, increased activation in a network of brain regions (left precentral, superior temporal, posterior cingulate, right middle temporal, and lingual cortices) correlated with poorer treatment outcomes following 10 weeks of outpatient substance abuse treatment (Kosten *et al.*, 2006). The greater response to drug cues in sensory, motor, and limbic cortical areas observed in users who relapsed compared to those who did not may underlie a vulnerability to cocaine abuse relapse that can be identified in early abstinence.

Opioids

Prolonged dependence on opioid compounds is associated with a broad range of neuropathologic changes, but there is little evidence for major

anatomical abnormalities (see Büttner and colleagues, 2000, for a review). There are instances where the brains of opioid-dependent individuals contain hypoxic–ischemic changes, lesions, and abscesses; although these findings are frequently attributed to drug-induced respiratory problems, detrimental effects of adulterants mixed with the drug, or infections resulting from unsterile injections (Büttner *et al.*, 2000). Evidence from single photon emission computed tomography (SPECT) studies in adults with opioid dependence indicates cerebral perfusion defects in the frontal, parietal and temporal cortices that show partial improvement with prolonged abstinence (Rose *et al.*, 1996). Structural MRI has shown wider Sylvian fissures and enlarged ventricles in opioid-dependent patients compared to healthy non-users, suggesting some cerebral atrophy associated with chronic opioid use (Kivisaari *et al.*, 2004). Although most domains of neuropsychological functioning do not seem to be significantly impaired in opioid users, deficits in verbal fluency and cognitive flexibility have been observed, with evidence for recovery of cognitive ability during continued abstinence (Davis *et al.*, 2002).

In the first fMRI study of cognitive ability in opioid dependence, performance on a response inhibition task elicited diminished activation of the anterior cingulate cortex compared to healthy controls (Forman *et al.*, 2004). In addition, opioid-dependent individuals failed to exhibit a strong relationship between brain activation and error rate performance that was demonstrated in the control group. The authors concluded that this disruption in error-related anterior cingulate activity may contribute to behavioral impulsivity in opioid addiction. Similar findings were reported by Lee and colleagues, who suggested that, among heroin users, attenuated activity in the anterior cingulate region and the left inferior frontal gyrus during performance of a go–no-go task reflected inefficient self-monitoring and cognitive control (Lee *et al.*, 2005). Among non-users, a network of structures was activated during response inhibition (including the medial prefrontal cortex, the anterior cingulate cortex, the inferior frontal gyrus, and the insula) that showed marked hypo-activation among heroin users (Fu *et al.*, 2008). In a combined MR spectroscopy and event-related fMRI study that required participants to perform a target detection task while ignoring multiple sources of cognitive interference, opioid-dependent individuals exhibited increased task-related activation in frontal, parietal and cerebellar regions and reduced concentrations of N-acetylaspartate and glutamate/glutamine in the anterior cingulate cortex compared to healthy controls (Yücel et al., 2007). Replicating findings from previous studies, the investigators also found that an expected correlation between anterior cingulate activation and behavioral performance measures was not observed in the opioid-dependent group. Taken together, these findings indicate biochemical and physiological abnormalities of the anterior cingulate that may require the compensatory recruitment of fronto-parietal and cerebellar involvement in the attempt to exert inhibitory control following opioid addiction.

To compare drug craving induced by opioid cues to a naturalistic craving, Xiao and colleagues examined the neural response of abstinent heroin users who were temporarily deprived of water as they viewed drug-related and water-related cues (Xiao et al., 2006). They found that water-related cues elicited the expected activation in the anterior cingulate region, whereas the drug-related cues elicited activation in a broader network including the inferior frontal cortex, the fusiform gyrus, and the cerebellum. The findings suggested that opioid craving involves neural substrates that may differ from those supporting basic physiological drives. When undergoing a methadone treatment program, heroin addicts demonstrated a heightened response to drug-related cues compared to neutral cues across several brain areas (orbitofrontal cortex, anterior cingulate cortex, hippocampal regions, insula, and the right amygdala) just prior to receiving a daily methadone dose (Langleben et al., 2008). After receiving methadone, the users exhibited a decrease in activation in all areas previously sensitive to drug-related cues except for the anterior cingulate and the orbitofrontal cortices that suggested a continued vulnerability to craving even after receiving methadone treatment. In an interesting study of abstinent opioid users who were presented with drug-related and emotional cues, Xu and colleagues compared fMRI activation before and after administering electroacupuncture therapy to the participants (Xu et al., 2008). Prior to electroacupuncture, opioid users exhibited the expected heightened activation of various brain regions (dorsolateral frontal regions, anterior cingulate cortex, inferior/superior parietal lobule, and fusiform gyrus) in response to the drug-related cues compared to

emotional cues. However, after receiving electroacupuncture treatment, the opioid group demonstrated a decrease in activation associated with drug-related cues and a more normalized, increased neural response to the emotional cues.

MDMA

MDMA (3, 4-methylenedioxymethamphetamine) is a substance with complex pharmacological properties that can have a broad range of effects on the brain (see Cowan, 2007, for review). There are multiple preparations of MDMA (sometimes referred to as "Ecstasy") that result in numerous forms of the drug, each with slightly different chemical compositions (Tanner-Smith, 2006). MDMA use is associated with degeneration of serotonergic pathways characterized by global and regional reductions of serotonin receptor and reuptake transporter levels across subcortical and cortical regions (Cowan, 2007). Chronic MDMA users exhibit a range of mild to moderate cognitive deficits, with learning and memory showing the greatest impairment (Zakzanis et al., 2007).

While performing a working memory task, MDMA users demonstrated heightened activation of the prefrontal cortex, hippocampus, and basal ganglia compared to non-users (Moeller et al., 2004). This greater activation in a network of structures supporting working memory and sustained attention may have reflected an inefficient neural response among MDMA users. Another study using an n-back test of working memory had more equivocal findings (Daumann et al., 2003a). A conservative statistical threshold found no differences in brain activation between MDMA users and non-users. However, when a liberal criterion was applied, MDMA users exhibited increased activation in the right parietal cortex and decreased response in the left frontal and temporal regions. In a follow-up study, the investigators found that this parietal activation, which was directly related to higher doses of MDMA, was greater 18 months after baseline testing in individuals who continued to use MDMA compared to those who remained abstinent (Daumann et al., 2004).

To assess hippocampal functioning in MDMA use, Daumann and colleagues (2005) compared the neural response of users and non-users during performance of an encoding and retrieval task. They found that although both groups performed equally well on memory functioning, the MDMA users

437

displayed diminished and more spatially restricted activation in the left hippocampus compared to non-users. In contrast, adolescent MDMA users exhibited greater activation of the left hippocampus during a working memory task compared to age-matched controls (Jacobsen *et al.*, 2004a). In addition, longer durations of abstinence correlated with lower levels of activation in the hippocampus, suggesting a potential recovery of function with sustained abstinence from MDMA. These findings provide evidence for hippocampal dysfunction that may have resulted from the effects of MDMA toxicity on serotonergic neurons targeting the hippocampus.

Due to the high rates of polysubstance abuse among MDMA users, disentangling the cognitive and neural sequelae that are solely attributable to MDMA can pose some difficulties. Using regression analyses, Jager and colleagues (2008) assessed the independent effects of MDMA and other drugs while assessing neurocognitive function of polysubstance users. Of the three cognitive domains that were tested in an fMRI paradigm, two (working memory and attention) were unaffected by MDMA use, while the remaining domain (associative memory) showed impairment as a function of MDMA use that was correlated with lower activation of the left dorsolateral prefrontal cortex and increased activation of the right middle occipital gyrus. In a study investigating the effects of pure MDMA use on working memory, participants were grouped into three categories: MDMA users with no other substance use history, MDMA users with concomitant polysubstance use, and non-using controls (Daumann *et al.*, 2003b). Performance on a working memory task was equivalent in all three groups, but only the pure MDMA group showed decreased activation in the inferior temporal gyrus, the angular gyrus and the striate cortex compared to the other two groups. Taken together, these studies indicate MDMA use is associated with altered neural responses that can be uniquely attributed to MDMA toxicity but which may be modulated by the presence of polysubstance use.

Nicotine

Reward pathways in the brain are strongly activated by nicotine, which binds to receptors on dopaminergic cell bodies resulting in increased dopamine levels in the nucleus accumbens (Ray *et al.*, 2008). Structural

MRI studies of cigarette smokers have found smaller gray matter volumes in broad areas of the frontal lobe, occipital lobe, and medial temporal regions compared to non-smokers (Gallinat *et al.*, 2006). Importantly, many of the harmful neurological effects of cigarettes are not solely due to nicotine, but are also linked to the oxidative stress, inflammation, and atherosclerotic processes resulting from exposure to tobacco smoke (Swan and Lessov-Schlaggar, 2007). Although acute doses of nicotine have been shown to improve cognitive functioning (Potter and Newhouse, 2008), nicotine withdrawal is associated with slowed information processing, disruption of working memory, and other cognitive deficits (Blake and Smith, 1997; Snyder *et al.*, 1989).

While requiring smokers to perform an *n*-back working memory task with varying degrees of cognitive load, Xu and colleagues found that activity in the left dorsal lateral prefrontal cortex showed an expected increase with task difficulty when participants were allowed to smoke on the day of the experiment (Xu *et al.*, 2005). However, when participants were required to abstain from smoking for 14–16 h prior to testing, the same dorsal lateral prefrontal region maintained a heightened level of activation, regardless of task difficulty. This finding suggests that working memory processing was less efficient during abstinence from nicotine. A subsequent study by the same authors found that after a night of abstinence, smokers who were allowed a cigarette prior to testing exhibited a pattern of brain activation that resembled the neural response of healthy controls during a working memory task (Xu *et al.*, 2006). Similar to findings in adults, adolescent smokers performing a working memory task exhibit increased activation in left prefrontal cortex as well as left inferior parietal lobe following a period of abstinence (Jacobsen *et al.*, 2007a). Thus, the reduction in cortical efficiency associated with nicotine abstinence may develop fairly rapidly given that it is observable in adolescents who have been smoking cigarettes for far shorter durations than adult smokers. With as little as one hour of smoking deprivation, the neural effects of nicotine withdrawal have been observed in smokers performing a cognitive interference task that elicited greater activation in the right prefrontal cortex compared to an ad-lib smoking condition that allowed participants to smoke just prior to being tested (Xu *et al.*, 2007).

A number of studies have evaluated cue reactivity in nicotine-dependent individuals. Typically, abstinent smokers are presented with smoking-related visual cues (pictures, video, virtual environment simulation) that result in greater activation of visuospatial, attention, and reward circuitry compared to neutral cues (Brody *et al.*, 2007; David *et al.*, 2005; Due *et al.*, 2002; J. H. Lee *et al.*, 2005). The neural response to smoking cues has shown correlations with subjective reports of craving and expectancy to smoke (McBride *et al.*, 2006; McClernon *et al.*, 2005) and is sometimes moderated by gender and ethnicity (McClernon *et al.*, 2007; Okuyemi *et al.*, 2006). Despite the varying durations of abstinence in these studies, there is consistent evidence that cue-induced craving activates nicotine reward pathways involving prefrontal, anterior cingulate, and limbic regions.

Summary

fMRI studies conducted in the past decade have greatly expanded our understanding of how the chronic heavy use of alcohol and other drugs affect brain systems subserving cognitive functioning and reward processing, and have pointed toward neural features linked with the probability of favorable treatment response. Across alcohol, cannabis, stimulants, and opioids, we see that cognitive challenges such as working memory and executive control tasks tend to reveal activation patterns suggestive of neural compensation. That is, those with SUD may perform adequately on the task but tend to show some areas of less response (i.e. failure to engage) and other areas of greater response (i.e. compensation). Across substances, presentation of addiction-relevant cues evokes increased activation, particularly in reward (nucleus accumbens), limbic (amygdala), and the executive processing regions with strong limbic connections (e.g. prefrontal and anterior cingulate). During treatment, particularly high cue reactivity and particularly low response to cognitive or decision-making tasks has been linked to elevated risk for relapse. Differential results across substance types may pertain to sociodemographic factors, direct and indirect neurotoxic effects of use and withdrawal from each substance, and the long-term effects of each compound on cerebrovasculature. Please see Table 30.1 for a detailed presentation of findings from different fMRI paradigms across substances of abuse.

Several important methodological issues are critical for future studies in this area. First, polysubstance use is common, so studies either need to have multiple comparison groups (e.g. users of MDMA, users of the same substances taken by the MDMA users but no history of MDMA use, and non-users), or large samples and a careful collection of continuous measures of each drug class so that statistical covariation (including of potential interaction effects) can be employed. Second, the duration of abstinence at the time of the fMRI is critical to consider, as results could be attributed to intoxication, withdrawal, early recovery, or to long-term effects depending on how much time had elapsed since the most recent substance use. Related to this issue is verification of self-reported substance use, where multiple sources (e.g. self-report, collateral report, and biological confirmation) of data are recommended. Third, inferences about causality cannot be drawn from cross-sectional comparisons of users and non-users, as a multitude of features that predate the substance use (e.g. family history, prenatal substance exposure, traumatic brain injury, conduct disorder, inhibition deficits, mood disorders) may account for findings. Longitudinal studies are helpful for ascertaining whether changes in substance use are followed by changes in BOLD response patterns. Finally, most substances of abuse adversely affect cerebrovasculature, but through different mechanisms, and such compromise should be ruled out prior to drawing conclusions about observed BOLD response abnormalities.

> **Box 30.2. Summary points**
> - fMRI activation in SUD populations has been related to cognitive function, reward circuitry, and treatment response.
> - Despite normal performance on some cognitive tasks, individuals with SUD have shown a combination of weakened neural response in some brain areas, and an increased compensatory response in other areas.
> - Duration of abstinence at the time of neuroimaging can determine whether fMRI findings are associated with effects of intoxication, withdrawal, or chronic use.
> - Drug-induced changes in cerebrovasculature should be ruled out when investigating fMRI activation in substance abuse.

Acknowledgments

This work was made possible by grants from the National Institute on Drug Abuse (1R01 DA021182–03, 1 P20 DA024194–02) and the National Institute on Alcohol Abuse and Alcoholism (5R01 AA13419–07).

Table 30.1 Summary of fMRI studies on individuals with substance use disorders

Substance	Cognitive domain	Neural correlates	Findings
Alcohol	Spatial working memory	Frontal parietal pathways	Decreased activation of frontal regions (Pfefferbaum et al., 2001; Tapert et al., 2001, 2004a) and the dorsal "where" stream (Pfefferbaum et al., 2001; Rosenbloom et al., 2007) and increased activation of inferior regions/ventral "what" stream, reflecting the use of an alternative strategy/neural network (Pfefferbaum et al., 2001; Tapert et al., 2004a).
	Verbal working memory	Left frontal lobe, right cerebellum	Inefficient hyperactivation of verbal working memory circuitry, along with compensatory recruitment of widespread bilateral cortical areas (Desmond et al., 2003).
	Cue reactivity	Prefrontal cortex, ventral striatum, anterior cingulate	Heightened response of attention, working memory, and decision-making pathways specific to reward processing and reinforcement of pleasurable behavior (George et al., 2001; Tapert et al., 2003, 2004a; Wrase et al., 2002).
		Limbic regions	Increased activation of centers of emotional craving that impact learned associations (Myrick et al., 2004; Schneider et al., 2001; Tapert et al., 2003).
	Emotional responsiveness	Anterior cingulate	Decreased activation in a region important for integrating emotional and cognitive information (Salloum et al., 2007).
		Parahippocampal gyrus	Increased response to emotionally negative stimuli of the ventral "what" stream that returned to normal when alcohol cue was present (Gilman and Hommer, 2008).
Cannabis	Spatial working memory	Prefrontal cortex, anterior cingulate	Greater response in expected medial and frontal networks supporting task performance (Kanayama et al., 2004; Padula et al., 2007; Schweinsburg et al., 2008) with recruitment of additional cortical areas to compensate or support alternative strategies (Padula et al., 2007).
	Auditory working memory	Hippocampus	Dysfunctionally high activation during mnemonic processing (Jacobsen et al., 2004b).
	Visual working memory	Prefrontal cortex, anterior cingulate	Normal to diminished response of prefrontal regions with compensatory hyperactivation seen in the anterior cingulate (Yurgelun-Todd et al., 1999) and parietal regions (Jager et al., 2006) suggesting burdensome task demands.
	Learning and memory retrieval	Middle frontal and parahippocampal regions	Reduced activation in attentional networks during learning and heightened response in memory formation circuitry (Jacobsen et al., 2007b; Nestor et al., 2008).
	Recognition memory	Parahippocampal regions	Weakened response of memory circuitry (Jager et al., 2007).
	Executive control	Prefrontal cortex, anterior cingulate	Recruitment of bilateral, dorsolateral prefrontal and parietal cortical areas to achieve adequate performance; diminished activation of error monitoring (anterior cingulate) (Gruber and Yurgelun-Todd, 2005; Tapert et al., 2007).

Table 30.1 (cont.)

Substance	Cognitive domain	Neural correlates	Findings
Stimulants	Executive control	Anterior cingulate, insula, prefrontal cortex	Hypoactivation of frontal executive systems that is unable to adapt to changes in cognitive load (Hester and Garavan, 2004; Kaufman *et al.*, 2003; Paulus *et al.*, 2002) and correlates with poor planning (Paulus *et al.*, 2003) and increased relapse risk (Paulus *et al.*, 2005).
	Cue reactivity	Prefrontal cortex, anterior cingulate, parietal lobes	Hyperactivation of medial frontal attentional systems related to reward processing (Garavan *et al.*, 2000; Risinger *et al.*, 2005; Wexler *et al.*, 2001).
		Caudate nucleus, Limbic regions	Craving-related activation in areas overlapping with networks supporting sexual drive and emotion regulation (Garavan *et al.*, 2000; Risinger *et al.*, 2005; Wexler *et al.*, 2001).
	Emotional responsiveness	Anterior cingulate	Increased activation reflecting over-attentiveness to negative stimuli when viewing emotional cues (Goldstein *et al.*, 2007; Payer *et al.*, 2007).
			Decreased activation during stressful guided imagery reflecting failure to exert cognitive control (Sinha *et al.*, 2005).
Opioids	Executive control	Anterior cingulate, inferior frontal gyrus	Reduced activation of response inhibition networks (Forman *et al.*, 2004; Fu *et al.*, 2008; T. M. C. Lee *et al.*, 2005) resulting in compensatory recruitment of parietal and cerebellar regions (Yücel *et al.*, 2007).
	Cue reactivity	Anterior cingulate, orbitofrontal cortex, fusiform gyrus	Increased activation of craving circuitry in addition to broader involvement of multiple cortical regions (Langleben *et al.*, 2008; Xiao *et al.*, 2006; Xu *et al.*, 2008).
MDMA	Working memory	Prefrontal cortex, hippocampus	Heightened activation of sustained attention and working memory networks reflecting an inefficient neural response (Jacobsen *et al.*, 2004a; Moeller *et al.*, 2004).
		Temporal regions	Decreased activation possibly reflecting damage to serotonergic pathways (Daumann *et al.*, 2003a; 2003b).
	Learning and memory retrieval	Hippocampus, prefrontal cortex	Diminished activation of memory-formation circuitry (Daumann *et al.*, 2005; Jager *et al.*, 2008).
Nicotine	Working memory	Left prefrontal cortex	Increased activation of sustained attention circuitry suggesting inefficient neural response, even with reduced task difficulty (Jacobsen *et al.*, 2007a; Xu *et al.*, 2005).
	Executive control	Right prefrontal cortex	Greater activation when task performance requires filtering of interfering information (Xu *et al.*, 2007).
	Cue reactivity	Prefrontal cortex, anterior cingulate, limbic regions	Increased activation of visuospatial, attention, and reward circuitry (Brody *et al.*, 2007; David *et al.*, 2005; Due *et al.*, 2002; J. H. Lee *et al.*, 2005).

References

American Psychiatric Association. 1994. *DSM-IV: Diagnostic and Statistical Manual of Mental Disorders – 4th Edition.* Washington, DC: APA.

Beatty W W, Katzung V M, Moreland V J and Nixon S J. 1995. Neuropsychological performance of recently abstinent alcoholics and cocaine abusers. *Drug Alcohol Depend* **37**, 247–53.

Berry J, Van Gorp W G, Herzberg D S, *et al.* 1993. Neuropsychological deficits in abstinent cocaine abusers: Preliminary findings after two weeks of abstinence. *Drug Alcohol Depend* **32**, 231–7.

Blake J and Smith A. 1997. Effects of smoking and smoking deprivation on the articulatory loop of working memory. *Hum Psychopharmacol* **12**, 259–64.

Block R I, O'Leary D S, Hichwa R D, *et al.* 2000. Cerebellar hypoactivity in frequent marijuana users. *Neuroreport* **11**, 749–53.

Brody A L, Mandelkern M A, Olmstead R E, *et al.* 2007. Neural substrates of resisting craving during cigarette cue exposure. *Biol Psychiatry* **62**, 642–51.

Büttner A, Mall G, Penning R and Weis S. 2000. The neuropathology of heroin abuse. *Foren Sci Int* **113**, 435–42.

Chang L and Chronicle E P. 2007. Functional imaging studies in cannabis users. *The Neuroscientist* **13**, 422.

Chang L, Ernst T, Speck O, *et al.* 2002. Perfusion MRI and computerized cognitive test abnormalities in abstinent methamphetamine users. *Psychiatry Res Neuroimag* **114**, 65–79.

Chang L, Yakupov R, Cloak C and Ernst T. 2006. Marijuana use is associated with a reorganized visual–attention network and cerebellar hypoactivation. *Brain* **129**, 1096.

Cowan R L. 2007. Neuroimaging research in human MDMA users: A review. *Psychopharmacology* **189**, 539–56.

Daumann J, Fimm B, Willmes K, Thron A and Gouzoulis-Mayfrank E. 2003a. Cerebral activation in abstinent ecstasy (MDMA) users during a working memory task: A functional magnetic resonance imaging (fMRI) study. *Cogn Brain Res* **16**, 479–87.

Daumann J, Fischermann T, Heekeren K, Henke K, Thron A and Gouzoulis-Mayfrank E. 2005. Memory-related hippocampal dysfunction in poly-drug ecstasy (3, 4-methylenedioxymethamphetamine) users. *Psychopharmacology* **180**, 607–11.

Daumann J, Fischermann T, Heekeren K, Thron A and Gouzoulis-Mayfrank E. 2004. Neural mechanisms of working memory in ecstasy (MDMA) users who continue or discontinue ecstasy and amphetamine use: Evidence from an 18-month longitudinal functional magnetic resonance imaging study. *Biol Psychiatry* **56**, 349–55.

Daumann J, Schnitker R, Weidemann J, Schnell K, Thron A and Gouzoulis-Mayfrank E. 2003b. Neural correlates of working memory in pure and polyvalent ecstasy (MDMA) users. *Neuroreport* **14**, 1983.

David S P, Munafn M R, Johansen-Berg H, *et al.* 2005. Ventral striatum/nucleus accumbens activation to smoking-related pictorial cues in smokers and nonsmokers: A functional magnetic resonance imaging study. *Biol Psychiatry* **58**, 488–94.

Davis P E, Liddiard H and McMillan T M. 2002. Neuropsychological deficits and opiate abuse. *Drug Alcohol Depend* **67**, 105–08.

Desmond J E, Chen S H A, DeRosa E, Pryor M R, Pfefferbaum A and Sullivan E V. 2003. Increased frontocerebellar activation in alcoholics during verbal working memory: An fMRI study. *Neuroimage* **19**, 1510–20.

Due D L, Huettel S A, Hall W G and Rubin D C. 2002. Activation in mesolimbic and visuospatial neural circuits elicited by smoking cues: Evidence from functional magnetic resonance imaging. *Am J Psychiatry* **159**, 954–60.

Forman S D, Dougherty G G, Casey B J, *et al.* 2004. Opiate addicts lack error-dependent activation of rostral anterior cingulate. *Biol Psychiatry* **55**, 531–7.

Franklin T R, Acton P D, Maldjian J A, *et al.* 2002. Decreased gray matter concentration in the insular, orbitofrontal, cingulate, and temporal cortices of cocaine patients. *Biol Psychiatry* **51**, 134–42.

Fu L P, Bi G H, Zou Z T, *et al.* 2008. Impaired response inhibition function in abstinent heroin dependents: An fMRI study. *Neurosci Lett* **438**, 322–6.

Gallinat J, Meisenzahl E, Jacobsen L K, *et al.* 2006. Smoking and structural brain deficits: A volumetric MR investigation. *Eur J Neurosci* **24**, 1744–50.

Garavan H, Pankiewicz J, Bloom A, *et al.* 2000. Cue-induced cocaine craving: Neuroanatomical specificity for drug users and drug stimuli. *Am J Psychiatry* **157**, 1789–98.

George M S, Anton R F, Bloomer C, *et al.* 2001. Activation of prefrontal cortex and anterior thalamus in alcoholic subjects on exposure to alcohol-specific cues. *Arch Gen Psychiatry* **58**, 345–52.

Gilman J M and Hommer D W. 2008. Modulation of brain response to emotional images by alcohol cues in alcohol-dependent patients. *Addiction Biol* **13**, 423–34.

Goldstein R Z, Tomasi D, Rajaram S, *et al.* 2007. Role of the anterior cingulate and medial orbitofrontal cortex in processing drug cues in cocaine addiction. *Neuroscience* **144**, 1153–9.

Gruber S A and Yurgelun-Todd D A. 2005. Neuroimaging of marijuana smokers during inhibitory processing: A pilot investigation. *Cogn Brain Res* **23**, 107–18.

Grüsser S M, Wrase J, Klein S, *et al.* 2004. Cue-induced activation of the striatum and medial prefrontal cortex is associated with subsequent relapse in abstinent alcoholics. *Psychopharmacology* **175**, 296–302.

Heinz A, Wrase J, Kahnt T, *et al.* 2007. Brain activation elicited by affectively positive stimuli is associated with a lower risk of relapse in detoxified alcoholic subjects. *Alcohol Clin Exp Res* **31**, 1138–47.

Hester R and Garavan H. 2004. Executive dysfunction in cocaine addiction: Evidence for discordant frontal, cingulate, and cerebellar activity. *J Neurosci* **24**, 11 017–22.

Jacobsen L K, Mencl W E, Constable R T, Westerveld M and Pugh K R. 2007a. Impact of smoking abstinence on working memory neurocircuitry in adolescent daily tobacco smokers. *Psychopharmacology* **193**, 557–66.

Jacobsen L K, Mencl W E, Pugh K R, Skudlarski P and Krystal J H. 2004a. Preliminary evidence of hippocampal dysfunction in adolescent MDMA ("ecstasy") users: Possible relationship to neurotoxic effects. *Psychopharmacology (Berl)* **173**, 383–90.

Jacobsen L K, Mencl W E, Westerveld M and Pugh K R. 2004b. Impact of cannabis use on brain function in adolescents. *Ann N Y Acad Sci* **1021**, 384–90.

Jacobsen L K, Pugh K R, Constable R T, Westerveld M and Mencl W E. 2007b. Functional correlates of verbal memory deficits emerging during nicotine withdrawal in abstinent adolescent cannabis users. *Biol Psychiatry* **61**, 31–40.

Jaffe J H, Cascella N G, Kumor K M and Sherer M A. 1989. Cocaine-induced cocaine craving. *Psychopharmacology* **97**, 59–64.

Jager G, de Win M M L, van der Tweel I, *et al.* 2008. Assessment of cognitive brain function in ecstasy users and contributions of other drugs of abuse: Results from an fMRI study. *Neuropsychopharmacology* **33**, 247.

Jager G, Kahn R S, Van Den Brink W, Van Ree J M and Ramsey N F. 2006. Long-term effects of frequent cannabis use on working memory and attention: An fMRI study. *Psychopharmacology* **185**, 358–68.

Jager G, Van Hell H H, De Win M M L, *et al.* 2007. Effects of frequent cannabis use on hippocampal activity during an associative memory task. *Eur Neuropsychopharmacol* **17**, 289–97.

Kanayama G, Rogowska J, Pope H G, Gruber S A and Yurgelun Todd D A. 2004. Spatial working memory in heavy cannabis users: A functional magnetic resonance imaging study. *Psychopharmacology* **176**, 239–47.

Kaufman J N, Ross T J, Stein E A and Garavan H. 2003. Cingulate hypoactivity in cocaine users during a GO-NOGO task as revealed by event-related functional magnetic resonance imaging. *J Neurosci* **23**, 7839–43.

Kivisaari R, Kähkönen S, Puuskari V, Jokela O, Rapeli P and Autti T. 2004. Magnetic resonance imaging of severe, long-term, opiate-abuse patients without neurologic symptoms may show enlarged cerebrospinal spaces but no signs of brain pathology of vascular origin. *Arch Med Res* **35**, 395–400.

Kosten T R, Scanley B E, Tucker K A, *et al.* 2006. Cue-induced brain activity changes and relapse in cocaine-dependent patients. *Neuropsychopharmacology* **31**, 644–50.

Langleben D D, Ruparel K, Elman I, *et al.* 2008. Acute effect of methadone maintenance dose on brain fMRI response to heroin-related cues. *Am J Psychiatry* **165**, 390.

Lee J H, Lim Y, Wiederhold B K and Graham S J. 2005. A functional magnetic resonance imaging (fMRI) study of cue-induced smoking craving in virtual environments. *Appl Psychophysiol Biofeedb* **30**, 195–204.

Lee T M C, Zhou W, Luo X, Yuen K S L, Ruan X and Weng X. 2005. Neural activity associated with cognitive regulation in heroin users: A fMRI study. *Neurosci Lett* **382**, 211–6.

Lundqvist T, Jonsson S and Warkentin S. 2001. Frontal lobe dysfunction in long-term cannabis users. *Neurotoxicol Teratol* **23**, 437–43.

Matochik J A, Eldreth D A, Cadet J L and Bolla K I. 2005. Altered brain tissue composition in heavy marijuana users. *Drug Alcohol Depend* **77**, 23–30.

McBride D, Barrett S P, Kelly J T, Aw A and Dagher A. 2006. Clinical research effects of expectancy and abstinence on the neural response to smoking cues in cigarette smokers: An fMRI study. *Neuropsychopharmacology* **31**, 2728–38.

McClernon F J, Hiott F B, Huettel S A and Rose J E. 2005. Abstinence-induced changes in self-report craving correlate with event-related fMRI responses to smoking cues. *Neuropsychopharmacology* **30**, 1940.

McClernon F J, Kozink R V and Rose J E. 2007. Individual differences in nicotine dependence, withdrawal symptoms, and sex predict transient fMRI-BOLD responses to smoking cues. *Neuropsychopharmacology* **33**, 2148.

Medina K L, Hanson K L, Schweinsburg A D, Cohen-Zion M, Nagel B J and Tapert S F. 2007. Neuropsychological functioning in adolescent marijuana users: Subtle deficits detectable after a month of abstinence. *J Int Neuropsychol Soc* **13**, 807–20.

Moeller F G, Steinberg J L, Dougherty D M, Narayana P A, Kramer L A and Renshaw P F. 2004. Functional MRI study of working memory in MDMA users. *Psychopharmacology* **177**, 185–94.

443

Myrick H, Anton R F, Li X, *et al.* 2004. Differential brain activity in alcoholics and social drinkers to alcohol cues: Relationship to craving. *Neuropsychopharmacology* **29**, 393–402.

Nestor L, Roberts G, Garavan H and Hester R. 2008. Deficits in learning and memory: Parahippocampal hyperactivity and frontocortical hypoactivity in cannabis users. *Neuroimage* **40**, 1328–39.

Okuyemi K S, Powell J N, Savage C R, *et al.* 2006. Enhanced cue-elicited brain activation in African American compared with Caucasian smokers: An fMRI study. *Addiction Biol* **11**, 97–106.

Padula C B, Schweinsburg A D and Tapert S F. 2007. Spatial working memory performance and fMRI activation interactions in abstinent adolescent marijuana users. *Psychol Addict Behav* **21**, 478.

Paulus M P, Hozack N, Frank L, Brown G G and Schuckit M A. 2003. Decision making by methamphetamine-dependent subjects is associated with error-rate-independent decrease in prefrontal and parietal activation. *Biol Psychiatry* **53**, 65–74.

Paulus M P, Hozack N E, Zauscher B E, *et al.* 2002. Behavioral and functional neuroimaging evidence for prefrontal dysfunction in methamphetamine-dependent subjects. *Neuropsychopharmacology* **26**, 53–63.

Paulus M P, Tapert S F and Schuckit M A. 2005. Neural activation patterns of methamphetamine-dependent subjects during decision making predict relapse. *Arch Gen Psychiatry* **62**, 761–8.

Payer D E, Lieberman M D, Monterosso J R, Xu J, Fong T W and London E D. 2007. Differences in cortical activity between methamphetamine-dependent and healthy individuals performing a facial affect matching task. *Drug Alcohol Depend* **93**, 93–102.

Pfefferbaum A, Desmond J E, Galloway C, Menon V, Glover G H and Sullivan E V. 2001. Reorganization of frontal systems used by alcoholics for spatial working memory: An fMRI study. *Neuroimage* **14**, 7–20.

Pfefferbaum A, Sullivan E V, Mathalon D H and Lim K O. 1997. Frontal lobe volume loss observed with magnetic resonance imaging in older chronic alcoholics. *Alcohol Clin Exp Res* **21**, 521–9.

Pillay S S, Rogowska J, Kanayama G, *et al.* 2008. Cannabis and motor function: fMRI changes following 28 days of discontinuation. *Exp Clin Psychopharmacol* **16**, 22.

Pillay S S, Rogowska J, Kanayama G, *et al.* 2004. Neurophysiology of motor function following cannabis discontinuation in chronic cannabis smokers: An fMRI study. *Drug Alcohol Depend* **76**, 261–71.

Pope H G and Yurgelun-Todd D. 1996. The residual cognitive effects of heavy marijuana use in college students. *JAMA* **275**, 521–7.

Pope J H G, Gruber A J, Hudson J I, Huestis M A and Yurgelun-Todd D. 2001. Neuropsychological performance in long-term cannabis users. *Am Med Assoc* **58**, 909–15.

Potter A S and Newhouse P A. 2008. Acute nicotine improves cognitive deficits in young adults with attention-deficit/hyperactivity disorder. *Pharmacol Biochem Behav* **88**, 407–17.

Quickfall J and Crockford D. 2006. Brain neuroimaging in cannabis use: A review. *J Neuropsychiatry Clin Neurosci* **18**, 318.

Ray R, Loughead J, Wang Z, *et al.* 2008. Neuroimaging, genetics and the treatment of nicotine addiction. *Behav Brain Res* **193**, 159–69.

Risinger R C, Salmeron B J, Ross T J, *et al.* 2005. Neural correlates of high and craving during cocaine self-administration using BOLD fMRI. *Neuroimage* **26**, 1097–108.

Rose J S, Branchey M, Buydens-Branchey L, *et al.* 1996. Cerebral perfusion in early and late opiate withdrawal: A technetium-99m-HMPAO SPECT study. *Psychiatry Res Neuroimag* **67**, 39–47.

Rosenbloom M J, Sullivan E V, Sassoon S A, *et al.* 2007. Alcoholism, HIV infection, and their comorbidity: Factors affecting self-rated health-related quality of life. *J Stud Alcohol* **68**, 115–25.

Salloum J B, Ramchandani V A, Bodurka J, *et al.* 2007. Blunted rostral anterior cingulate response during a simplified decoding task of negative emotional facial expressions in alcoholic patients. *Alcohol Clin Exp Res* **31**, 1490–504.

Schneider F, Habel U, Wagner M, *et al.* 2001. Subcortical correlates of craving in recently abstinent alcoholic patients. *Am J Psychiatry* **158**, 1075–83.

Schweinsburg A D, Nagel B J, Schweinsburg B C, Park A, Theilmann R J and Tapert S F. 2008. Abstinent adolescent marijuana users show altered fMRI response during spatial working memory. *Psychiatry Res Neuroimag* **163**, 40–51.

Scott J C, Woods S P, Matt G E, *et al.* 2007. Neurocognitive effects of methamphetamine: A critical review and meta-analysis. *Neuropsychol Rev* **17**, 275–97.

Sinha R, Lacadie C, Skudlarski P, *et al.* 2005. Neural activity associated with stress-induced cocaine craving: A functional magnetic resonance imaging study. *Psychopharmacology (Berl)* **183**, 171–80.

Snyder F R, Davis F C and Henningfield J E. 1989. The tobacco withdrawal syndrome: Performance decrements assessed on a computerized test battery. *Drug Alcohol Depend* **23**, 259–66.

Solowij N and Battisti R. 2008. The chronic effects of cannabis on memory in humans: A review. *Curr Drug Abuse Rev* **1**, 81–98.

Solowij N, Michie P T and Fox A M. 1995. Differential impairments of selective attention due to frequency and duration of cannabis use. *Biol Psychiatry* **37**, 731–9.

Strickland T L. 1993. Cerebral perfusion and neuropsychological consequences of chronic cocaine use. *Am Neuropsych Assoc* **5**, 419–27.

Substance Abuse and Mental Health Services Administration (SAMHSA). 2008. *Results from the 2007 National Survey on Drug Use and Health: National Findings* (NSDUH Series H-34, DHHS Publication No. SMA 08-4343). Rockville, MD.

Swan G E and Lessov-Schlaggar C N. 2007. The effects of tobacco smoke and nicotine on cognition and the brain. *Neuropsychol Rev* **17**, 259–73.

Tanner-Smith E E. 2006. Pharmacological content of tablets sold as "ecstasy": Results from an online testing service. *Drug Alcohol Depend* **83**, 247–54.

Tapert S F, Brown G G, Baratta M V and Brown S A. 2004a. fMRI BOLD response to alcohol stimuli in alcohol dependent young women. *Addict Behav* **29**, 33–50.

Tapert S F, Brown G G, Kindermann S, Cheung E H, Frank L R and Brown S A. 2001. fMRI measurement of brain dysfunction in alcohol-dependent young women. *Alcohol Clin Exp Res* **25**, 236–45.

Tapert S F, Cheung E H, Brown G G, et al. 2003. Neural response to alcohol stimuli in adolescents with alcohol use disorder. *Arch Gen Psychiatry* **60**, 727–35.

Tapert S F, Schweinsburg A D, Barlett V C, et al. 2004b. Blood oxygen level dependent response and spatial working memory in adolescents with alcohol use disorders. *Alcohol Clin Exp Res* **28**, 1577–86.

Tapert S F, Schweinsburg A, Drummond S, et al. 2007. Functional MRI of inhibitory processing in abstinent adolescent marijuana users. *Psychopharmacology* **194**, 173–83.

Thompson P M, Hayashi K M, Simon S L, et al. 2004. Structural abnormalities in the brains of human subjects who use methamphetamine. *J Neurosci* **24**, 6028–36.

Toomey R, Lyons M J, Eisen S A, et al. 2003. A twin study of the neuropsychological consequences of stimulant abuse. *Am Med Assoc* **60**, 303–10.

Volkow N D, Chang L, Wang G J, et al. 2001. Association of dopamine transporter reduction with psychomotor impairment in methamphetamine abusers. *Am J Psychiatry* **158**, 377–82.

Volkow N D, Fowler J S, Wang G J, et al. 1993. Decreased dopamine D2 receptor availability is associated with reduced frontal metabolism in cocaine abusers. *Synapse* **14**(2), 169–77.

Wexler B E, Gottschalk C H, Fulbright R K, et al. 2001. Functional magnetic resonance imaging of cocaine craving. *Am J Psychiatry* **158**, 86–95.

Wrase J, Grüsser S M, Klein S, et al. 2002. Development of alcohol-associated cues and cue-induced brain activation in alcoholics. *Eur Psychiatry* **17**, 287–91.

Xiao Z, Lee T, Zhang J X, et al. 2006. Thirsty heroin addicts show different fMRI activations when exposed to water-related and drug-related cues. *Drug Alcohol Depend* **83**, 157–62.

Xu J, Mendrek A, Cohen M S, et al. 2005. Brain activity in cigarette smokers performing a working memory task: Effect of smoking abstinence. *Biol Psychiatry* **58**, 143–50.

Xu J, Mendrek A, Cohen M S, et al. 2006. Effects of acute smoking on brain activity vary with abstinence in smokers performing the N-Back Task: A preliminary study. *Psychiatry Res Neuroimag* **148**, 103–09.

Xu J, Mendrek A, Cohen M S, et al. 2007. Effect of cigarette smoking on prefrontal cortical function in nondeprived smokers performing the stroop task. *Neuropsychopharmacology* **32**, 1421–8.

Xu P, Jiang Y, Geng D, Wang Y and Lu G. 2008. *A fMRI Study on Electroacupuncture Intervening Heroin Abstainers' Cognitive Attention*. Paper presented at the 7th Asian-Pacific Conference on Medical and Biological Engineering, Beijing, China.

Yücel M, Lubman D I, Harrison B J, et al. 2007. A combined spectroscopic and functional MRI investigation of the dorsal anterior cingulate region in opiate addiction. *Mol Psychiatry* **12**, 691–702.

Yurgelun-Todd D, Gruber A J, Hanson R A, Baird A A, Renshaw P F and Pope H G Jr. 1999. *Residual Effects of Marijuana Use: A fMRI Study*. Paper presented at the Problems of Drug Dependence 1998: Proceedings of the 60th Annual Scientific Meeting of the College on Problems of Drug Dependence, Bethesda, MD.

Zakzanis K K, Campbell Z and Jovanovski D. 2007. The neuropsychology of ecstasy (MDMA) use: A quantitative review. *Hum Psychopharmacol* **22**, 427–35.

Molecular imaging of substance abuse

Brian C. Schweinsburg, Alecia D. Dager Schweinsburg and Graeme F. Mason

Introduction

The use of substances for psychoactive effects dates to antiquity with evidence in archaeological finds of alcohol-related intoxication and possibly ritualistic use of *Nymphaea caerulea* in ancient Egypt and alcohol abuse in classic Greek and Roman culture. While a variety of legal and illicit substances are used for their mind-altering effects, the misuse of drugs and alcohol can result in a constellation of behavioral and physiologic consequences that comprise addiction, which is often considered to be a cyclic process associated with chronic relapse. Koob and Le Moal (2001) outlined a continuum of allostasis to pathology as an individual experiences the rewarding properties of drugs, transitions to dependence, develops addiction, and enters periods of protracted abstinence. Circuitry including cortical–thalamo-striatal loops, the reward system, and stress system contribute to a reward system allostatic state that reflects long-term deviation from normal brain states that ultimately can lead to pathologic change (Koob and Le Moal, 2001). While there are a number of potential individual and environmental differences associated with vulnerabilities in the transition to drug and alcohol-related brain pathology (allostatic load), a core neurobiological feature of the continuum is altered neurochemistry among neural pathways.

Scope of the addiction problem

A five-year population survey of civilian, non-institutionalized United States residents aged 12 or older revealed substantial use of drugs and alcohol (Substance Abuse and Mental Health Services Administration (SAMHSA), 2008). Based on survey estimates, 22.3 million persons (9.0% of the United States population aged 12 years or older) met Diagnostic and Statistical Manual of Mental Disorders, 4th edition (DSM-IV) criteria for substance dependence or abuse in the past year; 3.2 million individuals were classified with dependence on or abuse of both alcohol and illicit drugs; 3.7 million were dependent on or abused illicit drugs but not alcohol; and 15.5 million were dependent on or abused alcohol but not illicit drugs. Males aged 12 or older had nearly twice the rate of substance use disorders compared to females (12.5 versus 5.7%). However, male and female youths aged 12–17 showed similar rates (7.7%). The percent estimate of illicit drug use during the past month in youths aged 12–17 (9.5%) has remained relatively stable since 2005, and was significantly lower in 2007 compared to 2002–2004. However, 19.7% of young adults aged 18–25 used illicit drugs in the past month in 2007, which reflects a generally stable pattern of use from 2002 to 2007, but a statistically larger percentage than those aged 12–17. Further, the National Survey on Drug Use and Health revealed that the 18–25 cohort were the most likely to use tobacco products during the past month (41.8%), in the context of 70.9 million United States residents aged 12 or older using tobacco products over the past month in the year 2007.

The transition from drug or alcohol use initiation to a substance use disorder is a complex pathway involving, but certainly not limited to, genetics (e.g. family history), age at first use, and character traits, to highlight a few. Further, the National Comorbidity Survey Replication revealed a significant level of association indicating comorbidity between drug and/or alcohol dependence and psychiatric disorders including social phobia, generalized anxiety disorder, manic/hypomanic disorder, attention deficit hyperactivity disorder, intermittent explosive disorder, major depressive disorder, dysthymia, and post-traumatic stress disorder (Kessler *et al.*, 2005).

Even relatively conservative estimates of the economic cost of alcohol and drug abuse in 1995 were staggering. Adjusted population estimated costs were 276 billion dollars for alcohol and drug-related health care expenditures, impact on productivity (e.g. illness, premature death, crime/victims), and other losses associated with motor vehicle accidents and the impact on the criminal justice system (NIDA and NIAAA, 1998).

The neurobehavioral characterization of addiction encompasses a broad spectrum of features. Typically it includes character traits such as sensation-seeking and impulsivity, as well as altered behavior, such as compulsiveness. Associated neuropsychological disruptions include executive dysfunction, for example. Structural and functional brain abnormalities include brain volume loss, altered white matter pathway integrity, and dysfunctional neural networks. In line with a neurobiological model of addiction, altered neurochemistry remains at the core of the acute and chronic addictive process that is so disruptive to individuals, their families, and the public. This underscores the importance of describing the addiction process through careful in-vivo neurochemical investigation, and it is fortunate that there exist today powerful imaging tools to enhance understanding of human addiction. Box 1 summarizes the overarching aims of the review.

Box 31.1. Substance abuse review aims

1. Provide an overview of the most commonly used methods for studying the neurochemistry of human addiction in-vivo.
2. Describe the current literature highlighting neurochemical changes associated with both illicit and non-illicit substances of abuse.
3. Summarize findings in a neurobiological context and report considerations for future work.

Review summary points

1. A variety of methods are now in use to study diverse aspects of neurochemistry in the living human brain.
2. Legal and illegal substances have some common effects on neurochemistry of function and identifiers of neuronal health such as NAA. However, each substance has its own variations that make it unique in its effects on the brain.

---

3. Future studies will include some improvements in technology but are likely to profit enormously from collaborative, interdisciplinary approaches that include neuroimaging, genetics, and pharmacology.

In-vivo neurochemical measurements

Positron emission tomography (PET)

One might think of PET and SPECT (single-photon emission computed tomography) as inside-out X-rays or CT scans. X-rays and CT use a beam of gamma radiation external to the head, shining it on the head so that the bones and other tissues of varying density cast a range of shadows on film or other detector on the opposite side of the body. PET, however, makes use of radioactive compounds that are injected into the body and shine X-rays outward from whatever their location. By detecting the radiation from angles all around the body, it is possible to create a three-dimensional reconstruction of where the radiation is most highly concentrated. Therefore, SPECT and PET provide images of how particular radioactive chemicals are distributed through the body, and in particular, within regions of the brain.

PET and SPECT differ from one another in that SPECT uses one X-ray per molecule, and PET uses two. The radioactive isotopes used for PET emit positrons, which are positively charged electrons, a form of anti-matter. A positron travels randomly for up to a few millimeters until it encounters an electron, at which point the electron and positron, matter and anti-matter, annihilate one another. From the site of the collision, two X rays are emitted in almost exactly opposite directions. The PET camera has radiation detectors around the head, and a count is registered when two X-rays are detected simultaneously $180°$ apart. Background radiation is a source of noise in PET and SPECT imaging, and the requirement that detection be simultaneous at opposite detectors decreases the likelihood of random counts and increases the spatial resolution of the detection, with machines available with resolution of 4–5 mm.

PET can be used for many purposes. The most common application for the brain is the measurement of the uptake of the glucose. Under most circumstances, glucose provides the primary fuel for brain energy metabolism, and it passes across the blood–brain barrier on a passive transporter. Once in the brain, within 1–2 s, the glucose diffuses throughout the brain water space, and its first step in metabolism

447

is the addition of a phosphate group. There exists an analog of glucose, deoxyglucose, which once phosphorylated is almost entirely trapped in the brain and cannot be metabolized further. By injecting radiolabeled deoxyglucose and mapping the radioactivity in the brain, one can measure how quickly various regions of the brain are using glucose, as developed in pioneering work by Louis Sokoloff and colleagues in 1977, and adapted and validated for use in humans in 1979 by Michael Phelps and coworkers with the positron emitter fluorine-18 in fluoro-deoxyglucose (FDG) (Phelps et al., 1979).

Other useful compounds are carbon-11 (^{11}C) and oxygen-15 (^{15}O), because those elements are common in many biological compounds. For example, instead of the glucose analog FDG, it is possible to use glucose labeled with ^{11}C, which is chemically identical to naturally occurring glucose in the body. Oxygen-15 (^{15}O) can be used to create labeled water and image its uptake into the brain tissue as a measure of blood flow. A technical difficulty with some isotopes, including ^{11}C and ^{15}O, is their short radiological half-life, 20 min and 122 s, respectively. Facilities that use such short-lived isotopes must have a cyclotron on site to generate the isotopes immediately before each measurement.

These and other radioisotopes can be used to create ligands, called radioligands, used to study dopamine release, dopamine receptor binding, and many other systems that are of interest for substance abuse.

For any of the neurotransmitter systems, the strategy to evaluate the receptor density is to inject the radiotracer and measure how much radioactivity results in each pixel of the brain image. The strategy to assess the amount of neurotransmitter released to bind to receptors is to administer a ligand that binds to the appropriate receptors, image the radioactivity, and then administer a drug that causes a release of the neurotransmitter. Upon release of the neurotransmitter, the neurotransmitters will displace a fraction of the radioactive ligand from the receptors, thereby decreasing radioactivity in that area of the image. An example is the measurement of dopamine release that occurs with a dose of cocaine.

The general approach is comparative. That is, to evaluate the effects of cocaine use on dopamine receptor binding, one might measure dopamine receptor binding in a group of subjects who habitually use cocaine and in a group of appropriately matched subjects who do not use cocaine. To evaluate the effects of acute ethanol administration on metabolism as measured by FDG–glucose, one might measure glucose metabolism in a group of subjects and then repeat the measurement after giving a dose of ethanol. In some cases, it is desirable to wait a period of time long enough to allow the radioactivity from the first study to be reduced either by radioactive decay or excretion from the body.

Often, radioligands are analogs of the natural neurotransmitter under study. Development of the radioligands can require years to synthesize and test a wide range of compounds for efficacy and toxicity. Requirements of an effective radioligand are numerous and stringent. The requirements include appropriate binding affinity: binding should be sufficient for the radioligand to attach to the receptor in subpharmaceutical doses and remain there long enough to acquire the images. If the radioligand is intended for competitive binding studies with neurotransmitter release, then binding must also be weak enough to allow the neurotransmitter to displace the radioligand. The radioligand must have the ability to enter the brain, either in the form administered or as a metabolized product. Transfer into the brain may require a transporter, or it may demand appropriate lipophilicity to pass through the blood–brain barrier. Many molecules must usually be screened to meet the many requirements of a radioligand for PET or SPECT.

PET researchers have developed techniques to study various aspects of the neurotransmitter systems. For dopamine, targets include type D1-like and D2-like receptors, the synaptic dopamine transporter, the vesicular dopamine transporter, and the dopamine-degrading enzymes monoamine oxidase A and monoamine oxidase B (reviewed in Lindsey et al., 2005; Elsinga et al., 2006). The serotonergic system has been studied from the perspective of serotonin transporters and serotonin receptors, with a variety of compounds synthesized for imaging of serotonin transporters and 5-HT1A and 5-HT2A receptors (Hesse et al., 2004). Opioid receptor mapping has been achieved with chemicals with specificity for different receptor subtypes: ligands exist that are used for μ, or μ/δ/κ, and μ/κ receptor subtypes (Henriksen and Willoch, 2008). More recently, cannabinoid receptors have received growing attention from the neuroimaging community (Lindsey et al., 2005), and several tracers for measurement of cannabinoid receptors have been developed to the point of testing in humans (Horti and Van Laere, 2008). The GABAergic system has been subject to study for some time using SPECT and PET, using receptors that have varying degrees of specificity by for subtypes of the benzodiazepine receptor (Katsifis and Kassiou, 2004). Glutamate, by far the most abundant neurotransmitter in the human brain, provides a large and largely understudied target in neuroimaging, with ligands under development or in use for metabotropic glutamate receptors (Wang et al., 2007; Sanchez-Pernaute et al., 2008), AMPA receptors (Arstad et al., 2006; Gao et al., 2006), and NMDA receptors (Waterhouse et al., 2004; Stone et al., 2006; Biegon et al., 2007).

In all cases, there are trade-offs to be made among the ligands. ^{18}F has a longer half-life than ^{11}C and is therefore easier to use in many cases, but depending on the system under study, a given ^{18}F tracer may have binding affinity or specificity that is inferior to those of another tracer that has been synthesized with ^{11}C. A SPECT tracer with ^{123}I, with its long half-life, may show promise, but with its single photon will yield lower precision than the double-photon obtained with PET and a positron emitter. Each tracer has its own strengths and weaknesses that must be assessed for a given application.

^{1}H magnetic resonance imaging and spectroscopy (MRI and MRS)

MRI and MRS have their basis in the detection of atomic nuclei with spin, such as the nuclei of hydrogen (found abundantly in water, fat, and other neurochemicals). Although the detection is of the atomic nucleus, there is no ionizing radiation as is found with X-rays, radioactive decay, or nuclear power generation. For MRI, a person lies in a magnetic field that is typically tens of thousands of times more powerful than the magnetic field of the Earth. The nuclei that have spin, such as hydrogen, orient themselves either with or against the orientation of the large magnetic field, which people often call North–South when speaking of magnets. A very slight majority of the nuclei, far less than 1%, orient themselves with the magnetic field, and a burst of radio energy, typically on the order of a few thousandths of a second, is transmitted to the person in the region of interest, which in the case of this chapter is the brain. That disturbs the orientation of that tiny majority of nuclei, and then they return a signal of radio energy on the order of microvolts, and it is that signal that yields MRI and MRS. MRI is based on the localization of the signal in different parts of the head, often with resolution of 1 mm or better.

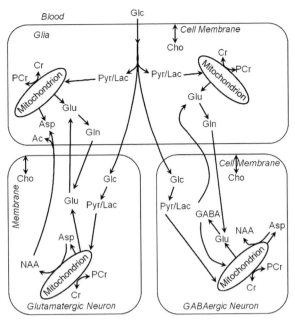

Figure 31.1 Many of the neurochemicals detected by MRS. Ac, acetate; Asp, aspartate; Cho, choline, phosphocholine, and glycerophosphocholine; Cr, creatine; PCr, phosphocreatine; GABA, gamma-amino-butyric acid; Glc, glucose; Glu, glutamate; Gln, glutamine; NAA, N-acetylaspartate; Pyr, pyruvate; Lac, lactate. Pyruvate is not typically detected in the brain with ^{1}H MRS, but lactate sometimes is and, when elevated, often indicates an energetic problem. Intercellular cycles are known to exist for glutamate, glutamine, and GABA, and evidence suggests a cycle for NAA, as well.

MRI of many types can be used to study neurobiology. Structural MRI yields views of the brain that appear similar to what one might find in an anatomy book, although the techniques of acquisition can be modified to emphasize particular features of interest, such as fluid pockets (e.g. in multiple sclerosis) or beds of blood vessels (e.g. to study tumor pathology). Diffusion tensor imaging (DTI) has been developed to measure the characteristics of diffusion in the tissue, which can be used to track fibers or observe the process of breakdown of tissue structure over the course of diseases. Functional MRI (fMRI) is used heavily today to detect regional changes in brain activity by measuring changes in signal intensity that depend on blood flow, blood volume, and oxygen extraction in the living, working brain.

MRS typically yields much coarser spatial resolution than MRI, but provides identification of multiple neurochemicals at the same time. That is because the precise frequency at which the signal returns from the brain depends on the type of chemical in which the nucleus resides. For example, hydrogen nuclei in glutamate

449

yield a signal whose frequency differs slightly from that of glutamine. Nuclei in fat yield a signal whose frequency is generally distinct from that of water.

Choline (Cho) that is detected by MRS is believed to be associated primarily with membrane metabolism, appearing either by transport into the brain (Michel *et al.*, 2006), or via synthesis *de novo* from phosphatidyl ethanolamine using *S*-adenosylmethionine as a methyl donor (Blusztajn *et al.*, 2008). Although choline is used for the generation of acetylcholine, the quantity of acetylcholine is so low that it forms an undetectably small component of what is seen by MRS.

The synthesis of creatine (Cr), derived from arginine, also requires *S*-adenosylmethionine as a methyl donor, or creatine can be transported into the brain from the blood stream (Braissant *et al.*, 2001). Once in the brain, creatine is phosphorylated to generate phosphocreatine as a reserve of high-energy phosphate for the maintenance of levels of ATP. The creatine signal observed with MRS in vivo represents an unresolved combination of creatine and phosphocreatine, although in well-prepared acquisitions from high-quality extracts, creatine and phosphocreatine can be distinguished from one another.

The synthesis of *N*-acetylaspartate (NAA) by the methylation of aspartate with acetylCoA, is catalyzed by aspartate-*N*-acetyltransferase, which is found most abundantly in association with mitochondria (Patel and Clark, 1979; Truckenmiller *et al.*, 1985; Ariyannura *et al.*, 2008). Because the enzyme to degrade NAA resides in glia (Truckenmiller *et al.*, 1985; Chakraborty *et al.*, 2001), and neurons contain at least the great majority of NAA, it is believed that the synthesis of NAA occurs primarily in neurons. The primary purposes of NAA remain to be determined, although diverse purposes been proposed. Clinically, its level appears to represent neuronal viability, perhaps as a marker of mitochondrial soundness.

Myo-inositol in the MRS field is regarded primarily as a compound used to regulate brain osmolarity (this role is reviewed in a study of *myo*-inositol transport (Silver *et al.*, 2002)). *Myo*-inositol also plays a role in phosphoinositide metabolism (Brockerhoff and Ballou, 1962) and, therefore, intracellular signaling (Pacheco and Jope, 1996). Generally, elevations in MR-detected levels of *myo*-inositol are associated with pathology.

Glutamate, glutamine, and γ-aminobutyric acid (GABA) are related structurally to one another and to brain energy metabolism. Glutamate is an excitatory transmitter that is derived from α-ketoglutarate, an intermediate of the oxidative metabolism via the Krebs cycle. Glutamine synthetase catalyzes the conversion of glutamate to glutamine, and glutamate decarboxylase mediates the modification of glutamate to form the inhibitory transmitter GABA. Most studies of MRS of brain today acquire data under conditions that do not resolve the three metabolites from one another, yielding a composite signal that is by convention called Glx. The separate detection of glutamate, glutamine, and GABA becomes easier at higher magnetic fields and with strategies to isolate the signals from one another. Examples of selective strategies are J-editing (Rothman *et al.*, 1993), echo time averaging (TE-averaging) (Hurd *et al.*, 2004), and strategic choices of acquisition parameters (Choi *et al.*, 2006).

Underlying the metabolites are macromolecules, including protein resonances. Under conditions common to many psychiatric MRS studies, the macromolecules are present in significant quantities and contribute significantly to measurements of Glx (Behar and Ogino, 1993). Strategies have been developed to characterize the macromolecular resonances for each MRS acquisition method, and it is crucial to do so if Glx or any of its components are to be assessed.

^{13}C MRS

The explanation of MRS referred in its examples to an application entirely to the detection of the hydrogen nucleus (^{1}H). However, there exist many nuclei with spin, including phosphorus-31 (^{31}P), which yields information about high-energy compounds involved in metabolism, as well as other neurochemicals. The nuclei of other elements such as lithium, sodium, and oxygen-17 (^{17}O) have also been detected for various purposes. One atom that is most complementary to ^{1}H studies of neuroenergetics and neurotransmission is carbon-13 (^{13}C).

^{13}C comprises 1% of the naturally occurring carbon in the human body, is not radioactive, and has spin, so ^{13}C can be detected with MRS. Most carbon has the form carbon-12 (^{12}C) and is invisible to MRS. The safety of consumption of ^{13}C coupled with its low natural occurrence in the human body means that one can administer natural compounds such as sugar, enriched with ^{13}C, and follow the fate of that ^{13}C as it appears in the brain and is converted to various products that MRS can then detect. If one administers ^{13}C-enriched sugar to a patient and then uses MRS to detect ^{13}C in the brain, one will first observe the appearance of the sugar in the brain, followed by ^{13}C enrichment of glutamate, glutamine, and other neurochemicals. If ^{13}C appears in these various compounds more quickly in one condition than another, even though the sugar gets to the brain in a similar amount of time, then one can determine that those compounds are being produced more quickly. Therefore, by tracking the appearance of ^{13}C-labeled neurochemicals over the course of one or a few hours, it is possible to measure rates of metabolic processes.

A major metabolic focus of interest is neurochemical signaling. There are two major cell types in the brain, neurons and glia. Neurons transmit electrical impulses and communicate with each other by release of neurotransmitters. Glia surround the neurons and maintain a stable extracellular environment as well as providing the neurons with key substrates. The glutamate/glutamine cycle is a metabolic pathway shared between neurons and glia. In this pathway, glutamate released by the neuron as a neurotransmitter is taken up by surrounding glial cells, then converted to glutamine. Glutamine is not neuroactive, and is released by the glia for uptake by the neurons to replace lost glutamate. Measurement of the glutamate/glutamine cycle is of particular interest because it is a direct measurement of glutamate neurotransmission, which is the major excitatory neurotransmitter pathway in the cerebral cortex. Neuronal glucose oxidation by the Krebs cycle is the main source of energy for the brain, and impairment of the Krebs cycle is a symptom of several neurological and psychiatric diseases.

^{13}C MRS has the unique ability to measure both of these critical pathways simultaneously and non-invasively. [13]C is a non-radioactive isotope of carbon with a natural abundance of 1.1%. If metabolic substrates such as glucose are enriched with ^{13}C, then as the glucose is consumed by the brain, products such as glutamate, glutamine, and GABA become labeled. By tracking the labeling of these compounds in the brain over the course of a 2-h infusion, as has been done in hundreds of human measurements in the Yale MR Center and other institutions, one can determine rates of glucose oxidation and glutamate–glutamine neurotransmitter cycling, and GABA synthesis.

Drugs of abuse

Methamphetamine

Methamphetamine abuse impacts the brain in multiple, sometimes overlapping ways. One established line of research has been to examine the cerebrovascular effects of the drug. Methamphetamine has been found to result in microinfarctions, hemorrhagic lesions, and/or vasculitis (Bostwick, 1981; Cahill et al., 1981). This type of cerebrovascular damage is observed to be widespread resulting in global cerebral hypometabolism or hypoperfusion (Kao et al., 1994; Iyo et al., 1997; Alhassoon et al., 2001). On the other hand, the neurochemical impact of methamphetamine appears to be more selective. Due to its direct effect on dopaminergic neurotransmission, studies of methamphetamine have found significant damage in fronto-striatal and thalamic pathways (Wang et al., 2004). A well-documented finding from this body of literature is the significant loss of striatal dopamine transporters, which are considered markers of dopaminergic terminals (Wang et al., 2004). Some researchers have found that dopamine terminal damage is associated with motor and verbal learning deficits (Volkow et al., 2001) and is reversible with long-term abstinence (Volkow et al., 2001b).

^{1}H MRS in-vivo has been used to explore the effect of methamphetamine on NAA, choline, myo-inositol (MI) and creatine. These studies have found reductions in NAA (Ernst et al., 2000; Taylor et al., 2000; Nordahl et al., 2002), increased myo-inositol (Ernst et al., 2000), elevated choline (Ernst et al., 2000), and decreased creatine + phosphocreatine (Ernst et al., 2000; Sekine et al., 2002) in a diverse set of regions. Researchers have attributed changes in these metabolites to neuronal injury or death, astrocytosis, membrane changes, and alterations in energy metabolism in the brain. Although some of these findings are regional (e.g. decreased NAA in basal ganglia and frontal white matter, increased myo-inositol in the frontal gray matter), it is not clear whether the findings are specific to these regions or simply reflect changes that potentially affect other regions of the brain as well.

Using rodent models of methamphetamine abuse, researchers have reported significant damage to dopamine terminals and changes in glutamatergic neurotransmission (Eisch et al., 1992; Pu and Vorhees 1995; Cass, 1997; Fleckenstein et al., 2000). The mechanisms underlying these changes have received considerable attention, with many studies suggesting important roles for excitotoxicity and accumulation of reactive oxygen species, as well as other factors (Farfel and Seiden, 1995; Davison et al., 1996; Stephans and Yamamoto, 1996; Larsen et al., 2002). These studies are the foundation for acute models of methamphetamine-related injury.

451

Eisch *et al.* (1996) reported on ^{3}H-mazindol binding to striatal dopamine transporters and ^{3}H-glutamate binding to glutamate receptors in the striatum and cortex one week and one month after methamphetamine infusion. Findings indicate that a neurotoxic regimen of methamphetamine results in long-lasting injury to striatal dopamine terminals but reversible decreases in glutamate receptor binding. This and other research from the animal literature (Eisch *et al.*, 1996; Yamamoto *et al.*, 1999) supports the notion that the brain is involved in a neuroadaptive process during acute methamphetamine exposure, withdrawal, and abstinence.

In contrast to the multiple studies that have examined the effect of methamphetamine on dopaminergic neurons in humans, there have been very few in-vivo studies examining the impact of the drug on non-dopaminergic systems (Volkow *et al.*, 2001c). This is despite the fact that there is evidence that methamphetamine abuse might impact brain regions that are not significantly innervated by dopaminergic pathways. For example, Volkow and colleagues (2001c) found significant hypermetabolism in the parietal lobe of methamphetamine dependent patients. Based on animal research that had found increases in glutamatergic receptors in the parietal cortex of rats (Eisch *et al.*, 1996), Volkow and colleagues speculated on whether such an increase in receptors would make the parietal lobe sensitive to glutamatergic excitotoxicity. In addition, they questioned whether the regional impact of methamphetamine might be similar to the effect of the drug on pyramidal glutamatergic cells in the parietal cortex of rats (Commins and Seiden, 1986; Ryan *et al.*, 1990).

While the mechanisms have not been fully characterized, animal studies form the foundation for understanding the complex phenomenon of neuroadaptation after drug abstinence. It may be the case that the neurochemical changes during methamphetamine abstinence parallel other models of neuroadaptation after withdrawal (e.g. alcoholism). If this is the case, the neurochemical signature during acute methamphetamine use and during abstinence is likely to be different. Whereas an excitotoxic process is implicated in methamphetamine-related neuronal injury during acute use, longer-term abstinence (>one month) may be associated with the opposite effect. For example, Yamamoto and colleagues show that after seven days of abstinence, rats displayed decreased cortical glutamate release (Yamamoto *et al.*, 1999).

Opioids

Few studies have examined opioid receptor binding in humans, and thus the relationship between the neurochemical underpinnings of intoxication and the transition to prolonged use remains largely unclear. Methadone maintenance among former heroin users has been associated with decreased striatal mu- and kappa-opioid receptor binding (Kling *et al.*, 2000). Similarly, others have characterized a dose-dependent reduction in mu receptor binding during buprenorphine maintenance, particularly in frontal, striatal, and limbic regions (Zubieta *et al.*, 2000; Greenwald *et al.*, 2003). Buprenorphine maintenance is also associated with reduced mu-opioid receptor availability (Greenwald *et al.*, 2007). In one preliminary study, mu-opioid receptor binding was characterized using ^{11}C-carfentanil PET among three heroin-dependent individuals both during buprenorphine maintenance and after 2 weeks of detoxification (Zubieta *et al.*, 2000). During detoxification, heroin users demonstrated increased mu receptor binding compared to non-users in inferior prefrontal cortex and anterior cingulate, which could suggest upregulation of opioid receptors in heroin dependence. However, the small sample of only three heroin users should be noted when interpreting results.

The endogenous opioid system may have a general role in substance dependence. For instance, cocaine-dependent men showed increased carfentanil binding, indicating increased mu-opioid receptor density, in the caudate, thalamus, anterior cingulate, and frontal and temporal cortices (Zubieta *et al.*, 1996). There has also been question as to whether chronic opioid use is associated with altered reward system functioning. A recent PET study examined striatal dopamine transporter availability in 11 former heroin users, 10 former users undergoing methadone maintenance, and 10 non-users (Shi *et al.*, 2008). Compared to non-users, methadone-maintained individuals showed reduced dopamine transporter function in bilateral caudate and putamen, while abstinent heroin users demonstrated lower dopamine transporter function in bilateral caudate alone. These results could suggest recovery of function with prolonged abstinence from opioids. In addition, anxiety level was correlated to dopamine transporter density in the caudate among methadone maintenance subjects, while there was no relationship between dopamine transporter density and craving in either opioid-dependent group. Thus, it appears that reduced in heroin craving among methadone users may not be related to striatal dopamine functioning.

There is scant evidence on brain metabolite levels among individuals with opioid dependence. One proton MRS study characterized metabolites in individuals with heroin dependence during methadone maintenance. Heroin-dependent subjects demonstrated diminished absolute concentrations of NAA in medial frontal gray matter. No differences were found for choline or creatine, nor in NAA levels in medial frontal gray matter, lateral frontal white or gray matter (Haselhorst et al., 2002).

Nicotine

Nicotine acts through a variety of mechanisms and diverse neurotransmitters to alter dopamine release in the brain. It causes release of dopamine (Brody et al., 2004), and the nicotine is an important factor for that release (Brody et al., 2009). Nicotine also exerts diverse effects on GABAergic neurons and their interactions with glutamatergic and dopaminergic neurons. In the cortex, GABAergic neurons exert their inhibitory powers on glutamatergic neurons locally, including those glutamatergic neurons that project from anywhere in the cortex to the striatum, where the glutamatergic projections stimulate dopaminergic neurons. Striatal GABAergic neurons locally inhibit dopaminergic neurons, which project to the nucleus accumbens. One action of nicotine is to stimulate GABAergic activity through nicotinic acetylcholine receptors (nAChRs) for several minutes and then receptor desensitization reverses this effect, which actually inhibits ongoing cholinergic inputs. Both activation and desensitization of nAChRs likely contribute to the circuit and behavioral effects of nicotine, but the impact of each of these is unknown. In rat midbrain tissue slice experiments, nAChR desensitization leads to disinhibition of the dopamine neurons through suppression of GABA neuron excitability (Mansvelder et al., 2002). Similar disinhibition of cortical pyramidal neurons by desensitization of nAChRs on GABA neurons may occur, but this would be preceded by an increase in GABA neuron activity and enhanced GABA release. A recent study in rat prefrontal cortex slices suggests that nAChR excitation of GABA interneurons enhances GABAergic drive onto pyramidal neurons. Under these conditions, stronger synaptic inputs to the pyramidal neurons are necessary to induce LTP, which means that the synaptic inputs that are reinforced must have a higher signal-to-noise ratio (Couey et al., 2007).

Nicotine has been shown to increase the release of GABA in a variety of brain regions and conditions, at readily attainable levels of nicotine (McGehee and Role, 1996). For a useful review of the neurochemistry of nicotine interactions with these neurotransmitter systems, see Watkins et al. (2000). The release of tritiated glutamate was increased in rat cerebellar slices through the action of nicotine on α_7 acetylcholine receptor activation (Markus et al., 2003), and the effect could be blocked with α-bungarotoxin (Markus et al., 2004). In preparations of prefrontal cortical slices of rat brain, nicotine induced glutamate release, with the observation lacking in mice that lacked the β_2-nAChR subunit (Lambe et al., 2003). Also in primary hippocampal neuronal cultures, nicotine-induced glutamatergic neurotransmission has been observed, as well as stimulation of release of GABA (Gray et al., 1996; Radcliffe and Dani, 1998; Radcliffe et al., 1999). Likewise, nicotine-induced GABA release has been observed in slices of human cerebral cortex (Alkondon et al., 2000).

Studies of smoking to examine neurochemical damage to the brain, rather than nicotine in particular, have shown that smoking exerts apparently deleterious effects on the neurochemicals NAA and choline in recovering alcoholics (Gazdzinski et al., 2008), although it is uncertain whether the effects arise from nicotine in particular or the broader effects of smoking.

Although nicotine affects many systems, it is possible that its breadth of impact presents greater opportunities for treatment of addiction than would be possible if its effects were more focused.

MDMA

There is considerable variability in purity of the ingredient methylenedioxymethamphetamine (MDMA) in Ecstasy pills, presenting methodological challenges for researching the effects of this drug. In addition, much of the neuroimaging work related to MDMA use has focused on the possible neurotoxic impact of chronic exposure, rather than the acute neurochemical effects that may contribute to continued use and dependence. One PET study of MDMA administration demonstrated reduced glucose metabolism in bilateral frontal cortex, but increased glucose metabolism in bilateral cerebellum and right putamen (Reneman *et al.*, 2002a).

Both PET and SPECT studies have reported reduced serotonin transporter (SERT) levels throughout the brain among current users (for review, see Cowan, 2007), with similar results produced by different ligands (McCann *et al.*, 2005). Reductions in prefrontal and parietal SERT levels appear associated with learning and memory decrements among current users (McCann *et al.*, 2008). However, one group described continued verbal learning decrements following discontinuation of use, despite normalization of SERT levels (Thomasius *et al.*, 2003, 2006), questioning the behavioral implications of these serotonin system changes. The question of mood dysregulation among chronic MDMA users has remained equivocal, and recent evidence has not supported a relationship between SERT availability and mood (de Win *et al.*, 2004; Thomasius *et al.*, 2006).

Although most radioligand imaging among MDMA users has focused on SERT levels, a few studies have explored alterations in other receptor systems. One group has used SPECT imaging to characterize the effects of chronic MDMA use on post-synaptic serotonin receptors. Current MDMA users demonstrated reduced serotonin-2A receptor levels in frontal, parietal, and occipital cortex (Reneman *et al.*, 2002a). Dopamine systems have also been investigated. One study found higher [^{123}I]-CIT binding in the striatum of current MDMA users, reflecting increased dopamine transporter levels (Reneman *et al.*, 2000b), while others have found no difference in dopamine transporter binding (McCann *et al.*, 2008).

A preliminary PET study identified diminished resting glucose metabolism among MDMA users within the amygdala, hippocampus, and prefrontal cortex (Obrocki *et al.*, 1999). Utilizing PET, reduced glucose metabolism was observed in the striatum, amygdala, and cingulate among current users (Buchert *et al.*, 2001). This effect was more pronounced among individuals who began use before the age of 18.

MRS studies of MDMA use have presented some inconsistent findings. One group has reported increased parietal white matter *myo*-inositol related to lifetime use, but no difference in NAA/Cr in frontal, occipital, and parietal regions (Chang *et al.*, 1999). A study of polydrug-abusing MDMA users also failed to observe significant reductions in NAA/Cr in cortical regions, and a trend toward lower NAA/Cr in the

hippocampus (Daumann *et al.*, 2004). More recently, an MRSI study demonstrated no differences in absolute concentrations of occipital NAA or *myo*-inositol among MDMA users compared to controls, although small sample size and a gender imbalance may have influenced results (Cowan *et al.*, 2007). An extension of this work found no relationship between degree of MDMA use and metabolite levels (Cowan *et al.*, 2009). However, others have observed reduced NAA among MDMA users. Reneman and colleagues (2002c) characterized reduced NAA/Cr and NAA/Cho in frontal cortex, with degree of exposure negatively correlated to NAA ratios. No differences were found in midline occipital gray or parietal white matter NAA ratios or in *myo*-inositol ratios. Another study by the same group identified reduced prefrontal gray matter NAA/Cr that was associated with poorer verbal delayed recall among MDMA users, although no relationship was found with immediate recall (Reneman *et al.*, 2001). Overall, MRS findings have been relatively subtle, which could imply that this technique is less sensitive to detecting neurotoxicity related to MDMA use.

Although much research has indicated neurochemical abnormalities among MDMA users, the question of whether these effects predate the onset of use remains difficult to answer. In a recent prospective multi-modal neuroimaging study, 188 young adults who were at risk for MDMA use were scanned both before MDMA initiation and again one to three years later (de Win *et al.*, 2008). At follow-up, those who initiated use demonstrated no differences in SERT binding or MRS metabolite ratios compared to individuals who remained Ecstasy-naive. This study suggests that initiation of Ecstasy use may not cause neurochemical abnormalities among novel low-dose users.

While mounting evidence indicates serotonergic system damage among current MDMA users, recent work has suggested the possibility of normalization during protracted abstinence. With relative consistency across a variety of cross-sectional and longitudinal designs, former users have exhibited normalized SERT binding (for review, see Gouzoulis-Mayfrank and Daumann, 2006; Cowan, 2007). Further supporting the possibility of recovery, studies have characterized a positive correlation between duration of MDMA abstinence and SERT binding (Semple *et al.*, 1999; Buchert *et al.*, 2004). There is also preliminary evidence of normalization of serotonin-2A receptor densities. In a cross-sectional SPECT study, recent users exhibited reduced binding throughout the cortex, but users who had been abstinent at least two months demonstrated altered binding only in occipital cortex (Reneman *et al.*, 2002a). Moreover, there was a positive correlation between binding and abstinence duration.

Cannabinoids

Marijuana is the most widely used illicit substance in the United States (SAMHSA, 2008), and researchers have been attempting to describe its influence on the brain for decades. Much in-vivo imaging work has focused on neurocognition among marijuana users, yet less attention has been given to the possible neurochemical impact of marijuana use in humans. In addition, research on the effects of cannabinoids presents unique methodological considerations because cannabinoid metabolites can remain detectable in the urine for several weeks among heavy users (Ellis *et al.*, 1985), and may continue to affect neural functioning beyond the stage of acute intoxication. Thus, it is important to consider length of abstinence among study participants in order to determine whether results represent acute, residual, or persisting alterations in neural functioning.

Acutely, marijuana primarily exerts its psychoactive effects via stimulation of CB1 receptors by Δ-9-tetrahydrocannabinol (THC). Autoradiographic investigations have revealed the greatest distribution of CB1 receptors in the basal ganglia, hippocampus, cerebellum, and association cortices, including prefrontal cortex and cingulate gyrus (Herkenham *et al.*, 1990; Glass *et al.*, 1997; Eggan and Lewis, 2007). In-vivo imaging of the cannabinoid system is under recent development (cf. Lindsey *et al.*, 2005), and new ligands are beginning to be tested (Burns *et al.*, 2007; Hamill *et al.*, 2009). A case report SPECT study indicated an increase in striatal dopamine release following marijuana use, as a participant in a schizophrenia research study surreptitiously used between scans (Voruganti *et al.*, 2001). More recently and in a controlled environment, a raclopride PET study demonstrated dopamine release in the human ventral striatum following inhalation of THC (Bossong *et al.*, 2009). This provides preliminary evidence that marijuana, like other drugs of abuse, causes striatal dopamine release consistent with the neurochemical model of reward response in addiction. There is also evidence that cannabinoids modulate other neurotransmitter systems (for review, see Lopez-Moreno *et al.*, 2008); however, this has not yet been demonstrated in-vivo in humans.

Acute THC administration increases cerebellar glucose metabolism in both non-users (Volkow *et al.* 1991, 1996) and individuals with cannabis dependence (Volkow *et al.*, 1996). In addition, dependent individuals demonstrated increased glucose metabolism in orbitofrontal cortex, prefrontal cortex, and basal ganglia (Volkow *et al.*, 1996), which are regions densely packed with CB1 receptors.

Among chronic users, one PET study has revealed reduced resting cerebellar glucose metabolism (Volkow *et al.*, 1996). Recent investigations have also begun utilizing proton MRS to characterize neurochemical functioning in chronic marijuana users. Chang and colleagues (2006) scanned individuals with histories of heavy marijuana use with and without HIV, localizing voxels in frontal white matter, parietal white matter, basal ganglia, thalamus, cerebellar vermix, and occipital gray matter. Independent of HIV status, marijuana use was associated with decreased NAA, choline, and glutamate in the basal ganglia, and increased creatine in the thalamus. HIV-negative marijuana users also demonstrated reduced *myo*-inositol compared to controls. In a ^{1}H MRSI study, a group of current heavy cannabis-using males exhibited lower dorsolateral prefrontal NAA/Cr than controls (Hermann *et al.*, 2007). A recent ^{1}H MRS study examined metabolite levels among polydrug MDMA users, and examined the relationship between metabolite levels and exposure to MDMA, cannabis, alcohol, or cocaine (Cowan *et al.*, 2009). Only the degree of marijuana involvement showed a relationship with reductions in inferior frontal/insula NAA/Cr.

The question of neurochemical recovery in heavy marijuana users has begun to be explored. Sevy and colleagues measured raclopride and FDG binding among marijuana dependent individuals who had been abstinent at least 12 weeks (Sevy *et al.*, 2008). Results indicated similar striatal D2/D3 receptor availability between groups. Cerebral glucose metabolism was reduced in orbitofrontal cortex, precuneus, and putatmen; no relationship was found between D2/D3 availability and glucose metabolism. These results indicate lasting alterations in glucose metabolism, but normal dopamine functioning. In the ^{1}H MRS study by Chang and colleagues (2006), a large proportion of marijuana users had been abstinent for months or even years. Although length of abstinence was not specifically examined in relation to brain metabolite levels, it is possible that altered neurochemistry observed in this study represents changes that persist with abstinence.

Alcohol

MRS investigations have revealed chemical pathology in the brains of alcoholic individuals. Decreased levels of NAA have been found in the frontal lobes (Fein *et al.*, 1994; Jagannathan *et al.*, 1996; Bendszus *et al.*, 2001; Schweinsburg and *et al.*, 2001, 2003), thalamus (Jagannathan *et al.*, 1996), and cerebellum (Jagannathan *et al.*, 1996; Seitz *et al.*, 1999; Bendszus *et al.*, 2001) of abstinent alcoholics. The reductions in NAA found in these studies are generally thought to reflect neuronal injury or death. In addition, elevated *myo*-inositol has been reported in brain white matter (Schweinsburg *et al.*, 2001). The damage may result from nutritional problems such as thiamine deficiencies (Pfefferbaum *et al.*, 2007), but other factors can certainly contribute significantly (Zahr *et al.*, 2009).

Several MRS studies have examined the impact of sobriety on brain metabolites. Martin and colleagues (1995) found reduced levels of choline/NAA in the cerebellar vermis of recently detoxified alcoholics. Individuals who maintained sobriety showed improvements in this ratio, and the authors concluded that this may indicate "remyelination or reversal of partial cholinergic deafferentation". Similar choline results were found in the cerebellum by Bendszus and colleagues (2001). Increased frontal lobe (Bendszus *et al.*, 2001) and cerebellar (Bendszus *et al.*, 2001; Parks *et al.*, 2002) NAA levels have been observed after approximately 30 days sober. In a preliminary study, *myo*-inositol was significantly elevated in a midline frontal gray matter and right thalamus region of interest in recently detoxified alcoholics (Schweinsburg *et al.*, 2000). However, a small group of individuals who had maintained long-term abstinence from alcohol had concentrations of *myo*-inositol that closely reflected control values. These results suggest reversible astrocyte proliferation and/or an osmolar response to alcohol-induced cell shrinkage.

In further support of a model of energy inefficiency associated with alcohol use and alcoholism, positron emission tomography (PET) studies using fluorodeoxyglucose (FDG) have revealed reductions in resting glucose metabolism. Glucose is oxidized to carbon dioxide and water in a series of reactions that yield a fundamental energy source ATP. In a recent quantitative PET study, healthy volunteers displayed substantial reductions in whole brain and regional glucose metabolism during an alcohol challenge (Wang *et al.*, 2003). The largest reductions were in occipital cortex with large changes in parietal lobes as well. An earlier study showed similar findings, and a small group of alcoholics evidenced even greater decreases than controls (Volkow *et al.*, 1990). Abstinent alcoholics generally demonstrate glucose hypometabolism (Wik *et al.*, 1988; Gilman *et al.*, 1990; Volkow *et al.*, 1992, 1994; Johnson-Greene *et al.*, 1997; Dao-Castellana *et al.*, 1998), with evidence of recovery during short-term (Volkow *et al.*, 1992, 1994) and long-term (Johnson-Greene *et al.*, 1997) abstinence. The frontal lobes may be particularly vulnerable to alcoholism-related glucose hypometabolism, and reduced metabolism is reportedly correlated with tests of frontal lobe functioning (Adams *et al.*, 1993). The reduction in glucose metabolism may be paired with reduced production of ATP by mitochondria. Given the links between NAA synthesis and glucose metabolism (Moreno *et al.*, 2001) and the evidence provided by previous PET studies, the observed reductions in NAA during short-term sobriety and subsequent increases during protracted abstinence suggest that chronic, heavy alcohol consumption may lead to alterations in cerebral energy metabolism.

As mentioned earlier in this chapter, smoking is associated with compromised functional and neurochemical recovery in alcoholics (Gazdzinski *et al.*, 2008). With respect to neurotransmission, smoking and non-smoking alcoholics show different time-dependent changes in brain GABA levels after the onset of sobriety (Mason *et al.*, 2006). This may be due to different adaptations of acetylcholine receptors (Staley *et al.*, 2006), GABA receptors (Staley *et al.*, 2005), or other aspects of diverse neurotransmitter systems.

Factors that moderate substance use

One important moderating factor to consider is gender. There are gender differences in the prevalence of substance use, with rates generally higher among men (SAMHSA, 2006). There are also gender differences in physiological response to intoxication. For example, lower percent body water and slower alcohol metabolism lead to greater alcohol intoxication among women. Gender differences in response to acute and long-term exposure may be subserved by neurochemical differences as well.

Conclusions

Physicists, engineers, mathematicians, chemists, biologists, biochemists, physiologists, and clinicians from a range of fields have worked in teams at institutions around the world to create the methods and applications that have led to current neurochemical findings about substance abuse. At this point, information exists that show structural, chemical, and functional alterations from legal and illicit substances. Some of the changes appear to be outright damage, while others are likely to be adaptive. To carry the research further, developments are under way to improve spatial resolution of the imaging methods or to enhance the ability to differentiate similar chemicals that are detected by MRS. New radiochemicals are constantly in development to achieve greater sensitivity and specificity for given aspects of particular neurotransmitter systems. However, an approach has been appearing more often: multi-modal experiments.

Increasingly, neuroimaging scientists are working together in groups within and between institutions to study similar patients or the same patients using various methods at their disposal. For example, one may explore structural changes in the brains of methamphetamine abusers with the use of diffusion imaging and then evaluate neurochemical changes in areas of abnormalities by the use of MRS and PET. Such studies are expensive but yield richer information than would be obtained by performing all three measurements as completely separate operations.

Another recent entry into the field of neurochemistry is genetics. Studies are now being designed in the context of substance abuse to explore the relationships of the precise form of certain genes with function and neurochemistry. For example, it is now possible to perform genotyping of a family and then measure aspects of brain structure, function, and chemistry in the same people to compare to what was found with the genes. This type of work also requires a constructive collaborative environment of the sort used for multi-modal imaging projects.

A third tool for research on substance abuse is pharmacology. Today there exists a rich arsenal of medications that are designed to target particular aspects of neurochemistry, and they can be used to test hypotheses. If neurochemical imaging shows that dopamine is probably the primary target of an illicit substance, and a medication is given with the goal of an opposite effect on dopamine, one can measure if the neurochemical effect was reversed. At the same time, functional and behavioral aspects of the substance and the medication's effects can be studied.

In summary, the future of neurochemical research on substance abuse will probably entail group efforts to evaluate several aspects of brain function.

References

Adams K M, Gilman S, Koeppe R A, et al. 1993. Neuropsychological deficits are correlated with frontal hypometabolism in positron emission tomography studies of older alcoholic patients. *Alcohol Clin Exp Res* **17**, 205–10.

Alhassoon O M, Dupont R M, Schweinsburg B C, Taylor M J, Patterson T L and Grant I. 2001. Regional cerebral blood flow in cocaine- versus methamphetamine-dependent patients with a history of alcoholism. *Int J Neuropsychopharmacol* **4**, 105–12.

Alkondon M, Pereira E F, Eisenberg H M and Albuquerque E X. 2000. Nicotinic receptor activation in human cerebral cortical interneurons: A mechanism for inhibition and disinhibition of neuronal networks. *J Neurosci* **20**, 66–75.

Ariyannura P S, Madhavaraoa C N and Namboodiri A M A. 2008. N-acetylaspartate synthesis in the brain: Mitochondria vs. microsomes. *Brain Res* **1227**, 34–41.

Arstad E, Gitto R, Chimirri A, et al. 2006. Closing in on the AMPA receptor: Synthesis and evaluation of 2-acetyl-1-(4'-chlorophenyl)-6-methoxy-7-[^{11}C] methoxy-1,2,3,4-tetrahydroisoquinoline as a potential PET tracer. *Bioorg Med Chem* **14**, 4712–7.

Behar K L and Ogino T. 1993. Characterization of macromolecule resonances in the 1H NMR spectrum of rat brain. *Magn Reson Med* **30**, 38–44.

Bendszus M, Weijers H G, Wiesbeck G, et al. 2001. Sequential MR imaging and proton MR spectroscopy in patients who underwent recent detoxification for chronic alcoholism: Correlation with clinical and neuropsychological data. *Am J Neuroradiol* **22**, 1926–32.

Biegon A, Gibbs A, Alvarado M, Ono M and Taylor S. 2007. In vitro and in vivo characterization of [3H]CNS-5161 – A use-dependent ligand for the N-methyl-D-aspartate receptor in rat brain. *Synapse* **61**, 577–86.

Blusztajn J K, Liscovitch M and Richardson U I. 2008. Synthesis of acetylcholine from choline derived from phosphatidylcholine in a human neuronal cell line. *Proc Natl Acad Sci USA* **84**, 5474–7.

Bossong M G, van Berckel B N, Boellaard R, et al. 2009. Delta 9-tetrahydrocannabinol induces dopamine release in the human striatum. *Neuropsychopharmacology* **34**, 759–66.

457

Bostwick D G. 1981. Amphetamine induced cerebral vasculitis. *Hum Pathol* **12**, 1031–3.

Braissant O, Henry H, Loup M, Eilers B and Bachmann C. 2001. Endogenous synthesis and transport of creatine in the rat brain: An in situ hybridization study. *Mol Brain Res* **86**, 193–201.

Brockerhoff H and Ballou C E. 1962. On the metabolism of the brain phosphoinositide complex. *J Biol Chem* **237**, 1764–8.

Brody A L, Mandelkern M A, Olmstead R E, *et al.* 2009. Ventral striatal dopamine release in response to smoking a regular vs a denicotinized cigarette. *Neuropsychopharmacology* **34**, 282–9.

Brody A L, Olmstead R E, London E D, *et al.* 2004. Smoking-induced ventral striatum dopamine release. *Am J Psychiatry* **161**, 1211–8.

Buchert R, Obrocki J, Thomasius R, *et al.* 2001. Long-term effects of "ecstasy" abuse on the human brain studied by FDG PET. *Nucl Med Commun* **22**, 889–97.

Buchert R, Thomasius R, Wilke F, *et al.* 2004. A voxel-based PET investigation of the long-term effects of "ecstasy" consumption on brain serotonin transporters. *Am J Psychiatry* **161**, 1181–9.

Burns H D, Van Laere K, Sanabria-Bohorquez S, *et al.* 2007. [18F]MK-9470, a positron emission tomography (PET) tracer for in vivo human PET brain imaging of the cannabinoid-1 receptor. *Proc Natl Acad Sci U S A* **104**, 9800–05.

Cahill D W, Knipp H and Mosser J. 1981. Intracranial hemorrhage with amphetamine abuse. *Neurology* **31**, 1058–9.

Cass W A. 1997. Decreases in evoked overflow of dopamine in rat striatum after neurotoxic doses of methamphetamine. *J Pharmacol Exp Ther* **280**, 105–13.

Chakraborty G, Mekala P, Yahya D, Wu G and Ledeen R W. 2001. Intraneuronal N-acetylaspartate supplies acetyl groups for myelin lipid synthesis: evidence for myelin-associated aspartoacylase. *J Neurochem* **78**. 736–45.

Chang L, Cloak C, Yakupov R and Ernst T. 2006. Combined and independent effects of chronic marijuana use and HIV on brain metabolites. *J Neuroimmune Pharmacol* **1**, 65–76.

Chang L, Ernst T, Grob C S and Poland R E. 1999. Cerebral (1)H MRS alterations in recreational 3, 4-methylenedioxymethamphetamine (MDMA, "ecstasy") users. *J Magn Reson Imaging* **10**, 521–6.

Choi C, Coupland N J, Bhardwaj P P, Malykhin N, Gheorghiu D and Allen P S. 2006. Measurement of brain glutamate and glutamine by spectrally-selective refocusing at 3 Tesla. *Magn Reson Med* **55**, 997–1005.

Commins D L and Seiden L S. 1986. Alpha-methyltyrosine blocks methylamphetamine-induced degeneration in the rat somatosensory cortex. *Brain Res* **365**, 15–20.

Couey J J, Meredith R M, Spijker S, *et al.* 2007. Distributed network actions by nicotine increase the threshold for spike-timing-dependent plasticity in prefrontal cortex. *Neuron* **54**, 73–87.

Cowan R L. 2007. Neuroimaging research in human MDMA users: A review. *Psychopharmacology (Berl)* **189**, 539–56.

Cowan R L, Bolo N R, Dietrich M, Haga E, Lukas S E and Renshaw P F. 2007. Occipital cortical proton MRS at 4 Tesla in human moderate MDMA polydrug users. *Psychiatry Res* **155**, 179–88.

Cowan R L, Joers J M and Dietrich M S. 2009. N-acetylaspartate (NAA) correlates inversely with cannabis use in a frontal language processing region of neocortex in MDMA (Ecstasy) polydrug users: A 3 T magnetic resonance spectroscopy study. *Pharmacol Biochem Behav* **92**, 105–10.

Dao-Castellana M H, Samson Y, Legault F, *et al.* 1998. Frontal dysfunction in neurologically normal chronic alcoholic subjects: Metabolic and neuropsychological findings. *Psychol Med* **28**, 1039–48.

Daumann J, Fischermann T, Pilatus U, Thron A, Moeller-Hartmann W and Gouzoulis-Mayfrank E. 2004. Proton magnetic resonance spectroscopy in ecstasy (MDMA) users. *Neurosci Lett* **362**, 113–6.

Davison F D, Sweeney B J and Scaravilli F. 1996. Mitochondrial DNA levels in the brain of HIV-positive patients after zidovudine therapy. *J Neurol* **243**, 648–51.

de Win M M, Jager G, Booij J, *et al.* 2008. Sustained effects of ecstasy on the human brain: A prospective neuroimaging study in novel users. *Brain* **131**, 2936–45.

de Win M M, Reneman L, Reitsma J B, den Heeten G J, Booij J and van den Brink W. 2004. Mood disorders and serotonin transporter density in ecstasy users – The influence of long-term abstention, dose, and gender. *Psychopharmacology (Berl)* **173**, 376–82.

Eggan S M and Lewis D A. 2007. Immunocytochemical distribution of the cannabinoid CB1 receptor in the primate neocortex: A regional and laminar analysis. *Cerebral Cortex* **17**, 175–52.

Eisch A J, Gaffney M, Weihmuller F B, O'Dell S J and Marshall J F. 1992. Striatal subregions are differentially vulnerable to the neurotoxic effects of methamphetamine. *Brain Res* **598**, 321–6.

Eisch A J, O'Dell S J and Marshall J F. 1996. Striatal and cortical NMDA receptors are altered by a neurotoxic regimen of methamphetamine. *Synapse* **22**, 217–25.

Ellis G M Jr, Mann M A, Judson B A, Schramm N T and Tashchian A. 1985. Excretion patterns of cannabinoid metabolites after last use in a group of chronic users. *Clin Pharmacol Therap* **38**, 572–8.

Elsinga P H, Hatano K and Ishiwata K. 2006. PET tracers for imaging of the dopaminergic system. *Curr Med Chem* **13**, 2139–53.

Ernst T, Chang L, Leonido-Yee M and Speck O. 2000. Evidence for long-term neurotoxicity associated with methamphetamine abuse: A 1H MRS study. *Neurology* **54**, 1344–9.

Farfel G M and Seiden L S. 1995. Role of hypothermia in the mechanism of protection against serotonergic toxicity. II. Experiments with methamphetamine, *p*-chloroamphetamine, fenfluramine, dizocilpine and dextromethorphan. *J Pharmacol Exp Ther* **272**, 868–75.

Fein G, Meyerhoff D J, Discalfani V, *et al.* 1994. ¹H magnetic resonance spectroscopic imaging separates neuronal from glial changes in alcohol-related brain atrophy. In Lancaster F E (Ed.) *Alcohol and Glial Cells*. Bethesda, MD: National Institutes of Health, **27**, 227–41.

Fleckenstein A E, Gibb J W and Hanson G R. 2000. Differential effects of stimulants on monoaminergic transporters: Pharmacological consequences and implications for neurotoxicity. *Eur J Pharmacol* **406**, 1–13.

Gao M, Kong D, Clearfield A and Zheng Q-H. 2006. Synthesis of carbon-11 and fluorine-18 labeled *N*-acetyl-1-aryl-6,7-dimethoxy-1,2,3,4-tetrahydroisoquinoline derivatives as new potential PET AMPA receptor ligands. *Bioorg Med Chem Lett* **16**, 2229–33.

Gazdzinski S, Durazzo T C, Yeh P -H, Hardin D, Banys P and Meyerhoff D J. 2008. Chronic cigarette smoking modulates injury and short-term recovery of the medial temporal lobe in alcoholics. *Psychiatry Res* **162**, 133–45.

Gilman S, Adams K, Koeppe R A, *et al.* 1990. Cerebellar and frontal hypometabolism in alcoholic cerebellar degeneration studied with positron emission tomography. *Ann Neurol* **28**, 775–85.

Glass M, Dragunow M and Faull R L. 1997. Cannabinoid receptors in the human brain: A detailed anatomical and quantitative autoradiographic study in the fetal, neonatal and adult human brain. *Neuroscience* **77**, 299–318.

Gouzoulis-Mayfrank E and Daumann J. 2006. Neurotoxicity of methylenedioxyamphetamines (MDMA; ecstasy) in humans: How strong is the evidence for persistent brain damage? *Addiction* **101**, 348–61.

Gray R, Rajan A S, Radcliffe K A, Yakehiro M and Dani J A. 1996. Hippocampal synaptic transmission enhanced by low concentrations of nicotine. *Nature* **383**, 713–6.

Greenwald M, Johanson C -E, Bueller J, *et al.* 2007. Buprenorphine duration of action: Mu-opioid receptor availability and pharmacokinetic and behavioral indices. *Biol Psychiatry* **61**, 101–10.

Greenwald M K, Johanson C-E, Moody D E, *et al.* 2003. Effects of buprenorphine maintenance dose on mu-opioid receptor availability, plasma concentrations, and antagonist blockade in heroin-dependent volunteers. *Neuropsychopharmacology* **28**, 2000–9.

Hamill T G, Lin L S, Hagmann W, *et al.* 2009. PET imaging studies in rhesus monkey with the cannabinoid-1 (CB1) receptor ligand [(11)C]CB-119. *Mol Imaging Biol* **11**, 246–52.

Haselhorst R, Dursteler-MacFarland K M, Scheffler K, *et al.* 2002. Frontocortical *N*-acetylaspartate reduction associated with long-term i.v. heroin use. *Neurology* **58**, 305–07.

Henriksen G and Willoch F. 2008. Imaging of opioid receptors in the central nervous system. *Brain* **131**, 1171–96.

Herkenham M, Lynn A B, Little M D, *et al.* 1990. Cannabinoid receptor localization in brain. *Proc Natl Acad Sci USA* **87**, 1932–6.

Hermann D, Sartorius A, Welzel H, *et al.* 2007. Dorsolateral prefrontal cortex *N*-acetylaspartate/total creatine (NAA/tCr) loss in male recreational cannabis users. *Biol Psychiatry* **61**, 1281–9.

Hesse S, Barthel H, Schwarz J, Sabri O and Muller U. 2004. Advances in in vivo imaging of serotonergic neurons in neuropsychiatric disorders. *Neurosci Biobehav Rev* **28**, 547–63. [Erratum, *Neurosci Biobehav Rev*, 2005, **29**, 1119.]

Horti A G and Van Laere K. 2008. Development of radioligands for in vivo imaging of type 1 cannabinoid receptors (CB1) in human brain. *Curr Pharmaceut Des* **14**, 3363–83.

Hurd R, Sailasuta N, Srinivasan R, Vigneron D B, Pelletier D and Nelson S J. 2004. Measurement of brain glutamate using TE-averaged PRESS at 3T. *Magn Reson Med* **51**, 435–40.

Iyo M, Namba H, Yanagisawa M, Hirai S, Yui N and Fukui S. 1997. Abnormal cerebral perfusion in chronic methamphetamine abusers: A study using 99MTc-HMPAO and SPECT. *Prog Neuropsychopharmacol Biol Psychiatry* **21**, 789–96.

Jagannathan N R, Desai N G, *et al.* 1996. Brain metabolite changes in alcoholism: An in vivo proton magnetic resonance spectroscopy (MRS) study. *Magn Res Imag* **14**, 553–7.

Johnson-Greene D, Adams K M, Gilman S, *et al.* 1997. Effects of abstinence and relapse upon neuropsychological function and cerebral glucose metabolism in severe chronic alcoholism. *J Clin Exp Neuropsychol* **19**, 378–85.

Kao C H, Wang S J and Yeh S H. 1994. Presentation of regional cerebral blood flow in amphetamine abusers by 99Tcm-HMPAO brain SPECT. *Nucl Med Commun* **15**, 94–8.

Katsifis A and Kassiou M. 2004. Development of radioligands for in vivo imaging of GABA(A)-benzodiazepine receptors. *Mini-Rev Med Chem* **4**, 909–21.

Kessler R C, Chiu W T, Demler O, Merikangas K R and Walters E E. 2005. Prevalence, severity, and comorbidity of 12-month DSM-IV disorders in the National Comorbidity Survey Replication. *Arch Gen Psychiatry* **62**, 617–27.

Kling M A, Carson R E, Borg L, *et al.* 2000. Opioid receptor imaging with positron emission tomography and [(18)F] cyclofoxy in long-term, methadone-treated former heroin addicts. *J Pharmacol Exp Therap* **295**, 1070–6.

Koob G F and Le Moal M. 2001. Drug addiction, dysregulation of reward, and allostasis. *Neuropsychopharmacology* **24**, 97–129.

Lambe E K, Picciotto M R and Aghajanian G K. 2003. Nicotine induces glutamate release from thalamocortical terminals in prefrontal cortex. *Neuropsychopharmacology* **28**, 216–25.

Larsen K E, Fon E A, Hastings T G, Edwards R H and Sulzer D. 2002. Methamphetamine-induced degeneration of dopaminergic neurons involves autophagy and upregulation of dopamine synthesis. *J Neurosci* **22**, 8951–60.

Lindsey K P, Glaser S T and Gatley S J. 2005. Imaging of the brain cannabinoid system. *Handb Exp Pharmacol* **168**, 425–43.

Lopez-Moreno J A, Gonzalez-Cuevas G, Moreno G and Navarro M. 2008. The pharmacology of the endocannabinoid system: Functional and structural interactions with other neurotransmitter systems and their repercussions in behavioral addiction. *Addict Biol* **13**, 160–87.

Mansvelder H D, Keath J R and McGehee D S. 2002. Synaptic mechanisms underlie nicotine-induced excitability of brain reward areas. *Neuron* **33**, 905–19.

Markus R P, Reno L A C, Zago W and Markus R P. 2004. Release of [(3)H]-L-glutamate by stimulation of nicotinic acetylcholine receptors in rat cerebellar slices. *Neuroscience* **124**, 647–53.

Markus R P, Santos J M, Zago W and Reno L A C. 2003. Melatonin nocturnal surge modulates nicotinic receptors and nicotine-induced [3H]glutamate release in rat cerebellum slices. *J Pharmacol Exp Therap* **305**, 525–30.

Martin P R, Gibbs S J, *et al.* 1995. Brain proton magnetic resonance spectroscopy studies in recently abstinent alcoholics. *Alcohol Clin Exp Res* **19**, 1078–82.

Mason G F, Petrakis I L, de Graaf R A, *et al.* 2006. Cortical GABA levels and the recovery from alcohol dependence: Preliminary evidence of modification by cigarette smoking. *Biol Psychiatry* **59**, 85–93.

McCann U D, Szabo Z, Seckin E, *et al.* 2005. Quantitative PET studies of the serotonin transporter in MDMA users and controls using [11C]McN5652 and [11C]DASB. *Neuropsychopharmacology* **30**, 1741–50.

McCann U D, Szabo Z, Vranesic M, *et al.* 2008. Positron emission tomographic studies of brain dopamine and serotonin transporters in abstinent (+/−)3,4-methylenedioxymethamphetamine ("ecstasy") users: Relationship to cognitive performance. *Psychopharmacology (Berl)* **200**, 439–50.

McGehee D S and Role L W. 1996. Presynaptic ionotropic receptors. *Curr Opin Neurobiol* **6**, 342–9.

Michel V, Yuan Z, Ramsubir S and Bakovic M. 2006. Choline transport for phospholipid synthesis. *Exp Biol Med* **231**, 490–504.

Moreno A, Ross B D, *et al.* 2001. Direct determination of the *N*-acetyl-L-aspartate synthesis rate in the human brain by (13)C MRS and [1-(13)C]glucose infusion. *J Neurochem* **77**, 347–50.

NIDA and NIAAA. 1998. The economic costs of alcohol and drug abuse in the United States – 1992. *NIH Publication Number* **98**-4327.

Nordahl T E, Salo R, Possin K, *et al.* 2002. Low *N*-acetyl-aspartate and high choline in the anterior cingulum of recently abstinent methamphetamine-dependent subjects: A preliminary proton MRS study. Magnetic resonance spectroscopy. *Psychiatry Res* **116**, 43–52.

Obrocki J, Buchert R, Vaterlein O, Thomasius R, Beyer W and Schiemann T. 1999. Ecstasy – Long-term effects on the human central nervous system revealed by positron emission tomography. *Br J Psychiatry* **175**, 186–8.

Pacheco M A and Jope R S. 1996. Phosphoinositide signaling in human brain. *Progr Neurobiol* **50**, 255–73.

Parks M H, Dawant B M, Riddle W R, *et al.* 2002. Longitudinal brain metabolic characterization of chronic alcoholics with proton magnetic resonance spectroscopy. *Alcohol Clin Exp Res* **26**, 1368–80.

Patel T B and Clark J B. 1979. Synthesis of *N*-acetyl-L-aspartate by rat brain mitochondria and its involvement in mitochondrial/cytosolic carbon transport. *Biochem J* **184**, 539–46.

Pfefferbaum A, Adalsteinsson E, Bell R L and Sullivan E V. 2007. Development and resolution of brain lesions caused by pyrithiamine- and dietary-induced thiamine deficiency and alcohol exposure in the alcohol-preferring rat: A longitudinal magnetic resonance imaging and spectroscopy study. *Neuropsychopharmacology* **32**, 1159–77.

Phelps M E, Huang S C, Hoffman E J, Selin C, Sokoloff L and Kuhl D E. 1979. Tomographic measurement of local cerebral glucose metabolic rate in humans with

(F-18)2-fluoro-2-deoxy-D-glucose: Validation of method. *Ann Neurol* **6**, 371–88.

Pu C and Vorhees C V. 1995. Protective effects of MK-801 on methamphetamine-induced depletion of dopaminergic and serotonergic terminals and striatal astrocytic response: An immunohistochemical study. *Synapse* **19**, 97–104.

Radcliffe K A and Dani J A. 1998. Nicotinic stimulation produces multiple forms of increased glutamatergic synaptic transmission. *J Neurosci* **18**, 7075–83.

Radcliffe K A, Fisher J L, Gray R and Dani J A. 1999. Nicotinic modulation of glutamate and GABA synaptic transmission of hippocampal neurons. *Ann N Y Acad Sci* **868**, 591–610.

Reneman L, Booij J, Lavalaye J, *et al.* 2002b. Use of amphetamine by recreational users of ecstasy (MDMA) is associated with reduced striatal dopamine transporter densities: A [123I]beta-CIT SPECT study – Preliminary report. *Psychopharmacology (Berl)* **159**, 335–40.

Reneman L, Endert E, de Bruin K, *et al.* 2002a. The acute and chronic effects of MDMA ("ecstasy") on cortical 5-HT2A receptors in rat and human brain. *Neuropsychopharmacology* **26**, 387–96.

Reneman L, Majoie C B, Flick H and den Heeten G J. 2002c. Reduced *N*-acetylaspartate levels in the frontal cortex of 3,4-methylenedioxymethamphetamine (Ecstasy) users: Preliminary results. *Am J Neuroradiol* **23**, 231–7.

Reneman L, Majoie C B, Schmand B, van den Brink W and den Heeten G J. 2001. Prefrontal *N*-acetylaspartate is strongly associated with memory performance in (abstinent) ecstasy users: Preliminary report. *Biol Psychiatry* **50**, 550–4.

Rothman D L, Petroff O A, Behar K L and Mattson R H. 1993. Localized 1H NMR measurements of gamma-aminobutyric acid in human brain in vivo. *Proc Natl Acad Sci USA* **90**, 5662–6.

Ryan L J, Linder J C, Martone M E and Groves P M. 1990. Histological and ultrastructural evidence that D-amphetamine causes degeneration in neostriatum and frontal cortex of rats. *Brain Res* **518**, 67–77.

SAMHSA. 2006. Results from the 2005. National Survey on Drug Use and Health: National Findings. *NSDUM Series H-30*. Rockville, MD, Office of Applied Studies.

SAMHSA. 2008. Results from the 2007 National Survey on Drug Use and Health: National Findings. *NSDUH Series H-34*. Rockville, MD, Office of Applied Studies.

Sanchez-Pernaute R, Wang J Q, Kuruppu D, *et al.* 2008. Enhanced binding of metabotropic glutamate receptor type 5 (mGluR5) PET tracers in the brain of parkinsonian primates. *Neuroimage* **42**, 248–51.

Schweinsburg B C, Alhassoon O M, Taylor M J, *et al.* 2003. Effects of alcoholism and gender on brain metabolism. *Am J Psychiatry* **160**, 1180–3.

Schweinsburg B C, Taylor M J, Alhassoon O M, *et al.* 2001. Chemical pathology in brain white matter of recently detoxified alcoholics: A 1H magnetic resonance spectroscopy investigation of alcohol-associated frontal lobe injury. *Alcohol Clin Exp Res* **25**, 924–34.

Schweinsburg B C, Taylor M J, Videen J S, *et al.* 2000. Elevated myo-inositol in gray matter of recently detoxified but not long-term abstinent alcoholics: A preliminary MR spectroscopy study. *Alcohol Clin Exp Res* **24**, 699–705.

Seitz D, Widmann U, Seeger U, *et al.* 1999. Localized proton magnetic resonance spectroscopy of the cerebellum in detoxifying alcoholics. *Alcohol Clin Exp Res* **23**, 158–63.

Sekine Y, Minabe Y, Kawai M, *et al.* 2002. Metabolite alterations in basal ganglia associated with methamphetamine-related psychiatric symptoms. A proton MRS study. *Neuropsychopharmacology* **27**, 453–61.

Semple D M, Ebmeier K P, Glabus M F, O'Carroll R E and Johnstone E C. 1999. Reduced in vivo binding to the serotonin transporter in the cerebral cortex of MDMA ("ecstasy") users. *Br J Psychiatry* **175**, 63–9.

Sevy S, Smith G S, Ma Y, *et al.* 2008. Cerebral glucose metabolism and D2/D3 receptor availability in young adults with cannabis dependence measured with positron emission tomography. *Psychopharmacology (Berl)* **197**, 549–56.

Shi J, Zhao L-Y, Copersino M L, *et al.* 2008. PET imaging of dopamine transporter and drug craving during methadone maintenance treatment and after prolonged abstinence in heroin users. *Eur J Pharmacol* **579**, 160–6.

Silver S M, Schroeder B M and Sterns R H. 2002. Brain uptake of myoinositol after exogenous administration. *J Am Soc Nephrol* **13**, 1255–60.

Sokoloff L, Reivich M, Kennedy C, *et al.* 1977. The [14C]-deoxyglucose method for the measurement of local cerebral glucose utilization: Theory, procedure, and normal values in the conscious and anesthetized albino rat. *J Neurochem* **28**, 879–916.

Staley J K, Gottschalk C, Petrakis I L, *et al.* 2005. Cortical gamma-aminobutyric acid type A-benzodiazepine receptors in recovery from alcohol dependence: Relationship to features of alcohol dependence and cigarette smoking. *Arch Gen Psychiatry* **62**, 877–88.

Staley J K, Krishnan-Sarin S, Cosgrove K P, *et al.* 2006. Human tobacco smokers in early abstinence have higher levels of β₂*nicotinic acetylcholine receptors than nonsmokers. *J Neurosci* **26**, 8707–14.

Stephans S and Yamamoto B. 1996. Methamphetamines pretreatment and the vulnerability of the striatum to methamphetamine neurotoxicity. *Neuroscience* **72**, 593–600.

Stone J M, Erlandsson K, Arstad E, *et al.* 2006. Ketamine displaces the novel NMDA receptor SPET probe [(123)I]CNS-1261 in humans in vivo. *Nucl Med Biol* **33**, 239–43.

Taylor M J, Alhassoon O M, Schweinsburg B C, Videen J S and Grant I. 2000. MR spectroscopy in HIV and stimulant dependence HNRC Group. HIV Neurobehavioral Research Center. *J Int Neuropsychol Soc* **6**, 83–5.

Thomasius R, Petersen K, Buchert R, *et al.* 2003. Mood, cognition and serotonin transporter availability in current and former ecstasy (MDMA) users. *Psychopharmacology (Berl)* **167**, 85–96.

Thomasius R, Zapletalova P, Petersen K, *et al.* 2006. Mood, cognition and serotonin transporter availability in current and former ecstasy (MDMA) users: The longitudinal perspective. *J Psychopharmacol* **20**, 211–25.

Truckenmiller M E, Namboodiri M A, Brownstein M J and Neale J H. 1985. *N*-Acetylation of L-aspartate in the nervous system: Differential distribution of a specific enzyme. *J Neurochem* **45**, 1658–62.

Volkow N D, Chang L, Wang G J, *et al.* 2001a. Loss of dopamine transporters in methamphetamine abusers recovers with protracted abstinence. *J Neurosci* **21**, 9414–8.

Volkow N D, Chang L, Wang G J, *et al.* 2001b. Higher cortical and lower subcortical metabolism in detoxified methamphetamine abusers. *Am J Psychiatry* **158**, 383–9.

Volkow N D, Chang L, Wang G J, *et al.* 2001c. Association of dopamine transporter reduction with psychomotor impairment in methamphetamine abusers. *Am J Psychiatry* **158**, 377–82.

Volkow N D, Gillespie H, Mullani N, *et al.* 1991. Cerebellar metabolic activation by delta-9-tetrahydro-cannabinol in human brain: A study with positron emission tomography and 18F-2-fluoro-2-deoxyglucose. *Psychiatry Res* **40**, 69–78.

Volkow N D, Gillespie H, Mullani N, *et al.* 1996. Brain glucose metabolism in chronic marijuana users at baseline and during marijuana intoxication. *Psychiatry Res Neuroimag* **67**, 29–38.

Volkow N D, Hitzemann R, Wang G J, *et al.* 1992. Decreased brain metabolism in neurologically intact healthy alcoholics. *Am J Psychiatry* **149**, 1016–22.

Volkow N D, Hitzemann R, Wolf A P, *et al.* 1990. Acute effects of ethanol on regional brain glucose metabolism and transport. *Psychiatry Res* **35**, 39–48.

Volkow N D, Wang G J, Hitzemann R, *et al.* 1994. Recovery of brain glucose metabolism in detoxified alcoholics. *Am J Psychiatry* **151**, 178–83.

Voruganti L N, Slomka P, Zabel P, Mattar A and Awad A G. 2001. Cannabis induced dopamine release: An in-vivo SPECT study. *Psychiatry Res* **107**, 173–7.

Wang G J, Volkow N D, Chang L, *et al.* 2004. Partial recovery of brain metabolism in methamphetamine abusers after protracted abstinence. *Am J Psychiatry* **161**, 242–8.

Wang J-Q, Tueckmantel W, Zhu A, Pellegrino D and Brownell A-L. 2007. Synthesis and preliminary biological evaluation of 3-[(18)F]fluoro-5-(2-pyridinylethynyl)benzonitrile as a PET radiotracer for imaging metabotropic glutamate receptor subtype 5. *Synapse* **61**, 951–61.

Wang G J, Volkow N D, Fowler J S, *et al.* 2003. Alcohol intoxication induces greater reductions in brain metabolism in male than in female subjects. *Alcohol Clin Exp Res* **27**, 909–17.

Waterhouse R N, Slifstein M, Dumont F, *et al.* 2004. In vivo evaluation of [11C]*N*-(2-chloro-5-thiomethylphenyl)-*N*'-(3-methoxy-phenyl)-*N*'-methylguanidine ([11C]GMOM) as a potential PET radiotracer for the PCP/NMDA receptor. *Nucl Med Biol* **31**, 939–48.

Watkins S S, Koob G F and Markou A. 2000. Neural mechanisms underlying nicotine addiction: Acute positive reinforcement and withdrawal. *Nicotine Tobacco Res* **2**, 19–37.

Wik G, Borg S, Sjogren I, *et al.* 1988. PET determination of regional cerebral glucose metabolism in alcohol-dependent men and healthy controls using 11C-glucose. *Acta Psychiatr Scand* **78**, 234–41.

Yamamoto H, Kitamura N, Lin X H, *et al.* 1999. Differential changes in glutamatergic transmission via *N*-methyl-D-aspartate receptors in the hippocampus and striatum of rats behaviourally sensitized to methamphetamine. *Int J Neuropsychopharmacol* **2**, 155–63.

Zahr N M, Mayer D, Vinco S, *et al.* 2009. In vivo evidence for alcohol-induced neurochemical changes in rat brain without protracted withdrawal, pronounced thiamine deficiency, or severe liver damage. *Neuropsychopharmacology* **34**, 1427–42.

Zubieta J, Greenwald M K, Lombardi U, *et al.* 2000. Buprenorphine-induced changes in mu-opioid receptor availability in male heroin-dependent volunteers: A preliminary study. *Neuropsychopharmacology* **23**, 326–34.

Zubieta J K, Gorelick D A, Stauffer R, Ravert H T, Dannals R F and Frost J J. 1996. Increased mu opioid receptor binding detected by PET in cocaine-dependent men is associated with cocaine craving. *Nat Med* **2**, 1225–9.

Neuroimaging offers a unique window into brain structure and physiology not otherwise available in living persons. Alcohol and other substances of abuse change the brain, and these changes themselves may contribute to maintenance of the disorders. Thus, it is often hard to know whether the brain alterations observed in patients with alcohol and substance abuse are cause or effect. Their clinical trajectories are classically ones of exacerbations and remissions, with some unfortunate individuals ending in death. With animal models we can manipulate many factors out of experimental control in humans; with humans we are limited to naturalistic observations following the course of the disorder. Yet, with longitudinal observations through remissions and exacerbations, some of the cause and effect mystery can be resolved.

The three preceding chapters set forth reviews of major neuroimaging approaches to the problem – structural integrity with computed tomography (CT) and magnetic resonance imaging (MRI), physiological response to cognitive and motor challenge with functional MRI (fMRI), metabolic and neurotransmitter function with positron emission tomography (PET) and single-photo emission computed tomography (SPECT), and metabolite assays with MR spectroscopy. Each of the approaches has strengths and limitations and they should all be considered complementary to each other. Done well, each requires substantial technical sophistication.

Among the insights we can potentially gain from in-vivo human neuroimaging regarding alcohol and substance abuse disorders are characterization of neuropathology; factors modulating or contributing to the onset, course, and maintenance of misuse; the scope and limits of recovery; and possible benefits of selective substance use (see Box 32.1).

Characterization

Magnetic resonance neuroimaging is uniquely suited for the delineation of the nature of alcohol and substance abuse induced neuropathology. Relevant characterization includes the specific patterns of sparing and loss of brain structures; the tissue type, quality, and microstructural integrity of affected loci; and global and regional cerebrovascular status. The ability to define the unique and common neuropathology attendant to the abuse of various substances has the potential to define specific neuropathology that may be of diagnostic, prognostic, and treatment relevance. Finally, brain structure–function studies can shed light on selective neural substrates of cognitive and motor functions and dysfunctions.

Modulators

Family history and genome analysis studies hold promise for elucidating the role of genetic contributions to susceptibility or resistance to brain damage from substances of abuse. However, as human conditions, substance abuse disorders are not merely pharmacological toxicities but comprise constellations of behaviors (e.g. quantity and frequency of consumption), comorbidities (e.g. polysubstance use, somatic pathology such as hepatic disease, HIV infection, and endogenous psychiatric comorbidities such as depression), and environmental factors (e.g. social and psychological deprivation, malnutrition, cigarette smoking). There is ample evidence that some substance abuse disorders, for example alcoholism, are "complex genetic disorders" and prototypic consequences of gene–environment interactions; the neuroimages of individuals with alcoholism are the product of both their genes and their environment.

Course and maintenance

Alcoholism especially is a lifelong disorder that interacts with the dynamic changes that occur in the brain throughout the life span from adolescence to senescence. As with normal development and aging, the neuroadaptive processes that are invoked to compensate for pathological compromise of function are amenable to longitudinal elucidation with neuroimaging. Conversely, rather than being adaptive, these neural changes may contribute to the furtherance of abuse, inducing self-perpetuating disorders. Study of individuals at risk but before the onset of substance abuse could allow the disentangling of the problem of determining what neuropathology is cause and what is effect. And once abuse and craving have developed, functional neuroimaging may be the ultimate brain structure–function investigative tool to determine the brain loci responsible for continued abuse.

Recovery

Functional MR studies of craving during abstinence, together with characterization of the degree and locus of macro- and microstructural neuropathology, could provide predictors of prognosis for relapse and recovery. Indeed, the nature of compensation and limits of rehabilitation depend on the degree to which there is brain repair with abstinence and progressive damage with continued abuse. Rehabilitative schemes should be directed towards functional sparing in compensation for known loss.

Benefits of use (not of abuse)

Finally, there are potential beneficial effects of many abused substances. When used judiciously, not all substances of abuse are necessarily detrimental to human health and well-being. Opiates are used to reduce pain; psychostimulants, including nicotine (although not delivered through tobacco smoke), are used to maintain alertness in dangerous battle conditions; marijuana is used for nausea control and appetite stimulation; and alcohol in moderation has cardiovascular and cerebrovascular protective properties demonstrable with neuroimaging.

Conclusion

The neuroimaging window into the brain structure and physiology of alcohol and other substances abuse disorders has already provided a wealth of insight into the characterization of common and specific neuropathology. The future potential and challenge for human neuroimaging of substance abuse disorders is to contribute to the understanding of the underlying mechanisms of maintenance, relapse, injury, and repair.

Acknowledgment

This work was supported by NIH grants AA005965, AA012388, AA017347

Box 32.1.   What can be learned about alcohol and substance abuse from in vivo human neuroimaging?

- CHARACTERIZATION
  - Neuropathology – Unique and Common
  - Diagnostic specificity
  - Substrates of selective cognitive and motor dysfunctions
- MODULATION
  - Genetic susceptibility or resistance to damage
  - Environmental contributions
  - Somatic pathology
  - Polysubstance
  - Psychiatric comorbidities
- COURSE AND MAINTENANCE
  - Lifetime dynamic course
  - Neuroadaptation
  - Self-perpetuating disorders
  - Craving
- RECOVERY
  - Repair with abstinence
  - Compensatory mechanisms
  - Time course
- BENEFICIAL EFFECTS OF USE (NOT OF ABUSE)
  - Somatic
  - Behavioral
  - Social

Neuroimaging of anorexia and bulimia

Guido K. W. Frank and Michael D. H. Rollin

Introduction

The conceptual framework of the pathophysiology and etiology of the eating disorders (EDs) anorexia nervosa (AN), bulimia nervosa (BN) as well as the emerging ED binge eating disorder (BED), has undergone significant changes in the past few decades. Brain imaging techniques now give us the opportunity to assess regional brain activity and neuroreceptor function in-vivo in humans, and thus may help us understand how neuronal circuits are related to behavior and pathophysiology.

A host of neuroimaging tools is now available for ED research. Structural imaging techniques such as computer tomography (CT) and radiation-free magnetic resonance imaging (MRI) provide information on gross structural abnormalities. Magnetic resonance spectroscopy (MRS) can detect brain chemicals containing choline, aspartate and others, which are involved in brain neurotransmission. Positron emission tomography (PET), single photon emission computed tomography (SPECT) and functional magnetic resonance imaging (fMRI) are used to assess brain activity thought to be associated with changes in regional cerebral blood flow (rCBF). In addition, neurotransmitter receptor function and regional cerebral glucose metabolism (rCGM) can be assessed with PET and SPECT and radioligands. Electroencephalography (EEG) and evoked potentials (EPs) record neuronal electrical activity, and quantitative electroencephalography (qEEG) employs spectral analysis of EEG data from multiple-electrode, whole-head recordings and provides better spatial resolution compared to the traditional EEG. Recent advances in the field of brain research using neuroscience-based imaging paradigms have made great progress with respect to emotional and cognitive processes that

may be altered in psychiatric illness. For example, a lot has been learned about brain pathways that are involved in fear-provoking stimuli (Ohman *et al.*, 2007), induction of abnormal mood states (Konarski *et al.*, 2007), processing of food and other rewarding stimuli (Chau *et al.*, 2004), cognitive flexibility (Alvarez and Emory, 2006), and numerous other areas with potentially direct relevance to eating disorders. In comparison with, for instance, psychosis or depression research, the body of neurobiologic research in EDs is relatively small, but nevertheless significant advances have been made over the past 10 years to shed light on biological brain processes that may be part of the pathophysiology of AN, BN and BED.

Of importance when reviewing ED research are state-related factors. The ill state of the EDs, particularly of AN, can be accompanied by severe metabolic, electrolyte, and endocrine disturbances (Task Force on DSM-IV, 1994). As such, research in ill EDs is always potentially confounded by these effects. We have taken care to indicate where studies have examined the ill state versus recovered state of these illnesses, as this may help to somewhat disentangle findings related to starvation versus traits related to the underlying pathophysiology of the illness. Even in recovered subjects, however, it has to be taken into consideration that observed differences may represent either premorbid traits contributing to the development of the illness, or a consequence of having been previously ill.

Anorexia nervosa

AN is a disorder that usually begins during adolescence, most commonly in females, and is associated with an intense fear of gaining weight, feeling fat despite being underweight, emaciation, and amenorrhea. The hallmark sign of low weight is defined as a body mass index (BMI, weight in kilograms/height in meters^2) of <17.5. A restricting type (AN-R), marked by food restriction and usually over-exercising, has been distinguished from a binge-eating/purging type (AN-B/P), where afflicted individuals regularly overeat and then use measures such as self-induced vomiting, laxatives or diuretics in order to lose or not gain weight (Task Force on DSM-IV, 1994). Comorbid depression and anxiety disorders are common (Bulik *et al.*, 1997).

CT and MRI studies

CT and MRI studies generally show that underweight AN subjects tend to have enlarged sulci and ventricles and decreased brain mass (Kornreich *et al.*, 1991; Hentschel *et al.*, 1995, 1997). While these alterations shift towards normal with weight restoration, it has been questioned to what extent they normalize (Golden *et al.*, 1996; Swayze *et al.*, 1996). It is also not clear whether these changes during the ill state are primarily related to changes in gray (GM) or white matter (WM), or to the extracellular space. Moreover, it remains uncertain whether these are generalized brain changes or are specific to particular brain regions. Katzman's group (Katzman and Colangelo, 1996) found reduced total GM and WM as well as enlarged cerebrospinal fluid (CSF) volume during the ill state in 13 adolescent AN women. By contrast, in a cohort of ill AN, BN and control women (CW), Husain assessed the midsagittal plane acquired by MRI, finding reduced midbrain and thalamic size in AN, but no GM alterations (Husain *et al.*, 1992). Lambe compared 12 *recovered* AN (defined as BMI > 17.0 kg/m^2, regular menses > 6 months) to 13 ill AN and 18 controls, and found that they had reduced GM and increased CSF volume compared to controls, but greater GM and smaller CSF space compared to ill AN subjects (Lambe *et al.*, 1997). Furthermore, a longitudinal study on 6 women studied during the ill state and after weight recovery (mean 16 months) showed that WM volume was recovered after weight recovery, but a GM deficit persisted as well as increased CSF space (Katzman *et al.*, 1997). More recently, Mühlau demonstrated a modest decrease in global GM volume after recovery from AN ($n = 22$) compared to controls (Mühlau *et al.*, 2007). In addition, there was a persistent significant decrease in anterior cingulate cortex

(ACC) volume that correlated with past lowest BMI. It is unclear, but possible that this finding represents a cortical injury due to a period of severe malnourishment, or alternatively a state of only partial recovery. A recent analysis of MRIs of 12 female and six male AN subjects, obtained in the mid 1990s, again found a persistent decrease in ACC volume after recovery, and furthermore, the degree to which ACC volume was restored with recovery was positively correlated with sustained remission from AN symptoms (McCormick *et al.*, 2008). However, Wagner *et al.* (2006) performed the largest study in recovered ED subjects, including 30 AN (14 AN-R, 16 AN-B/P), and found no significant alterations in GM, WM, or CSF volumes. Furthermore, most recently, a case series of 12 ill adolescent AN subjects again revealed global GM loss that at seven month follow-up had completely reversed (Castro-Fornieles *et al.*, 2009). Thus it appears that these volume abnormalities are likely state-related, and normalize with long-term recovery.

The reason for even these transient changes in brain volume is also not known. Some data suggest that cortisol may contribute to brain alterations. Katzman and Colangelo (1996) found that urinary free cortisol was positively correlated with CSF volume, and inversely with GM volume. AN subjects are known to have increased CSF cortisol (Gwirtsman *et al.*, 1989). Thus it is possible that hypercortisolemia may play a role in reduced brain mass in ill AN subjects, maybe through its catabolic or fluid-homeostatic effects (Ganong, 2005). On the other hand, reduced mesial temporal cortex (amygdalo-hippocampal complex) size in ill AN subjects did not show a relationship with hormonal levels including urinary free cortisol in the past (Giordano *et al.*, 2001). It is unclear if this finding was confined to the mesial temporal cortex or ubiquitous, making its interpretation difficult.

The question of whether alterations in brain mass contribute to cognitive or mood changes in ill AN subjects has not been well studied. Kingston *et al.* (1996) combined structural imaging with psychological assessments (including anxiety, depression, attention, memory) in 46 AN inpatients before and after weight gain, compared to controls. No significant correlations were found, suggesting either no specificity of disturbance that can be related to specific behavior, or simply inefficient analysis methods. Similarly, Connan correlated hippocampal volume in ill AN subjects with cognitive testing, and while finding a decrease in hippocampal volume in the AN group, found no correlation between cognitive performance and hippocampal volume loss (Connan *et al.*, 2006).

In summary, these studies tend to indicate that during the ill state, a GM and probably WM volume loss or shrinkage occur that at least partially recover with weight restoration. Those structural alterations are relatively non-specific, and behavioral correlates have not been discovered.

MRS studies

MRS can give information on nerve cell damage by assessing brain metabolites such as choline, *N*-acetyl-aspartate (NAA), phosphorus, and *myo*-inositol. MRS studies in juvenile AN subjects found higher choline-containing compounds relative to total creatine and lower ratios of NAA relative to choline in WM (Hentschel *et al.*, 1999; Schlemmer *et al.*, 1998). Those changes were interpreted to indicate altered cell membrane turnover, as they were reversible with recovery (Mockel *et al.*, 1999). Two studies (Rzanny *et al.*, 2003; Roser *et al.*, 1999) showed reduced brain phospholipids that positively correlated with BMI, also suggesting a state-dependent phenomenon. The latter study also found BMI positively correlated with frontal cortex *myo*-inositol, which is a part of the serotonin (5-HT) second messenger neurotransmission system (Leonard, 1994) and could be consistent with reduced 5-HT activity in ill AN subjects (Kaye *et al.*, 2000). Castro-Fornieles *et al.* (2007), in a longitudinal study, found state-dependent changes in NAA, glutamate/glutamine, and *myo*-inositol that again resolved with recovery from illness, further indicating that metabolic alterations are state-dependent and do not represent pathogenetic traits. These metabolic alterations are likely to be related to the neuronal insults suffered from starvation.

PET and SPECT studies, resting condition

Most studies that have assessed "resting" brain activity in AN subjects have used SPECT. Gordon *et al.* (1997) found that 13 of 15 ill AN had unilateral temporal lobe hypoperfusion that persisted in the subjects studied after weight restoration. Kuruoglu and colleagues studied two ill AN subjects with bilateral hypoperfusion in frontal, temporal, and parietal regions which normalized after three months of remission (Kuruoglu *et al.*, 1998). Takano *et al.* (2001) found hypoperfusion in 14 ill AN subjects, in the medial prefrontal cortex and ACC and hyperperfusion in the thalamus and

amygdalo-hippocampal complex. In a study by Chowdhury, 15 ill adolescent AN subjects had unilateral temporoparietal and frontal lobe hypoperfusion (Chowdhury *et al.*, 2003), and Rastam and colleagues found temporo parietal and orbitofrontal hypoperfusion in ill and recovered AN subjects (Rastam *et al.*, 2001). These studies, demonstrating abnormal rCBF in ill AN subjects, have, however, been challenged by a recent study that found no such abnormality when a partial volume correction, i.e. a correction for brain volume reduction seen in ill AN subjects, was applied during image processing (Bailer *et al.*, 2007b). This is in contrast to the previous rCBF studies, and suggests that prior findings of reduced rCBF in AN subjects could have been a confounded result due to brain volumetric alterations in AN subjects (Katzman *et al.*, 1997). Kojima and coworkers demonstrated a persistent decrease in rCBF in the ACC after weight recovery among 12 AN-R subjects (Kojima *et al.*, 2005). Matsumoto *et al.* (2006) studied 3 AN-R and 5 AN-B/P subjects before and after weight recovery, finding increases in rCBF in several regions after inpatient treatment. The same study found a significant correlation between low interoceptive awareness score on Eating Disorders Inventory-3 (EDI-3) and decreased perfusion of right dorsolateral prefrontal cortex, which is implicated in emotional self-awareness, a trait that has long been proposed as abnormal in AN (Bruch, 1962). After long-term recovery, Frank *et al.* (2007) found no persistent alterations in cerebral perfusion in 10 recovered AN-R and 9 recovered AN-B/P subjects, indicating that such abnormalities recover with illness recovery.

Fewer studies have assessed glucose metabolism using PET. Delvenne *et al.* studied 20 ill AN subjects who showed frontal and parietal hypometabolism compared to controls, which normalized with weight gain (Delvenne *et al.*, 1995, 1996, 1997a, 1997b). But here too, no correction for brain volume changes was applied, and the results would need to be confirmed in a partial volume corrected sample.

Taken together, brain activity studies in AN in the resting condition most frequently suggest alterations of the temporal, parietal or cingulate cortex during the ill state, and a few studies suggest persistent alterations in those areas after weight gain. It remains unclear whether cerebral perfusion changes truly exist or are just a technical confound due to brain volume abnormalities. If there is in fact reduced rCBF or glucose metabolism in ill and recovered AN, that could be a potentially important finding given that the mesial temporal cortex is implicated in emotional processing, and increased anxiety in AN could be related to altered amygdala function. However, at this point reduced rCBF after recovery and even during the ill state may be less likely (Bailer *et al.*, 2007b; Frank *et al.*, 2007).

Two studies (Frank *et al.*, 2007; Yonezawa *et al.*, 2008) have compared ill AN-R and AN-B/P subjects using SPECT, and have found no significant differences in rCBF between the two groups, suggesting that cerebral blood flow is not part of pathophysiology that distinguishes the two AN subtypes. Interestingly, Goethals and colleagues demonstrated an absence of rCBF differences between diagnoses among 31 AN-R, 16 AN-B/P, and 20 BN subjects, but showed that among all diagnoses, rCBF results in prefrontal and parietal areas were positively correlated with measures of body dissatisfaction and ineffectiveness as measured by EDI-3 (Goethals *et al.*, 2007).

EEG, EPs, and qEEG

EDs have been studied by EEG since at least 1955 (Martin, 1955). Since that time, much of the EEG work has focused on sleep and eating disorders. Early work confirmed the clinical finding that AN is accompanied by insomnia and early awakening (Crisp *et al.*, 1967; Lacey *et al.*, 1975). A complete overview of sleep EEG in AN is beyond the scope of this volume and we focus in this review on more specific AN- related symptoms.

Evoked potentials (EPs), or event-related potentials (ERPs), are specific activations in time and location, generated by response to sensory stimuli, and measured by electrophysiologic recording. Variations in these activations' amplitudes provide evidence of the nature of cortical response to the associated stimuli. Bradley *et al.* (1997) engaged 20 ill AN adolescents in both a verbal and a non-verbal memory task, and found increased latency and decreased amplitude of the P300 activation, which is associated with attention, processing capacity and memory integration; this alteration suggests slowness and inefficiency in the memory task performance. In follow-up with eight recovered AN subjects, there was partial but incomplete improvement of this parameter compared to controls, suggesting the possibility of a memory-related cognitive processing impairment in AN apart from nutritional status. Another study ($N = 12$) used a

sensory-filtering paradigm to assess P300 response to shape recognition. In controls, stimuli that appeared frequently would eventually yield a low-amplitude P300 response, suggestive of processing accommodation to repetition; however, AN subjects showed a consistently elevated P300 response suggestive of hyperarousal (Dodin and Nandrino, 2003).

Pieters *et al.* (2007) studied another ERP of interest, the error-related negativity (ERN), which is a discrete drop in amplitude recorded following a response error; thought to be part of an error-monitoring mechanism to enhance learning. Among controls, "perfectionism", as a psychological trait measured by questionnaire, was correlated with a higher magnitude (more negative) ERN, as might be expected, during a simple visual processing task ("flankers task"). Among AN subjects, perfectionism scores were higher, consistent with prior research (Kaye *et al.*, 1995), and AN subjects made fewer errors than their control counterparts. Paradoxically, however, AN subjects showed a *weaker* ERN than did controls in the anterior cingulate cortex (ACC) area, when error rate was included as a covariate, suggesting less prominent error monitoring among AN subjects in the ACC. The significance of this surprising finding is unclear; the authors conjectured that AN may recruit other cerebral structures in their error monitoring, such that the activation measured by ERN is only part of their error-monitoring mechanism. Interestingly, fMRI studies have identified ACC as the likely generator of the ERN signal (Carter *et al.*, 1998; Kiehl *et al.*, 2000), and a number of fMRI studies have shown significant alterations in ACC activation in EDs (see below).

Pollatos *et al.* (2008) studied visual identification of emotional state of faces by 12 AN females, and their associated visual EPs (VEPs). This study found AN subjects performed worse than controls in the task of correctly identifying the emotional valence of the faces. The amplitude of the N200 VEP, which is associated with processing of unfamiliar stimuli, was increased in response to all emotional categories of faces. This may suggest that AN subjects require more attentional resources in order to decode the emotional states of others. The P300 response, on the other hand, was decreased in amplitude to faces with negative valence (fear, anger, disgust), but *increased* to neutral faces. The authors posit that this reflects AN subjects working harder to resolve the emotional valence of the more ambiguous condition, as representative of a possible disturbance in social cognition.

Quantitative EEG (qEEG) studies have recently come to prominence as another functional assessment method. A standard qEEG setup involves a 19-channel recording scheme with electrodes regularly distributed according to the International 10–20 system (Grunwald et al., 2004; Klem et al., 1999). Grunwald and colleagues gave ill AN subjects a tactile exploration task and measured theta-frequency band power on each hemisphere, finding an asymmetry in theta power in both resting and active states in ill AN but not in CW subjects; furthermore, the active (but not resting) asymmetry persisted into recovery at follow-up testing. The significance of the global asymmetry is not obvious, but may reflect diffuse whole-hemispheric dysfunction in AN; the authors posit that this reflects a trait hyperarousal (leading to desynchronization and lower amplitude) of the right hemisphere. Alternatively, this finding may develop as a result of starvation and persist as a scar effect, with preferential preservation of the dominant left hemisphere function. The second qEEG study (Rodriguez et al., 2007) included AN-R, AN-B/P, and BN subjects, who were not recovered but past the acute phase of the illness (5–47 days post hospital admission). That study found decreased alpha frequency power in central, parietal, occipital, and temporal/limbic areas. Loss of amplitude in the main arousal-related frequency bands (alpha, beta, theta) suggests synaptic dysfunction and neuronal damage (Besthorn et al., 1997; Jelic et al., 1996; Moretti et al., 2004). The pathogenesis of the findings is unclear, but may be related in part to starvation, persistent electrolyte imbalance, and presence of psychotropic medication.

Task-activation studies using PET, SPECT, and fMRI (Table 33.1)

Functional brain imaging is performed in conjunction with paradigms and tasks that are meant to elicit areas of brain activation that might be specific for AN pathophysiology. Many different paradigms have been used over the past years, with PET and SPECT comprising the earlier work and fMRI achieving prominence more recently.

Eating custard cake showed increased brain activity in AN subjects compared to controls using SPECT in frontal, occipital, parietal and temporal areas (Nozoe et al., 1993, 1995). Food imagination on SPECT showed that AN-B/P subjects had greater right-sided parietal and prefrontal activation compared to controls and AN-R subjects (Naruo et al., 2000). Gordon found, using PET, that in AN subjects high-calorie foods provoked anxiety and led to greater temporo-occipital activation when compared to low calorie foods (Gordon et al., 2001). Ellison et al., using fMRI, also found that visual high-calorie presentation elicited high anxiety in AN subjects together with left mesial temporal as well as left insular and bilateral ACC activity (Ellison et al., 1998). These results could be consistent with anxiety provocation and related limbic activation (LeDoux, 2003). Uher et al. (2003) used pictures of food and non-food aversive emotional stimuli to assess ill and recovered AN subjects. Food images stimulated medial prefrontal and ACC in both recovered and ill AN subjects, but lateral prefrontal regions only in recovered AN subjects; in controls, food pictures were associated with occipital, basal ganglia and lateral prefrontal activation. Aversive non-food stimuli activated occipital and dorsolateral prefrontal cortex in all three subject groups. In recovered AN subjects, prefrontal cortex, ACC and cerebellum were more highly activated compared to both controls and chronic AN subjects after food presentation. This suggested that higher ACC and medial prefrontal cortex activity in both ill and recovered AN subjects compared to CW subjects may be a trait marker for AN. These are areas of executive function, decision-making, error-monitoring and also reward expectancy. Such alterations could suggest heightened vigilance or processing activity in response to visual food stimuli. Taken together, these studies suggest that the prefrontal cortex is active in the capacity to appropriately or inappropriately restrict food, possibly via heightened fear-related activation and anxious cognitions followed by related decision-making, such as food restriction.

Santel et al. (2006) compared AN-R subjects with CW subjects confronted by food images in both hungry and satiated states. They noted a decrease in inferior parietal lobule (IPL) activation among satiated AN subjects, and furthermore, the magnitude of decrease correlated with illness severity. The IPL is composed of both the primary somatosensory and sensory association cortices, so this finding suggests a decrease in sensory sensitivity, or increased habituation, to food images in ill AN subjects, which could indicate a pathogenetic mechanism that facilitates fasting or restriction. In turn, in the hungry state, AN subjects showed decreased activation to food

Table 33.1 Neuroreceptor and functional activation studies in anorexia nervosa (AN); nl, normal; ▼, decreased compared to controls; ▲, increased compared to controls; AN-R, anorexia nervosa, restricting type; AN-BP, anorexia nervosa, binge eating–purging type; AN*, diagnostic subgroup not distinguished with respect to results; REC, recovered. PET, positron emission tomography; SPECT, single-photon emission computed tomography; fMRI, functional MRI 5-HT, serotonin; DA, dopamine; ILL, illness; REC, recovered

Year	Author	Method	Activation	ILL	REC	N	Frontal Cortex left	Frontal Cortex right	Temporal Cortex with Amygdala left	Temporal Cortex with Amygdala right	Cingulate Cortex left	Cingulate Cortex right	Parietal Cortex left	Parietal Cortex right	Occipital Cortex right	Insula left	Insula right	Striatum left	Striatum right	Dorsal raphe
AN neurotransmitter–receptor studies																				
2002	Frank et al.	PET	5-HT₂ₐ		AN-R	16				▼		▼		▼			▼			
2003	Audenaert et al.	SPECT	5-HT₂ₐ	AN*		15		▼				▼		▼			▼			
2004	Bailer et al.	PET	5-HT₂ₐ		AN-BP	10				▼				▼			▼			
2005	Bailer et al.	PET	5-HT₁ₐ		AN-R	13	nl		nl		nl	▼	nl	▼	nl	nl	nl	nl	nl	nl
2005	Bailer et al.	PET	5-HT₁ₐ	AN-BP		12	▲		▲		▲		▲						▲	▲
2005	Frank et al.	PET	DA D₂/D₃		AN*	10	▲				▲								▲	
2007	Bailer et al.	PET	5-HT₁ₐ	AN*		15	▲		▲	▲	▲		▲	▲						▲
2007	Bailer et al.	PET	5-HT₂ₐ	AN*		15	nl		nl		nl		nl		nl	nl	nl	nl	nl	nl
2008	Galusca et al.	PET	5-HT₁ₐ		AN-R	8		▲	▲			▲	▲							
2008	Galusca et al.	PET	5-HT₁ₐ	AN-R		9		▲	▲	▲		▲	▲							
AN functional activation studies																				
1995	Nozoe et al.	SPECT	Eating food	AN*		8				▲		▲	▲				▲			
2000	Naruo et al.	SPECT	Food images	AN-R		7							▲		▲					
2000	Naruo et al.	SPECT	Food images	AN-BP		7		▲							▲					

Year	Author	Method	Task	Group	N
2001	Gordon et al.	PET rCBF	Food images	AN*	8
1998	Ellison et al.	fMRI	Food images	AN*	6
2002	Seeger et al.	fMRI	Body image	AN*	3
2003	Wagner et al.	fMRI	Body image	AN-R	15
2003	Uher et al.	fMRI	Food images	AN-R	AN-R
2004	Uher et al.	fMRI	Food image	AN, BN*	26
2004	Uher et al.	fMRI	Food image	AN*	16
2005	Uher et al.	fMRI	Body image	AN-R, AN-BP	13
2006	Santel et al.	fMRI	Food images: hungry vs. satiad	AN*	13
2007	Wagner et al.	fMRI	Monetary reward task	AN-R	13
2008	Redgrave et al.	fMRI	Emotional Stroop task: "thin" valence	AN*	6
2008	Redgrave et al.	fMRI	Emotional Stroop task: "fat" valence	AN*	6
2008	Sachdev et al.	fMRI	Self vs. non-self images	AN*	10
2008	Wagner et al.	fMRI	10% sucrose, water	AN-R	16

(a)

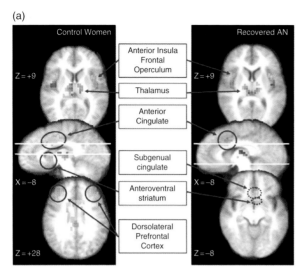

A. Main effect response to sequential Sucrose stimulation versus baseline; p = 0.005, 8 voxel minimal contiguity; both groups show thalamus and anterior cingulate in addition to bilateral frontal operculum/anterior insula activation; Control Women (CW) showed left sided anteroventral striatal activation, while Recovered Anorexia Nervosa (AN) had left subgenual cingulate activation that extended into the anteroventral striatum; CW also showed dorsolateral prefrontal brain activation.

(b)

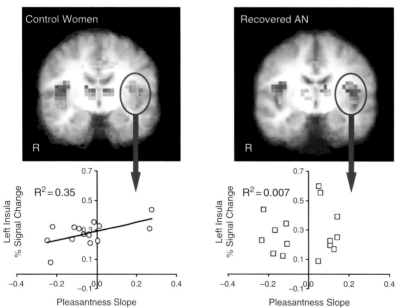

B. Pleasantness ratings positively predicted left insula/frontal operculum (FO/AI) main effect activation in the sequential Sucrose condition in CW. In contrast, pleasantness ratings did not correlate with left FO/AI main effect activation in RAN.

Figure 33.1 Preliminary results from a confirmation study (Frank *et al.*, unpublished data) indicate similar qualitative response to sucrose across groups of 15 recovered anorexia nervosa (RAN) and control women (CW) [A], but a lack of pleasantness rating correlation in RAN with insula activation as compared to the CW [B], and direct comparison of CW and RAN indicates reduced brain response in RAN in frontal cortex, insula and striatum to sucrose application [C].

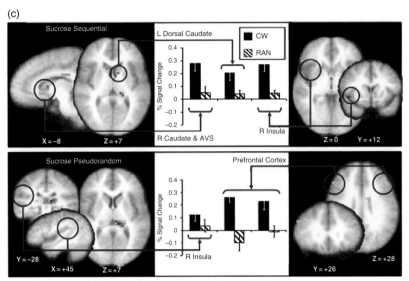

C. Comparison maps of Sucrose conditions across groups. Recovered AN subjects (RAN) show less brain response compared to controls (CW) for Sucrose application in the caudate, insula and prefrontal cortex.

Figure 33.1 (cont.)

stimuli in the occipital cortex compared to CW, which may indicate a learned or innate attentional bias away from food stimuli in the hungry state in AN subjects, which again would facilitate fasting.

Neurophysiologic responses to taste stimuli are in the early stages of investigation. Wagner et al. (2008) used a 10% sucrose solution and water in recovered AN-R subjects and found decreased ACC, insula, and striatal activation to both taste stimuli. Furthermore, self-report of pleasantness of the taste stimulus and activation in these brain regions were only correlated in controls. A confirmation study (Frank et al., unpublished data, Figure 33.1) similarly found reduced brain response to sucrose in recovered AN subjects compared to controls, and a lack of a correlation of pleasantness rating for sucrose with insula activation. This suggests a possible difference in the processing of tastes between AN-R and CW subjects. The insula is implicated both in early processing of sensory stimuli as well as reward associations (Craig, 2002). The ACC, as above, is implicated in reward anticipation and executive function (Bush et al., 2002). It is an interesting contrast that ACC is activated by visual food stimuli in AN subjects in Uher's study above, whereas its activation is decreased by gustatory stimuli in this study; this may represent a difference in stimulus saliency and anticipation versus actual stimulus-receipt processing. ACC activation was also found to be decreased in response to sweet stimuli among BN subjects (Frank et al., 2006) (see below), despite the very different behavioral approaches to food seen in the phenotypes of AN-R versus BN. The response of AN-B/P to similar stimuli remains to be seen. However, a major problem with those studies is that since the taste stimuli were readily distinguishable, it is not clear what the impact of cognitive restraint may have been with respect to reward activation control. In fact, pilot data from our lab (Frank et al., unpublished data) indicate that when ill AN subjects receive sweet taste solution unexpectedly, they show an even greater brain response in dopamine-related brain regions compared to controls. This serves to demonstrate that cognitive-emotional processes and underlying pathogenetic processes have yet to be disentangled.

Body image distortion is an integral part of AN pathophysiology and is part of its diagnostic criteria (Task Force on DSM-IV, 1994). In a small pilot study confronting three AN subjects and three CW with their own digitally distorted body images using a computer-based video technique and fMRI (Seeger et al., 2002), AN had greater activation in the brainstem, right-sided amygdala and fusiform gyrus, again suggesting anxiety related to the body experience that is reflected by amygdala activity. However, in a follow up study in a larger and more homogeneous sample using the same paradigm, Wagner et al. (2003) found no amygdala activation, but a hyper-responsiveness in brain areas belonging to the frontal visual system and the attention network (Brodmann area [BA] 9) as well as intraparietal lobule (IPL, BA 40), including the anterior part of the intraparietal sulcus. The latter areas are specifically involved in visuo spatial processing. More broadly, the parietal lobes are implicated in body schema integration and body ownership (Giummarra *et al.*, 2008). This finding makes the involvement of the brain anxiety circuit less clear, but suggests that perceptual alterations may be related directly to the mechanisms of body image construction. Another study that used line drawings of body shapes found reduced occipitotemporal (lateral fusiform gyrus) and parietal cortex activation in AN subjects compared to controls and BN subjects (Uher *et al.*, 2005). Interestingly, the AN subjects rated both underweight as well as overweight pictures as highly aversive and the reduced activation in those face and body recognition regions (Adolphs, 2002) may indicate a general aversion to body-related topics and a probably cognitively driven reduced brain response.

The amount of research in body image-related issues in AN is sparse; studies in controls may help develop new paradigms. In a study in a group of CW only found left amygdala activation in relation to unpleasant body-related words, as well as contra lateral parahippocampal activation that was negatively related to the Eating Disorders Inventory-2 (EDI-2) score (Shirao *et al.*, 2003). The same group compared healthy control women with matched males in the same body-related word paradigm, and again found increased left amygdala activation among only the women, whereas the men showed increased activity in medial prefrontal cortex and hippocampus (Shirao *et al.*, 2005). Thus young women, with or without AN, may have somewhat similar – probably learned – anxiety reactions to stimuli related to body image, which may help to explain in neurobiological terms why women are so much more susceptible to AN than men.

Related to body image distortion, Sachdev *et al.* (2008) studied brain response to images of self versus non-self in ill AN-R and AN-B/P versus CW subjects. This study found decreased activation in frontal, insula, precuneus and occipital regions for AN subjects compared to CW when faced with self-images; responses to other-images were similar. This suggests a potential variation in attention to or interpretation of self-images in AN. One might have expected a greater activation for AN subjects given their extreme

sensitivity to their own appearance; however, a conflation of self/other processing in AN patients might help maintain unrealistic ideas and expectations about their own bodies, and the undue influence of appearances of others and media imagery (Borzekowski and Robinson, 2005). A study of 18 CW aged 18–35 years examined activations as women actively compared images of themselves to slim fashion models; this revealed activity in both body shape-related areas including lateral fusiform gyri, right IPL, right lateral prefrontal and left ACC. Furthermore, activations in basal ganglia and amygdala were correlated with a self-report of anxiety generated by the task (Friederich *et al.*, 2007). Thus even in healthy women, both body image and anxiety mechanisms are implicated in the emotionally laden task of comparison to social ideals.

Rather than image stimuli, a recent small study on mostly AN-B/P subjects versus CW used words that were either neutral or associated with fatness or thinness, in a Stroop task, in which subjects respond to a word stimulus according to the color a word is printed in rather than the word itself, as a test of selective attention and executive function. This found in AN a behavioral attention bias toward the fat/thin valence words, as well as unique activation patterns for each valence condition, with increases in left frontal and left insula–temporo parietal junction activation with the thin valence, and decreases in left frontal and right parietal activation in the fat valence (Redgrave *et al.*, 2008). Notably absent was a variation in amygdala response, which might have been expected from other studies. This pattern calls further into question the significance of the emotional response to body image-related issues, while suggesting greater significance in mechanisms of body image construction and self-perception. Further study into these mechanisms will be crucial to understanding this important part of AN pathophysiology.

A developing area of AN imaging attempts to look directly at the neurophysiology of psychological trait markers. Heightened anxious traits are well-established in AN, and dopamine-mediated reward pathways have been implicated (see below). Wagner *et al.* (2007) used a monetary win/loss paradigm and found among recovered AN women a relationship between trait anxiety and response to wins and losses in the caudate. Furthermore, AN women had similar responses to positive and negative feedback in the anteroventral striatum, whereas controls' responses differed between positive and negative conditions. The overall striatal response was greater in the recovered AN women compared to controls. These findings suggest a variation in reward processing, and potentially a conflation between positive and negative stimuli that may help to explain the AN subject's ability to effectively restrict food and maintain anhedonia.

It is difficult to compare these studies as the imaging modalities and tasks are not consistent and the groups of subjects are small. Still, it appears that cingulate and prefrontal activity are frequently different between AN and CW subjects. Those regions may be over-activated when confronted with anxiety-provoking food-related stimuli. Such a heightened vigilance is probably related to anxious body and fear-of-fatness cognitions, followed by actions in order to avoid weight gain. On the other hand, AN subjects may respond less to taste and other reward stimuli, which may help to be able to restrict food intake, especially neurobiologically "rewarding" foods. The results from the other imaging studies are not conclusive. However, it appears that AN subjects do have altered self-perception related brain activation, and this may suggest incorrect processing of, and maybe abnormal feedback from, the body periphery, which in turn may allow over-valued ideas of thinness to control the self-image.

Receptor imaging studies (Table 33.1)

Neurotransmitters such as serotonin (5-HT) or dopamine (DA) are distributed throughout the brain via specific neuronal pathways. Their influence on behavior is believed to be via action on specific receptors in, for example, the midbrain, the basal ganglia and neocortex. Radioligands exist for several of the 5-HT receptor types. One of the most commonly assessed receptor types is the 5-HT2A receptor, which is involved in the regulation of feeding, mood, and anxiety, and in antidepressant action (Barnes and Sharp, 1999). Four studies have assessed 5-HT2A receptor binding in ill and recovered AN women. Ill subjects showed reduced binding in the left frontal, bilateral parietal and occipital cortex (Audenaert et al., 2003). Recovered AN-R subjects also had reduced 5-HT2A binding, most strongly in mesial temporal and parietal cortical areas as well as in the cingulate cortex (Frank et al., 2002). In another study, women recovered from AN-B/P had reduced 5-HT2A binding relative to controls in the left subgenual cingulate, left parietal, and right occipital cortex (Bailer

et al., 2004). In that study 5-HT2A binding was positively related to harm avoidance and negatively to novelty seeking in cingulate and temporal regions, with negative relationships between 5-HT2A binding and drive for thinness. A later study by the same group (Bailer et al., 2007b) found normal 5-HT2A binding in ill AN subjects, but replicated the correlation between 5-HT2A activity and harm avoidance.

The 5-HT2A findings further highlight the possibility of disturbances of the ACC and mesial temporal cortex in AN. Since these disturbances persist after recovery, it is possible they are trait disturbances. The ACC receives afferents from the amygdala and has direct projections to the premotor frontal cortex and other limbic regions. It plays a crucial role in initiation of and motivation for goal-directed behaviors (Devinsky et al., 1995) as well as computation of the future value of potentially rewarding stimuli (Richmond et al., 2003). In turn, the amygdala mediates the interpretation of fear and the representation of emotional stimuli values (LeDoux, 2003). One could hypothesize that AN subjects have disturbed processing of the valence of stimuli, resulting in poor flexibility in re-evaluating the actual danger of those stimuli and reduced adaptation to new situations. This could lead to altered reward prediction and reduced drive to approach food rewards. Future studies will need to determine whether relationships between 5-HT2A receptor activity and measures for anxiety such as harm avoidance can be replicated and expanded upon.

Another major serotonin receptor type is the 5-HT1A receptor. The Bailer study mentioned above (Bailer et al., 2007b), as well as an earlier study from the same group (Bailer et al., 2005), both examined 5-HT1A, which is found throughout the forebrain as well as in the midbrain raphe nuclei. The 2005 study of recovered AN-R, recovered AN-B/P, and recovered BN subjects found an increase in 5-HT1A availability in the dorsal raphe and throughout the cortex in the AN-B/P and BN groups, but not in the AN-R group, raising the possibility of alternative pathogenetic pathways for binging/purging versus restricting behavior. The group's 2007 study (Bailer et al., 2007b) in ill AN-R and AN-B/P subjects, however, found increased 5-HT1A activity in similar regions in both subtypes of AN, complicating the issue of this receptor's potential role in pathogenesis of the disease. Most recently, Galusca et al. (2008) examined 5-HT1A binding in ill and recovered AN-R subjects, finding similar profiles in both ill and recovered of increased binding potential in frontal, temporal, parietal, and amygdala regions. The consistency of diffuse increase in 5-HT1A receptor activity across these studies and levels of recovery suggests a potential trait disturbance in the serotonergic system.

Another study examined the serotonin transporter (5-HT-T) activity among recovered AN-R, AN-B/P, and BN subjects (Bailer *et al.*, 2007a). Each group revealed a distinct pattern of activity of this transporter in dorsal raphe and anteroventral striatum, with AN-R > AN-B/P and AN-B/P < BN (neocortical binding could not be assessed due to a lack of specificity of the radioligand). This finding suggests one possible explanation for the variability in the affective traits associated with the different eating disorder subtypes, but subgroups have been small and replication is needed.

Only one study has so far examined dopamine receptor (D2/D3) activity in AN subjects. Frank *et al.* (2005) found increased dopamine activity in the anteroventral striatum among recovered AN subjects. This finding suggests an upregulation of dopamine receptors, which may correspond to a prior finding of decreased CSF concentrations of dopamine metabolite in AN subjects (Kaye *et al.*, 1999). Specifically, high dopamine D2 receptor binding together with low brain dopamine (Kaye *et al.*, 1999) could be related to an inflexible dopamine system and low motivation to approach presented rewards in AN (Kelley, 2004). Dopamine is implicated in the reward and addiction system, with decreased dopamine receptor activity associated with both addiction and obesity (Wang *et al.*, 2004). As such, thus the inverse finding in AN may help to account for both food restriction as well as the anhedonic and avoidant drive frequently seen in AN.

Bulimia nervosa

BN is characterized by recurrent binge eating – eating large amounts of food in a relatively short period of time – followed by behaviors to counteract weight gain, such as self-induced vomiting, use of laxatives or diuretics, or excessive exercise. The purging type may use all of those methods to prevent weight gain, while the non-purging subtype engages only in food restriction and/or excessive exercise in order to not gain weight. Individuals with BN are at normal or often high-normal weight and present with a fear of gaining weight, as well as food and body weight-related preoccupations. BN subjects also frequently restrict food, but still ingest sufficient

amounts to not be underweight. BN is frequently associated with major depression, anxiety disorders, and substance abuse (Task Force on DSM-IV, 1994); poor impulse control, mood instability, and self-harming behavior also frequently co-occur (Task Force on DSM-IV, 1994; Steiger and Bruce, 2007; Svirko and Hawton, 2007).

CT and MRI studies

Only a few structural studies have been performed in BN subjects. Pituitary abnormalities have been suggested (Doraiswamy *et al.*, 1991), as well as cerebral atrophy (Laessle *et al.*, 1989; Hoffman *et al.*, 1989) and ventricular enlargement (Krieg *et al.*, 1987, 1989; Kiriike *et al.*, 1990). No conclusions on etiology or impact on behavior of those structural lesions have yet been drawn (Laessle *et al.*, 1989), since those measures may be short-term and dependent on nutritional intake (Puri *et al.*, 1999). As mentioned above, Wagner *et al.* (2006) studied 10 recovered BN subjects and found no persistent changes in gray or white matter or CSF volumes. Because BN is not marked by the same degree of starvation as AN, the lack of structural changes seen in BN subjects may suggest that those changes seen in AN subjects are in fact related strictly to the starvation state rather than underlying pathogenetic traits.

MRS studies

A mixed group of AN and BN subjects had reduced prefrontal myo-inositol and lipid compounds (Roser *et al.*, 1999; Rost *et al.*, 1999) compared to controls. However, a differentiation of AN- or BN-related brain behavior was not performed, and the implication on the clinical picture remains to be explored.

PET and SPECT studies, resting condition

Similar to brain glucose metabolism findings in AN, rCGM in the resting state was reduced globally in BN compared to controls, with significantly reduced rCGM in the parietal cortex using PET (Delvenne *et al.*, 1997c). Interestingly, depressive symptoms in a BN group correlated with rCGM in the left anterolateral cortex in one study (Andreason *et al.*, 1992). This finding has not been replicated. However, another study investigating brain activity in BN versus depressed subjects (Hagman *et al.*, 1990) found that BN subjects had reduced right frontal activation compared to CW and depressed subjects, but depressed subjects had reduced basal ganglia activity, supporting different pathophysiology for BN and depression. In 9 recovered (mean 57 months) BN subjects, rCBF was similar compared to 12 CW but correlated negatively with length of recovery (Frank *et al.*, 2000), which could reflect either a scarring effect or possibly a return to premorbid lower rCBF. A follow-up study found no rCBF alterations in recovered BN subjects (Frank *et al.*, 2007).

It therefore appears that rCBF and rCGM alterations during the ill state remit with recovery, although pre- or post-illness alterations cannot be completely excluded based on the available data. Furthermore, BN and depression may be distinguished by different patterns of brain activity, which is important considering the frequent overlap in depressive symptoms.

Task-activation studies using SPECT, fMRI (Table 33.2)

Nozoe *et al.* (1995) (SPECT) found that BN subjects had greater right inferior frontal and left temporal blood flow compared to controls before a meal, but similar activity after. BN subjects have increased subjective liking for sweet stimuli compared to controls (Drewnowski *et al.*, 1987), and therefore may have altered processing of taste stimuli. More recently, an fMRI study using a glucose taste paradigm versus a control solution found in recovered subjects with bulimic symptoms (seven BN and three AN-B/P) reduced ACC activity compared to six CW (Frank *et al.*, 2006). The ACC is an area that is involved in error monitoring but also in the anticipation of reward (Richmond *et al.*, 2003). In this paradigm, where subjects knew which taste stimulus to expect, higher activity in controls could suggest higher reward expectation by controls than anticipated by BN type subjects. On the other hand, Schienle and colleagues (2009) compared 14 BN and BED subjects, finding a relative increase in activation of the ACC in BN subjects confronted with images of food, as well as an increase in insula signal. It is possible that the insula activation represents emotional arousal by the image, whereas the ACC activation acts as a counterbalance to that response, as the ACC is implicated in selection of emotional attention and control of sympathetic autonomic arousal (Critchley *et al.*, 2002; Phan *et al.*, 2002). New pilot data (Oberndorfer *et al.*, submitted) compared sweet taste stimuli in BN compared to CW subjects, and found that BN subjects have increased insula and striatal

response to the stimuli. Such a biologic "over-responsiveness" might be associated with a vulnerability to overeat. But these results have to be confirmed.

One study has explored body image perception in BN (Uher *et al.*, 2005). In a small sample ($n = 9$), BN subjects were compared to AN and CW and presented with line drawings of body shapes (underweight, normal and overweight). Similarly to AN, BN subjects had reduced lateral fusiform gyrus activation, and comparably to AN high aversion ratings to any body shape. Thus, reduced brain activation may have been an aversion-driven restraint in brain response in that group. However, this area of research needs more sophisticated approaches to disentangle the various cognitive-emotional versus biologic aspects of brain response when studying body image perception and distortion.

Faris and colleagues have suggested a theory for the pathogenesis of BN, based on dysfunction/hyperactivity of the afferents of the vagus nerve. They have previously demonstrated reduction in binging/purging in BN by blocking vagal nerve transmission from the viscera with the drug ondansetron (Faris *et al.*, 2000). More recently, they studied PET scans in 18 healthy CW subjects undergoing artificial gastric distention, notably finding activity in left inferior frontal, bilateral opercula (frontal), left insula, and right ACC (Stephan *et al.*, 2003). The authors suggest that given these regions of activity, most notably ACC, the subjective experience of gastric distention might have a profound emotional component that could in turn contribute to the pathophysiology of binging and purging.

Receptor imaging studies (Table 33.2)

A few neurotransmitter–receptor studies have been done in BN subjects. Kaye *et al.* (2001) found reduced orbitofrontal 5-HT2A receptor binding in recovered BN subjects. Orbitofrontal alterations could reflect behavioral disturbances in BN that include impulsiveness and altered emotional processing (Steiger *et al.*, 2001). Altered orbitofrontal activity as found in borderline personality disorder (Soloff *et al.*, 2003) could indicate a common area for impulse control disturbance. In addition, in the Kaye *et al.* (2001) study, BN women failed to show common correlations of age and 5-HT2A binding. This finding raises the possibility that BN women may have alterations of developmental mechanisms of the 5-HT system. Another study reported reduced 5-HT transporter binding in thalamus and hypothalamus in ill BN subjects (Tauscher *et al.*,

477

Table 33.2 Neuroreceptor and functional activation studies in bulimia nervosa (BN) and binge eating disorder (BED); nl, normal; ▲, increased compared to controls; ▼, decreased compared to controls; BN, bulimia nervosa; REC, recovered. PET, positron emission tomography; SPECT, single photon emission computed tomography; fMRI, functional MRI 5-HT, serotonin; DA, dopamine

Year	Author	Method	Activation	ILL	REC	N	Frontal Cortex left	Frontal Cortex right	Temporal Cortex with Amygdala left	Temporal Cortex with Amygdala right	Cingulate Cortex left	Cingulate Cortex right	Parietal Cortex left	Parietal Cortex right	Occipital Cortex left	Occipital Cortex right	Insula left	Insula right	Striatum	Dorsal raphe
BN neurotransmitter–receptor studies																				
2001	Tauscher et al.	SPECT	5-HT-T	BN		10														
2001	Kaye et al.	PET	5-HT$_{2A}$		BN	9		▼												
2004	Tiihonen et al.	PET	5-HT$_{1A}$	BN		8	▲				▲		▲		▲					
2007	Bailer et al.	PET	5-HT-T		BN	9														
BN functional activation studies																				
1995	Nozoe et al.	SPECT	Eating food	BN		5														
2004	Uher et al.	fMRI	Food image	BN		10	▼													
2005	Uher et al.	fMRI	Body image	BN		9				▼				▼						
2006	Frank et al.	fMRI	Glucose		BN	10						▲				▲				
2008	Schienle et al.	fMRI	Food, disgust, neutral images	BN		14						▲ (food)								
BED functional activation studies																				
2006	Geliebter et al.	fMRI	Visual/Auditory food stimulation	BED, thin		5														
2006	Geliebter et al.	fMRI	Visual/Auditory food stimulation	BED, obese		5	▲													
2008	Schienle et al.	fMRI	Food, disgust, neutral images	BED		17	▲ (food)										▲ (food)			

2001). The 5-HT system has consistently been shown to be disturbed in EDs, and reduced 5-HT transporter when ill may be related to altered brain 5-HT function, such as reduced 5-HT activity during the ill state (Jimerson *et al.*, 1992). Reduced 5-HT2A activity *after recovery* could reflect a trait disturbance involved in alterations of mood, anxiety and impulse control. Most recently, increased 5-HT1A receptor binding was found by Tiihonen *et al.* (2004) using PET in ill BN subjects in all studied brain regions, but most prominently in prefrontal, cingulate and a parietal cortex area. Central serotonin function is inversely related to BN severity (Jimerson *et al.*, 1992) and increased 5-HT1A receptor binding could be a negative-feedback upregulation. Higher 5-HT1A binding could also be related to the well-known phenomenon that BN patients require higher doses of selective 5-HT reuptake inhibitors compared to, for example, patients being treated for depression. However, those 5-HT receptor alterations and their implications on treatment will have to be mechanistically studied and the findings replicated.

Binge eating disorder

BED is a proposed diagnostic category for DSM (Task Force on DSM-IV, 1994). BED is characterized by BN-like binging symptoms, except that no compensatory measures are used. Very little is known about brain activity in BED. Karhunen and colleagues found that there may be a lateralization of blood flow in BED, with higher activity in the left hemisphere compared to theright in response to visual food presentation (Karhunen *et al.*, 2000). Also, there was a linear correlation of hunger with left frontal/prefrontal cortical activity. The same group found reduced 5-HT-T binding in the midbrain (Kuikka *et al.*, 2001), which improved with fluoxetine and group psychotherapy (Tammela *et al.*, 2003), suggesting, at least in part, state-dependent serotonergic alterations. Interestingly, a study of the 5-HT transporter in six subjects with night eating syndrome (NES), which is characterized by increased late-night eating in non-binge portions, showed *increased* serotonin transporter binding in the midbrain (Lundgren *et al.*, 2008). This preliminary contrast with BED suggests that the appetitive drives in binging versus nocturnal eating are represented by very different pathologies.

One fMRI study in BED (Geliebter *et al.*, 2006) compared thin BED and obese BED subjects with matched thin and obese controls, with food-related visual and auditory stimuli. This study found activation differences only in the obese binge eaters, who exhibited increased activity in the frontal pre-central region, near the premotor area that is associated with planning and mouth movements, which suggests that the food stimuli brought about motor planning associated with eating in these subjects. In the study of Schienle *et al.* (2009) comparing BN and BED, increased activation of orbitofrontal cortex was found for BED subjects compared to BN and controls. Furthermore, strength of this activation correlated with self-reported reward-responsiveness. The orbitofrontal cortex is implicated in secondary gustatory processing and may reflect hedonic values of food (Rolls *et al.*, 1989), and is involved in determining the reward value of food (Kringelbach, 2004). However, future studies will need to test behaviors in relation to specific brain response in order to draw meaningful conclusions for the pathophysiology of BED.

Research in other conditions may help to illuminate the pathophysiology of binge eating. Recently, the prefrontal cortex was implicated in the capacity to lose or maintain weight; Le *et al.* (2007) compared obese women with lean and formerly obese women, finding that only the currently obese had decreased activity in the left dorsolateral prefrontal cortex as measured by PET. However, such studies need to be followed up with paradigms that test emotional and cognitive aspects of behavior control and their implications for the clinical presentation. A recent prospective study of 32 patients with neurodegenerative diseases of different types were observed in a free-feeding condition. Of these, six were found to compulsively binge after reporting satiety. All six of those were independently clinically diagnosed with fronto-temporal dementia (FTD), a specific form of neuro-degenerative dementia. When compared with the rest of the neurodegenerative cohort, the structural MRI of binge eaters revealed significant atrophy of the right ventral insula, right striatum, and right orbitofrontal cortex (Woolley *et al.*, 2007). Dysfunction in these areas may contribute to binging behavior. A second MRI study of FTD found that among 16 male subjects with the disorder, a specific decrease in gray matter volume of bilateral posterolateral orbitofrontal cortex was associated with the symptom of hyperphagia (Whitwell *et al.*, 2007). As such, orbitofrontal cortex in particular, from this and the studies above, appears to be implicated in the binging process, although what exact role it plays in binging remains to be clarified.

In summary, very little brain imaging work in BED has been done, but the available results indicate possible serotonin abnormalities during the ill state, and the orbitofrontal cortex and insula may be target regions for future research.

Conclusion

Until recently, the assessment of psychiatric disorders has relied on subjective reports from patients, and biologic research has been limited by the inaccessibility of the living human brain. The emergence of brain imaging techniques enables us to assess brain function in-vivo and assess human behavior in conjunction with biological correlates. The new imaging methods give hope to the prospect of identifying biologic markers that will help categorize the EDs AN and BN and, in turn, identify more effective treatments that could reduce morbidity associated with these frequently debilitating and deadly illnesses. The above-reviewed brain imaging studies in AN, BN and BED have identified the following aspects for future ED research.

Studying EDs is complicated due to a relatively small prevalence and the many state-related (e.g. hormonal, nutritional) disturbances associated with these illnesses. Thus, it is difficult to assess factors that may be trait related and possibly premorbid. Studying subjects after long-term recovery may be our closest approximation to studying subjects premorbidly. That approach, however, carries uncertainty as to whether the results obtained are truly premorbid conditions, or represent a "scar" from the illness. Ideally, studies during the ill state correct for state dependent confounds (such as partial volume correction for reversible brain reductions) but test disorder-specific behaviors in relation to specific functional brain abnormalities.

The common global reductions of gray and white matter in ill AN subjects remit at least in part with recovery, and ill BN subjects may have similar changes. It is possible that the explanation for reduction in brain mass when ill may be brain protein, fat, or fluid loss secondary to emaciation and dehydration. However, since some ED studies found relationships of brain volume with cortisol levels as well as cortisol related to brain cell death (Lee et al., 2002), it remains to be assessed whether hypercortisolemia in ill AN subjects is truly contributing to those findings.

Resting rCBF and rCGM in AN and BN subjects showed mostly a general reduced cortical activity in the ill state that is most pronounced in temporal, parietal or cingulate cortex. Very limited data suggest some persistence of these findings after recovery in both AN and BN, although more recent study of recovered subjects disagree and do not suggest that rCBF/cCGM studies should be made a main focus of future research.

Functional MRI studies using visual stimuli of food or body image in AN have had variegated approaches and outcomes. Broadly, their results have most often implicated involvement of prefrontal, ACC, temporal and parietal cortices, with exaggerated brain response to anxiety-provoking food stimuli. In contrast, readily distinguishable taste stimuli indicate a general reduction of brain response in recovered AN subjects. Whether reduced brain response to otherwise rewarding stimuli is cognitively or more biologically driven will be an important next step in AN research. One of the few task activation studies in BN suggests altered ACC and cuneus activity in response to a sweet taste stimulus. This finding suggests that the decision-making network as well as reward pathways may be differently activated in those tasks in BN. However, those studies still have to be replicated.

The receptor imaging studies that are available at this point in AN show that reduced 5-HT2A and increased 5-HT1A receptor binding occurs in the ill state. After recovery, this appears to normalize in AN-R, but subjects with binging/purging symptoms may continue to have increased 5-HT1A receptor binding. BN subjects showed reduced 5-HT2A receptor activity when recovered, and reduced 5-HT transporter binding when ill, and they may have increased 5-HT1A receptor binding during the ill state. Such findings of 5-HT disturbances in ill and recovered subjects with EDs strongly suggest a trait disturbance of the 5-HT system. Altered 5-HT receptor activity could be related to emotional disturbances such as increased depressive symptoms or anxiety. However, the exact mechanisms of neuroreceptor–behavior interactions needs further study.

Few studies have been done in EDs in comparison to depressive disorders or OCD. The overlap and comorbidity of both major depression and OCD with EDs require studies that will directly compare those disorders. EDs, and in particular AN, are frequently debilitating with a high mortality. Studies comparing psychiatric disorders will help to find common pathways and distinct areas of disturbance that may identify targets for successful drug interventions.

Lastly, the combination of various imaging techniques such as fMRI and ERP may hold the promise of relating real time neuronal activity with behavior and good spatial localization. And new techniques will enable new types of imaging studies in EDs. For example, manganese-enhanced MRI (MEMRI), which uses manganese ion as a blood flow-related contrast medium, was recently used to track binding of the appetite-stimulating gut hormone ghrelin and the appetite-suppressing peptide YY_{3-36} in mouse brains, allowing for examination of the time course of hormone binding in the hypothalamus versus appetitive behavior (Kuo *et al.*, 2007). Tracking the brain–hormone link in humans will unfold a new wrinkle in the evolving study of EDs.

Taken together, the last few decades have shown significant advances in the study of ED neurobiology, but the specific relationships between ED traits and behaviors and brain function remain obscure. This will be the task of the next generation of brain imaging studies in EDs.

Box 33.1. **Main research findings**

- Neurotransmitter receptor studies have repeatedly implicated serotonin abnormalities in ill and recovered eating disorder subjects, suggesting that serotonin system abnormalities are a trait disturbance in EDs.
- Functional brain imaging studies with challenge tasks indicate a heightened arousal and anxiety response to visual food presentation, but actual food/taste stimulus presentation tends to result in a reduced brain response.
- ED subjects may have a biologic under-responsiveness to food stimuli, or – maybe more likely – control cognitively aspects of the reward system and thus are able to maintain food restriction.

References

Adolphs R. 2002. Recognizing emotion from facial expressions: Psychological and neurological mechanisms. *Behav Cogn Neurosci Rev* **1**, 21–62.

Alvarez J A and Emory E. 2006. Executive function and the frontal lobes: A meta-analytic review. *Neuropsychol Rev* **16**, 17–42.

Andreason P J, Altemus M, Zametkin A J, King A C, Lucinio J and Cohen R M. 1992. Regional cerebral glucose metabolism in bulimia nervosa. *Am J Psychiatry* **149**, 1506–13.

Audenaert K, Van Laere K, Dumont F, *et al.* 2003. Decreased 5-HT2a receptor binding in patients with anorexia nervosa. *J Nucl Med* **44**, 163–9.

Bailer U F, Frank G K, Henry S E, *et al.* 2007a. Serotonin transporter binding after recovery from eating disorders. *Psychopharmacology* **195**, 315–24.

Bailer U F, Frank G K, Henry S E, *et al.* 2007b. Exaggerated 5-HT1A but normal 5-HT2A receptor activity in individuals ill with anorexia nervosa. *Biol Psychiatry* **61**, 1090–9.

Bailer U F, Frank G K, Henry S E, *et al.* 2005. Altered brain serotonin 5-HT1A receptor binding after recovery from anorexia nervosa measured by positron emission tomography and [carbonyl^{11}C]WAY-100635. *Arch Gen Psychiatry* **62**, 1032–41.

Bailer U F, Price J C, Meltzer C C, *et al.* 2004. Altered 5-HT (2A) receptor binding after recovery from bulimia-type anorexia nervosa: Relationships to harm avoidance and drive for thinness. *Neuropsychopharmacology* **29**, 1143–55.

Barnes N M and Sharp T. 1999. A review of central 5-HT receptors and their function. *Neuropharmacology* **38**, 1083–152.

Besthorn C, Zerfass R, Geiger-Kabisch C, *et al.* 1997. Discrimination of Alzheimer's disease and normal aging by EEG data. *Electroencephalogr Clin Neurophysiol* **103**, 241–8.

Borzekowski D L and Robinson T N. 2005. The remote, the mouse, and the no. 2 pencil: The household media environment and academic achievement among third grade students. *Arch Pediatr Adolesc Med* **159**, 607–13.

Bradley S J, Taylor M J, Rovet J F, *et al.* 1997. Assessment of brain function in adolescent anorexia nervosa before and after weight gain. *J Clin Exp Neuropsychol* **19**, 20–33.

Bruch H. 1962. Perceptual and conceptual disturbances in anorexia nervosa. *Psychosom Med* **24**, 187–94.

Bulik C M, Sullivan P F, Fear J L and Joyce P R. 1997. Eating disorders and antecedent anxiety disorders: A controlled study. *Acta Psychiatr Scand* **96**, 101–7.

Bush G, Vogt B A, Holmes J, *et al.* 2002. Dorsal anterior cingulate cortex: A role in reward-based decision making. *Proc Natl Acad Sci USA* **99**, 523–8.

Carter C S, Braver T S, Barch D M, Botvinick M M, Noll D and Cohen J D. 1998. Anterior cingulate cortex, error detection, and the online monitoring of performance. *Science* **280**, 747–9.

Castro-Fornieles J, Bargallo N, Lazaro L, *et al.* 2009. A cross-sectional and follow-up voxel-based morphometric MRI study in adolescent anorexia nervosa. *J Psychiatr Res* **43**, 331–40.

Castro-Fornieles J, Bargallo N, Lazaro L, *et al.* 2007. Adolescent anorexia nervosa: Cross-sectional and follow-up frontal gray matter disturbances detected with proton magnetic resonance spectroscopy. *J Psychiatr Res* **41**, 952–8.

Chau D T, Roth R M and Green A I. 2004. The neural circuitry of reward and its relevance to psychiatric disorders. *Curr Psychiatry Rep* **6**, 391–9.

Chowdhury U, Gordon I, Lask B, Watkins B, Watt H and Christie D. 2003. Early-onset anorexia nervosa: Is there evidence of limbic system imbalance? *Int J Eat Disord* **33**, 388–96.

Connan F, Murphy F, Connor S E, *et al.* 2006. Hippocampal volume and cognitive function in anorexia nervosa. *Psychiatry Res* **146**, 117–25.

Craig A D. 2002. How do you feel? Interoception: The sense of the physiological condition of the body. *Nat Rev Neurosci* **3**, 655–66.

Crisp A H, Fenton G W and Scotton L. 1967. The electroencephalogram in anorexia nervosa. *Electroencephalogr Clin Neurophysiol* **23**, 490.

Critchley H D, Mathias C J and Dolan R J. 2002. Fear conditioning in humans: The influence of awareness and autonomic arousal on functional neuroanatomy. *Neuron* **33**, 653–63.

Delvenne V, Goldman S, Biver F, De Maertalaer V, Wikler D, Damhaut P and Lotstra F. 1997a. Brain hypometabolism of glucose in low-weight depressed patients and in anorectic patients: A consequence of starvation? *J Affect Disord* **44**, 69–77.

Delvenne V, Goldman S, De Maertelaer V, Simon Y, Luxen A and Lotstra F. 1996. Brain hypometabolism of glucose in anorexia nervosa: Normalization after weight gain. *Biol Psychiatry* **40**, 761–8.

Delvenne V, Goldman S, De Maertelaer V, Wikler D, Damhaut P and Lotstra F. 1997b. Brain glucose metabolism in anorexia nervosa and affective disorders: Influence of weight loss or depressive symptomatology. *Psychiatry Res* **74**, 83–92.

Delvenne V, Goldman S, Simon Y, De Maertelaer V and Lotstra F. 1997c. Brain hypometabolism of glucose in bulimia nervosa. *Int J Eat Disord* **21**, 313–20.

Delvenne V, Lotstra F, Goldman S, *et al.* 1995. Brain hypometabolism of glucose in anorexia nervosa: A PET scan study. *Biol Psychiatry* **37**, 161–9.

Devinsky O, Morrell M J and Vogt B A. 1995. Contributions of anterior cingulate cortex to behaviour. *Brain* **118**, 279–306.

Dodin V and Nandrino J L. 2003. Cognitive processing of anorexic patients in recognition tasks: An event-related potentials study. *Int J Eat Disord* **33**, 299–307.

Doraiswamy P M, Krishnan K R, Boyko O B, *et al.* 1991. Pituitary abnormalities in eating disorders: Further evidence from MRI studies. *Progr Neuro-Psychopharmacol Biol Psychiatry* **15**, 351–6.

Drewnowski A, Bellisle F, Aimez P and Remy B. 1987. Taste and bulimia. *Physiol Behav* **41**, 621–6.

Ellison Z, Foong J, Howard R, Bullmore E, Williams S and Treasure J. 1998. Functional anatomy of calorie fear in anorexia nervosa. *Lancet* **352**, 1192.

Faris P L, Kim S W, Meller W H, *et al.* 2000. Effect of decreasing afferent vagal activity with ondansetron on symptoms of bulimia nervosa: A randomised, double-blind trial. *Lancet* **355**, 792–7.

Frank G K, Bailer U F, Henry S E, *et al.* 2005. Increased dopamine D2/D3 receptor binding after recovery from anorexia nervosa measured by positron emission tomography and [11C]raclopride. *Biol Psychiatry* **58**, 908–12.

Frank G K, Bailer U F, Meltzer C C, *et al.* 2007. Regional cerebral blood flow after recovery from anorexia or bulimia nervosa. *Int J Eat Disord* **40**, 488–92.

Frank G K, Kaye W H, Greer P, Meltzer C C and Price J C. 2000. Regional cerebral blood flow after recovery from bulimia nervosa. *Psychiatry Res* **100**, 31–9.

Frank G K, Kaye W H, Meltzer C C, *et al.* 2002. Reduced 5-HT2A receptor binding after recovery from anorexia nervosa. *Biol Psychiatry* **52**, 896–906.

Frank G K, Wagner A, Achenbach S, *et al.* 2006. Altered brain activity in women recovered from bulimic-type eating disorders after a glucose challenge: A pilot study. *Int J Eat Disord* **39**, 76–9.

Friederich H C, Uher R, Brooks S, *et al.* 2007. I'm not as slim as that girl: Neural bases of body shape self-comparison to media images. *Neuroimage* **37**, 674–81.

Galusca B, Costes N, Zito N G, *et al.* 2008. Organic background of restrictive-type anorexia nervosa suggested by increased serotonin 1A receptor binding in right frontotemporal cortex of both lean and recovered patients: [18F]MPPF PET scan study. *Biol Psychiatry* **64**, 1009–13.

Ganong W. 2005. *Review of Medical Physiology.* New York, NY: The McGraw-Hill Companies, Inc.

Geliebter A, Ladell T, Logan M, *et al.* 2006. Responsivity to food stimuli in obese and lean binge eaters using functional MRI. *Appetite* **46**, 31–5. [Erratum appears in *Appetite*, 2006; **46**, 395. Note: Schweider, Tzipporah [corrected to Schneider, Tzipporah].]

Giordano G D, Renzetti P, Parodi R C, *et al.* 2001. Volume measurement with magnetic resonance imaging of hippocampus–amygdala formation in patients with anorexia nervosa. *J Endocrinol Invest* **24**, 510–4.

Giummarra M J, Gibson S J, Georgiou-Karistianis N and Bradshaw J L. 2008. Mechanisms underlying embodiment, disembodiment and loss of embodiment. *Neurosci Biobehav Rev* 32, 143–60.

Goethals I, Vervaet M, Audenaert K, Jacobs F, Ham H and Van Heeringen C. 2007. Does regional brain perfusion correlate with eating disorder symptoms in anorexia and bulimia nervosa patients? *J Psychiatr Res* 41, 1005–11.

Golden N H, Ashtari M, Kohn M R, *et al*. 1996. Reversibility of cerebral ventricular enlargement in anorexia nervosa, demonstrated by quantitative magnetic resonance imaging. *J Pediatr* 128, 296–301.

Gordon C M, Dougherty D D, Fischman A J, *et al*. 2001. Neural substrates of anorexia nervosa: A behavioral challenge study with positron emission tomography. *J Pediatr* 139, 51–7.

Gordon I, Lask B, Bryant-Waugh R, Christie D and Timimi S. 1997. Childhood-onset anorexia nervosa: Towards identifying a biological substrate. *Int J Eat Disord* 22, 159–65.

Grunwald M, Weiss T, Assmann B, *et al*. 2004. Stable asymmetric interhemispheric theta power in patients with anorexia nervosa during haptic perception even after weight gain: A longitudinal study. *J Clin Exp Neuropsychol* 26, 608–20.

Gwirtsman H E, Kaye W H, George D T, Jimerson D C, Ebert M H and Gold P W. 1989. Central and peripheral ACTH and cortisol levels in anorexia nervosa and bulimia. *Arch Gen Psychiatry* 46, 61–9.

Hagman J O, Buchsbaum M S, Wu, J C, Rao S J, Reynolds C A and Blinder B J. 1990. Comparison of regional brain metabolism in bulimia nervosa and affective disorder assessed with positron emission tomography. *J Affect Disord* 19, 153–62.

Hentschel F, Besthorn C and Schmidt M H. 1997. Die fraktale Dimension als Bildbearbeitungsparameter im CT bei Anorexia nervosa vor und nach Therapie. *Zeitschrift fur Kinder- und Jugendpsychiatrie und Psychotherapie* 25, 201–06.

Hentschel F, Schmidbauer M, Detzner U, Blanz B and Schmidt M H. 1995. Reversible Hirnvolumenanderungen bei der Anorexia nervosa. *Zeitschrift fur Kinder- und Jugendpsychiatrie und Psychotherapie* 23, 104–12.

Hentschel J, Mockel R, Schlemmer H P, *et al*. 1999. 1H-MR-Spektroskopie bei Anorexia nervosa: charakteristische Unterschiede zwischen Patienten und gesunden Probanden. *ROFO-Fortschritte auf dem Gebiet der Rontgenstrahlen und der Bildgebenden V* 170, 284–9.

Hoffman G W, Ellinwood E H Jr, Rockwell W J, Herfkens R J, Nishita J K and Guthrie L F. 1989. Cerebral atrophy in bulimia. *Biol Psychiatry* 25, 894–902.

Husain M M, Black K J, Doraiswamy P M, *et al*. 1992. Subcortical brain anatomy in anorexia and bulimia. *Biol Psychiatry* 31, 735–8.

Jelic V, Shigeta M, Julin P, Almkvist O, Winblad B and Wahlund L O. 1996. Quantitative electroencephalography power and coherence in Alzheimer's disease and mild cognitive impairment. *Dementia* 7, 314–23.

Jimerson D C, Lesem M D, Kaye W H and Brewerton T D. 1992. Low serotonin and dopamine metabolite concentrations in cerebrospinal fluid from bulimic patients with frequent binge episodes. *Arch Gen Psychiatry*, 49, 132–8.

Karhunen L J, Vanninen E J, Kuikka J T, Lappalainen R I, Tiihonen J and Uusitupa M I. 2000. Regional cerebral blood flow during exposure to food in obese binge eating women. *Psychiatry Res* 99, 29–42.

Katzman D K and Colangelo J J. 1996. Cerebral gray matter and white matter volume deficits in adolescent girls with anorexia nervosa. *Hlth Law Canada* 16, 110–4.

Katzman D K, Kaptein S, Kirsh C, *et al*. 1997. A longitudinal magnetic resonance imaging study of brain changes in adolescents with anorexia nervosa. *Compr Psychiatry* 38, 321–6.

Kaye W H, Bastiani A M and Moss H. 1995. Cognitive style of patients with anorexia nervosa and bulimia nervosa. *Int J Eat Disord* 18, 287–90.

Kaye W H, Frank G K and McConaha C. 1999. Altered dopamine activity after recovery from restricting-type anorexia nervosa. *Neuropsychopharmacology* 21, 503–06.

Kaye W H, Frank G K, Meltzer C C, *et al*. 2001. Altered serotonin 2A receptor activity in women who have recovered from bulimia nervosa. *Am J Psychiatry* 158, 1152–5.

Kaye W H, Klump K L, Frank G K and Strober M. 2000. Anorexia and bulimia nervosa. *Annu Rev Med* 51, 299–313.

Kelley A E. 2004. Ventral striatal control of appetitive motivation: Role in ingestive behavior and reward-related learning. *Neurosci Biobehav Rev* 27, 765–76.

Kiehl K A, Liddle P F and Hopfinger J B. 2000. Error processing and the rostral anterior cingulate: An event-related fMRI study. *Psychophysiology* 37, 216–23.

Kingston K, Szmukler G, Andrewes D, Tress B and Desmond P. 1996. Neuropsychological and structural brain changes in anorexia nervosa before and after refeeding. *Psychol Med* 26, 15–28.

Kiriike N, Nishiwaki S, Nagata T, Inoue Y, Inoue K and Kawakita Y. 1990. Ventricular enlargement in normal weight bulimia. *Acta Psychiatr Scand* 82, 264–6.

Klem G H, Luders H O, Jasper H H and Elger C. 1999. The ten-twenty electrode system of the International Federation.

483

The International Federation of Clinical Neurophysiology. *Electroencephalogr Clin Neurophysiol Suppl* **52**, 3–6.

Kojima S, Nagai N, Nakabeppu Y, *et al.* 2005. Comparison of regional cerebral blood flow in patients with anorexia nervosa before and after weight gain. *Psychiatry Res* **140**, 251–8.

Konarski J Z, McIntyre R S, Soczynska J K and Kennedy S H. 2007. Neuroimaging approaches in mood disorders: Technique and clinical implications. *Ann Clin Psychiatry* **19**, 265–77.

Kornreich L, Shapira A, Horev G, Danziger Y, Tyano S and Mimouni M. 1991. CT and MR evaluation of the brain in patients with anorexia nervosa. *Am J Neuroradiol* **12**, 1213–6.

Krieg J C, Backmund H and Pirke K M. 1987. Cranial computed tomography findings in bulimia. *Acta Psychiatrica Scand* **75**, 144–9.

Krieg J C, Lauer C and Pirke K M. 1989. Structural brain abnormalities in patients with bulimia nervosa. *Psychiatry Res* **27**, 39–48.

Kringelbach M L. 2004. Food for thought: Hedonic experience beyond homeostasis in the human brain. *Neuroscience* **126**, 807–19.

Kuikka J T, Tammela L, Karhunen L, *et al.* 2001. Reduced serotonin transporter binding in binge eating women. *Psychopharmacology* **155**, 310–4.

Kuo Y T, Parkinson J R, Chaudhri O B, *et al.* 2007. The temporal sequence of gut peptide CNS interactions tracked in vivo by magnetic resonance imaging. *J Neurosci* **27**, 12 341–8.

Kuruoglu A C, Kapucu O, Atasever T, Arikan Z, Isik E and Unlu M. 1998. Technetium-99m-HMPAO brain SPECT in anorexia nervosa. *J Nucl Med* **39**, 304–06.

Lacey J H, Crisp A H, Kalucy R S, Hartmann M K and Chien C N. 1975. Weight gain and the sleeping electroencephalogram: Study of 10 patients with anorexia nervosa. *Br Med J* **4**, 556–8.

Laessle R G, Krieg J C, Fichter M M and Pirke K M. 1989. Cerebral atrophy and vigilance performance in patients with anorexia nervosa and bulimia nervosa. *Neuropsychobiology* **21**, 187–91.

Lambe E K, Katzman D K, Mikulis D J, Kennedy S H and Zipursky R B. 1997. Cerebral gray matter volume deficits after weight recovery from anorexia nervosa. *Arch Gen Psychiatry* **54**, 537–42.

Le D S, Pannacciulli N, Chen K, *et al.* 2007. Less activation in the left dorsolateral prefrontal cortex in the reanalysis of the response to a meal in obese than in lean women and its association with successful weight loss. *Am J Clin Nutr* **86**, 573–9.

Ledoux J. 2003. The emotional brain, fear, and the amygdala. *Cell Mol Neurobiol* **23**, 727–38.

Lee A L, Ogle W O and Sapolsky R M. 2002. Stress and depression: Possible links to neuron death in the hippocampus. *Bipolar Disord* **4**, 117–28.

Leonard B E. 1994. Serotonin receptors – Where are they going? *Int Clin Psychopharmacol* **9** (Suppl 1), 7–17.

Lundgren J D, Newberg A B, Allison K C, Wintering N A, Ploessl K and Stunkard A J. 2008. 123I-ADAM SPECT imaging of serotonin transporter binding in patients with night eating syndrome: A preliminary report. *Psychiatry Res* **162**, 214–20.

Martin F. 1955. Pathological neurological and psychiatric aspects of some deficiency manifestations with digestive and neuro-endocrine disorders. II. Studies of the changes in the central nervous system in two cases of anorexia (so-called anorexia nervosa) in young girls. *Helv Med Acta* **22**, 522–9.

Matsumoto R, Kitabayashi Y, Narumoto J, *et al.* 2006. Regional cerebral blood flow changes associated with interoceptive awareness in the recovery process of anorexia nervosa. *Prog Neuropsychopharmacol Biol Psychiatry* **30**, 1265–70.

McCormick L M, Keel P K, Brumm M C, *et al.* 2008. Implications of starvation-induced change in right dorsal anterior cingulate volume in anorexia nervosa. *Int J Eat Disord* **41**, 602–10.

Mockel R, Schlemmer H P, Guckel F, *et al.* 1999. 1H-MR-Spektroskopie bei Anorexia nervosa: reversible zerebrale Metabolitenanderungen. *ROFO-Fortschritte auf dem Gebiet der Rontgenstrahlen und der Bildgebenden V* **170**, 371–7.

Moretti D V, Babiloni C, Binetti G, *et al.* 2004. Individual analysis of EEG frequency and band power in mild Alzheimer's disease. *Clin Neurophysiol* **115**, 299–308.

Muhlau M, Gaser C, Ilg R, *et al.* 2007. Gray matter decrease of the anterior cingulate cortex in anorexia nervosa. *Am J Psychiatry* **164**, 1850–7.

Naruo T, Nakabeppu Y, Sagiyama K, *et al.* 2000. Characteristic regional cerebral blood flow patterns in anorexia nervosa patients with binge/purge behavior. *Am J Psychiatry* **157**, 1520–2.

Nozoe S, Naruo T, Nakabeppu Y, *et al.* 1993. Changes in regional cerebral blood flow in patients with anorexia nervosa detected through single photon emission tomography imaging. *Biol Psychiatry* **34**, 578–80.

Nozoe S, Naruo T, Yonekura R, *et al.* 1995. Comparison of regional cerebral blood flow in patients with eating disorders. *Brain Res Bull* **36**, 251–5.

Ohman A, Carlsson K, Lundqvist D and Ingvar M. 2007. On the unconscious subcortical origin of human fear. *Physiol Behav* **92**, 180–5.

Phan K L, Wager T, Taylor S F and Liberzon I. 2002. Functional neuroanatomy of emotion: A meta-analysis of emotion activation studies in PET and fMRI. *Neuroimage* **16**, 331–48.

Pieters G L, De Bruijn E R, Maas Y, *et al.* 2007. Action monitoring and perfectionism in anorexia nervosa. *Brain Cogn* **63**, 42–50.

Pollatos O, Herbert B M, Schandry R and Gramann K. 2008. Impaired central processing of emotional faces in anorexia nervosa. *Psychosom Med* **70**, 701–08.

Puri B K, Lewis H J, Saeed N and Davey N J. 1999. Volumetric change of the lateral ventricles in the human brain following glucose loading. *Exp Physiol* **84**, 223–6.

Rastam M, Bjure J, Vestergren E, *et al.* 2001. Regional cerebral blood flow in weight-restored anorexia nervosa: A preliminary study. *Dev Med Child Neurol* **43**, 239–42.

Redgrave G W, Bakker A, Bello N T, *et al.* 2008. Differential brain activation in anorexia nervosa to Fat and Thin words during a Stroop task. *Neuroreport* **19**, 1181–5.

Richmond B J, Liu Z and Shidara M. 2003. Neuroscience. Predicting future rewards. *Science* **301**, 189–80.

Rodriguez G, Babiloni C, Brugnolo A, *et al.* 2007. Cortical sources of awake scalp EEG in eating disorders. *Clin Neurophysiol* **118**, 1213–22.

Rolls E T, Sienkiewicz Z J and Yaxley S. 1989. Hunger modulates the responses to gustatory stimuli of single neurons in the caudolateral orbitofrontal cortex of the macaque monkey. *Eur J Neurosci* **1**, 53–60.

Roser W, Bubl R, Buergin D, Seelig J, Radue E W and Rost B. 1999. Metabolic changes in the brain of patients with anorexia and bulimia nervosa as detected by proton magnetic resonance spectroscopy. *Int J Eat Disord* **26**, 119–36.

Rost B, Roser W, Bubl R, Radue E W and Buergin D. 1999. MRS of the brain in patients with anorexia or bulimia nervosa. *Hosp Med (London)* **60**, 474–6.

Rzanny R, Freesmeyer D, Reichenbach J R, *et al.* 2003. 31P-MRS des Hirns bei Anorexia nervosa: Charakteristische Unterschiede in den Spektren von Patienten und gesunden Vergleichspersonen. *ROFO-Fortschritte auf dem Gebiet der Rontgenstrahlen und der Bildgebenden V* **175**, 75–82.

Sachdev P, Mondraty N, Wen W, *et al.* 2008. Brains of anorexia nervosa patients process self-images differently from non-self-images: An fMRI study. *Neuropsychologia* **46**, 2161–8.

Santel S, Baving L, Krauel K, *et al.* 2006. Hunger and satiety in anorexia nervosa: fMRI during cognitive processing of food pictures. *Brain Res* **1114**, 138–48.

Schienle A, Schafer A, Hermann A and Vaitl D. 2009. Binge-eating disorder: Reward sensitivity and brain activation to images of food. *Biol Psychiatry* **65**, 654–61.

Schlemmer H P, Mockel R, Marcus A, *et al.* 1998. Proton magnetic resonance spectroscopy in acute, juvenile anorexia nervosa. *Psychiatry Res* **82**, 171–9.

Seeger G, Braus D F, Ruf M, Goldberger U and Schmidt M H. 2002. Body image distortion reveals amygdala activation in patients with anorexia nervosa – A functional magnetic resonance imaging study. *Neurosci Lett* **326**, 25–8.

Shirao N, Okamoto Y, Mantani T, *et al.* 2005. Gender differences in brain activity generated by unpleasant word stimuli concerning body image: An fMRI study. *Br J Psychiatry* **186**, 48–53.

Shirao N, Okamoto Y, Okada G, Okamoto Y and Yamawaki S. 2003. Temporomesial activation in young females associated with unpleasant words concerning body image. *Neuropsychobiology* **48**, 136–42.

Soloff P H, Meltzer C C, Becker C, Greer P J, Kelly T M and Constantine D. 2003. Impulsivity and prefrontal hypometabolism in borderline personality disorder. *Psychiatry Res* **123**, 153–63.

Steiger H and Bruce K R. 2007. Phenotypes, endophenotypes, and genotypes in bulimia spectrum eating disorders. *Can J Psychiatry* **52**, 220–7.

Steiger H, Young S N, Kin N M, *et al.* 2001. Implications of impulsive and affective symptoms for serotonin function in bulimia nervosa. *Psychol Med* **31**, 85–95.

Stephan E, Pardo J V, Faris P L, *et al.* 2003. Functional neuroimaging of gastric distention. *J Gastrointest Surg* **7**, 740–9.

Svirko E and Hawton K. 2007. Self-injurious behavior and eating disorders: The extent and nature of the association. *Suicide Life Threat Behav* **37**, 409–21.

Swayze V W 2nd, Andersen A, Arndt S, *et al.* 1996. Reversibility of brain tissue loss in anorexia nervosa assessed with a computerized Talairach 3-D proportional grid. *Psychol Med* **26**, 381–90.

Takano A, Shiga T, Kitagawa N, *et al.* 2001. Abnormal neuronal network in anorexia nervosa studied with I-123-IMP SPECT. *Psychiatry Res* **107**, 45–50.

Tammela L I, Rissanen A, Kuikka J T, *et al.* 2003. Treatment improves serotonin transporter binding and reduces binge eating. *Psychopharmacology* **170**, 89–93.

Task Force On DSM-IV. 1994. *Diagnostic and Statistical Manual of Mental Disorders DSM-IV-TR (Text Revision)*, Washington DC:, American Psychiatric Press.

Tauscher J, Pirker W, Willeit M, *et al.* 2001. [123I] beta-CIT and single photon emission computed tomography reveal reduced brain serotonin transporter availability in bulimia nervosa. *Biol Psychiatry* **49**, 326–32.

Tiihonen J, Keski-Rahkonen A, Lopponen M, *et al.* 2004. Brain serotonin 1A receptor binding in bulimia nervosa. *Biol Psychiatry* **55**, 871–3.

Uher R, Brammer M J, Murphy T, *et al.* 2003. Recovery and chronicity in anorexia nervosa: Brain activity associated with differential outcomes. *Biol Psychiatry* **54**, 934–42.

Uher R, Murphy T, Friederich H C, *et al.* 2005. Functional neuroanatomy of body shape perception in healthy and eating-disordered women. *Biol Psychiatry* **58**, 990–7.

Wagner A, Aizenstein H, Mazurkewicz L, *et al.* 2008. Altered insula response to taste stimuli in individuals recovered from restricting-type anorexia nervosa. *Neuropsychopharmacology* **33**, 513–23.

Wagner A, Aizenstein H, Venkatraman V K, *et al.* 2007. Altered reward processing in women recovered from anorexia nervosa. *Am J Psychiatry* **164**, 1842–9.

Wagner A, Greer P, Bailer U F, *et al.* 2006. Normal brain tissue volumes after long-term recovery in anorexia and bulimia nervosa. *Biol Psychiatry* **59**, 291–3.

Wagner A, Ruf M, Braus D F and Schmidt M H. 2003. Neuronal activity changes and body image distortion in anorexia nervosa. *Neuroreport* **14**, 2193–7.

Wang G J, Volkow N D, Thanos P K and Fowler J S. 2004. Similarity between obesity and drug addiction as assessed by neurofunctional imaging: A concept review. *J Addict Dis* **23**, 39–53.

Whitwell J L, Sampson E L, Loy C T, *et al.* 2007. VBM signatures of abnormal eating behaviours in frontotemporal lobar degeneration. *Neuroimage* **35**, 207–13.

Woolley J D, Gorno-Tempini M L, Seeley W W, *et al.* 2007. Binge eating is associated with right orbitofrontal–insular–striatal atrophy in frontotemporal dementia. *Neurology* **69**, 1424–33.

Yonezawa H, Otagaki Y, Miyake Y, Okamoto Y and Yamawaki S. 2008. No differences are seen in the regional cerebral blood flow in the restricting type of anorexia nervosa compared with the binge eating/purging type. *Psychiatry Clin Neurosci* **62**, 26–33.

Gene-Jack Wang, Nora D. Volkow, Joanna S. Fowler and Panayotis K. Thanos

Abstract

Obesity is a major public health problem affecting increasingly large numbers of people worldwide. Although it reflects an imbalance between energy intake and expenditure, the core pathophysiological mechanisms responsible for maintaining this balance are not well understood. It is of particular relevance that the maintenance of normal weight requires the coordination of peripheral signals of hunger and satiety and brain responses to either procure and consume food or to stop eating after a meal. Brain imaging studies show that obese individuals have significant deficits in regulation of energy homeostasis (i.e. delayed response to peripheral metabolic signals in the hypothalamus) and the brain circuits that regulate normal eating behavior (i.e. hunger, satiety, motivation, reward, emotion, learning, memory and inhibitory control). Because of the complexity and multi-factorial nature of obesity and eating disorders, future progress will be facilitated by a transdisciplinary approach which integrates modern imaging tools with new knowledge on behavior and genetics to guide the development of effective preventive and therapeutic approaches.

Introduction

According to the National Center for Chronic Disease Prevention and Health Promotion, an epidemic of obesity has developed in the United States during the past 30 years. Obesity is defined as an excessively high amount of body fat or adipose tissue in relation to lean body mass (Stunkard and Wadden, 1993). Health effects can be related to both the amount of body fat (or adiposity) as well as to the distribution of fat throughout the body and the size of local adipose tissue deposits. Local fat deposits can be imaged using standard techniques such as magnetic resonance imaging (MRI). The standard measure of obesity is the Body Mass Index (BMI), which is defined as a person's body mass in kilograms divided by the square of his or her height in meters. The BMI is more highly correlated with body fat than any other indicator of height and weight.

Recent results of the National Center for Health Statistics (NCHS) 2006 indicate that an estimated 34% of US adults aged 20–74 are obese, which is defined as having a BMI of more than 30. More than 72 million Americans are obese (Ogden et al., 2006), and about 32.7% of adults are overweight (BMI between 25 and 29). It is particularly worrisome that approximately 17% of children and adolescents are now overweight, and this percentage has doubled since the early 1970s (Ogden et al., 2007b). Although the prevalence of obesity is leveling off in women, children and adolescents, it is increasing in men (Ogden et al., 2007a, 2008).

The Centers for Disease Control and Prevention (CDC) estimates that: "as many as 47 million Americans may exhibit a cluster of medical conditions (a 'metabolic syndrome') characterized by insulin resistance and the presence of obesity, abdominal fat, high blood sugar and triglycerides, high blood cholesterol, and high blood pressure." This syndrome may result from poor diet and insufficient physical activity, conditions that are now common in childhood. Overweight and obese individuals (BMI of 25 and above) are at increased risk for conditions that include: hypertension; hyper-cholesterolemia; type 2 diabetes; insulin resistance, glucose intolerance; coronary heart disease; angina pectoris; congestive heart failure; stroke; cholecystitis; cholelithiasis; gout; osteoarthritis;

Understanding Neuropsychiatric Disorders, ed. M. E. Shenton and B. I. Turetsky. Published by Cambridge University Press.

obstructive sleep apnea and respiratory problems; some types of cancer (endometrium, breast, prostate, and colon); complications of pregnancy; poor female reproductive health (i.e. menstrual irregularities, infertility, irregular ovulation); bladder control problems (i.e. stress incontinence); uric acid nephrolithiasis, and psychological disorders (i.e. depression, eating disorders, distorted body image, and low self esteem) (Ogden *et al.*, 2007b).

Obesity can derive from a variety of causes (i.e. genetic, culture, nutrition intake, physical activity; Bessesen, 2008). Although maintenance of an appropriate body weight requires balance between caloric intake and physical activity, genetic factors play an important role in both energy requirements and general activity levels. Most notably, obesity is 10 times more prevalent in persons whose parents, brothers, or sisters are obese. Studies in identical twins have clearly demonstrated that genetics play a major role (Segal and Allison, 2002). For example, non-identical twins raised together were less similar in weight than identical twins raised apart. However, despite the importance of genetics, it is likely that the changes in the environment are the main contributors to the rapid escalation and magnitude of the obesity epidemic in recent decades. The nature and nurture interactions associated with obesity are thought to occur after conception but before birth. Maternal nutritional imbalance and metabolic disturbances during pregnancy could affect gene expression and contribute to the development of obesity and diabetes mellitus of offspring in later life (Catalano and Ehrenberg, 2006). Recent experiments have shown nutritional exposures, stress or disease state after birth may also result in lifelong remodeling of gene expression (Gallou-Kabani and Junien, 2005).

Environmental and cultural influences are of particular relevance. In modern society, food is not only widely available, but also increasingly more varied and palatable. Nonetheless, the net effect of these influences on overweight and obesity and on morbidity and mortality is difficult to quantify. It is likely that a gene–environment interaction(s), in which genetically susceptible individuals respond to an environment with increased availability of palatable energy-dense foods and reduced opportunities for energy expenditure, contribute to the current high prevalence of obesity (Mietus-Snyder and Lustig, 2008). Learned behaviors also play a large role in determining whether people become overweight or obese, and

interventions in this area are the basis of most prevention and treatment strategies. Surgical treatment of obesity is becoming more common, and great efforts are being directed towards developing pharmacological approaches. In the meantime, the high prevalence of obesity and associated ailments underscores an urgent need to understand the mechanisms that predispose individuals towards excessive body weight, and to develop comprehensive efforts directed at prevention and treatment. In the last decade, functional brain imaging techniques have been used to investigate the neurochemical and functional mechanisms associated with food reward and with overeating and obesity.

Application of functional and neurochemical brain imaging for ingestive behavior and obesity

Positron emission tomography (PET) and single photon emission computed tomography (SPECT) are imaging methods that measure the distribution and movement of radiolabeled compounds in the living human and animal body. With these methods, it is possible to measure the distribution and concentration of many receptors, transporters and enzymes in the human brain as well as cerebral blood flow (Zipursky *et al.*, 2007). With PET it is also possible to measure regional brain glucose metabolism using 2-deoxy-2-[^{18}F]fluoro-D-glucose (FDG), a radiotracer that is now widely available though regional radiopharmacies.

Functional magnetic resonance imaging (fMRI) has provided measurement to assess changes in neural activity levels in the brain in response to various stimulations. fMRI measures the vascular correlate of neuronal activity via the blood oxygen level-dependent (BOLD) signal. BOLD-fMRI is the most commonly used technique to study brain function in humans non-invasively. For activated regions, the local increases of cerebral blood flow and volume largely exceed the local increase in oxygen consumption, producing a decrease in paramagnetic deoxyhemoglobin concentration, which increases the homogeneity of the local magnetic field, and consequently the local MRI signal. This dynamic signal increase is the basis of the BOLD contrast (Ogawa *et al.*, 1990, 1993; Kim *et al.*, 1993; Turner *et al.*, 1993). The BOLD signal consists of both micro and

488

macro vascular components (Duong *et al.*, 2003). The BOLD effect arising from the capillary bed reflects local increases of synaptic activity (Ugurbil *et al.*, 1999). The BOLD signals arising from large veins and pial veins, on the other hand, significantly reduce spatial localization in fMRI studies, because these draining veins can extend from several to tens of millimeters from the activation sites (Menon, 2002).

Brain imaging of peripheral signals in obesity

Food ingestion is modulated by needs for nutrition, pleasure, and responses to stress. Food ingestion is modulated by both peripheral and central signals. Several factors were known to regulate eating behavior include glucose, fatty acids, insulin and gut hormones/peptides. Peripheral hormone signals that originate from the gut (i.e. ghrelin, peptide YY_{3-36}, glucagon-like peptide 1, cholecystokinin), from the adipose tissues (i.e. leptin, adiponectin) and from the pancreas (insulin) continually inform the brain about the status of acute hunger and satiety (Cummings and Overduin, 2007). Neurons in the hypothalamus express receptors for these peptide hormones. These neurons mediate the actions of the gut hormones that reflect energy content in the body and coordinate eating behaviors and food intake to maintain energy homeostasis. The hypothalamus and its various circuits, including orexin and melanin concentrating hormone-producing neurons in the lateral hypothalamus, as well as neuropeptide Y/agouti-related protein and alpha-melanocyte stimulating hormone producing neurons in the arctuate nucleus, are thought to be the principal homeostatic brain regions responsible for the regulation of body weight (Morrison and Berthoud, 2007). Numerous studies have shown damage involving the hypothalamic neurons induced hyperphagia and obesity (reviewed in King, 2006).

Functional neuroimaging techniques have been used to assess the link between intake of food ingredients (i.e. glucose) and changes in hypothalamus and to compare responses in lean and obese individuals. Several fMRI studies reported transient changes of the BOLD signals in the hypothalamus after administration of glucose in rats and humans. Drinking of glucose solution in fasting healthy volunteers revealed a dose-dependent prolonged decreased BOLD signal in the hypothalamus. The decreased fMRI signal

started shortly after drinking began (4–10 min) and lasted for 30 min (Liu *et al.*, 2000; Matsuda *et al.*, 1999; Smeets *et al.*, 2005). However, the obese subjects have much higher plasma insulin levels after glucose ingestion, and the magnitude of inhibition of responses in the hypothalamus is lower than in lean subjects. The time to reach the maximal inhibition effects in the hypothalamus is also much longer in obese than in lean subjects (Matsuda *et al.*, 1999). The impaired responses in hypothalamus to glucose ingestion might be a contribution factor or a consequence of overeating in obese individuals.

Glucose ingestion also triggers the release of several gut peptides such as peptide YY_{3-36} (PYY), and glucagon-like peptide 1 (GLP-1), which act in the hypothalamus to induce satiety (Batterham *et al.*, 2003). Plasma PYY levels increase in proportion to the caloric intake after eating. A human fMRI study showed BOLD signal in hypothalamus predicted food intake in the fasting state when circulating levels of PYY were low. Intravenous infusion of PYY to reach plasma concentrations equivalent to that of postprandial state minimized the response of the hypothalamus to eating behavior (Batterham *et al.*, 2007). Subjects with reduced postprandial PYY release exhibit lower satiety which would be predicted to promote the development and or maintenance of obesity (Karra *et al.*, 2009). An animal in-vivo functional imaging using manganese-enhanced MRI revealed that GLP-1 inhibits neuronal activity in the hypothalamus of rats. The inhibition of fMRI signal in hypothalamic neuron was more effective by drinking glucose solution orally than via intravenous infusion (Parkinson *et al.*, 2009).

Adipocytes modulate the influx of dietary fat and secrete a variety of hormones (e.g. leptin). Leptin signals to the brain the level of body fat stores and induces weight loss by suppressing food intake and increasing metabolic rate (Myers *et al.*, 2008). It is also involved in the neuroendocrine response to starvation, energy expenditure and reproduction (initiation of human puberty) (Ross and Desai, 2005). Leptin-deficient mammals including humans are usually hyperphagic, which is reversed with leptin-replacement therapy (Morton *et al.*, 2006; Zhang *et al.*, 1994). Direct injection of leptin into the cerebral ventricle or hypothalamus of animals lacking leptin inhibited food intake and decreased body weight and fat (Zhang *et al.*, 1994).

FMRI-BOLD has been used to map brain responses while viewing food in genetically leptin-deficient

489

human subjects. These studies revealed that viewing food images elicited a desire to eat even when the subjects had just eaten. After leptin replacement, viewing images of favorite food elicited a desire to eat only during fasting (Farooqi *et al.*, 2007). The brain images showed the leptin treatment suppressed activity in response to food cue in the striatum, a brain region involved in reward and motivation (see following sections). Baicy *et al.* also reported in a group of genetically leptin-deficient adults that leptin replacement decreased food intake and weight and the decrement was associated with suppressed activity in brain regions related to hunger (i.e. insula, parietal and temporal cortices) and enhanced activation in regions related to satiety (i.e. prefrontal cortex) in response to food cue (Baicy *et al.*, 2007). Nevertheless there are very few humans with leptin deficiency. The common forms of obesity in humans are associated with leptin resistance (failure of high leptin levels to suppress feeding and mediate weight loss; Lustig, 2006; Myers *et al.*, 2008). High levels of leptin in obese patients have been posited to be due to leptin receptor signaling defects, downstream blockade in neuronal circuits, and defects in leptin transport across the blood–brain barrier (Banks, 2008; Morrison, 2008). Leptin resistance in the hypothalamus invokes the starvation pathway and promotes food intake. Leptin is also a critical hormone that alters metabolism during caloric restriction in human (Ahima and Lazar, 2008; Ahima *et al.*, 1996). Decreased leptin levels in a weight-reduced state can reduce energy expenditure and promote weight gain.

Obese individuals often have enlarged adipocytes with a reduced buffering capacity for fat storage. The dysfunction of adipose tissue (particularly abdominal fat) plays an important role in the development of insulin resistance. Insulin shares a common central signaling pathway with leptin that regulates energy homeostasis through the hypothalamus. Insulin levels reflect short-term changes in energy intake, whereas leptin levels reflect energy balance over a longer period of time (Ahima and Lazar, 2008). Insulin also acts as an endogenous leptin antagonist. Suppression of insulin ameliorates leptin resistance. Chronically, increases in insulin (i.e. insulin resistance) impede leptin signal transduction and promote obesity. High plasma levels of insulin and glucose due to insulin resistance are believed to be the origin of metabolic syndrome and type 2 diabetes. Studies using fMRI-BOLD showed subjects with type 2

diabetes while viewing high-energy food pictures increased responses in insula, orbitofrontal cortex (OFC) and striatum, which are brain regions involved in interoception, motivation and emotion (Chechlacz *et al.*, 2009). These findings are in part similar to the brain imaging studies observed in obese individuals, which are discussed in the following sections.

In contrast to PYY or leptin, ghrelin normally increases during fasting and drops after a meal (Berthoud, 2008). The hunger peptide, ghrelin increases food intake and body weight by stimulating neurons in the hypothalamus. When ghrelin is administered intravenously to healthy volunteers during fMRI, their response to food stimuli (pictures) increased in regions of the brain, including the amygdala, OFC, anterior insula, and striatum (Malik *et al.*, 2008). The effects of ghrelin on the amygdala and OFC are associated with self-reports of hunger. This observation provides evidence that ghrelin influences the brain regions involving hedonic and incentive response, which are beyond nutritional needs. Fasting ghrelin levels are lower in obese individuals and fail to decline after a meal, which may contribute to their overeating (Wren, 2008).

Neurobiology of eating behavior

Eating is a highly reinforcing behavior (Wise, 2006). In fact, some ingredients in palatable food (i.e. sugar, corn oil) are compulsively consumed, and this loss of control over food intake is similar to what is observed with compulsive consumption of substances of abuse (Rada *et al.*, 2005; Liang *et al.*, 2006). Behavioral studies show similarities among certain patterns of overeating and other excessive behaviors such as drinking too much alcohol and compulsive gambling. These behaviors activate brain circuitry that involves reward, motivation, decision-making, learning, and memory. Indeed, ingestion of sugar induces brain release of opioids and dopamine (DA), which are neurotransmitters traditionally associated with the rewarding effects of drugs of abuse. In certain conditions (i.e. intermittent, excessive sugar intake) rats can display behavioral and neurochemical changes that resemble those observed in animal models of drug dependence (Avena *et al.*, 2008). From an evolutionary perspective, animals would benefit from a neural mechanism (circuitry) that supports an animal's ability to pursue natural rewards (food, water, sex). However, these circuits are sometimes dysfunctional, leading to various types of disorders.

Endogenous opioids are expressed throughout the limbic system and contribute to processing of reinforcing signals, and palatable foods increases endogenous opioid gene expression (Will *et al.*, 2003). Furthermore, injection of mu-opioid agonists in the nucleus accumbens potentiates the intake of palatable foods (Woolley *et al.*, 2006). Opioid antagonists, on the other hand, reduce food ratings of pleasantness without affecting hunger (Yeomans and Gray, 1997). It is likely that the opioid system is involved with the liking and the pleasurable responses to food that might promote the intake of highly palatable foods such as those consumed in a diet high in fat and sugar (Will *et al.*, 2006).

Other neurotransmitters (e.g. acetylcholine, GABA, serotonin and glutamine) are also involved in eating behaviors (Kelley *et al.*, 2005). For example, acetylcholine and DA play opposite roles in the nucleus accumbens (NAcc) in feeding behavior. DA in the NAcc can increase appetite, but as feeding slows down toward to the end of a meal, extracellular acetylcholine increases (Avena *et al.*, 2006). In addition, other mechanisms modulate eating behavior such as stress, which increases consumption of high-energy food (Dallman *et al.*, 2003), also contribute to obesity (Adam and Epel, 2007). Neurotransmitter imaging studies for obesity and overeating behaviors in humans have mostly investigated the DA system, and a few studies have also assessed the serotonin system and we review them in the following sections.

Eating behavior and brain DA system

DA is a neurotransmitter known to play a major role in motivation that is involved with reward and prediction of reward. The mesocorticolimbic DA system projects from the ventral tegmental area to the nucleus accumbens (NAcc), with inputs from various components of the limbic system including the amygdala, hippocampus, hypothalamus, striatum, OFC, and the prefrontal cortex. DA has been shown to mediate the reinforcing effects of natural rewards (i.e. sucrose) (Smith, 2004). DA pathways make food more reinforcing and are also associated with the reinforcing responses to drugs of abuse (i.e. alcohol, methamphetamine, cocaine, heroine; Di Chiara and Bassareo, 2007). The mesencephalic DA system regulates pleasurable and motivating responses to food intake and stimuli (Volkow *et al.*, 2008a; Volkow and Wise, 2005), which affects and alters behavioral

components of energy homeostasis. The mesencephalic DA system can respond to food stimuli even in the presence of postprandial satiety factors (Batterham *et al.*, 2007). When that occurs, the regulation of eating behavior can be switched from a homeostatic state to an hedonic corticolimbic state.

DA regulates food intake via the mesolimbic circuitry apparently by modulating appetitive motivational processes (Wise, 2006). There are projections from the NAcc to the hypothalamus that directly regulate feeding (Baldo and Kelley, 2007). Other forebrain DA projections are also involved. DAnergic pathways are critical for survival since they help influence the fundamental drive for eating. Brain DA systems are necessary for wanting incentives, which is a distinct component of motivation and reinforcement (Robinson *et al.*, 2007). It is one of the natural reinforcing mechanisms that motivate an animal to perform a given behavior such as seeking food. The mesolimbic DA system mediates incentive learning and reinforcement mechanisms associated with positive reward, such as palatable food in a hungry animal (Robinson *et al.*, 2007).

DAnergic neurotransmission is mediated by five distinct receptor subtypes, which are classified into two main classes of receptors termed D1-like (D1 and D5) and D2-like (D2, D3 and D4). In the case of drug self-administration, activation of D2-like receptors has been shown to mediate the incentive to seek further cocaine reinforcement in animals. In contrast, D1-like receptors mediate a reduction in the drive to seek further cocaine reinforcement (Self *et al.*, 1996). Both the D1- and D2-like receptors act synergistically when regulating feeding behaviors. Nevertheless, the precise involvement of DA receptor subtypes in mediating eating behavior is still not clear. DA D1-like receptors play a role in motivation to work for reward-related learning and translation of new reward to action (Trevitt *et al.*, 2001; Fiorino *et al.*, 1993). No human imaging studies have assessed the involvement of D1 receptors on eating behaviors. Animal studies showed that infusion of DA D1 receptor antagonists in the NAcc shell impaired associative gustatory (i.e. taste) learning and blunted the rewarding effects of palatable food (Fenu *et al.*, 2001). Selective D1 receptor agonist can enhance preference of high-palpability food over regular maintenance diet (Cooper and Al-Naser, 2006). The role of DA D5 receptors on eating behaviors is not established due to the lack of selective ligands that can discriminate between D1 and D5 receptors.

491

The D2 receptors have been associated with feeding and addictive behaviors in animal and human studies. D2 receptors play a role in reward seeking, prediction, expectation and motivation (Wise, 2006). Food seeking is initiated by hunger; however, it is food-predictive cues that activate DA cell firing and motivate animals (Watanabe *et al.*, 2001). Many animal studies have evaluated mixed D2/D3 receptor antagonists or agonists on food-seeking behaviors (Missale *et al.*, 1998). D2 receptor antagonists block food seeking behaviors that depend on history association (reinforcement) between the cues and the reward they predict as well as on palatable foods (McFarland and Ettenberg, 1998). When food is no longer priming and rewarding for an animal, D2 agonists can be used to reinstate extinguished reward-seeking behavior (Wise *et al.*, 1990). Human imaging studies of eating behaviors have mainly used PET studies with [^{11}C]raclopride, a reversible DA D2/D3 receptor radioligand, which binds at D2 receptors and D3 receptors with similar affinity and which is sensitive to changes in extracellular DA. A human PET study with [^{11}C]raclopride that measured DA release in the striatum following consumption of a favorite food showed the amount of DA release was correlated with the ratings of meal pleasantness (Small *et al.*, 2003). Food deprivation potentiates the rewarding effects of food (Cameron *et al.*, 2008). During fasting, the role of DA is not selective for food, but rather signals the salience for a variety of potential biological rewards and cues that predict rewards (Carr, 2007). Chronic food deprivation also potentiates the rewarding effects of most addictive drugs (Carr, 2002). The striatum, OFC and amygdala, which are brain regions that receive DA projections are activated during the expectation of food (Schultz, 2004). In fact, using PET and [^{11}C]raclopride to evaluate changes in extracellular DA in striatum in response to food cues (presentation of palatable food) in food-deprived subjects, we showed significant increases in extracellular DA in the dorsal striatum but not in the ventral striatum (where the NAcc is located) (Volkow *et al.*, 2002). The DA increases were significantly correlated with the increases in self-reports of hunger and desire for food. These results provided evidence of conditioned-cue reaction in the dorsal striatum. The involvement of DA in the dorsal striatum appears to be crucial for enabling the motivation required to consume the food that is necessary for survival (Sotak *et al.*, 2005; Palmiter, 2008). It is

different from the activation in the NAcc, which may related more to motivation associated with food palatability (Szczypka *et al.*, 2001; Wise, 2006).

It has been postulated that D3 receptors might be involved in drug dependence and addiction (Heidbreder *et al.*, 2005). Recently, several selective D3 receptor antagonists have been developed. These antagonists have higher selectivity for the D3 receptor compared to other DA receptors (Heidbreder *et al.*, 2005). Administration of a selective D3 receptor antagonist prevented nicotine-triggered relapse to nicotine-seeking behavior (Andreoli *et al.*, 2003). It also attenuated sucrose-seeking behavior induced by sucrose-associated cue reintroduction in the rodent (Cervo *et al.*, 2007). We have also shown that D3 receptor antagonists decrease food intake in rats (Thanos *et al.*, 2008b). Several selective D3 receptor PET radioligands have been developed (Hocke *et al.*, 2008; Narendran *et al.*, 2006; Prante *et al.*, 2008), but none to our knowledge has been used to investigate eating behavior and obesity in humans. The D4 receptors are predominantly located in cortical regions in both pyramidal and GABAergic cells (Mrzljak *et al.*, 1996), in striatal neurons and in hypothalamus (Rivera *et al.*, 2002). It is believed that D4 receptors act as an inhibitory post-synaptic receptor controlling the neurons of the frontal cortex and striatum (Oak *et al.*, 2000). These receptors may play a role influencing satiety (Huang *et al.*, 2005).

Imaging the interaction between peripheral metabolic signals and eating behavior

Many peripheral metabolic signals directly or indirectly interact with brain DA pathways. Highly palatable foods can override internal homeostatic mechanisms through action on brain DA pathways and lead to overeating and obesity (Batterham *et al.*, 2007). Simple carbohydrates such as sugar are a major nutritional source and contribute to about a quarter of total energy intake. Animal studies have demonstrated that glucose modulates DA neuronal activity in the ventral tegmental area and substantia nigra directly. The midbrain DA neurons also interact with insulin, leptin and ghrelin (Palmiter, 2007; Myers *et al.*, 2008; Abizaid *et al.*, 2006). Ghrelin activates DA neurons; whereas leptin and insulin inhibit them. Food restriction increases circulating ghrelin released from the stomach and activates the mesolimbic system increasing DA release in the NAcc (Abizaid *et al.*, 2006). An fMRI study showed that infusion of ghrelin to healthy subjects enhanced activation to food cues in brain regions involved in hedonic and incentive responses (Malik *et al.*, 2008).

Insulin stimulates glucose metabolism directly, functioning as a neurotransmitter or stimulating neuronal glucose uptake indirectly. There is evidence that brain insulin plays a role in feeding behavior, sensory processing and cognitive function (Brody *et al.*, 2004; Rotte *et al.*, 2005; Schultes *et al.*, 2005). Laboratory animals with disruption of brain insulin receptors show enhanced feeding (Bruning *et al.*, 2000). A recent human study using PET-FDG showed that brain insulin resistance co-exists in subjects with peripheral insulin resistance, especially in the striatum and insula (regions that relate to appetite and reward; Anthony *et al.*, 2006). These brain regions in subjects with insulin resistance may require much higher levels of insulin to experience the reward and the interoceptive sensations of eating.

Leptin also plays a role in regulating eating behavior in part through regulation of the DA pathway (but also the cannabinoid system). An fMRI study showed leptin could diminish food reward and enhance the response to satiety signals generated during food consumption through the modulation of neuronal activity in the striatum in leptin-deficient human subjects (Farooqi *et al.*, 2007). Recently, we showed evidence that leptin modulated D2R expression in the mouse striatum, and that these effects were genotype/phenotype-dependent (Pfaffly *et al.*, 2010). In addition, it was recently shown that leptin plays an important role in modulating adaptation responses of the DA system with respect to chronic food restriction (Thanos *et al.*, 2008c). Thus insulin and leptin can act complementarily to modify the DA pathway and alter eating behaviors. Leptin and insulin resistance in the brain DA pathways makes food intake a more potent reward and promotes palatable food intake (Figlewicz *et al.*, 2006).

Imaging sensory experience of food and its relation to eating behaviors

Sensory processing of food and food-related cues plays an important role in the motivation for food, and it is especially important in the selection of a varied diet. Sensory inputs of taste, vision, olfaction,

temperature and texture are first sent to the primary sensory cortices (i.e. insula, primary visual cortex, pyriform, primary somatosensory cortex) and then to the OFC and amygdala (Rolls, 2007). The hedonic reward value of food is closely linked to the sensory perception of the food. The relation of DA in these brain regions during sensory perception of food will be discussed.

Insular cortex

The insular cortex is involved in the interceptive sense of the body and in emotional awareness (Craig, 2003). The connection between stomach and brain were assessed using fMRI and balloon extension, which mimicked the gastric distension that occurs during normal food intake. Gastric distension activated the posterior insula, which may reflect its role in the awareness of body state (Wang *et al.*, 2008). Indeed, in smokers, damage to the insula disrupts their physiological urge to smoke (Naqvi *et al.*, 2007). Moreover, a recent study in rats reported that the administration of a hypocretin receptor antagonist into the insula decreases nicotine self-administration (Hollander *et al.*, 2008). The insula is the primary gustatory area, which participates in many aspects of eating behavior such as taste. DA plays an important role in the tasting of palatable foods, which is mediated through the insula (Hajnal and Norgren, 2005). Animal studies have shown that tasting sucrose increases DA release in the NAcc (Hajnal *et al.*, 2004). Lesions in the ventral tegmental area reduced consumption of a preferred sucrose solution (Shimura *et al.*, 2002). Human imaging studies have shown that tasting palatable foods activated the insula and midbrain areas (Del Parigi *et al.*, 2005; Frank *et al.*, 2008). However, the human brain can distinguish the calorie content of the sweet solution unconsciously. For example, when normal weight women tasted sweetener with calories (sucrose), both the insula and DAnergic midbrain areas were activated, whereas when they tasted sweetener without calories (sucralose), they only activated the insula (Frank *et al.*, 2008). Obese subjects have greater activation in the insula than normal controls when tasting a liquid meal that consists of sugar and fat (Del Parigi *et al.*, 2005). In contrast, subjects that have recovered from anorexia nervosa show less activation in the insula when tasting sucrose and no association of feelings of pleasantness with insular activation as observed in the normal controls (Wagner *et al.*, 2008). It is likely that dysregulation of the insula in response to the taste might be involved in disturbances in appetite regulation. Recently, research in de Araujo's laboratory has shown for the first time the expression of the taste receptor genes Tas1r1, Tas1r2 and Tas1r3, and their associated G-protein genes, in the mammalian brain (Ren *et al.*, 2009). Neuronal expression of taste genes was detected in different nutrient-sensing forebrain regions. These results suggested that the G-protein coupled sweet receptor T1R2/T1R3 is a brain glucosensor (Ren *et al.*, 2009).

Somatosensory cortex

There is limited literature that addresses the role of the primary somatosensory cortex in food intake and obesity. Activation of the somatosensory cortex was reported in an imaging study of normal weight women during the viewing of images of high-caloric foods (Killgore *et al.*, 2003). Using PET and FDG to measure regional brain glucose metabolism (marker of brain function), we showed that morbidly obese subjects had higher than normal baseline metabolism in the somatosensory cortex (Figure 34.1) (Wang *et al.*, 2002). There is evidence that the somatosensory cortex influences brain DA activity (Huttunen *et al.*, 2003; Rossini *et al.*, 1995), including regulating amphetamine-induced striatal DA release (Chen *et al.*, 2008b). DA also modulates the somatosensory cortex in the human brain (Kuo *et al.*, 2008). Moreover, we recently showed an association between the availability of striatal D2 receptors and glucose metabolism in the somatosensory cortex of obese subjects (Volkow *et al.*, 2008b). Since DA stimulation signals saliency and facilitates conditioning (Zink *et al.*, 2003), DA's modulation of the somatosensory cortex to food stimuli might enhance their saliency, which is likely to play a role in the formation of conditioned associations between food and food-related environmental cues.

Orbitofrontal cortex (OFC)

The OFC, which is in part regulated by DA as well as serotonin activity, is a key brain region for controlling behaviors and for salience attribution including the value of food (Rolls and McCabe, 2007; Grabenhorst *et al.*, 2008). As such, it determines the pleasantness and palatability of food as a function of its context. Using PET and FDG in normal weight individuals, we

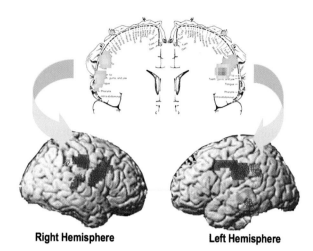

Right Hemisphere   Left Hemisphere

Figure 34.1 Color-coded statistical parametric mapping (SPM) result displayed in a coronal plane with a superimposed diagram of the somatosensory homunculus with its corresponding three-dimensional (3D) rendered SPM images show the areas with higher metabolism in obese than in lean subjects. The areas that are significantly higher are displayed in red and are superimposed into the surface of 3D reconstructed brain MRI images (grayscale). Obese subjects have higher metabolism than lean subjects in the somatosensory areas where the mouth, lips and tongue are represented. (Adapted from Wang *et al.*, 2002.)

showed that exposure to food cues (using the same paradigm as that with which we showed that cues increase DA in dorsal striatum) increased metabolism in OFC, and that these increases were associated with the perception of hunger and the desire for food (Wang *et al.*, 2004). The enhanced OFC activation by the food stimulation is likely to reflect downstream DAnergic effects, and is likely to participate in DA's involvement in the drive for food consumption. The OFC participates in learning stimulus-reinforcement associations and conditioning (Cox *et al.*, 2005; Gallagher *et al.*, 1999). It also participates in conditioned cues-elicited feeding (Weingarten, 1983). Thus its activation secondary to food-induced DA stimulation could result in an intense motivation to consume food. Dysfunction of the OFC is associated with compulsive behaviors including overeating (Machado and Bachevalier, 2007). This is relevant because food-induced conditioned responses very likely contribute to overeating irrespective of hunger signals (Ogden and Wardle, 1990).

Amygdala

The amygdala is another brain region involved in eating behaviors. More specifically, there is evidence that it is involved with learning and recognition of the biological significance of objects during food procurement (Petrovich and Gallagher, 2003). Extracellular DA levels in the amygdala were increased in a preclinical study of food intake after a brief period of fasting (Fallon *et al.*, 2007). Functional neuroimaging studies using PET and functional magnetic resonance imaging (fMRI) have shown activation of the amygdala with food-related stimuli, tastes and odors (Del Parigi *et al.*, 2002; Small and Prescott, 2005; Smeets *et al.*, 2006). The amygdala is also involved with the emotional component of food intake. Stress-induced amygdala activation can be dampened by the ingestion of energy-dense food (Dallman *et al.*, 2003). The amygdala receives interoceptive signals from the visceral organs. In an fMRI study in which we assessed the brain activation response to gastric distention, we showed an association between activation in the amygdala and subjective feelings of fullness (Wang *et al.*, 2008). We also found that the subjects with higher BMI had less amygdalar activation during gastric distention. It is likely that perception mediated by the amygdala could influence the content and volumes of food consumed in a given meal.

Imaging the connection between personality and overeating behavior

Eating behavior can be triggered by internal signals of an energy deficit or by external cues. External cues such as smelling, viewing or tasting of appetizing foods can trigger a desire to eat even without the subjective feeling of hunger (Burton *et al.*, 2007). The sensitivity to food cues can be variable among individuals. Using fMRI, Passamonti *et al.* (2009) showed that individual sensitivity to viewing appetizing food was associated with changes in brain connectivity between the striatum, amygdala, anterior cingulate and premotor cortex. Individuals who were more sensitive to the external food cues had a greater increase in their subjective feeling of hunger in the presence of appetizing food. The differences in sensitivity to food cues were positively associated with the connectivity between ventral striatum and amygdala when viewing appetizing food, as well as the connectivity between ventral stratum and the premotor cortex, which is involved with the preparation for oral movement. The differences in sensitivity were negatively correlated with connection between the anterior cingulate gyrus and OFC, which is associated with

coding of the reward value of food. These results implied that individuals with higher sensitivity to food cues had increased risk to overeat when exposed to an environment with constant exposure to food stimuli (e.g. advertisements and food displays).

An individual's experience to food reward also plays an important role on eating behaviors. Animal studies showed that anticipating an impending reward from food intake activated mesotelencephalic DA neurons, and the DA activation in the NAcc was greater when conditioned stimuli that signaled food receipt than after delivery of an unexpected meal (Blackburn *et al.*, 1989; Kiyatkin and Gratton, 1994; Schultz *et al.*, 1993). In an experimental environment, individuals who worked harder to earn a preferred snack in a task that permitted later consumption had a stronger association with the intakes of the preferred food and with total calorie intake than with the subjective perception of pleasantness for the chosen food. It is likely that anticipated reward from food intake is a stronger indicator of caloric intake than the actual reward experience (Epstein *et al.*, 2004). The individual difference in anticipation and motivation for food might lead to difference in food intake. Obese individuals experience greater food reward from anticipation and consumption and are more motivated to eat than normal body weight subjects (Epstein *et al.*, 2007). In fact, an fMRI study of adolescent girls showed obese girls had greater activation in insula and gustatory somatosensory cortex than lean girls in response to anticipated food intake and to actual consumption of food. These are the brain regions that related to the sensory and hedonic aspect of the food. However, the obese girls also had decreased activation in caudate nucleus in response to food consumption that might indicate a dysfunctioning DA system, which increases the risk of overeating (Stice *et al.*, 2008b).

Brain imaging studies of binge eating disorder

Binge eating disorder (BED) is characterized by episodes of eating an objectively large amount of food and feelings of loss of control (American Psychiatric Association, 1994). It occurs in about 0.7–4% of the general population and in about 30% of obese subjects attending weight control programs (Dymek-Valentine *et al.*, 2004). Obese binge eaters eat significantly more calories than obese non-binge eaters when asked to eat as much as they want or simply to eat normally (Goldfein *et al.*, 1993; Yanovski *et al.*, 1993). Obese binge eaters have high relapse rates during weight control programs and experience their disorder for long periods of time. A high prevalence of BED (30–80%) was reported among morbidly obese subjects who have undergone bariatric surgery (Niego *et al.*, 2007). The eating disturbances persist (6–26%) in many of the same patients after surgery and are correlated with weight regain (Burgmer *et al.*, 2005; Sallet *et al.*, 2007). Obese binge eaters lost less excess body weight than obese non-BED obese subjects after bariatric surgery (Wolnerhanssen *et al.*, 2008; Colles *et al.*, 2008). There is evidence that alteration in brain monoaminergic system might play a role in BED (Jimerson *et al.*, 1992; Leibowitz and Alexander, 1998). Bulimic patients with frequent binging episodes have lower serotonin and DA metabolite concentrations in cerebral spinal fluid (Jimerson *et al.*, 1992).

Several functional neuroimaging studies have been used to investigate brain response to visual food cue stimulation in BED subjects. Karhunen *et al.* (2000) used SPECT to observe cerebral blood flow changes in individual with clinical relevant BED symptomatology during food stimulation. Following overnight fasting, the obese female binge eaters had greater left prefrontal and left frontal activation than non-BED obese female subjects following exposure to freshly cooked food (without consumption). This activation was correlated with feelings of hunger. Using fMRI, Geliebter and colleagues found obese binge eaters had greater activation in premotor cortex adjacent to the oral region compare to non-obese binge eaters when viewing high-caloric food. The scans were performed after intake of a standard meal. It was suggested the activation might reflect oral movement preparation for food consumption even after the meal (Geliebter *et al.*, 2006). A recent fMRI study investigated the association between brain activitation and reward sensitivity during viewing of food pictures in non-obese female binge eaters and in non-binge eaters (Schienle *et al.*, 2009). All of the subjects experienced pleasant feelings while viewing the food pictures and activation of OFC was observed in both groups of subjects, with the BED showing greater OFC activation than non-BED. Enhanced activation in frontal and prefrontal regions, which are highly associated with DA and serotonergic innervation in the binge eaters, suggested a trait disturbance in these neurotransmitters in the etiology of BED.

The role of the serotonergic system on BED has been mainly documented in clinical and drug treatment studies (Grilo *et al.*, 2006; Capasso *et al.*, 2009). Kuikka *et al.* used SPECT and ^{123}I labeled nor-β-CIT, a radioligand that labels serotonin transporters to compare obese BED and obese non-BED control women (Kuikka *et al.*, 2001). The BED had lower serotonin transporter availability in the midbrain than did the control women. Serotonergic dysregulation was implicated in depression, and decreased serotonin transporters in the midbrain were also observed in subjects with major depression (Staley *et al.*, 1998). Similar results were reported in subjects with bulimia nervosa using SPECT and ^{123}I labeled β-CIT, which showed low levels of serotonin transporters in hypothalamus and thalamus in subjects with the longer duration of illness (Tauscher *et al.*, 2001). These imaging studies suggest serotonergic dysfunction in BED subjects may contribute to sequential periods of binge eating and depression.

Brain DA system and obesity

The involvement of DA in overeating and obesity has also been reported in rodent models of obesity (Meguid *et al.*, 2000; Hamdi *et al.*, 1992; Geiger *et al.*, 2008; Bina and Cincotta, 2000). DA plays a role in pathological feeding behavior, since low levels of DA may interfere with the drive and motivation to eat. Human genetic studies show a higher prevalence of individuals with the A1 allele of *Taq*1A (A1/A1 or A1/A2) are more likely to be obese than those without this allele (Noble *et al.*, 1991; Spitz *et al.*, 2000; Epstein *et al.*, 2007). The individuals with at least one A1 allele of *Taq*1A restriction fragment length polymorphism has been linked with lower levels of D2R (Jonsson *et al.*, 1999; Ritchie and Noble, 2003; Tupala *et al.*, 2003). Nevertheless, a SPECT study did not replicate the finding, which might imply that SPECT did not have sufficient resolution to detect the difference (Laruelle *et al.*, 1998). Variants of the human obesity gene and the D2R gene have been examined in relationship to obesity (Noble *et al.*, 1994). These two polymorphisms together account for about 20% of the variance in BMI; the association is particularly found in younger women (Comings *et al.*, 1996). The study suggested that these individuals might overeat to compensate for hypofunctioning DA system.

BED and/or obese subjects who carry the A1 allele of *Taq*1A have a relatively high degree of reward sensitivity (Davis *et al.*, 2008b). Both BED individuals and non-BED obese subjects are more reward-sensitive, have greater impulsivity and more addictive personality traits than normal body weight non-BED subjects (Davis *et al.*, 2008a). This sensitivity to reward in the obese subjects is positively related to overeating behavior and to a preference for sweet and fatty food (Davis *et al.*, 2007). It is consistent with the finding in binge eaters with frequent binge episodes who are reported to have low DA metabolite concentrations in cerebrospinal fluid (Jimerson *et al.*, 1992). A recent fMRI by Stice *et al.* (2008a) found striatal activation in response to food intake is related to body weight changes and these changes were associated with the D2R gene. Individuals with the *Taq*1A A1 allele showed less activation in striatal regions during food stimulation. These individuals also had higher BMI and were susceptible to future weight gain. These results indicated that low DA brain activity (either due to decreased DA release or to decreased stimulation of post-synaptic DA receptors) might be associated with dysfunctional eating patterns.

Molecular imaging of brain DA system on obesity

The DA system has been targeted for therapy of obesity. Treatment with DA agonists in obese rodents induced weight loss, presumably through DA D2-like and DA D1-like receptor activation (Pijl, 2003). Humans chronically treated with antipsychotic drugs (D2R antagonists) are at a greater risk of weight gain and obesity, which is mediated in part by blockade of D2R (Wise, 2006). Administration of DA agonists in obese mice normalizes their hyperphagia (Bina and Cincotta, 2000). Our PET studies with [^{11}C]raclopride have documented a reduction in striatal D2/D3 receptor availability in obese subjects (Wang *et al.*, 2001). The BMI of the obese subjects was between 42 and 60 (body weight: 274–416 lb), and their body weight remained stable prior to the study. The scans were done after subjects fasted for at least 17 h and were done under resting conditions (no stimulation, eyes open, minimal noise exposure). In obese subjects but not in controls, D2/D3 receptor availability was inversely related to BMI (Figure 34.2).

To assess whether low D2/D3 receptors in obesity reflected the consequences of food over-consumption as opposed to a vulnerability that preceded obesity, we assessed the effect of food intake on D2/D3 receptor

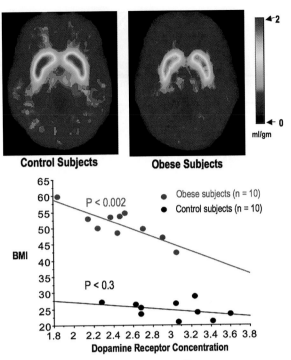

Figure 34.2 Group-averaged images of [^{11}C]raclopride PET scans for obese and control subjects at the level of the basal ganglia. The images are scaled with respect to the maximum value (distribution volume) obtained on the control subjects and presented using the rainbow scale. Red represents the highest value (2.0) and dark violet represents the lowest value (0 ml/g). The obese subjects have lower D2R availability as compared to the control subjects. Linear regression between D2R availability (Bmax/Kd) and body mass index (BMI) shows D2R availability levels were inversely related to BMI in the obese subjects but not in the control subjects. (Adapted from Wang *et al.*, 2001.)

in Zucker rats (a genetically leptin-deficient rodent model of obesity) using autoradiography (Thanos *et al.*, 2008c). The animals had free access to food for 3 months and the D2/D3 receptor levels were evaluated at 4 months of age. Results showed that Zucker obese (fa/fa) rats had lower D2/D3 receptor levels than the lean (Fa/Fa or Fa/fa) rats, and that food restriction increased D2/D3 receptors both in the lean and the obese rats, indicating that low D2/D3 reflects in part the consequences of food over-consumption. Similar to the human study, we also found an inverse correlation of D2/D3 receptor levels and body weight in these obese rats. The relationship between BMI and brain DA transporter (DAT) levels has also been investigated. Rodent studies demonstrated significant decreases in DAT densities in the striatum of obese mice (Huang *et al.*, 2006; Geiger *et al.*, 2008). In humans, a recent study using single photon emission

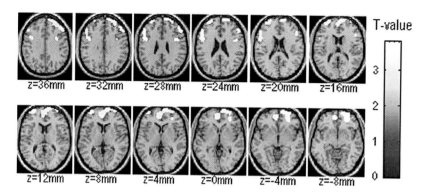

Figure 34.3 Color-coded SPM images show the areas where absolute metabolic measures are negatively associated with BMI. The brain areas that are associated with BMI are displayed in yellow and are superimposed into the brain MRI structural images (grayscale). Subjects with higher BMI have lower prefrontal metabolic measures (Adapted from Volkow et al., 2009.)

tomography (SPECT) and [^{99m}Tc] TRODAT-1 to study 50 Asians (BMI: 18.7–30.6) in resting state showed that BMI was inversely associated with striatal DAT availability (Chen et al., 2008a). These studies suggest the involvement of an understimulated DA system in excessive weight gain. Since the DA pathways have been implicated in reward (predict reward) and motivation, these studies suggest that deficiency in DA pathways may lead to pathological eating as a means to compensate for an understimulated reward system.

Inhibitory control and obesity

Impaired inhibitory control may contribute to behavioral disorders such as addiction and pathological overeating. We evaluated the responses of the brain when subjects were exposed to appealing food either with or without a prior directive to suppress the desire for food (cognitive inhibition) (Wang et al., 2009). Regional brain metabolic responses to food stimulation with and without cognitive inhibition were assessed with PET and FDG. Specifically with cognitive inhibition as compared with no inhibition male subjects (but not females) showed significant decreases in anterior cingulate gyrus, left OFC, left amygdala, right striatum. These regions, which decreased metabolism, had been shown by prior studies to be activated by food stimuli when presented via pictures, smells, taste, recall or a combination of these (Wang et al., 2004; Delamater, 2007). The suppressed activation of the OFC with inhibition was also associated with decreases in self-reports of hunger, which corroborates the involvement of this region in processing the conscious awareness of the drive to eat. This finding suggests a mechanism by which cognitive inhibition decreases the desire for food.

Individuals with dysfunction in the prefrontal cortex can have higher risk for obesity. In fact, we assessed brain glucose metabolism with PET and FDG in a group of healthy volunteer (BMI range 19–37 kg/m^2) during baseline condition (no stimulation) (Volkow et al., 2009). We found a significant negative correlation between BMI and metabolic activity in prefrontal regions, but not in other cortical or subcortical regions (Figure 34.3). The metabolism in these prefrontal regions was positively associated with performance in tests of memory and executive function. These findings suggest that the deleterious effects of excessive weight on cognitive function in healthy individuals may be mediated in part via its association with decreased activity of prefrontal regions.

There are several genes related to DA transmission that play important roles in drug reward and inhibitory control (Hurd, 2006). For example, polymorphisms in the D2 receptor gene in healthy subjects are associated with behavioral measures of inhibitory control. Individuals with the gene variant that is linked with lower D2 receptor expression had lower inhibitory control than individuals with the gene variant associated with higher D2 receptor expression (Klein et al., 2007). These behavioral responses are associated with differences in activation of the anterior cingulate gyrus and dorsolateral prefrontal cortex, which are brain regions that have been implicated in various components of inhibitory control (Dalley et al., 2004). Prefrontal regions also participate in the inhibition of tendencies for inappropriate behavioral responses (Goldstein and Volkow, 2002). The significant association between D2R availability and metabolism in prefrontal regions is observed in our studies in drug-addicted subjects (cocaine, methamphetamine and alcohol) (Volkow et al., 1993, 2001,

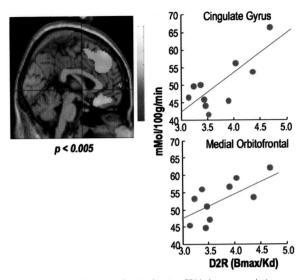

p < 0.005

Figure 34.4 Brain map obtained using SPM shows correlation between D2R availability and brain metabolism in obese subjects. The areas that metabolic measures are significantly correlated with D2R availability are displayed in orange and superimposed into a sagittal plane of brain MRI images (grayscale). The association between DA D2 receptors and metabolism in orbitofrontal cortices and cingulate gyrus suggests that D2 receptor-mediated dysregulation of regions implicated in inhibitory control may underlie the inability to control their food intake despite their conscious attempts to do so. (Adapted from Volkow et al., 2008b.)

2007). We found that the reduction in D2R availability in these subjects was associated with decreased metabolism in prefrontal cortical regions (Volkow et al., 2008b) (Figure 34.4), which are involved in regulating impulse control, self-monitoring and goal-directed behaviors (Grace et al., 2007; Brewer and Potenza, 2008). A similar observation was documented in individuals at high familial risk for alcoholism (Volkow et al., 2006). These behaviors could influence the ability of an individual to self-regulate his/her eating behavior. In fact, damage to the prefrontal cortex (i.e. Gourmand syndrome) can cause overeating and weight gain (Regard and Landis, 1997). Diffuse hypoperfusion of prefrontal cortex was identified using SPECT in overeating conditions (e.g. Kleine–Levine syndrome) (Arias et al., 2002). Previous work with PET using [^{11}C]raclopride, [^{11}C] d-threo-methylphenidate (to measure DAT availability) and FDG to evaluate the association between DA activity and brain metabolism in morbidly obese subjects (BMI > 40 kg/m^2) found that D2/D3 receptor but not DAT were associated with glucose metabolism in dorsolateral prefrontal, OFC and cingulate cortices (Volkow et al., 2008b). The findings suggested that

D2/D3 receptor-mediated dysregulation of regions implicated in inhibitory control in the obese subjects might underlie their inability to control food intake despite their conscious attempts to do so. This led us to consider the possibility that the low D2/D3 receptor modulation of the risk for overeating in the obese subjects could also be driven by its regulation of the prefrontal cortex.

Memory and obesity

The susceptibility to gain weight is in part due to the variability in individual responses to environmental triggers, such as caloric content of food. The intense desire to eat a specific food or food craving is an important factor influencing appetite control. Food craving is a learned appetite for energy through the reinforcing effects of eating a specific food when hungry (Rolls and McCabe, 2007). It is a very common event that is frequently reported across all ages. Nevertheless, food craving can also be induced by food cues and sensory stimulation regardless of the state of satiety indicating that conditioning is independent of the metabolic need for food (Fedoroff et al., 2003). Functional brain imaging studies have shown that the desire to eat a specific food was associated with activation of the hippocampus, which is likely to reflect its involvement in storing and retrieving the memories for the desired food (Pelchat et al., 2004; Thanos et al., 2008a).

The hippocampus connects with brain regions involved in satiety and hunger signals including the hypothalamus and insula. Using imaging studies with implantable gastric stimulator and balloon gastric distention methods, we showed activation of the hippocampus presumably from downstream stimulation of the vagus nerve and the solitary nucleus (Wang et al., 2006, 2008). In these studies we found that the activation of the hippocampus was associated with a sensation of fullness (Figure 34.5). The findings suggest a functional connection between the hippocampus and peripheral organs such as the stomach in the regulation of food intake. The hippocampus also modulates the saliency of stimuli through regulation of DA release in the NAcc (Berridge and Robinson, 1998), and is involved in incentive motivation (Tracy et al., 2001). It also regulates activity in prefrontal regions involved with inhibitory control (Peleg-Raibstein et al., 2005). Using imaging methodology, Del Parigi et al. showed that tasting a liquid meal

499

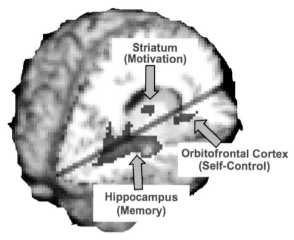

Figure 34.5 Brain scans in obese subjects reveal higher metabolism in brain reward pathways when a "stomach stimulator" is turned on to simulate fullness vs. off. The 3D rendered SPM images show the areas with higher metabolism when the "stomach stimulator" is turned on. The areas that are significantly higher are displayed in red and are superimposed into 3D reconstructed brain MRI images (grayscale). (Adapted from Wang et al., 2006.)

resulted in decreased activity in the posterior hippocampus in obese and previously obese but not in lean subjects. Persistence of abnormal neuronal response in the hippocampus in the previously obese was associated with their susceptibility to relapse. These findings implicate the hippocampus in the neurobiology of obesity (Del Parigi et al., 2004). Obese subjects are reported to crave energy-dense foods that make them susceptible to gain weight (Gilhooly et al., 2007).

Application of brain imaging to drug discovery and treatment of obesity

There are a number of targets for drug therapies of obesity. Many small molecules and peptides that target the hypothalamus have been reported to increase satiety, reduce food intake and balance energy homeostasis in rodent models (Harrold and Halford, 2006; Aronne and Thornton-Jones, 2007). However, some of these molecules when tested on clinical trials failed to show meaningful weight loss (Erondu et al., 2007). Functional neuroimaging techniques play a role in assessing the efficacy of the medication when the human subjects are in conditioned food stimulation or in predicting the efficacy of the medication in satiated state. For example:

(1) Leptin showed promising results for the treatment of animal and human subjects with leptin

deficiency. Nevertheless, most of the obese human subjects have high leptin levels and not leptin deficiency. Leptin as an anti-obesity treatment agent was called into question. However, recent studies showed that low doses of leptin when given after weight loss in obese subjects could restore energy expenditures (i.e. increasing skeletal muscle work efficiency, sympathetic nervous system tone, thyroid function) and help maintain the reduction in body weight (Rosenbaum et al., 2005).

An imaging study with fMRI-BOLD was used to assess the brain responses to visual food stimulation under different weight conditions and leptin levels (i.e. usual weight, 10% weight reduction and after leptin treatment) in obese subjects (Rosenbaum et al., 2008). At the initial weight, visual food stimuli increased activity in brain regions involved in energy homeostasis and emotional memory of food intake (i.e. hypothalamus, amygdala, hippocampus, parahippocampus, cingulate gyrus, frontal and parietal cortices). The weight reduction state was associated with increased activity in the brain stem, parahippocampus, putamen as well as frontal and temporal regions, which involved in motivation and decision-making functions. The leptin treatment reversed the brain activation to the pattern in the initial weight state. This finding suggests that leptin modulates the reward and executive control responses to visual food stimuli, and that the replacement of leptin can facilitate the maintenance of weight loss. These results also suggest that some obese individuals with relatively lower leptin levels might benefit from leptin replacement therapy.

(2) Peptide YY_{3-36} (PYY), a physiological gut-derived satiety signaling peptide, has shown promising results in increasing satiety and reducing food intake in humans (Batterham et al., 2003). An fMRI study was used to assess the mechanism of PYY in modulating neural activity related to hedonic, cognitive and homeostatic pathways in human subjects and to predict the efficacy of PYY in inducing satiety. In this study, the fasting participants were infused with PYY or saline during 90 min of fMRI scanning (Batterham et al., 2007). The fMRI signal changes in the hypothalamus and OFC extracted from time series data were compared with subsequent caloric intake for each subject on the PYY and saline

days. On the saline day when the subjects were fasted and had lower plasma levels of PYY, the change in the hypothalamus correlated with subsequent caloric intake. In contrast, on the PYY day when high plasma levels of PYY mimicked the fed state, the changes in the OFC predicted caloric intake independently of meal-related sensory experience, whereas hypothalamic signal changes did not. Thus functional imaging studies provide a tool to assess the efficacy of the medication in the fasted and fed states. In this case, eating behaviors could be easily switched from a homeostatic state to an hedonic corticolimbic state by treatment with PPY alone. Therefore the strategy to treat obesity should also include agents that modulate the hedonic state of food intake.

Concluding remarks

Obesity reflects an imbalance between energy intake and expenditure that is mediated by the interaction of energy homeostasis and hedonic food intake behavior. Brain imaging studies show that obese individuals have significant deficits in regulation of energy homeostasis (i.e. delayed response to peripheral metabolic signals in the hypothalamus) and circuits that regulate abnormal eating behavior (i.e. motivation, reward, emotion, learning, memory and inhibitory control). These brain imaging studies have the potential to facilitate understanding the mechanisms underlying obesity and overeating behaviors and provide scientific bases for the assessment of the efficacy of drug treatments and for the development of novel pharmacological approaches. A key limitation to progress in this area is that a core pathophysiological abnormality that underlies obesity has yet to be identified. However, overeating behaviors and obesity are likely heterogeneous disorders (Hainer et al., 2008). Therefore, future brain imaging studies might be applied to investigate the interaction between peripheral signals and hedonic pathways, as well as to assess the efficacy of drug treatments, surgical therapy and lifestyle changes (e.g. diet control and aerobic exercise). In addition to PYY and leptin, several peptides (e.g. GLP-1) as well as medications with DA properties (DA reuptake inhibitors, e.g. Bupropion), opioid antagonists (e.g. Naltrexone) or combination of other drugs that modulate DA and GABA activity (e.g. Zonisamide, Topiramate) have been reported to promote weight loss in obese subjects (Gadde et al., 2003, 2007; Stenlof et al., 2007; Bessesen, 2008; Aronne and Thornton-Jones, 2007). The efficacy and mechanisms of these medications can be assessed by functional neuroimaging techniques. Future progress will also require the development of better neuroimaging methods and a wider variety of radiotracers to image the growing number of molecular targets that have been implicated in obesity and other eating disorders (Aronne and Thornton-Jones, 2007).

Acknowledgments

This study was supported in part by grants from the US Department of Energy OBER (DE-ACO2–76CH00016), National Institute on Drug Abuse (RO1DA06891, RO1DA6278 & R21DA018457), National Institute on Mental Health (RO1MH66961), National Institute on Alcohol Abuse and Alcoholism (RO1AA9481 and Y1AA3009) and by the GCRC at University Hospital Stony Brook (NIH MO1RR010710). The authors also thank the scientific and technical staffs at the Brookhaven Center for Translational Neuroimaging for their support of these research studies as well as the individuals who volunteered for these studies.

> **Box 34.1.** Most significant findings of functional neuroimaging studies in obesity and overeating behavior
>
> - Peripheral metabolic signals in obese individuals
>   Delayed response to glucose in the hypothalamus.
>   Reduced postprandial peptide YY release and exhibited lower satiety.
>   Failure to decrease ghrelin after a meal.
>   Decreased leptin levels in weight-reduced state could promote weight gain.
> - Brain dopamine pathway and overeating behavior
>   Consumption of a favorite food induced dopamine release in the striatum.
>   Exposure to food-cues induced striatal dopamine release and increased orbitofrontal metabolism, which has a downstream dopaminergic effect.
>   Obese individuals had a reduction in striatal D2/D3 receptor availability.
> - Prefrontal function and overeating behavior
>   In non-obese individuals during a food cue, cognitive inhibition could decrease activity in prefrontal and in orbitofrontal cortices.
>   Greater body mass index was correlated with decreased prefrontal activity.

In obese individuals, decreases in striatal D2/D3 receptor availability were associated with decreases in prefrontal metabolic activity.

- Memory and overeating behavior
  Desire to eat a specific food was associated with activation of the hippocampus.

  Activation of the hippocampus was associated with a sensation of fullness.

  Obese and previously obese individuals decreased activity in the posterior hippocampus when tasting a liquid meal.

References

Abizaid A, Liu Z W, Andrews Z B, *et al.* 2006. Ghrelin modulates the activity and synaptic input organization of midbrain dopamine neurons while promoting appetite. *J Clin Invest* **116**, 3229–39.

Adam T C and Epel E S. 2007. Stress, eating and the reward system. *Physiol Behav* **91**, 449–58.

Ahima R S and Lazar M A. 2008. Adipokines and the peripheral and neural control of energy balance. *Mol Endocrinol* **22**, 1023–31.

Ahima R S, Prabakaran D, Mantzoros C, *et al.* 1996. Role of leptin in the neuroendocrine response to fasting. *Nature* **382**, 250–2.

American Psychiatric Association. 1994. *Diagnostic and Statistical Manual of Mental Disorders, 4th Edition.* Washington, DC: American Psychatric Association, 729–31.

Andreoli M, Tessari M, Pilla M, Valerio E, Hagan J J and Heidbreder C A. 2003. Selective antagonism at dopamine D3 receptors prevents nicotine-triggered relapse to nicotine-seeking behavior. *Neuropsychopharmacology* **28**, 1272–80.

Anthony K, Reed L J, Dunn J T, *et al.* 2006. Attenuation of insulin-evoked responses in brain networks controlling appetite and reward in insulin resistance: The cerebral basis for impaired control of food intake in metabolic syndrome? *Diabetes* **55**, 2986–92.

Arias M, Crespo Iglesias J M, Perez J, Requena-Caballero I, Sesar-Ignacio A and Peleteiro-Fernandez M. 2002. Kleine–Levin syndrome: Contribution of brain SPECT in diagnosis. *Rev Neurol* **35**, 531–3.

Aronne L J and Thornton-Jones Z D. 2007. New targets for obesity pharmacotherapy. *Clin Pharmacol Ther* **81**, 748–52.

Avena N M, Rada P and Hoebel B G. 2008. Evidence for sugar addiction: Behavioral and neurochemical effects of intermittent, excessive sugar intake. *Neurosci Biobehav Rev* **32**, 20–39.

Avena N M, Rada P, Moise N and Hoebel B G. 2006. Sucrose sham feeding on a binge schedule releases accumbens dopamine repeatedly and eliminates the acetylcholine satiety response. *Neuroscience* **139**, 813–20.

Baicy K, London E D, Monterosso J, *et al.* 2007. Leptin replacement alters brain response to food cues in genetically leptin-deficient adults. *Proc Natl Acad Sci U S A* **104**, 18 276–9.

Baldo B A and Kelley A E. 2007. Discrete neurochemical coding of distinguishable motivational processes: Insights from nucleus accumbens control of feeding. *Psychopharmacology (Berl)* **191**, 439–59.

Banks W A. 2008. The blood–brain barrier as a cause of obesity. *Curr Pharm Des* **14**, 1606–14.

Batterham R L, Cohen M A, Ellis S M, *et al.* 2003. Inhibition of food intake in obese subjects by peptide YY3–36. *N Engl J Med* **349**, 941–8.

Batterham R L, Ffytche D H, Rosenthal J M, *et al.* 2007. PYY modulation of cortical and hypothalamic brain areas predicts feeding behaviour in humans. *Nature* **450**, 106–09.

Berridge K C and Robinson T E. 1998. What is the role of dopamine in reward: Hedonic impact, reward learning, or incentive salience? *Brain Res Rev* **28**, 309–69.

Berthoud H R. 2008. Vagal and hormonal gut–brain communication: From satiation to satisfaction. *Neurogastroenterol Motil* **20** (Suppl 1), 64–72.

Bessesen D H. 2008. Update on obesity. *J Clin Endocrinol Metab* **93**, 2027–34.

Bina K G and Cincotta A H. 2000. Dopaminergic agonists normalize elevated hypothalamic neuropeptide Y and corticotropin-releasing hormone, body weight gain, and hyperglycemia in ob/ob mice. *Neuroendocrinology* **71**, 68–78.

Blackburn J R, Phillips A G, Jakubovic A and Fibiger H C. 1989. Dopamine and preparatory behavior: II. A neurochemical analysis. *Behav Neurosci* **103**, 15–23.

Brewer J A and Potenza M N. 2008. The neurobiology and genetics of impulse control disorders: Relationships to drug addictions. *Biochem Pharmacol* **75**, 63–75.

Brody S, Keller U, Degen L, Cox D J and Schachinger H. 2004. Selective processing of food words during insulin-induced hypoglycemia in healthy humans. *Psychopharmacology (Berl)* **173**, 217–20.

Bruning J C, Gautam D, Burks D J, *et al.* 2000. Role of brain insulin receptor in control of body weight and reproduction. *Science* **289**, 2122–5.

Burgmer R, Grigutsch K, Zipfel S, *et al.* 2005. The influence of eating behavior and eating pathology on weight loss after gastric restriction operations. *Obes Surg* **15**, 684–91.

Burton P, Smit H J and Lightowler H J. 2007. The influence of restrained and external eating patterns on overeating. *Appetite* **49**, 191–7.

Cameron J D, Goldfield G S, Cyr M J and Doucet E. 2008. The effects of prolonged caloric restriction leading to weight-loss on food hedonics and reinforcement. *Physiol Behav* **94**, 474–80.

Capasso A, Petrella C and Milano W. 2009. Pharmacological profile of SSRIs and SNRIs in the treatment of eating disorders. *Curr Clin Pharmacol* **4**, 78–83.

Carr K D. 2002. Augmentation of drug reward by chronic food restriction: Behavioral evidence and underlying mechanisms. *Physiol Behav* **76**, 353–64.

Carr K D. 2007. Chronic food restriction: Enhancing effects on drug reward and striatal cell signaling. *Physiol Behav* **91**, 459–72.

Catalano P M and Ehrenberg H M. 2006. The short- and long-term implications of maternal obesity on the mother and her offspring. *Br J Obstet Gynaecol* **113**, 1126–33.

Cervo L, Cocco A, Petrella C and Heidbreder C A. 2007. Selective antagonism at dopamine D3 receptors attenuates cocaine-seeking behaviour in the rat. *Int J Neuropsychopharmacol* **10**, 167–81.

Chechlacz M, Rotshtein P, Klamer S, *et al.* 2009. Diabetes dietary management alters responses to food pictures in brain regions associated with motivation and emotion: a functional magnetic resonance imaging study. *Diabetologia* **52**, 524–33.

Chen P S, Yang Y K, Yeh T L, *et al.* 2008a. Correlation between body mass index and striatal dopamine transporter availability in healthy volunteers – A SPECT study. *Neuroimage* **40**, 275–9.

Chen Y I, Ren J, Wang F N, *et al.* 2008b. Inhibition of stimulated dopamine release and hemodynamic response in the brain through electrical stimulation of rat forepaw. *Neurosci Lett* **431**, 231–5.

Colles S L, Dixon J B and O'Brien P E. 2008. Grazing and loss of control related to eating: Two high-risk factors following bariatric surgery. *Obesity (Silver Spring)* **16**, 615–22.

Comings D E, Gade R, MacMurray J P, Muhleman D and Peters W R. 1996. Genetic variants of the human obesity (OB) gene: Association with body mass index in young women, psychiatric symptoms, and interaction with the dopamine D2 receptor (DRD2) gene. *Mol Psychiatry* **1**, 325–35.

Cooper S J and Al-Naser H A. 2006. Dopaminergic control of food choice: contrasting effects of SKF 38393 and quinpirole on high-palatability food preference in the rat. *Neuropharmacology* **50**, 953–63.

Cox S M, Andrade A and Johnsrude I S. 2005. Learning to like: A role for human orbitofrontal cortex in conditioned reward. *J Neurosci* **25**, 2733–40.

Craig A D. 2003. Interoception: The sense of the physiological condition of the body. *Curr Opin Neurobiol* **13**, 500–05.

Cummings D E and Overduin J. 2007. Gastrointestinal regulation of food intake. *J Clin Invest* **117**, 13–23.

Dalley J W, Cardinal R N and Robbins T W. 2004. Prefrontal executive and cognitive functions in rodents: Neural and neurochemical substrates. *Neurosci Biobehav Rev* **28**, 771–84.

Dallman M F, Pecoraro N, Akana S F, *et al.* 2003. Chronic stress and obesity: A new view of "comfort food". *Proc Natl Acad Sci U S A* **100**, 11 696–701.

Davis C, Levitan R D, Carter J, *et al.* 2008a. Personality and eating behaviors: A case-control study of binge eating disorder. *Int J Eat Disord* **41**, 243–50.

Davis C, Levitan R D, Kaplan A S, *et al.* 2008b. Reward sensitivity and the D2 dopamine receptor gene: A case-control study of binge eating disorder. *Prog Neuropsychopharmacol Biol Psychiatry* **32**, 620–8.

Davis C, Patte K, Levitan R, Reid C, Tweed S and Curtis C. 2007. From motivation to behaviour: A model of reward sensitivity, overeating, and food preferences in the risk profile for obesity. *Appetite* **48**, 12–9.

Delamater A R. 2007. The role of the orbitofrontal cortex in sensory-specific encoding of associations in pavlovian and instrumental conditioning. *Ann N Y Acad Sci* **1121**, 152–73.

Del Parigi A, Chen K, Salbe A D, *et al.* 2002. Tasting a liquid meal after a prolonged fast is associated with preferential activation of the left hemisphere. *Neuroreport* **13**, 1141–5.

Del Parigi A, Chen K, Salbe A D, *et al.* 2004. Persistence of abnormal neural responses to a meal in postobese individuals. *Int J Obes Relat Metab Disord* **28**, 370–7.

Del Parigi A, Chen K, Salbe A D, Reiman E M and Tataranni P A. 2005. Sensory experience of food and obesity: a positron emission tomography study of the brain regions affected by tasting a liquid meal after a prolonged fast. *Neuroimage*, **24**, 436–43.

Di Chiara G and Bassareo V. 2007. Reward system and addiction: What dopamine does and doesn't do. *Curr Opin Pharmacol* **7**, 69–76.

Duong T, Yacoub E, Adriany G, Hu X, Ugurbil K and Kim S. 2003. Microvascular BOLD contribution at 4 and 7 T in the human brain: Gradient-echo and spin-echo fMRI with suppression of blood effects. *Magn Res Med* **49**, 1019–27.

Dymek-Valentine M, Rienecke-Hoste R and Alverdy J. 2004. Assessment of binge eating disorder in morbidly obese patients evaluated for gastric bypass: SCID versus QEWP-R. *Eat Weight Disord* **9**, 211–6.

Epstein L H, Temple J L, Neaderhiser B J, Salis R J, Erbe R W and Leddy J J. 2007. Food reinforcement, the dopamine D2 receptor genotype, and energy intake in obese and nonobese humans. *Behav Neurosci* **121**, 877–86.

503

Epstein L H, Wright S M, Paluch R A, *et al*. 2004. Food hedonics and reinforcement as determinants of laboratory food intake in smokers. *Physiol Behav* **81**, 511–7.

Erondu N, Addy C, Lu K, *et al*. 2007. NPY5R antagonism does not augment the weight loss efficacy of orlistat or sibutramine. *Obesity (Silver Spring)* **15**, 2027–42.

Fallon S, Shearman E, Sershen H and Lajtha A. 2007. Food reward-induced neurotransmitter changes in cognitive brain regions. *Neurochem Res* **32**, 1772–82.

Farooqi I S, Bullmore E, Keogh J, Gillard J, O'Rahilly S and Fletcher P C. 2007. Leptin regulates striatal regions and human eating behavior. *Science* **317**, 1355.

Fedoroff I, Polivy J and Herman C P. 2003. The specificity of restrained versus unrestrained eaters' responses to food cues: General desire to eat, or craving for the cued food? *Appetite* **41**, 7–13.

Fenu S, Bassareo V and Di Chiara G. 2001. A role for dopamine D1 receptors of the nucleus accumbens shell in conditioned taste aversion learning. *J Neurosci* **21**, 6897–904.

Figlewicz D P, Bennett J L, Naleid A M, Davis C and Grimm J W. 2006. Intraventricular insulin and leptin decrease sucrose self-administration in rats. *Physiol Behav* **89**, 611–6.

Fiorino D F, Coury A, Fibiger H C and Phillips A G. 1993. Electrical stimulation of reward sites in the ventral tegmental area increases dopamine transmission in the nucleus accumbens of the rat. *Behav Brain Res* **55**, 131–41.

Frank G K, Oberndorfer T A, Simmons A N, *et al*. 2008. Sucrose activates human taste pathways differently from artificial sweetener. *Neuroimage* **39**, 1559–69.

Gadde K M, Franciscy D M, Wagner H R 2nd and Krishnan K R. 2003. Zonisamide for weight loss in obese adults: A randomized controlled trial. *JAMA* **289**, 1820–5.

Gadde K M, Yonish G M, Foust M S and Wagner H R. 2007. Combination therapy of zonisamide and bupropion for weight reduction in obese women: A preliminary, randomized, open-label study. *J Clin Psychiatry* **68**, 1226–9.

Gallagher M, McMahan R W and Schoenbaum G. 1999. Orbitofrontal cortex and representation of incentive value in associative learning. *J Neurosci* **19**, 6610–4.

Gallou-Kabani C and Junien C. 2005. Nutritional epigenomics of metabolic syndrome: New perspective against the epidemic. *Diabetes* **54**, 1899–906.

Geiger B M, Behr G G, Frank L E, *et al*. 2008. Evidence for defective mesolimbic dopamine exocytosis in obesity-prone rats. *Faseb J* **22**, 2740–6.

Geliebter A, Ladell T, Logan M, Schneider T, Sharafi M and Hirsch J. 2006. Responsivity to food stimuli in obese and lean binge eaters using functional MRI. *Appetite* **46**, 31–5.

Gilhooly C H, Das S K, Golden J K, *et al*. 2007. Food cravings and energy regulation: The characteristics of craved foods and their relationship with eating behaviors and weight change during 6 months of dietary energy restriction. *Int J Obes (Lond)* **31**, 1849–58.

Goldfein J A, Walsh B T, Lachaussee J L, Kissileff H R and Devlin M J. 1993. Eating behavior in binge eating disorder. *Int J Eat Disord* **14**, 427–31.

Goldstein R Z and Volkow N D. 2002. Drug addiction and its underlying neurobiological basis: Neuroimaging evidence for the involvement of the frontal cortex. *Am J Psychiatry* **159**, 1642–52.

Grabenhorst F, Rolls E T and Bilderbeck A. 2008. How cognition modulates affective responses to taste and flavor: Top-down influences on the orbitofrontal and pregenual cingulate cortices. *Cereb Cortex* **18**, 1549–59.

Grace A A, Floresco S B, Goto Y and Lodge D J. 2007. Regulation of firing of dopaminergic neurons and control of goal-directed behaviors. *Trends Neurosci* **30**, 220–7.

Grilo C M, Masheb R M and Wilson G T. 2006. Rapid response to treatment for binge eating disorder. *J Consult Clin Psychol* **74**, 602–13.

Hainer V, Toplak H and Mitrakou A. 2008. Treatment modalities of obesity: What fits whom? *Diabetes Care* **31** (Suppl 2), S269–77.

Hajnal A and Norgren R. 2005. Taste pathways that mediate accumbens dopamine release by sapid sucrose. *Physiol Behav* **84**, 363–9.

Hajnal A, Smith G P and Norgren R. 2004. Oral sucrose stimulation increases accumbens dopamine in the rat. *Am J Physiol Regul Integr Comp Physiol* **286**, R31–7.

Hamdi A, Porter J and Prasad C. 1992. Decreased striatal D2 dopamine receptors in obese Zucker rats: Changes during aging. *Brain Res* **589**, 338–40.

Harrold J A and Halford J C. 2006. The hypothalamus and obesity. *Recent Patents CNS Drug Discov* **1**, 305–14.

Heidbreder C A, Gardner E L, Xi Z X, *et al*. 2005. The role of central dopamine D3 receptors in drug addiction: A review of pharmacological evidence. *Brain Res Brain Res Rev* **49**, 77–105.

Hocke C, Prante O, Salama I, *et al*. 2008. 18F-Labeled FAUC 346 and BP 897 derivatives as subtype-selective potential PET radioligands for the dopamine D3 receptor. *Chem Med Chem* **3**, 788–93.

Hollander J A, Lu Q, Cameron M D, Kamenecka T M and Kenny P J. 2008. Insular hypocretin transmission regulates nicotine reward. *Proc Natl Acad Sci U S A* **105**, 19 480–5.

Huang X F, Yu Y, Zavitsanou K, Han M and Storlien L. 2005. Differential expression of dopamine D2 and

D4 receptor and tyrosine hydroxylase mRNA in mice prone, or resistant, to chronic high-fat diet-induced obesity. *Brain Res Mol Brain Res* **135**, 150–61.

Huang X F, Zavitsanou K, Huang X, *et al.* 2006. Dopamine transporter and D2 receptor binding densities in mice prone or resistant to chronic high fat diet-induced obesity. *Behav Brain Res* **175**, 415–9.

Hurd Y L. 2006. Perspectives on current directions in the neurobiology of addiction disorders relevant to genetic risk factors. *CNS Spectr* **11**, 855–62.

Huttunen J, Kahkonen S, Kaakkola S, Ahveninen J and Pekkonen E. 2003. Effects of an acute D2-dopaminergic blockade on the somatosensory cortical responses in healthy humans: Evidence from evoked magnetic fields. *Neuroreport* **14**, 1609–12.

Jimerson D C, Lesem M D, Kaye W H and Brewerton T D. 1992. Low serotonin and dopamine metabolite concentrations in cerebrospinal fluid from bulimic patients with frequent binge episodes. *Arch Gen Psychiatry* **49**, 132–8.

Jonsson E G, Nothen M M, Grunhage F, *et al.* 1999. Polymorphisms in the dopamine D2 receptor gene and their relationships to striatal dopamine receptor density of healthy volunteers. *Mol Psychiatry* **4**, 290–6.

Karhunen L J, Vanninen E J, Kuikka J T, Lappalainen R I, Tiihonen J and Uusitupa M I. 2000. Regional cerebral blood flow during exposure to food in obese binge eating women. *Psychiatry Res* **99**, 29–42.

Karra E, Chandarana K and Batterham R L. 2009. The role of peptide YY in appetite regulation and obesity. *J Physiol* **587**, 19–25.

Kelley A E, Baldo B A, Pratt W E and Will M J. 2005. Corticostriatal-hypothalamic circuitry and food motivation: Integration of energy, action and reward. *Physiol Behav* **86**, 773–95.

Killgore W D, Young A D, Femia L A, Bogorodzki P, Rogowska J and Yurgelun-Todd D A. 2003. Cortical and limbic activation during viewing of high- versus low-calorie foods. *Neuroimage* **19**, 1381–94.

Kim S G, Ashe J, Hendrich K, *et al.* 1993. Functional magnetic resonance imaging of motor cortex: Hemispheric asymmetry and handedness. *Science* **261**, 615–7.

King B M. 2006. The rise, fall, and resurrection of the ventromedial hypothalamus in the regulation of feeding behavior and body weight. *Physiol Behav* **87**, 221–44.

Kiyatkin E A and Gratton A. 1994. Electrochemical monitoring of extracellular dopamine in nucleus accumbens of rats lever-pressing for food. *Brain Res* **652**, 225–34.

Klein T A, Neumann J, Reuter M, Hennig J, Von Cramon D Y and Ullsperger M. 2007. Genetically determined differences in learning from errors. *Science* **318**, 1642–5.

Kuikka J T, Tammela L, Karhunen L, *et al.* 2001. Reduced serotonin transporter binding in binge eating women. *Psychopharmacology (Berl)* **155**, 310–4.

Kuo M F, Paulus W and Nitsche M A. 2008. Boosting focally-induced brain plasticity by dopamine. *Cereb Cortex* **18**, 648–51.

Laruelle M, Gelernter J and Innis R B. 1998. D2 receptors binding potential is not affected by Taq1 polymorphism at the D2 receptor gene. *Mol Psychiatry* **3**, 261–5.

Leibowitz S F and Alexander J T. 1998. Hypothalamic serotonin in control of eating behavior, meal size, and body weight. *Biol Psychiatry* **44**, 851–64.

Liang N C, Hajnal A and Norgren R. 2006. Sham feeding corn oil increases accumbens dopamine in the rat. *Am J Physiol Regul Integr Comp Physiol* **291**, R1236–9.

Liu Y, Gao J H, Liu H L and Fox P T. 2000. The temporal response of the brain after eating revealed by functional MRI. *Nature* **405**, 1058–62.

Lustig R H. 2006. Childhood obesity: behavioral aberration or biochemical drive? Reinterpreting the First Law of Thermodynamics. *Nat Clin Pract Endocrinol Metab* **2**, 447–58.

Machado C J and Bachevalier J. 2007. The effects of selective amygdala, orbital frontal cortex or hippocampal formation lesions on reward assessment in nonhuman primates. *Eur J Neurosci* **25**, 2885–904.

Malik S, McGlone F, Bedrossian D and Dagher A. 2008. Ghrelin modulates brain activity in areas that control appetitive behavior. *Cell Metab* **7**, 400–9.

Matsuda M, Liu Y, Mahankali S, *et al.* 1999. Altered hypothalamic function in response to glucose ingestion in obese humans. *Diabetes* **48**, 1801–6.

McFarland K and Ettenberg A. 1998. Haloperidol does not affect motivational processes in an operant runway model of food-seeking behavior. *Behav Neurosci* **112**, 630–5.

Meguid M M, Fetissov S O, Blaha V and Yang Z J. 2000. Dopamine and serotonin VMN release is related to feeding status in obese and lean Zucker rats. *Neuroreport* **11**, 2069–72.

Menon R. 2002. Postacquisition suppression of large-vessel BOLD signals in high-resolution fMRI. *Magn Res Med* **47**, 1–9.

Mietus-Snyder M L and Lustig R H. 2008. Childhood obesity: Adrift in the "limbic triangle". *Annu Rev Med* **59**, 147–62.

Missale C, Nash S R, Robinson S W, Jaber M and Caron M G. 1998. Dopamine receptors: From structure to function. *Physiol Rev* **78**, 189–225.

Morrison C D. 2008. Leptin resistance and the response to positive energy balance. *Physiol Behav* **94**, 660–3.

Morrison C D and Berthoud H R. 2007. Neurobiology of nutrition and obesity. *Nutr Rev* **65**, 517–34.

Morton G J, Cummings D E, Baskin D G, Barsh G S and Schwartz M W. 2006. Central nervous system control of food intake and body weight. *Nature* **443**, 289–95.

Mrzljak L, Bergson C, Pappy M, Huff R, Levenson R and Goldman-Rakic P S. 1996. Localization of dopamine D4 receptors in GABAergic neurons of the primate brain. *Nature* **381**, 245–8.

Myers M G, Cowley M A and Munzberg H. 2008. Mechanisms of leptin action and leptin resistance. *Annu Rev Physiol* **70**, 537–56.

Naqvi N H, Rudrauf D, Damasio H and Bechara A. 2007. Damage to the insula disrupts addiction to cigarette smoking. *Science* **315**, 531–4.

Narendran R, Slifstein M, Guillin O, et al. 2006. Dopamine (D2/3) receptor agonist positron emission tomography radiotracer [11C]-(+)-PHNO is a D3 receptor preferring agonist in vivo. *Synapse* **60**, 485–95.

Niego S H, Kofman M D, Weiss J J and Geliebter A. 2007. Binge eating in the bariatric surgery population: A review of the literature. *Int J Eat Disord* **40**, 349–59.

Noble E P, Blum K, Ritchie T, Montgomery A and Sheridan P J. 1991. Allelic association of the D2 dopamine receptor gene with receptor-binding characteristics in alcoholism. *Arch Gen Psychiatry* **48**, 648–54.

Noble E P, Noble R E, Ritchie T, et al. 1994. D2 dopamine receptor gene and obesity. *Int J Eat Disord* **15**, 205–17.

Oak J N, Oldenhof J and Van Tol H H. 2000. The dopamine D(4) receptor: One decade of research. *Eur J Pharmacol* **405**, 303–27.

Ogawa S, Lee T M, Kay A R and Tank D W. 1990. Brain magnetic resonance imaging with contrast dependent on blood oxygenation. *Proc Natl Acad Sci U S A* **87**, 9868–72.

Ogawa S, Menon R S, Tank D W, et al. 1993. Functional brain mapping by blood oxygenation level-dependent contrast magnetic resonance imaging. A comparison of signal characteristics with a biophysical model. *Biophys J* **64**, 803–12.

Ogden C L, Carroll M D, Curtin L R, et al. 2006. Prevalence of overweight and obesity in the United States, 1999–2004. *JAMA* **295**, 1549–55.

Ogden C L, Carroll M D and Flegal K M. 2008. High body mass index for age among US children and adolescents, 2003–2006. *JAMA* **299**, 2401–5.

Ogden C L, Carroll M D, McDowell M A and Flegal K M. 2007a. Obesity among adults in the United States – No change since 2003–2004. *NCHS Data Brief No 1*. Hyattsville, MD: National Center for Health Statistics.

Ogden C L, Yanovski S Z, Carroll M D and Flegal K M. 2007b. The epidemiology of obesity. *Gastroenterology* **132**, 2087–102.

Ogden J and Wardle J. 1990. Cognitive restraint and sensitivity to cues for hunger and satiety. *Physiol Behav* **47**, 477–81.

Palmiter R D. 2007. Is dopamine a physiologically relevant mediator of feeding behavior? *Trends Neurosci* **30**, 375–81.

Palmiter R D. 2008. Dopamine signaling in the dorsal striatum is essential for motivated behaviors: Lessons from dopamine-deficient mice. *Ann N Y Acad Sci* **1129**, 35–46.

Parkinson J R, Chaudhri O B, Kuo Y T, et al. 2009. Differential patterns of neuronal activation in the brainstem and hypothalamus following peripheral injection of GLP-1, oxyntomodulin and lithium chloride in mice detected by manganese-enhanced magnetic resonance imaging (MEMRI). *Neuroimage* **44**, 1022–31.

Passamonti L, Rowe J B, Schwarzbauer C, Ewbank M P, Von Dem Hagen E and Calder A J. 2009. Personality predicts the brain's response to viewing appetizing foods: The neural basis of a risk factor for overeating. *J Neurosci* **29**, 43–51.

Pelchat M L, Johnson A, Chan R, Valdez J and Ragland J D. 2004. Images of desire: Food-craving activation during fMRI. *Neuroimage* **23**, 1486–93.

Peleg-Raibstein D, Pezze M A, Ferger B, et al. 2005. Activation of dopaminergic neurotransmission in the medial prefrontal cortex by N-methyl-D-aspartate stimulation of the ventral hippocampus in rats. *Neuroscience* **132**, 219–32.

Petrovich G D and Gallagher M. 2003. Amygdala subsystems and control of feeding behavior by learned cues. *Ann N Y Acad Sci* **985**, 251–62.

Pfaffly J, Michaelides M, Wang G J, Pessin J E, Volkow N D and Thanos P K. 2010. Leptin increases striatal dopamine D2 receptor (D2R) binding in leptin-deficient obese (ob/ob) mice. *Synapse* **64**, 503–10.

Pijl H. 2003. Reduced dopaminergic tone in hypothalamic neural circuits: expression of a "thrifty" genotype underlying the metabolic syndrome? *Eur J Pharmacol* **480**, 125–31.

Prante O, Tietze R, Hocke C, et al. 2008. Synthesis, radiofluorination, and in vitro evaluation of pyrazolo [1,5-a]pyridine-based dopamine D4 receptor ligands: Discovery of an inverse agonist radioligand for PET. *J Med Chem* **51**, 1800–10.

Rada P, Avena N M and Hoebel B G. 2005. Daily bingeing on sugar repeatedly releases dopamine in the accumbens shell. *Neuroscience* **134**, 737–44.

Regard M and Landis T. 1997. "Gourmand syndrome": Eating passion associated with right anterior lesions. *Neurology* **48**, 1185–90.

Ren X, Zhou L, Terwilliger R, Newton S S and De Araujo I E. 2009. Sweet taste signaling functions as a hypothalamic glucose sensor. *Front Integr Neurosci* **3**, 12.

Ritchie T and Noble E P. 2003. Association of seven polymorphisms of the D2 dopamine receptor gene with brain receptor-binding characteristics. *Neurochem Res* **28**, 73–82.

Rivera A, Cuellar B, Giron F J, Grandy D K, De la Calle A and Moratalla R. 2002. Dopamine D4 receptors are heterogeneously distributed in the striosomes/matrix compartments of the striatum. *J Neurochem* **80**, 219–29.

Robinson S, Rainwater A J, Hnasko T S and Palmiter R D. 2007. Viral restoration of dopamine signaling to the dorsal striatum restores instrumental conditioning to dopamine-deficient mice. *Psychopharmacology (Berl)* **191**, 567–78.

Rolls E T. 2007. Sensory processing in the brain related to the control of food intake. *Proc Nutr Soc* **66**, 96–112.

Rolls E T and McCabe, C. 2007. Enhanced affective brain representations of chocolate in cravers vs. non-cravers. *Eur J Neurosci* **26**, 1067–76.

Rosenbaum M, Goldsmith R, Bloomfield D, et al. 2005. Low-dose leptin reverses skeletal muscle, autonomic, and neuroendocrine adaptations to maintenance of reduced weight. *J Clin Invest* **115**, 3579–86.

Rosenbaum M, Sy M, Pavlovich K, Leibel R L and Hirsch J. 2008. Leptin reverses weight loss-induced changes in regional neural activity responses to visual food stimuli. *J Clin Invest* **118**, 2583–91.

Ross M G and Desai M. 2005. Gestational programming: Population survival effects of drought and famine during pregnancy. *Am J Physiol Regul Integr Comp Physiol* **288**, R25–33.

Rossini P M, Bassetti M A and Pasqualetti P. 1995. Median nerve somatosensory evoked potentials. Apomorphine-induced transient potentiation of frontal components in Parkinson's disease and in parkinsonism. *Electroencephalogr Clin Neurophysiol* **96**, 236–47.

Rotte M, Baerecke C, Pottag G, et al. 2005. Insulin affects the neuronal response in the medial temporal lobe in humans. *Neuroendocrinology* **81**, 49–55.

Sallet P C, Sallet J A, Dixon J B, et al. 2007. Eating behavior as a prognostic factor for weight loss after gastric bypass. *Obes Surg* **17**, 445–51.

Schienle A, Schafer A, Hermann A and Vaitl D. 2009. Binge-eating disorder: Reward sensitivity and brain activation to images of food. *Biol Psychiatry* **65**, 654–61.

Schultes B, Peters A, Kern W, et al. 2005. Processing of food stimuli is selectively enhanced during insulin-induced hypoglycemia in healthy men. *Psychoneuroendocrinology* **30**, 496–504.

Schultz W. 2004. Neural coding of basic reward terms of animal learning theory, game theory, microeconomics and behavioural ecology. *Curr Opin Neurobiol* **14**, 139–47.

Schultz W, Apicella P and Ljungberg T. 1993. Responses of monkey dopamine neurons to reward and conditioned stimuli during successive steps of learning a delayed response task. *J Neurosci* **13**, 900–13.

Segal N L and Allison D B. 2002. Twins and virtual twins: Bases of relative body weight revisited. *Int J Obes Relat Metab Disord* **26**, 437–41.

Self D W, Barnhart W J, Lehman D A and Nestler E J. 1996. Opposite modulation of cocaine-seeking behavior by D1- and D2-like dopamine receptor agonists. *Science* **271**, 1586–9.

Shimura T, Kamada Y and Yamamoto T. 2002. Ventral tegmental lesions reduce overconsumption of normally preferred taste fluid in rats. *Behav Brain Res* **134**, 123–30.

Small D M, Jones-Gotman M and Dagher A. 2003. Feeding-induced dopamine release in dorsal striatum correlates with meal pleasantness ratings in healthy human volunteers. *Neuroimage* **19**, 1709–15.

Small D M and Prescott J. 2005. Odor/taste integration and the perception of flavor. *Exp Brain Res* **166**, 345–57.

Smeets P A, De Graaf C, Stafleu A, Van Osch M J, Nievelstein R A and Van Der Grond J. 2006. Effect of satiety on brain activation during chocolate tasting in men and women. *Am J Clin Nutr* **83**, 1297–305.

Smeets P A, De Graaf C, Stafleu A, Van Osch M J and Van Der Grond J. 2005. Functional MRI of human hypothalamic responses following glucose ingestion. *Neuroimage* **24**, 363–8.

Smith G P. 2004. Accumbens dopamine mediates the rewarding effect of orosensory stimulation by sucrose. *Appetite* **43**, 11–3.

Sotak B N, Hnasko T S, Robinson S, Kremer E J and Palmiter R D. 2005. Dysregulation of dopamine signaling in the dorsal striatum inhibits feeding. *Brain Res* **1061**, 88–96.

Spitz M R, Duphorne C M, Detry M A, et al. 2000. Dietary intake of isothiocyanates: evidence of a joint effect with glutathione S-transferase polymorphisms in lung cancer risk. *Cancer Epidemiol Biomarkers Prev* **9**, 1017–20.

Staley J K, Malison R T and Innis R B. 1998. Imaging of the serotonergic system: Interactions of neuroanatomical and functional abnormalities of depression. *Biol Psychiatry* **44**, 534–49.

Stenlof K, Rossner S, Vercruysse F, Kumar A, Fitchet M and Sjostrom L. 2007. Topiramate in the treatment of obese subjects with drug-naive type 2 diabetes. *Diabetes Obes Metab* **9**, 360–8.

507

Stice E, Spoor S, Bohon C and Small D M. 2008a. Relation between obesity and blunted striatal response to food is moderated by TaqIA A1 allele. *Science* **322**, 449–52.

Stice E, Spoor S, Bohon C, Veldhuizen M G and Small D M. 2008b. Relation of reward from food intake and anticipated food intake to obesity: A functional magnetic resonance imaging study. *J Abnorm Psychol* **117**, 924–35.

Stunkard A J and Wadden T A. 1993. *Obesity Theory and Therapy* (2nd ed.). New York, NY: Raven Press.

Szczypka M S, Kwok K, Brot M D, *et al.* 2001. Dopamine production in the caudate putamen restores feeding in dopamine-deficient mice. *Neuron* **30**, 819–28.

Tauscher J, Pirker W, Willeit M, *et al.* 2001. [123I] beta-CIT and single photon emission computed tomography reveal reduced brain serotonin transporter availability in bulimia nervosa. *Biol Psychiatry* **49**, 326–32.

Thanos P K, Michaelides M, Gispert J D, *et al.* 2008a. Differences in response to food stimuli in a rat model of obesity: In-vivo assessment of brain glucose metabolism. *Int J Obes (Lond)* **32**, 1171–9.

Thanos P K, Michaelides M, Ho C W, *et al.* 2008b. The effects of two highly selective dopamine D3 receptor antagonists (SB-277011A and NGB-2904) on food self-administration in a rodent model of obesity. *Pharmacol Biochem Behav* **89**, 499–507.

Thanos P K, Michaelides M, Piyis Y K, Wang G J and Volkow N D. 2008c. Food restriction markedly increases dopamine D2 receptor (D2R) in a rat model of obesity as assessed with in-vivo muPET imaging ([11C] raclopride) and in-vitro ([3H] spiperone) autoradiography. *Synapse* **62**, 50–61.

Tracy A L, Jarrard L E and Davidson T L. 2001. The hippocampus and motivation revisited: Appetite and activity. *Behav Brain Res* **127**, 13–23.

Trevitt J T, Carlson B B, Nowend K and Salamone J D. 2001. Substantia nigra pars reticulata is a highly potent site of action for the behavioral effects of the D1 antagonist SCH 23390 in the rat. *Psychopharmacology (Berl)* **156**, 32–41.

Tupala E, Hall H, Mantere T, Rasanen P, Sarkioja T and Tiihonen J. 2003. Dopamine receptors and transporters in the brain reward circuits of type 1 and 2 alcoholics measured with human whole hemisphere autoradiography. *Neuroimage* **19**, 145–55.

Turner R, Jezzard P, Wen H, *et al.* 1993. Functional mapping of the human visual cortex at 4 and 1.5 Tesla using deoxygenation contrast EPI. *Magn Res Med* **29**, 277–9.

Ugurbil K, Hu X, Chen W, Zhu X, Kim S and Georgopoulos A. 1999. Functional mapping in the human brain using high magnetic fields. *Phil Trans R Soc Lond B* **354**, 1195–213.

Volkow N D, Chang L, Wang G J, *et al.* 2001. Low level of brain dopamine D2 receptors in methamphetamine abusers: Association with metabolism in the orbitofrontal cortex. *Am J Psychiatry* **158**, 2015–21.

Volkow N D, Fowler J S, Wang G J, *et al.* 1993. Decreased dopamine D2 receptor availability is associated with reduced frontal metabolism in cocaine abusers. *Synapse* **14**, 169–77.

Volkow N D, Wang G J, Begleiter H, *et al.* 2006. High levels of dopamine D2 receptors in unaffected members of alcoholic families: Possible protective factors. *Arch Gen Psychiatry* **63**, 999–1008.

Volkow N D, Wang G J, Fowler J S, *et al.* 2002. "Nonhedonic" food motivation in humans involves dopamine in the dorsal striatum and methylphenidate amplifies this effect. *Synapse* **44**, 175–80.

Volkow N D, Wang G J, Fowler J S and Telang F. 2008a. Overlapping neuronal circuits in addiction and obesity: Evidence of systems pathology. *Phil Trans R Soc Lond B Biol Sci* **363**, 3191–200.

Volkow N D, Wang G J, Telang F, *et al.* 2009. Inverse association between BMI and prefrontal metabolic activity in healthy adults. *Obesity (Silver Spring)* **17**, 60–5.

Volkow N D, Wang G J, Telang F, *et al.* 2007. Profound decreases in dopamine release in striatum in detoxified alcoholics: Possible orbitofrontal involvement. *J Neurosci* **27**, 12 700–06.

Volkow N D, Wang G J, Telang F, *et al.* 2008b. Low dopamine striatal D2 receptors are associated with prefrontal metabolism in obese subjects: Possible contributing factors. *Neuroimage* **42**, 1537–43.

Volkow N D and Wise R A. 2005. How can drug addiction help us understand obesity? *Nat Neurosci* **8**, 555–60.

Wagner A, Aizenstein H, Mazurkewicz L, *et al.* 2008. Altered insula response to taste stimuli in individuals recovered from restricting-type anorexia nervosa. *Neuropsychopharmacology* **33**, 513–23.

Wang G J, Tomasi D, Backus W, *et al.* 2008. Gastric distention activates satiety circuitry in the human brain. *Neuroimage* **39**, 1824–31.

Wang G J, Volkow N D, Felder C, *et al.* 2002. Enhanced resting activity of the oral somatosensory cortex in obese subjects. *Neuroreport* **13**, 1151–5.

Wang G J, Volkow N D, Logan J, *et al.* 2001. Brain dopamine and obesity. *Lancet* **357**, 354–7.

Wang G J, Volkow N D, Telang F, *et al.* 2004. Exposure to appetitive food stimuli markedly activates the human brain. *Neuroimage* **21**, 1790–7.

Wang G J, Volkow N D, Telang F, *et al.* 2009. Evidence of gender differences in the ability to inhibit brain activation elicited by food stimulation. *Proc Natl Acad Sci U S A* **106**, 1249–54.

Wang G J, Yang J, Volkow N D, *et al.* 2006. Gastric stimulation in obese subjects activates the hippocampus and other regions involved in brain reward circuitry. *Proc Natl Acad Sci U S A* **103**, 15 641–5.

Watanabe M, Cromwell H C, Tremblay L, Hollerman J R, Hikosaka K and Schultz W. 2001. Behavioral reactions reflecting differential reward expectations in monkeys. *Exp Brain Res* **140**, 511–8.

Weingarten H P. 1983. Conditioned cues elicit feeding in sated rats: A role for learning in meal initiation. *Science* **220**, 431–3.

Will M J, Franzblau E B and Kelley A E. 2003. Nucleus accumbens mu-opioids regulate intake of a high-fat diet via activation of a distributed brain network. *J Neurosci* **23**, 2882–8.

Will M J, Pratt W E and Kelley A E. 2006. Pharmacological characterization of high-fat feeding induced by opioid stimulation of the ventral striatum. *Physiol Behav* **89**, 226–34.

Wise R A. 2006. Role of brain dopamine in food reward and reinforcement. *Phil Trans R Soc Lond B Biol Sci* **361**, 1149–58.

Wise R A, Murray A and Bozarth M A. 1990. Bromocriptine self-administration and bromocriptine-reinstatement of cocaine-trained and heroin-trained lever pressing in rats. *Psychopharmacology (Berl)* **100**, 355–60.

Wolnerhanssen B K, Peters T, Kern B, *et al.* 2008. Predictors of outcome in treatment of morbid obesity by laparoscopic adjustable gastric banding: Results of a prospective study of 380 patients. *Surg Obes Relat Dis* **4**, 500–06.

Woolley J D, Lee B S and Fields H L. 2006. Nucleus accumbens opioids regulate flavor-based preferences in food consumption. *Neuroscience* **143**, 309–17.

Wren A M. 2008. Gut and hormones and obesity. *Front Horm Res* **36**, 165–81.

Yanovski S Z, Nelson J E, Dubbert B K and Spitzer R L. 1993. Association of binge eating disorder and psychiatric comorbidity in obese subjects. *Am J Psychiatry* **150**, 1472–9.

Yeomans M R and Gray R W. 1997. Effects of naltrexone on food intake and changes in subjective appetite during eating: Evidence for opioid involvement in the appetizer effect. *Physiol Behav* **62**, 15–21.

Zhang Y, Proenca R, Maffei M, Barone M, Leopold L and Friedman J M. 1994. Positional cloning of the mouse obese gene and its human homologue. *Nature* **372**, 425–32.

Zink C F, Pagnoni G, Martin M E, Dhamala M and Berns G S. 2003. Human striatal response to salient nonrewarding stimuli. *J Neurosci* **23**, 8092–7.

Zipursky R B, Meyer J H and Verhoeff N P. 2007. PET and SPECT imaging in psychiatric disorders. *Can J Psychiatry* **52**, 146–57.

Neuroimaging of eating disorders: commentary

Janet Treasure

Introduction

The preceding two chapters synthesize the evidence from imaging studies which explore normal eating behavior, and the clinical manifestations of disturbed eating behavior ranging from obesity through to anorexia nervosa. Both chapters have been written by individuals with a high level of expertise and they contain a wealth of information. For those of us struggling to keep up and assimilate this knowledge base, it is easy to get lost in the detail. I have therefore introduced a simple diagram to help to navigate a path through this information. In this diagram the central control of appetite is simplified into three basic elements (Figure 35.1).

First, there is the *homeostatic system* (Nutrostat) centered mainly in the brain stem and hypothalamus that integrates metabolic markers (insulin, leptin, PYY, ghrelin, etc.), and information from the gastrointestinal tract, and has outputs such as hunger, fullness and autonomic nervous activity. The neurotransmitters involved include MCH, alpha MSH, agouti-related peptide, orexin and neuropeptide Y. Second, there is the *drive and reward system* (Hedonic) centered within the mesolimbic system and striatum, which registers the salience and reward value associated with food and is involved in signaling the drive to eat. This has inputs from sensory organs and the hippocampus. The key neurotransmitters in this system are dopamine and opioids. The third

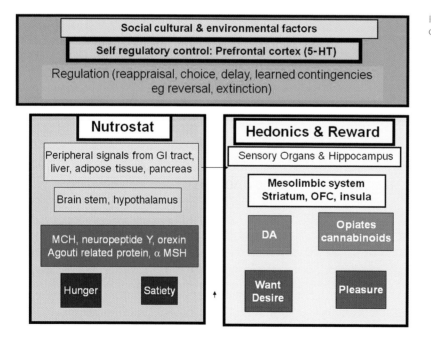

Figure 35.1 A simplified model of the central control of appetite.

Understanding Neuropsychiatric Disorders, ed. M. E. Shenton and B. I. Turetsky. Published by Cambridge University Press.
© Cambridge University Press 2011.

system, the *self-regulatory system*, includes fronto-striatal circuits involving 5-HT, amongst other neurotransmitters. This exerts control over the other more reflexive, automatic components and serves to integrate appetite into a personal and societal framework.

The mechanisms involved within the nutrostat and hedonic components of the model shown on the diagram have been derived from laboratory work with animals. In man, the cortical, deliberative component plays a more dominant role. The function of this system includes choices, costs, learning and decision making. An imbalance between these three components may explain some of the clinical variation in eating behaviors.

How brain imaging has clarified understanding about the central control of appetite in Man

Hedonic and metabolic systems

Scanning work in humans has for the most part validated most of the elements within this model. In his chapter, Wang has elaborated upon this and only brief highlights are reiterated here.

Glucose, insulin and other GI-related hormones modulate brain appetite systems by mechanisms involving both the hedonic and nutrostat systems. For example, fluxes in blood sugar parallel changes in metabolism within the hypothalamus (Liu et al., 2000; Smeets et al., 2005). PYY reduces eating behavior and hypothalamic activation by food (Batterham et al., 2007). Conversely, when ghrelin (a hormone increased by fasting) is administered intravenously, the metabolic response to pictures of food is increased in the areas of the brain associated with the hedonic system such as the amygdala, orbito- frontal cortex, anterior insula and striatum (Malik et al., 2008).

The role of dopamine (DA) as a key neurochemical in the hedonic system has been confirmed by several studies. For example, the presentation of palatable foods to fasting humans is associated with an increase in DA in the dorsal striatum (Volkow et al., 2002). Furthermore, the amount of dopamine released is associated with the pleasure experienced (Small et al., 2003). Tasting palatable foods also activates the insula and midbrain areas (Frank et al., 2008), and gastric distension modulates activity in the posterior insula (Wang et al., 2008).

Obesity

People with obesity (who are a heterogeneous group) appear to have problems within all three components from the model. For example, people with obesity appear to have deficits in the nutrostat system with a delayed response to peripheral metabolic signals in the hypothalamus (Matsuda et al., 1999).

Scanning studies designed to interrogate reward function and dopamine pathways in obesity have led to fascinating findings. Obese subjects have higher metabolism in the somatosensory areas related to the mouth, tongue and lips (Wang et al., 2002), and greater activation in reward centers when a device to mimic fullness is switched on in the stomach (Wang et al., 2008). These findings suggest that elements of the hedonic response to food are more active in obesity.

There is an inverse linear relationship between dopamine receptor (DA2) levels and BMI in people with a BMI over 40 (Wang et al., 2001). This reduction in dopamine receptors is associated with lower metabolic measures in the prefrontal area (Volkow et al., 2009). Thus it is possible that dopamine may be implicated in the loss of regulatory control overeating in obesity (Volkow et al., 2008).

Studies of people with specific syndromes associated with obesity also offer interesting insights into the central control of appetite. People with Prader Willi syndrome who satiate poorly to a meal have reduced medial orbitofrontal activity (Hinton et al., 2006), and those people with congenital leptin deficiency have the activation of the limbic system in response to food cues reduced by leptin replacement (Baicy et al., 2007; Farooqi et al., 2007). This suggests that overeating in both of these syndromes is associated with abnormalities in brain function.

Eating disorders

As is well argued by Frank, there can be problems interpreting some of the results of scanning studies in people with eating disorders, as food restriction alters brain structure with the loss of gray and white matter. In order to overcome this difficulty, several groups have studied patients after recovery, as for the most part brain mass is restored following weight gain (Castro-Fornieles et al., 2009; McCormick et al., 2008).

The neurochemistry and functional anatomy of the brain has been explored. Brain monoamine function in eating disorders has been studied both in the acute state and after recovery using specific ligands with PET technology. Changes in monamine receptor density have been found both in the prefrontal regulatory control areas and the mesostriatal areas of the hedonic system. 5-HT1A receptors in the prefrontal cortex are increased especially in the acute state but also after recovery (Bailer *et al.*, 2005, 2007b; Galusca *et al.*, 2008). In the striatum, 5-HTT receptors are increased in the restricting form anorexia nervosa after recovery, whereas they appear to be decreased in the binge purge form (Bailer *et al.*, 2007a) and dopamine receptors (DA2) are also increased after recovery in anorexia nervosa (Frank *et al.*, 2005). In summary, people with eating disorders have key abnormalities in monoamine function in both the hedonic and the regulatory regions, and this may contribute to the abnormal patterns of eating behaviors.

The functional changes elicited by specific eating disorder stimuli (food and body) and more general aspects of the psychopathology (reward, and self-regulatory control) have also been examined. Food-related imagery increases activity in the frontal and limbic areas of people with eating disorders (Naruo *et al.*, 2000; Gordon *et al.*, 2001; Ellison *et al.*, 1998; Uher *et al.*, 2003, personal communication; Uher *et al.*, 2004; Schienle *et al.*, 2009; Geliebter *et al.*, 2006). On the other hand, the metabolic response to the taste of sucrose/glucose in the insula and striatal circuits is reduced in anorexia nervosa (Frank *et al.*, 2006; Wagner *et al.*, 2008). Thus anticipation of food appears highly salient, whereas the consumption is less salient or rewarding.

Activation to body image cues varies according to the contextual aspects of the stimulus. In general, body-related cues do not activate the same frontal/limbic circuits as do food cues; rather, there is activation in the insula and occipital/parietal regions (Uher *et al.*, 2005; Redgrave *et al.*, 2008; Sachdev *et al.*, 2008; Wagner *et al.*, 2003; Seeger *et al.*, 2002). The insula is known to be a bridge between information from the body and the limbic system, producing an emotional context for sensory experience.

People with anorexia nervosa and those with bulimia nervosa fail to have different activation patterns in the ventral striatum to reward or non-reward in a guessing game (Wagner *et al.*, 2007, 2010). This suggests that the reward system in general and not just to food is dysfunctional.

People in the acute phase of anorexia nervosa have deficits in executive function with poor set shifting (Roberts *et al.*, 2007). This is associated with greater activation in the frontal regulatory regions and less activation in the striatum to a set-shifting task, suggesting that this task requires greater effortful control (Zastrow *et al.*, 2009). People with bulimia nervosa also have decreased activity in the neural systems that mediate self-regulatory control to the Simon task in the inferior lateral prefrontal cortex on both sides and mid-dorsal striatum (Marsh *et al.*, 2009). This suggests that there is a difficulty in self-regulation and control in people with eating disorders which leads to rigidity.

In the following section I try to integrate some of the current findings and develop some hypothetical models which may explain some the clinical varieties of eating and hopefully may suggest future research directions. At the present time these are speculative, although they do fit with some of the information discovered from the research into brain scanning described in these two chapters. I start with a model for eating disorders, as these are more homogeneous and are set more firmly within the framework of psychology and psychiatry.

A model of brain function in eating disorders

In this section, I have developed a hypothetical model of eating disorders which could be used as the basis for further research. For the sake of simplicity, the model is limited to appetite control, although the inclusion of other aspects of brain function characteristic of people with eating disorders, such as a tendency to anxiety and compulsive behaviors, should also be included in a more complete model. A diagram illustrating the underlying processes is shown in Figure 35.2.

The hypothesis is that the subcortical appetite system (hedonic and nutrostat) in people at risk for anorexia nervosa is set to attain less reward from food and there is a a lower set point with tighter control around it. This disposition to leanness is a familial trait (Hebebrand and Remschmidt, 1995). In contrast, those at risk of binge eating have a greater reward from food with a set point which is more loosely regulated in the direction of weight gain. Thus there is a tendency to overeat and be overweight. Restriction, a key eating disorder behavior, results from a choice to impose regulatory control over subcortical areas.

However, over time, continued dietary restriction produces nutritional and emotional consequences that adversely impacts on the function of the regulatory control system. This reduces the control over the

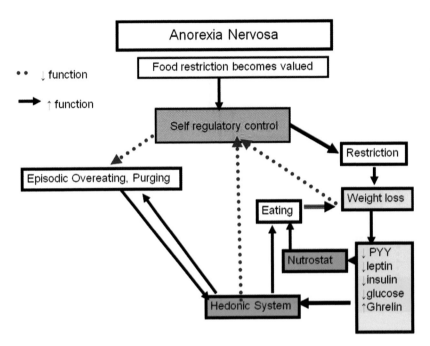

Figure 35.2 A putative model describing the development of anorexia nervosa. In a proportion of cases, binge eating develops because of decreases in the self-regulatory control and increased sensitivity in the hedonic system.

hedonic and the nutrostat systems. This means that these subcortical regions (the amygdala and basal ganglia and ventromedial prefrontal cortex) are freed from inhibition. Moreover, the level of inhibition needed to regulate the lower sytems escalates with weight loss because homeostatic mechanisms to maintain weight at the set point swing into action and produce activation in the nutrostat and hedonic systems. For example, dopamine function within the hedonic system may be modulated by the decrease in PPY and leptin and increases in ghrelin. This means that food becomes more rewarding. Also lower levels of glucose and insulin adjust the output of the nutrostat system.

In addition to these homeostatic pathways, some eating disorder behaviors themselves have a specific impact on the control of appetite. This is exemplified by models of binge eating in laboratory rodents. Scientists have replicated in the laboratory the conditions implicated in the exponential increase of binge eating, i.e. food restriction, gastric drainage, stress and intermittent access to highly palatable food and produced "food addiction" (Avena et al., 2008; Avena, 2007). Not only do these animals "binge" eat, but they also show withdrawal effects, a propensity to relapse after a time, and cross-tolerance to alcohol and cocaine. Thus the hedonic system becomes more sensitive to food. There is individual variation in the propensity to develop these changes.

This sensitization of brain reward systems in combination with the decreased capacity of the regulatory system may explain the switch from extreme restriction to bulimic behavior which commonly occurs within the first three years of the development of anorexia nervosa (Eddy et al., 2008; Wentz et al., 2009).

The decrease in self-regulatory function may explain the increase in avoidance, behavioral inhibition and compulsive behaviors, as these also become more dominant as they become freed from regulatory control.

A model of brain function in obesity

Obesity is a heterogeneous condition and is beyond the scope of this chapter to produce a model that can account for all the various subtypes. In Figure 35.3, a simple model is depicted which accounts for a proportion of cases. The hypothesis is that the nutrostat and the hedonic system are set towards an increased sensitivity to the reward of food. In part, this may be innate or it may be acquired through learning. This disposition leads to weight gain. Amongst the negative consequences of weight gain stigma and low self esteem can reduce functioning of the self-regulation centre and also reduce the range of possible rewarding activities by making

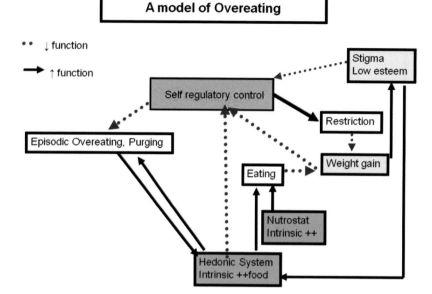

A model of Overeating

•• ↓ function

➤ ↑ function

Self regulatory control

Stigma Low esteem

Restriction

Episodic Overeating, Purging

Weight gain

Eating

Nutrostat Intrinsic ++

Hedonic System Intrinsic ++food

Figure 35.3 The development of overeating.

social connection a source of pain rather than pleasure. Thus food becomes the main source of solace and security and there is less ability to inhibit this behavior, resulting in a vicious circle.

Overall conclusions

Overall, there appears to be a coherence developing in the central models of the control of appetite from animals to man and into the clinical areas. Both obesity and the eating disorders are associated with abnormal functioning in regulatory control areas and in the hedonic systems. Furthermore, the pattern of monoamine functioning in these areas is abnormal. In this chapter, I have speculated as to how innate vulnerabilities and acquired changes may allow these varieties of abnormal eating behavior to occur. It is to be hoped that further interrogation of these systems and translating some of the findings in to treatment might improve the outcome of these conditions.

References

Avena N M. 2007. Examining the addictive-like properties of binge eating using an animal model of sugar dependence. *Exp Clin Psychopharmacol* **15**, 481–91.

Avena N M, Rada P and Hoebel B G. 2008. Evidence for sugar addiction: Behavioral and neurochemical effects of intermittent, excessive sugar intake. *Neurosci Biobehav Rev* **32**, 20–39.

Baicy K, London E D, Monterosso J, *et al.* 2007. Leptin replacement alters brain response to food cues in genetically leptin-deficient adults. *Proc Natl Acad Sci U S A* **104**, 18 276–9.

Bailer U F, Frank G K, Henry S E, *et al.* 2007a. Serotonin transporter binding after recovery from eating disorders. *Psychopharmacology (Berl)* **195**, 315–24.

Bailer U F, Frank G K, Henry S E, *et al.* 2007b. Exaggerated 5-HT1A but normal 5-HT2A receptor activity in individuals ill with anorexia nervosa. *Biol Psychiatry* **61**, 1090–9.

Bailer U F, Frank G K, Henry S E, *et al.* 2005. Altered brain serotonin 5-HT1A receptor binding after recovery from anorexia nervosa measured by positron emission tomography and [carbonyl11C]WAY-100635. *Arch Gen Psychiatry* **62**, 1032–41.

Batterham R L, Ffytche D H, Rosenthal J M, *et al.* 2007. PYY modulation of cortical and hypothalamic brain areas predicts feeding behaviour in humans. *Nature* **450**, 106–09.

Castro-Fornieles J, Bargallo N, Lazaro L, *et al.* 2009. A cross-sectional and follow-up voxel-based morphometric MRI study in adolescent anorexia nervosa. *J Psychiatr Res* **43**, 331–40.

Eddy K T, Dorer D J, Franko D L, Tahilani K, Thompson-Brenner H and Herzog D B. 2008. Diagnostic crossover in anorexia nervosa and bulimia nervosa: Implications for DSM-V. *Am J Psychiatry* **165**, 245–50.

Ellison Z, Foong J, Howard R, Bullmore E, Williams S, and Treasure J. 1998. Functional anatomy of calorie fear in anorexia nervosa. *Lancet* **352**, 1192.

Farooqi I S, Bullmore E, Keogh J, Gillard J, O'Rahilly S, and Fletcher P C. 2007. Leptin regulates striatal regions and human eating behavior. *Science* **317**, 1355.

Frank G K, Bailer U F, Henry S E, *et al.* 2005. Increased dopamine D2/D3 receptor binding after recovery from anorexia nervosa measured by positron emission tomography and [(11)C]raclopride. *Biol Psychiatry* **32**, 755–61.

Frank G K, Oberndorfer T.A, Simmons A N, *et al.* 2008. Sucrose activates human taste pathways differently from artificial sweetener. *Neuroimage* **39**, 1559–69.

Frank G K, Wagner A, Achenbach S, *et al.* 2006. Altered brain activity in women recovered from bulimic-type eating disorders after a glucose challenge: A pilot study. *Int J Eat Disord* **39**, 76–9.

Galusca B, Costes N, Zito N G, *et al.* 2008. Organic background of restrictive-type anorexia nervosa suggested by increased serotonin 1A receptor binding in right frontotemporal cortex of both lean and recovered patients: [18F]MPPF PET scan study. *Biol Psychiatry* **64**, 1009–13.

Geliebter A, Ladell T, Logan M, Schneider T, Sharafi M and Hirsch J. 2006. Responsivity to food stimuli in obese and lean binge eaters using functional MRI. *Appetite* **46**, 31–5.

Gordon C M, Dougherty D D, Fischman A J, *et al.* 2001. Neural substrates of anorexia nervosa: A behavioral challenge study with positron emission tomography. *J Pediatr* **139**, 51–7.

Hebebrand J and Remschmidt H. 1995. Anorexia nervosa viewed as an extreme weight condition: Genetic implications. *Hum Genet* **95**, 1–11.

Hinton E C, Holland A J, Gellatly M S, *et al.* 2006. Neural representations of hunger and satiety in Prader-Willi syndrome. *Int J Obes (Lond)* **30**, 313–21.

Liu Y, Gao J H, Liu H L and Fox P T. 2000. The temporal response of the brain after eating revealed by functional MRI. *Nature* **405**, 1058–62.

Malik S, McGlone F, Bedrossian D and Dagher A. 2008. Ghrelin modulates brain activity in areas that control appetitive behavior. *Cell Metab* **7**, 400–9.

Marsh R, Steinglass J E, Gerber A J, *et al.* 2009. Deficient activity in the neural systems that mediate self-regulatory control in bulimia nervosa. *Arch Gen Psychiatry* **66**, 51–63.

Matsuda M, Liu Y. Mahankali S, *et al.* 1999. Altered hypothalamic function in response to glucose ingestion in obese humans. *Diabetes* **48**, 1801–06.

McCormick L M, Keel P K, Brumm M C, *et al.* 2008. Implications of starvation-induced change in right dorsal anterior cingulate volume in anorexia nervosa. *Int J Eat Disord* **41**, 602–10.

Naruo T, Nakabeppu Y, Sagiyama K, *et al.* 2000. Characteristic regional cerebral blood flow patterns in anorexia nervosa patients with binge/purge behavior. *Am J Psychiatry* **157**, 1520–2.

Redgrave G W, Bakker A, Bello N T, *et al.* 2008. Differential brain activation in anorexia nervosa to Fat and Thin words during a Stroop task. *Neuroreport* **19**, 1181–5.

Roberts M E, Tchanturia K, Stahl D, Southgate L and Treasure J. 2007. A systematic review and meta-analysis of set-shifting ability in eating disorders. *Psychol Med* **37**, 1075–84.

Sachdev P, Mondraty N, Wen W and Gulliford K. 2008. Brains of anorexia nervosa patients process self-images differently from non-self-images: An fMRI study. *Neuropsychologia* **46**, 2161–8.

Schienle A, Schafer A, Hermann A and Vaitl D. 2009. Binge-eating disorder: Reward sensitivity and brain activation to images of food. *Biol Psychiatry* **65**, 654–61.

Seeger G, Braus D F, Ruf M, Goldberger U and Schmidt M H. 2002. Body image distortion reveals amygdala activation in patients with anorexia nervosa – A functional magnetic resonance imaging study. *Neurosci Lett* **326**, 25–8.

Small D M, Jones-Gotman M and Dagher A. 2003. Feeding-induced dopamine release in dorsal striatum correlates with meal pleasantness ratings in healthy human volunteers. *Neuroimage* **19**, 1709–15.

Smeets P A, de G C, Stafleu A, van Osch M J and van der Grond J. 2005. Functional magnetic resonance imaging of human hypothalamic responses to sweet taste and calories. *Am J Clin Nutr* **82**, 1011–6.

Uher R, Murphy T, Brammer M J, *et al.* 2004. Medial prefrontal cortex activity associated with symptom provocation in eating disorders. *Am J Psychiatry* **161**, 1238–46.

Uher R, Murphy T, Friederich H C, *et al.* 2005. Functional neuroanatomy of body shape perception in healthy and eating-disordered women. *Biol Psychiatry* **58**, 990–7.

Volkow N D, Wang G J, Fowler J S, *et al.* 2002. "Nonhedonic" food motivation in humans involves dopamine in the dorsal striatum and methylphenidate amplifies this effect. *Synapse* **44**, 175–80.

Volkow N D, Wang G J, Fowler J S and Telang F. 2008. Overlapping neuronal circuits in addiction and obesity: Evidence of systems pathology. *Phil Trans R Soc Lond B Biol Sci* **363**, 3191–200.

Volkow N D, Wang G J, Telang F, *et al.* 2009. Inverse association between BMI and prefrontal metabolic activity in healthy adults. *Obesity (Silver Spring)* **17**, 60–5.

Wagner A, Aizenstein H, Mazurkewicz L, *et al.* 2008. Altered insula response to taste stimuli in individuals recovered from restricting-type anorexia nervosa. *Neuropsychopharmacology* **33**, 513–23.

Wagner A, Aizenstein H, Venkatraman V K, *et al.* 2010. Altered striatal response to reward in bulimia nervosa after recovery. *Int J Eat Disord* **45**, 289–94.

Wagner A, Aizenstein H, Venkatraman V K, *et al.* 2007. Altered reward processing in women recovered from anorexia nervosa. *Am J Psychiatry* **164**, 1842–9.

Wagner A, Ruf M, Braus D F and Schmidt M H. 2003. Neuronal activity changes and body image distortion in anorexia nervosa. *Neuroreport* **14**, 2193–7.

Wang G J, Tomasi D, Backus W, *et al.* 2008. Gastric distention activates satiety circuitry in the human brain. *Neuroimage* **39**, 1824–31.

Wang G J, Volkow N D, Felder C, *et al.* 2002. Enhanced resting activity of the oral somatosensory cortex in obese subjects. *Neuroreport* **13**, 1151–5.

Wang G J Volkow N D, Logan J, *et al.* 2001. Brain dopamine and obesity. *Lancet* **357**, 354–7.

Wentz E, Gillberg I C, Anckarsater H, Gillberg C and Rastam M. 2009. Adolescent-onset anorexia nervosa: 18-year outcome. *Br J Psychiatry* **194**, 168–74.

Zastrow A, Kaiser S, Stippich C, *et al.* 2009. Neural correlates of impaired cognitive-behavioral flexibility in anorexia nervosa. *Am J Psychiatry* **166**, 608–16.

36

Neuroimaging of autism spectrum disorders

John D. Herrington and Robert T. Schultz

The past two decades of neuroimaging research on developmental disabilities appear to reflect the development of the field of neuroimaging itself. The vast majority of magnetic resonance imaging (MRI) studies on developmental disabilities have come from *modular* perspectives of brain function – where specific areas are associated with specific mental operations, developmental patterns, and clinical symptoms. More recently, it has become clear that, although critical, modular perspectives ought not to obscure the importance of *distributed* perspectives, where cognitive functions are implemented via complex interactions between multiple brain areas.

This chapter reviews MRI findings on developmental disabilities that arise from both modular and distributed perspectives on brain function, although the former clearly represent the majority of existing data. The chapter will focus exclusively on autism-spectrum disorders (ASD, including the diagnoses of autism, Asperger's Syndrome, and Pervasive Developmental Disorder – Not Otherwise Specified).[1] Some of the most recent and exciting developments in the neurobiology of ASD relate to abnormal functional and structural connectivity – in particular, findings of decreased long-range connectivity between brain areas. We conclude the chapter by discussing important futures avenues, with particular emphasis on study designs and techniques that are capable of integrating data from multiple sources.

The autism spectrum

The classic "triad" of autism includes (1) delayed or impaired communication abilities, (2) diminished social skills and social isolation, and (3) repetitive behaviors or restricted interest repertoires. These symptoms typically emerge early in development (noticeable by age 2 or 3) and are generally lifelong

(Volkmar *et al.*, 2005). In addition to the triad, ASDs are associated with a number of other serious conditions, including mental retardation and seizure disorders. Although other biological abnormalities (such as tuberous sclerosis) confer risk for autistic symptoms, no specific abnormality has proven causal in a majority of cases (see Bailey *et al.*, 1996; Abrahams and Geschwind, 2008).

There is growing appreciation for the diverse manifestations of these symptoms and the disorder's very broad functional range – from a complete absence of daily living skills to only subtle differences in behavior. The inclusion of the diagnosis of Asperger's Disorder (AD) in the DSM-IV reflects the recognition that a large number of individuals with significant social skill deficits fail to show delayed language (whereas language delays are part of the autism diagnosis). The diagnosis of Pervasive Developmental Disorder – Not Otherwise Specified captures cases who have some but not all of the symptoms of autism or AD.

The etiology of ASD remains elusive. The data covered in this chapter represent attempts to identify critical brain mechanisms of ASD – attempts that have proven both fruitful and incomplete. The etiology of ASD can, of course, be examined from other levels, including genetics. Although rarely integrated with studies of brain mechanisms, research on the genetics of ASDs bear directly on our understanding of relevant brain mechanisms. The studies reviewed in this chapter do not formally include genetics; however, it is important to note that ASD does appear highly genetically mediated, in ways that may prove critical to MRI findings. The concordance rate for ASD in monozygotic twins is considerably higher (80–90%) than in dizygotic twins (10–20%;

Bailey *et al.*, 1995; Burmeister *et al.*, 2008). The relative risk of a child being diagnosed with autism is 25 times the population average in families that already have one affected sibling (Jorde *et al.*, 1991; O'Roak and State, 2008). Even in the absence of multiple affected children, parents and other immediate family members will often show mild, subsyndromal manifestations of autism – the so-called broader autism phenotype (Piven *et al.*, 1997).

The relationship between these genetics findings and those from neuroimaging has come increasing into focus. In the last two years, there have been several reports on the contribution of rare genetic variants to ASD risk, including sequence and structural variants (i.e. copy number variants; Glessner *et al.*, 2009; O'Roak and State, 2008; Sebat, 2007; Wang *et al.*, 2009). Many of these rare variants involve genes that impact the growth and development of the synapse (i.e. the neuroligands, neurexin, contactin-associated proteins, among others). These findings bear directly on recent accounts of long-range connectivity deficits in ASD (described below).

Abnormal brain size and cellular architecture in ASD

The observation that individuals with autism tend to have enlarged heads dates back to the origin of the diagnosis itself (Kanner, 1943). Although many subsequent studies of head circumference have confirmed this observation, it did not receive much attention until recently, as MRI technology permitted the widespread measurement of in-vivo brain volume and morphology. A pioneering study by Piven *et al.* (1995) reported brain volume measurements from 22 individuals with autism and 20 controls. The average total tissue volume of individuals in the autism group was 85 ml larger than the control group. This increase manifested as both brain tissue and ventricular enlargement. Several studies now show that brain and head size are normal at birth (Lainhart, 2006; Hazlett *et al.*, 2005), but undergo a period of exuberant growth around 1 year of age (Courchesne *et al.*, 2001; Hazlett *et al.*, 2005). There appears to be a shifting of the entire brain size/head size distribution toward large size, with about 20% of those with ASD having brain sizes that average about 5% larger than normal ones accounting for age and IQ, meeting the 97th percentile criterion for macrocephaly (Lainhart, 2006; Redcay and Courchesne, 2005).

Although white matter (WM) size reductions have been shown in some tracts (such as the corpus callosum; see Chung *et al.*, 2004; Egass *et al.*, 1995; Piven *et al.*, 1997), several studies have found that the WM compartment is disproportionately enlarged in autism (Courchesne *et al.*, 2001; Herbert *et al.*, 2003). Allometric models of cerebral development suggest that doubling the number of minicolumns (defined below) supports a fourfold increase in neuronal connectivity, potentially generating a fourfold increase in some WM areas (Casanova *et al.*, 2002). In other words, WM increases may reflect increased neuronal number in ASD. It seems counterintuitive that *increases* in brain size and neuron count might be associated with the profound deficits of autism. However, our accumulated knowledge of typical brain development, alongside theoretical models of increased brain size (e.g. Ringo, 1991), clearly indicate that abnormally increased WM likely reflects suboptimal signal transfer, particularly between distant structures.

Although MRI has played a critical role in our understanding of brain size in ASD, it does not allow for the inspection of small-scale neuronal organization, as in post-mortem studies. An increasing number of post-mortem studies are identifying cellular abnormalities in ASD. We will highlight only one of these findings, as it pertains directly to recent connectivity data from fMRI. Casanova and colleagues (2002, 2006) now have two post-mortem studies of select cortical areas with abnormal minicolumnar structure. Minicolumns are comprised of sets of radially oriented neurons that play a critical role in neural information processing (Casanova *et al.*, 2006). Minicolumns appear significantly increased in number and reduced in width in autism. This finding is consistent with the observed WM increase in ASD. Moreover, they found that neuronal cell size was decreased, and speculated that this would give rise to an abundance of short range fibers only, since longer fibers require larger cell bodies to support their metabolic needs. Using MRI parcellation schemes, Herbert *et al.* (2003) found that WM increases were especially pronounced in the more superficial layers of WM, and argued that this is consistent with an overabundance of short-range fibers, and a decrease of long-range fibers. Thus, there is an interesting convergence of data suggesting that autism may involve an overabundance of short-range fiber connections and a decrease of long-range connections.

ASD and language systems

Considerations of communication and language in ASD are more complicated than suggested by a cursory read of DSM-IV criteria (APA, 2000). Delays in speech development are a defining feature of autism. However, it is not strictly necessary for these delays to manifest as language impairments after the first few years of life. While impaired *communication* skills represent a core diagnostic symptom of autism, formal *language* impairments in ASD are only variably present, and are not part of the core phenotype. Indeed, it is not clear that autism speech delays inevitably lead to functional language impairments. Studies of language functioning in autism later in childhood reveal only subtle and inconsistent formal "language" difficulties (Groen *et al.*, 2008; Kjelgaard and Tager-Flusberg, 2001; Tager-Flusberg *et al.*, 2005). Importantly, formal aspects of language are correlated with IQ, and matching study groups on IQ greatly diminishes language effects.

Nevertheless, language is impaired or absent in a sizeable fraction of ASD cases. One of the most common deficit areas, and one of the only language deficit areas that has proven independent from IQ deficits, relates to pragmatics (Colle *et al.*, 2008; Ghaziuddin and Gerstein, 1996). There is an entire literature documenting the relationships between social interactions during early childhood and the development of language skills. Theory of Mind skills (ToM, discussed in more detail below) have been linked to the development of language. In this regard, language deficits may be a consequence of what we consider to be more of a core or universal ASD deficit (i.e. ToM).

Because of what is known about the neural basis of language, hypotheses on the nature of ASD language deficits have been highly focused – namely, on Broca's and Wernicke's areas. ASD abnormalities have been identified in both of these areas via structural MRI (sMRI) (Herbert *et al.*, 2003) and hemodynamic imaging (for review, see Schultz and Robins, 2005). Some data indicate that the typical left-hemisphere asymmetry of language functions (among right-handers) is shifted rightward (Müller *et al.*, 1999; Boddaert *et al.*, 2003). These data are supported by a structural MRI study indicating a more rightward bias in the size of language areas (Herbert *et al.*, 2002).

Some evidence indicates that observed abnormalities in language areas may reflect different processing styles, rather than deficits per se. In particular, Just

et al. (2004) showed decreased left Broca's area activity during a sentence comprehension task, but also an increase in activity in Wernicke's area. The authors concluded that this pattern may reflect a bias away from the integration of word meaning within the sentences, and towards an in-depth processing of individuals words. This conclusion is consistent with theories of overall cognitive style in ASD (such as weak central coherence theory, discussed below).

ASD and visual information processes

A recurring debate within the autism research community centers on whether the complex profiles of the disorder emerge from deficits in broad systems, or from circumscribed ones that have radiating effects (for more detailed considerations of this topic, see Belmonte *et al.*, 2004a; Schultz, 2005). The theoretical underpinnings of such debates are often thornier than they first appear – to what extent can system-wide brain abnormalities emerge from focal ones? Which brain systems might represent specific impairment loci, versus downstream effects of abnormalities in other areas? Do progressions from discrete abnormalities to broader ones follow specific developmental trajectories that are themselves instrumental?

Data on visual information processing deficits in ASD kindle many of these debates, as visual information (gestures, facial expressions, etc.) is often pivotal to social understanding. Indeed, it has been pointed out that congenital blindness, although associated with outcomes that are clearly distinct from autism, entails social behavior that resembles ASD in many respects (Hobson and Bishop, 2003). Findings on basic visual information processing deficits in ASD have proven particularly compelling, and may in fact play an etiological role in the disorder (Schultz, 2005).

Low-level visual information processing systems

Visual information processing has always been a topic of great interest to ASD researchers, as individuals with ASD often show preserved and sometimes enhanced visual abilities. Particularly compelling is the observation that individuals with ASD often perform relatively well on tasks requiring the disambiguation of stimulus parts from a larger whole (Frith, 1989; Shah and Frith, 1983, 1993). These findings directly inform theories on the etiology of ASD – namely, weak central coherence theory, which associates ASD with a diminished capacity to perceive broad, coherent patterns of information in the environment (Frith, 1989). Evidence in support of this theory comes from, for example, the embedded figures task, where one must locate a small figure embedded in a larger one. Individuals with ASD have shown normal or above-normal performance on this task, despite deficits in other visual and cognitive domains (Shah and Frith, 1983). For this task, the tendency to perceive and process the entire stimulus may actually interfere with the critical task – to find a particular piece of that stimulus. Hence, the failure to attend to the entire stimulus may leave individuals with ASD at an advantage.

Other visual processes nevertheless appear diminished in ASD. For example, some evidence indicates that individuals with ASD show a diminished capacity to perceive global, coherent motion, as measured by random dot kinematograms (RDKs) and related stimuli (see Dakin and Frith, 2005). A deficit in this area is of particular interest to the clinical phenomenology of ASD, as motion perception is critical to disambiguation of objects within scenes, including other individuals (their gestures, body language, etc.). As pointed out by Dakin and Frith (2005), data on global motion perception in ASD are made problematic by the use of paradigms where *local* motion is poorly controlled (see Barlow and Tripathy, 1997, for a consideration of local motion in RDKs). However, in lieu of more direct evidence of local motion processing deficits in ASD (see Bertone et al., 2003; Bertone and Faubert, 2006; Pellicano et al., 2005; Pellicano and Gibson, 2008), the weight of the existing data seems to favor a global motion deficit.

As depth of processing increases (moving anteriorly along dorsal and ventral streams), additional visual processing abnormalities become evident. For example, numerous studies have established that the integration of complex motion vectors across space is implemented by the human homolog of the monkey area MT+, often referred to as MT+/V5 (Cowey et al., 2006; Dumoulin et al., 2000; Herrington et al., 2007; Newsome and Pare, 1988). The complex kinematics of human movement (including highly configural, pendular motion) exemplify this type of visual input. Numerous studies of biological motion have used point-light (PL) displays, where a moving human form is represented entirely by small number of dots placed in locations corresponding to the major

joints of the body. When stationary, these dots may not be readily identifiable as a human representation; however, when made to move like a person, the human form immediately becomes obvious (Johansson, 1973).

Herrington et al. (2007) were among the first to examine brain activity during PL biological motion perception among individuals with ASD. A sample of individuals with Asperger's Disorder and age- and IQ-matched controls were asked to indicate whether a PL figure appeared to be walking to the left or right. When completing the task, decreased AD activity was observed in multiple posterior areas including MT+/V5 (see Figure 36.1). Furthermore, the two groups did not differ in MT+/V5 activity during a control condition where the same dots were presented in scrambled form. This suggests that the difference appears specific to the configural processing demands elicited by a human form (although it remains to be seen whether other, highly configural stimuli may invoke similar effects).

Despite these intriguing findings, there is still considerable debate surrounding whether ASD is associated with abnormal function in basic visual processing areas. Ultimately the debate may turn less on the localization of specific visual cortex deficits in ASD, and more on the identification of particular levels of cognitive complexity where differences arise. For example, Bertone and colleagues (2003, 2006) argue that individuals with ASD have intact first-order (luminance-based), but impaired second-order (contrast-based) motion processors. Although this would seem to implicate some areas of the dorsal stream (i.e. V2 and V3) and not others (i.e. V1), to our knowledge there have been no MRI studies directly testing this hypothesis.

Fusiform gyrus and person perception

Visual information processing deficits in ASD emerge more robustly in brain areas that are responsive to specific classes of objects – namely, those related to people. A large literature yields consistent evidence that individuals with ASD are selectively impaired in their ability to recognize face identity and facial expressions (reviewed in Schultz, 2005; Wolf et al., 2008). Importantly, the visual impairment is specific to people, as individuals with ASD are not impaired in other types of complex objects, such as buildings or furniture (Grelotti et al., 2002; Wolf et al., 2008). Face

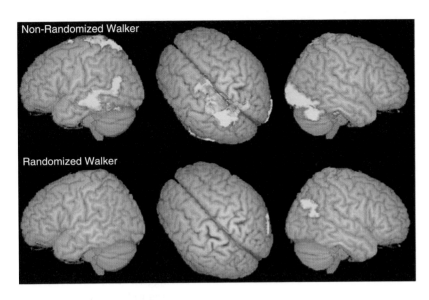

Non-Randomized Walker

Randomized Walker

Figure 36.1 Abnormal patterns of temporal lobe activity in ASD during the perception of a point-light walking figure. Areas of reduced brain activity among individuals with Asperger's Disorder during the randomized and fully coherent walking conditions. The statistical maps represent the comparison of brain activity between the two groups for the contrast of fully coherent walker versus fixation (top) and randomized walker vs. fixation (bottom). Activations in yellow represent clusters of activity that are significantly lower for the ASD group as compared to controls. The widespread decreases in temporal lobe activity for the ASD group appear for the fully coherent motion perception condition, and largely disappear for the randomized walker condition. Taken with permission from Herrington et al. (2007).

perception can be divided into the recognition of identity via structural facial features, and recognition of the affective state of another (independent of their identity) via the shape of individual features and dynamic changes in their relative distance. Both types of perception are necessary in navigating the social world, although they appear to be mediated by somewhat different systems. Person identification is critically dependent on portions of the fusiform gyrus (FG), an area on the underside of the temporal lobes (Kanwisher et al., 1997; Kanwisher, 2000; Puce et al., 1995). A medial portion of FG appears particularly responsive to faces processing; this area is typically referred to as the fusiform face area (FFA). In the first neuroimaging study of face recognition in ASD, we found selective hypoactivation of FG in ASD (Schultz et al., 2000). FG hypoactivation has now been replicated by 9 other labs (see Schultz and Robins, 2005).

Although the FG deficit is among the most established neurobiological findings in ASD, it remains unclear how this deficit develops. It is important to note that individuals with ASD not only show diminished face processing abilities, but are also generally less interested in attending to facial information (Klin et al., 2002; Sasson et al., 2008). Although interest and ability in certain skills would appear to be highly overlapping (e.g. those who are interested in knitting are likely to have above-average knitting skills), they are not reducible to one another, and may influence one another dynamically. Schultz (2005) proposed a model

whereby FG deficits in ASD arise from an initial decrease in the social and emotional salience of faces (which in turn stems from abnormalities in amygdala function). As a consequence, these individuals have less experience interpreting facial information, leaving areas involved in face computations underdeveloped. Ultimately, this leads to diminished social intelligence and awareness.

This model is supported primarily by findings reviewed in this chapter on FG, amygdala, and their connectivity. Unfortunately, the vast majority of these findings come from teenage samples or older, whereas the progression of amygdala-mediated salience to FG function likely begins in infancy, long before one generally receives an ASD diagnosis. This presents a formidable methodological challenge for research on person information processing deficits in ASD. Researchers are increasingly focusing on studies of brain structure among infants at elevated risk for ASD – those with an older sibling on the spectrum – in order to understand better the developmental origins of the social deficit. Although measures of functional brain activity remains largely out of reach for this age group, other measures such as eyetracking are gaining widespread prominence as tools to measure attentional biases at very young ages (for example, see Jones et al., 2008; Klin et al., 2009). In the future, these tools can be combined with structural MRI and diffusion tensor imaging (DTI) to get a more complete picture of what is happening in the brains of infants as ASD clinical symptoms emerge.

Superior temporal sulcus and the processing of faces and gestures

A large number of (mostly non-clinical) studies have established the role of superior temporal sulcus (STS) in various aspects of social perception. This area appears responsive to the perception of a variety of human movements, including limb motion, dynamic facial expression, and shifts in eye gaze (Adolphs, 2003; Allison et al., 2000; Haxby et al., 2000; Pelphrey et al., 2004; Robins et al., 2009; Thompson et al., 2007). As the STS receives inputs from numerous sensory and limbic/paralimbic areas, it has been conceptualized as an integration area for perceptual information (Barnes and Pandya, 1992; Milner, 2006; Oram and Perrett, 1996; Selzer and Pandya, 1994). In fact, STS is a key node of the "mirror neuron system" (MNS) – a network of structures implicated in imitation and social perception (discussed in more detail below).

Although these functions are of direct clinical relevance to ASD, few published functional imaging studies have tested for STS abnormalities in this population (see studies discussed in the MNS section of this chapter). However, MRI data on this topic are beginning to emerge. Using voxel-based morphometry, Boddaert et al. (2004) reported decreased STS gray matter concentration in ASD. Their data have recently been corroborated by Lee et al. (2007), who observed degradation in STS WM structure using multiple indices from DTI (FA, axial and radial diffusivity). Finally, although the recent sMRI study of Bigler et al. (2007) focuses on language processes (and not visual perception), their finding of diminished superior temporal gyrus structure in ASD constitutes further evidence for local abnormalities. Collectivity, these data have proven sufficient to lead some researchers to conclude that STS dysfunction plays a significant role in ASD symptoms (Redcay, 2008; Ziibovicius et al., 2006). Lastly, Herrington et al. (2007) observed decreased STS activity in ASD during human movement perception. More functional imaging studies are needed to clarify our understanding of STS function in ASD.

ASD and social intelligence

A central agenda in ASD brain imaging research has been the identification of brain regions involved in social functions. Many of these studies examine social intelligence from the perspective of "Theory of Mind" (ToM) – the ability to infer another's mental state (Baron-Cohen and Tager-Flusberg, 2000). Deficits in ToM are a cardinal characteristic of autism, distinguishing it from, for example, specific forms of mental retardation such as Williams Syndrome. There has always been some debate regarding the specificity and cognitive modularity of ToM (i.e. is ToM a distinct cognitive process, or does it emerge from numerous others, and if the latter, which?). As a case in point, the aforementioned data on FG in ASD could just as easily be included in this section. Nevertheless, some form or other of ToM plays a role in virtually every comprehensive account of the clinical profile of ASD, a role that is often considered distinct from established deficits in "lower-level" cognitive processes.

Ambiguities surrounding the cognitive specificity of ToM are at the center of MRI research of this topic, if not always explicitly addressed. In particular, there is considerable theoretical (and likely neural) overlap between the constructs of social intelligence and emotion. Many paradigms that tap ToM abilities do so via the identification of another person's emotional state. Take, for example, functional MRI (fMRI) studies of facial expression or eye gaze interpretation in ASD, such as Baron-Cohen et al. (1999; article chosen at random from many illustrating this point). Although conceived as a study of social functions, their data on abnormal amygdala function in ASD can just as easily be interpreted strictly in terms of emotion processes. Neurobiological studies of emotion have their own rich history, vocabulary, theoretical landscape (i.e. emotional identification versus emotional expression, versus emotional experience, versus emotion regulation, each putatively associated with distinct and overlapping brain areas). In studies such as that of Baron-Cohen et al. (1999), the invocation of emotion constructs does not directly challenge the utility of theories such as ToM; rather, they bring into focus a somewhat different set of theoretical questions. Perhaps foremost among them: to what extent are social skill deficits in ASD a consequence of a dysregulation of emotion processes, particularly those concerning emotion identification? Few studies have directly addressed this question. This is unfortunate, as studies on the neural correlates of ToM in ASD may prove highly revealing about the manner in which humans make contact with their social environments.

Amygdala

Research on the role of amygdala in social and emotional functions dates back more than a half-century (Kluver and Bucy, 1939). The evidence accumulated during this time points most clearly to an account of amygdala function that involves social and emotional surveillance (i.e. monitoring the environment for socially and emotionally salient information) and emotional experience (particularly negative affect and fear conditioning; see Zald, 2003).

Our understanding of the role of amygdala deficits in ASD has evolved considerably over the past decade. Decreased amygdala activity has been observed in ASD across multiple studies involving face or eye stimuli (Ashwin *et al.*, 2007; Baron-Cohen *et al.*, 1999; Critchley *et al.*, 2000; Dapretto *et al.*, 2006; Hadjikhani *et al.*, 2007; Pelphrey *et al.*, 2007; Pinkham *et al.*, 2008). These studies complement a handful of volumetric (Aylward *et al.*, 1999; Howard *et al.*, 2000; Juranek *et al.*, 2006) and post-mortem (Bailey *et al.*, 1998; Bauman and Kemper, 1994; Kemper and Bauman, 1998) studies showing amygdala anomalies in ASD (though there is some inconsistency among studies regarding the precise nature of the abnormality, e.g. larger or smaller volume). Indeed, the available data and theoretical compatibility of amygdala dysfunction accounts have led some to tie it closely with the core etiology of ASD (see Baron-Cohen *et al.*, 2000; Schultz *et al.*, 2000a).

However, amygdala accounts of ASD have proven less complete than they may appear. In particular, they leave unanswered some important questions about the status of emotion processes (both emotion perception and experience) in ASD. Numerous studies have associated *increased* amygdala function with negative affect in depression and anxiety (see Davidson *et al.*, 2002). Although most clinical accounts of the core ASD symptoms fail to mention depression and anxiety, there is growing recognition that individuals with ASD experience significantly elevated rates of both (Stewart *et al.*, 2006; Sukhodolsky *et al.*, 2008). This presents a sort of contradiction – on the one hand, individuals with ASD show signs of decreased amygdala activity (based on decreased social salience), and on the other hand, one might predict an increase (based on the presence of elevated negative affect).

Some attempts have been made to reconcile this discrepancy via the consideration of abnormal attention processes in ASD. Dalton *et al.* (2005) recently reported that amygdala signal in an ASD group during face perception was positively correlated with the amount of time spent fixating on the eyes. They argued that amygdala function in ASD may in fact be more intact than expected. Furthermore, they suggest that ASD participants in prior studies may have shown amygdala decreases not due to any fundamental neuropathology, but from inattention to, or possibly avoidance of, emotionally salient parts of their environment (e.g. the eyes; also see Dalton *et al.*, 2007).

Their findings warrant replication for multiple reasons. First, one aspect of this study has often been misunderstood; although fMRI and eye gaze data were collected simultaneously, they were not directly compared, as might be done via the use of eye gaze data as an explanatory variable in a whole-brain generalized linear model (GLM) analysis. Such an analysis would arguably be more robust in interpreting eye gaze/amygdala relationships. Second, participants were not characterized in terms of co-occurring mood or anxiety symptoms that might have affected amygdala function. Nevertheless, if replicated, their results will have a number of implications for future MRI studies on social information processes in ASD. Minimally, they draw attention to the importance of monitoring attentional resource allocation during ToM studies, to confirm that observed deficits are not merely a consequence of inattention. More broadly, it would shake up a number of assumptions about the subcortical (e.g. amygdala) pathogenesis of ASD that are frequently taken for granted.

At any rate, there remains a piece missing from the amygdala account of ASD: how to account for symptoms of negative affect and emotion dysregulation. Unfortunately, at present we can say little about how negative affect, ASD and amygdala function may be related, as almost no MRI studies of ASD formally measure depression or anxiety. One noteworthy exception is a recent study by Juranek *et al.* (2006) reporting a significant correlation between increased amygdala volume and a coarse measure of negative affect – the Externalizing subscale of the Child Behavior Checklist. It is possible that, rather than representing a broad ASD endophenotype, amygdala function may actually represent an important individual difference variable, capturing variance in both internal emotional experiences and in social–emotional contact with others.

Medial prefrontal cortex

Converging evidence from multiple experimental tasks and sensory domains points to a role for medial prefrontal cortex (mPFC) in aspects of ToM and perspective taking (see Schultz and Robins, 2005). Much of these data come from studies of ASD, where mPFC activity is typically decreased. Although studies vary, most localize this decrease to somewhere within Brodmann areas 8 or 9. For example, Gallagher et al. (2000) presented a sample of individuals with ASD and a control group a series of cartoons where the thoughts and intentions of specific characters had to be inferred. The ASD sample demonstrated decreased mPFC activity for those cartoons requiring mental state inferences, but not for control cartoons requiring non-mental state inferences.

An interesting line of research on ToM focuses on the tendency for most people to anthropomorphize objects and shapes that move in an apparently deliberate fashion. Evidence for this phenomenon originated with Heider and Simmel (1944), who created animations depicting geometric shapes moving in a manner that suggested specific gestures and emotions, such as aggression and playfulness. Klin (2000) developed an assessment around these videos, called the Social Attribution Task (SAT). He showed that individuals with ASD were less likely to make social inferences about these videos, and more likely to interpret them in strictly mechanistic ways.

Schultz et al. (2003) used a modified SAT to identify ToM brain areas in a non-clinical sample. As a control condition, participants observed the shapes moving in a non-interactive manner. They identified a number of areas showing increased activity during the social animation condition, including FG, STS, amygdala, and mPFC (these results were recently replicated by Vanderwal et al., 2008). In another study, Schultz et al. (2008; in preparation) show decreased activity in each of these areas in an ASD sample. Castelli et al. (2000, 2002) have also reported decreased mPFC activity in and ASD sample using a variation on the Heider and Simmel task.

Castelli et al. (2002) conclude that the mPFC, along with temporal areas, "can be considered the rudiments of the mentalizing network of the brain, independent of task and modality" (p. 1846). This conclusion alludes to an important topic among social neuroscientists in this field – the degree to which mPFC functions as a discrete module

subserving ToM, or instead implements some subordinate process that need not be specific to ToM at all. A few studies to date indicate that mPFC plays a role in social perspective-taking during the comprehension of verbal information. In one of the first mPFC studies on ASD, Fletcher et al. (1995) used brief social stories requiring inferences about different characters and events (presented as text on a screen; also see Happé et al., 1996). Similar stimuli were used by Gallagher et al. (2000) in a study using a non-clinical sample; they found increased mPFC activity during the social versus non-social story comprehension. Nieminen-Von Wendt et al. (2003) reported decreased mPFC activity in ASD during an aurally presented variation of Happé's social stories task.

Despite Castelli et al.'s conclusion and the aforementioned studies, the link between mPFC and ToM requires more refined cognitive theories about how individuals make social inferences. The convergence of data from both visual and language-based tasks lends some credence to the notion of ToM-specific functions, but it is less clear whether ToM deficits in ASD may be ancillary to other cognitive impairments, particularly with the domain of executive functions. In the words of Frith and Frith (2000), "there is clearly a need for more studies of patients with circumscribed lesions and for the development of test materials for which difficulties with mentalizing can be distinguished from more general problems of understanding" (p. 342).

ASD, imitation, and the mirror neuron system

There has recently been considerable speculation regarding the relationship between ASD symptoms and a constellation of brain areas referred to as the mirror neuron system (MNS). MNS has proven responsive to both the perception and implementation of specific body movements. Research in this area was pioneered by Gallese et al. (1996), who measured single cells in macaque area F5 (premotor cortex; the homolog of the human inferior frontal gyrus). They found that certain cells within F5 responded both when observing specific body movements and when implementing those same movements. Neurons with this "mirroring" property have also been identified in inferior parietal and superior temporal cortices (see Fogassi et al., 2005; Keysers and

Gazzola, 2006). Together, these three areas comprise what is typically regarded as the MNS. Human neuroimaging studies quickly followed the non-human primate work, homing in on an analogous set of brain structures.

Over the past decade there has been much speculation regarding the function and developmental trajectory of MNS. Numerous researchers have proposed that these cells may work together to process information regarding movements and gestures (Carr *et al.*, 2003, Dapretto *et al.*, 2006; Fogassi *et al.*, 2005; Gallese *et al.*, 2004). If so, this role has provocative implications for how people use their personal experience of movement to interpret other people's movements, and possibly vice versa (Hurley and Chater, 2005). More recently, scientists have begun to speculate that the MNS may play a role in the interpretation of social information (Rogers and Williams, 2006; Hurley and Chater, 2005).

If MNS does support social communication, it follows that it may function abnormally in ASD – as has indeed been proposed by a number of researchers (see Gallese, 2006). There are a growing number of electrophysiology and hemodynamic imaging papers supporting a link between ASD and abnormal MNS function (Bernier *et al.*, 2007; Dapretto *et al.*, 2006; Hadjikhani *et al.*, 2006; Nishitani *et al.*, 2004; Oberman *et al.*, 2005; Théoret *et al.*, 2005; Williams *et al.*, 2006). However, this is clearly a nascent area of inquiry, with critical questions remaining unanswered.

ASD studies aside, there are growing theoretical concerns about the precise function of MNS. Despite the numerous reports tying MNS functions to social understanding, almost no studies have robustly tested this. In a recent review of MNS and action understanding, Hickock (2009) argued MNS activity may reflect either a "pure Pavlovian association" or mere "sensory-motor pairings". Indeed, MNS studies typically involve passive perception or tasks that require decisions that have little or nothing to do with social understanding per se. Those tasks that may have a social perceptual component – such as facial expression perception – often involve static displays where task demands are minimal (as in Dapretto *et al.*, 2006). The lack of data on this topic leaves open the possibility that MNS activity may indeed be understandable as a sort of neural reflex, without any clear association with action understanding.

Herrington *et al.* (in preparation) recently addressed this issue by devising a task in which

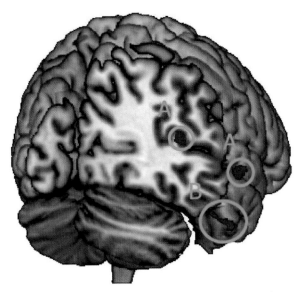

Figure 36.2 Accuracy on a human movement judgment task is associated with increased activity within Superior Temporal Sulcus (labeled A) and inferior temporal gyrus (labeled B). STS has proven responsive to a variety of human movements (see Puce and Perrett, 2003) and is counted among nodes of the "mirror neuron system" (Keysers and Gazzola, 2006). Taken with permission from Herrington *et al.* (in preparation).

responses to simple movement varied from trial to trial. Their study required participants to judge the direction in which a series of point-light figures were walking. The task was made challenging by perturbing the dot trajectories, deliberately inducing errors in participant responses. Although both the STS and inferior temporal gyrus (ITG) components of MNS were responsive to the walking figure condition (compared to a control stimulus), walking figure task accuracy predicted activation in STS but not ITG (see Figure 36.2). These data provide some of the first evidence directly linking MNS activity to the accurate perception of human actions, while also suggesting that MNS nodes might prove somewhat heterogeneous in this function.

A second limitation on MNS theory relates to the literature on imitation deficits in ASD. A key premise behind MNS theories of ASD concerns the role that childhood imitation plays in fostering the understanding of social gestures (see Rogers and Williams, 2006). A presumptive causal chain behind this premise starts with an MNS deficit, which leads to an imitation deficit, which ultimately inhibits social development and understanding. The difficulty with this causal chain is that the literature on imitation deficits in ASD is fairly equivocal – deficits emerge in some functional domains and not others, and may be restricted in large part to spontaneous imitation only (Rogers and Williams, 2006). Hamilton *et al.* (2007) illustrated this in a study using a variety of basic imitation tasks that were selected specifically for their relation to putative MNS functions. They found no performance differences among individuals with ASD on these tasks. On the other hand, Bernier *et al.* (2007) used a more challenging imitation measure and found robust imitation differences between ASD and control samples, which in turn predicted MNS activity. These studies ultimately point to the importance of identifying the specific parameters surrounding possible MNS abnormalities in ASD, including the influences of attention and motivation.

ASD and brain connectivity

The relatively high spatial resolution of MRI lends itself very well to the isolation of specific brain structures. However, a focus on localized structure and function may obscure emergent properties of cortical networks. ASD researchers using MRI have grown increasingly worried that, much like someone on a darkened street who looks for his missing keys exclusively under the nearest lamppost, researchers may rely too heavily on the most obvious uses of MRI technology. Future research on the neurobiology of ASD is more likely to prove fruitful if it is guided by the principles of the systems we hope to understand, and not the tools we use to understand them. These principles clearly favor the analysis of distributed cortical systems (Belmonte *et al.*, 2004a). MRI can measure such systems in multiple ways – namely, through sMRI and DTI-based measures of cortical volume and organization, and estimates of the interrelatedness of brain imaging signals across time.

Connectivity between fusiform gyrus, amygdala, and superior temporal gyrus

Two of the aforementioned brain areas – FG and amygdala – share extensive structural and functional connections (Amaral and Price, 1984). Their respective roles appear distinct but overlapping – whereas FG and STG/STS are tuned to the perception of distinct person identities, the amygdala serves as a rapid encoding system for emotionally arousing percepts, including expressions (see Zald, 2003). Their

independent roles have been emphasized in studies where individuals with FG lesions still remain capable of completing facial affect discriminating tasks (Tranel *et al.*, 1988; Wada and Yamamoto, 2001).

However, FG and amygdala appear functionally as well as structurally connected. We and others hypothesize that FG activity is enhanced by input from the amygdala (Morris *et al.*, 1998a, 1998b; Schultz, 2005; Vuilleumier *et al.*, 2004). Data in support of this hypothesis have come primarily from lesion studies (Anderson and Phelps, 2001; Vuilleumier *et al.*, 2004). To date, few experiments on this topic have used functional connectivity analyses (this represents an important next step in this line of research). We have found an increased correlation between amygdala and FG activity during a face identification task (relative to house identification) in a non-clinical sample (Schultz *et al.*, 2005). Furthermore, connectivity between FG and amygdala was significantly greater for control participants compared to an ASD sample.

Data on FG/amygdala connectivity are also beginning to emerge from DTI studies. Jou *et al.* (2007) compared fractional anisotrophy (FA) data from 10 individuals with ASD and 10 controls (matched for age and IQ). The ASD group showed decreased FA (indicating reduced WM integrity) along the corpus callosum (CC), superior longitudinal fasciculus (SLF), and inferior longitudinal fasciculus (ILF). As ILF connects FG and amygdala, an FA reduction in this area strongly suggests abnormal connectivity between these regions. Two other studies have provided evidence for abnormal FG/amygdala connectivity in ASD. Barnea-Goraly *et al.* (2004) reported reduced FA in an ASD sample along the medial temporal gyrus, directly adjacent to the FG. Although the authors do not provide tractography data on their sample, their cluster appears proximal to ILF and inferior fronto-occipital fasciculus. Also using FA, Keller *et al.* (2007) reported decreased WM integrity in the posterior limb of the right internal capsule. This area covers a number of WM tracts, including SLF and ILF.

Long-range connectivity

Converging evidence indicates that long-range connectivity is particularly susceptible in ASD. Numerous MRI studies suggest decreased corpus callosum (CC) integrity in ASD (Alexander *et al.*, 2007; Barnea-Goraly *et al.*, 2004; Herbert *et al.*, 2004; Jou *et al.*, 2007). The CC is a key communication channel between the two hemispheres, composed of large quantities of long-range fibers (Witelson, 1989). The implications of this abnormality are extremely broad, as numerous cognitive operations require the coordination of both hemispheres (see Banich, 2004). In a recent DTI study, Alexander *et al.* (2007) reported that increased radial diffusivity in CC (reflecting decreased WM organization) was inversely correlated with processing speed and overall performance on neuropsychological measures, though only for individuals with ASD. Radial diffusivity was also related to degree of social impairment, as measured by the Social Reciprocity Scale. CC abnormalities have also been indicated by fMRI. Just *et al.* (2004) measured brain activity during a sentence comprehension task, and found decreased inter-hemispheric connectivity between multiple language structures. Together, these findings make a strong case for CC abnormalities in ASD, though the degree to which such abnormalities are specific to ASD remains largely unknown.

Long-range connectivity abnormalities have also been identified within hemispheres. An early hemodynamic imaging (positron emission tomography; PET) study showed reduced inter-regional correlations in persons with autism, suggesting reduced functional integration and connectivity (Horwitz *et al.*, 1988). In recent years there have been at least six reports using fMRI that also find reduced levels of functional connectivity at longer distances. Just and colleagues have numerous papers showing that fMRI activation time series of widely spaced cortical processing nodes are less well synchronized in ASD (Cherkassky *et al.*, 2006; Just *et al.*, 2004, 2007; Kana *et al.*, 2006; Koshino *et al.*, 2005). Reduced long-range synchronization is also consistent with a prior PET study in autism during a theory of mind experiment (Castelli *et al.*, 2002).

These findings fit particularly well with the ASD clinical profile. Belmonte *et al.* (2004b) outline how the local/long-distance connection imbalance can result in the broad tuning of perceptual functions such that seemingly miniscule information in the environment ends up co-opting broader-band cognitive processes. In principle, the imbalance can encompass symptoms at multiple levels of analysis, from abnormal motion coherence thresholds to comorbid seizure disorders. The possible behavior manifestations appear consistent with weak central coherence theory, where resources that might be allocated to the holistic processing of stimuli or semantic meanings

are instead allocated to fragments of these (Belmonte *et al.*, 2004a; Frith, 1989).

Clearly, these findings warrant more detailed analysis. In particular, accounts of long- and short-range connectivity differences may ultimately prove too coarse – how precisely does one delineate and categorize these connections (e.g. "long" versus "short" range), and how well do the delineations conform to known processes of neuronal development? Are there particular long- and short-range systems that are affected, or do they vary from person to person, tracking individual differences in behavior? As described below, the answers to these questions will likely necessitate the more widespread use of sophisticated analytic approaches that can identify and distinguish between neural systems on multiple scales.

Neuroimaging studies of ASD: future directions

Despite two decades of brain imaging data, the field has yet to converge on specific, robust models of core ASD pathobiology – although several attractive candidate models described in this chapter can serve as a heuristic guide to future research. When reviewing these data, it is easy to become bewildered by the variety of brain structures and processes that have been identified, and the difficulty in determining which are etiological versus epiphenomenal. However, recent years have witnessed great strides in ASD model development – strides that bode well for the future prospects of identifying ASD biomarkers. In particular, the convergence of genetic, sMRI, fMRI and DTI data on WM abnormalities and connectivity disruption suggest that the field is learning how to fruitfully integrate data from multiple sources. Indeed, the pursuit of connectivity accounts of ASD is likely to feature prominently in the next decade of research.

This section concerns itself with areas in which the field of ASD brain research is likely to grow. Note the decidedly methodological thrust to this summary – it is our view that the future of this field lies in large part in the advancement of analytic techniques that can more effectively extract information from the complex signals provided by MRI.

Functional connectivity

It is important to note that fMRI signals have some inherent disadvantages with respect to connectivity measurement. While the typical sampling rate of fMRI is somewhat faster than changes in blood oxygenation, these changes are themselves orders of magnitude slower than the time-scale of connectivity between neurons. Nevertheless, the use of fMRI connectivity analyses has become increasingly widespread. The most straightforward analysis of connectivity continues to be multiple regression, where voxel-by-voxel activity is predicted by the interaction of an experimental task and a specific brain region of interest (Friston *et al.*, 1997). Although not without its complications, it is computationally equivalent to what is carried out in almost every fMRI study; we hope to see it used even more routinely in studies of ASD.

Although connectivity analyses promise to enrich our general understanding of brain function, it seems particularly well-suited to the study of ASD. Of particular interest is connectivity between nodes of the social brain, including amygdala, fusiform gyrus, superior temporal gyrus/sulcus, and portions of prefrontal cortex. Although the field of ASD research has played a critical role in expanding our understanding of what these brain areas do, very little is know about how they function vis-à-vis one another.

fMRI pattern analysis

Functional imaging analyses typically involve "massively univariate" statistics – the repeated application of GLM-based analyses predicting signal from individual voxels throughout the brain. Newer methods are emerging that can look at entire samples of voxels in a multivariate framework that may ultimately prove more sensitive and specific for categorizing ASD subtypes and symptoms. Some of these methods have already refined our understanding of modularity in the brain, particularly within visual cortex (Haxby *et al.*, 2000, 2001, 2002; Norman *et al.*, 2006). The work of Haxby *et al.* has shown that the "on" or "off" brain responses researchers typically report for basic fMRI cognitive tasks can be superimposed on more complex patterns of activity, where constellations of tissue that appear dedicated to one function actually play roles in other functions as well (see Norman *et al.*, 2006). Haxby's findings emerged from the application of pattern analysis to fMRI data. Pattern analysis involves the selection and weighting of a set of input "features" in the development of a

classification model. In the case of fMRI, input features are composed of a set of voxels chosen either a priori or by some other technique, such as traditional per-voxel GLM (although much more sophisticated feature selection procedures are available). The classification model is then validated by testing its validity and reliability in predicting subsequent observations (e.g. additional blocks of data within an fMRI run).

The relevance of this technique to ASD research comes into focus when one considers the pattern of findings on ventral stream abnormalities in ASD. Some evidence indicates that facial recognition deficits in ASD stem not from a lesion-like absence of FG function, but from a reallocation of FG and adjacent areas to other visual tasks in a manner that may ultimately prove inefficient (Grelotti *et al.*, 2005; Schultz *et al.*, 2000b). Pattern analysis appears particularly well-equipped to further test this hypothesis, although it has not yet been used in this way.

Multi-modal pattern analysis

The "features" that are submitted to pattern analysis need not consist entirely of data from any one imaging technique. A growing literature has used pattern classification to categorize individuals as belonging to specific clinical groups based on a combination of multiple indices derived from sMRI and/or DTI (Davatzikos *et al.*, 2008; Fan *et al.*, 2008; Verma *et al.*, 2008; Wang and Verma, unpublished data). A key advantage of this approach is that it is able to simultaneously select those channels and features (such as discrete brain areas) that maximally predict one's group membership (e.g. ASD or control). Data from fMRI (such as parameter estimate maps) can easily be included in this type of analysis. This technique may prove extremely useful in identifying the specific MRI modalities (fMRI, DTI, etc.) that capture the most relevant information about brain abnormalities in ASD.

The integration of genetics

Recent genetic advances suggest that abnormal intracellular communication may represent an endophenotype of ASD (Glessner *et al.*, 2009; Jamain *et al.*, 2003; O'Roak and State, 2008; Sebat, 2007; Wang *et al.*, in press). However, no ASD studies to date have combined genetics and MRI data.

Techniques have been developed that allow for the integration of fMRI data and large arrays of genetic information. Liu *et al.* (2009) used an approach called parallel independent component analysis (ICA) to isolate fMRI and single nucleotide polymorphism (SNP) factors that varied as a function of group (in their case, schizophrenia versus control). Their approach used independent components from the separate modalities to inform and constrain the calculation of final factors across both modalities. Their data isolated a subset of 10 SNPs and signal from a parietal lobe cluster that differed significantly between the groups. This type of analysis seems extremely well suited to research on the neurobiology of ASD, where numerous common and rare genetic variations are likely to play a role.

The spectra of individual differences

Throughout this chapter, the autism-spectrum disorders have often been treated as if they represented a unitary construct. This is clearly not the case (Geschwind, 2008). The three diagnoses that encompass ASD represent one particular clinical dimension; there are a great many others. The increasing use of the term ASD instead of actual (DSM-IV) diagnoses themselves reflects the profound ambiguity among autism researchers regarding what categories are suitable to capture the variety of presenting symptoms.

A key agenda of future research on ASD should be to use neuroimaging to further define the underlying dimensions of autism. For example, it may be that issues of general intelligence in ASD relate to abnormal long-range connectivity between structures and hemispheres, but that this very abnormality interacts with regional connections to enhance certain specific abilities (perhaps explaining savant skills). It is possible that this interaction is itself mediated by the superposition of specific genetic profiles within a given individual – one that influences long-range axonal development, and another that enhances local relationships between pyramidal cells. The important point here is not whether these particular speculations ought to be pursued (although we feel that this would prove fruitful), but rather, to illustrate that, rather than looking at single functions among small samples of individuals, neuroimaging studies of ASD will benefit from approaches that consider multiple aspects of the disorder simultaneously.

In an influential article on the study of environmental contributions to genetically mediated disorders, Rutter *et al.* (2001) highlighted the importance of designs that involve very large numbers of participants and research strategies, likely spanning multiple research sites. We would argue that the complexity of polygenetic conditions like autism, with numerous important loci and gene-by-gene interactions, indeed necessitates a large allocation of resources. Endeavors such as the Autism Genetic Resource Exchange (Geschwind *et al.*, 2001) reflect this growing necessity. As is often the case, the challenge becomes one of resource availability. In some respects, this pursuit has gotten much easier as technology and MRI availability have advanced – it is considerably quicker to acquire sMRI and DTI data than it was only a few years ago, and advances in computational power allow for much faster analysis throughput.

However, there is one area in which it is hard to imagine significant resource advances in the short term – the critical step of ASD phenotyping and diagnosis. Gold-standard research assessments on ASD minimally rely on the Autism Diagnostic Observation Schedule (Lord *et al.*, 2000) and the Autism Diagnostic Inventory – Revised (Lord *et al.*, 1994). Together, these instruments typically take 2–4 h to administer, and should be used to inform diagnosis by a clinical expert, an additional time and resource burden. When one adds to this numerous other dimensional measures of ASD symptomatology, the marginal time required by trained staff and clinicians often reaches two days or more. Add to this the resources required for broad participant recruitment, and the difficulty many individuals with developmental disabilities have laying still in an MRI machine for an hour or more, and large-scale imaging studies of ASD quickly seem daunting. Ultimately, multidimensional studies of ASDs will benefit greatly from widespread collaboration between scientists and labs.

Box 36.1. The key nodes of the "social brain"

- Amygdala
- Fusiform gyrus
- Superior temporal sulcus/gyrus
- Ventromedial prefrontal cortex (VMPFC)

Box 36.2. A hypothetical cascade: from genes to brain systems

Level of analysis	Findings
Genes	• Common and rare variants influencing synaptic development (Abrahams and Geschwind, 2008; Bucan *et al.*, 2009; Glessner *et al.*, 2009; Wang *et al.*, in press).
Neurons	• Abnormal minicolumn structure (Casanova *et al.*, 2002, 2006).
Pathways	• Broad patterns of increased white matter (Courchesne *et al.*, 2001; Herbert *et al.*, 2003).
	• Focal patterns of decreased white matter (e.g. corpus callosum; Chung *et al.*, 2004; Egass *et al.*, 1995; Piven *et al.*, 1997).
Brain connectivity	• Decreased long-range connectivity between neurons (Cherkassky *et al.*, 2006; Just *et al.*, 2004, 2007; Kana *et al.*, 2006; Koshino *et al.*, 2005).

References

Abrahams B S and Geschwind D H. 2008. Advances in autism genetics: On the threshold of a new neurobiology. *Nat Rev Genet* **9**, 341–55.

Adolphs R. 2003. Cognitive neuroscience of human social behaviour. *Nat Rev Neurosci* **4**, 165–78.

Alexander A L, Lee J E, Lazar M, *et al.* 2007. Diffusion tensor imaging of the corpus callosum in Autism. *Neuroimage* **34**, 61–73.

Allison T, Puce A, and McCarthy G. 2000. Social perception from visual cues: Role of the STS region. *Trends Cogn Sci* **4**, 267–78.

Amaral D G and Price J L. 1984. Amygdalo-cortical projections in the monkey (*Macaca fascicularis*). *J Comp Neurol* **230**, 465–96.

American Psychiatric Association. 2000. *Diagnostic and Statistical Manual of Mental Disorders DSM-IV-TR Fourth Edition (Text Revision)*. Washington, DC: American Psychiatric Association.

Anderson A K and Phelps E A. 2001. Lesions of the human amygdala impair enhanced perception of emotionally salient events. *Nature* **411**, 305–09.

Armstrong D D. 2001. Rett syndrome neuropathology review 2000. *Brain Dev* **23** (Suppl 1), S72–6.

Ashwin C, Baron-Cohen S, Wheelwright S, O'Riordan M and Bullmore E T. 2007. Differential activation of the amygdala and the "social brain" during fearful face-processing in Asperger Syndrome. *Neuropsychologia* **45**, 2–14.

Aylward E H, Minshew N J, Goldstein G, *et al.* 1999. MRI volumes of amygdala and hippocampus in non-mentally retarded autistic adolescents and adults. *Neurology* **53**, 2145–50.

Bailey A, Le Couteur A, Gottesman I, *et al.* 1995. Autism as a strongly genetic disorder: Evidence from a British twin study. *Psychol Med* **25**, 63–77.

Bailey A, Luthert P, Dean A, *et al.* 1998. A clinicopathological study of autism. *Brain* **121**, 889–905.

Bailey A, Phillips W and Rutter M. 1996. Autism: Towards an integration of clinical, genetic, neuropsychological, and neurobiological perspectives. *J Child Psychol Psychiatry All Discip* **37**, 89–126.

Banich M. 2004. *Cognitive Neuroscience and Neuropsychology*. Boston, MA: Houghton Mifflin,

Barlow H and Tripathy S P. 1997. Correspondence noise and signal pooling in the detection of coherent visual motion. *J Neurosci* **17**, 7954–66.

Barnea-Goraly N, Kwon H, Menon V, Eliez S, Lotspeich L and Reiss A L. 2004. White matter structure in autism: Preliminary evidence from diffusion tensor imaging. *Biol Psychiatry* **55**, 323–6.

Barnes C L and Pandya D N. 1992. Efferent cortical connections of multimodal cortex of the superior temporal sulcus in the rhesus monkey. *J Comp Neurol* **318**, 222–44.

Baron-Cohen S, Ring H A, Wheelwright S, *et al.* 1999. Social intelligence in the normal and autistic brain: An fMRI study. *Eur J Neurosci* **11**, 1891–8.

Baron-Cohen S, Ring H, Bullmore E, Wheelwright S, Ashwin C and Williams S. 2000. The amygdala theory of autism. *Neurosci Biobehav Rev* **24**, 355–64.

Baron-Cohen S and Tager-Flusberg H. 2000. *Understanding Other Minds: Perspectives from Developmental Cognitive Neuroscience*. New York: Oxford University Press, p. 530.

Bauman M and Kemper T. 1994. *The Neurobiology of Autism*. Baltimore, MD: Johns Hopkins University Press.

Belmonte M K, Cook E H, Anderson G M, *et al.* 2004a. Autism as a disorder of neural information processing: directions for research and targets for therapy. *Mol Psychiatry* **9**(7), 646–63.

Belmonte M K, Allen G, Beckel-Mitchener A, Boulanger L M, Carper R A and Webb S J. 2004b. Autism and abnormal development of brain connectivity. *J Neurosci* **24**, 9228–31.

Bernier R, Dawson G, Webb S and Murias M. 2007. EEG mu rhythm and imitation impairments in individuals with autism spectrum disorder. *Brain Cogn* **64**, 228–37.

Bertone A and Faubert J. 2006. Demonstrations of decreased sensitivity to complex motion information not enough to propose an autism-specific neural etiology. *J Autism Devptl Disord* **36**, 55–64.

Bertone A, Mottron L, Jelenic P and Faubert J. 2003. Motion perception in autism: A "complex" issue. *J Cogn Neurosci* **15**, 218–25.

Bigler E D, Mortensen S, Neeley E S, *et al.* 2007. Superior temporal gyrus, language function, and autism. *Devptl Neuropsychol* **31**, 217–38.

Boddaert N, Chabane N, Gervais H, *et al.* 2004. Superior temporal sulcus anatomical abnormalities in childhood autism: A voxel-based morphometry MRI study. *Neuroimage* **23**, 364–9.

Boddaert N, Belin P, Chabane N, *et al.* 2003. Perception of complex sounds: Abnormal pattern of cortical activation in autism. *Am J Psychiatry* **160**, 2057–60.

Bucan M, Abrahams B S, Wang K, *et al.* 2009. Genome-wide analyses of exonic copy number variants in a family-based study point to novel autism susceptibility genes. *PLoS Genet* **5**, e1000536.

Burmeister M, McInnis M G and Zöllner S. 2008. Psychiatric genetics: Progress amid controversy. *Nat Rev Genet* **9**, 527–40.

Carr L, Iacoboni M, Dubeau M, Mazziotta J C and Lenzi G L. 2003. Neural mechanisms of empathy in humans: A relay from neural systems for imitation to limbic areas. *Proc Natl Acad Sci U S A*, **100**, 5497–502.

Casanova M F, Buxhoeveden D P, Switala A E and Roy E. 2002. Minicolumnar pathology in autism. *Neurology* **58**, 428–32.

Casanova M F, van Kooten I A J, Switala A E, *et al.* 2006. Minicolumnar abnormalities in autism. *Acta Neuropathol* **112**, 287–303.

Castelli F, Happe F, Frith U and Frith C. 2000. Movement and mind: A functional imaging study of perception and interpretation of complex intentional movement patterns. *Neuroimage* **12**, 314–25.

Castelli F, Frith C, Happé F and Frith U. 2002. Autism, Asperger syndrome and brain mechanisms for the attribution of mental states to animated shapes. *Brain* **125**, 1839–49.

Cherkassky V L, Kana R K, Keller T A and Just M A. 2006. Functional connectivity in a baseline resting-state network in autism. *Neuroreport* **17**, 1687–90.

Chung M K, Dalton K M, Alexander A L and Davidson R J. 2004. Less white matter concentration in autism: 2D voxel-based morphometry. *Neuroimage* **23**, 242–51.

Colle L, Baron-Cohen S, Wheelwright S and van der Lely H K J. 2008. Narrative discourse in adults with high-functioning autism or Asperger syndrome. *J Autism Devptl Disord* **38**, 28–40.

Courchesne E, Karns C M, Davis H R, *et al.* 2001. Unusual brain growth patterns in early life in patients with autistic disorder: An MRI study. *Neurology* **57**, 245–54.

Cowey A, Campana G, Walsh V and Vaina L M. 2006. The role of human extra-striate visual areas V5/MT and V2/V3 in the perception of the direction of global motion: A transcranial magnetic stimulation study. *Exp Brain Res* **171**, 558–62.

Critchley H, Daly E, Bullmore E, *et al.* 2000. The functional neuroanatomy of social behaviour: Changes in cerebral blood flow when people with autistic disorder process facial expressions. *Brain* **123**, 2203–12.

Dakin S and Frith U. 2005. Vagaries of visual perception in autism. *Neuron* **48**, 497–507.

Dalton K M, Nacewicz B M, Alexander A L and Davidson R J. 2007. Gaze-fixation, brain activation, and amygdala volume in unaffected siblings of individuals with autism. *Biol Psychiatry* **61**, 512–20.

Dalton K M, Nacewicz B M, Johnstone T, *et al.* 2005. Gaze fixation and the neural circuitry of face processing in autism. *Nat Neurosci* **8**, 519–26.

Dapretto M, Davies M S, Pfeifer J H, *et al.* 2006. Understanding emotions in others: Mirror neuron dysfunction in children with autism spectrum disorders. *Nat Neurosci* **9**, 28–30.

Davatzikos C, Fan Y, Wu X, Shen D and Resnick S M. 2008. Detection of prodromal Alzheimer's disease via pattern classification of magnetic resonance imaging. *Neurobiol Aging* **29**, 514–23.

Davidson R, Lewis D, Alloy L, *et al.* 2002. Neural and behavioral substrates of mood and mood regulation. *Biol Psychiatry* **52**, 478–502.

Dumoulin S, Bittar R, Kabani N, *et al.* 2000. A new anatomical landmark for reliable identification of human area V5/MT: A quantitative analysis of sulcal patterning. *Cerebral Cortex* **10**, 454–63.

Egass B, Courchesne E and Saitoh O. 1995. Reduced size of corpus callosum in autism. *Arch Neurol* **52**, 794–801.

Fan Y, Batmanghelich N, Clark C M and Davatzikos C. 2008. Spatial patterns of brain atrophy in MCI patients, identified via high-dimensional pattern classification, predict subsequent cognitive decline. *Neuroimage* **39**, 1731–43.

Fletcher P, Happe F, Frith U, *et al.* 1995. Other minds in the brain: A functional imaging study of "theory of mind" in story comprehension. *Cognition* **57**, 109–28.

Fogassi L, Ferrari P F, Gesierich B, Rozzi S, Chersi F and Rizzolatti G. 2005. Parietal lobe: From action

531

organization to intention understanding. *Science* **308**, 662–7.

Friston K, Buechel C, Fink G, Morris J, Rolls E and Dolan R. 1997. Psychophysiological and modulatory interactions in neuroimaging. *Neuroimage* **6**, 218–29.

Frith C and Frith U. 2000. Understanding other minds: Perspectives from developmental cognitive neuroscience. In Baron-Cohen, S and Tager-Flusberg H (Eds.) *Understanding Other Minds: Perspectives from Developmental Cognitive Neuroscience* (2nd ed.). New York, NY: Oxford University Press, pp. 334–56.

Frith U. 1989. *Autism: Explaining the Enigma*. Oxford, UK: Basil Blackwell.

Gallagher H, Happe F, Brunswick N, Fletcher P, Frith U and Frith C. 2000. Reading the mind in cartoons and stories: An fMRI study of "theory of the mind" in verbal and nonverbal tasks. *Neuropsychologia* **38**, 11–21.

Gallese V. 2006. Intentional attunement: A neurophysiological perspective on social cognition and its disruption in autism. *Brain Res* **1079**, 15–24.

Gallese V, Fadiga L, Fogassi L and Rizzolatti G. 1996. Action recognition in the premotor cortex. *Brain* **119**, 593–609.

Gallese V, Keysers C and Rizzolatti G. 2004. A unifying view of the basis of social cognition. *Trends Cogn Sci* **8**, 396–403.

Geschwind D H. 2008. Autism: Many genes, common pathways? *Cell* **135**, 391–5.

Geschwind D H, Sowinski J, Lord C, *et al.* 2001. The autism genetic resource exchange: A resource for the study of autism and related neuropsychiatric conditions. *Am J Human Genet* **69**, 463–6.

Ghaziuddin M and Gerstein L. 1996. Pedantic speaking style differentiates Asperger syndrome from high-functioning autism. *J Autism Devptl Disord* **26**, 585–95.

Glessner J T, Wang K, Cai G, *et al.* 2009. Autism genome-wide copy number variation reveals ubiquitin and neuronal genes. *Nature* **459**, 569–73.

Grelotti D, Gauthier I and Schultz R. 2002. Social interest and the development of cortical face specialization: What autism teaches us about face processing. *Devptl Psychobiol* **40**, 213–25.

Grelotti D J, Klin A J, Gauthier I, *et al.* 2005. fMRI activation of the fusiform gyrus and amygdala to cartoon characters but not to faces in a boy with autism. *Neuropsychologia* **43**, 373–85.

Groen W B, Zwiers M P, van der Gaag R and Buitelaar J K. 2008. The phenotype and neural correlates of language in autism: An integrative review. *Neurosci Biobehav Rev* **32**, 1416–25.

Hadjikhani N, Joseph R M, Snyder J and Tager-Flusberg H. 2006. Anatomical differences in the mirror neuron system and social cognition network in autism. *Cerebral Cortex* **16**, 1276–82.

Hadjikhani N, Joseph R M, Snyder J, and Tager-Flusberg H. 2007. Abnormal activation of the social brain during face perception in autism. *Hum Brain Mapp* **28**, 441–9.

Hamilton A F D C, Brindley R M and Frith U. 2007. Imitation and action understanding in autistic spectrum disorders: How valid is the hypothesis of a deficit in the mirror neuron system? *Neuropsychologia* **45**, 1859–68.

Happe F, Ehlers S, Fletcher P, *et al.* 1996. "Theory of mind" in the brain: Evidence from a PET scan study of Asperger syndrome. *Neuroreport* **8**, 197–201.

Haxby J, Hoffman E and Gobbini M. 2000. The distributed human neural system for face perception. *Trends Cogn Sci* **4**, 223–33.

Haxby J, Gobbini M, Furey M, Ishai A, Schouten J and Pietrini P. 2001. Distributed and overlapping representations of faces and objects in ventral temporal cortex. *Science* **293**, 2425–30.

Haxby J, Hoffman E and Gobbini M. 2002. Human neural systems for face recognition and social communication. *Biol Psychiatry* **51**, 59–67.

Hazlett H C, Poe M, Gerig G, *et al.* 2005. Magnetic resonance imaging and head circumference study of brain size in autism: Birth through age 2 years. *Arch Gen Psychiatry* **62**, 1366–76.

Heider F and Simmel M. 1944. An experimental study of apparent behavior. *Am J Psychol* **57**, 243–59.

Herbert M R, Harris G J, Adrien K T, *et al.* 2002. Abnormal asymmetry in language association cortex in autism. *Ann Neurol* **52**, 588–96.

Herbert M R, Ziegler D A, Deutsch C K, *et al.* 2003. Dissociations of cerebral cortex, subcortical and cerebral white matter volumes in autistic boys. *Brain J Neurol* **126**, 1182–92.

Herbert M R, Ziegler D A, Makris N, *et al.* 2004. Localization of white matter volume increase in autism and developmental language disorder. *Ann Neurol* **55**, 530–40.

Herrington J D, Baron-Cohen S, Wheelwright S J, *et al.* 2007. The role of MT+/V5 during biological motion perception in Asperger Syndrome: An fMRI study. *Res Autism Spectr Disord* **1**, 14–27.

Herrington J, Nymberg C and Schultz R T. In preparation. Biological motion task performance predicts superior temporal sulcus activity.

Hickok G. 2009. Eight problems for the mirror neuron theory of action understanding in monkeys and humans. *J Cogn Neurosci* **21**, 1229–43.

Hobson R P and Bishop M. 2003. The pathogenesis of autism: Insights from congenital blindness. *Phil Trans R Soc Lond Series B Biol Sci* **358**, 335–44.

Horwitz B, Rumsey J M, Grady C L and Rapoport S I. 1988. The cerebral metabolic landscape in autism. Intercorrelations of regional glucose utilization. *Arch Neurol* **45**, 749–55.

Howard M A, Cowell P E, Boucher J, *et al.* 2000. Convergent neuroanatomical and behavioural evidence of an amygdala hypothesis of autism. *Neuroreport* **11**, 2931–5.

Hurley S and Chater N. 2005. *Perspectives on Imitation: From Neuroscience to Social Science (Vol. 1)*. Cambridge, MA: MIT Press.

Jamain S, Quach H, Betancur C, *et al.* 2003. Mutations of the X-linked genes encoding neuroligins NLGN3 and NLGN4 are associated with autism. *Nat Genet* **34**, 27–9.

Johansson G. 1973. Visual perception of biological motion and a model for its analysis. *Percept Psychophys* **14**, 201–11.

Jones W, Carr K and Klin A. 2008. Absence of preferential looking to the eyes of approaching adults predicts level of social disability in 2-year-old toddlers with autism spectrum disorder. *Arch Gen Psychiatry* **65**, 946–54.

Jorde L B, Hasstedt S J, Ritvo E R, *et al.* 1991. Complex segregation analysis of autism. *Am J Human Genet* **49**, 932–8.

Jou R, Paterson S, Jackowski A, *et al.* 2007. Abnormalities in white matter structure in autism spectrum disorders detected by diffusion tensor imaging. *Biol Psychiatry* **61**, 217S.

Juranek J, Filipek P A, Berenji G R, Modahl C, Osann K and Spence M A. 2006. Association between amygdala volume and anxiety level: Magnetic resonance imaging (MRI) study in autistic children. *J Child Neurol* **21**, 1051–8.

Just M A, Cherkassky V L, Keller T A, Kana R K and Minshew N J. 2007. Functional and anatomical cortical underconnectivity in autism: Evidence from an FMRI study of an executive function task and corpus callosum morphometry. *Cerebral Cortex* **17**, 951–61.

Just M A, Cherkassky V L, Keller T A and Minshew N J. 2004. Cortical activation and synchronization during sentence comprehension in high-functioning autism: Evidence of underconnectivity. *Brain J Neurol* **127**, 1811–21.

Kana R K, Keller T A, Cherkassky V L, Minshew N J and Just M A. 2006. Sentence comprehension in autism: Thinking in pictures with decreased functional connectivity. *Brain J Neurol* **129**, 2484–93.

Kanner L. 1943. Autistic disturbances of affective contact. *Nerv Child* **2**, 217–50.

Kanwisher N. 2000. Domain specificity in face perception. *Nat Neurosci* **3**, 759–63.

Kanwisher N, McDermott J and Chun M. 1997. The fusiform face area: A module in human extrastriate cortex specialized for face perception. *J Neurosci* **17**, 4302–11.

Keller T A, Kana R K and Just M A. 2007. A developmental study of the structural integrity of white matter in autism. *Neuroreport* **18**, 23–7.

Kemper T L and Bauman M. 1998. Neuropathology of infantile autism. *J Neuropathol Exp Neurol* **57**, 645–52.

Keysers C and Gazzola V. 2006. Towards a unifying neural theory of social cognition. *Progr Brain Res* **156**, 379–401.

Kjelgaard M M and Tager-Flusberg H. 2001. An investigation of language impairment in autism: implications for genetic subgroups. *Lang Cogn Proc* **16**, 287–308.

Klin A. 2000. Attributing social meaning to ambiguous visual stimuli in higher-functioning autism and Asperger syndrome: The Social Attribution Task. *J Child Psychol Psychiatry All Disc* **41**, 831–46.

Klin A, Jones W, Schultz R, Volkmar F and Cohen D. 2002. Defining and quantifying the social phenotype in autism. *Am J Psychiatry* **159**, 909–16.

Klin A, Lin D J, Gorrindo P, Ramsay G and Jones W. 2009. Two-year-olds with autism orient to non-social contingencies rather than biological motion. *Nature* **459**, 257–61.

Kluver H and Bucy P. 1939. Preliminary analysis of functions of the temporal lobes in monkeys. *Arch Neurol Psychiatry* **42**, 979–1000.

Koshino H, Carpenter P A, Minshew N J, Cherkassky V L, Keller T A and Just M A. 2005. Functional connectivity in an fMRI working memory task in high-functioning autism. *Neuroimage* **24**, 810–21.

Lainhart J E. 2006. Advances in autism neuroimaging research for the clinician and geneticist. *Am J Med Genet Part C Semin Med Genet*, **142C**, 33–9.

Lee J E, Bigler E D, Alexander A L, *et al.* 2007. Diffusion tensor imaging of white matter in the superior temporal gyrus and temporal stem in autism. *Neurosci Lett* **424**, 127–32.

Liu J, Pearlson G, Windemuth A, Ruano G, Perrone-Bizzozero N I and Calhoun V. 2009. Combining fMRI and SNP data to investigate connections between brain function and genetics using parallel ICA. *Hum Brain Mapp* **30**, 241–55.

Lord C, Risi S, Lambrecht L, *et al.* 2000. The autism diagnostic observation schedule-generic: A standard measure of social and communication deficits associated with the spectrum of autism. *J Autism Devptl Disord* **30**, 205–23.

Lord C, Rutter M and Le Couteur A. 1994. Autism Diagnostic Interview-Revised: A revised version of a diagnostic interview for caregivers of individuals with possible pervasive developmental disorders. *J Autism Devptl Disord* **24**, 659–85.

Milner A D. 2006. *The Visual Brain in Action* (2nd ed.). Oxford, UK: Oxford University Press.

Morris J, Friston K, Buchel C, *et al.* 1998a. A neuromodulatory role for the human amygdala in processing emotional facial expressions. *Brain* **121**, 47–57.

Morris J, Ohman A and Dolan R. 1998b. Conscious and unconscious emotional learning in the human amygdala. *Nature* **393**, 467–70.

Morris J, Ohman A and Dolan R. 1999. A subcortical pathway to the right amygdala mediating "unseen" fear. *Proc Natl Acad Sci U S A* **96**, 1680–5.

Müller R A, Behen M E, Rothermel R D, *et al.* 1999. Brain mapping of language and auditory perception in high-functioning autistic adults: A PET study. *J Autism Devptl Disord* **29**, 19–31.

Newsome W and Pare E. 1988. A selective impairment of motion perception following lesions of the middle temporal visual area (MT). *J Neurosci* **8**, 2201–11.

Nieminen-von Wendt T, Metsähonkala L, Kulomäki T, *et al.* 2003. Changes in cerebral blood flow in Asperger syndrome during theory of mind tasks presented by the auditory route. *Eur Child Adolesc Psychiatry* **12**, 178–89.

Nishitani N, Avikainen S and Hari R. 2004. Abnormal imitation-related cortical activation sequences in Asperger's syndrome. *Ann Neurol* **55**, 558–62.

Norman K A, Polyn S M, Detre G J and Haxby J V. 2006. Beyond mind-reading: multi-voxel pattern analysis of fMRI data. *Trends Cogn Sci* **10**, 424–30.

Oberman L M, Hubbard E M, McCleery J P, Altschuler E L, Ramachandran V S and Pineda J A. 2005. EEG evidence for mirror neuron dysfunction in autism spectrum disorders. *Cogn Brain Res* **24**, 190–8.

Oram M W and Perrett D I. 1996. Integration of form and motion in the anterior superior temporal polysensory area (STPa) of the Macaque monkey. *J Neurophysiol* **76**, 109–29.

O'Roak B J and State M W. 2008. Autism genetics: Strategies, challenges, and opportunities. *Autism Res Off J Int Soc Autism Res* **1**, 4–17.

Pellicano E and Gibson L Y. 2008. Investigating the functional integrity of the dorsal visual pathway in autism and dyslexia. *Neuropsychologia* **46**, 2593–6.

Pellicano E, Gibson L, Maybery M, Durkin K, and Badcock D R. 2005. Abnormal global processing along the dorsal visual pathway in autism: A possible mechanism for weak visuospatial coherence? *Neuropsychologia* **43**, 1044–53.

Pelphrey K A, Morris J P, McCarthy G and Labar K S. 2007. Perception of dynamic changes in facial affect and identity in autism. *Soc Cogn Affect Neurosci* **2**, 140–9.

Pelphrey K A, Viola R J and McCarthy G. 2004. When strangers pass: Processing of mutual and averted social gaze in the superior temporal sulcus. *Psycholog Sci* **15**, 598–603.

Pinkham A E, Hopfinger J B, Pelphrey K A, Piven J and Penn D L. 2008. Neural bases for impaired social cognition in schizophrenia and autism spectrum disorders. *Schizophr Res* **99**, 164–75.

Piven J, Arndt S, Bailey J, Havercamp S, Andreasen N C and Palmer P. 1995. An MRI study of brain size in autism. *Am J Psychiatry* **152**, 1145–9.

Piven J, Palmer P, Jacobi D, Childress D and Arndt S. 1997. Broader autism phenotype: Evidence from a family history study of multiple-incidence autism families. *Am J Psychiatry* **154**, 185–90.

Puce A, Allison T, Gore J C and McCarthy G. 1995. Face-sensitive regions in human extrastriate cortex studied by functional MRI. *J Neurophysiol* **74**, 1192–9.

Puce A and Perrett D. 2003. Electrophysiology and brain imaging of biological motion. *Phil Trans R Soc Lond Series B Biol Sci* **358**, 435–45.

Redcay E. 2008. The superior temporal sulcus performs a common function for social and speech perception: Implications for the emergence of autism. *Neurosci Biobehav Rev* **32**, 123–42.

Redcay E and Courchesne E. 2005. When is the brain enlarged in autism? A meta-analysis of all brain size reports. *Biol Psychiatry* **58**, 1–9.

Ringo J L. 1991. Neuronal interconnection as a function of brain size. *Brain Behav Evol* **38**, 1–6.

Robins D L, Hunyadi E and Schultz R T. 2009. Superior temporal activation in response to dynamic audio-visual emotional cues. *Brain Cogn* **69**, 269–78.

Rogers S and Williams J G. 2006. *Imitation and the Social Mind: Autism and Typical Development*. New York, NY: Guilford Press.

Rutter M, Pickles A, Murray R and Eaves L. 2001. Testing hypotheses on specific environmental causal effects on behavior. *Psychol Bull* **127**, 291–324.

Sasson N J, Turner-Brown L M, Holtzclaw T N, Lam K S L and Bodfish J W. 2008. Children with autism demonstrate circumscribed attention during passive viewing of complex social and nonsocial picture arrays. *Autism Res* **1**, 31–42.

Schultz R T. 2005. Developmental deficits in social perception in autism: The role of the amygdala and fusiform face area. *Int J Devptl Neurosci* **23**, 125–41.

Schultz R T, Gauthier I, Klin A, *et al.* 2000b. Abnormal ventral temporal cortical activity during face discrimination among individuals with autism and Asperger syndrome. *Arch Gen Psychiatry* **57**, 331–40.

Schultz R T, Grelotti D, Klin A, *et al.* 2003. The role of the fusiform face area in social cognition: Implications for the pathobiology of autism. *Phil Trans R Soc London B* **358**, 415–27.

Schultz R T, Grupe D W, Hunyadi E, Jones W, Wolf J M and Hoyt E. 2008. *The Effect of Task Differences on FFA Activity in Autism Spectrum Disorders.* Paper Presented at the International Meeting for Autism Research, London, UK, May 2008.

Schultz R T, Hunyadi E, Conners C and Pasley B. 2005. *fMRI Study of Facial Expression Perception in Autism: The Amygdala, Fusiform Face Area and their Functional Connectivity.* Paper presented at the annual meeting of the Organization for Human Brain Mapping, 12–16 June 2005.

Schultz R T and Robins D. 2005. Functional neuroimaging studies of autism spectrum disorders. In Volkmar F, Klin A (Eds.), *Handbook of Autism and Pervasive Developmental Disorders* (3rd ed.). New York, NY: John Wiley and Sons. pp. 515–22.

Schultz R T, Romanski L M and Tsatsanis K D. 2000a. Neurofunctional models of autistic disorder and Asperger syndrome: Clues from neuroimaging. In Klin A, Volkmar F, Sparrow S (Eds.), *Asperger Syndrome.* New York, NY: Guilford Press, pp. 172–209.

Sebat J. 2007. Major changes in our DNA lead to major changes in our thinking. *Nat Genet* **39** (7 Suppl), S3–5.

Seltzer B and Pandya D N. 1994. Parietal, temporal, and occipital projections to cortex of the superior temporal sulcus in the rhesus monkey: A retrograde tracer study. *J Comp Neurol* **343**, 445–63.

Shah A and Frith U. 1983. An islet of ability in autistic children: A research note. *J Child Psychol Psychiatry All Discip* **24**, 613–20.

Shah A and Frith U. 1993. Why do autistic individuals show superior performance on the block design task? *J Child Psychol Psychiatry All Discip* **34**, 1351–64.

Stewart M E, Barnard L, Pearson J, Hasan R and O'Brien G. 2006. Presentation of depression in autism and Asperger syndrome: A review. *Autism Int J Res Pract* **10**, 103–16.

Sukhodolsky D G, Scahill L, Gadow K D, *et al.* 2008. Parent-rated anxiety symptoms in children with pervasive developmental disorders: Frequency and association with core autism symptoms and cognitive functioning. *J Abnorm Child Psychol* **36**, 117–28.

Tager-Flusberg H, Paul R and Lord C. 2005. Language and communication in autism. In: Volkmar F, Klin A (Eds.) *Handbook of Autism and Pervasive Developmental Disorders* (3rd ed.). New York, NY: John Wiley and Sons, pp. 335–64.

Théoret H, Halligan E, Kobayashi M, Fregni F, Tager-Flusberg H and Pascual-Leone A. 2005. Impaired motor facilitation during action observation in individuals with autism spectrum disorder. *Curr Biol* **15**, R84–5.

Thompson J C, Hardee J E, Panayiotou A, Crewther D and Puce A. 2007. Common and distinct brain activation to viewing dynamic sequences of face and hand movements. *Neuroimage* **37**, 966–73.

Tranel D, Damasio A R and Damasio H. 1988. Intact recognition of facial expression, gender, and age in patients with impaired recognition of face identity. *Neurology* **38**, 690–6.

Vanderwal T, Hunyadi E, Grupe D W, Connors C M and Schultz R T. 2008. Self, mother and abstract other: An fMRI study of reflective social processing. *Neuroimage* **41**, 1437–46.

Verma R, Zacharaki E I, Ou Y, *et al.* 2008. Multiparametric tissue characterization of brain neoplasms and their recurrence using pattern classification of MR images. *Acad Radiol* **15**, 966–77.

Volkmar F R, Paul R, Klin A and Cohen D. 2005. *Handbook of Autism and Pervasive Developmental Disorders, Vol. 1: Diagnosis, Development, Neurobiology, and Behavior.* Hoboken, NJ: John Wiley and Sons.

Vuilleumier P, Richardson M P, Armony J L, Driver J and Dolan R J. 2004. Distant influences of amygdala lesion on visual cortical activation during emotional face processing. *Nat Neurosci* **7**, 1271–8.

Wada Y and Yamamoto T. 2001. Selective impairment of facial recognition due to a haematoma restricted to the right fusiform and lateral occipital region. *J Neurol Neurosurg Psychiatry* **71**, 254–7.

Wang K, Zhang H, Bucan M, *et al.* 2009. Common genetic variation in the intergenic region between CDH10 and CDH9 is associated with susceptibility to autism spectrum disorders. *Nature* **459**, 528–33.

Williams J H G, Waiter G D, Gilchrist A, Perrett D I, Murray A D and Whiten A. 2006. Neural mechanisms of imitation and 'mirror neuron' functioning in autistic spectrum disorder. *Neuropsychologia* **44**, 610–21.

Witelson S F. 1989. Hand and sex differences in the isthmus and genu of the human corpus callosum. A postmortem morphological study. *Brain* **112**, 799–835.

Wolf J M, Tanaka J W, Klaiman C, *et al.* 2008. Specific impairment of face-processing abilities in children with autism spectrum disorder using the Let's Face It! skills battery. *Autism Res* **1**, 329–40.

Zald D. 2003. The human amygdala and the emotional evaluation of sensory stimuli. *Brain Res Rev* **41**, 88–123.

Zilbovicius M, Meresse I, Chabane N, Brunelle F, Samson Y and Boddaert N. 2006. Autism, the superior temporal sulcus and social perception. *Trends Neurosci* **29**, 359–66.

Endnote

1. For discussions of the neurobiology of Rett Syndrome, see Armstrong (2000). The other (and final) Pervasive Development Disorder not discussed here is Childhood Disintegrative Disorder (CDD). Almost no neuroimaging studies of the disorder have been carried out on CDD, likely due to ongoing concerns about the nosology and construct validity of the disorder.

Chapter 37

Neuroimaging of Williams–Beuren syndrome

Andreia Santos and Andreas Meyer-Lindenberg

Introduction

In the last decades, studying genetic neuropsychiatric syndromes at multiple levels has proven to be a powerful means for elucidating the pathways of both typical and atypical neurodevelopment. Within this context, Williams–Beuren syndrome, or Williams syndrome (WS) for short, has been established as model syndrome of special interest to investigate gene–brain–behavior relationships and a "unique window to genetic contributions to neural function" (Meyer-Lindenberg *et al.*, 2006, p. 391).

WS is a relatively rare neurodevelopmental disorder characterized by a combination of distinctive clinical, cognitive, behavioral, genetic and neuroanatomical features. It was first described in the early 1960s by two groups of cardiologists as a condition involving a constellation of cardiovascular abnormalities, hypercalcemia, peculiar facial "elfin-like" features, and mild to moderate mental retardation (Beuren *et al.*, 1962; Williams *et al.*, 1961).

Insights into the nature of WS culminated in the mid 1990s with the identification of the genetic cause, a so-called microdeletion (see below, Genetic profile). Since then, several neuroimaging studies, using a wide range of new imaging techniques, have attempted to uncover the structural and functional neural substrates of WS, providing an emerging understanding of brain mechanisms mediating between genetic variation and cognitive-behavioral phenotypes in humans.

The aim of this chapter is to review imaging studies delineating the unique neuropsychiatric features of WS, as well as recent advances in investigating the neural substrates of the disorder, which have provided significant contributions to unraveling the impact of a specific genetic defect on brain structure and function.

Williams syndrome – an "odd" syndrome

Clinical profile

WS is a genetic disorder caused by a hemideletion on chromosome 7 (see further details below). Its estimated prevalence ranges from 1 in 20,000 (Morris *et al.*, 1988) to 1 in 7500 (Strømme *et al.*, 2002) live births, which means that WS could account for 6% of all cases of mental retardation of genetic origin (Strømme *et al.*, 2002).

Clinical features of WS include a typical craniofacial dysmorphology (e.g. pouting lips, wide mouth, spaced teeth, broad brow, full cheeks, short upturned nose, flat nasal bridge, full nasal tip; Hammond *et al.*, 2005), growth retardation, and cardiovascular abnormalities, such as supravalvular aortic stenosis (present in ~80% of individuals with WS) and a narrowing of the aorta (AAP, 2001). Furthermore, individuals with WS often present several neurological symptoms, including hyperreflexia, visual symptoms (e.g. strabismus, nystagmus; Chapman *et al.*, 1996; Morris, 2006), hearing abnormalities (e.g. abnormal sensitivities to classes of sounds (hyperacusis); fearfulness to specific sounds (auditory allodynia); sensorineural hearing loss; Cherniske *et al.*, 2004; Levitin *et al.*, 2005; Marler *et al.*, 2005) and coordination difficulties (e.g. trouble walking down a staircase). Endocrine (e.g. transient hypercalcemia and impaired glucose tolerance), gastrointestinal (e.g. constipation, prolapse and diverticula), and orthopedic (e.g. scoliosis or joint contractures) symptoms are also commonly reported in WS (Morris, 2006), together with connective tissue disorders, failure to thrive in infancy and premature aging (Korenberg *et al.*, 2008; Morris and Mervis, 2000).

Understanding Neuropsychiatric Disorders, ed. M. E. Shenton and B. I. Turetsky. Published by Cambridge University Press.
© Cambridge University Press 2011.

Of central interest for neuropsychology, psychiatry and therefore, in the end, neuroimaging, the WS deletion further results in an array of cognitive and behavioral abnormalities, which have attracted a great deal of research over the past decades.

Behavioral profile

The hallmark of WS behavior is undoubtedly their high sociability. Most of the individuals with WS exhibit an intriguing mix of social attributes. From early development they are unusually friendly, interact easily and show no fear of strangers (e.g. Jones et al., 2000). They also appear highly empathetic (Klein-Tasman and Mervis, 2003) and show enhanced emotional empathy relative to other developmentally delayed individuals (Tager-Flusberg and Sullivan, 2000). Finally, they tend to be socially fearless and extremely outgoing to the point of being called hypersociable (e.g. Jones et al., 2000). For a long time, this notion of hypersociability and the idea of an "intact" social "module" in WS prevailed (e.g. Bellugi et al., 1994; Karmiloff-Smith et al., 1995). This was believed to underlie strengths in specific domains such as face processing, language and theory of mind (e.g. Karmiloff-Smith et al., 1995). Yet, the panorama is not always that positive and clear, since the social fearlessness and gregariousness of individuals with WS goes along with notable deficiencies in the pragmatic aspects of social behavior. For instance, individuals with WS show substantial problems in social adjustment (Gosch and Pankau, 1994), poor social judgment (Einfield et al., 1997; Gosch and Pankau, 1997) and social decision-making (Fidler et al., 2007), and they tend to be socially isolated in the school environment (Udwin and Yule, 1991). As a consequence, their social behavior is often maladapted and characterized by overfriendliness, oversensivity and poor peer relations (e.g. Laing et al., 2002). Although sociability, empathy and overfriendliness are integral features of WS, such data challenge the assumption that sociability is a unitary trait entirely spared in WS.

In remarkable contrast to the absent social fear, pervasive, intense and persistent non-social fears (e.g. Blomberg et al., 2006), anticipatory anxiety, and specific phobias are often described in individuals with WS (Dykens, 2003; Einfield et al., 1997) but are not, in themselves, unique to the WS behavioral phenotype, since they also be found in individuals with other disorders that result in mental retardation (e.g. VanLieshout et al., 1998). The intensity of these symptoms varies significantly across individuals. Some WS individuals may be "on edge", uneasy, or worried, whereas others may be beset with phobias and panic attacks (Scheiber, 2000). Attention deficit hyperactivity disorder (ADHD, predominantly inattentive type or combined type) is also common (>50%) in children and adolescents with WS (Leyfer et al., 2006).

While the WS behavioral profile concerns overt behavior, the WS cognitive profile concerns the cognitive processes underlying the overt behavior. This distinction is important as different cognitive processes may underlie similar behavioral expressions (Karmiloff-Smith, 1998).

Cognitive profile

The WS cognitive profile is characterized by co-existing strengths and deficits – not only between (e.g. verbal and visuospatial) but also within (e.g. visuoperceptual and visuoconstructive) domains.

A fundamental stable phenotype in WS is a severe visuospatial construction deficit, which concerns the inability to construct a whole from parts, such as in a puzzle. The most impaired performance is clinically observed on block design (Wechsler scales, see below) and drawing tasks (Bellugi et al., 1988; Mervis et al., 1999). Performance on such tasks is characterized by a lack of global organization: individual elements are not integrated accurately into the global form (Bellugi et al., 1988). By contrast, at the level of visuo-perception, the WS pattern of global and local processing resembles that of typically developing controls (Deruelle et al., 2006; Farran et al., 2001, 2003; Rondan et al., 2008). Surprisingly, weakness in visuoconstructive, visuomotor and visuospatial working memory tasks (Atkinson et al., 2001; Bellugi et al., 2000; Farran et al., 2003) contrasts with near-normal abilities to identify objects and faces (e.g. Landau et al., 2006; Paul et al., 2002; Tager-Flusberg et al., 2003; Wang et al., 1995).

In contradistinction, it was proposed until recently that language abilities are relatively spared in WS. Relative strengths in lexical development (Bello et al., 2004), verbal working memory (Jarrold et al., 1998; Vicari et al., 1996; Wang and Bellugi, 1994), socially engaging use of prosody, discourse and narrative skills (Karmiloff-Smith et al., 1995; Reilly et al., 2004) seem all to have served to augment an overall impression of linguistic strength (for a critical review see Brock, 2007; Mervis *et al.*, 2003b). However, it is now clear that language development in WS mostly follows a delayed and atypical path (for a review, see Karmiloff-Smith *et al.*, 2003), and more recent studies have shown qualitatively different patterns of deficit within both language and visuospatial cognition (for a review see Brock, 2007; Farran and Jarrold, 2003).

Finally, the WS cognitive profile is characterized by mild to moderate mental retardation, with mean IQ scores (inferred from standardized measures of intelligence, such as the Wechsler scales) falling about two standard deviations below the general population mean (e.g. Udwin *et al.*, 1987). Typical of WS are significant differences between mean scores at the verbal and the performance subtests (which usually contain a visuoconstructive component), often reaching 14 points (Howlin *et al.*, 1998; Udwin and Yule, 1991). Indeed, close observation of the IQ scores in WS suggest that it is not a unitary condition characterized by homogeneous slowness of cognitive development, but by a variety of conditions in which some cognitive functions may be more disrupted than others (for a review see Santos *et al.*, 2007a).

Importantly, for the purpose of this review, there is consistent evidence showing that IQ and brain structure are correlated. For instance, a negative correlation between gray matter volume and IQ has been found in typically developing children and adolescents, with IQ explaining 9–15% of the variance in gray matter volume (Reiss *et al.*, 1996; Wilke *et al.*, 2003). Although global, this association appears to be more pronounced between gray matter volumes of the prefrontal and cingulated cortices and IQ (Reiss *et al.*, 1996; Wilke *et al.*, 2003), and mild between subcortical and cerebellar gray matter and IQ (Reiss *et al.*, 1996). Moreover, IQ has been found negatively correlated to parietal volume (Reiss *et al.*, 1996), and linked to cortical folding patterns in humans (Thompson *et al.*, 2001). Putatively, the strong association between IQ and brain structure is mediated by genetic factors, since, for instance, gray matter volumes seem to be highly hereditary (Pennington *et al.*, 2000; Reiss *et al.*, 1996; Wilke *et al.*, 2003). This creates issues for WS research, because if one studies participants with WS and reduced IQ compared to either healthy controls or a group with mental retardation of other cause(s), variance will be introduced either by the IQ difference itself or by the

pathology underlying the IQ reduction in the comparison group. Our approach to this problem has been to study exceptional participants with WS and normal-range IQ, which allow a comparison to truly healthy controls. This strategy, however, while fruitful, depends on the assumption that these subjects are representative of WS in general (Meyer-Lindenberg *et al.*, 2006). WS provides a privileged setting to elucidate genetic influences on brain organization, as well as on complex brain functions.

Genetic profile

WS is a genomic disorder caused by the absence of some 26 contiguous genes on chromosome band 7q11.23 in one of the two chromosomes 7 (Donnai and Karmiloff-Smith, 2000; Ewart *et al.*, 1993; Korenberg *et al.*, 2000; Peoples *et al.*, 2000), leading to a gene dosage effect which includes the gene for elastin (*ELN*) in over 96% of individuals with WS (Lowery *et al.*, 1995). The microdeletion is due to a hemizygous deletion during meiosis (Urbán *et al.*, 1996), related to that of repetitive sequences flanking the region (Korenberg *et al.*, 2000). Because the genes involved in WS are known, and the dosage of at least some of these genes is clearly abnormal, the study of neural mechanisms in WS affords a privileged setting to understand genetic influences on complex brain functions in a "bottom-up" way.

Since the early 1990s, WS diagnosis is determined by detecting the absence of one copy of the *ELN* gene using the fluorescent in-situ hybridization (FISH) test. The FISH is a cytogenetic method that detects complex and cryptic chromosomal rearrangements, and thus plays an important role in the investigation of unsolved cases of mental retardation and multiple anomalies (e.g. WS, Prader-Willi, DiGeorge syndrome; Sukarova-Angelovska *et al.*, 2007).

The size of the deletion is approximately 1.5–1.8 megabases of genomic DNA, with little variance across most individuals (Lowery *et al.*, 1995). Yet, occasionally individuals with WS are identified who have smaller deletions – such cases are potentially very useful as a way of providing clues to the roles of specific genes in the behavioral expression of the syndrome.

Brain structure

Several studies have aimed to determine structural changes of the brain in WS. Early post-mortem studies have indicated cytoarchitectonic anomalies in primary visual areas in WS, including increased cell packing density, abnormal neuronal organization, clustering and orientation, as well as reduced volume of posterior forebrain areas (Galaburda *et al.*, 1994, 2001, 2002). Interestingly, these latest differences were interpreted as possibly related to the visuospatial deficits in WS (Galaburda *et al.*, 2002). Further early gross anatomical analyses revealed reduced brain size, short central sulcus, a lack of asymmetry in the planum temporale (Galaburda and Bellugi, 2000), and an increased incidence of neurodevelopmental abnormalities such as Chiari I malformations (e.g. Pober and Filiano, 1995; Wang *et al.*, 1992b). Both increased neocerebellar vermis (Jernigan and Bellugi, 1990), normal cerebellar size (Jernigan and Bellugi, 1990), and normal neocerebellar tonsils (Wang *et al.*, 1992b) have been reported in WS individuals. However, these initial studies have mostly used chronological age-matched individuals with Down syndrome as a comparison group (e.g. Jernigan and Bellugi, 1990; Jernigan *et al.*, 1993; Wang *et al.*, 1992b). Since 1993, most studies have rather used typically developing age- and gender-matched controls, thus somewhat reducing the ambiguity inherent in using a control group that suffers from a different neurogenetic syndrome, but still raising the problem of discrepant IQ.

Studies using high-resolution magnetic resonance imaging (MRI) have found significant brain differences between WS and typically developing individuals. These include volumetric decreases in cerebral gray (approximately 11%) and white matters (approximately 18%) of the thalamus, occipital and parietal lobes (relative to frontal regions), along with a relative increase in the size of the amygdala and superior temporal and orbitofrontal gyri in WS relative to typical controls (Reiss *et al.*, 2004; Thompson *et al.*, 2005). These anatomical abnormalities were found to co-exist with relative preservations in the auditory cortex (Holinger *et al.*, 2005) and cerebellum (Jones *et al.*, 2002). Interestingly, the most pronounced reductions (in occipital and parietal regions relative to frontal regions; Reiss *et al.*, 2004) suggest that cortical patterning genes (Bishop *et al.*, 2000) play a role in the developmental neuropathology of WS. Several genes, such as *CYLN2* and *LIMK1*, are implicated in neurodevelopment. In addition, it may be that the deleted transcription factor II-I (*TFII-I*) genes influence cortical patterning in WS because they regulate goosecoid, a protein that modulates anatomical patterning

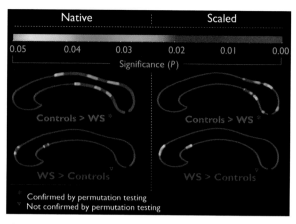

Figure 37.1 Group differences in callosal thickness. Illustrated are regions of significant differences in callosal thickness between WS patients and controls. The color bar encodes the *P* value associated with the *t*-test performed at each distance value from upper and lower callosal boundaries. Permutation tests were significant for the comparison of controls > WS (both in native and scaled space), but not significant for the findings of WS > controls. Results shown in the left panel are based on analyses in native space; findings on the right refer to scaled space. Reproduced, with permission, from Luders *et al.* (2007).

in vertebrate embryos (Ku *et al.*, 2005). Further, *CYLN2* and *LIMK1* have been implicated in cellular and axonal motility, which could impact on cortical patterning.

Insights from analyses of regional volume have been extended by analyses of cortical shape showing reduced overall curvature of the brain (Schmitt *et al.*, 2001a), as well as abnormally increased gyrification in parietal and occipital lobes (Schmitt *et al.*, 2002) and the temporoparietal zone (Thompson *et al.*, 2005) in WS. Unusual brain shape has also been found in the hippocampus (Meyer-Lindenberg *et al.*, 2005b), the central sulcus (Jackowski and Schultz, 2005) and the corpus callosum (Luders *et al.*, 2007; Schmitt *et al.*, 2001b; see Figure 37.1). These latter data concern both the shape (less curved) and the volume (reduced), with anterior callosal sections being relatively spared, while the splenium and the isthmus were found reduced in size (Schmitt *et al.*, 2001b; Tomaiuolo *et al.*, 2002).

Significant advances in our understanding of the structural basis of WS have come from the application of voxel-based morphometry (VBM), which allows the study of genetic variation without restriction to anatomical boundaries. Meyer-Lindenberg and colleagues (2004) identified circumscribed symmetrical reductions in gray matter volume in

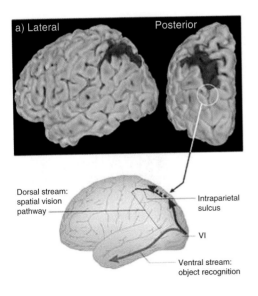

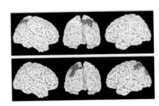

Figure 37.2 Left panel: Spatial relationship between area found to be structurally abnormal with voxel-based morphometry (yellow), and two tasks tapping into the function of the dorsal visual stream (red and blue) in high-functioning participants with Williams syndrome (WS) compared with controls during fMRI. Overlapping regions in the parietal lobule are colored purple, showing consistent functional abnormalities in the dorsal visual stream directly adjacent to the structural abnormality. Lower panel shows location of proposed functional–structural impairment in the dorsal stream at the intraparietal sulcus. V1, primary visual cortex. Right panel: Significant hypoactivation in the parietal lobe of people with WS compared with controls in the square completion visuoconstruction task during fMRI, showing dorsal visual stream impairment. Reproduced, with permission, from Meyer-Lindenberg et al. (2004).

high-functioning individuals with WS in three particular regions: in the region of the dorsal occipitoparietal sulcus/vertical part of the intraparietal sulcus, in the hypothalamic area around the third ventricule, and in the orbitofrontal region (Meyer-Lindenberg et al., 2004). Evidence for reduced gray matter volume in the parietal sulcus is consistent with previous studies on WS individuals with mental retardation showing abnormal gyrification in the parietal lobe (Schmitt et al., 2002) and with fMRI findings for hypofunction in this region during visual processing, suggesting deficient input from the parietal sulcus into the later dorsal stream (Meyer-Lindenberg et al., 2004, see Figure 37.2).

Further morphometric studies have shown significant volume reductions in the occipital cortex and thalamus (Reiss et al., 2004), which are regions known to play a role in visuospatial processing (Logothetis, 1999; Zeki, 2001). In line with the hypothesis of visual system abnormalities in WS, Reiss and coworkers (2004) also found reduced gray matter density in bilateral parahippocampal gyri, extending across the midbrain tectum (superior and inferior colliculi) and in superior parietal and occipital regions known to be important components of the primate visual brain. According to evidence in non-human primates (Lawler and Cowey, 1986), the reduced volume and gray matter density in the thalamus and superior colliculus may contribute to WS visual deficits

(Atkinson et al., 2001), as well as to WS individuals' unusually "intense" gaze when interacting with others (Mervis et al., 2003a). Likewise, abnormalities in the parahippocampal region possibly relate to deficits in visual–spatial processing (Aguirre et al., 1998; Epstein and Kanwisher, 1998) and memory (Davachi et al., 2003; Ranganath and D'Esposito, 2001) in WS. Finally, there is some evidence that anomalous posterior cortical development in individuals with WS is most pronounced in the superior parietal lobule, which is significantly reduced relative to controls, even after controlling for total cerebral volume (Eckert et al., 2005).

While VBM studies of WS have produced consistent findings of reduced posterior parietal gray matter compared to typical individuals, different findings have been reported for the hypothalamus and orbitofrontal gray matter regions (Meyer-Lindenberg et al., 2004; Reiss et al., 2004). In a recent study using deformation based-morphometry analyses, Eckert and colleagues (2006b) argued that this discrepancy was due to methodological differences during imaging pre-processing, since both findings of the NIH cohort were replicated by the Stanford group when Jacobian modulation of the images, which allows an estimate of regional volume, was used (Eckert et al., 2006b). In line with robust previous findings, this study reported anomalous orbitofrontal cortex (Meyer-Lindenberg et al., 2004) and posterior

541

parietal development and in WS (e.g. Eckert *et al.*, 2005; Meyer-Lindenberg *et al.*, 2004; Kippenhan *et al.*, 2005; Reiss *et al.*, 2004; Schmitt *et al.*, 2002; Thompson *et al.*, 2005).

Furthermore, recent findings indicate that WS is associated with atypical sulcal/gyral patterning. For instance, atypical central sulcus (Galaburda *et al.*, 2001; Jackowski, and Schultz, 2005) and Sylvian fissure (Eckert *et al.*, 2006a), as well as increased gyrification, particularly in posterior cortical regions (Schmitt *et al.*, 2001a) have been reported. Moreover, one particular case report showed oligogyric microcephaly with a simplified gyral pattern, mostly in the parietal lobe, where shallow parietal sulci were observed, in a 19-month-old infant with WS (Faravelli *et al.*, 2003). Although unusual, this finding is relevant, as there are few studies examining WS infants or early childhood brains. Using a novel method (curvature-based approach) to analyze gyrification, Gaser and colleagues (2006) have shown increased gyrification bilaterally in occipital regions and over the cuneus in WS individuals relative to age-matched controls. With respect to gyrification asymmetry, small but numerous clusters of leftward asymmetry or diminished rightward asymmetry, across the medial cortical surface were found in WS (Gaser *et al.*, 2006).

Further studies using surface-based analyses – a method that can cope with the complexity of convolutions and the high degree of individual variability within the normal population – have revealed several localized folding abnormalities in WS individuals, arranged in a broad dorsoposterior to ventroanterior swath, which was unusually symmetric in the two hemispheres (Van Essen *et al.*, 2006). In addition, many of these abnormalities were found to occur in pairs, involving a control-deeper region near the fundus of a sulcus and a nearby WS-deeper region near the crowd of a gyrus. Discrete folding abnormalities were also observed in cortical areas associated with multiple sensory modalities, as well as regions implicated in cognitive and emotional behavior, together with reduced hemispheric asymmetry in the temporal cortex. Findings of this study suggest intriguing correspondence with several aspects of the WS behavioral profile. For instance, prominent folding abnormalities in the dorsal parietal cortex involved regions typically engaged in visuospatial and attentional processing (e.g. Meyer-Lindenberg *et al.*, 2004; Eckert *et al.*, 2005), as well as folding abnormality in the hippocampal region overlaps with

a region showing functional and structural abnormalities in WS (e.g. Meyer-Lindenberg *et al.*, 2005b). Other examples for this correspondence come from fMRI studies reporting altered activations during gaze discrimination (Mobbs *et al.*, 2004), auditory perception (Levitin *et al.*, 2004b), visuospatial contruction and spatial location processing (Meyer-Lindenberg *et al.*, 2004) in several regions that overlap with the folding abnormalities found in WS (Van Essen *et al.*, 2006).

Kippenhan and coworkers (2005), using a different surface-based method to measure sulcal depth, also found significant depth reductions in the parietal sulcus, in particular in the left parietal sulcus (8.5 mm), as well as significant reductions in the left orbitofrontal region and in the left collateral sulcus in high-functioning individuals with WS. In this study, sulcal depth findings in the intraparietal/occipitoparietal sulcus were found to correspond closely to measures of reduced gray matter volume in the same area (Meyer-Lindenberg *et al.*, 2004; Reiss *et al.*, 2004), suggesting that the gray matter volume loss and abnormal sulcal geometry may be related. Together with functional imaging (e.g. Meyer-Lindenberg *et al.*, 2004; Mobbs *et al.*, 2004; Eckert *et al.*, 2005) and neuropsychological evidence (e.g. Mervis *et al.*, 2000; Atkinson *et al.*, 2003), these findings provide compelling converging evidence that the parietal sulcus is involved in the pathophysiology of WS (Kippenhan *et al.*, 2005).

Because the WS deletion includes genes that regulate cytoskeletal dynamics in neurons, especially *LIMK1* and *CYLN2*, WS offers a privileged opportunity to investigate the role of these genes in the formation of white matter tracks. Recently, the first study has appeared investigating this issue. Using diffusion tensor imaging (DTI), Marenco and colleagues (2007) reported alterations in white matter fiber directionality, deviation in posterior fiber track course and reduced lateralisation of fiber coherence in individuals with WS (Marenco *et al.*, 2007; see Figure 37.3). Findings were consistent with a reduction in cortical fibers in intraparietal/parietal regions implicated in the visuoconstructive deficit of WS.

In agreement with this, another DTI study examining white matter integrity in the dorsal and ventral streams in individuals with WS showed significant associations between higher fractional anisotropy and visuoconstructive deficits in WS (Hoeft *et al.*, 2007). Importantly, differences in white matter tissue

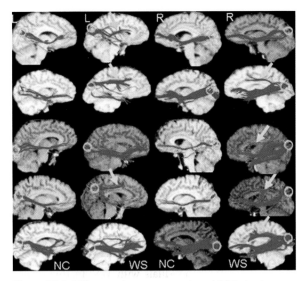

Figure 37.3 Differences between controls and WS in tracts connecting to the intraparietal sulcus and the ventral portion of the cingulum bundle. The yellow arrows indicate fiber tracts coursing rostrally to the corpus callosum, which were never present in controls (normal first and third columns) but present in four of five individuals with WS (second and fourth columns), especially in the right hemisphere ($P < 0.05$). Reproduced, with permission, from Marenco et al., 2007.

in individuals with WS led to the hypothesis that haploinsufficiency in the WS region plays a major role during the later stages of neuronal migration. Redirected fibers that would ordinarily develop into U-fibers or cross the midline in the dorsal portions of the corpus callosum become unable to reach their natural target and therefore deviate longitudinally, giving rise to altered fiber tracts and orientation of white matter (Marenco et al., 2007). In addition, evidence for altered laterality of anisotropy in WS (Marenco et al., 2007) suggest an abnormality either in the differential timing of hemispheric development of the white matter fibers or of differential quantity of fibers formed in the two hemispheres.

Taken together, these studies provide important information to guide future investigations of postmortem brain tissue in WS, knockout mouse models of WS-related genes, and individuals with small deletions in the WS critical region. Furthermore, these studies reveal critical differences in WS' brain structure and have helped clarifying the atypical neural substrate and type of brain processing in WS. Interestingly, it has been suggested that some of these anatomical findings may concur with behavioral features of WS. For instance, Santos and colleagues (2007b) have found atypical development of functions that

depend on callosal integrity (interhemispheric communication and hemispheric asymmetry) in children and adults with WS, possibly related to structural callosal abnormalities. Furthermore, convergent evidence suggests that the reduced intraparietal sulcal depth (Kippenhan et al., 2005), volume reduction in this region (Meyer-Lindenberg et al., 2004) and reductions in parietal/occipital volumes (Chiang et al., 2007) underlie the well-known visuospatial deficits in this condition. Direct evidence from multi-modal imaging and path analysis for this latter proposal was found by Meyer-Lindenberg et al. (2004).

On the other hand, apparent sparing of the volume of limbic structures, together with alterations in prefrontal structures regulating amygdala, may underlie hypersociability and relative strengths in affective functions (Jernigan et al., 1993; Reiss et al., 2000).

Using a signal detection methodology, Gothelf and colleagues (2008) have recently suggested that aberrant morphology of the ventral anterior prefrontal cortex in adolescents and young adults with WS might be related to the social-affective language use typically observed in this population. This interpretation is also consistent with a recent study using tensor-based morphometry (TBM), suggesting that relatively preserved or even enlarged frontal lobes, amygdala and cingulate gyrus may be related to unusual affect regulation and language production in WS (Chiang et al., 2007). A recent study using VBM in children with WS has also found correlations between inattention and volumetric differences in the frontal lobes, caudate nucleus and cerebellum, and between hyperactivity and differences in the left temporal and parietal lobes and cerebellum (Campbell et al., 2009), pointing to currently uncharacterized frontostriatal and frontocerebellar involvement that may be important for comorbities of WS.

While structural neuroimaging studies have brought forth significant advances for the understanding of anatomo-behavioral correlates in WS, the functional implications of abnormal structure require studies using functional neuroimaging. We now turn to this subject area.

Function

Many functional MRI (fMRI) studies on WS have focused on the neural basis of disturbed visuospatial cognition – a hallmark, yet fractioned, feature of the disorder (e.g. Frangiskakis *et al.*, 1996). There is increasing evidence for a dissociation between visuo-constructive and visuoperceptual abilities in WS (e.g. Farran and Jarrold, 2003), with increased perform-ance on tasks involving purely visual processing abil-ities, such as visual closure abilities (e.g. Deruelle 2006), than on visuoconstructive tasks requiring mental imagery and the integration of visual and motor components (e.g. Farran *et al.*, 2001). The current view of the visual system – marked by the functional and anatomical dissociation between a ventral stream specialized for perception and a dorsal stream specialized for action (Milner and Goodale, 1995) – has been proposed to account for this dissoci-ation between visuoconstructive and visuoperceptual functioning in WS. The theory that the ventral path-way (projecting from primary visual cortex to the temporal lobe) is primarily dedicated to perceptual recognition of shape, form, objects and faces, and the dorsal pathway (projecting from primary visual cortex to the parietal lobe) is specialized for process-ing spatial information and in visuomotor planning has received strong support from both animal research (e.g. Ungerleider and Mishkin, 1982), func-tional neuroimaging (Haxby *et al.*, 1999), and neuro-psychological studies on patients with localized brain damage (e.g. Milner and Goodale, 1995).

Recent studies on a wide range of developmental disorders have also shown that the distinction between a ventral visual system governing object perception and a dorsal system governing visuospatial processing has neurodevelopmental relevance. Developmental anomalies (e.g. hemiplegia, fragile X syndrome, autism, dyslexia) disrupt the two visual processing streams differently, with greater impairments on dorsal- than ventral-stream functions (e.g. visuocon-structive and visuoperceptual tasks, respectively; Gunn *et al.*, 2002; Hansen *et al.*, 2001; Kogan *et al.*, 2004; Spencer *et al.*, 2000). Neuropsychologically, the profile of abilities in WS is characterized by visual abilities subserved by the ventral stream, such as face recognition, that are relatively well developed, whereas those subserved by the dorsal stream, such as visuo-spatial manipulation, are markedly impaired. It has been consistently demonstrated that children and adults with WS show greater performance deficits in motion- (dorsal stream-dependent task) than in form-coherence tasks, known to be dorsal and ventral-stream dependent, respectively (Atkinson *et al.*, 1997, 2003, 2006). These findings suggest that the dorsal

visual pathway may be more modifiable by atypical input and/or experience than the ventral visual pathway and support the idea of a dorsal-stream vul-nerability in WS (Atkinson, 2000). While the two pathways show numerous interactions (Van Essen *et al.*, 1992), and the differentiation of roles between them is not straightforward, several authors (Atkinson *et al.*, 2003; Galaburda *et al.*, 2002; Nakamura *et al.*, 2001; Paul *et al.*, 2002) have hypothesized that the neural basis of the visuospatial construction deficit in WS might lie in the dorsal stream.

In order to test this hypothesis, Meyer-Lindenberg and colleagues (2004) conducted a series of fMRI experiments designed to assess visual system func-tions hierarchically. In this study, 13 individuals with genetically confirmed WS but normal general intelli-gence were compared to (IQ, gender and age) matched healthy subjects. Two tasks were included in this study: a square completion and an attention to object or location task. Both fMRI experiments showed normal ventral system activation but consist-ent hypoactivation in the dorsal visual stream in WS participants. In addition, results of path analyses sug-gested that a deficient input from the parietal sulcus into the lateral dorsal stream was could account for the hypoactivity observed in these regions. In other words, it was argued that a localized structural anom-aly in the intraparietal sulcus (consistent with previ-ous evidence for bilaterally reduced gray matter volume and sulcal depth) was associated with hypoac-tivity in directly adjacent parietal regions during spatial localization and visuospatial construction in WS (see Figure 37.2). Based on these findings, the authors argued that some genes in the WS deletion might be implicated in visuospatial constructive cog-nition through an impact on intraparietal sulcus (Meyer-Lindenberg *et al.*, 2004).

Visuospatial processing in WS has also been explored in relation to the local processing bias hypothesis. This processing style refers to the percep-tion of individual elements of an image, whilst attending to the image as a whole figure is referred to as global processing. It is now widely accepted that both typically developing children (e.g. Kimchi, 1990) and adults (e.g. Fagot and Deruelle, 1997; Navon, 1977) perceive information at the global level (i.e. the contour of the shape) faster than at the local level (i.e. the elements that compose the shape). By con-trast, in visuoconstructive tasks, individuals with WS tend to focus more on the parts or local elements of a stimulus, while ignoring or attending less to global information (e.g. Bihrle *et al.*, 1989). Evidence for increased attention to local information has been observed in the Block Design task and in drawings by individuals with WS. For example, when assembling cubes in the Block Design task, individuals with WS tend to reproduce local rather than global information (e.g. Bellugi *et al.*, 1994). In drawings of objects, individuals with WS usually attend to details of the figure and tend to have difficulty processing the outline (e.g. Wang and Bellugi, 1994). A strong bias toward local processing has also been found in tasks involving the copying of hierarchical figures. For instance, when drawing figures of a large letter made up of smaller letters, individuals with WS were significantly better at reproducing the smaller shapes than at depicting the global shape making up the figure (e.g. Bihrle *et al.*, 1989).

Global processing abilities in WS were recently investigated using fMRI (Mobbs *et al.*, 2007a). In this study, 10 genetically diagnosed individuals with WS were compared to 10 typically developing (gender and age) matched controls. Results revealed that individuals with WS were less accurate and showed reduced activation in the visual and parietal cortices when performing the global processing task. The authors also found relatively normal activation in the ventral occipitotemporal cortex, but increased activation in several posterior thalamic nuclei in WS individuals relative to controls. In line with previous studies, these findings suggest that a dorsal, but not ventral, stream dysfunction underlies atypical visuospatial cognition in WS, including global processing deficits (Mobbs *et al.*, 2007a).

There is evidence that face and house stimuli have different relevance to spatial cognition, with faces preferentially activating the ventral stream and houses being rather processed by both ventral and dorsal streams (Grill-Spector, 2003). Based on this idea, Meyer-Lindenberg and colleagues (2005b) conducted an fMRI study examining functional reactivity of the hippocampal formation during passive viewing of face and house stimuli in nine high-functioning individuals with WS relative to (IQ and age) matched controls. Indeed, both positron emission tomography (PET) and fMRI findings in this study supported hypofunction in the intraparietal sulcus and parietal lobe. Recently, Sarpal and colleagues (2008) have also used this passive face- and house-viewing paradigm to investigate further neural interactions of ventral

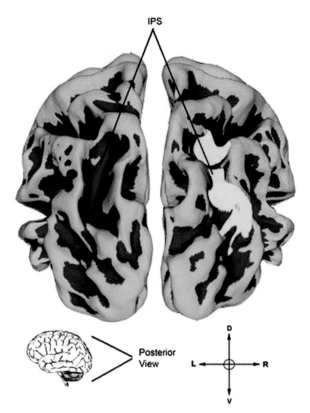

Figure 37.4 Activation difference between groups during house viewing in the right intraparietal sulcus (IPS; $P < 0.05$, corrected). No differences were observed between groups during face stimuli viewing. Reproduced, with permission, from Sarpal *et al.* (2008).

stream areas in WS. In particular, the authors focused on the parahippocampal gyrus and the fusiform gyrus, which are thought to respond in a selective manner to stimuli depicting places and faces, respectively (e.g. Aguirre *et al.*, 1998; Kanwisher *et al.*, 1997). This study included the same participants as Meyer-Lindenberg *et al.* (2004 and 2005b). Consistent with previous neuroimaging findings and behavioral accounts for relatively spared face processing in WS (e.g. Paul *et al.*, 2002; Tager-Flusberg *et al.*, 2003), no differences were found between the WS and the control groups in ventral stream activation during face viewing. However, the WS group showed not only abnormal activation in the intraparietal sulcus during house viewing, but also abnormal interaction of this region with ventral visual areas (see Figure 37.4).

In addition, significantly decreased functional connectivity was found between the parahippocampal place area and the intraparietal sulcus for the WS group, whereas the control group showed a tight

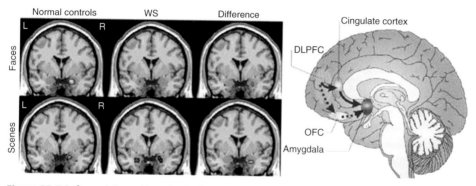

Figure 37.5 Left panel: Amygdala activation ($p < 0.05$, corrected for multiple comparisons) for face and scene stimuli. First column, normal controls; second column, high-functioning participants with Williams syndrome; third column, significant differences between groups (blue NC > WS, red WS > NC) in the amygdala. Right panel: Schema depicting key regions for social cognition and emotional regulation affected in WS: amygdala, OFC, DLPFC and cingulate cortex. Left panel reproduced, with permission, from Meyer-Lindenberg *et al.* (2005a). Right panel adapted, with permission, from Meyer-Lindenberg *et al.* (2006).

functional coupling between these two areas. Further reductions in functional connectivity between ventral areas and areas implicated in visuospatial constructive, executive and emotional functions that depend on visual information input, were also found for the WS group.

A further domain where subjects with WS show marked impairment is delayed memory as well as spatial orientation, both of which are hippocampally dependent. To test the hypothesis of hippocampal dysfunction in WS, Meyer-Lindenberg *et al.* (2005b) studied activity during encoding of face and house stimuli, hypothesizing that house viewing, which has been linked to spatial function, would be abnormal in this group. Confirming this hypothesis, results showed no differential hippocampal formation activation to either stimulus in WS individuals, while for controls faces elicited greater activation patterns than houses. Together with marked hypoperfusion in the hippocampal formation in PET, these findings revealed a primary hippocampal dysfunction in WS (Meyer-Lindenberg *et al.*, 2005b) and launched the idea that the WS region contains genes implicated in hippocampal function.

At the behavior level, individuals with WS do show intriguing social features including overfriendliness, overuse of social engagement devises (e.g. eye contact), increased empathy and drive towards social interaction, positive interpersonal bias and social disinhibition (Bellugi *et al.*, 1999; Jones *et al.*, 2000; Klein-Tasman and Mervis, 2003; Mervis and Klein-Tasman, 2000). Of particular interest for research is the lack of social fear observed in individuals with WS, who show no fear of strangers, nor even people they objectively consider as not approachable (Frigerio *et al.*, 2006), together with non-social anxiety, specific phobia and excessive worrying (e.g. Bellugi *et al.*, 1999). There is indeed evidence that socially protective neural processing and dissociable systems for social and non-social fear lie in the amygdala (Adolphs, 2003; Prather *et al.*, 2001). Based on this idea, Meyer-Lindenberg and colleagues (2005a) conducted a study focusing on amygdala functioning and regulation in individuals with WS relative to controls (same participants as Meyer-Lindenberg *et al.*, 2004, 2005b; Sarpal *et al.*, 2008). This study included two tasks requiring processing of threatening stimuli, either faces or scenes, known to engage amygdala (Hariri *et al.*, 2002). Interestingly, these two tasks brought forth significant group differences in amygdala activation. Relative to controls, individuals with WS showed reduced amygdala activation for threatening faces but increased amygdala activation for threatening scenes (see Figure 37.5). Both results were found to be clearly in agreement with the WS atypical social profile: diminished amygdala reactivity to threatening faces being putatively related to absence of fear of strangers and consequent social disinhibition, and abnormally increased reactivity to threatening scenes suggesting a potential mechanism for excessive non-social anxiety (e.g. specific phobias) in WS. Similar reactivity differences as a function of the task were also found in the prefrontal cortex, where controls differentially activated orbitofrontal, dorsolateral- and medial–prefrontal cortex for threatening faces, while WS

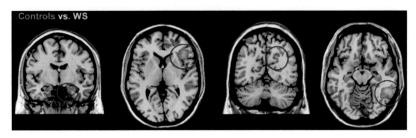

Figure 37.6 Results from the between-groups comparisons in right amygdala, right inferior frontal gyrus, right intraparietal sulcus and right middle temporal gyrus (from left to right, respectively). Greater FFA connectivity was observed in control than WS participants in bilateral amygdala and right inferior frontal gyrus. The bilateral intraparietal sulcus exhibited significantly greater parahippocampal place area connectivity in controls than in participants with WS. Participants with WS showed significantly more parahippocampal place area connectivity than controls with posterior regions, including middle temporal gyrus. Reproduced, with permission, from Sarpal et al. (2008).

individuals showed a task-invariant pattern of activation. Given that both medial–prefrontal and orbito-frontal cortex are densely interconnected with amygdala and dorsolateral–prefrontal cortex and have been implicated in the regulation of amygdala regulation, these findings provide evidence for a dysregulation of amygdala-prefrontal systems (involved in social and non-social fear signalling; e.g. Schultz, 2005) in WS, which may account for the gregarious behavioral profile, the lack of socially related fear, and the presence of non-social anxieties commonly reported in this condition (Meyer-Lindenberg et al., 2005a).

The recent study by Sarpal et al. (2008) further showed significant reductions in functional connectivity between the fusiform face area (FFA) and the amygdala and prefrontal cortex (see Figure 37.6), areas possibly involved in the hypersocial symptoms of WS, suggesting that also the afferent flow of face-emotion related information into amygdala is impaired in WS. Very recently, the finding of reduced amygdala activation to fearful social visual stimuli was replicated in a group of subjects with WS and mental retardation (Haas et al., 2009). This study also showed increased activation to positive stimuli (happy faces), adding a new facet to the neural mechanisms underlying prosocial behavior in WS, and suggesting that dysregulation of amygdala by prefrontal cortex may lead to changed activation profiles not only between socially relevant and less relevant stimuli, but also across a range of stimulus valence.

For a long time, media and families have held the idea that individuals with WS have an unusual musical talent. Empirical studies have indeed shown that individuals with WS outperform individuals with other neurodevelopmental disorders (autism and Down syndrome) in musical accomplishment,

engagement and interest (Levitin et al., 2004). Moreover, they were found to display greater emotional responses to music, manifest interest in music at an earlier age, spend more time listening to music and to be more engaged in musical activities than others (Levitin et al., 2004, 2005). There is nevertheless no clear evidence for increased musical ability in WS, as in most tests their performance does not seem to be better than that of typically developing individuals (Levitin et al., 2004). Also, Deruelle and colleagues (2005) have reported atypical music perception strategies in children with WS relative to typically developing controls. At the neural level, significant differences in brain activation have been found between WS and control groups, with regions implicated in auditory processing of music and noise in typically developing individuals (e.g. superior temporal and middle temporal gyri) not being consistently activated in the WS group (Levitin et al., 2003). Rather, increased activation in the right amygdala and a widely distributed network of activation in cortical and subcortical structures was found for this group during music processing.

Finally, Mobbs and colleagues (2007b) have explored the neurobiological systems that underlie response inhibition and attention deficits in WS using fMRI. Although this study did not reveal group differences in accuracy, significant differences were found in brain activation patterns between WS and (age and gender) matched typically developing individuals. Relative to controls, individuals with WS have shown reduced activation in the striatum, dorsolateral prefrontal, and dorsal anterior cingulate cortices (Mobbs et al., 2007b), suggesting abnormalities in critical cortical and subcortical structures involved in behavioral inhibition in WS, possibly at the origin of deficits in response inhibition and the unusual social phenotype of this disorder.

Conclusion

Taken together, these studies provide evidence for atypical brain structure and function in WS suggesting that brains of individuals with WS develop differently from the outset, which probably has subtle but widespread repercussions at the cognitive and behavioral levels. These studies revealed that MRI techniques, by offering the possibility to study brain structure, regional activation (fMRI) and white matter tracks (DTI), are a powerful tool to investigate neural correlates in WS. These techniques allow us to capture images of the brain and to define tissue types, activation levels and connectivity. There are, however, limitations to the use of MRI to investigate WS in many participants, in particular due to the fact that most individuals present mental retardation. Even if, contrary to initial reports (e.g. Bellugi *et al.*, 1988), recent studies indicate that severe mental impairment is rare in WS (Mervis and Klein-Tasman, 2000), the intellectual impairment characterizing the disorder limits WS individuals to perform consistently during testing. Certain paradigms used in fMRI studies are thus impossible to use with WS individuals due to their level of difficulty. In addition, it is often difficult to obtain usable images, because children with intellectual impairment have more problems in staying still in an MRI scanner thus resulting in movement artifacts. This can be avoided by selecting normal-intelligence participants with WS (e.g. Meyer-Lindenberg *et al.*, 2004, 2005a, 2005b, 2006), who can cooperate with extensive cognitive and imaging procedures and be appropriately compared with typically developing controls.

Despite these limitations, studies using MRI to investigate WS have provided important insights into brain mechanisms underlying atypical behavior and cognitive functioning. These findings form a springboard for future research, which needs to move towards a detailed and mechanistic inquiry into specific neural and genetic mechanisms of neuropsychiatric syndromes. The mapping of fundamental molecular events to specific neurobiological substrates and phenotypic correlates may ultimately enable the identification of relationships between genetic etiology, cognitive processes and behavioral outcomes of these still so sparsely understood syndromes. Findings of the studies reviewed here offer a systems-level characterization of genetically mediated abnormalities of neural interactions that can be probed for the identification of single-gene effects on brain maturation. Further studies focusing on whether and how single genes, or their interactions, in the WS deletion contribute to the emergence of separable neural systems abnormalities are indeed needed. Future research using animal models, examining atypical participants and, potentially, investigating variation in WS region genes in the general population holds the promise to uncover the links between genetic mechanisms and complex behavior, not only in WS, but also in the general population. Finally, we hope that findings from studies integrating MRI research with molecular, cellular, and behavioral methods will contribute to the development of specific and more effective clinical interventions for patients with neurogenetic disorders.

Acknowledgments

A. Santos was funded by the Fyssen Fondation (France) during the writing of this chapter.

Box 37.1. Summary

Williams syndrome (WS), a genetic microdeletion syndrome, has been established as a *unique window to genetic contributions to neural function*. This chapter reviews imaging studies showing atypical brain structure and function in WS and their possible implications at the cognitive and behavioral levels.

Brain structure in WS.
- Reduced overall brain size.
- Volumetric decreases in cerebral gray and white matters of the thalamus, occipital and parietal lobes (relative to frontal regions).
- Reductions in gray matter volume and depth in the intraparietal sulcus, a region that is important for visuospatial constructive function, and in orbitofrontal cortex.
- Relative increase in the size of the amygdala and superior temporal gyri.
- Abnormal sulcal/gyral patterning.
- Abnormal white matter fiber connectivity, especially in posterior fiber tract course.

Brain function
- Normal ventral visual stream activation but hypoactivation in the dorsal visual stream, possibly associated with structural anomalies in the intraparietal sulcus and severe deficits in visuospatial construction.

- Hypofunction in the intraparietal sulcus and parietal lobe and abnormal interaction of this region with ventral visual areas.
- Hypoactivation in the amygdala in response to threatening faces, but increased activity to threatening non-social stimuli, mirroring the behavioral profile of absence of fear from strangers and excessive non-social anxiety, respectively.
- Abnormal interactions between the amygdala and prefrontal regulatory regions, in particular the orbitofrontal cortex, areas critically involved in social processing.
- Reductions in functional connectivity between the fusiform face area and the amygadala and prefrontal cortex.
- Hypoactivation in the hippocampus associated with reduced blood flow, abnormal neuronal integrity marker NAA and abnormal shape.

References

Adolphs R. 2003. Cognitive neuroscience of human social behaviour. *Nat Rev Neurosci* **4**, 165–78.

Aguirre G K, Zarahn E and D'Esposito M. 1998. Neural components of topographical representation. *Proc Natl Acad Sci U S A* **95**, 839–46.

American Academy of Pediatrics. 2001. Health care supervision for children with Williams syndrome. *Pediatrics* **107**, 1192–204.

Atkinson J. 2000. *The Developing Visual Brain*. Oxford, UK: Oxford University Press.

Atkinson J, Anker S, Braddick O, Nokes L, Mason A and Braddick F. 2001. Visual and visuospatial development in young children with Williams syndrome. *Devptl Med Child Neurol* **43**, 330–7.

Atkinson J, Braddick O, Anker S, *et al.* 2003. Neurobiological models of visuospatial cognition in children with Williams syndrome: Measures of dorsal-stream and frontal function. *Devptl Neuropsychol* **23**, 139–72.

Atkinson J, Braddick O, Rose F E, Searcy Y M, Wattam-Bell J and Bellugi U. 2006. Dorsal-stream motion processing deficits persist into adulthood in Williams syndrome. *Neuropsychologia* **44**, 828–33.

Atkinson J, King J, Braddick O, Nokes L, Anker S and Braddick F. 1997. A specific deficit of dorsal stream function in Williams syndrome. *Neuroreport* **8** 1919–22.

Bello A, Capirci O and Volterra V. 2004. Lexical production in children with Williams syndrome: Spontaneous use of gesture in a naming task. *Neuropsychologia* **42**, 201–13.

Bellugi U, Adolphs R, Cassadi C and Chiles M. 1999. Towards the neural basis for hypersociability in a genetic syndrome. *Neuroreport* **10**, 1653–7.

Bellugi U, Lichtenberger L, Jones W, Lai Z and St. George M. 2000. I. The neurocognitve profile of Williams syndrome: A complex pattern of strengths and weaknesses. *J Cogn Neurosci* **12** (Suppl 1), 7–29.

Bellugi U, Sabo H and Vaid V. 1988. Spatial defects in children with Williams syndrome. In Stiles-Davis J, Kritchevsky M, Bellugi U (Eds.), *Spatial Cognition: Brain Bases and Development*. Hillsdale, NJ: Lawrence Erlbaum Associates, pp. 273–98.

Bellugi U, Wang P and Jernigan T. 1994. Higher cortical functions: Evidence from specific genetically based syndromes of disorder. In Broman S, Graffman J (Eds.), *Cognitive Deficits in Developmental Disorders: Implications for Brain Function*. Hillsdale, NJ: Lawrence Erlbaum, pp. 23–56.

Beuren A J, Apitz J and Harmjanz D. 1962. Supravalvular aortic stenosis in association with mental retardation and a certain facial appearance. *Circulation* **26**, 1235–40.

Bihrle A M, Bellugi U, Delis S and Marks S. 1989. Seeing the forest or the trees: Dissociation in visuospatial processing. *Brain Cogn* **11**, 37–49.

Bishop K M, Goudreau G and O'Leary D D. 2000. Regulation of area identity in the mammalian neocortex by Emx2 and Pax6. *Science* **288**, 344–9.

Blomberg S, Rosander M and Andersson G. 2006. Fears, hyperacusis and musicality in Williams syndrome. *Res Devptl Disabil* **27**, 668–80.

Brock J. 2007. Language abilities in Williams syndrome: A critical review. *Devpt Psychopathol* **19**, 97–127.

Campbell L E, Daly E, Toal F, *et al.* 2009. Brain structural differences associated with the behavioural phenotype in children with Williams syndrome. *Brain Res* **1258**, 96–107.

Chapman C A, De Plessis A and Pober B R. 1996. Neurologic findings in children and adults with Williams syndrome. *J Child Neurol* **11**, 63–5.

Cherniske E M, Carpenter T O, Klaiman C, *et al.* 2004. Multisystem study of 20 older adults with Williams syndrome. *Am J Med Genet* **131A**, 255–64.

Chiang M C, Reiss A L, Lee A D, *et al.* 2007. 3D pattern of brain abnormalities in Williams syndrome visualized using tensor-based morphometry. *Neuroimage* **36**, 1096–109.

Danoff S K, Taylor H E, Blackshaw S and Desiderio S. 2004. TFII-I, a candidate gene for Williams syndrome cognitive profile: Parallels between regional expression in mouse brain and human phenotype. *Neuroscience* **123**, 931–8.

Davachi L, Mitchell J P and Wagner A D. 2003. Multiple routes to memory: Distinct medial temporal lobe processes build item and source memories. *Proc Natl Acad Sci U S A* **100**, 2157–62.

Deruelle C, Rondan C, Livet M O and Mancini J. 2003. Exploring face processing in Williams syndrome. *Cogn Brain Behav* **7**, 157–72.

Deruelle C, Rondan C, Mancini J and Livet M O. 2006. Do children with Williams syndrome fail to process visual configural information? *Res Devptl Disabil* **27**, 243–53.

Deruelle C, Schön D, Rondan C and Mancini J. 2005. Global and local music perception in children with Williams syndrome. *Neuroreport* **16**, 631–4.

Donnai D and Karmiloff-Smith A. 2000. Williams syndrome: From genotype through to the cognitive phenotype. *Am J Med Genet Semin Med Genet* **97**, 164–71.

Dykens E M. 2003. Anxiety, fears, and phobias in persons with Williams syndrome. *Devptl Neuropsychol* **23**, 291–316.

Eckert M A, Galaburda A M, Karchemskiy A, *et al.* 2006a. Anomalous Sylvian fissure morphology in Williams syndrome. *Neuroimage* **33**, 39–45.

Eckert M A, Hu D, Eliez S, *et al.* 2005. Evidence for superior parietal impairment in Williams syndrome. *Neurology* **64**, 152–3.

Eckert M A, Tenforde A, Galaburda A M, *et al.* 2006b. To modulate or not to modulate: Differing results in uniquely shaped Williams syndrome brains. *Neuroimage* **32**, 1001–07.

Einfield S, Tonge B and Florio T. 1997. Behavioral and emotional disturbance in individuals with Williams syndrome. *Am J Mental Retard* **102**, 45–53.

Epstein R and Kanwisher N. 1998. A cortical representation of the local visual environment. *Nature* **392**, 598–601.

Ewart A K, Morris C A, Atkinson D, *et al.* 1993. Hemizygosity at the elastin locus in a developmental disorder, Williams syndrome. *Nat Genet* **5**, 11–6.

Fagot J and Deruelle C. 1997. Processing of global and local visual information and hemispheric specialization in humans (*Homo sapiens*) and baboons (*Papio papio*). *J Exp Psychol Hum Percept Perform* **23**, 429–42.

Faravelli F, D'Arrigo S, Bagnasco I, *et al.* 2003. Oligogyric microcephaly in a child with Williams syndrome. *Am J Med Genet A* **117**, 169–71.

Farran E K and Jarrold C. 2003. Visuospatial cognition in Williams syndrome: Reviewing and accounting for the strengths and weaknesses in performance. *Devptl Neuropsychol* **23**, 173–200.

Farran E K, Jarrold C and Gathercole S E. 2001. Block design performance in the Williams syndrome phenotype: A problem with mental imagery? *J Child Psychol Psychiatry* **42**, 719–28.

Farran E K, Jarrold C and Gathercole S E. 2003. Divided attention, selective attention and drawing: processing preferences in Williams syndrome are dependent on the task administered. *Neuropsychologia* **41**, 676–87.

Fidler D J, Hepburn S L, Most D E, Philofsky A and Rogers S J. 2007. Emotional responsivity in young children with Williams syndrome. *Am J Mental Retard* **112**, 194–206.

Frangiskakis J M, Ewart A K, Morris C A, *et al.* 1996. LIM-kinase1 hemizygosity implicated in impaired visuospatial constructive cognition. *Cell* **86**, 59–69.

Frigerio E, Burt D M, Gagliardi C, *et al.* 2006. Is everybody always my friend? Perception of approachability in Williams syndrome. *Neuropsychologia* **44**, 254–9.

Galaburda A M and Bellugi U. 2000. V. Multi-level analysis of cortical neuroanatomy in Williams syndrome. *J Cogn Neurosci* **12** (Suppl 1), 74–88.

Galaburda A M, Holinger D P, Bellugi U and Sherman G F. 2002. Williams syndrome: neuronal size and neuronal-packing density in primary visual cortex. *Arch Neurol* **59**, 1461–7.

Galaburda A M, Schmitt J E, Atlas S W, Eliez S, Bellugi U and Reiss A L. 2001. Dorsal forebrain anomaly in Williams syndrome. *Arch Neurol* **58**, 1865–9.

Galaburda A M, Wang P P, Bellugi U and Rossen M. 1994. Cytoarchitectonic anomalies in a genetically based disorder: Williams syndrome. *Neuroreport* **5**, 753–7.

Gaser C, Luders E, Thompson P M, *et al.* 2006. Increased local gyrification mapped in Williams syndrome. *Neuroimage* **33**, 46–54.

Gothelf D, Searcy Y M, Reilly J, *et al.* 2008. Association between cerebral shape and social use of language in Williams syndrome. *Am J Med Genet* **146**, 2753–61.

Gosch A and Pankau R. 1994. Social–emotional and behavioral adjustment in children with Williams–Beuren syndrome. *Am J Med Genet* **52**, 291–6.

Gosch A and Pankau R. 1997. Personality characteristics and behavioural problems in individuals of different ages with Williams syndrome. *Devptl Med Child Neurol* **39**, 327–533.

Grill-Spector, K. 2003. The neural basis of object perception. *Curr Opin Neurobiol* **13**, 159–66.

Gunn A, Cory E, Atkinson J, *et al.* 2002. Dorsal and ventral stream sensitivity in normal development and hemiplegia. *Neuroreport* **13**, 843–7.

Haas B W, Mills D, Yam A, Hoeft F, Bellugi U and Reiss A. 2009. Genetic influences on sociability: Heightened amygdala reactivity and event-related responses to positive social stimuli in Williams syndrome. *J Neurosci* **29**, 1132–49.

Hammond P, Hutton T J, Allanson J E, *et al.* 2005. Discriminating power of localized three-dimensional facial morphology. *Am J Hum Genet* **77**, 999–1010.

Hansen P C, Stein J F, Orde S R, Winter J L and Talcott J B. 2001. Are dyslexics' visual deficits limited to measures of dorsal stream function? *Neuroreport* **12**, 1527–30.

Hariri A R, Tessitore A, Mattay V S, Fera F and Weinberger D R. 2002. The amygdala response to emotional stimuli: A comparison of faces and scenes. *Neuroimage* **17**, 317–23.

Haxby J V, Ungerleider L G, Clark V P, Schouten J L, Hoffman E A and Martin A. 1999. The effect of face inversion on activity in human neural systems for face and object perception. *Neuron* **22**, 189–99.

Hoeft F, Barnea-Goraly N, Haas B W, *et al.* 2007. More is not always better: Increased fractional anisotropy of superior longitudinal fasciculus associated with poor visuospatial abilities in Williams syndrome. *J Neurosci* **27**, 11 960–5.

Holinger D P, Bellugi U, Mills D L, *et al.* 2005. Relative sparing of primary auditory cortex in Williams syndrome. *Brain Res* **1037**, 35–42.

Hoogenraad C C, Koekkoek B, Akhmanova A, *et al.* 2002. Targeted mutation of Cyln2 in the Williams syndrome critical region links CLIP-115 haploinsufficiency to neurodevelopmental abnormalities in mice. *Nat Genet* **32**, 116–27.

Howlin P, Davies M and Udwin O. 1998. Cognitive functioning in adults with Williams syndrome. *J Child Psychol Psychiatry* **39**, 183–9.

Jackowski A P and Schultz R T. 2005. Foreshortened dorsal extension of the central sulcus in Williams syndrome. *Cortex* **41**, 282–90.

Jarrold C, Baddeley A D and Hewes A K. 1998. Verbal and nonverbal abilities in the Williams syndrome phenotype: Evidence for diverging developmental trajectories. *J Child Psychol Psychiatry* **39**, 511–23.

Jernigan T L and Bellugi U. 1990. Anomalous brain morphology on magnetic resonance images in Williams syndrome and Down syndrome. *Arch Neurol* **47**, 529–33.

Jernigan T L, Bellugi U, Sowell E, Doherty S and Hesselink J R. 1993. Cerebral morphologic distinctions between Williams and Down syndromes. *Arch Neurol* **50**, 186–91.

Jones W, Bellugi U, Lai Z, *et al.* 2000. Hypersociability in Williams syndrome. *J Cogn Neurosci* **12** (Suppl 1), 30–46.

Jones W, Hesselink J, Courschene E, *et al.* 2002. Cerebellar abnormalities in infants and toddlers with Williams syndrome. *Devptl Med Child Neurol* **44**, 688–94.

Kanwisher N, McDermott J and Chun M M. 1997. The fusiform face area: A module in human extrastriate cortex specialized for face perception. *J Neurosci* **17**, 4302–11.

Karmiloff-Smith A. 1998. Development itself is the key to understanding developmental disorders. *Trends Cogn Sci* **2**, 389–98.

Karmiloff-Smith A, Brown J H, Grice S and Paterson S. 2003. Dethroning the myth: Cognitive dissociations and innate modularity in Williams syndrome. *Devptl Neuropsychol* **23**, 227–42.

Karmiloff-Smith A, Klima E, Bellugi U, Grant J and Baron-Cohen S. 1995. Is there a social module? Language, face-processing and theory of mind in Williams syndrome. *J Cogn Neurosci* **7**, 196–208.

Kimchi R. 1990. Children's perceptual organization of hierarchical visual patterns. *Eur J Cogn Psychol* **2**, 133–49.

Kippenhan J S, Olsen R K, Mervis C B, *et al.* 2005. Genetic contributions to human gyrification: Sulcal morphometry in Williams syndrome. *J Neurosci* **25**, 7840–6.

Klein-Tasman B P and Mervis C B. 2003. Distinctive personality characteristics of 8–9, and 10-year-olds with Williams syndrome. *Devptl Neuropsychol* **23**, 269–90.

Kogan C S, Boutet I, Cornish K, *et al.* 2004. Differential impact of the FMR1 gene on visual processing in fragile X syndrome. *Brain* **127**, 591–601.

Korenberg J R, Chen X N, Hirota H, *et al.* 2000. IV. Genome structure and cognitive map of Williams syndrome. *J Cogn Neurosci* **12** (Suppl 1), 89–107.

Korenberg J R, Dai L, Bellugi U, *et al.* 2008. Deletion of 7q11.23 Genes and Williams syndrome. In Epstein C J, Erickson R P, Wynshaw-Boris A (Eds.), *Inborn Errors of Development* (2nd ed.). New York, NY: Oxford University Press.

Ku M, Sokol S, Wu J, Tussie-Luna M, Roy A and Hata A. 2005. Positive, and negative regulation of the transforming growth factor beta/activin target gene goosecoid by the TFII-I family of transcripton factors. *Mol Cell Biol* **25**, 7144–57.

Laing E, Butterworth G, Ansari D, *et al.* 2002. Atypical development of language and social communication in toddlers with Williams syndrome. *Devptl Sci* **5**, 233–46.

Landau B, Hoffman J E and Kurz N. 2006. Object recognition with severe spatial deficits in Williams syndrome: Sparing and breakdown. *Cognition* **100**, 483–510.

Lawler K A and Cowey A. 1986. The effects of pretectal and superior collicular lesions on binocular vision. *Exp Brain Res* **63**, 402–08.

Levitin D J, Menon V, Schmitt J E, *et al.* 2003. Neural correlates of auditory perception in Williams syndrome: An fMRI study. *Neuroimage* **18**, 74–82.

Levitin D J, Cole K, Chiles M, Lai Z, Lincoln A and Bellugi U. 2004. Characterizing the musical phenotype in individuals with Williams Syndrome. *Child Neuropsychol* **10**, 223–47.

Levitin D J, Cole K, Lincoln A and Bellugi U. 2005. Aversion, awareness, and attraction: Investigating claims of hyperacusis in the Williams syndrome phenotype. *J Child Psychol Psychiatry* **46**, 514–23.

Leyfer O T, Woodruff-Borden J, Klein-Tasman B P, Fricke J S and Mervis C B. 2006. Prevalence of psychiatric disorders in 4 to 16-year-olds with Williams syndrome. *Am J Med Genet Neuropsychiatr Genet* **141**, 615–22.

Logothetis N K. 1999. Vision: A window on consciousness. *Sci Am* **281**, 69–75.

Lowery M C, Morris C A, Ewart A, *et al.* 1995. Strong correlation of elastin deletions, detected by FISH, with Williams syndrome. *Am J Hum Genet* **57**, 49–53.

Luders E, Di Paola M, Tomaiuolo F, *et al.* 2007. Callosal morphology in Williams syndrome: A new evaluation of shape and thickness. *Neuroreport* **18**, 203–07.

Marler J A, Elfenbein J L, Ryals B M, Urban Z and Netzloff M L. 2005. Sensorineural hearing loss in children and adults with Williams syndrome. *Am J Medl Genet* **138**, 318–27.

Marenco S, Siuta M A, Kippenhan J S, *et al.* 2007. Genetic contributions to white matter architecture revealed by diffusion tensor imaging in Williams syndrome. *Proc Natl Acad Sci U S A* **104**, 15 117–222.

Mervis C B and Klein-Tasman B P. 2000. Williams syndrome: Cognition, personality, and adaptive behaviour. *Mental Retard Devptl Disabil Res Rev* **6**, 148–58.

Mervis C B, Morris C A, Bertrand J and Robinson B F. 1999. Williams syndrome: Findings from an integrated program of research. In Tager-Flusberg H (Ed.), *Neurodevelopmental Disorders: Contributions to a New Framework from the Cognitive Neurosciences.* Cambridge, MA: MIT Press, pp. 65–110.

Mervis C B, Morris C A, Klein-Tasman B P, *et al.* 2003a. Attentional characteristics of infants and toddlers with Williams syndrome during triadic interactions. *Devptl Neuropsychol* **23**, 243–68.

Mervis C B, Robinson B, Bertrand J, Morris C A, Klein-Tasman B and Armstrong S. 2000. The Williams syndrome cognitive profile. *Brain Cogn* **44**, 604–28.

Mervis C B, Robinson B F, Rowe M L, Becerra A M and Klein-Tasman B P. 2003b. Language abilities of individuals with Williams syndrome. *Int Rev Res Mental Retard* **27**, 35–81.

Meyer-Lindenberg A, Hariri A R, Munoz K E, *et al.* 2005a. Neural correlates of genetically abnormal social cognition in Williams syndrome. *Nat Neurosci* **8**, 991–3.

Meyer-Lindenberg A, Kohn P, Mervis C B, *et al.* 2004. Neural basis of genetically determined visuospatial construction deficit in Williams syndrome. *Neuron* **43**, 623–31.

Meyer-Lindenberg A, Mervis C B and Berman K F. 2006. Neural mechanisms in Williams syndrome: A unique window to genetic influences on cognition and behaviour. *Nat Neurosci* **8**, 991–3.

Meyer-Lindenberg A, Mervis C B, Sarpal D, *et al.* 2005b. Functional, structural, and metabolic abnormalities of the hippocampal formation in Williams syndrome. *J Clin Invest* **115**, 1888–95.

Milner A D and Goodale M A. 1995. *The Visual Brain in Action.* Cambridge, UK: MIT Press.

Mobbs D, Eckert M A, Menon V, *et al.* 2007a. Reduced parietal and visual cortical activation during global processing in Williams syndrome. *Devptl Med Child Neurol* **49**, 433–8.

Mobbs D, Eckert M A, Mills D, *et al.* 2007b. Frontostriatal dysfunction during response inhibition in Williams syndrome. *Biol Psychiatry* **62**, 256–61.

Mobbs D, Garrett A S, Menon V, Rose F E, Bellugi U and Reiss A L. 2004. Anomalous brain activations during face and gaze processing in Williams syndrome. *Neurology* **62**, 2070–6.

Morris C A. 2006. The dysmorphology, genetics, and natural history of Williams–Beuren syndrome. In Morris C A, Lenhoff H M, Wang P P (Eds.), *Williams–Beuren Syndrome: Research, Evaluation and Treatment.* Baltimore, MD: Johns Hopkins University Press, pp. 3–17.

Morris C A, Demsey S A, Leonard C O, Dilts C and Blackburn B L. 1988. Natural history of Williams syndrome: Physical characteristics. *J Ped* **113**, 318–26.

Morris C A and Mervis C B. 2000. Williams syndrome and related disorders. *Annu Rev Genom Hum Genet* **1**, 461–84.

Nakamura M, Watanabe K, Matsumoto A, *et al.* 2001. Williams syndrome and deficiency in visuospatial recognition. *Devptl Med Child Neurol* **43**, 617–21.

Navon D. 1977. Forest before trees: The precedence of global features in visual perception. *Cogn Psychol* **9**, 353–83.

Paul B M, Stiles J, Passarotti A, Bavar N and Bellugi U. 2002. Face and place processing in Williams syndrome: Evidence for a dorsal–ventral dissociation. *Neuroreport* **13**, 1115–9.

Pennington B F, Filipek P A, Lefly D, *et al.* 2000. A twin MRI study of size variations in human brain. *J Cogn Neurosci* **12**, 223–32.

Peoples R, Franke Y, Wang Y K, *et al.* 2000. A physical map, including a BAC/PAC clone contig, of the Williams–Beuren syndrome – Deletion region at 7q11.23. *Am J Hum Genet* **66**, 47–68.

Pober B R and Filiano J J. 1995. Association of Chiari I malformation and Williams syndrome. *Ped Neurol* **12**, 84–8.

Prather M D, Lavenex P, Mauldin-Jourdain M L, *et al.* 2001. Increased social fear and decreased fear of objects in monkeys with neonatal amygdala lesions. *Neuroscience* **106**, 653–8.

Ranganath C and D'Esposito M. 2001. Medial temporal lobe activity associated with active maintenance of novel information. *Neuron* **31**, 865–73.

Reilly J, Losh M, Bellugi U and Wulfeck B. 2004. Frog, where are you? Narratives in children with specific language impairment, early focal brain injury, and Williams syndrome. *Brain Lang* 88, 229–47.

Reiss A L, Abrams M T, Singer H S, Ross J L and Denckla M B. 1996. Brain development, gender and IQ in children. A volumetric imaging study. *Brain* 119, 1763–74.

Reiss A L, Eckert M A, Rose F E, *et al.* 2004. An experiment of nature: Brain anatomy parallels cognition and behaviour in Williams Syndrome. *J Neurosci* 24, 5009–15.

Reiss A L, Eliez S, Schmitt J E, *et al.* 2000. IV. Neuroanatomy of Williams syndrome: A high-resolution MRI study. *J Cogn Neurosci* 12 (Suppl 1), 65–73.

Rondan C, Santos A, Mancini J, Livet M O and Deruelle C. 2008. Global and local processing in Williams syndrome: Drawing versus perceiving. *Child Neuropsychol* 14, 237–48.

Santos A, Milne D, Rosset D and Deruelle C. 2007a. Challenging symmetry on mental retardation: Evidence from Williams syndrome. In Heinz E B (Ed.), *Mental Retardation Research Advances*. New York, NY: Nova Science Publishers, pp. 147–74.

Santos A, Rondan C, Mancini J and Deruelle C. 2007b. Behavioural indexes of callosal functioning in Williams syndrome. *J Neuropsychol* 1, 189–200.

Sarpal D, Buchsbaum B R, Kohn P D, *et al.* (2008). A genetic model for understanding higher order visual processing: Functional interactions of the ventral visual stream in Williams syndrome. *Cerebral Cortex* 18, 2402–09.

Scheiber, B. 2000. *Fulfilling Dreams – Book 1. A Handbook for Parents of Williams Syndrome Children*. Clawson, MI: Williams Syndrome Association.

Schmitt J E, Eliez S, Bellugi U and Reiss A L. 2001a. Analysis of cerebral shape in Williams syndrome. *Arch Neurol* 58, 283–7.

Schmitt J E, Eliez S, Warsofsky I S, Bellugi U and Reiss A L. 2001b. Corpus callosum morphology of Williams syndrome: Relation to genetics and behaviour. *Devpt1 Med Child Neurol* 43, 155–9.

Schmitt J E, Watts K, Eliez S, Bellugi U, Galaburda A M and Reiss A L. 2002. Increased gyrification in Williams syndrome: Evidence using 3D MRI methods. *Devptl Med Child Neurol* 44, 292–5.

Schultz R T. 2005. Developmental deficits in social perception in autism: The role of the amygdala and fusiform face are. *Int J Devptl Neurosci* 23, 125–41.

Spencer J, O'Brien J, Riggs K, Braddick O, Atkinson J and Wattam-Bell J. 2000. Motion processing in autism: Evidence for a dorsal stream deficiency. *Neuroreport* 11, 2765–7.

Strømme P, Bjørnstad P G and Ramstad K. 2002. Prevalence estimation of Williams syndrome. *J Child Neurol* 17, 269–71.

Sukarova-Angelovska E, Piperkova K, Sredovska A, Ilieva G and Kocova M. 2007. Implementation of fluorescent in situ hybridization (FISH) as a method for detecting microdeletion syndromes – Our first experiments. *Prilozi* 28, 87–98.

Tager-Flusberg H, Plesa Skewerer D, Faja S and Joseph R M. 2003. People with Williams syndrome processes faces holistically. *Cognition* 89, 11–24.

Tager-Flusberg H and Sullivan K. 2000. A componential view of theory of mind: Evidence from Williams syndrome. *Cognition* 76, 59–90.

Thompson P M, Cannon T D, Narr K L, *et al.* 2001. Genetic influences on brain structure. *Nat Neurosci* 4, 1253–8.

Thompson P M, Lee A D, Dutton R A, *et al.* 2005. Abnormal cortical complexity and thickness profiles mapped in Williams syndrome. *J Neurosci* 25, 4146–58.

Tomaiuolo F, Di Paola M, Caravale B, Vicari S, Petrides M and Caltagirone C. 2002. Morphology and morphometry of the corpus callosum in Williams syndrome: A TI-weighted MRI study. *Neuroreport* 13, 2281–4.

Udwin O and Yule W. 1991. A cognitive and behavioural phenotype in Williams syndrome. *J Clin Exp Neuropsychol* 13, 232–44.

Udwin O, Yule W and Martin N. 1987. Cognitive abilities and behavioural characteristics of children with idiopathic infantile hypercalcaemia. *J Child Psychol Psychiatry All Discipl* 28, 297–309.

Ungerleider L and Mishkin M. 1982. Two cortical visual systems. In Ingle D J, Goodale M A, Mansfeld R J W (Eds.), *Analyses of visual behaviour*. Cambridge, MA: MIT Press, pp. 549–86.

Urbán Z, Helms C, Fekete G, *et al.* 1996. 7q11.23 deletions in Williams syndrome arise as a consequence of unequal meiotic crossover. *Am J Hum Genet* 59, 958–62.

Van Essen D.C, Anderson C H and Felleman D J. 1992. Information processing in the primate visual system: An integrated systems perspective. *Science* 255, 419–23.

Van Essen D C, Dierker D, Snyder A Z, Raichle M E, Reiss A L and Korenberg J. 2006. Symmetry of cortical folding abnormalities in Williams syndrome revealed by surface-based analyses. *J Neurosci* 26, 5470–83.

VanLieshout C, DeMeyer R, Curfs L and Fryns J. 1998. Family contexts, parental behavior, and personality profiles of children and adolescents with Prader-Willi, Fragile-X, or Williams syndrome. *J Child Psychol Psychiatry All Discipl* 39, 699–710.

Vicari S, Brizzolara D, Carlesimo G A, Pezzini G and Volterra V. 1996. Memory abilities in children with Williams syndrome. *Cortex* 32, 502–14.

Wang P P and Bellugi U. 1994. Evidence from two genetic syndromes for a dissociation between verbal and

553

visual–spatial short-term memory. *J Child Exp Neuropsychol* **162**, 317–22.

Wang P P, Doherty S, Hesselink J R and Bellugi U. 1992. Callosal morphology concurs with neurobehavioral and neuropathological findings in two neurodevelopmental disorders. *Arch Neurol* **49**, 407–11.

Wang P P, Doherty S, Rourke S B and Bellugi U. 1995. Unique profile of visuo-perceptual skills in a genetic syndrome. *Brain Cogn* **29**, 54–65.

Wang P P, Hesselink J R, Jernigan T L, Doherty S and Bellugi U. 1992. Specific neurobehavioral profile of Williams' syndrome is associated with neocerebellar hemispheric preservation. *Neurology* **42**, 1999–2002.

Wilke M, Sohn J H, Byars A W and Holland S K. 2003. Bright spots: Correlations of gray matter volume with IQ in a normal pediatric population. *Neuroimage* **20**, 202–15.

Williams J C P, Barret-Boyes B G and Lowe J B. 1961. Supravalvular aortic stenosis. *Circulation* **24**, 1311–8.

Zeki S. 2001. Localization and globalization in conscious vision. *Annu Rev Neurosci* **24**, 57–86.

Zhao C, Aviles C, Abel R A, Almli C R, McQuillen P and Pleasure S J. 2005. Hippocampal and visuospatial learning defects in mice with a deletion of frizzled 9, a gene in the Williams syndrome deletion interval. *Development* **132**, 2917–27.

Chapter 38

Neuroimaging of developmental disorders: commentary

Nancy J. Minshew

The two chapters in this section focus on two fascinating neurodevelopmental disorders – autism and Williams syndrome. Over the past 30 years, these disorders have risen from the obscurity of "undecipherable, enigmatic, rare" disorders to disorders that have and will contribute breakthrough understandings of gene–brain–cognition–behavior relationships. In the process, these disorders also turned out not to be as rare as initially thought.

The advances did not occur all at once, nor did they occur with broad foresight of the significance of these disorders for cognitive neuroscience and the clinical specialties. The advances came slowly in phases reflecting step-wise gains in methodology and technology. The investments supporting this research were meager, reflecting the perceived rarity of and general disinterest in neurodevelopmental disorders. This status did not change until decades of mostly small-sized cognitive studies had identified intriguing features of the cognitive profiles, similarly sized magnetic resonance imaging (MRI) and neuropathologic studies were sufficient to implicate disturbances in pre- and post-natal neuronal organizational and migrational events, and genetic discoveries closed the developmental neurobiologic loop. With the identification of genes came the beginning of the molecular pathophysiologies and the widespread conviction of the significance of these disorders for cognitive neuroscience and behavioral neuropsychiatry. It is now no longer accurate to say that little is known about the cause of autism or Williams syndrome, or that these are minor disorders. However, as we read these chapters, we do find that the price paid for small studies and limited research funding for decades is that many of the findings are inadequately defined or remain unclear after many years. Fortunately,

sufficient work had been completed by the time the genetic studies were conducted that it was possible to make general sense of how the genes discovered might relate to the brain and behavior in each syndrome. Much research remains to be done at every level of the pathophysiology to clearly define the mechanistic connections between the gene abnormalities, the brain's structural and functional alterations, the resulting differences in cognition and neurological function, and their relationship to behavior. This definition will empower treatment, as animal models are demonstrating, and the scientific and medical rewards of this research will extend far beyond these disorders. It is, therefore, time that the neurodevelopmental disorders be accorded their rightful place among the major neuropsychiatric disorders that have a serious impact on humans across the life span and have great potential for providing gene–brain–cognition–behavior insights with broad implications for skill deficits among "typical" individuals, acquired brain injuries, and degenerative disorders.

The first vital contribution in both of these neurodevelopmental disorders was the refinement of the diagnostic criteria and their reliable and valid operationalization in individuals with IQ scores in the normal range. The study of individuals without intellectual disability enabled identification of the unusual cognitive profiles in both disorders, as well as functional imaging with IQ-matched typical controls, thus avoiding the confound of controls with intellectual disability with its own cognitive diversity. The study of the high functioning end of the spectrum of both disorders as a research strategy was met with considerable resistance in the field, taking decades to overcome and even then it was not clear that the underlying principle of this strategy was appreciated.

Understanding Neuropsychiatric Disorders, ed. M. E. Shenton and B. I. Turetsky. Published by Cambridge University Press.
© Cambridge University Press 2011.

In Williams syndrome, it was not until the discovery of the genetic abnormality in the 7q11.23 region that the validity of studying individuals without intellectual disability was fully accepted, e.g. all individuals with Williams syndrome have a microdeletion at 7q11.23. In autism, the discovery of low- and high-functioning individuals with ASD among siblings and twins, and the discovery of variability in affectation among family members with the same gene, led to more acceptance of studying individuals without intellectual disability as a research strategy for gaining insight into the fundamental nature of the disorder. The clinical expansion of the ASD spectrum to the point that about 50% do not have intellectual disability has probably been just as influential in quelling the criticism of studying high functioning individuals with ASD. These examples are reminders that variation in severity is typical of most biologic disorders, and that variation in severity alone is rarely a sufficient basis for differentiating between disorders.

It is notable that both disorders are associated with a range of intellectual ability, signifying that intellectual disability is not a separate comorbid disorder in either condition, but part and parcel of the biology of each condition. According to the rules governing genetics, chance co-occurrence (prevalence of A × prevalence of B = chances of A&B), cannot explain the frequency of intellectual disability in these neurodevelopmental disorders. If not comorbidity, there needs to be a neurobiologic conceptualization of each disorder that accounts for the frequent expression of intellectual disability. In Williams syndrome, an explanation has been proposed first at the genetic level as a gene dosage effect. Ultimately, the impact of varying gene dose on cognition and behavior will be determined and the mechanisms will be understood for the variability in expression of the syndrome. In autism, an explanation has been articulated based on studies of the neuropsychological profile that demonstrated intact information acquisition abilities, intact or enhanced simple information processing abilities, and impaired higher order or complex information processing abilities (Minshew et al., 1992, 1997; Williams et al., 2006). The predictable outcome of progressive loss of complex information processing capacity is mental retardation with disproportionate loss of higher-order abilities (social, language, reasoning) and preservation or enhancement of simple or elementary information processing abilities, thus maintaining the unusual profile associated with

autism in low-functioning individuals. This characterization of the cognitive and neurological profile in autism is consistent with the broad involvement of the brain manifested by the increased total brain volume in children with ASD and the onset of early accelerated growth in head size at 9 months coincident with the onset of multi-domain signs (Dawson et al., 2007; Rogers, 2009).

Once a sufficient number of individuals with autism and Williams syndrome without intellectual disability (mental retardation) could be identified and matched to typical controls, it was possible to define the unique cognitive features of these two disorders and then begin the challenging process of establishing links between the cognitive features and the behavioral manifestations. This process was notable in both disorders for defining a *profile* of deficits and intact or enhanced abilities.

The strengths in both disorders defined these disorders as much as the deficits, but were ultimately appreciated to be accompanied by significant limitations. In Williams syndrome, the hallmark of fearless sociability and high degree of empathy were initially considered great strengths. When the children reached school age, their intense gaze and bold sociability became impaired social cognition and poor peer relationships, providing an example of how "too much" can be as dysfunctional as "too little". The social hallmark of autism was for a long time considered to be the opposite of Williams syndrome, i.e. a detachment or disinterest in people and lack of empathy. However, as the spectrum of behavior was more fully appreciated, the social impairment in autism was refined to specify impairment in the reciprocity of social interactions, embracing both those who fail to respond and those who respond excessively. The discovery of theory of mind deficits aided greatly in the understanding of the social impairment so that it could be understood in terms other than the absence of interactions. The development of social cognitive abilities will now aid the definition of the social impairments in Williams syndrome. The hallmark strengths of autism were the remarkable memory for minute or inconsequential details and the often superior visuospatial abilities. However, it quickly became apparent that their unusual perception and recall of details was accompanied by equally impaired common sense, reasoning and judgment, e.g. they cannot use these details to solve problems or cope in daily life.

Because of their strengths and their deficits, both disorders have been considered to have local processing strengths and global processing weaknesses, but as a result of different underlying cognitive and neurologic patterns. In Williams syndrome, there is a severe visuospatial construction deficit resulting in an inability to construct a whole from parts. Puzzle assembly and block design are poor, but face and object identification are normal. Interestingly, a global processing deficit was proposed for their difficulty with Block Design and H-S tasks (large letter filled with the same or different smaller letters) because of their difficulty perceiving the global outline and the large letter. The basis for this striking profile is the dissociation between an intact ventral visual processing stream and an impaired dorsal visual processing stream. The impaired dorsal stream processing accounts for both the visuospatial construction deficit and the global processing deficit. By comparison, individuals with autism often, although not always, do well on puzzles and Block Design, and poorly on face recognition and face emotion recognition, with nearly normal performance on object recognition. Enhanced local processing and/or impaired global processing deficits have been hypothesized to explain these findings in autism also (Kuschner et al., 2009). In autism, however, the hypothesis is that increased u-fibers, e.g. increased local connectivity, explains the enhanced local processing skills, and reduced cortico-cortical connectivity explains the global processing deficit. The application of the global processing deficit to two behavioral syndromes that are very different from a cognitive perspective, and even more different from a structural brain perspective and genetic perspective, highlights the extreme limitations of behaviorally based explanations for phenomena that originate at a genetic and brain level.

Neither of these syndromes has been reducible to a single primary deficit. In fact, this construct does not have validity for neurologic disorders, i.e. disorders of brain origin. Neurologic or brain dysfunction produces a pattern or profile of cognitive and neurologic findings that conform to the principle of the causative agent such as stroke, traumatic brain injury, and so on. The first step in assessing neurologic disorders is therefore to define carefully the profile of impairments and the profile of intact or enhanced abilities. Every major domain of function must be examined and the pattern within each domain must be examined to discern patterns that provide clues to the underlying pathophysiologic–neurobiologic process.[1] Volpe's (1998) chapters on the clinical manifestations of disorders of organogenesis, neuronal proliferation, neuronal organization, and neuronal migration and glial events provide a superb foundation for cognitive neuroscientists and clinicians to make links between developmental neurobiology and the clinical expressions of brain dysfunction. In Williams syndrome, the key was finding the selective involvement of dorsal visual stream processing with sparing of ventral stream processing. The faithful recurrence of such a cognitive profile accompanied by congenital malformations and dysmorphism classified this disorder as a disorder of brain development from the start. In autism, the key to recognizing autism as a disorder of neuronal organization from the beginning was the *profile* of deficits and intact abilities, which was first suggested in studies of IQ profiles, and Volpe's description of neuronal organization events as those events in brain development that result in the circuitry that supports those abilities that are most uniquely human.

Without this conceptual foundation, the awareness of the developmental neurobiologic origins of these disorders awaited critical clues provided by structural imaging studies. In the case of Williams syndrome, the abnormalities in cortical volume, thickness and gyrification involved posterior cerebral cortices corresponding to the disturbance in dorsal stream visual processing and in orbital frontal cortex related to the social difficulties. In autism, the increase in total brain volume composed of increased cortical gray matter (all lobes or all lobes except occipital) and increased cerebral white matter but not corpus callosum indicated a generalized cortical process. These findings drew the attention of neuroscientists, who immediately appreciated the implications of such growth disturbances. Current imaging studies are now examining cortical volume as a function of cortical thickness and surface area to discern differing neurodevelopmental processes (Raznahan et al., 2009) and exploring the impact of genotype on brain structure (Raznahan et al., 2009; Scott et al., 2009). The potential contributions of imaging research especially in combination with other modalities is on the brink of an entirely new world of discoveries (Church et al., 2009; Dosenbach et al., 2008).

It took some time for the neurobiologic significance of these findings to impact models of both disorders. The final push came from genetic discoveries.

In Williams syndrome, the genetic findings are relatively uniform in that every case has a hemizygous microdeletion in the same location on chromosome 7. However, how this microdeletion actually causes the syndrome and its variations is unknown – it is still a long way from gene to brain, but identification of the genes is the beginning of the molecular pathophysiology. In autism, 20–25 genes have been discovered, all related to the development of neuronal connections. These genes account for 15–20% of ASD cases. The progress on their molecular pathophysiology has been dramatic in only a few years. The rescue of adult animal models of some of these genes and the prevention of the development of seizures in tuberous sclerosis with mammalian target of rapamycin (mTor) inhibitors have provided proof of concept of the potential benefit of future neurobiologic interventions for those affected individuals who elect them.

In conclusion, these two disorders have illustrious histories that are both interesting and edifying. Hopefully, the lessons learned from them can be applied in the future to these and other neurodevelopmental disorders to hasten progress and the efficient use of all resources. For these two disorders, the next 5 and 10 years will witness the rapid growth of far more complex technologies and methods of data analyses to confront the enormous complexity of the brain, the genome, and the multi-modal data derived from their study.

References

Church J A, Fair D A, Dosenbach N U F, et al. 2009. Control networks in pediatric Tourette syndrome show immature and anomalous patterns of functional connectivity. Brain 132, 225–38.

Dawson G, Munson G, Webb S J, Nalty T, Abbott R and Toth K. 2007. Rate of head growth decelerates and symptoms worsen in the second year of life in autism. Biol Psychiatry 61, 458–64.

Dosenbach N U, Fair D A, Cohen A L, Schlaggar B L and Petersen S E. 2008. A dual networks architecture of top-down control. Trends Cogn Sci 12, 99–105.

Kuschner E, Bodner K and Minshew N J. 2009. Local versus global approaches to reproducing the Rey Osterrieth complex figure by children, adolescents and adults with high functioning autism. Autism Res 2, 348–58.

Minshew N J, Goldstein G and Siegel D J. 1997. Neuropsychologic functioning in autism: Profile of a complex information processing disorder. J Int Neuropsychol Soc 3, 303–16.

Minshew N J, Goldstein G, Muenz L R and Payton J B. 1992. Neuropsychological functioning in nonmentally retarded autistic individuals. J Clin Exp Neuropsychol 14, 749–61.

Raznahan A, Toro, R, Proitsi P, et al. 2009. A functional polymorphism of the brain derived neurotropic factor gene and cortical anatomy in autism spectrum disorder. J Neurodevelop Disord 1, 215–23.

Rogers S J. 2009. What are infant siblings teaching us about autism in infancy. Autism Res 2, 125–37.

Scott A A, Abraham B S, Alvarez-Retuerto A-I, et al. 2009. Genetic variation in CNTNAP2 modulates human frontal cortical connectivity. Abstract, Society for Neuroscience.

Volpe J J. 1998. Brain development unit. In Neurology of the newborn (5th ed.). Philadelphia, PA: Saunders-Elsevier, pp. 3–118.

Williams D L, Goldstein G and Minshew N J. 2006. Neuropsychologic functioning in children with autism: Further evidence for disordered complex information-processing. Child Neurol 12, 279–98.

Endnote

1. Even if the gene or developmental neurobiologic event has now been generally identified, the specifics of the mechanisms are not known. Each mechanism in the sequence between gene and behavior must be clearly defined and understood to empower intervention. In Williams syndrome, much remains to be done to characterize early development and outcome of social, affective, language, and communication skills. In autism, a more complete characterization of skills has been completed because of the focus on many potential single primary deficits. However, longitudinal studies of infant siblings at risk are providing vital new information; such studies and much more across the age span will be needed to sort out the sequence of brain events.

Index